An Atlas and Textbook of Diagnostic Ultrasonography of the Dog and Cat

An Atlas and Textbook of Diagnostic Ultrasonography of the Dog and Cat

Professor Cordula Poulsen Nautrup DrMedVet
Specialist in Veterinary Anatomy
Faculty of Veterinary Medicine
University of Munich, Munich, Germany

Dr Ralf Tobias DrMedVet
Specialist in Small Animals
School of Veterinary Medicine, Hannover, Germany

Edited by Dr Robert E. Cartee BA BS DVM MS
Associate Professor in the Department of Anatomy, Physiology and Pharmacology
College of Veterinary Medicine
Auburn University, Alabama, USA

Translation by Dr Katharina Hittmair DrMedVet
Radiologic Clinic
University of Veterinary Medicine, Vienna, Austria

Manson Publishing/The Veterinary Press

Fourth Impression 2007
Third Impression 2004
Second Impression 2001
Published in 2000 by Manson Publishing Ltd

ISBN-10: 1-874545-10-3
ISBN-13: 978-1-874545-10-1

A CIP catalogue record for this book is available from the British Library.

For full details of all Manson Publishing titles, please write to:
Manson Publishing Ltd
73 Corringham Road
London NW11 7DL, UK
Tel: +44(0)20 8905 5150
Fax: +44(0)20 8201 9233
www.mansonpublishing.com

Printed in Germany

CONTENTS

ACKNOWLEDGEMENTS

The anatomical sections, including the photographs, were prepared by Drs. F. Breiling (Lueneburg), A. Diekgerdes (Moringen), T. Lauxtermann (Oppenheim) and A. Lippert (Hannover) in their individual dissertations, and we are very grateful to them for their contributions. The majority of the technical illustrations were prepared by Ms. G. Poulsen Nautrup (Hannover). Most of the pictograms demonstrating transducer positions were kindly drawn for us by Dr. A. Diekgerdes (Moringen).

We would like to thank the following companies, and especially their employees, for their technical support and for helping us to work with the latest technical standards:

ATL-Advanced Technology Laboratories (Hamburg): Ms. E. Bayer, Mr. R. Fischer and Mr. B. Spenke.
Esaote Biomedica (Neufahrn): Mr. T. Roth.
Kretztechnik und Medisonic (Gelsenkirchen): Mr. E. Noeding and Mr. P.W. Quast.
Pameda Medizinische Systeme GmBH (Loerrach): Mr. H.R. Richli and Mr. R. Richli.
Physia GmBH Roentgen-Ultraschall (Neu-Isenburg): Mr. J. Eberspaecher and Mr. H. Gerhards.
Schering AG (Berlin): Dr. K. Foerster.
Siemens Medizinische Systeme (Erlangen): Mr. P. Harbert.
Sonotron GmBH (Cologne): Mr. A. Hoppe.
Toshiba Medical Systems (Neuss and Hannover): Mr. S. Bus and Ms. U. Jacob.

We are extremely grateful to many friends and colleagues for their suggestions and corrections, especially Dr. C. Bonneau, Dr. A. Gabriel (Hannover), Dr. M. Gerke (Hannover), Academic Director Dr. U. Kersten (Hannover), Dr. S. Lalla (Lampertheim), Dr. B. Morisse (Hannover), Academic Director Dr. Muenster (Hannover), Dr. I. Stephan (Hannover) and Ms. P. Wilmes (Wuppertal). Veterinarians Ms. U. Depken, Mr. F. Goeddenhenrich, Ms. I. Hanenberg, Ms. R. Kawauchi and Ms. I. Rohrweber contributed with their corrections of the proofs.

We would like to thank Dr. U. Oslage and Mr. H. Schmidt from Schlütersche, Verlag und Druckerei, in Hannover, for their superb cooperation and participation from the beginning to the publication of this textbook.

We would also like to acknowledge all those helpers not listed by name for their contributions toward improving this textbook.

Cordula Poulsen Nautrup and Ralf Tobias

Dedications

To my son Hendrik and my parents.
Cordula Poulsen Nautrup

To my father and in memory of my mother.
Ralf Tobias

To my children and my wife.
Robert E. Cartee

CONTRIBUTORS

Dr. Bettina Denkewitz DrMedVet
Department of Functional and Applied Anatomy
School of Medicine, Hannover
D-30623 Hannover

Dr. Jens Dieterich DrVetMed
Institute for Reproductive Medicine
School of Veterinary Medicine, Hannover
Buenteweg 17, D -30559 Hannover

Dr. Carolyn Döhner DrMedVet
Small Animal Clinic
School of Veterinary Medicine, Hannover
Bischofshofer Damm 15, D-30173 Hannover

Dr. Sabine Eggers DrMedVet
Luetjenburger Strasse 11, D-23714 Malente

Dr. Andreas Engelke DrMedVet
Small Animal Clinic
School of Veterinary Medicine, Hannover
Bischofshofer Damm 15, D-30173 Hannover

Dr. Gabriele Gassner DrMedVet
Small Animal Clinic
School of Veterinary Medicine, Hannover
Bischofshofer Damm 15, D-30173 Hannover

Professor Anne-Rose Günzel-Apel DrMedVet
Specialist in Veterinary Breeding Hygiene and Artificial Insemination
Institute for Reproductive Medicine
School of Veterinary Medicine, Hannover
Buenteweg 17, D -30559 Hannover

Dr. Barbara Güssregen DrMedVet
Specialist in Experimental Medicine
Department of Experimental Surgery
Technical University, Munich
Ismaninger Strasse 22, D-81675 Munich

Dr. Hans-Josef Heider DrMedVet DipECVO
Specialist in Small Animals and Veterinary Ophthalmology
Small Animal Clinic
School of Veterinary Medicine, Hannover
Bischofshofer Damm 15, D-30173 Hannover

Dr. Britta Heinze DrMedVet
Department of Reproductive Medicine
School of Veterinary Medicine, Hannover
Buenteweg 17, D -30559 Hannover

Dr. Julia Henke DrMedVet
Specialist in Experimental Medicine and Anaesthesiology
Department of Experimental Surgery
Technical University, Munich
Ismaninger Strasse 22, D-81675 Munich

Dr. Angelika Hörauf DrMedVet
Veterinary Specialist in Internal Medicine
Clinic for Small Animal Medicine
University of Zurich
Winterthurer Strasse 260, CH-8057 Zurich

Dr. Martin Janthur DrMedVet
Small Animal Clinic
School of Veterinary Medicine, Hannover
Bischofshofer Damm 15, D-30173 Hannover

Dr. Wolfgang Kästner DrMed
Specialist in Internal Medicine and Cardiology
Weinstrasse 20, D-30171 Hannover

Dr. Martin Köhle DrMedVet
Clinic for Small Animals and Out-Patients
Free University of Berlin
Oertzenweg 19b, D-14163 Berlin

Dr. Jan-Gerd Kresken DrMedVet
Specialist in Small Animals
Veterinary Clinic Kaiserberg
Wintgenstrasse 81-83, D-47058 Duisburg

Dr. Dirk Lüerssen DrMedVet
Specialist in Small Animals
Small Animal Practice Lüerssenhof
Hauptstrasse 71, D-30966 Hemmingen, OT Hiddestorf

Professor Cordula Poulsen Nautrup DrMedVet
Specialist in Veterinary Anatomy
Faculty of Veterinary Medicine
University of Munich
Veterinärstraße 13, D-80539 Munich

Dr. Adelheid Prüfer DrMedVet
Specialist in Small Animals
Small Animal Clinic
School of Veterinary Medicine, Hannover
Bischofshofer Damm 15, D-30173 Hannover

Dr. Sven Reese DrMedVet
Specialist in Veterinary Anatomy
Faculty of Veterinary Medicine
University of Munich
Veterinärstraße 13, D-80539 Munich

Dr. Danielle Schäfer DrMedVet
Biberacher Strasse 29, D-88427 Bad Schussenried

Dr. Sabine Scholz DrMedVet
Department of Functional and Applied Anatomy
School of Medicine, Hannover
D-30623 Hannover

Dr. Susanne Thamke DrMedVet
Product Manager for Veterinary Ultrasonography
Eichelscheider Strasse 8, D-66914 Waldmohr

Dr. Ralf Tobias DrMedVet
Specialist in Small Animals
Small Animal Clinic
School of Veterinary Medicine, Hannover
Bischofshofer Damm 15, D-30173 Hannover

Jörg Wefer DrMed
Clinic for Emergency Surgery
School of Medicine, Hannover
D-30623 Hannover

Professor Burkhard Wippermann DrMed
Specialist in Surgery and Emergency Surgery
Clinic for Emergency Surgery
School of Medicine, Hannover
D-30623 Hannover

FOREWORD

Diagnostic ultrasonography has developed at a rapid rate in the past decade. This technology has become an important part of all the specialty areas in clinical veterinary medicine, such as internal medicine, gynaecology and obstetrics, surgery, cardiology, gastroenterology, orthopaedics and ophthalmology.

The main feature of ultrasonography is its non-invasiveness and repeatability. Even hair coat removal has often become unnecessary. Constantly developing technology provides a variety of transducer systems, stand-off pads, automatic focusing, colour-coding and combinations of Doppler and B-mode ultrasonography. Almost all the organs and tissues of the patient are now accessible. Not surprisingly, this explosion of technology has led to a flood of publications. The American College of Veterinary Radiology, in association with the International Veterinary Radiology Association and the European Association of Veterinary Diagnostic Imaging, has responded to the demand for information with the publication of a dedicated veterinary ultrasonography magazine (*Veterinary Radiology and Ultrasound*).

The increasing significance of ultrasonography is recognized in veterinary schools, where the teaching in this field is now comparable to that in radiology. The number of students, a substantial curriculum and a limited faculty do not always allow practical work and studies on the patient. For this reason, a number of seminars on practical ultrasonographic techniques are offered as postgraduate and continuing education courses. These seminars are often lacking in information on in-depth theoretical background. Preparation and review of the subject matter in text and image are left to each individual.

This ultrasound book has filled a void in the veterinary medical literature, which has been lacking a work of this substance. Most of the existing textbooks on diagnostic ultrasound are usually limited to organ systems such as the gastrointestinal or genital tract. Since diagnostic ultrasound has recently become an integral part of many veterinary practices, a comprehensive textbook is needed to assist students as well as practising veterinarians. This task has been accomplished by a group of twenty-four veterinarians and two medical doctors, composed of university associates and experienced practitioners, who have pooled their experience and particular knowledge of diagnostic ultrasonography. The versatility and completeness of this textbook is best demonstrated by the list of authors, who come from various fields in veterinary medicine.

As with many other imaging methods, ultrasonography requires a precise knowledge of anatomy, a three-dimensional understanding and a great deal of practice. These characteristics are needed to create a complete image from the individual pictures and, in combination with pathological–anatomical knowledge, to reach a diagnosis. It is therefore very fortunate that the publication and compilation of this book is under the guidance of an anatomist (Professor Cordula Poulsen Nautrup) and a clinician (Dr. Ralf Tobias). Their cooperation has led to a fruitful synthesis of both the basic principles and the practical usefulness of ultrasonography.

The aim of the authors was to present the indications for ultrasonography, to show its limitations and pitfalls, and to illustrate the often considerable differences between dogs and cats. The reader must be made aware that ultrasonography is only one of many diagnostic tools.

More recent advances, such as colour-coded Doppler sonography, are introduced, discussed and compared with other imaging methods such as radiography, computed tomography and scintigraphy.

In order to provide the reader with information extending beyond this textbook, each chapter is followed by a comprehensive list of literature references, divided into 'cited references' and 'further reading'. Great care has been taken with the quality of the illustrations, each accompanied by an explanatory, intelligible line drawing. In this way an ultrasonographic beginner can easily become acquainted with the subject matter.

Diagnostic ultrasonography is a non-invasive imaging method, with few, if any, adverse effects on the patient or the sonographer. Ultrasound has become a critical diagnostic imaging method in veterinary medicine. This book will certainly be a contribution.

Ingo Nolte

PREFACE

Progress in ultrasonography during the past years has effectively changed diagnostics in veterinary medicine. Ultrasonography has fulfilled the wishes of many veterinarians to pursue extensive examination of almost all the organ systems, without side-effects, with minimal effort, repeatable at any time and with immediate results. Apart from its high efficiency, this method has also been promoted because of the acceptable costs and easy handling for experienced sonographers. With newer diagnostic tools, it is often easy to overestimate a technique as well as to use it indiscriminately.

Although there are presently numerous publications on specialized ultrasonographic subjects, a current, extensive textbook has been missing. This book encompasses information for ultrasonographic beginners, as well as meticulous scientific illustrations of difficult problems. It is meant for students in their clinical semesters, for veterinarians in continuing education, and also for colleagues with practical ultrasonographic experience. The comparison of two-dimensional ultrasonographic images and anatomical cross-sectional specimens helps the beginner to be sonographically orientated in the different body regions. Ultrasonography is not an isolated diagnostic method, which is why other imaging methods are specifically mentioned. Conventional and colour-coded Doppler echography is not limited to the cardiology chapter. The advanced sonographer is shown the newest developments in three-dimensional ultrasonography, various forms of interventional examinations and ultrasonographic monitoring of bone healing. The most important comprehensive veterinary and human medical publications are listed for further studies.

A comprehensive book of this kind must encompass the knowledge of many authors. The differing styles of the authors have been accommodated in order to create a book in which all the chapters have a similar format. It seemed very important to us to caption the ultrasound images clearly. Since the aesthetics of each sonogram should be preserved, drawings of all the ultrasound images were made, documenting the important findings. Abbreviations were not used in the line drawings, enabling easier reading.

This book should not only give quick, clear and extensive information on ultrasonography in the dog and cat, it should also give pleasure to the reader. We have strived to share our enthusiasm and to show the unique fascination in the aesthetics as well as the diagnostic meaning of this method.

In the nomenclature, German or germanized terms are used. In some cases the original terms have been used to avoid uncommon or unusual notations.

To produce an up-to-date book, we have endeavoured to improve some of the sonograms using the newest standards, almost up to the day of printing. This has been made possible by numerous institutions and companies providing us with the latest in technical equipment. An atlas and textbook on this developing diagnostic technique relies on dialogue with its readers. For this reason, we encourage suggestions for future improvements.

Cordula Poulsen Nautrup and Ralf Tobias

The authors of this text have designed and produced a textbook that can be used by the student as a good reference guide, by the beginner veterinary ultrasonographer as a handy guide, and by the more advanced sonographer for clarification of standard procedures and as an introduction to some very new and exciting areas of sonography.

The illustrations are both elucidating and artistically pleasing. By mixing excellent ultrasound scans and colour schematics the authors have succeeded in creating both an interesting and an easily read text. This is a textbook for readers who want to understand how ultrasound can help diagnose specific diseases without dwelling on each disease for too long. More importantly, the authors are more interested in teaching rather than in impressing the reader. Not many textbooks can do this, but this one is an exception. I have found it a great pleasure to help edit this English language translation and I believe that you, the reader, will be glad to have this book within easy reach. I do not believe it will spend any time gathering dust.

Robert E. Cartee

NOMENCLATURE AND ABBREVIATIONS

Nomenclature

This book uses terms from clinical use to designate organs and structures as well as their anatomy, physiology and pathology. The Latin organ and structure names are taken from the *Nomina Anatomica Veterinaria*, *Nomina Histologica* and *Nomina Embryologica Veterinaria* (1994*). The notations for diseases and lesions correspond with the common pathological terms. Individual names are not used.

Abbreviations

Apart from physical units, common abbreviations as well as those found in *the Nomina Anatomica Veterinaria*, *Nomina Histologica* and *Nomina Embryologica Veterinaria* (1994*) are used.

The numerous abbreviations found in English publications on ultrasound diagnostics are explained in the various chapters. Declinations and gender are not considered with the abbreviations. A double last letter refers to the plural.

a. = artery
caud. = caudal
cran. = cranial
dist. = distal
ln. = lymph node
m. = muscle
med. = medial
n. = nerve
dors. = dorsal
ext. = external
gl. = gland
int. = internal
lat. = lateral
lig. = ligament
prof. = profundus
r. = ramus
rostr. = rostral
supf. = superficial
v. = vein
ventr. = ventral

SI basic units and derived SI units

g = gram
J = joule
m = metre
N = newton
s = second
W = watt

Special units

db = decibel
h = hour
Hz = hertz
min = minute

SI prefixes

M- = mega- (× 1,000,000)
k- = kilo- (× 1,000)
c- = centi- (× 0.01)
m- = milli- (× 0.001)
μ- = micro- (× 0.000001)

**Nomina Anatomica Veterinaria.* 4th ed., *Nomina Histologica.* 2nd ed., *Nomina Embryologica Veterinaria* (1994). Publ. Int. Comm. Vet. Anat. Nomenclature of the World Assoc. Vet. Anat., Zurich, Ithaca, New York.

PART I GENERAL PRINCIPLES AND METHODOLOGY

1 Terminology and Historical Review

Cordula Poulsen Nautrup

Terminology

Imaging biological or medical structures with the help of high frequency sound waves is referred to as diagnostic ultrasound, sonography or echography (from Latin *sonus* = tone or sound; Greek *echo* = tone or sound; Greek *graphein* = write).

Sonography usually refers to real-time diagnostic ultrasonography of the abdominal and pelvic organs. Echography is used in combination with a designated organ and refers to local examinations. The terms echocardiography, echoencephalography and echo-ophthalmology are used for ultrasonographic images of the heart, the brain and the eye respectively.

Word combinations may also define the method used more clearly. Two-dimensional ultrasonography, displaying anatomical sections of the examined structures, is referred to as echotomography. Supplementary terms such as 'Doppler', 'duplex' and 'triplex', as in Doppler echography or duplex (triplex) sonography, indicate the additional use of the Doppler principle to measure blood flow parameters or the use of more than one or a combination of display modes.

History of Diagnostic Ultrasonography

The development of ultrasonographic imaging methods in biology and in veterinary and human medicine was relatively slow compared with that of radiographic methods. Radiographic imaging was implemented immediately after the discovery of x-rays.

Basic acoustic principles, such as reflection (= echo) or attenuation (= weakening of sound over a distance), have been noted for thousands of years. At the end of the 18th century, the German physicist Ernst F. F. Chladni (1758–1827) discovered the sounds of stringed instruments to be longitudinal waves. In 1842 the Austrian physicist Christian J. Doppler (1803–1853) described the optic and acoustic phenomenons, which were later named after him. Francis Galton (1822–1911), an English scientist, developed a whistle in the mid-19th century, which produced high frequency sounds up to 100 kHz.

Although there was sufficient scientific interest and relatively early attempts to produce ultrasound, high frequency sound waves could not be used as a diagnostic tool at the time. Most of the technical requirements, such as efficient transmitters, receivers and amplifiers, were missing.

At the beginning of the 20th century, after the sinking of the Titanic, increased research to locate and image invisible objects in water using ultrasound was initiated. Since marine employment was based mainly in the military, ultrasound technologies developed rapidly during the two World Wars.

During World War I the French physicist M. Paul Langevin (1872–1946) was able to produce ultrasound waves with a quartz crystal and transmit them in water. This method assisted in detecting submarines[27]. At the same time, Langevin unknowingly demonstrated the biological effects of ultrasound waves. The sound intensity during these experiments was so high that the fish, hit by these sound waves, died[10].

Apart from the civil and military employment, e.g. the SONAR method (sonar = sound navigation and ranging), industry discovered the use of ultrasound for material inspection. During the 1920s, 1930s and 1940s, the Russian S. J. Sokoloff[2, 40] and the American Floyd A. Firestone[11, 12] used this method to reveal material faults in metals and in rubber tyres. The development of medical diagnostic ultrasonography began shortly before World War II. The neurologist and army surgeon Karl T. Dussik[8] first published an essay on biological–medical application of high frequency sound in 1942. He displayed a lateral ventricle in a cerebral specimen and called this A-mode sonography 'hyperphonography'.

From the late 1940s to 1950s, diagnostic ultrasound was established simultaneously in various specialist institutions[16]. The pioneers in human medicine included John J. Wild[42], who differentiated sonographically between healthy and tumorous tissues, as well as Douglass H. Howry and Joseph H. Holmes[18, 19, 20], who produced two-dimensional sectional images of the neck and abdomen using the Compound method (see Compound Scan, page 40).

A-mode echocardiography was first used by Wolf-Dieter Keidel[23] to observe cardiac volume changes. Inge Edler and Carl H. Hertz[9, 15] later displayed atrial and ventricle wall movements with the help of ultrasound. Lars Leskell[28, 29] was the founder of clinical echoencephalography.

Eye examinations with the help of A-mode ultrasound were first published by G. Henry Mundt and William F. Hughes[31]. Numerous other publications on this subject appeared worldwide in the following years. The first two-dimensional echo-ophthalmograms were presented by Gilbert Baum[1]. One of the founders of gynaecological and obstetrical diagnostic ultrasonography was Ian Donald[6].

S. Satomura[39] published a paper on blood flow patterns working with the Doppler principle. The rapid development and improvement of Doppler systems led to a variety of applications in angiology and cardiology. Another big advance was the introduction of colour-coded Doppler echocardiography in the early 1980s. In this period the Japanese K. Namekawa[32, 33] and his group, as well as the Americans William J. Bommer and Larry Miller[3], colour coded cardiac blood flow and displayed it in a two-dimensional, real-time echocardiogram, using an ultrasound machine prototype.

1

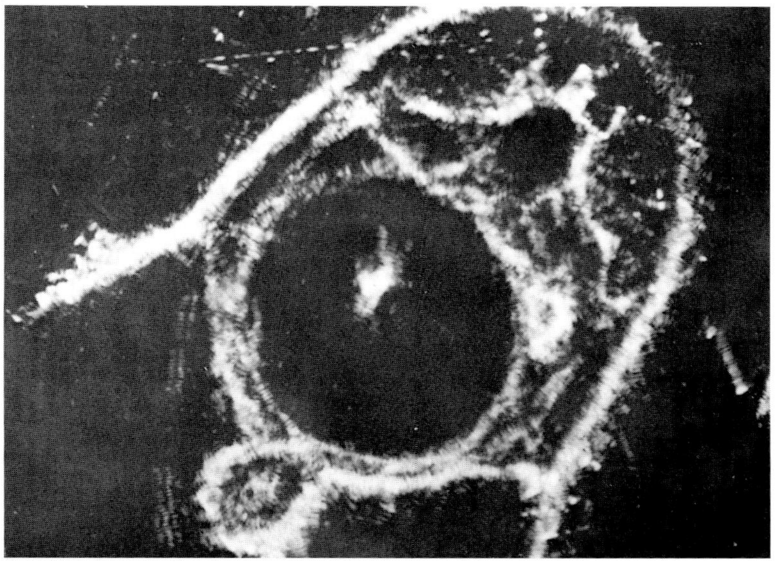

1 Two-dimensional ultrasound image (compound mode) of the pelvic region in a male dog, showing a vertebra, the filled urinary bladder and the penis.

[From Holmes JH (1974) Diagnostic ultrasound: historical perspective. In King DL (ed): *Diagnostic Ultrasound*, CV Mosby Company, St. Louis, p. 5, with permission of the Plenum Publishing Corp., New York. First published as Holmes JH and Howry DH (1963) Ultrasonic diagnosis of abdominal diseases. *Am. J. Dig. Dis.* **8**, 12–32.]

2

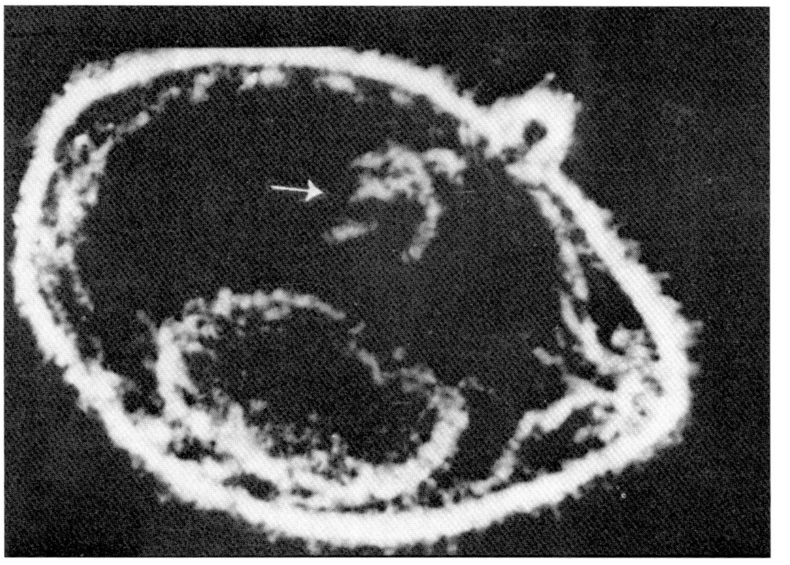

2 Two-dimensional ultrasound image (compound mode) of the cranial abdomen in a cat, showing stomach and liver including an abscess (arrow).

[From Holmes JH and Howry DH (1963) Ultrasonic diagnosis of abdominal diseases. *Am. J. Dig. Dis.* **8**, p. 18, with permission of the Plenum Publishing Corp., New York.]

From a veterinary point of view, two named pioneers of human ultrasonography must be mentioned. In the early 1960s, D. H. Howry and J. H. Holmes displayed abdominal organs in dogs and cats on evident echotomograms[17] (**1, 2**). Sonographic examination of animals, as well as of sick people, was difficult at the time, since the patients, depending on the indication, had to be almost entirely immersed in a water bath[16] (**3**).

In the 1950s, veterinary ultrasonography was used mainly to examine animal tissues and to determine slaughter animal composition and condition[41]. This ultrasonographic application is still a separate field today, although it is mainly used in farm animals, such as pigs and cows.

The first publication on veterinary diagnostic ultrasonography was by Ivan L. Lindahl[30] in 1966. Lindahl used A-mode ultrasonography to diagnose pregnancy in sheep (**4**). The first clinical ultrasonographic examinations of small animals were done in the late 1960s by Seth A. Koch[24] and Lionel F. Rubin[38]. They consisted of echo-ophthalmograms in dogs. Further efforts were made in sonographic pregnancy diagnosis using the Doppler principle. In 1970 both Leoyd C. Helper[14] and Ann-Marie Lamm[26] described the observation of beating hearts in canine fetuses with the help of ultrasound.

Numerous publications on one-dimensional (M-mode) echocardiography appeared in the late 1970s. A pioneer in the use

3

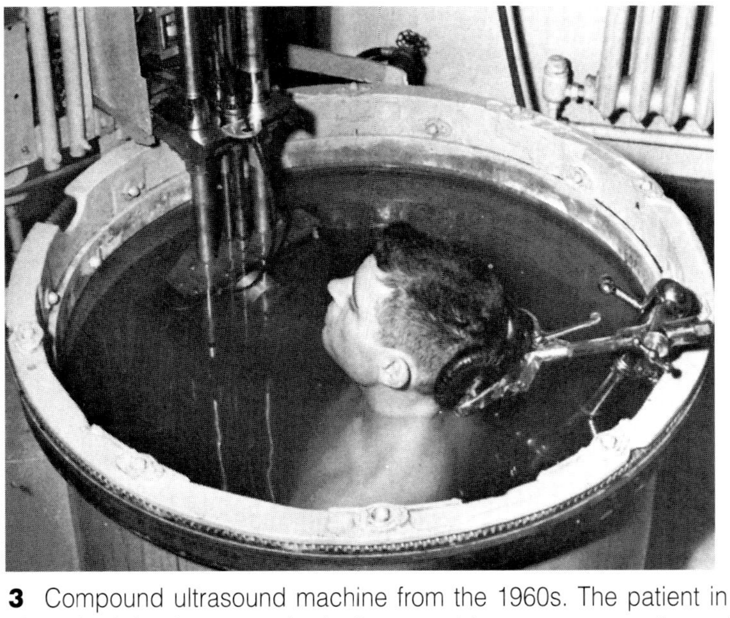

3 Compound ultrasound machine from the 1960s. The patient in this photo is sitting in a water bath. Sonographic transverse sections of the neck area are to be made. The transducer travels along the wall, just below the water surface, and around the patient. The images in **1** and **2** were produced with this or a similar system.

[From Holmes JH (1974) Diagnostic ultrasound: historical perspective. In King, D. L. (ed): *Diagnostic Ultrasound*, C. V. Mosby Company, St. Louis, p. 3, with permission of Mosby Year Book, St. Louis.]

4

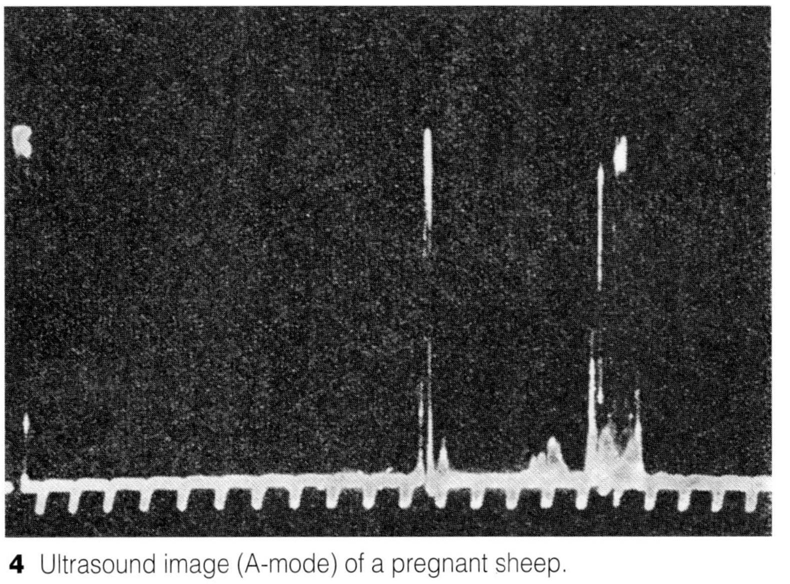

4 Ultrasound image (A-mode) of a pregnant sheep.

[Reprinted with permission from *Nature*, **212**, pp. 642–643; Copyright ©1966 Macmillan Magazines Limited.]

of this method in veterinary medicine was Frank S. Pipers[36, 37], who also applied this method in dogs and cats. Compound B-mode ultrasonographic images of abdominal organs in animals were published in the mid-1970s by A. Everette James and associates[21, 22]. After the development of two-dimensional real-time sonography in the early 1980s, abdominal ultrasonography became an established imaging method in dogs and cats. Robert E. Cartee[4, 5] and Thomas G. Nyland[34, 35] were two of the pioneers in this field.

While a simple Doppler method was already in use for pregnancy diagnosis (see above) in the early 1970s, it took 15 years until the Japanese Mitsuyoshi Hagio and Hiromitsu Otsuka[13] used pulsed-Doppler echocardiography clinically to examine cardiac haemodynamics in dogs. Three years later, in the early 1990s, Peter G. G. Darke[7] first described the significance of colour-coded Doppler echocardiography in the diagnosis of canine heart disease.

Although ultrasonography has been successfully applied in all fields of veterinary diagnostics in the past 27 years[25], it has just recently become a routine diagnostic method in many veterinary clinics and practices. In the past five and eight years, in German and English speaking countries respectively, the use of ultrasound is comparable to that of radiography.

References

1 Baum G and Greenwood I (1958) The application of ultrasonic locating techniques to ophthalmology. *Arch. Ophthal.* **60**, 263–279.

2 Bergmann L (1939) *Der Ultraschall.* 2nd Edn. VDI-Verlag, Berlin.

3 Bommer WJ and Miller L (1982) Real-time, two-dimensional color-flow Doppler: enhances Doppler flow imaging in the diagnosis of cardiovascular disease (abstr.). *Am. J. Cardiol.* **49**, 944.

4 Carter RE (1981) Diagnostic real-time ultrasonography of the liver of the dog and cat. *J. Am. Anim. Hosp. Assoc.* **17**, 731–737.

5 Cartee RE, Selcer BA and Patton CS (1980) Ultrasonographic diagnosis of renal disease in small animals. *J. Am. Vet. Med. Assoc.* **176**, 426–430.

6 Donald I, MacVicar J and Brown TG (1958) Investigation of abdominal masses by pulsed ultrasound. *Lancet* **1**, 1188–1195.

7 Darke PGG (1990) Doppler echocardiography in small animals. *Vet. Internat.* **2**, 3–13.

8 Dussik KT (1942) Über die Möglichkeit, hochfrequente mechanische Schwingungen als diagnostisches Hilfsmittel zu verwerten. *Zeitschr. gesamt. Neurol. Psych.* **174**, 153–168.

9 Edler I and Hertz CH (1954) The use of ultrasonic reflectoscope for the continuous recording of the movements of heart walls. *Kungl.Fysiografiska Sällskapet i Land Förhandlingar* **24**, 40–58.

10 Feigenbaum H (1976) *Echocardiography.* 2nd Edn. Lea & Febiger, Philadelphia.

11 Firestone FA (1945) The supersonic reflectoscope for interior inspection. *Metal Progress* **48**, 505–512.

12 Firestone FA (1946) The supersonic reflectoscope: an instrument for inspecting the interior of solid parts by means of sound waves. *J. Acoustical Soc. Am.* **17**, 287–299.

13 Hagio M and Otsuka H (1987) Pulsed Doppler echocardiography in normal dogs and calves, and three cases of valvular regurgitation. *Jpn. J. Vet. Sci.* **49**, 1113–1125.

14 Helper LC (1970) Diagnosis of pregnancy in the bitch with an ultrasonic Doppler instrument. *J. Am. Vet. Med. Assoc.* **156**, 60–62.

15 Hertz CH and Edler I (1956) Die Registrierung von Herzwandbewegungen mit Hilfe des Ultraschall-Impulsverfahrens. *Acustica* **6**, 361–364.

16 Holmes JH (1974) Diagnostic ultrasound: historical perspective. In: King DL (Ed.) *Diagnostic Ultrasound.* CV Mosby Company, Saint Louis, pp. 1–15.

17 Holmes JH and Howry DH (1963) Ultrasonic diagnosis of abdominal disease. *Am. J. Dig. Dis.* **8**, 12–32.

18 Holmes JH, Howry DH, Posakony GJ and Cushman CR (1954) The ultrasonic visualization of soft tissue structures in the body. *Trans. Am. Clin. Climat. Assoc.* **66**, 208–225.

19 Howry DH and Bliss WR (1952) Ultrasonic visualization of soft tissue structures of the body. *J. Lab. Clin. Med.* **40**, 579–592.

20 Howry DH, Stott DA and Bliss WR (1954) The ultrasonic visualization of carcinoma of the breast and other soft tissue structures. *Cancer* **7**, 354–358.

21 James AE, Sanders RC, Osterman FA, Novak GR and Bush RM (1975) Abdominal ultrasound in animals. *Seminars in Roentgenology* **10**, 323–328.

22 James AE, Osterman FO, Bush RM, Sheehan T, Novak G, Wight D and Sanders RC (1976) The use of compound B-mode ultrasound in abdominal disease of animals. *J. Am. Vet. Radiol. Soc.* **17**, 106–112.

23 Keidel W-D (1950) Über eine neue Methode zur Registrierung der Volumenänderungen des Herzens am Menschen. *Zeitschr. Kreislaufforschung* **39**, 257–271.

24 Koch SA and Rubin LF (1969) Diagnostic ultrasonography of the dog eye. *J. Small Anim.Pract.* **10**, 357–361.

25 Lamb CR, Stowater JL and Pipers FS (1988) The first twenty-one years of veterinary diagnostic ultrasound. *Vet. Radiol.* **29**, 37–45.

26 Lamm A-M (1970) Ultrasound diagnosis of pregnancy in the dog. *Acta Radiol.* **Suppl. 319**, 293–294.

27 Langevin MP (1928) Les ondes ultrasonores. *Rev. Gén. Électric* **23**, 626–634.

28 Leksell L (1955) Behandling av akuta skallskador och deras följdtillstånd. Kirurgisk behandling. *Nord. Med.* **15**, 1444.

29 Leksell L (1955/56) Echoencephalography. I. Detection of intracranial complications following head injury. *Acta Chir. Scand.* **110**, 301–315.

30 Lindhal IL (1966) Detection of pregnancy in sheep by means of ultrasound. *Nature* **212**, 642–643.

31 Mandt GH and Hughes WF (1956) Ultrasonics in ocular diagnosis. *Am. J. Ophthal.* **41**, 488–498.

32 Namekawa K, Kasai C, Tsukamoto M and Koyano A (1982) Real-time blood flow imaging system utilizing autocorrelation techniques. In: Lerski RA and Morley P (Eds.) *Ultrasound '82.* Pergamon Press, New York, Oxford, Toronto, pp. 203–208.

33 Namekawa K, Kasai, C, Omoto R, Kondo Y, Katabami T, Hidal T, Yoshikawa Y, Tsukamoto M, Yokote Y, Takamoto S and Koyano A (1983) Real-time, two-dimensional blood flow imaging using ultrasound Doppler. *J. Ultrasound Med. Biol.* **2 (Suppl.)**, 65.

34 Nyland TG and Bernard WV (1982) Application of abdominal ultrasound. *Calif. Vet.* **36**, 21–25.

35 Nyland TG, Park RD, Lattimer JC, Lebel JL and Miller CW (1981) Gray scale ultrasonography of the canine abdomen. *Vet. Radiol.* **22**, 220–227.

36 Pipers FS, Andrysco RM and Hamlin RL (1978) A totally noninvasive method for obtaining systolic time intervals in the dog. *Am. J. Vet. Res.* **39**, 1822–1826.

37 Pipers FS, Reef V and Hamlin RL (1979) Echocardiography in the domestic cat. *Am. J. Vet. Res.* **40**, 882–886.

38 Rubin LF and Koch SA (1968) Ocular diagnostic ultrasonography. *J. Am. Vet. Med. Assoc.* **153**, 1706–1716.

39 Satomura S (1959) Study of the flow patterns in peripheral arteries by ultrasonics. *J. Acoust. Soc. Jpn.* **15**, 151–158.

40 Sokoloff SJ (1929) Zur Frage der Fortpflanzung ultra-akustischer Schwingungen in verschiedenen Körpern. *Elektr. Nachrichten Technik* **6**, 454–461.

41 Temple RS, Stonaker HH and Howry D (1956) Ultrasonic and conductive methods for estimating fat thickness in live cattle. *Proc. Am. Soc. Anim. Prod. West Sec.* **7**, 477–479.

42 Wild JJ (1950) The use of ultrasonic pulses for the measurement of biologic tissues and the detection of tissue density changes. *Surgery* **27**, 183–188.

2 Physical Principles

Cordula Poulsen Nautrup

Ultrasound

Ultrasound is characterized by sound higher in frequency than the upper range of human hearing, which is 20,000 cycles per second (20 kHz). Frequencies up to 100 million cycles per second (100 MHz) have been achieved. Frequencies of 1–10 MHz, in some cases up to 20 MHz, are commonly used in medical diagnostics. Dogs and cats may perceive ultrasound of up to 100 kHz, but have not been reported to be disturbed by the commonly employed frequencies.

Sound waves are cyclic alterations of matter in time and space, caused by a force, in this case mechanical pressure. The material particles begin to be altered from a fixed state. This wave-like alteration is then transmitted at velocities characteristic of each medium. The particles are alternately compressed and rarefied (**5**).

A wavelength (λ) consists of the distance between compressed and rarefied particles in one cycle. Wavelengths are inversely proportional to frequencies (f) or cycles per second. High frequencies have shorter wavelengths and vice versa.

5

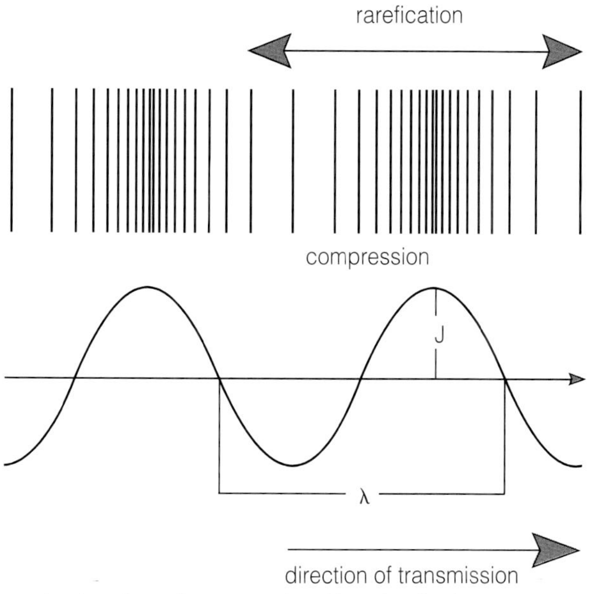

5 Schematic drawing of a transmitted longitudinal wave.

$$\lambda \sim 1/f \quad \lambda = c/f \quad \text{or} \quad c = \lambda \times f$$

[λ: wavelength; f: frequency; c: velocity]

Wavelengths can be calculated by this equation and are between 1.5 and 0.15 mm (at frequencies of 1–10 MHz and a mean velocity of 1,540 m/s in soft tissues) in medical diagnostics.

Waves with amplitudes in the transmitting direction are called longitudinal waves (**5**). Oscillations perpendicular to this direction are therefore transverse waves. Medical diagnostic ultrasonography uses only the longitudinal waves.

Interaction of Ultrasound Beams with Tissues

The basic acoustic principles, such as sound intensity, sound velocity and imedance, reflection, transmission, refraction, scatter, divergence and absorption, are also true for the interaction of ultrasound in biological tissues.

Sound Intensity, Velocity and Acoustic Impedance

The amplitude (J) of a two-dimensionally displayed sound wave (**5**) exemplifies the maximum extension of its oscillation. A higher amplitude may be attained by increasing the energy supply. In acoustics a high amplitude or high sound intensity is indicative of high sound volume. In real-time ultrasonography the higher the sound intensity the brighter the echoes will be on the monitor.

Sound velocity (c) is dependent on the wavelength and frequency of sound beams (see above). The density of the media in which the sound wave is transmitted also influences sound velocity.

Stiffness of the material is probably more important than density, but the two are interrelated by the formula for acoustic impedance.

Sound velocity varies in the body's soft tissues, with the exception of air-filled lung tissue, between 1,520 m/s (water) and 1,950 m/s (skin), the mean value being 1,540 m/s (*Table 1*).

Tissue characteristics, such as molecule connection and elementary substance inertia, counteract sound beam transmission and are referred to as sound wave resistance or acoustic impedance (*Table 1*). Acoustic impedance (Z) is defined as the product of the tissue's density (p) and propagation velocity (c):

$$Z = \rho \times c$$

[Z: acoustic impedance; ρ: tissue density; c: sound velocity]

Reflection, Transmission and Refraction

Tissues with impedance differences have acoustic interfaces that reflect sound waves with proportional intensity to the degree of difference in impedances.

Sound beams perpendicular to an interface at a 90 degree angle α will be reflected at a 90 degree angle β to the interface (α = β = 90 degrees). The sound receiver, scanner or transducer can register these echoes. The non-reflected sound beams continue transmitting through the new medium (**6**).

When the sound beam angle α is not 90 degrees, some of the reflected sound waves do not return directly to the transducer. The non-reflected sound waves travel through the new medium after altering their direction (angle γ), a fact which is referred to as refraction (**7**).

> Only sound beams perpendicular to an interface will produce ultrasound images that can be accurately assessed for their thickness and echogenicity (**8**).

The relationship of reflected to transmitted echo amplitude depends on the impedance difference of two tissues at an interface. At an interface with a high acoustic impedance nearly all sound intensity is reflected. Small differences in acoustic impedance will cause the reflected intensities to be small (*Table 1*).

Table 1 Sound velocity, acoustic impedance and attenuation in various substances and tissues at 37°C (98.6°F), as well as sound reflection at interfaces between water and a second medium.

Body tissue, medium	Sound velocity[7] (m/s)	Aoustic impedance[7] ×10⁶ (Ns/m³)	Attenuation of sound Intensity by absorption, divergence and scattering at 1 Mhz[7] (db/cm)	Reflected energy at interface with water with perpendicular beam[6] (%)
Skin	1,950	2.15	1.0	2.9
Fat	1,450	1.41	0.4	0.2
Muscle	1,570	1.68	0.7	0.4
Liver	1,560	1.65	0.6	0.3
Kidney	1,555	1.61	0.5	0.1
Brain	1,520	1.56	0.5	missing
Blood	1,560	1.56	0.1	0.1
Bone	2,200	7.30	5.0	42.0
Water	1,520	1.52	0.002	—
Air	345	0.00042	1.7	99.9

High acoustic impedance differences with total or almost complete reflection are caused by interfaces with gas or mineral. The body's soft tissues show only small differences in acoustic impedance (*Table 1*).

6

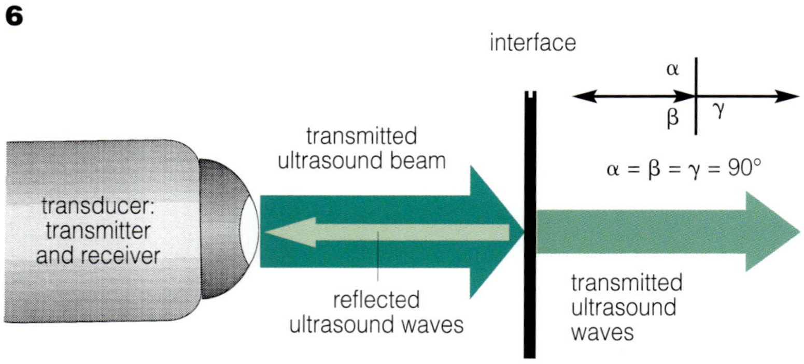

6 Schematic drawing of sound wave reflection and transmission perpendicular to an acoustic interface.

7

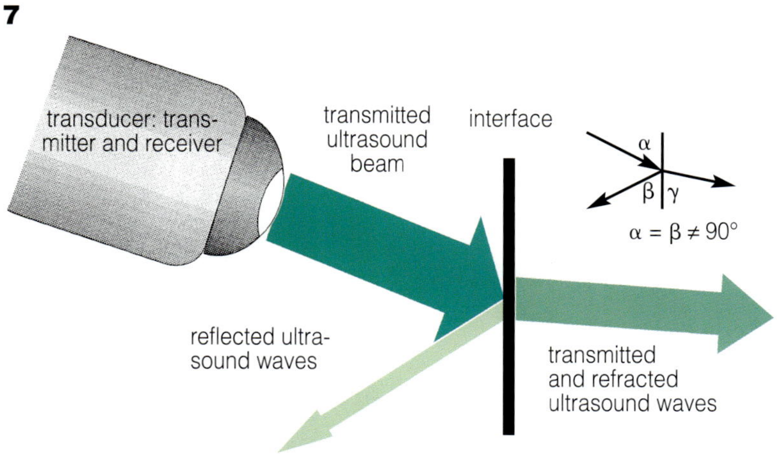

7 Schematic drawing of sound wave reflection and refraction at interface struck at an oblique angle.

Scattering, Absorption and Divergence

Ultrasound waves encountering small, uneven and inclined acoustic interfaces are diffusely reflected, also termed scattering (**9**).

Longitudinal waves travel straight through a homogeneous medium at a specific sound wave velocity. At the same time, part of the sound wave's mechanical energy is converted to other forms of energy (usually heat). This energy is no longer available for imaging.

> The decrease in sound energy and intensity through absorption is dependent upon the sound frequency and the tissue texture.

Absorption in soft tissues is relatively minor. Bones, calcifications and calculi show so-called 'acoustic shadowing' (see Acoustic Shadowing and Enhancement, page 70), due to the high attenuation and loss of energy distal to these textures.

Increased attenuation in soft tissues shows a linear correlation to higher frequencies. High frequencies lead to increased attenuation and decreased sound wave depth penetration (*Table 2*). In bones, attenuation becomes squared with each increase of frequency[5, 11].

Table 2 Frequency and penetration of ultrasound waves in soft tissues (c ~ 1,540 m/s).

Sound frequency	**1MHz**	**3.5 MHz**	**5 MHz**	**7.5 MHz**	**10MHz**	**15 MHz**
Soft tissue penetration	500 mm	150 mm	100 mm	70 mm	50 mm	10 mm

Sound beams meeting the outer areas of high attenuation tissues may cause an acoustic shadow (**10**). A similar shadow is also seen distal to rounded organ margins, e.g. kidneys or amniotic sacs. This phenomenon is due to reflection of the beam, not absorption (see **138**).

8

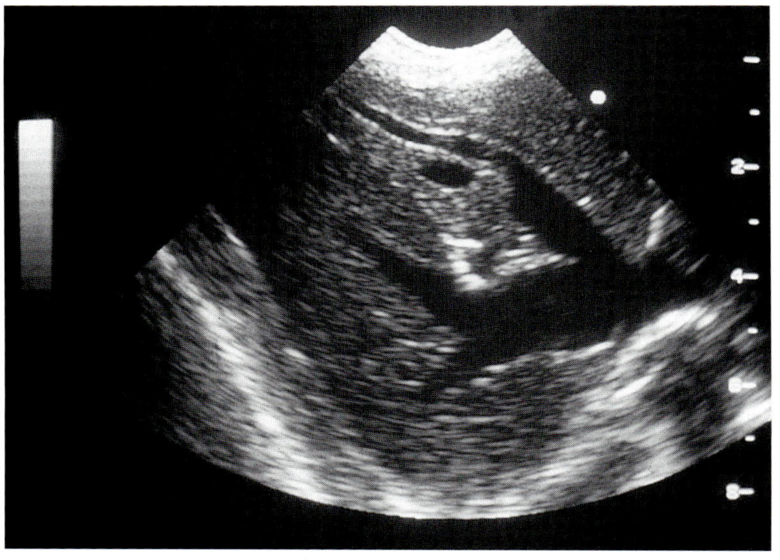

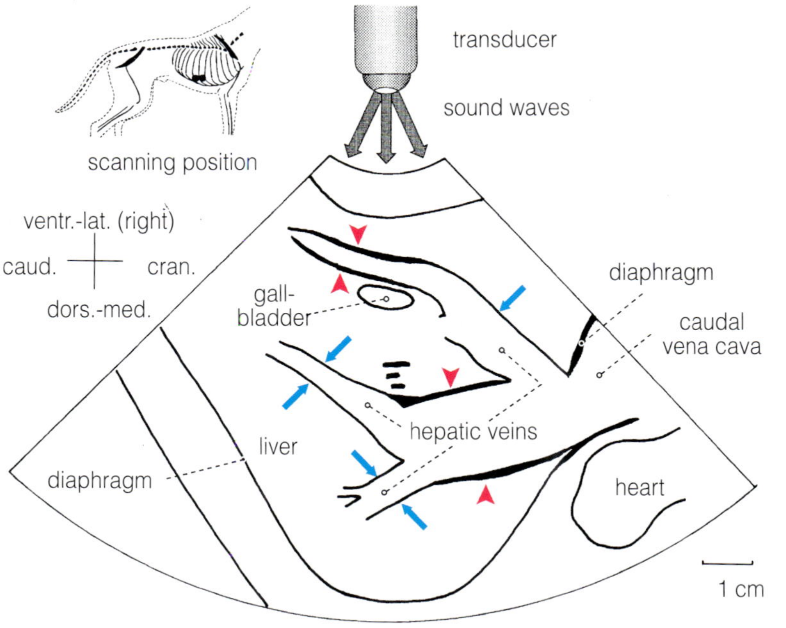

8 Ultrasound image of the liver in a dog; distinct image of hepatic vein walls (red arrow heads) with perpendicular sound beam and obscure or missing wall echoes with sound waves at an oblique angle.

9

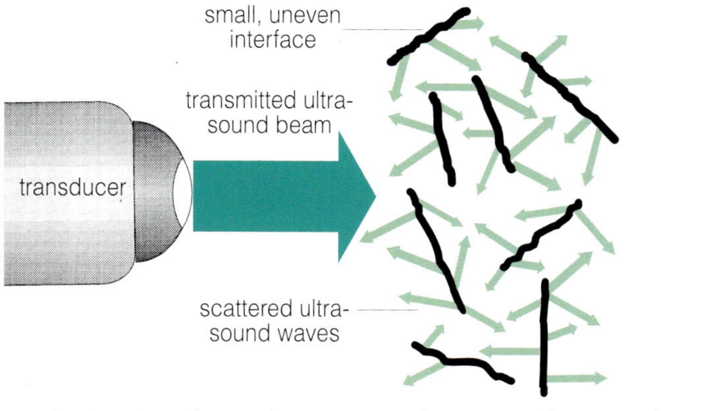

9 Schematic drawing of sound wave scattering at small, uneven interfaces.

10

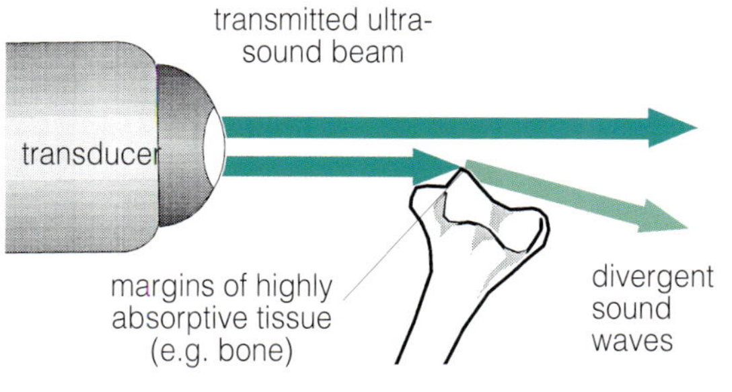

10 Schematic drawing of sound wave divergence of highly absorptive tissue margins (e.g. bone).

11

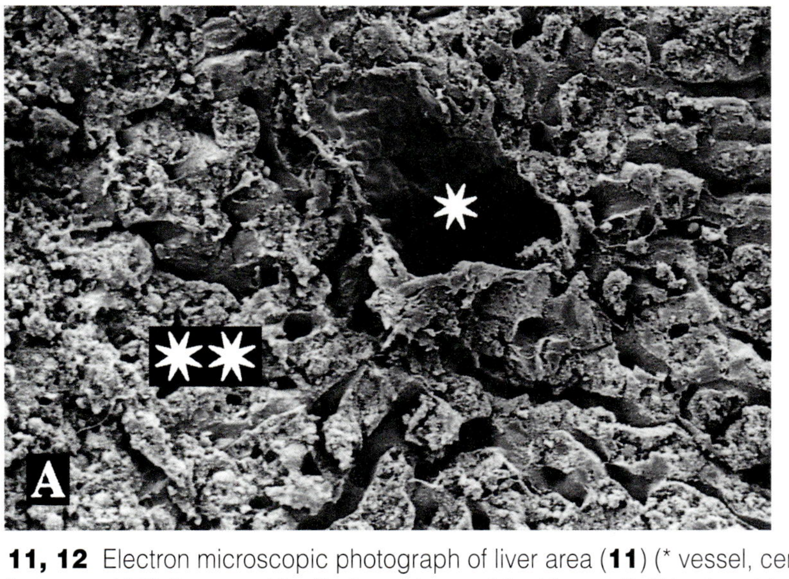

12

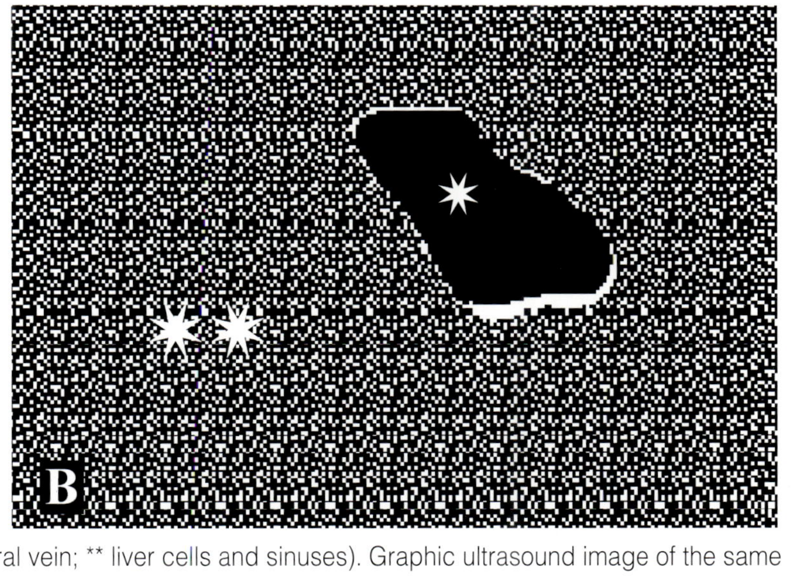

11, 12 Electron microscopic photograph of liver area (**11**) (* vessel, central vein; ** liver cells and sinuses). Graphic ultrasound image of the same liver area (**12**) (* geometric display of large object [vessel]; ** textured image of smaller structures [cells and sinuses]).

> Reflection, transmission and refraction are usually associated with relatively large objects, while scattering and divergence occur with smaller structures.

Large structures, such as organs with their inner structures, margins, vessels and neoplasia, are imaged according to the geometry of their interfaces with the help of ultrasound (11 *, 12 *, 13 *).

Finer tissue structures, e.g. capillaries and cells, which are smaller than an ultrasound wavelength, show distinct texture in which the separate echoes are not represented by an actual dot on the image. Various organ parenchyma are displayed by these artificial but typical textured images (11**, 12**, 13**). Fine parenchymal structures produce diffuse multiple echoes.

13

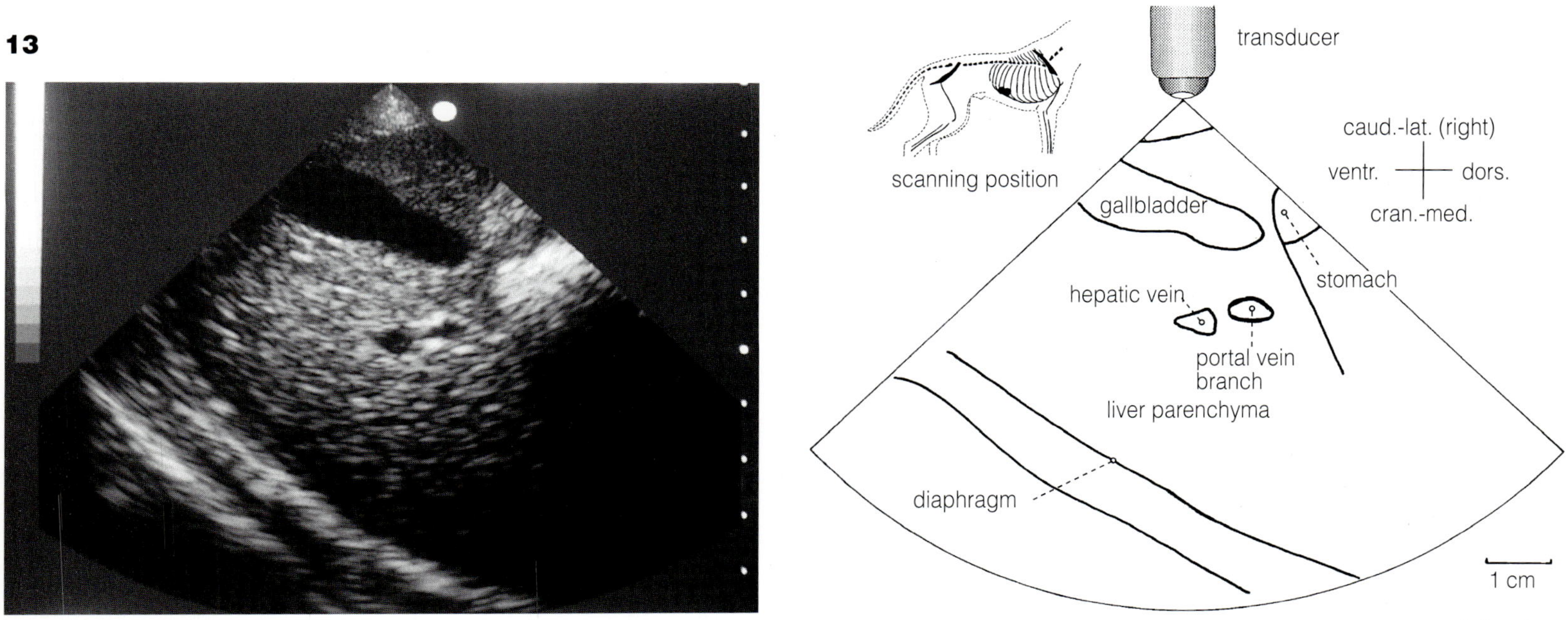

13 Ultrasound image of the liver in a dog with actual display of the gallbladder (*) and two vessels as well as a textured image of the liver parenchyma (**).

14

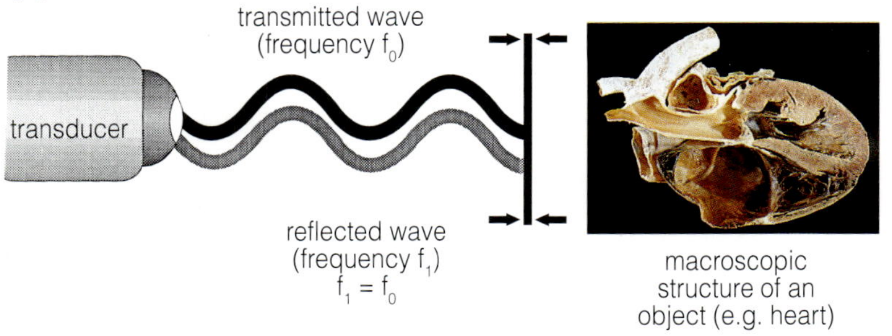

14 Schematic drawing of reflected sound waves from an immobile object.

15

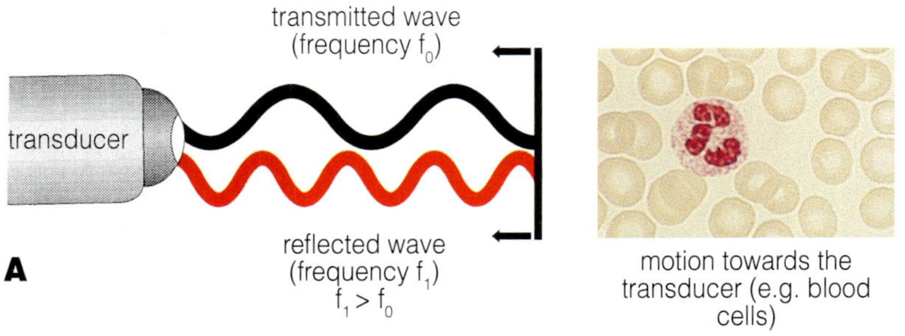

A

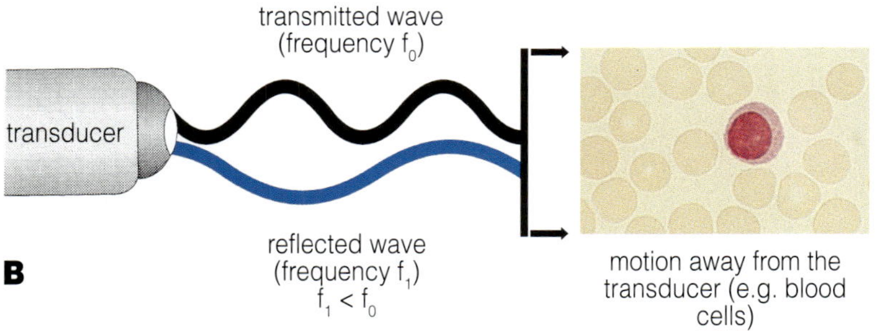

B

15 Schematic drawings of reflected sound waves from moving targets (e.g. blood cells). Motion towards the transducer (**A**); motion away from the transducer (**B**).

Doppler Effect

An ultrasound wave reflected from an immobile object has less energy than the original sound wave, although it has the same wavelength and frequency (**14**).

In contrast, sound wave reflection from a moving target results in a shift in frequency, the so-called 'Doppler shift' (**15A, B**).

The Doppler shift (f_d) is defined as the difference between the reflected 'new' frequency (f_1) and the transmitted 'original' frequency (f_0):

$$f_d = f_1 - f_0$$

The Doppler effect, named after its discoverer Christian J. Doppler (1803–1853), is well demonstrated in street traffic. The motor noise of a car or an airplane moving towards a person will not only become louder, but will also appear to have a higher pitch, which means that the frequency is higher. If the motion of the sound source is away from the person, the frequency will appear lower and the sound is fainter. The greater the velocity of the moving object, the greater the frequency shift, which is clearly higher in an airplane than in a car.

> In medical ultrasonography the Doppler effect is used to determine the relative direction and velocity of blood flow.

If blood cell motion is towards the transducer, the frequency of the reflected waves is higher than the transmitted sound. In this case the waves appear condensed ($f_1 > f_0$ and $f_d > 0$). Blood flow towards the transducer will be displayed above the zero baseline in conventional Doppler ultrasonography, and as shades of red in colour-flow Doppler (**15A, 16, 18**).

When blood flow is away from the transducer, the returning echoes will have a lower frequency than the transmitted sound. The waves appear extended ($f_1 < f_0$ and $f_d < 0$). In conventional Doppler ultrasonography this tracing will be displayed below the horizontal zero baseline, while it is represented as shades of blue in the colour Doppler display (**15B, 16, 17**).

The described choice of display modes, above or below the zero

16

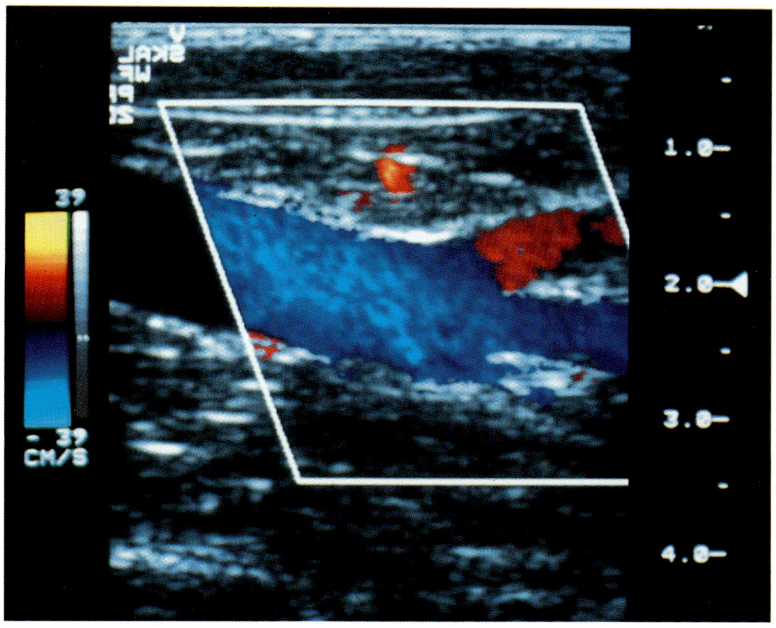

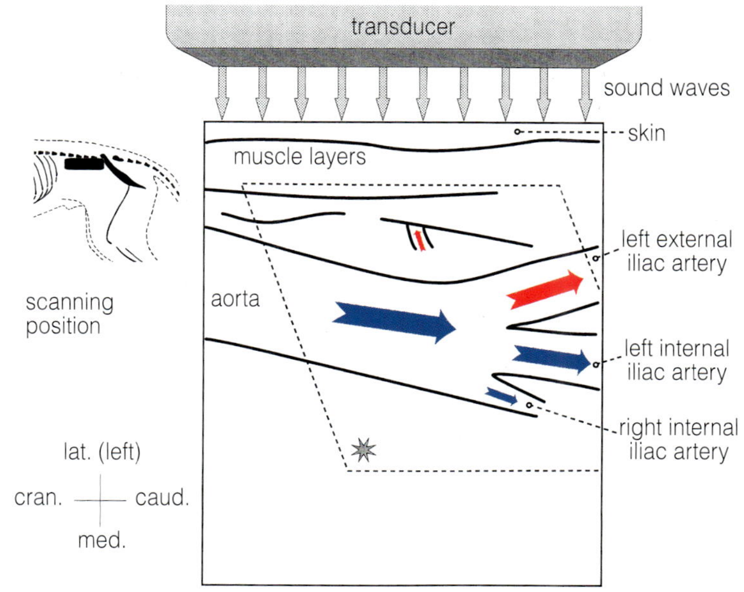

✳ The marked square represents the area in which blood flow is displayed by colour Doppler ultrasonography.

17

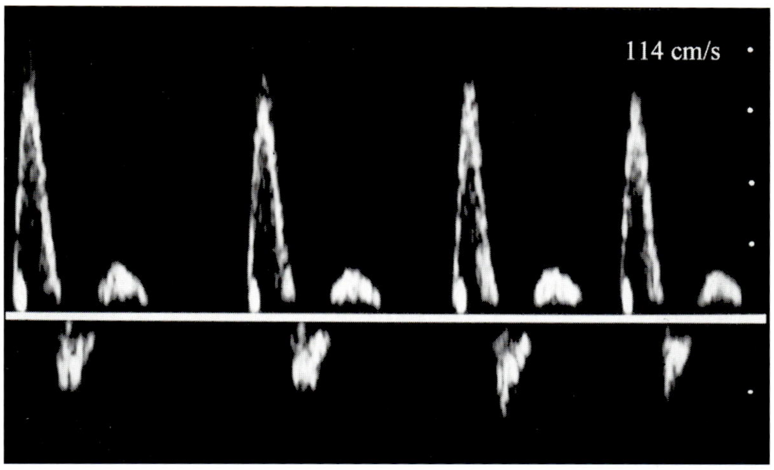

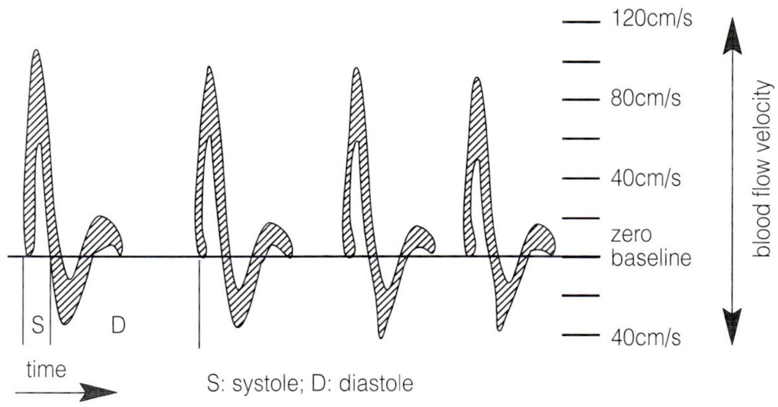

Blood flow in the external iliac artery
(predominantly towards the transducer)

18

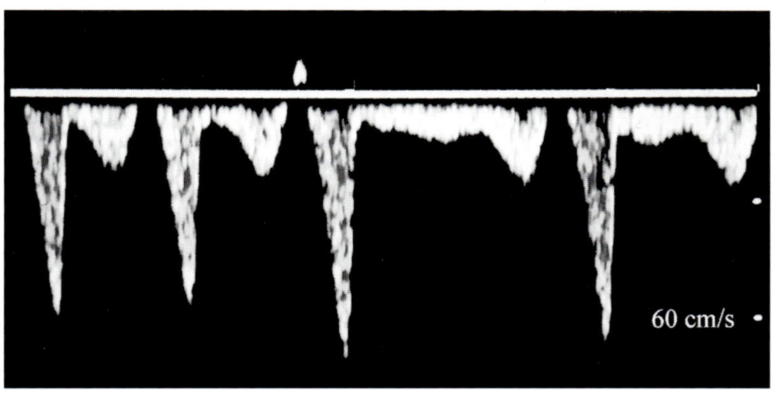

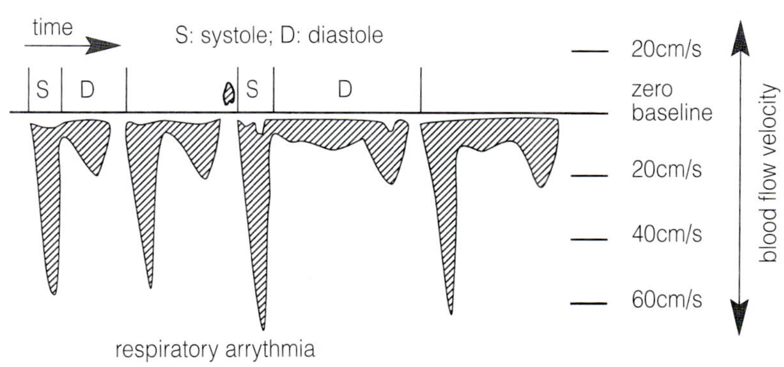

Blood flow in the internal iliac artery
(predominantly away from the transducer)

16–18 Arterial blood flow away from the transducer in the abdominal aorta and the internal iliac artery (**16**: blue colour; **18**: below the zero baseline) and arterial blood flow towards the transducer in the external iliac artery in a dog (**16**: red colour; **18**: above the zero baseline). Colour Doppler display (**16**) and conventional pulsed Doppler displays (**17, 18**). The blue colour in the aorta and the internal iliac artery represents relative direction of blood flow (**16**); this image is seen first during the examination.

19

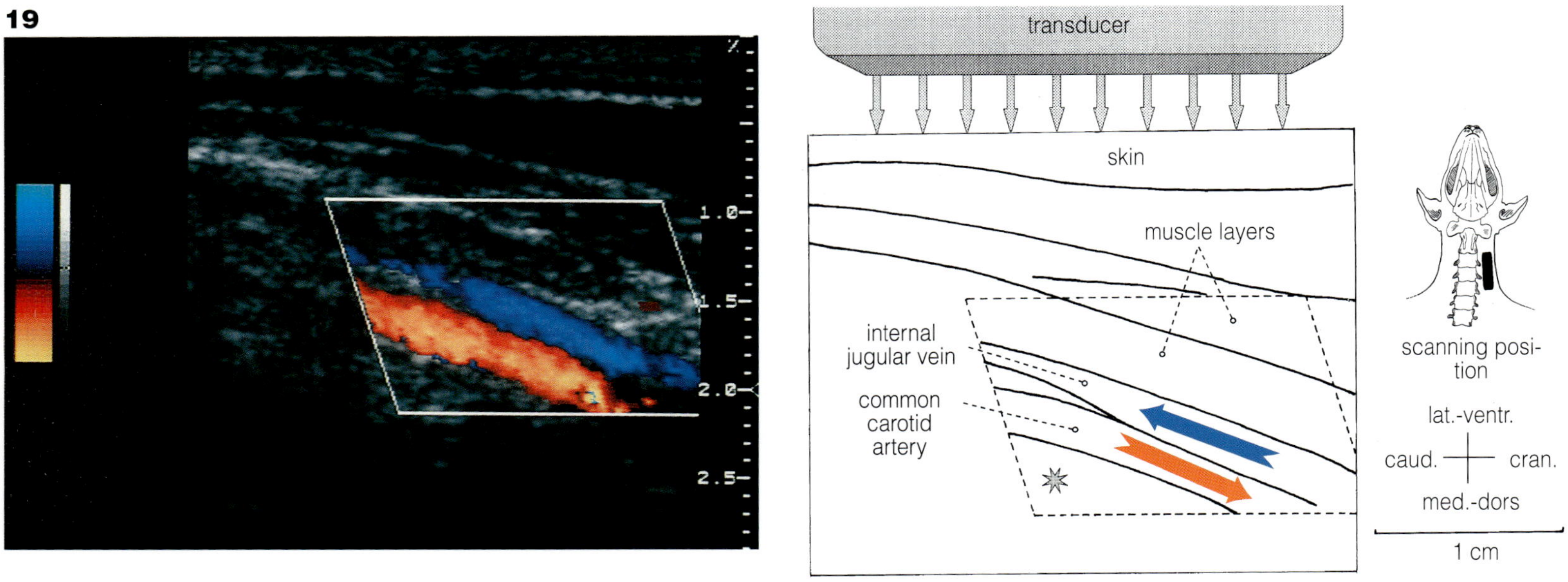

The marked square represents the area in which blood flow is displayed by colour Doppler ultrasonography.

20

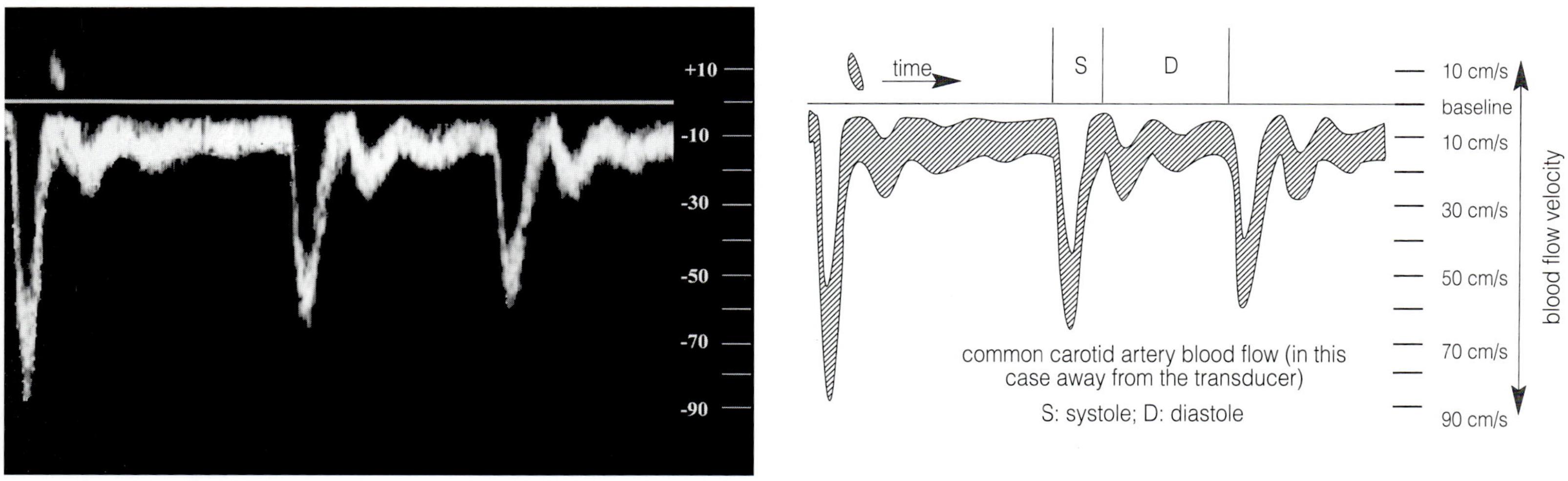

19, 20 Arterial blood flow away from the transducer in the common carotid artery, as well as venous blood flow towards the transducer in the internal jugular vein in a dog. Colour Doppler display (**19**): the adjusted colours correspond with the vessel type; blood flow in the common carotid artery is red, the internal jugular vein is blue. The colour bar on the left side of the image signifies colour flow direction. Conventional Doppler display (**20**): conventional pulsed-wave Doppler displays the common carotid artery tracing below the baseline, since blood flow is away from the transducer.

baseline, red or blue colour, are optional and may be changed at any time. They do not correspond with the wavelengths of coloured light (red: long wavelength; blue: short wavelength) and do not signify type of vessel (artery, vein) or blood quality (arterial or venous blood).

In modern angiology, for example, the original colour in a colour-coded Doppler spectrum is often changed later to conform with the vessel type, regardless of blood flow direction. Flow direction is indicated by a colour bar on the image (**19, 20**).

When the ultrasound beam cannot be projected parallel to blood flow, the Doppler shift depends on blood flow velocity (V) and on blood cell motion relative to the angle of the transmitted beam (cos q) and the sound velocity in tissues (c).

$$f_d = 2 \times f_0 \times \frac{V \times \cos\theta}{c}$$

[f_d: Doppler shift frequency; f_0: transmitted frequency; V: blood flow velocity; cos q: cosine of the angle θ between beam and blood flow; c: blood velocity (c = 1,560 m/s)]

The equation is rearranged to define blood flow velocity (V) as follows:

$$V = f_d \times \frac{c}{2 \times f_0 \times \cos\theta}$$

The most exact velocity recordings are obtained when the beam is orientated parallel to the blood flow, so that the incident beam angle θ is 0 degrees and $\cos\theta = 1$. Calculation errors are 0% in this case. At an angle of 45 degrees, flow velocity will be 29% too low, while at 60 degrees the error is 50%. Vessels travelling perpendicular to the transducer will not register blood flow in Doppler mode (angle $\theta = 90$ degrees $\rightarrow \cos\theta = 0$) (**24**).

The development of extremely sensitive instrumentation and methods to determine blood flow should compensate for this weakness.

Doppler shift frequencies are within the hearing range 0–20 kHz. The frequency shifts are therefore not only visually presented, but also audible. High velocity blood flows with high Doppler shifts produce loud sounds, while low velocity flows cause low noises.

> For exact velocity recordings, the incident beam should be orientated parallel to the blood flow and a correction factor must be applied for angle variation (**21–23**).

21

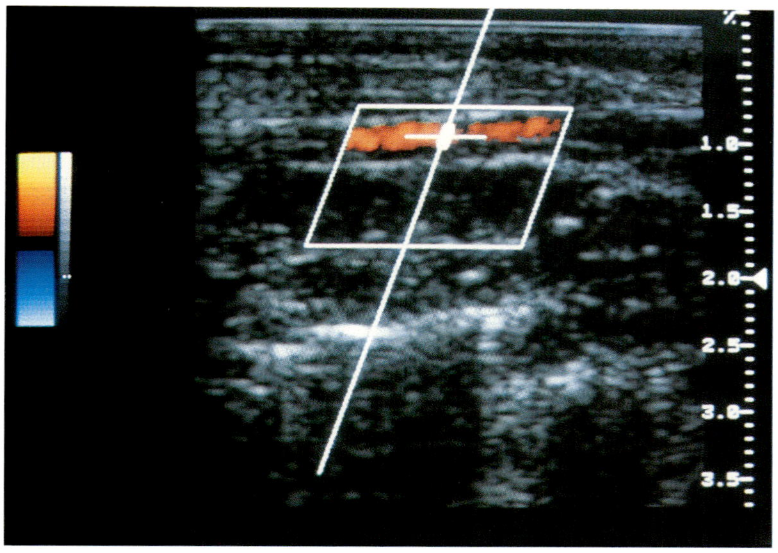

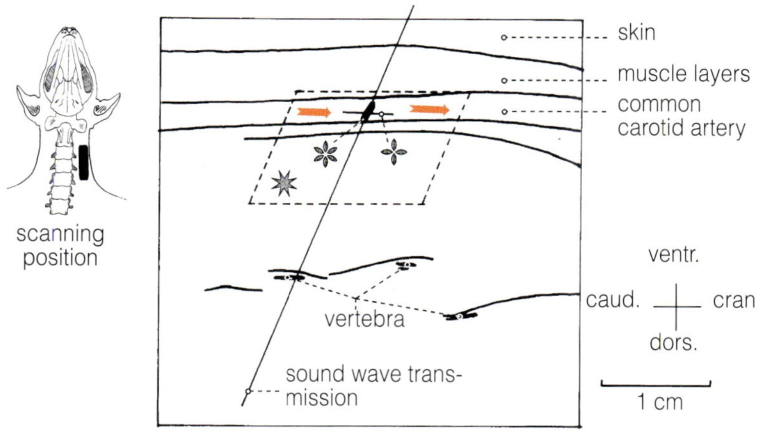

✳ The marked square represents the area in which blood flow is displayed by colour Doppler ultrasonography.

✳ The sample volume lies in the area in which blood flow is identified by pulsed-wave Doppler.

✧ The cursor through the sample shows the flow angle to the sound beam, which is represented by the long line.

22

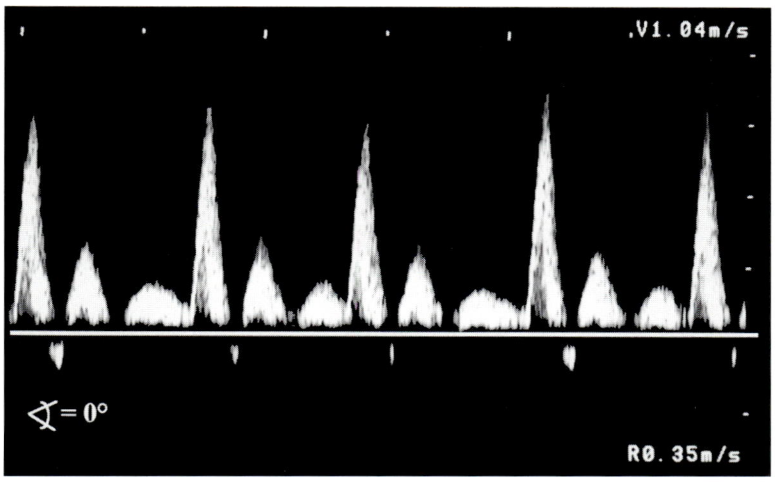

23

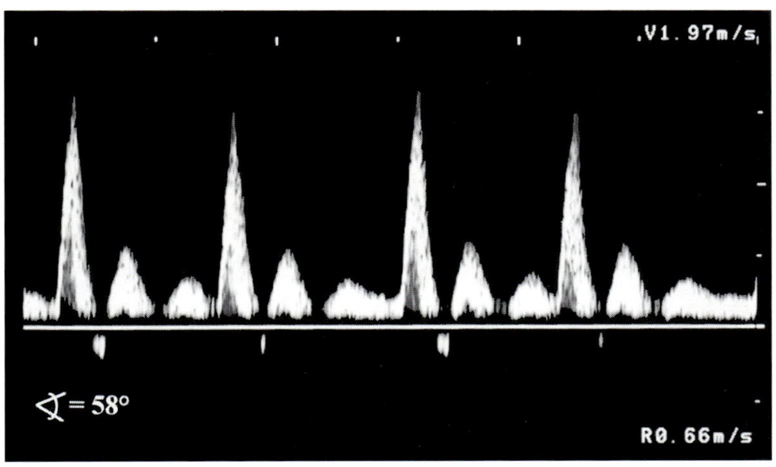

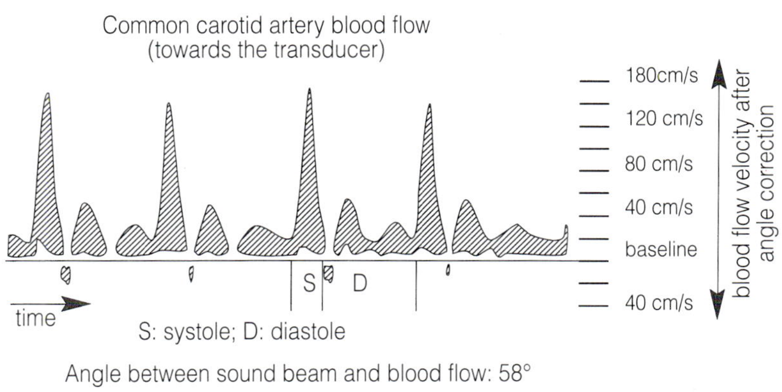

21–23 Arterial blood flow in the common carotid artery of a dog. Colour Doppler display (**21**): blood flow is towards the transducer, not parallel to the beam, but at a 58 degree angle. Pulsed-wave Doppler display (**22, 23**): blood flow measurements in the common carotid artery show a maximum velocity of 80 cm/s without angle correction (**22**) and 160 cm/s with angle correction (**23**).

24

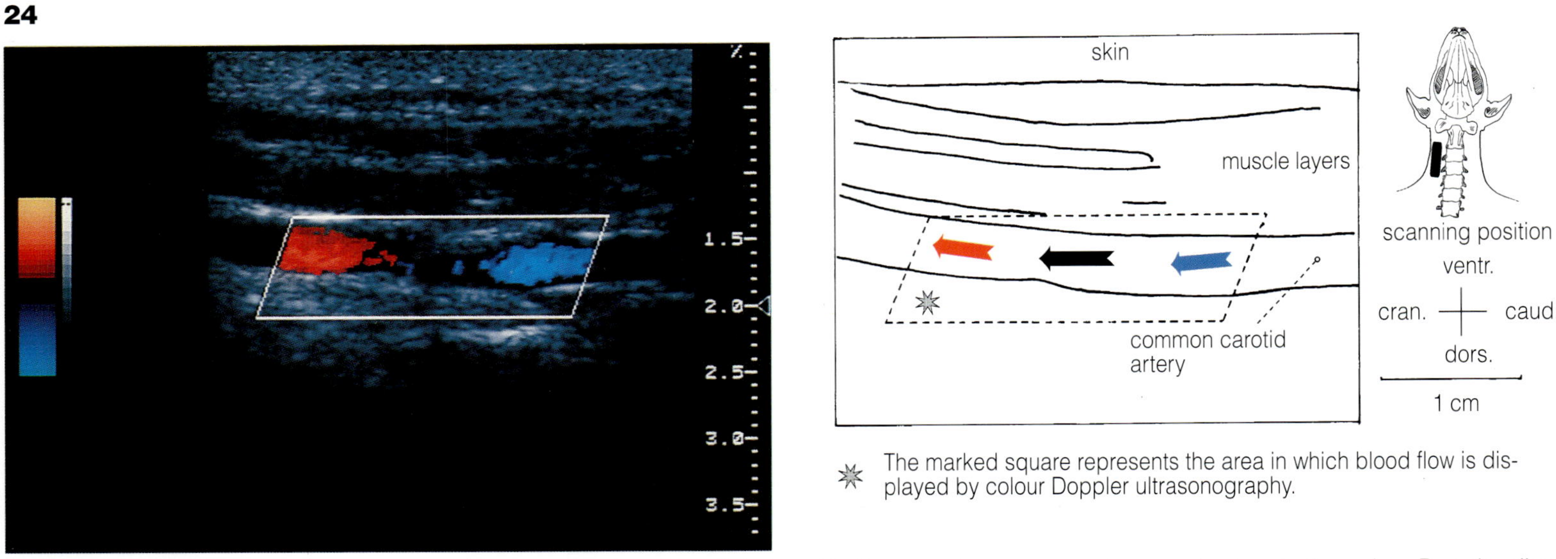

✳ The marked square represents the area in which blood flow is displayed by colour Doppler ultrasonography.

24 Arterial blood flow in the common carotid artery of a dog. The slight bend in the vessel produces a change of colour in the colour Doppler display, depending on the blood flow angle to the sound beam. Flow in the caudal portion of the common carotid artery is away from the transducer and is, therefore, blue. There are no flow tracings in the middle part, since the blood flow is perpendicular to the beam ($\cos\theta = V = 0$). The red colour in the cranial part shows blood flow towards the transducer.

Doppler Frequency Spectrum

Since blood cells do not all travel at the same flow velocity, registered Doppler signals are displayed as a frequency spectrum.

The frequency spectrum is narrow when similar flow velocities of blood cells are recorded, and the Doppler signal makes a clear, whistling noise. A wide frequency spectrum, however, sounds harsher and hisses.

Doppler spectral tracings are graphically displayed by separating the multifrequency signals into 'bins' of different frequencies. This is done through digital calculations following the fast Fourier transformation or an analog Chirp-Z transformation[3,4].

Because of limited time, spectral tracings do not analyze individual frequencies (Doppler shifts), but rather entire frequency segments.

> The Doppler spectral display determines three parameters:
>
> - The frequency spectrum or velocites and flow directions of blood cells.
> - Blood flow volume.
> - Blood flow velocity as a function of time.

These parameters are plotted on a two-dimensional graph (25–27):

- In conventional Doppler ultrasonography, blood cell velocity or frequency shift is displayed along the vertical axis (y-axis). With colour Doppler, this parameter is estimated by the colour shown. Apart from the velocities, the direction of blood flow is also imaged.
- Either blood flow volume or the Doppler signal amplitude or noise is displayed as varying shades of grey or colours.
- The Doppler signal as a function of time is plotted on the horizontal or x-axis in conventional Doppler and as an image change in colour Doppler.

Biological Effects of Ultrasound

The biological effects are mechanical, thermal and chemical[6,8,9,10].

Mechanical Effects

Ultrasound causes mechanical vibrations in tissues. The particles are compressed (pressure phase) and then dispersed (suction phase). Small cavities form in fluids during the suction phase and disappear in the pressure phase. This phenomenon is described as cavitation in gas-free fluids and pseudocavitation in fluids with gas.

The amount of cavitation and pseudocavitation depends on the frequency and the intensity (sound energy per area). High frequencies combined with high intensities have great mechanical effects. There are no confirmed adverse effects or mechanical damage to cell membranes or chromosomes by exposure to diagnostic levels of ultrasound.

Therapeutic ultrasound, which applies higher intensities than diagnostic sonography, uses these mechanical forces for generation of heat or, in a more sophisticated application, for the destruction of renal calculi (lithotripsy).

Thermal Effects

Thermal effects of ultrasound are due to ultrasound energy absorption and its transformation into heat. This effect is also dependent on sound frequency and intensity. Intensities used in diagnostic ultrasound are not thought to cause significant thermal effects. Beam characteristics and the heat reducing effect of vasculariza tion are thought to contribute to the lack of thermal effects, provided the vascular system is intact and moves the heat. Hyperthermia, however, is used in therapeutic ultrasonography.

25

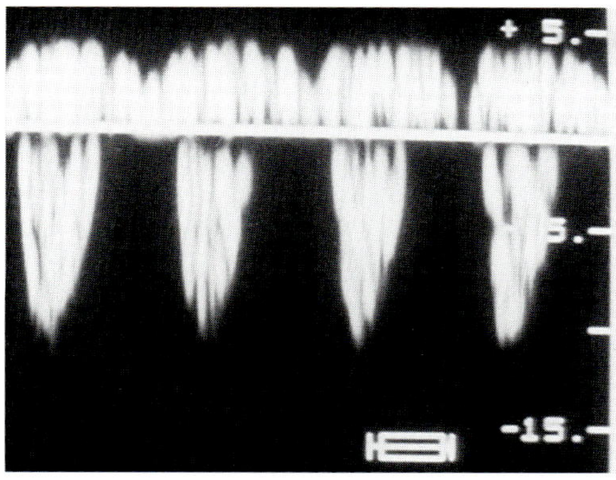

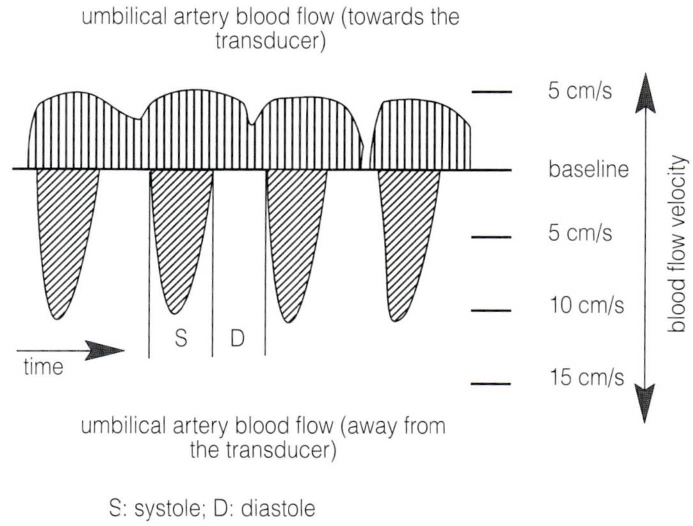

26

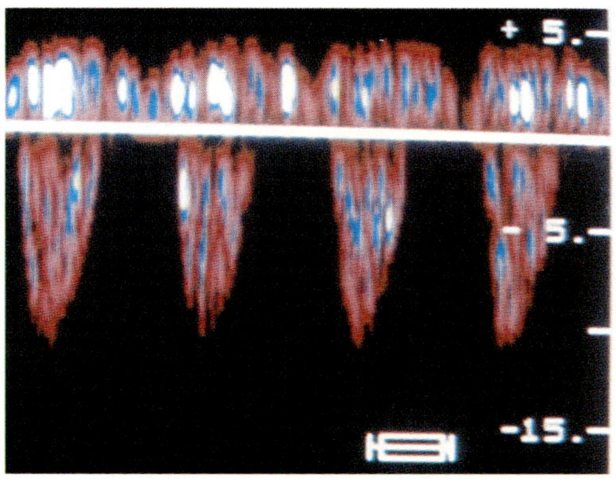

27

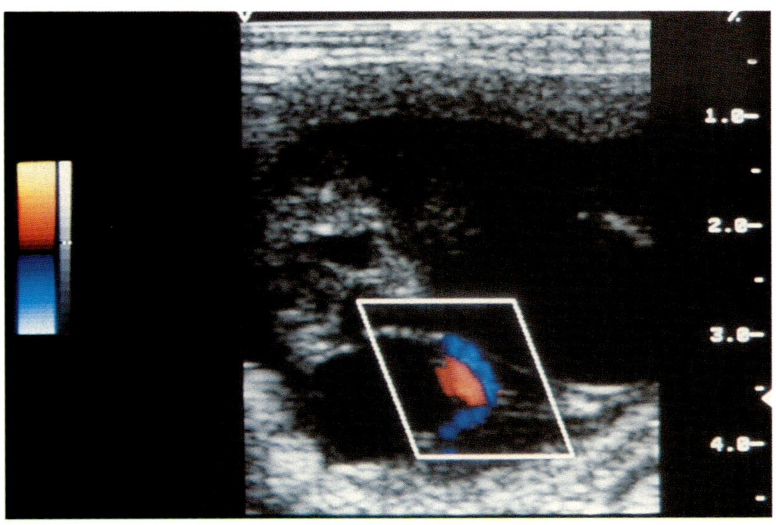

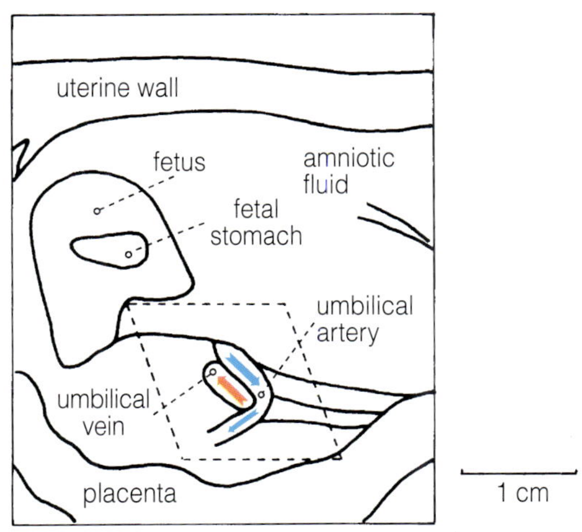

25–27 Doppler spectral tracings of umbilical arteries in cat fetuses, 32 days after conception (**25, 26**) and 35 days after breeding (**27**), displayed with pulsed-wave Doppler in black and white (**25**) and colour enriched (**26**), and with colour Doppler (**27**). The pulsed Doppler tracings (**25, 26**) show blood flow volumes in varying shades of grey or colour, while velocities are plotted along the vertical axis; volumes change from black (red) to grey (blue) and, finally, to white.

Chemical Effects

The chemical effects of ultrasound are oxidation, reduction and depolymerization. The ability of ultrasound to depolymerize macromolecules like polysaccharides, various proteins or isolated DNA, has been demonstrated experimentally. These adverse biological effects, however, are not found with diagnostic ultrasound[9].

> The effects of ultrasound depend on the frequency used, sound intensity and exposure.

High frequencies and high intensities have been shown to cause damage. Long exposure to ultrasound may lead to tissue lesions and necrosis, and even to teratogenic change, chromosomal damage and mutations. Numerous animal experiments and human statistics show that these adverse side-effects are not found with diagnostic ultrasound[10].

The American Institute of Ultrasound in Medicine (AIUM) published a paper in 1976 on these biological effects. The paper was rewritten in 1979 and the findings were confirmed in 1982. Until October 1978, no biological effects of ultrasound were noted with low MHz frequencies, when intensities less than

100 mW/cm^2 (spatial peak / temporal average[8, 10]) were applied to mammalian tissue. When exposure times of more than 1 second but less than 500 seconds are used, and exposure multiplied by intensity does not exceed 50 J/cm^2, higher intensities may be employed[1, 2, 10].

To avoid damage safely, intensities of over 100 mW/cm^2 (spatial peak/temporal average[8, 10]) should be applied for a limited time only (seconds or minutes).

The intensities approved for commercial, two-dimensional ultrasound systems in human medicine are around 10 mW/cm^2. Duplex ultrasonography, displaying both two-dimensional images and blood flow, may reach intensities of 60–90 mW/cm^2. Non-Doppler diagnostic ultrasound may be safely used continuously over a reasonably extended period.

Diagnostic ultrasonography is a safe method when using approved equipment.

Constant testing for adverse effects is done with any new and improved technique.

References

Cited References

1 AIUM Bioeffects Commitee (1976) Biological effects of ultrasonic energy on living mammals. *Ultrasound Med. Biol.* **2**, 351.

2 AIUM Bioeffects Commitee (1979) AIUM responds to EDA notice of intent for diagnostic ultrasound. *Reflections* **5**, 299.

3 Bubenheimer P and Kneisel GD (1989) *Doppler-Echokardiographie*. Verlag Edition Medizin, Weinheim.

4 Fehske W (1988) *Praxis der Konventionellen und Farbkodierten Doppler-Echokardiographie*. Verlag Hans Huber, Bern, Stuttgart, Toronto.

5 Hilz E (1969) *Physik and Technik der Ultraschall-Diagnostik*. Elektromedizin (Sonderausgabe), pp. 36–42.

6 Kaarmann H and Wessels G (1991) II–1 Physikalische Grandlagen. 10. Ergänzungslieferung. In: Braun B, Günther R and Schwerk W (Eds.) *Ultraschalldiagnostik. Lehrbuch und Atlas. Vol I.* Verlag Ecomed. Landsberg, München, Zürich.

7 Kossof G (1985) Physikalische Grandlagen und gerätetechnische Möglichkeiten des diagnostischen Ultraschalls. In: Hansmann M, Hackelöer B-J and Staudach A (Eds.) *Ultraschalldiagnostik in Geburtshilfe and Gynäkologie*. Springer Verlag, Berlin, Heidelberg, New York, Tokyo, pp. 1–13.

8 Rott HD (1981) Zur Frage der Schädigungsmöglichkeit durch diagnostischen Ultraschall. *Ultraschall* **2**, 56–64.

9 Rott HD (1982) Sicherheitsaspekte der Ultraschalldiagnostik. *Swiss Med.* **4**, 11–15.

10 Rott HD (1985) Sicherheitsaspekte der Ultraschalldiagnostik. In: Hansmann M, Hackelöer B-J and Staudach A (Eds.) *Ultraschalldiagnostik in Geburtshilfe und Gynäkologie*. Springer Verlag, Berlin, Heidelberg, New York, Tokyo, pp. 15–28.

11 Wessels G and Weber P (1983) II–1 Physikalische Grandlagen. In: Braun B, Günther R and Schwerk W (Eds.) *Ultraschalldiagnostik. Lehrbuch und Atlas. Vol I.* Verlag Ecomed. Landsberg, München, Zürich.

Additional Reading

Hill CR (Ed.) (1986) *Physical Principals of MedicalUultrasonics*. John Wiley, New York.

Kress H (1969) *Der Einfluß des Einfallswinkels bei der Ultraschall-Echo-Diagnostik*. Elektromedizin (Sonderausgabe), pp. 43–45.

Wells PNT (1975) *Physical Principles of Ultrasonic Diagnosis*. Academic Press London, New York.

Wells PNT (1977) *Biomedical Ultrasonics*. Academic Press, London.

3 Technical Principles

Cordula Poulsen Nautrup

Ultrasound Wave Production and Reception

Ultrasound wave production and reception is based on the piezoelectric characteristics of crystals (**28**). Piezoelectric crystals, stimulated by high-frequency electrical alternating voltage, are alternated and emit ultrasound waves. Reflected ultrasound waves, returning to the same crystal, produce voltage signals (reciprocal piezoelectric effect). In this way the crystal functions as both transmitter and receiver. Piezoelectric transducer crystals are manufactured using various ceramic compounds with quartz, zirconate and/or titanate[9].

The term 'transducer' describes its piezoelectric function of converting voltage to vibrations and vice versa. Other names commonly used include 'applicator', 'scanner' or 'probe' and refer to the transducers capability of transmitting and scanning.

Most modern ultrasound systems emit pulses that last for 1–2 μs[9] and 2–3 wavelengths[7]. 300–3,000 pulses are emitted per second.

Sound Beam Geometry

When stimulated by electrical pulses, piezoelectric ceramics emit so many ultrasound pulses that a spatial diameter is created, which can be characterized by sound beam geometry. The physical principles in Chapter 2 neglected this spatial diameter and described ultrasound pulses as lines. In reality this is not the case.

Sound beam resolution along the direction of sound transmission or axial pulse diameter is determined by the spatial pulse length (2–3 wavelengths; see above). Axial beam diameter is the same at any distance from the transducer for any given frequency.

Lateral beam width, however, is dependent on penetration depth and transducer shape. Beam geometry perpendicular to the direction of sound travel is described by a near field, a focal zone and a far field (**29A**).

The ultrasound beam has length (axial), width (spatial) and thickness (slice thickness). The length is infinite until all energy is redistributed. The width is determined by transducer shape and the thickness is determined by the aperture (**29B**).

In linear array systems or curved transducer crystals, the emitted sound waves traveling parallel in the near field interfere greatly with each other. Interfaces with similar echogenicities may have different echoes in the near field, due to sound wave obliteration and interference. An optimal laterally resolved image in this region is not possible because of beam width. An increase in frequency

28

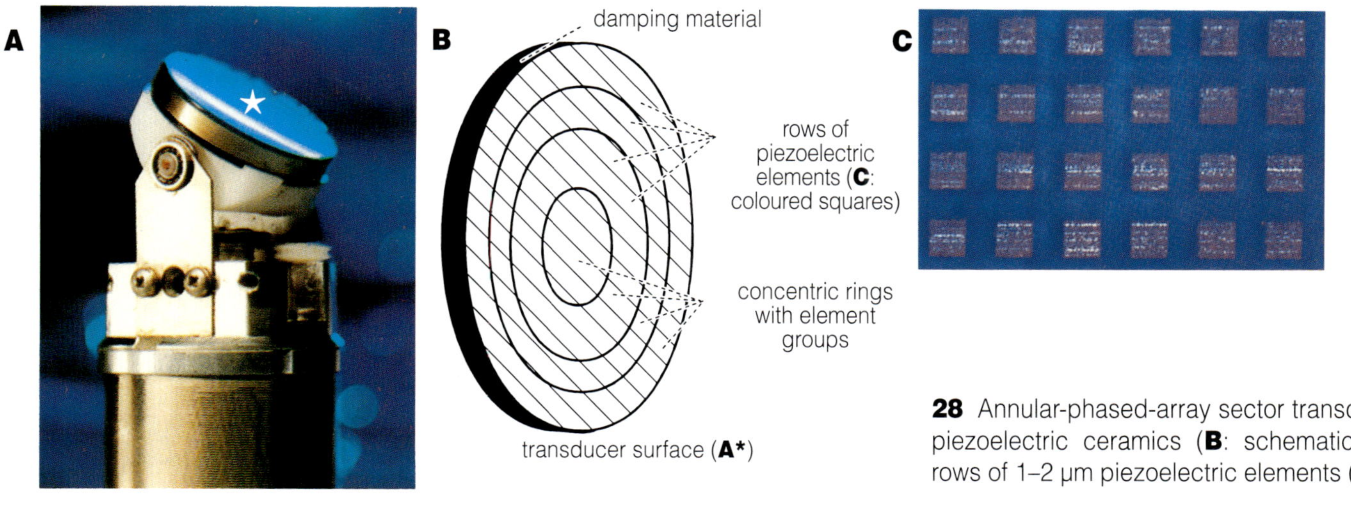

28 Annular-phased-array sector transducer (**A**) with modern piezoelectric ceramics (**B**: schematic drawing) containing rows of 1–2 μm piezoelectric elements (**C**: coloured squares).

29

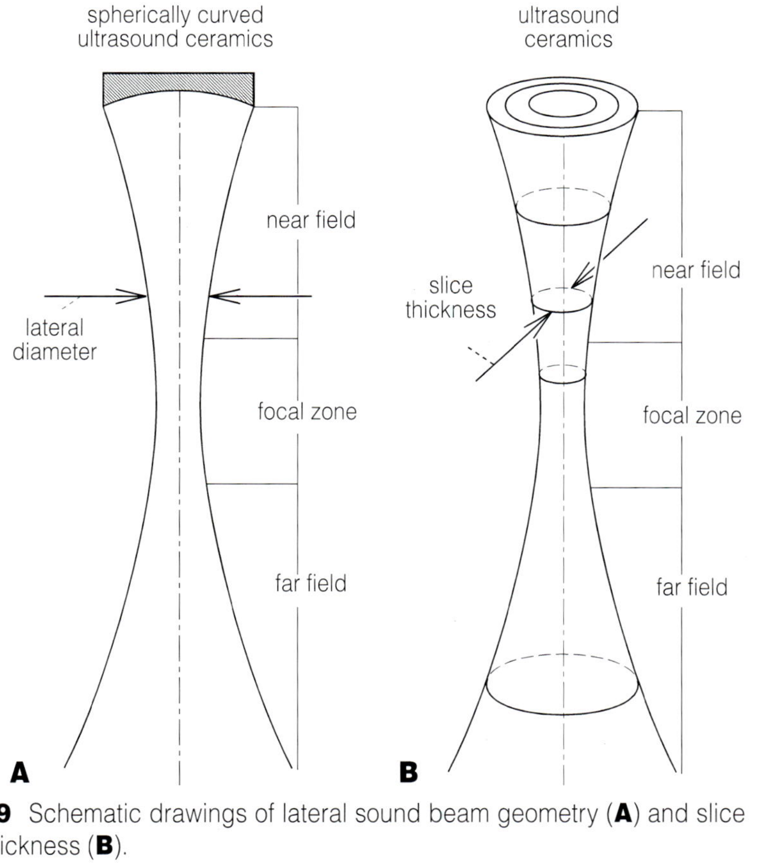

29 Schematic drawings of lateral sound beam geometry (**A**) and slice thickness (**B**).

30

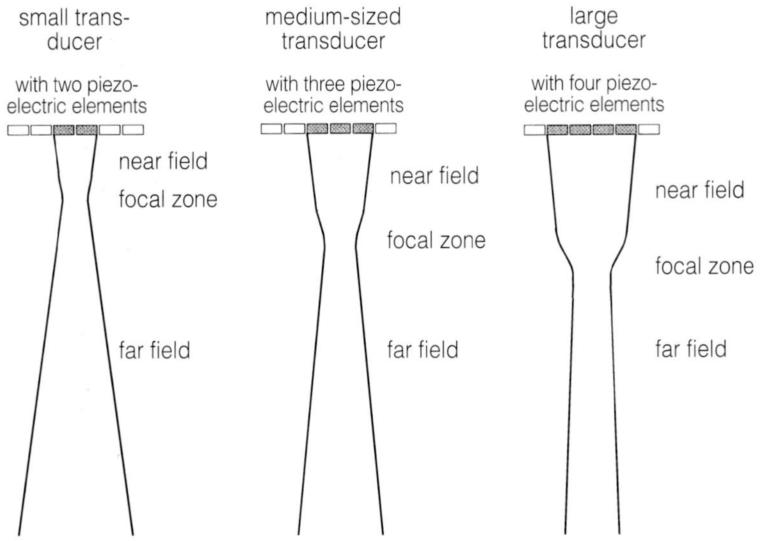

30 Schematic drawings of the sound beam diameter influenced by transducer size.

and a smaller transducer size will minimize the near field (30).

When using curved and focused transducers, the near field is followed by the focal zone. In this area the sound waves are bundled, the beam width is reduced and the intensity is increased. Lateral resolution is best in this small area (see Resolution). Higher frequencies and a larger transducer will reduce the beam width and increase the intensity in the focal zone (30).

The sound beam diverges in the far field distant to the transducer, which leads to a decrease in lateral resolution (see Resolution). Lower frequencies and a larger transducer will minimize the far field diameter (30).

It is not possible to produce an optimal sound beam geometry with a small and narrow near field, bundled focal zone and decreased far field diameter. An increase in frequency reduces the near field and decreases focal zone diameter, but increases the diameter in the far zone (30).

A stand-off pad (see page 56) may be used to move near field structures further from the transducer to a better imaging zone. In this way the object of interest is placed in the focal zone.

Mechanical and electronic focusing greatly improves the ultrasound image by decreasing the near field and reducing beam diameter in the focal zone (**31A–D**). Sound is mechanically focused by using a spherically curved ceramic surface (curved reflector) and/or an acoustic lens. Electronic focusing requires a number of piezoelectric crystals, which are pulsed in succession. The advantage of electronic focusing is in the multiple focal zones placed along the sound beam.

Focusing in a third plane, also called slice thickness focusing, is achieved by using lenses with linear- and curved-array transducers (**31D**). Annular-phased arrays (**31B**) are electronically steered by successive pulses with a time difference. This type of focusing produces an image with more contrast and brings out structural details.

Resolution

The axial resolution is determined by the ability to distinguish two structures separately along the axis of the sound beam. Lateral resolution refers to the minimum separation of two adjacent echoes perpendicular to the sound beam (**32A, 32B**).

Axial resolution is dependent on the spatial pulse length. The space between two interfaces must be large enough to allow for completion of the first reflection before echoes of the second interface reach the first (**33**). The separation of two reflectors must therefore be greater than half the pulse length multiplied by the propagation velocity of the tissue. *Table 3* gives the maximum axial resolution for different frequencies at mean sound velocity and a pulse length of two wavelengths.

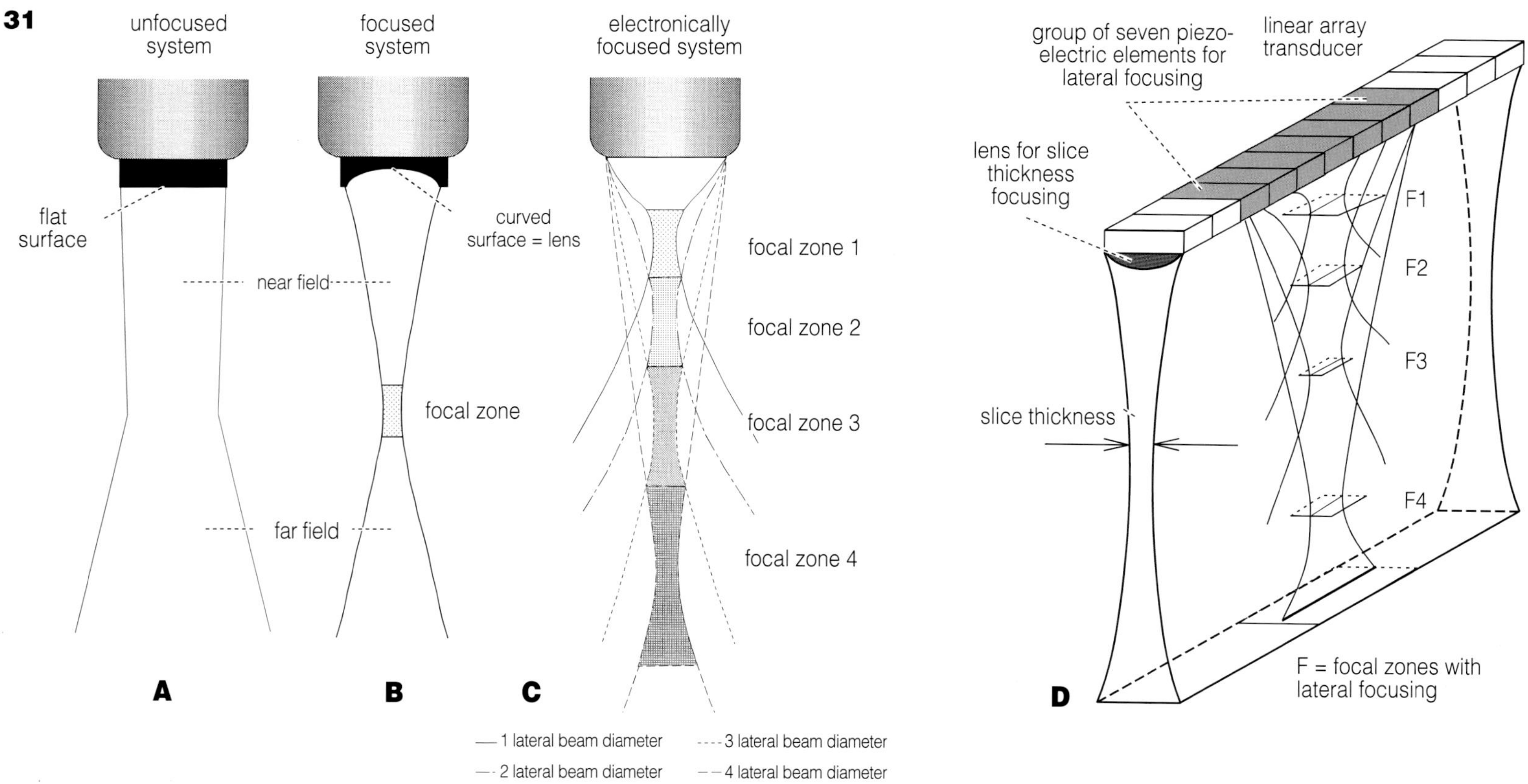

31 Schematic drawings of lateral beam diameter without focus (**A**), with mechanical focusing (**B**) and electronic focusing (**C, D**); slice thickness focusing with acoustic lenses (**D**).

Table 3 Frequency and maximum axial resolution in soft tissues (≈1,540 m/s).

Sound frequency	1 MHz	3.5 MHz	5 MHz	7.5 MHz	10 MHz	15 MHz
Maximum axial resolution in soft tissues	1. 5 mm	0.4 mm	0.3 mm	0.2 mm	0.15 mm	0.1 mm

Lateral resolution is determined by the sound beam diameter, which in turn is dependent on the ultrasound frequency, transducer diameter and penetration depth (see Sound Beam Geometry, page 31). Lateral resolution is best in the optimal focal zone, using a relatively large transducer, high frequency and adequate mechanical or electronic focusing. Axial resolution is usually two to three times superior to lateral resolution.

The maximum axial resolution in most 5 MHz transducers is 0.3–0.8 mm, while the size of distinguishable interfaces perpendicular to the sound beam is 0.6–1.6 mm. These structures are found only within the focal zone at a penetration depth of 40–70 mm. A higher frequency transducer will improve both axial and lateral resolution. Even 7.5–15 MHz transducers can only display macroscopic structures (interfaces) with a minimum size of 0.2–0.1 mm axially and 0.6–0.3 mm laterally.

High frequency transducers have high resolution but reduced depth penetration, while low frequency transducers have decreased resolution but good tissue penetration. Various applications of these transducers are listed in *Table 4* (page 35). The transitions are overlapping, so that a 5 MHz transducer with a near and far focus can be used in most cases.

Resolution and penetration are tested with the help of commercial phantoms (**34–40**). An easier and better method to test resolution and scanner controls (see Pre- and Postprocessing) is to use the sonographer's own body organs as a normal test object. To check resolution and near-field adjustments of medium to high frequency transducers (5 and 15 MHz), the accessible human thyroid gland, including the large cervical vessels, can be scanned (**41**). Medium to low frequency transducers (3.5–5 MHz) can be tested for resolution and scanner controls on the liver at the entrance of the hepatic veins into the caudal vena cava (**42**). The advantage of this method is in the use of natural body tissue as a test object. This 'phantom' is always available, and the scanner adjustments can generally be transferred to ultrasound examinations of dogs and cats.

Pre- and Postprocessing

Preprocessing

Preprocessing refers to all manipulations of emitted and reflected ultrasound signals before their conversion to analog or digital signals that produce an image on the monitor. These adjustments include intensity of sound output, time gain compensation, gain, enhancement, dynamic range and image integration.

Intensity of Sound Output

The intensity of an emitted ultrasound pulse can be reduced to 45–75% of the maximum 100 mW/cm^2 in most ultrasound machines. This low intensity output is usually sufficient with low frequencies and good imaging patients. In canine and feline ultrasonography, however, transducer frequencies of 5 MHz or higher are used, requiring full intensity output (100%) to produce an image.

32

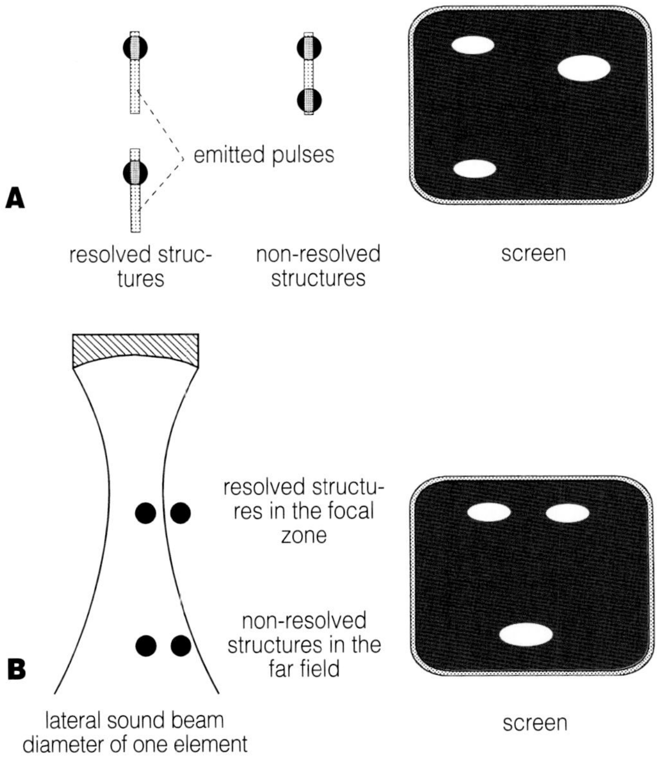

32 Schematic drawings of two structures with axial (**A**) and lateral (**B**) resolution.

33

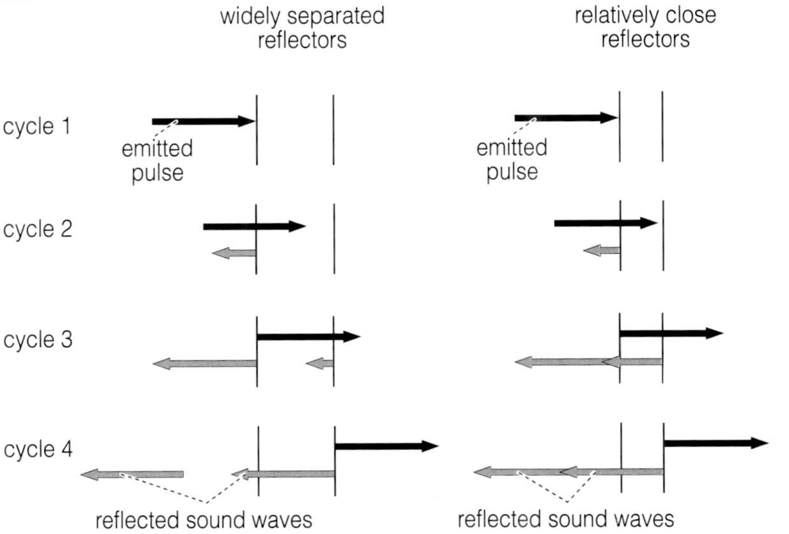

33 Schematic drawings of axial resolution dependent on reflector separation and pulse length.

34

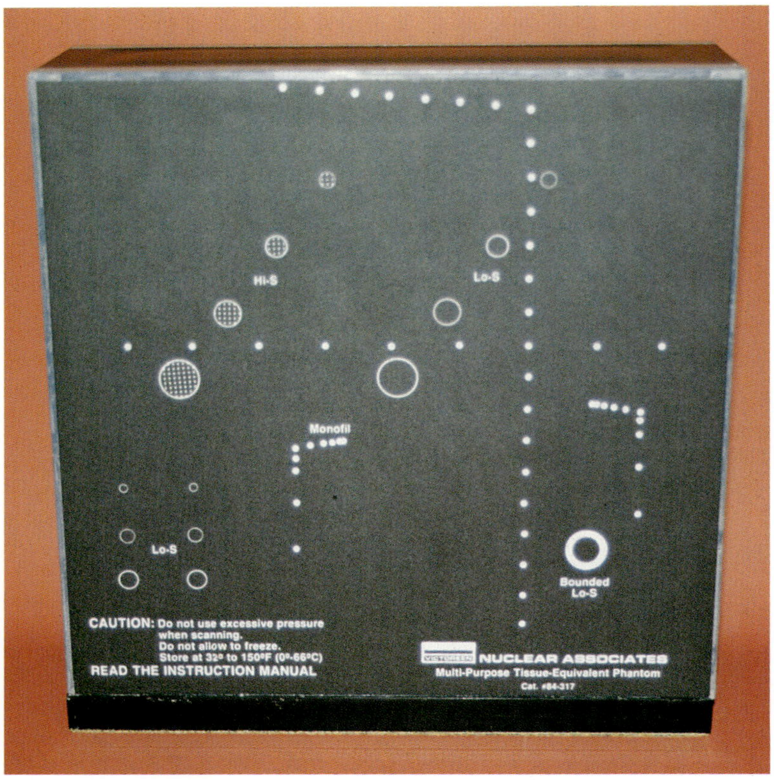

37

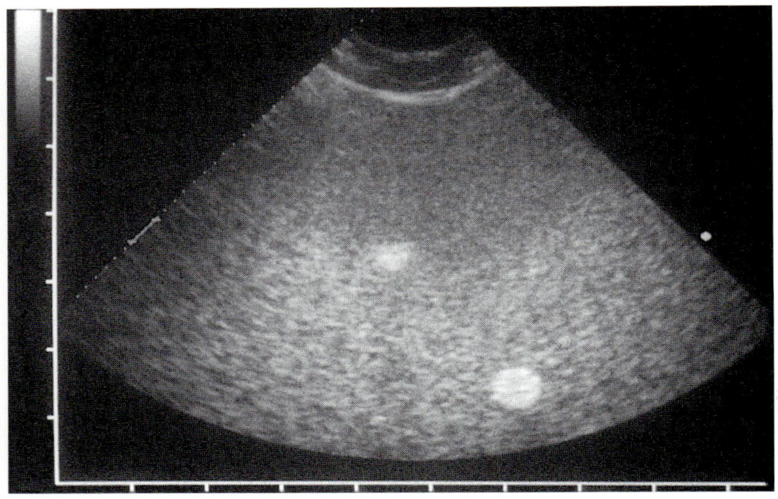

38

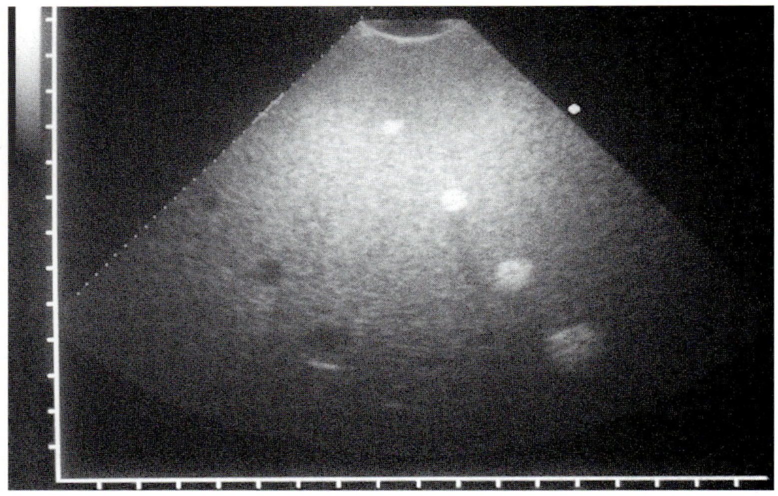

35

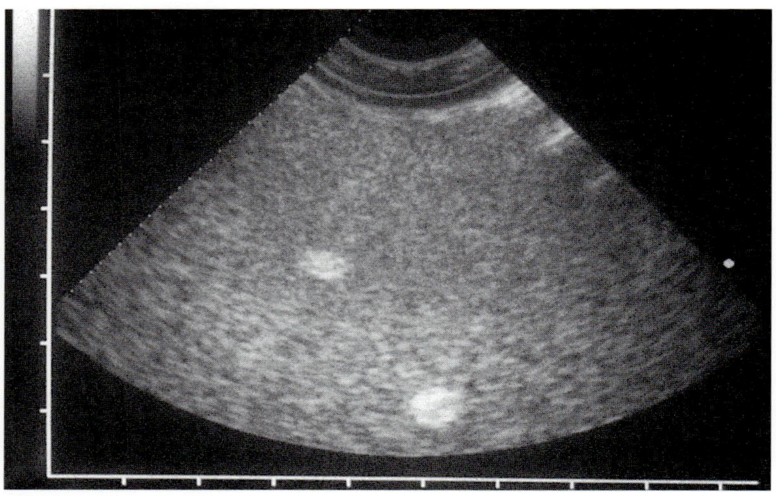

39

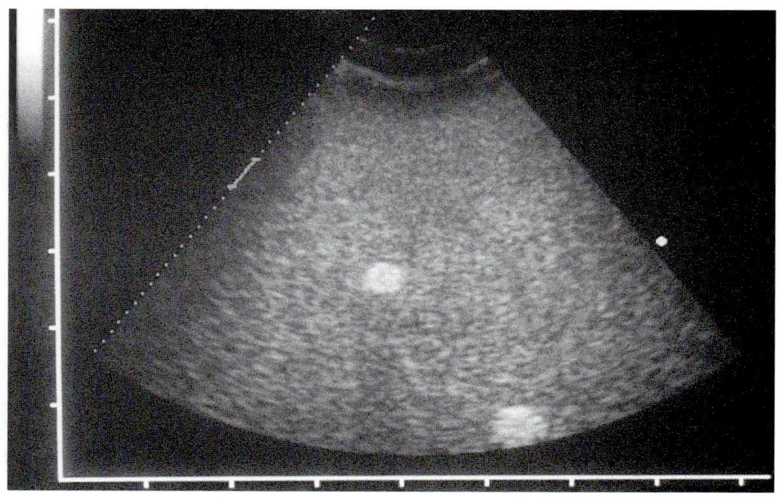

36

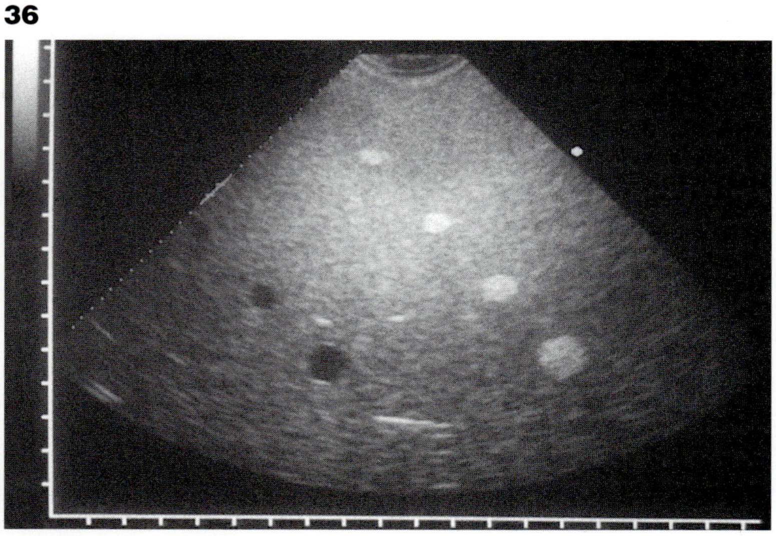

40

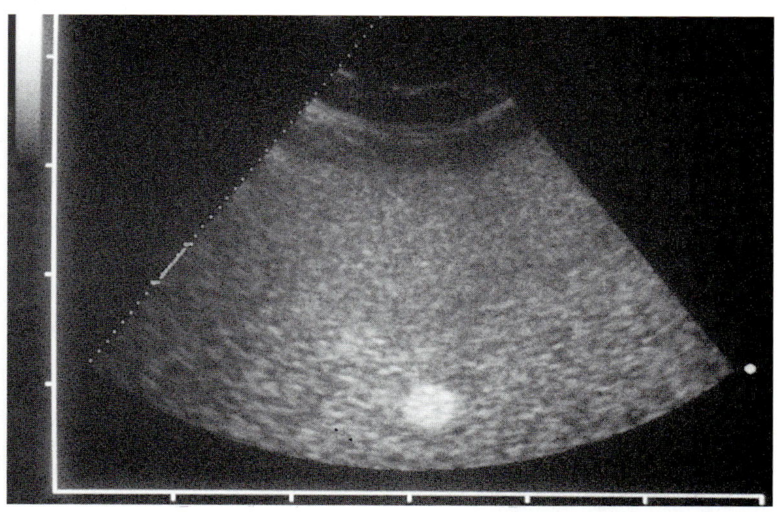

34–40 Ultrasound phantom (**34**: photo) with images using various frequencies and depths (**35, 36**: 3.5 MHz – 7 and 15 cm; **37, 38**: 5.0 MHz – 7 and 14 cm; **39, 40**: 7.5 MHz – 6 and 4 cm). Different resolutions at varying depths are dependent on transducer frequency.

Table 4 Review of various transducer frequency applications with overlapping transitions.

Transducer frequency	3.5 MHz	5 MHz	7.5 MHz	10 MHz
Applications	Large and medium-sized dogs: echocardiography, ultrasonography of late pregnancy.	Large dogs: abdominal ultrasonography. Medium-sized and small dogs: abdominal and cardiac ultrasonography. All dogs: pelvic ultrasonography, sonographic pregnancy diagnosis, echoencephalography, ultrasonography of the shoulder and hip joint.	Small dogs and cats: abdominal and cardiac ultrasonography. Medium-sized, small dogs and cats: pelvic ultrasongraphy, sonographic pregnancy diagnosis. Large dogs: cervical ultrasonography including thyroid, ultrasonography of superficial structures, i.e. skin, salivary glands, mammary glands, testicles, penis, and limb joints. Cats: echoencephalography. Puppies and kittens: abdominal, pelvic and cardiac ultrasonography and echoencephalography.	All dogs and cats: cervical ultrasonography including thyroid ultrasonography, echo-ophthalmography, ultrasonography of superficial structures, i.e. skin salivary glands, mammary glands, testicles and penis.

41

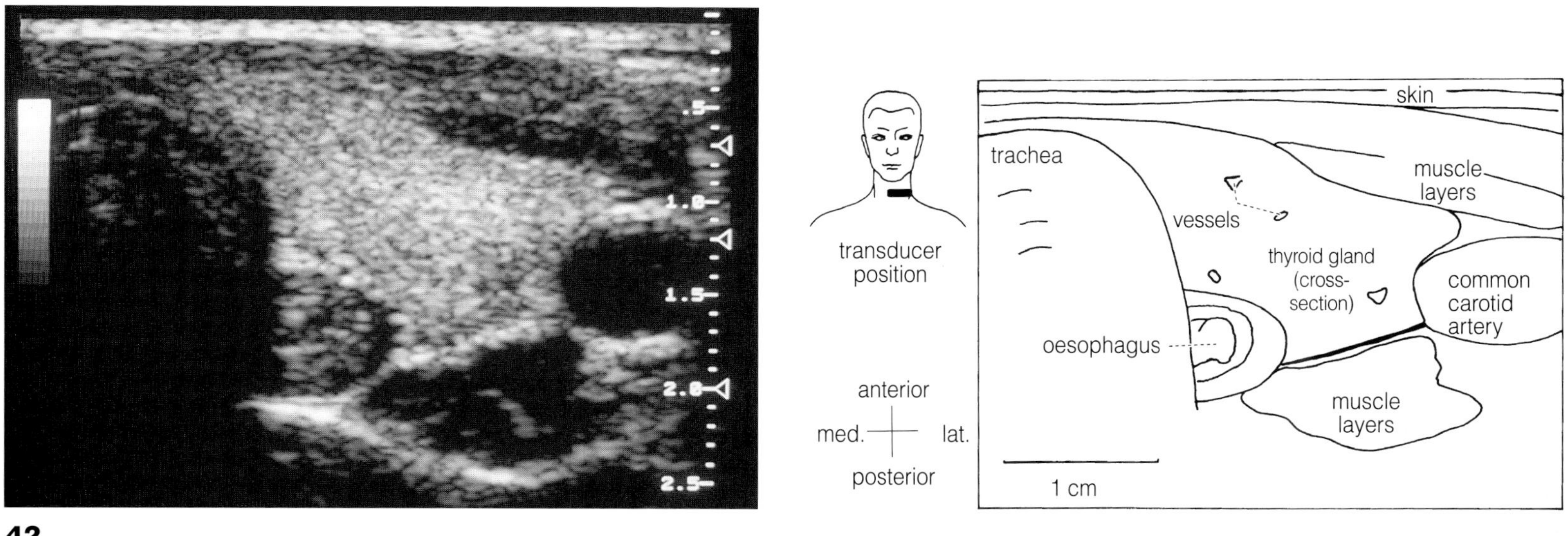

42

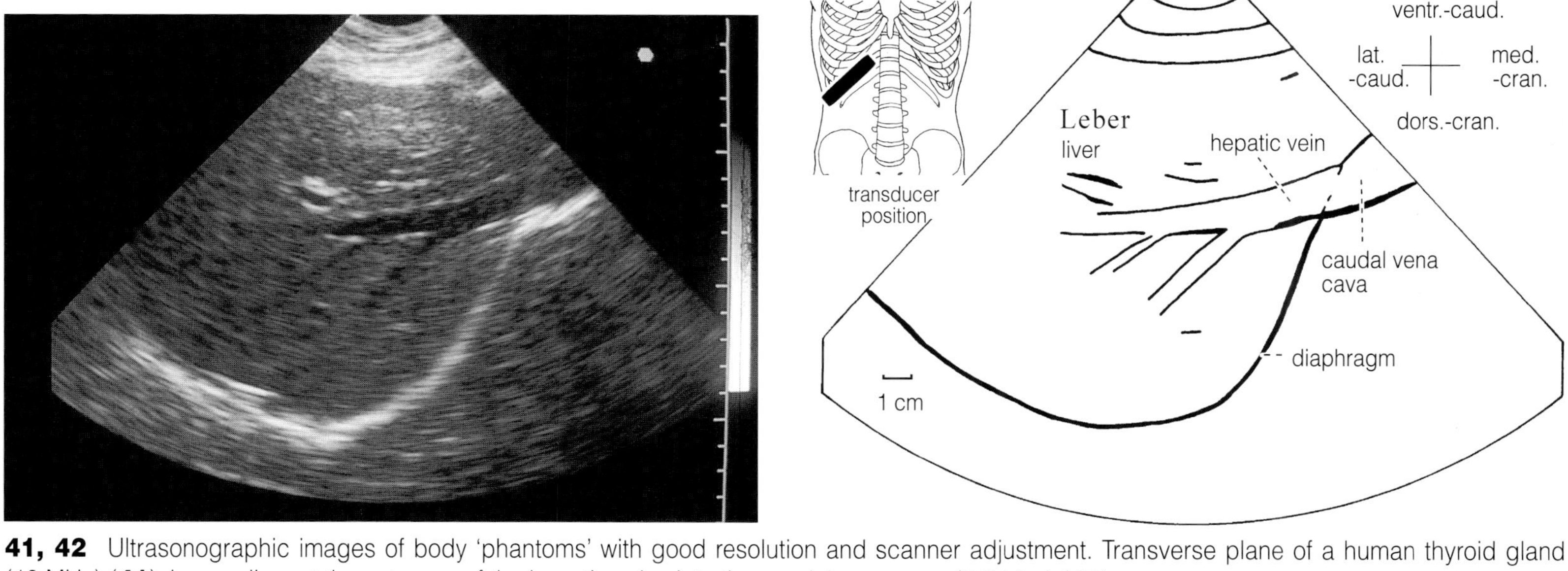

41, 42 Ultrasonographic images of body 'phantoms' with good resolution and scanner adjustment. Transverse plane of a human thyroid gland (10 MHz) (**41**); human liver at the entrance of the hepatic veins into the caudal vena cava (3.5 Mhz) (**42**).

43

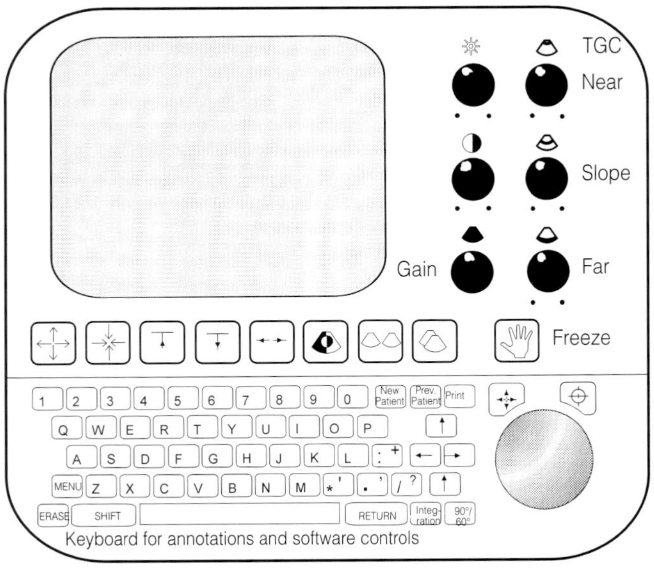

44

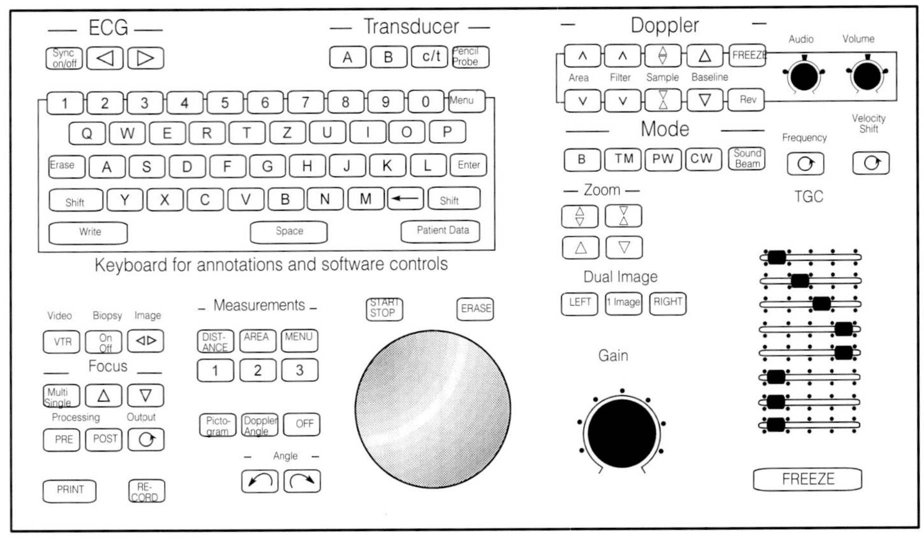

43, 44 Typical ultrasound scanner controls for two-dimensional real-time ultrasonography (**43**) and for two-dimensional ultrasonography in combination with Doppler echography (**44**).

45

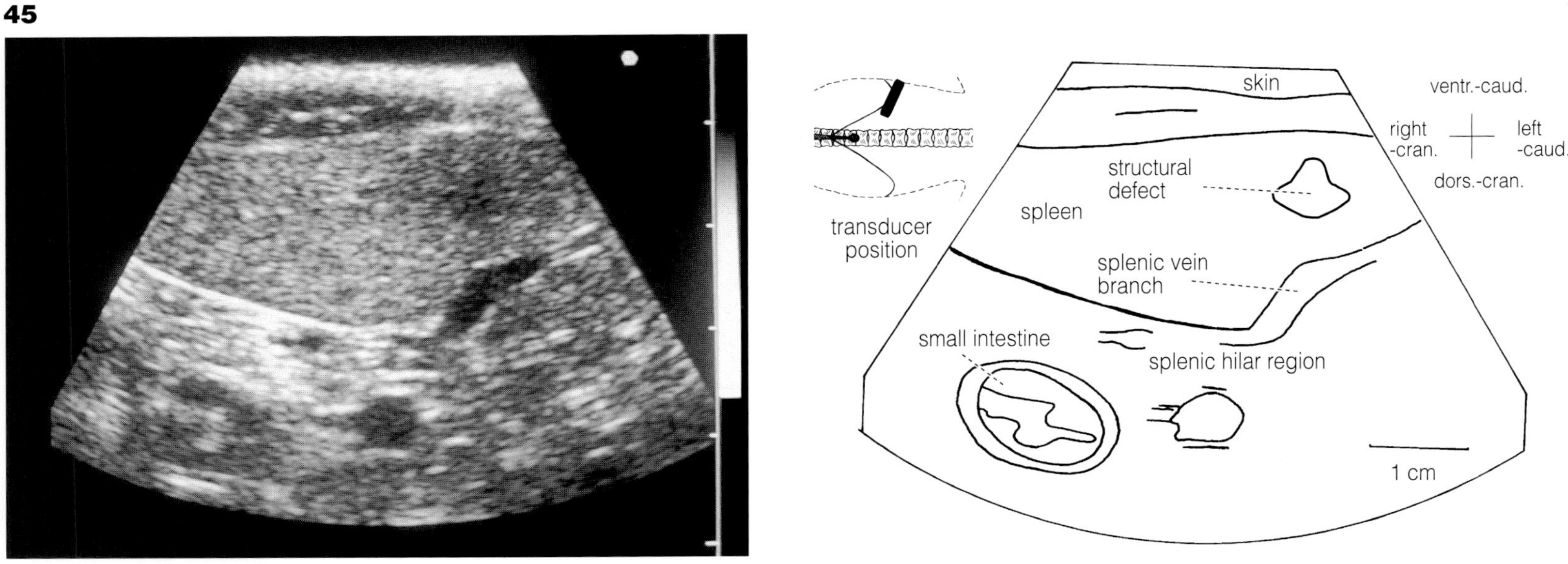

46

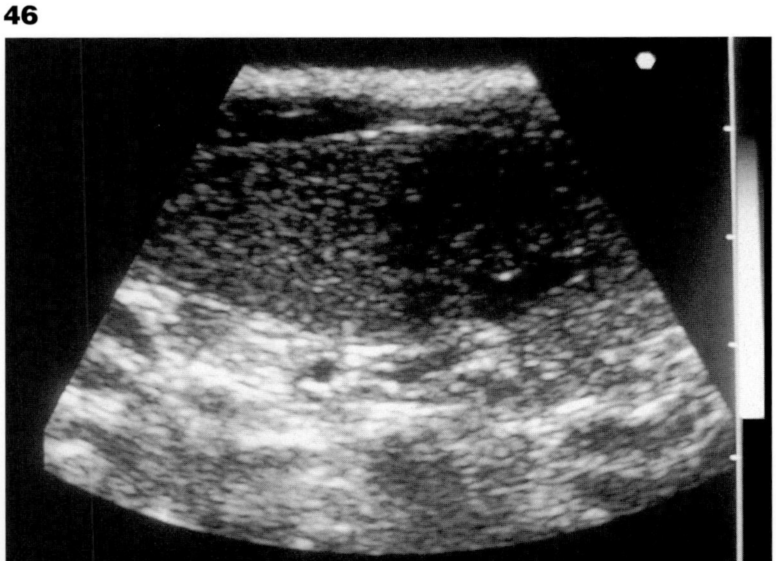

47

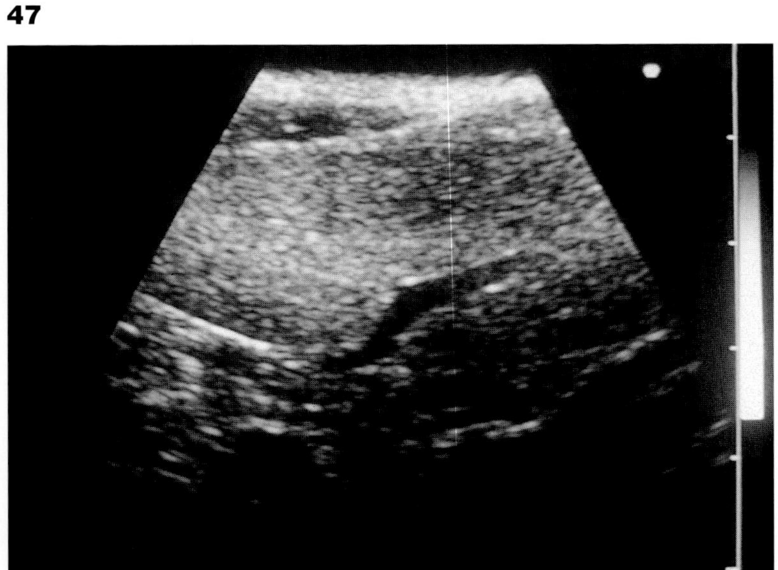

45–47 Different sonographic gain settings of a canine spleen. Correct setting (**45**); gain setting too low at the top, near field (**46**); gain setting too low at the bottom, far field (**47**). The images are not identical, because each preprocessing required a new ultrasound image.

Time Gain Compensation

Time gain compensation (TGC) equalizes weaker signals from deeper structures, caused by increased sound attenuation. This depth-dependent loss of intensity affects both emitted and reflected sound waves. Superficial structures are displayed better than deeper ones without any additional correction, although they have identical reflective qualities. The TGC controls are adapted for a median velocity, reflection, absorption and scattering. Increased or decreased attenuation is amplified manually for different tissues and depths.

Most commercial ultrasound scanners have at least three slide bars or knobs, consisting of a near gain, slope delay and far gain. Additional controls improve the image (**43, 44**).

Gain

The gain control allows for uniform amplification of all returning echoes from every tissue depth.

> Proper adjustment of preprocessing controls (intensity of sound output, TGC and gain) in a darkened room should produce an ultrasound image on the monitor with a wide range of grey values, including white and black (**45**).

Too high or too low gain settings will cause loss of detail and should be avoided (**46, 47**). Basic settings without a patient can be tested on an ultrasound phantom or on the sonographer's organs, such as the thyroid or liver (see Resolution, page 32). This basic control setting must then be adjusted for the individual patient. In abdominal ultrasonography a normal urinary bladder or a liver with gallbladder can be used for this purpose. The entire screen display should be uniformly bright with homogenous, anechoic (black) fluid-filled areas (urinary bladder and gallbladder).

Patients with reduced imaging or poor transducer-skin contact require an intensity of 100% and, frequently, a maximum gain and TGC setting.

Echoenhancement

Echoenhancement can amplify separate weaker signals, which makes these structures more prominent. A mean setting without grey level assignment is usually used for routine examinations.

Dynamic Range

The difference between the weakest and the strongest registered echo intensity is called the dynamic range. A high dynamic range will produce softer images with numerous grey shades, while a low dynamic range shows less grey shades and more contrast. Abdominal ultrasonography uses the maximum dynamic setting (70 dB), while a setting of 30 or 40 dB is appropriate for echocardiography.

Image Integration

Many ultrasound scanners offer image integration, which combines 1.2, 1.5 or 2 ultrasound images to make one whole image. This feature helps in detecting small structures or slight differences in tissue echogenicity (e.g. metastasis). At the same time the image appears softer or contrast poor. Image integration is useful for abdominal ultrasonography without organ movement. Images with organ or respiratory motion, such as the heart and liver, or fetal movement, are not suited for image integration. The low frame rate produces a blurred image. Ultrasound images without image integration are higher in contrast.

Postprocessing

Various postprocessing methods can improve an ultrasound image on the monitor. Grey shades can be accentuated, changed or replaced by colour (**48–51**). The grey scale can be mapped, compressed or expanded. The image can be contrast poor (softer) or high in contrast (hard).

48

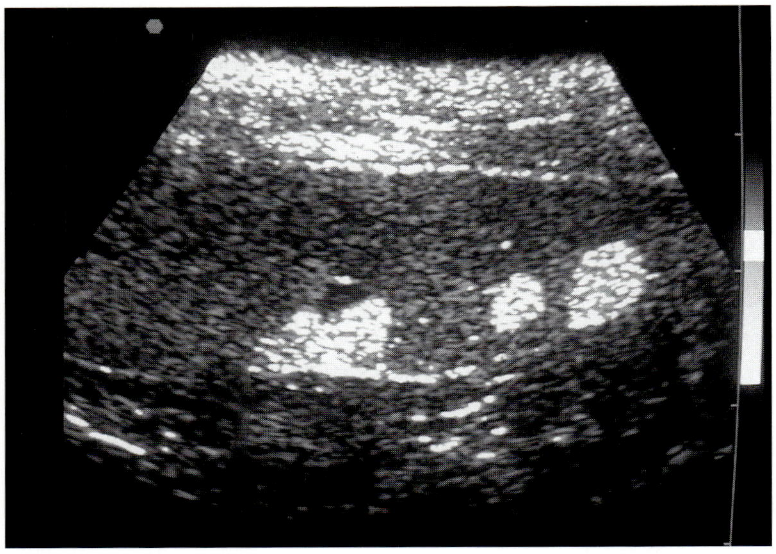

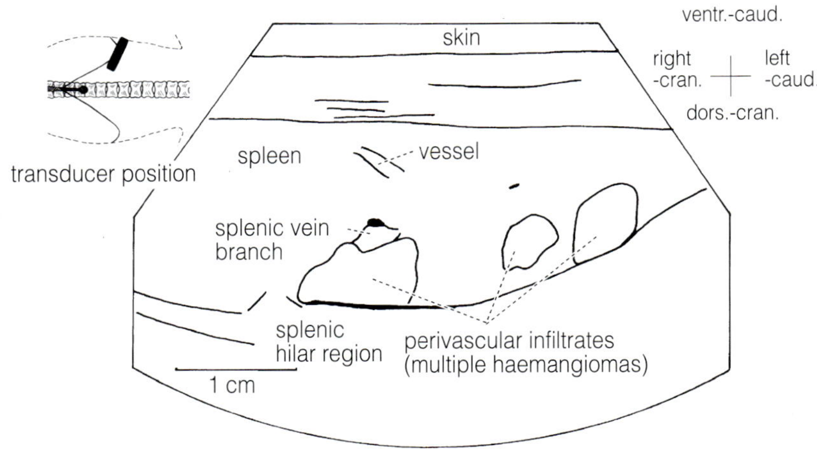

49

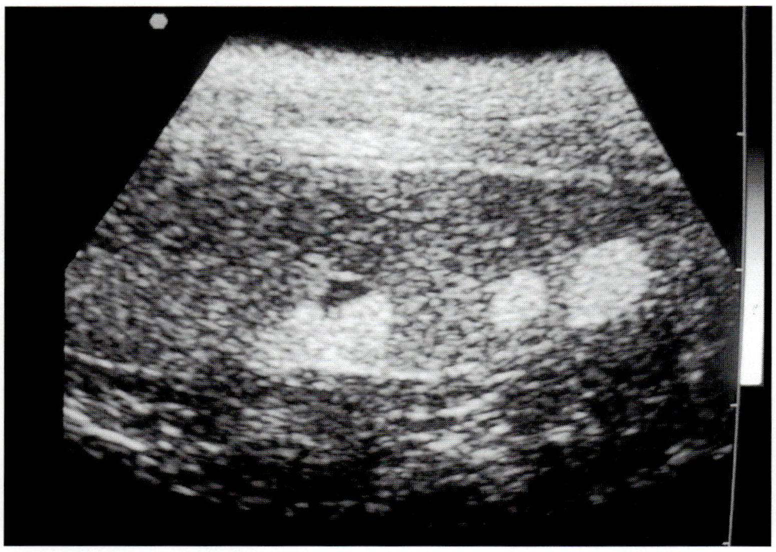

50

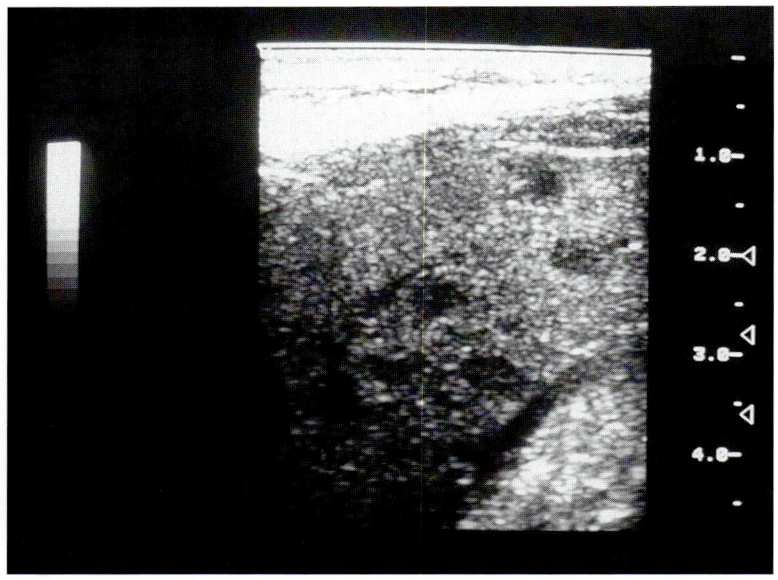

51

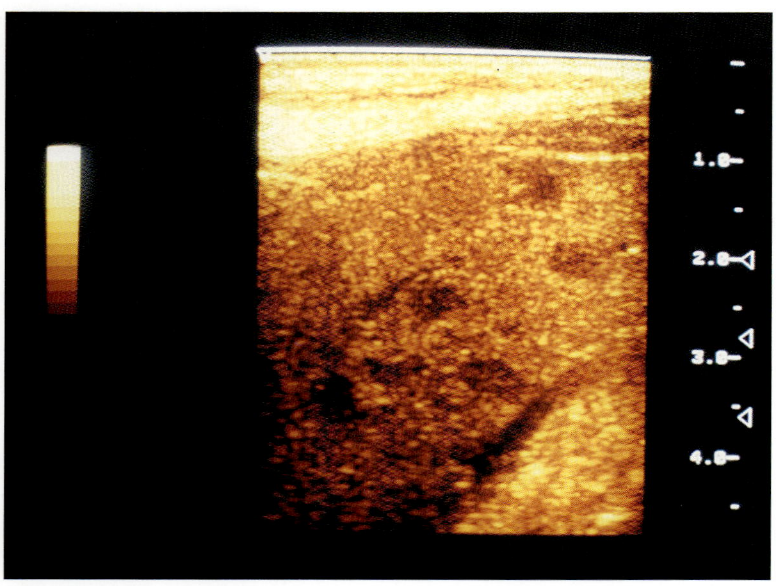

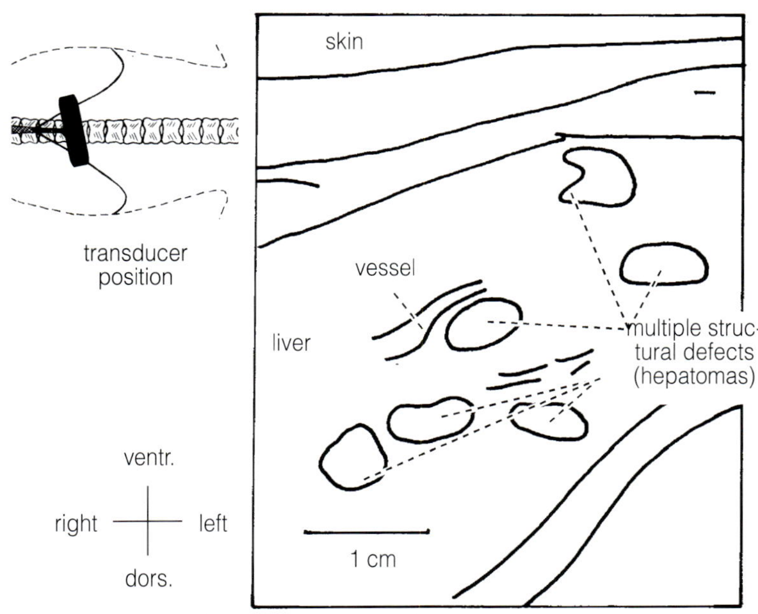

48–51 Sonographic postprocessing settings. Canine spleen with multiple haemangiomas after grey shade assignment (**48**) and normal display (**49**); canine liver with hepatomas after colour coding (**51**) and normal display (**50**).

A-Mode (Pulse-Echo-Mode)

In A-mode (amplitude mode) the reflecting interfaces are displayed along a baseline as vertical spikes with different amplitudes (52). The position of the spikes along this line represents the depth of the originating echo. In the mid 1960s it was used as the first successful ultrasonographic method for pregnancy diagnosis (4). More recently it has been used for echoencephalography and echo-ophthalmography.

B-Mode

B-mode (brightness mode) displays the returning echoes from a line or field as dots with varying brightness on the monitor (53). This mode displays interfaces, i.e. anatomical or pathological structures, in one- and two-dimensional ultrasound images. The amplitude of the returning echo is proportional to the brightness or grey scale on the monitor.

B-mode images are classified as either one- or two-dimensional, depending on the type of image displayed on the screen. Another B-mode classification considers the time needed to produce an image on the screen. These are divided into static modes and real-time methods. The two-dimensional compound mode, which requires a great deal of time to produce a monitor image, is a static method. The one-dimensional M-mode and the two-dimensional B-mode are referred to as real-time ultrasonography.

> For optimal ultrasonographic B-mode images, the ultrasound system should differentiate between as many grey levels as possible. (Modern ultrasound systems are designed with up to 256 grey shades.)

One-Dimensional B-Mode

A one-dimensional imaging method still used today is TM-mode (or M-mode) (T = time, M = motion). The echoes are traced along an axis and recorded on a vertical line on a monitor or strip chart. This B-mode also displays the echoes with varying brightness or grey levels. The tracings are recorded over time. The vertical axis displays the depth of the structures,

52, 53

52 A-Mode

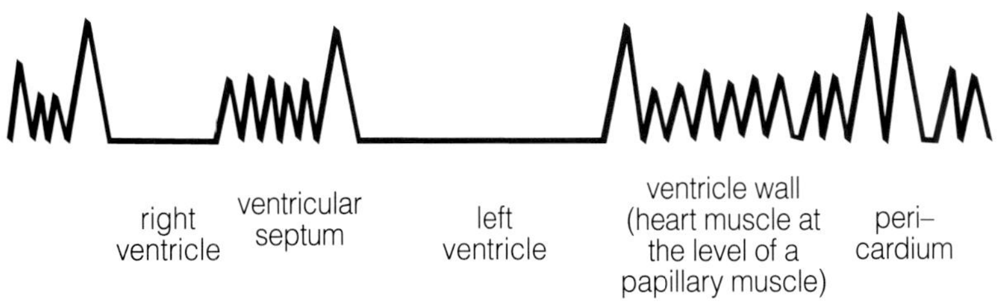

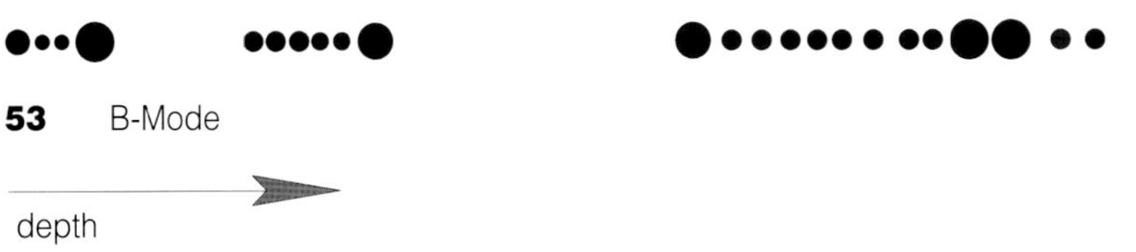

54

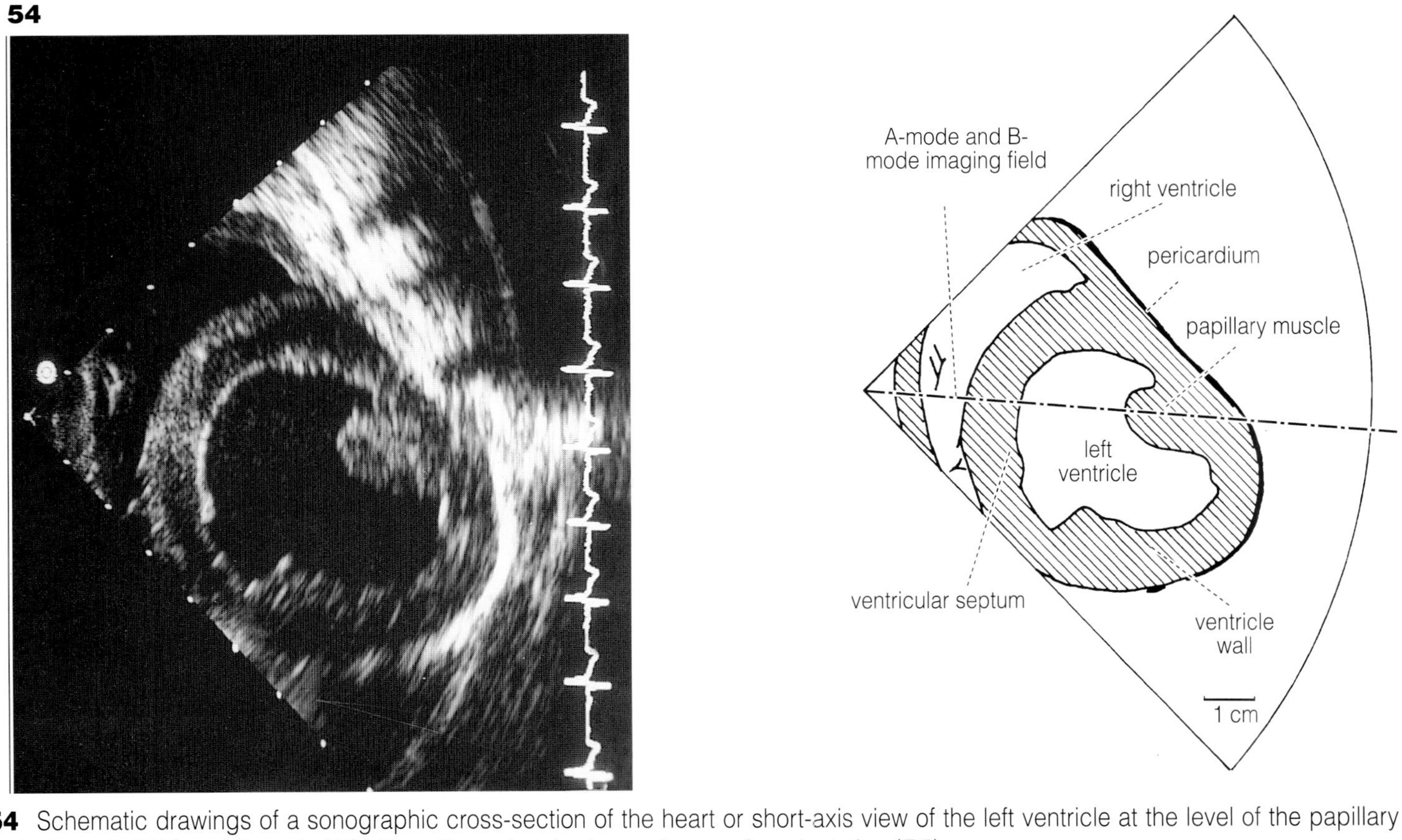

52–54 Schematic drawings of a sonographic cross-section of the heart or short-axis view of the left ventricle at the level of the papillary muscles shown in A-mode (**52**) and B-mode (**53**). Two-dimensional echocardiogram for orientation (**54**).

55

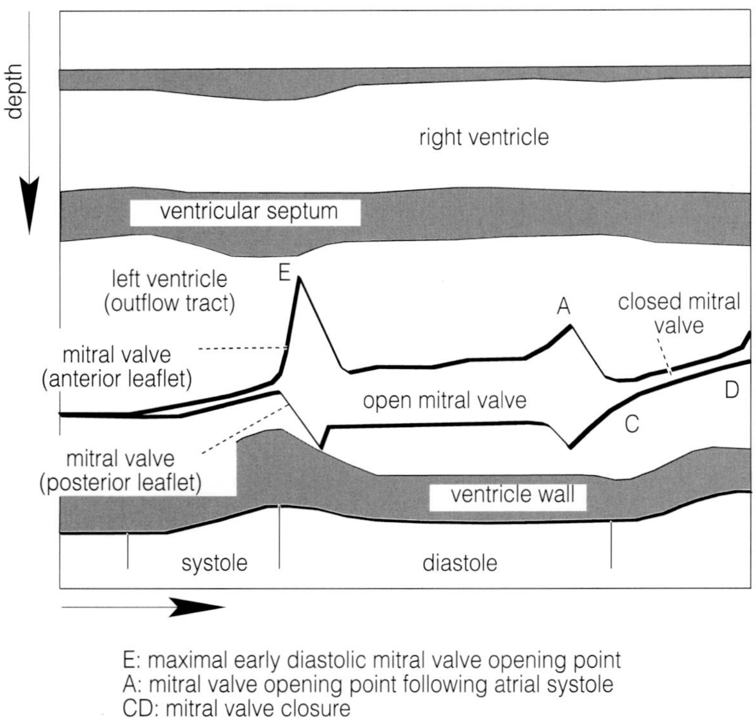

while time is recorded on the horizontal axis (**55–61**). TM-mode displays an echo-time diagram and the movement of structures. This mode is therefore often used in echocardiography. By moving the transducer, cardiac structures are displayed and the heart or vessel valves can be evaluated. This mode also measures systolic–diastolic, normal and pathological atrial and ventricular size, as well as wall thickness including the pericardium.

Two-Dimensional B-Mode

Two-dimensional B-mode includes the static compound scan and real-time ultrasonography.

Compound Scan

The compound mode assembles numerous one-dimensional scans into a two-dimensional ultrasound image. The echoes of structures along the sound beam axis are traced along a vertical line, similar to that in TM-mode. The transducer, mounted on an articulated arm, is moved manually over the region of interest. These

56

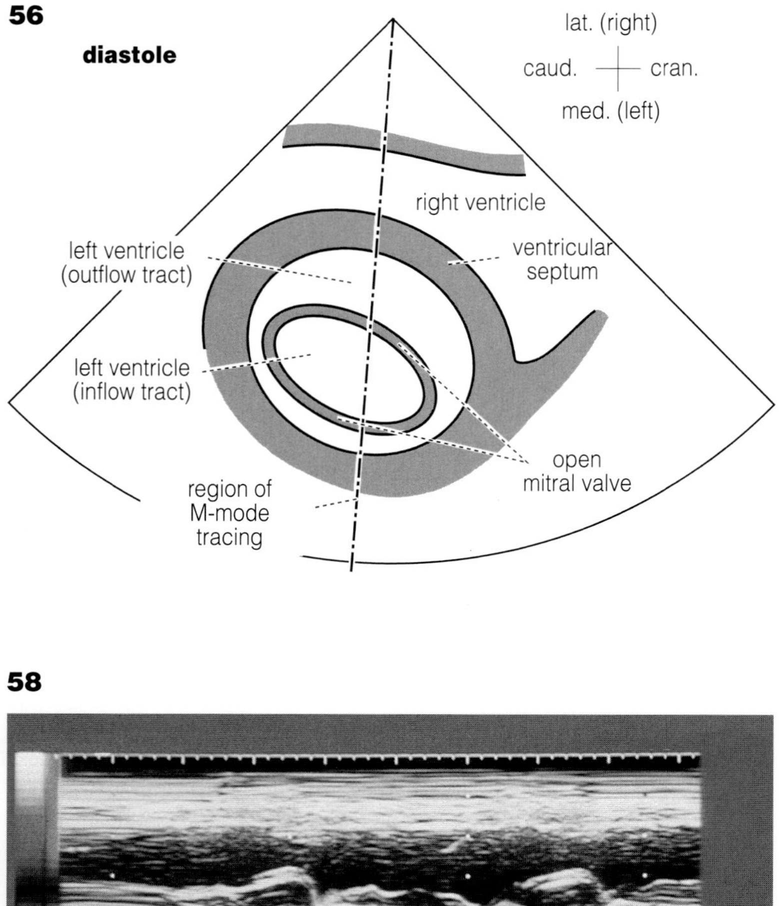

57

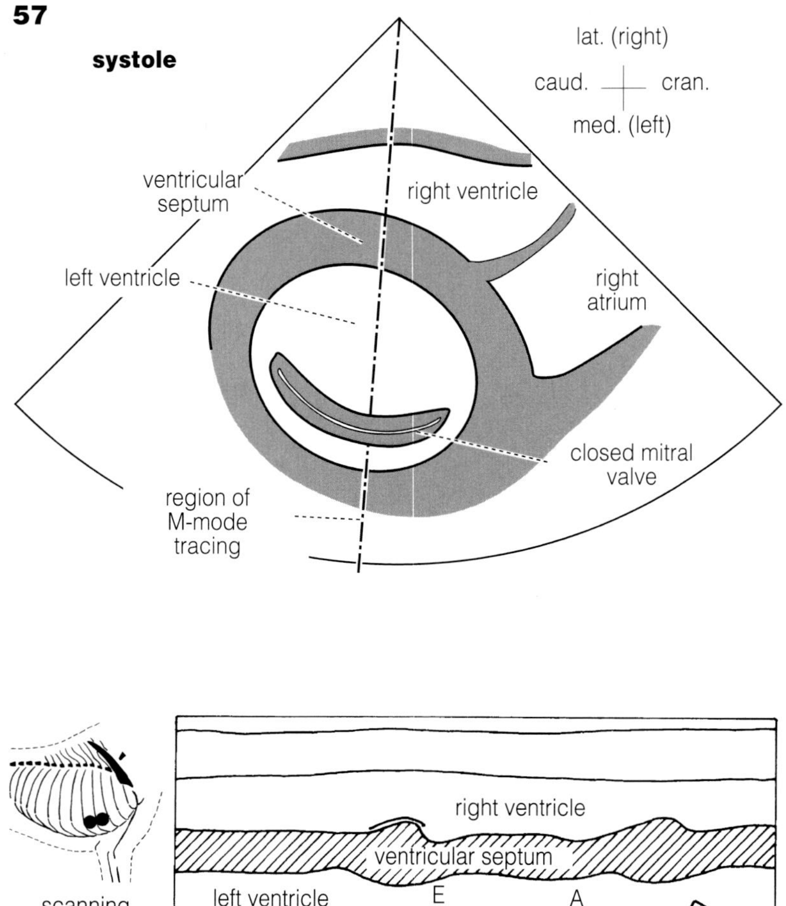

58

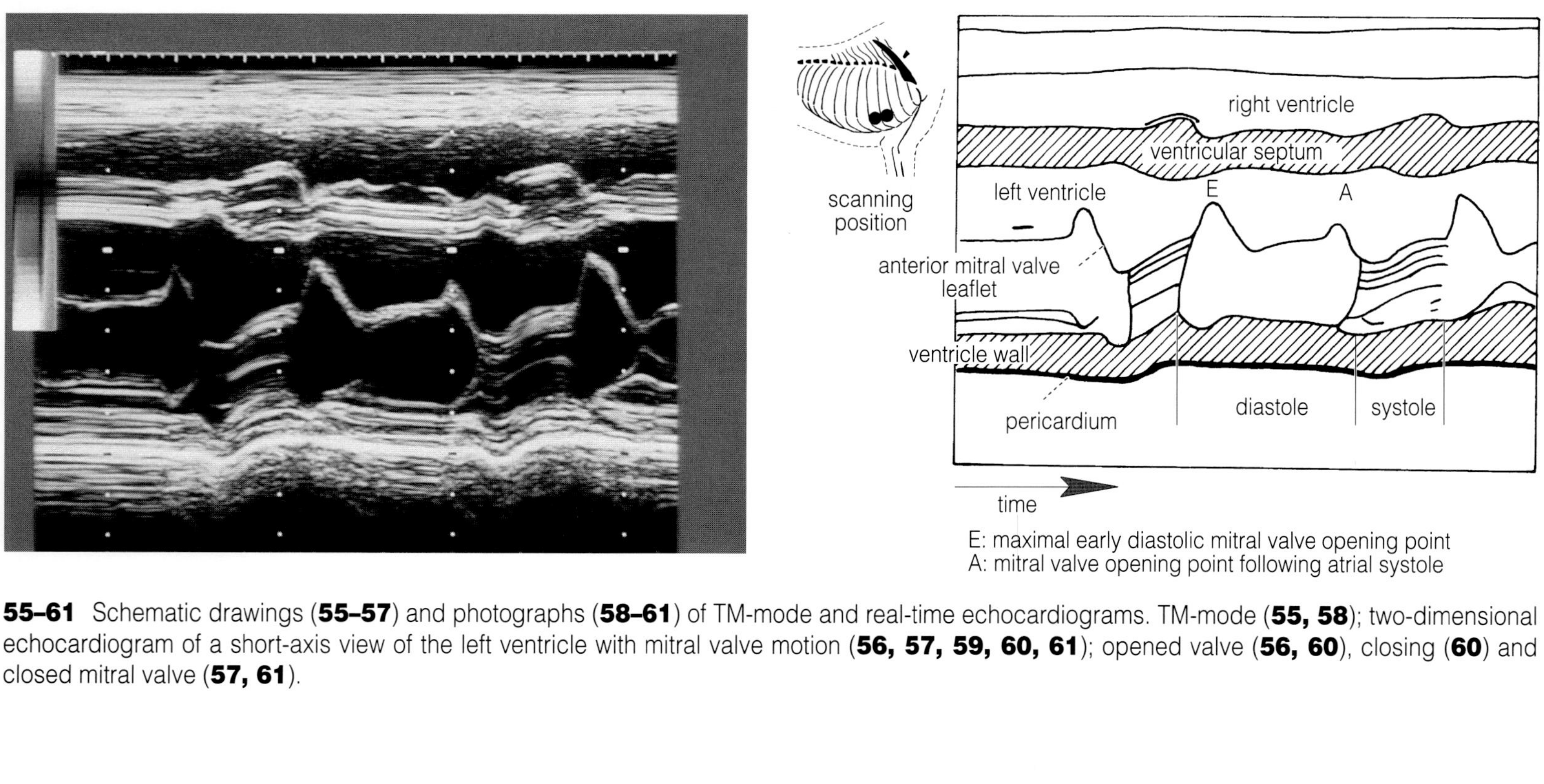

55–61 Schematic drawings (**55–57**) and photographs (**58–61**) of TM-mode and real-time echocardiograms. TM-mode (**55, 58**); two-dimensional echocardiogram of a short-axis view of the left ventricle with mitral valve motion (**56, 57, 59, 60, 61**); opened valve (**56, 60**), closing (**60**) and closed mitral valve (**57, 61**).

59

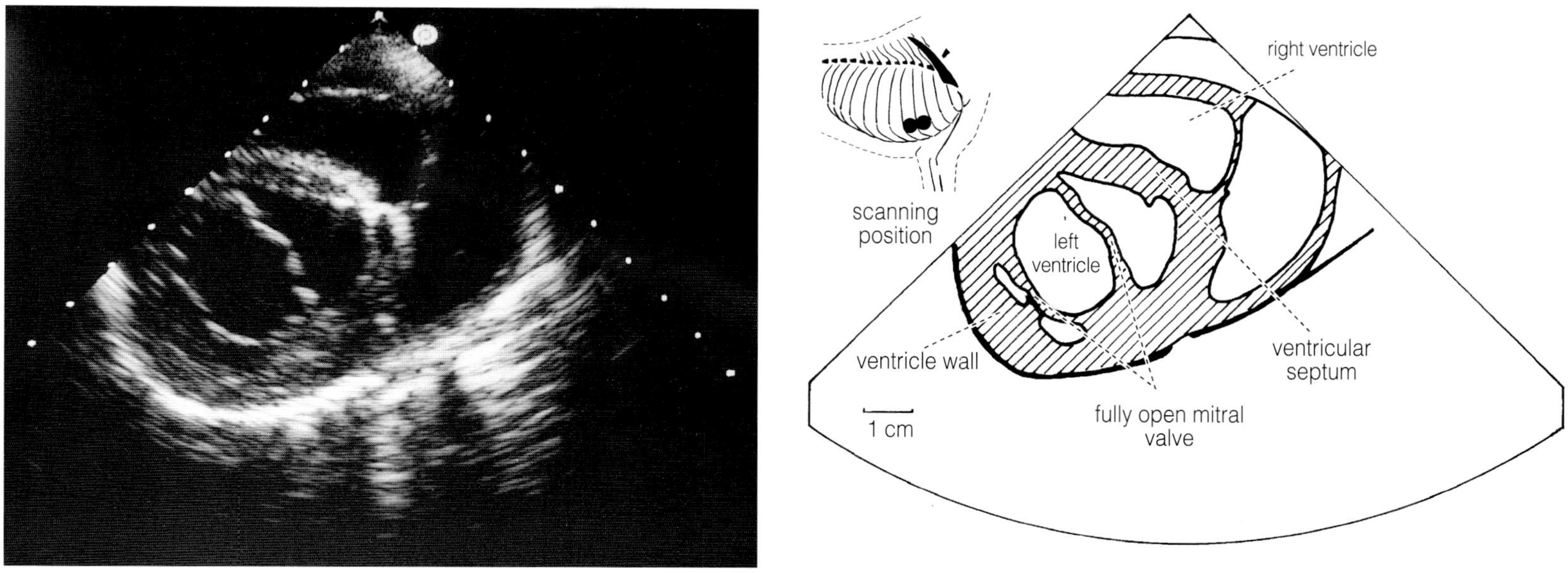
right ventricle
scanning position
left ventricle
ventricle wall
ventricular septum
1 cm
fully open mitral valve

60

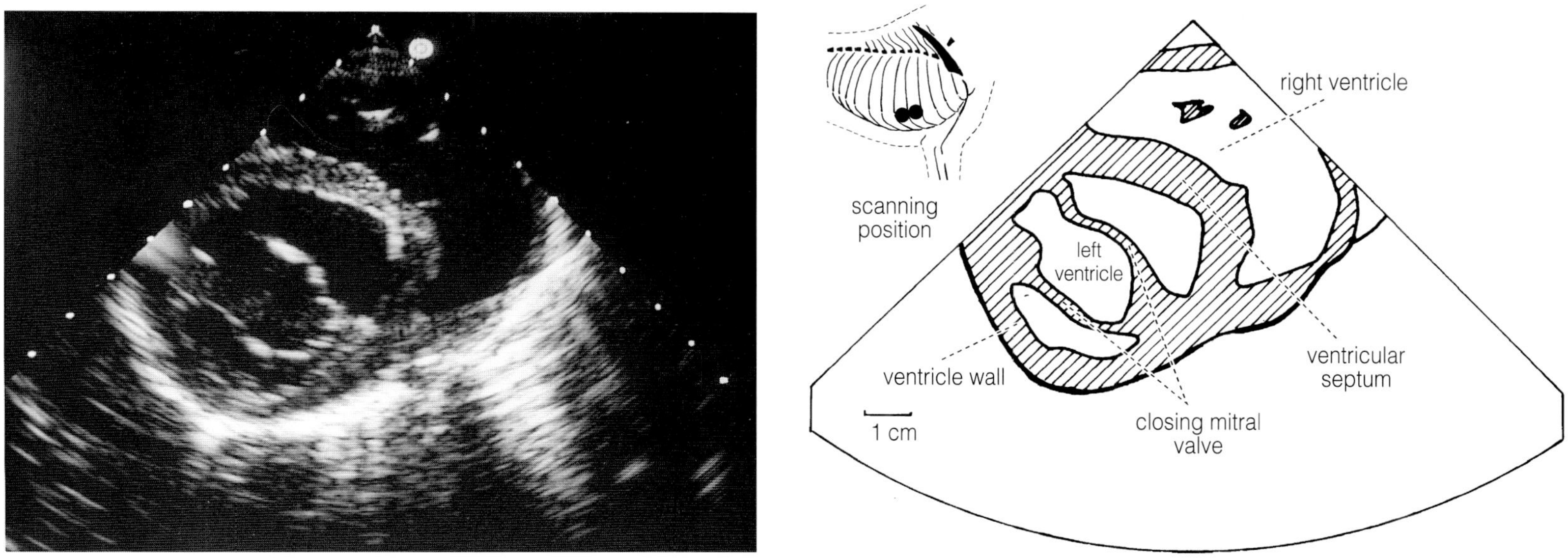
right ventricle
scanning position
left ventricle
ventricle wall
ventricular septum
1 cm
closing mitral valve

61

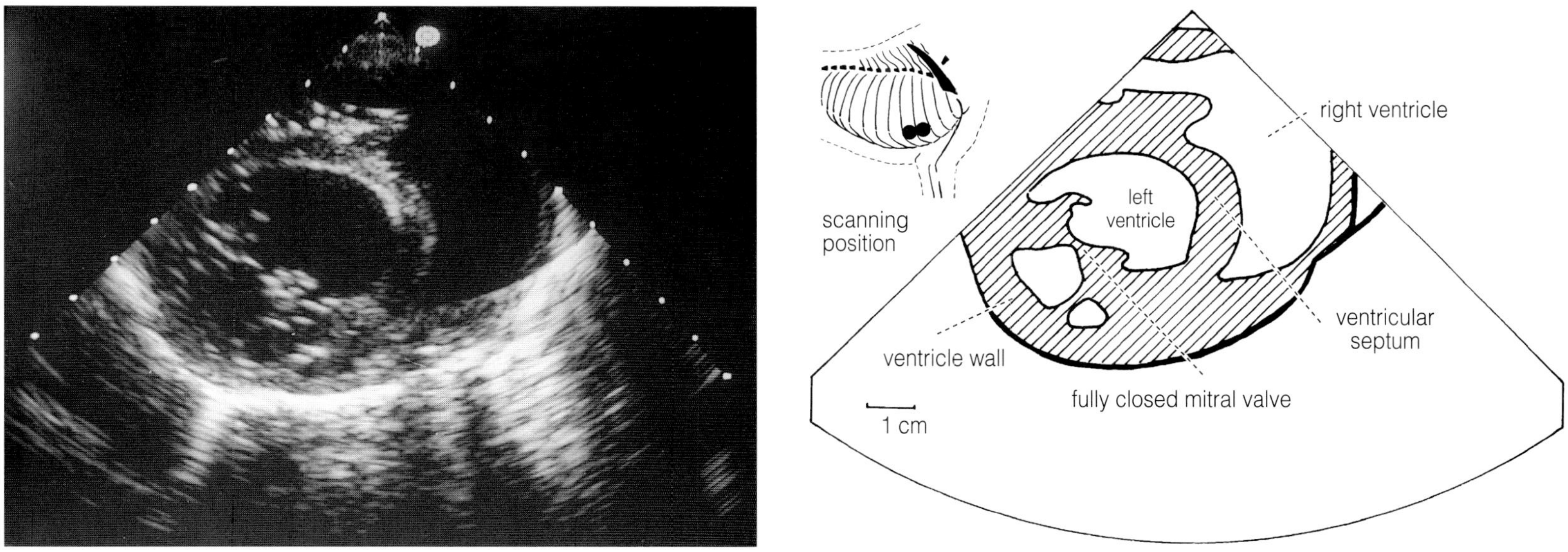
right ventricle
scanning position
left ventricle
ventricle wall
ventricular septum
1 cm
fully closed mitral valve

62

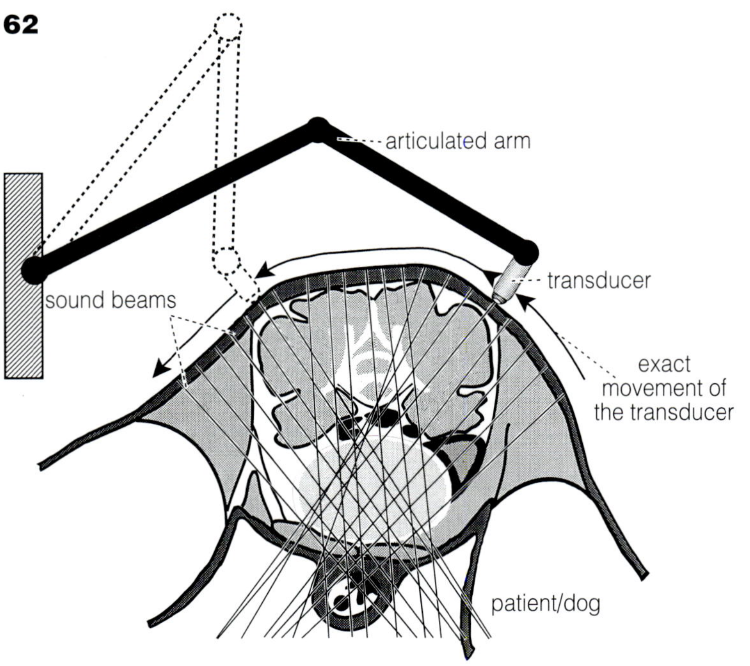

62 Schematic drawing of a compound scan (see **1**). Transverse view at the level of a filled canine urinary bladder.

one-dimensional scans from different views are compounded into a two-dimensional image (62). The advantage of this scanning method is the large field of view and good resolution. The disadvantage is the time-consuming procedure, which does not allow proper imaging of moving structures. In compound echocardiography the transmitting and receiving time must be closely correlated to the heart phase, which requires exact ECG triggering.

The first useful two-dimensional ultrasound images of canine and feline abdominal organs were produced with this compound mode (1, 2). Today it is of no diagnostic value.

Real-Time Ultrasonography

Twenty to fifty or more two-dimensional images are produced on the screen per second by reducing the time needed for echo production. This is a requirement for real-time scanning. The frame rate and image renewal time needed are dependent on the structures being examined. A slow frame rate and high scan line density are sufficient for static organs with minimal respiratory movement. Cardiological scans, on the other hand, need higher frame rates with at least 30 images per second.

Two-dimensional ultrasound examination or ultrasonography is the imaging method of choice in echocardiographic diagnostics. Ultrasonography assesses anatomical and pathological structures, including their movements, and allows for limited functional analysis. Additional methods are needed to determine organ function.

Compared to the compound mode described above, real-time images are not scanned manually but automatically. The beam may be steered mechanically or electronically. The resulting image is either a triangular or pie-shaped sector sonogram or a rectangular linear or parallel sonogram, depending on the transducer used. A combination of both is displayed as a trapezoid convex sonogram (63–68). The same classification applies to transducers.

63

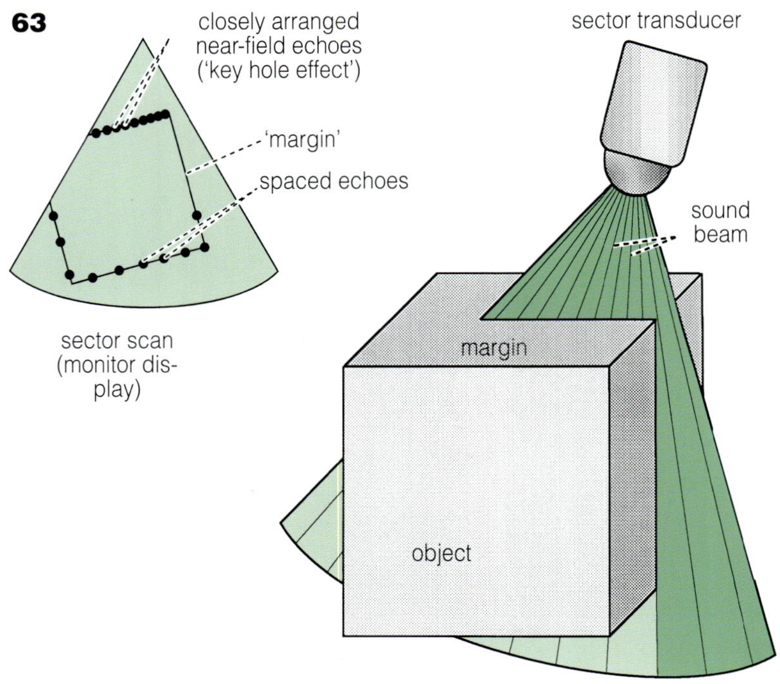

64

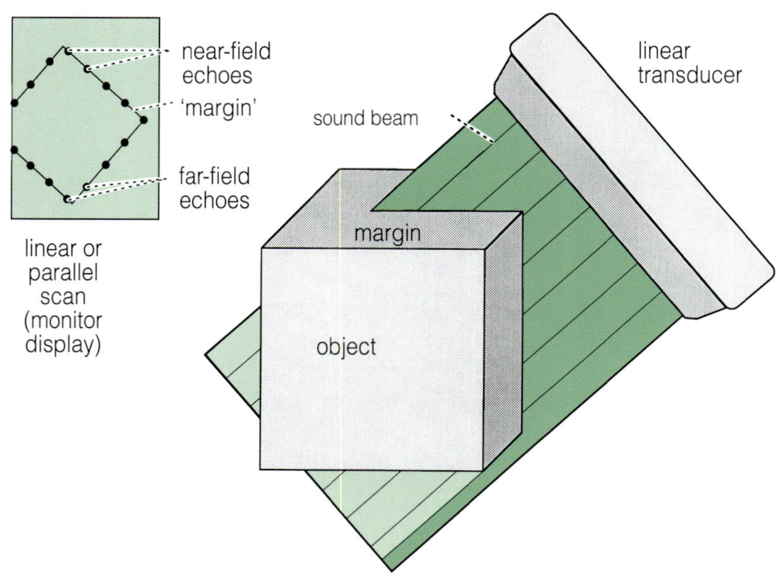

65

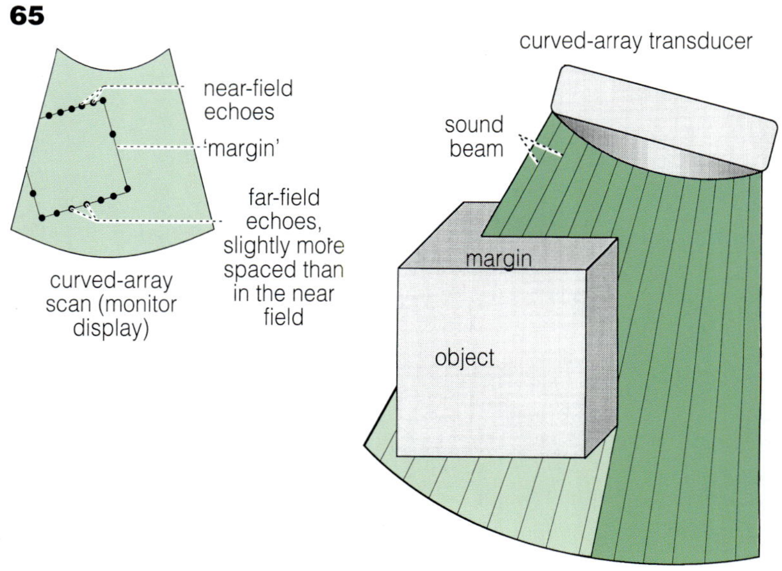

63–65 Schematic drawings of a sector (**63**), parallel (**64**) and convex sonogram (**65**).

66

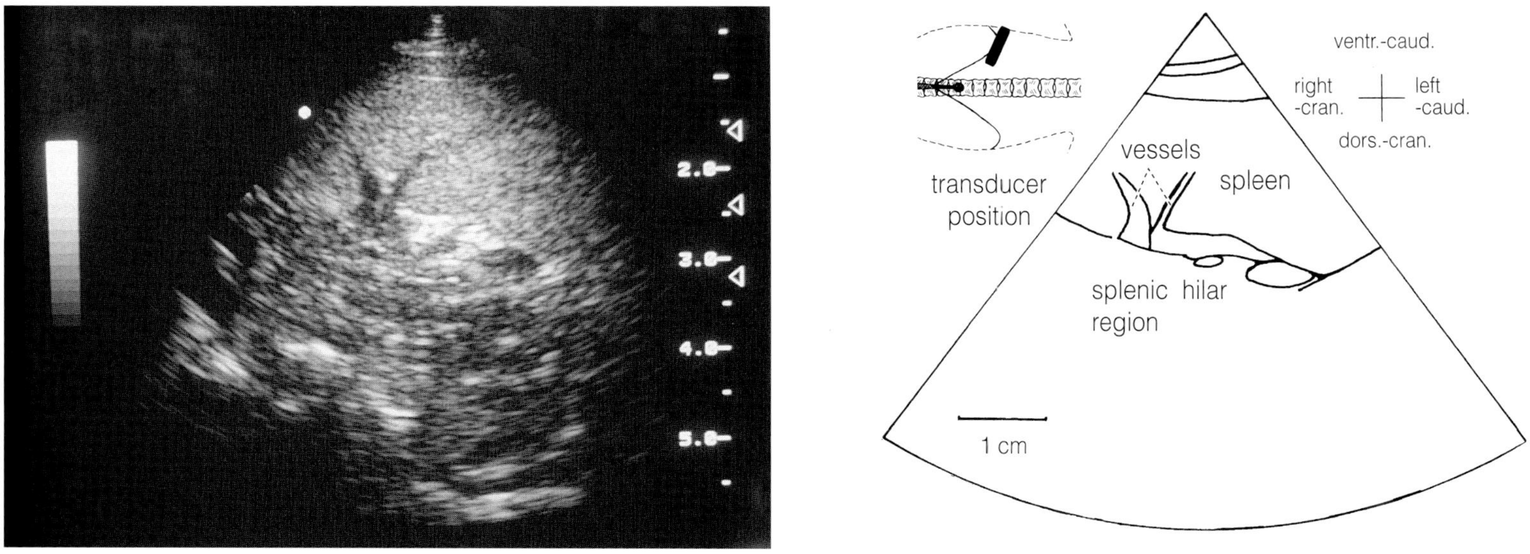

67

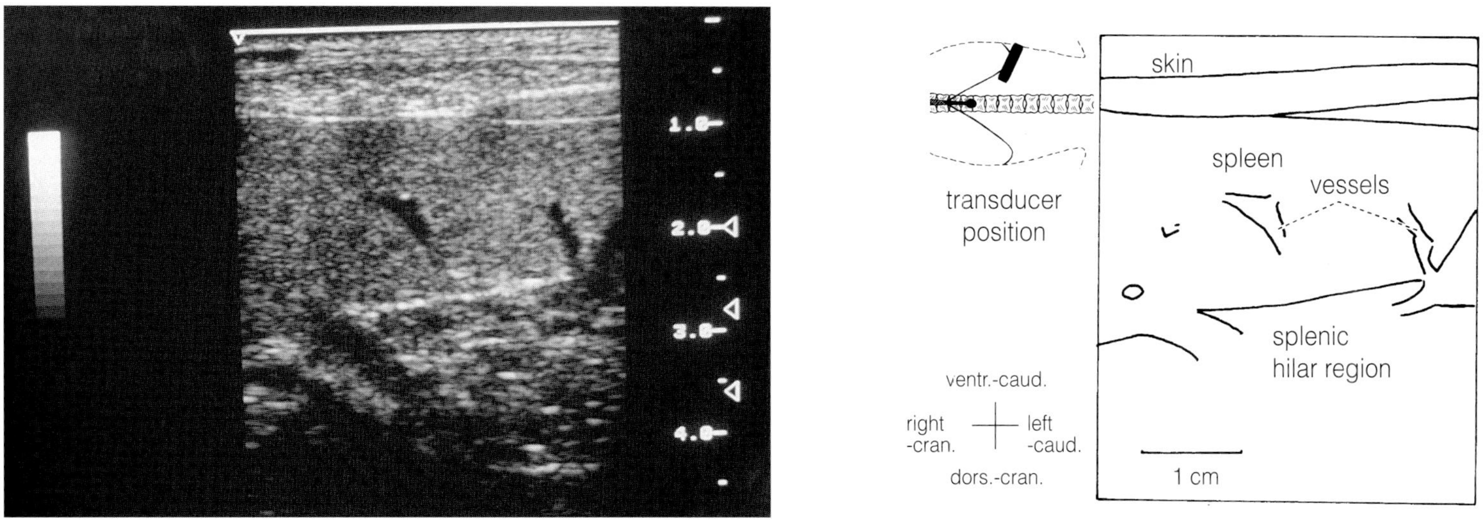

68

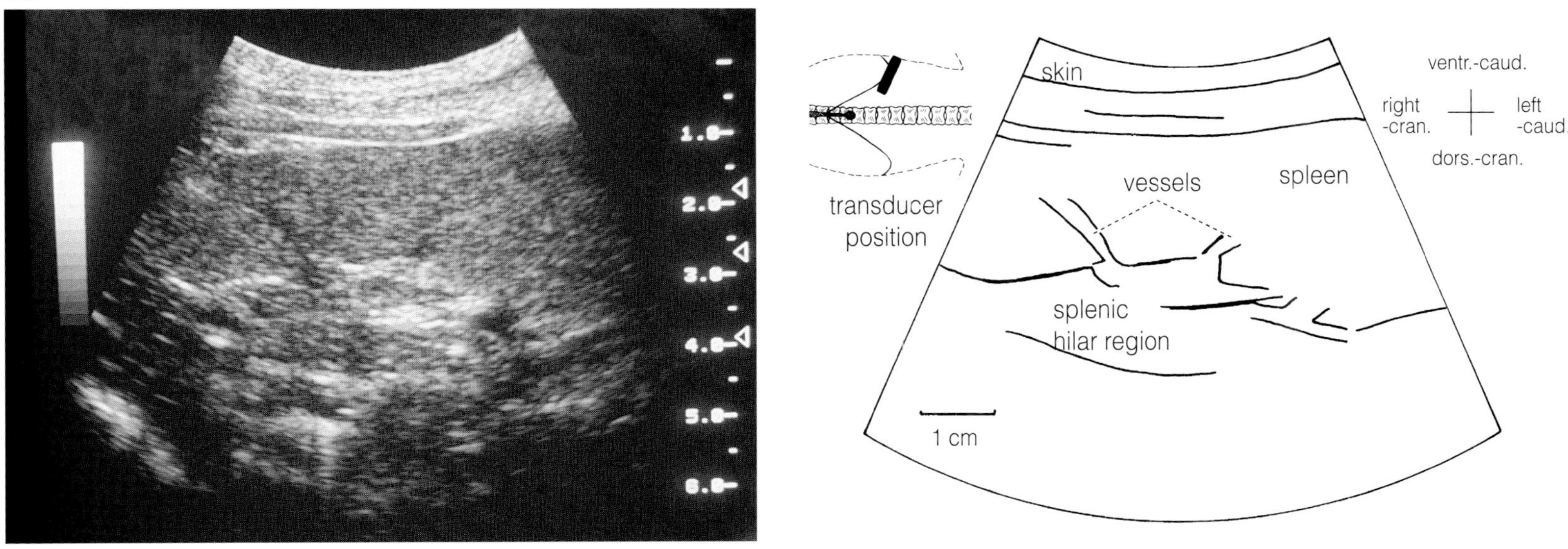

66–68 Comparative images of a canine spleen using a sector (**66**), linear (**67**) and curved-array transducer (**68**).

Sector Transducer – Sector Sonogram (63, 66, 69, 70)

Sector transducers produce a triangular or pie-shaped image. The scan line density of the display is higher in the near field, while the lines diverge in the far field.

Most commercial sector scanners are driven mechanically. One to eight piezoelectric crystals are mounted on the transducer and are either rotated in a circular motion or oscillated to-and-fro (**69**). After receiving an echo from a structure, the crystal sends the next pulse to produce a scan line. Because of the high velocity in soft tissues (c = 1,540 m/s), echoes from a depth of 10 cm return to the transducer 0.13 ms after being pulsed. An angle of 60–120 degrees can therefore be scanned within a short time.

Electronic sector scanners are made up of several ceramics, each holding numerous piezoelectric elements. These elements are arranged in a way to produce a sector view when pulsed. Triggering of these crystals must follow at exact sequences or phases, which is why these electronic transducers are called phased-array scanners.

The crystals in some newer sector scanners are mounted in an annular fashion. The circular sweep is steered by mechanical oscillation, while the elements are electronically focused by individual triggering. This mechanical as well as electronic scanner is referred to as an annular- (phased-) array transducer.

Sector transducers have the advantage of requiring only a small skin contact area, which allows for good contact even with small acoustic windows, such as the intercostal spaces. Sonographic examinations of the heart and complete views of the liver are therefore only possible with sector scanners. Hair coat removal is often not necessary with sector transducers. For sonographic beginners, interpretation of the triangular shape of a sector scan can be more difficult than a linear scan. Resolution in the near field is decreased by the scan line density and the narrow field of view. A stand-off pad is needed for scanning superficial structures (see Stand-Off Pads, page 56). Far field echoes are displayed as somewhat distorted.

69

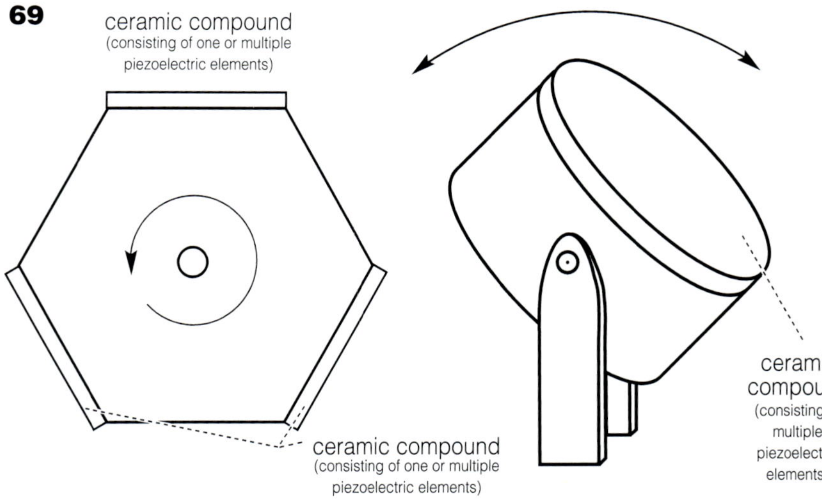

70

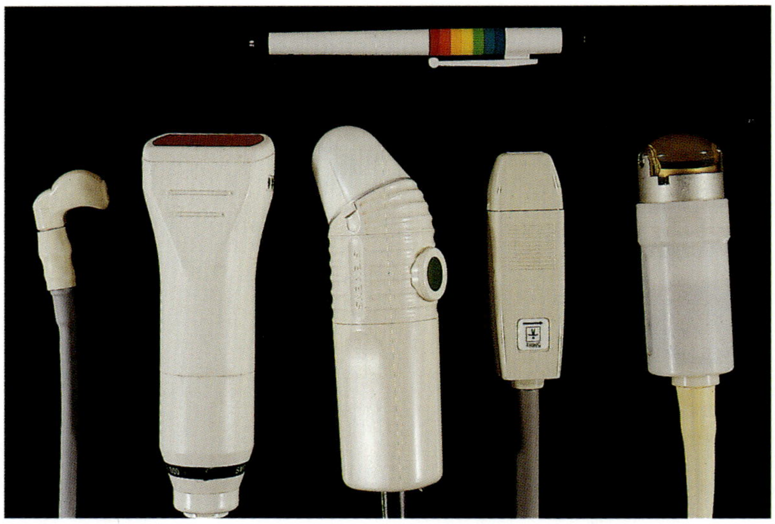

69, 70 Sector transducers. Schematic drawing of inner structure (**69**); sector transducer types (**70**).

Table 5 Comparison of transducer types; advantages and disadvantages as well as main applications. The use of these transducers is extended by applying a stand-off pad with sector scanners or using very small linear-array or curved-array tranducers.

	Sector transducer	Linear-array	Curved-array
Advantages	Small skin contact area.	High near-field resolution.	High near-field resolution.
Disadvantages	Decreased near-field resolution, diverging far field.	Large skin contact area.	Large skin contact area (smaller than linear-array), diverging far field.
Applications	Echocardiography, sonography of intrathoracic and intrapelvic abdominal organs; sonography of structures with small skin contact area: brain, eyes, testes and joints. Some small dogs, cats, and puppies with small skin contact areas (with stand-off pad).	Sonography of extrathoracic abdominal organs, cervical and cranial stuctures such as salivary glands, muscles; sonography of superficial structures: skin, mammary glands, penis, joints and tendons. Some small dogs, cats, and puppies requiring good near-field resolution.	Sonography of extrathoracic abdominal organs; sonographic pregnancy diagnosis.

71 72

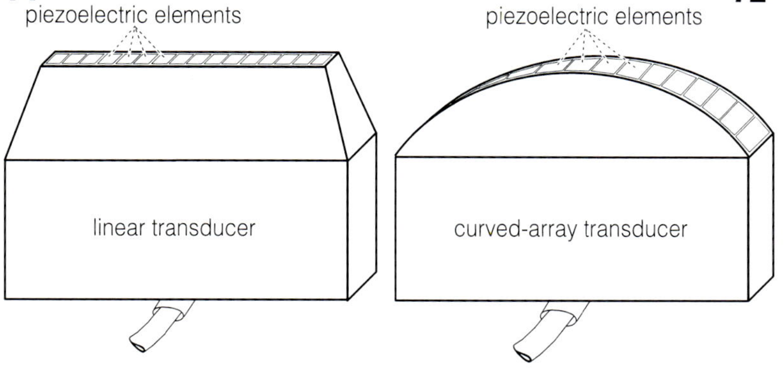

73

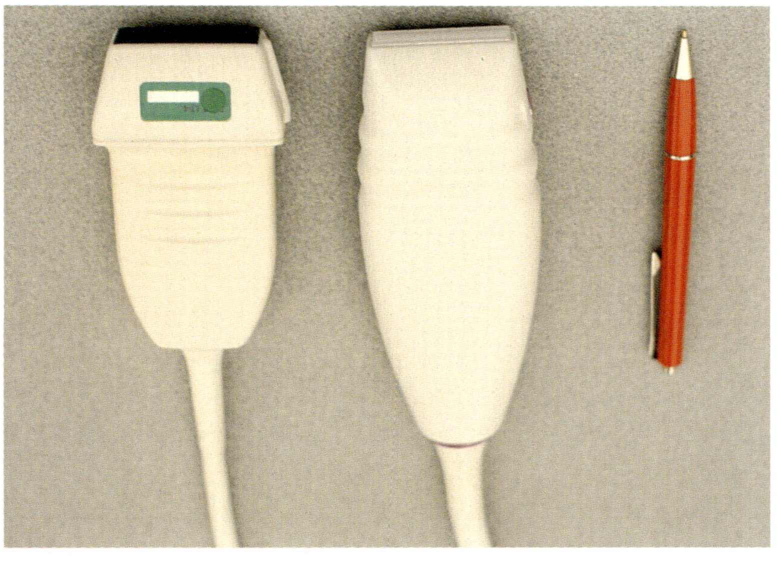

74

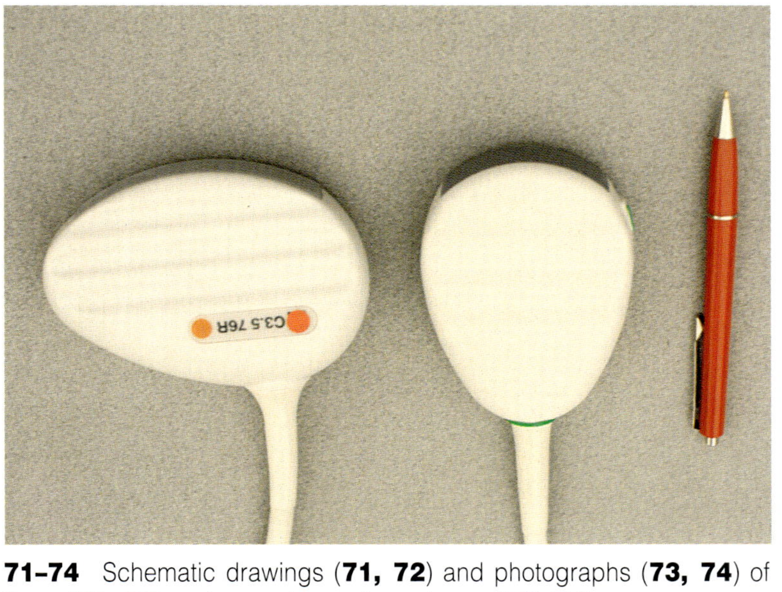

71–74 Schematic drawings (**71, 72**) and photographs (**73, 74**) of linear (**71, 73**) and curved-array transducers (**72, 74**).

Linear or Parallel Transducer – Parallel Sonogram (64, 67, 71, 73)

Linear transducers produce rectangular display formats; this means that the scan lines are arranged in a vertical, linear and parallel fashion.

The linear-array scanner has multiple crystals, which are arranged along a line (**71**). The shape of the linear transducer and parallel sonogram is rectangular.

The crystals are organized in groups that send out sound waves sequentially. This allows for a larger transmission and receiving unit, which improves sound beam geometry and lateral resolution. When the crystal groups overlap – group A may consist of crystal 1 through 5, and group B includes crystal 2 through 6 – the scan lines are arranged closer together. The number of elements also improves electronic focusing with numerous focal zones along the beam axis.

The main feature of linear transducers is their excellent near-field resolution. The rectangular images are easier to interpret. A disadvantage of this transducer type, which often limits its use, is the large skin contact area. Intercostal spaces cannot be used as acoustic windows with these scanners and hair coat removal is mandatory. The limitations of these transducers is seen even in shorter and smaller linear transducers, so-called small parts scanners.

Curved-Array Transducer – Convex Sonogram (65, 68, 72, 74)

Curved-array transducers are a combinination of both sector scanners and linear scanners. The crystals are arranged in a curved arc instead of a straight line (**72**). Focusing is electronic, similar to the linear-array tranducer.

The advantage of curved-array tranduces is the relatively good near-field resolution, with better skin contact than the linear-arrays. In some cases, hair coat clipping is therefore not necessary. This transducer type does not allow intercostal examinations.

The ideal transducer for all ultrasonographic examinations with good near-field and far-field resolution, good depth penetration and a small contact area does not exist. When choosing a transducer, compromises have to be made. The examination in question usually decides which transducer is used. Small linear-array and curved-array transducers are ideal for abdominal examinations, especially pregnancy diagnosis, but not for echocardiography (*Table* 5).

> An all-around transducer for both abdominal and cardiac examinations in dogs and cats is a 5 MHz sector transducer with near focus.

The small skin contact area of this sector transducer can be used for small dogs and cats, including puppies and kittens, and allows scanning through small acoustic windows without hair coat removal. Superficial structures can be scanned using a stand-off pad (see Stand-Off Pads, page 56).

Doppler Mode

Relative blood flow direction and flow velocity can be measured by applying the Doppler principle. This allows the sonographer to obtain information regarding cardiac haemodynamics, actual organ blood supply (see Interaction of Ultrasound Beams with Tissues, page 21) and information on vascular function.

Colour-coded Doppler ultrasonography has become an important factor in cardiovascular diagnostics. Continuous and pulsed-wave black-and-white Doppler mode are more commonly used.

Duplex Doppler ultrasonography (from Latin *duplex* = double) simultaneously uses real-time, two-dimensional ultrasonography or M-mode ultrasonography with a Doppler mode. Colour-coded Doppler ultrasonography simultaneously displays blood flows and real-time images. Pulsed-wave Doppler is also a part of duplex ultrasonography, although it can only be partially

75

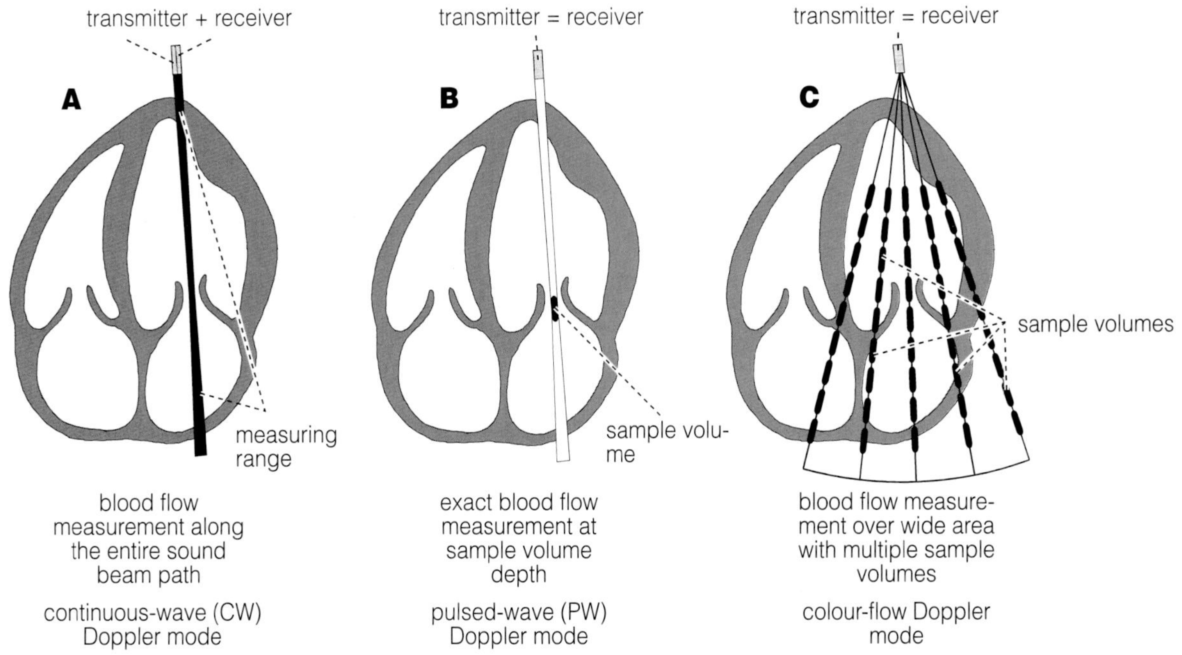

75 Schematic drawings of CW (**A**) and PW (**B**) Doppler modes as well as colour-flow Doppler sonography (**C**).

combined with two-dimensional sonography. First, the sample volume is placed in the real-time image, which is then frozen and switched to the spectral Doppler display. A number of ultrasound systems automatically update the real-time image by interrupting the Doppler display and displaying the new image. The position of the sample volume is checked periodically. Triplex ultrasonography combines real-time, two-dimensional images, pulsed Doppler, and colour-coded Doppler. This combination reduces image quality.

Continuous-Wave Doppler (CW Doppler)

Continuous-wave (CW) Doppler is a conventional method for determining blood flow. The transducer houses a transmitting and a receiving crystal. The transmitting element generates sound waves continuously, while another element receives reflections continuously from blood cells. CW Doppler is unable to determine and localize the origin or depth of an echo. The echoes are reflected from moving structures along the entire sound beam path (**75A**). The characteristic Doppler tracings for vessels and the heart can help to identify the structure within the beam path. Apart from peak velocities, which determine the spectral tracing, slower velocities are also recorded. Combinations of these tracings produce a Doppler spectral display (see Doppler Frequency Spectrum, page 28).

The main feature of CW ultrasonography is its ability to record very high blood flow velocities in the area of stenotic lesions. Simultaneous two-dimensional imaging is not possible during the CW tracing. This complicates blood flow measurements in restless animals, since the sound waves should always be parallel to the blood flow in the vessels or heart chambers (see Doppler Effect, page 24). These disadvantages of CW Doppler restrict its use in veterinary medicine. CW Doppler is applied mainly in cardiology to measure flow velocities and to determine the severity of valvular insufficiencies and stenoses (see Mitral and Aortic Valves, page 153).

Pulsed-Wave Doppler (PW Doppler)

Pulsed-wave (PW) Doppler is also part of conventional Doppler sonography. This mode uses only one piezoelectric element, which functions as both transmitter and receiver. The crystal emits short sound pulses and is switched to a receiving mode after a certain time. The received echo is registered at a specific depth (**75B**). A new signal is emitted after an echo is received. The time delay for an echo to return to the transducer is determined by the distance between the crystal and the area of the blood flow tracing.

The maximum number of pulses generated per second is called pulse repetition frequency (PRF). The PRF is proportional to the mean velocity (c = 1,540 m/s) and inversely proportional to two times the depth (2R):

$$PRF = \frac{c}{2R}$$

[PRF: pulse repetition frequency; c: mean sound wave velocity in soft tissues (c = 1,540 m/s); R: sample volume depth]

When the distance between a vessel and the transducer is, e.g. 10 cm, the sample volume depth (R) is 0.1 m and the PRF is 7,700/s or 7.7 kHz. The maximum PFR determines the registered maximum blood flow velocity (see Aliasing and Nyquist Limit, page 48).

The advantages of PW Doppler are range resolution and angle correction. This enables blood flow measurements within limits in vessels that are not parallel to the beam axis (see Doppler Effect, page 24; **21–23**). Blood flow tracings must be recorded at various locations to analyze haemodynamic changes and lesions. This can be time consuming and may not be tolerated by some dogs and cats. Another disadvantage of PW Doppler is its inability to trace high velocities in severe stenotic lesions or insufficiencies.

The velocities in CW and Doppler modes are traced along the vertical axis, while time is plotted on the horizontal axis. The spectral tracing above the zero baseline indicates blood flow towards the transducer. A tracing below the baseline indicates flow directed away from the transducer (see Doppler Effect, page 24; **17, 20**).

The difference between the transmitted and received frequencies is known as the Doppler shift and lies within the audible range between 0 and 16 kHz. The characteristic acoustic signals of heart and vascular structures indicate normal and pathological blood flow to the experienced sonographer. The noise is occasionally not tolerated by the animals and must be turned down, turned off or received by head phones.

Table 6 Comparison of different sonographic and Doppler methods according to function, advantages and disadvantages as well as the main applications.

	TM-mode	Two-dimensional real-time sonography	CW-Doppler mode	PW-Doppler mode	Colour-flow Doppler mode
Function	Displays motion and specific interfaces.	Displays morphology.	Displays blood flow in entire line of inquiry; quantitative and qualitative.	Displays blood flow in specific areas; quantitative and qualitative.	Displays blood flow; qualitative.
Advantages	Evaluates moving structures over time. Displays areas difficult to access.	Evaluates normal and pathological tissues and organs. Topographical view of cross-sectional anatomy.	Records very high blood flow velocities. Haemodynamic evaluation of stenotic lesions, insufficiencies or obstructions.	Sample volume choice. Angle correction possible. Evaluation of maximum velocity tracing (spectral display).	Simultaneous image of blood flow and TM-mode or blood flow and two-dimensional real-time. Very sensitive method; detects vessels not found in two-dimensional images. Displays turbulences. Quick and easy method.
Disadvantages	No evaluation of tissues and non-moving organs.	No functional diagnosis. No evaluation of air-filled lung tissue. Displays bone surfaces only.	No depth selection. Blind but parallel sonography of heart areas.	Relatively slow velocities only. Time consuming with several flow measurements.	No quantitative evaluation of flow velocities. Records only relatively slow velocities. Reduced resolution over time. Instrumentation expensive at present.
Applications	Echocardiography only, including fetal heart examinations. Displays ventricles and atria with regard to size and diastolic size variations. Atrioventricular and heart valves with regard to motion and opening; diagnose stenotic lesions.	Sonography of soft tissues of the body except air-filled lungs. Macroscopic evaluation of anatomical cross-sections depending on image quality and resolution.	Used almost exclusively in echocardiography. Measuring high velocities in stenotic lesions and insufficiencies. Quantifying severity of stenotic lesion by determining gradient (see Doppler Echocardiography, page 137).	All areas of cardiovascular diagnostics. Functional perfusion diagnostics.	All areas of cardio-vascular diagnostics. Functional perfusion diagnostics. Orientation for PW Doppler sample volume placement.

Colour-Flow Doppler

Colour-flow Doppler is the only real duplex mode that simultaneously displays both colour-coded blood flow spectrums and one- or two-dimensional sonograms. Colour-coded Doppler echography is also a pulsed-wave method, encompassing the advantages and disadvantages of PW Doppler sonography mentioned above. The blood velocities are not traced by a sample volume, but rather over a wide area of the field and displayed on the image (**75C**).

Normal laminar blood flow directed towards the transducer is colour coded in reds, while flow away from the transducer is represented by shades of blue (see Doppler Effect, page 24; **16, 19**). Turbulent flow is represented by a third colour, either greens or yellows (see Laminar and Turbulent Flows, page 64; **127**. Flow Velocities in Doppler Echocardiography, page 141; *Table 19*).

Colour-flow Doppler sonography is the most practical method for veterinary cardiovascular diagnostics, although it is the most expensive. The method allows a quick and easy haemodynamic interpretation, even with uncooperative animals. The colours are easily recognizable, and blood flows can be traced to structures displayed on the TM-mode or two-dimensional sonogram. This enables a definitive diagnosis to be reached. Vessels not found on high-resolution, two-dimensional images can be differentiated with the extremely sensitive colour-flow Doppler mode. Colour-coded Doppler sonography is capable of detecting lesions such as ventricular septal defects, atrial septal defects and patent ductus arteriosus, all of which may not be detected with conventional PW Doppler sonography.

Aliasing and Nyquist Limit

As mentioned earlier, PW Doppler and colour-flow Doppler methods are able to record and measure only relatively slow blood flow velocities. The reason for this is the so-called 'aliasing' phenomenon. The term is derived from the Latin word '*alias*' meaning 'different' or 'other'.

Aliasing is comparable to the stroboscope effect on films, exemplified by wheels standing still or rotating backwards on stagecoaches in Western movies. The actual direction of wheel rotation is seen only when the wheel rotates less than half-way during one frame. When the wheel rotates fully in one frame, it appears to stop; if the rotation is more than half-way around, but less than a full turn, the wheel appears to rotate backwards (**76**). A high sampling rate or multiple frames per second will detect high rotating velocities. The range at which direction **and** rotation are still perceived is called the Nyquist limit.

PW and colour-flow Doppler sonography does not receive echoes from blood cells continuously, which leads to this 'stroboscope effect' or aliasing.

High velocity measurements require a high sampling rate or a high pulse repetition frequency (PRF). The Doppler shift (fd_{max}, see Doppler Effect, page 24) can only be determined when it is less than half the maximum PRF.

$$|fd_{max}| < \frac{1}{2} \times PRF \quad \text{or} \quad |fd_{max}| < \frac{c}{4\,R}, \quad \text{and } PRF = \frac{c}{2\,R}$$

[fd_{max} : maximum frequency shift; PRF: pulse repetition frequency; c: mean velocity in soft tissues (c = 1,540 m/s); R: depth]

The Nyquist limit represents the maximum registered Doppler shift. In order to measure high velocities, the Nyquist limit should be as high as possible,

The following equations are valid (see Doppler Effect, page 24):

$$fd_{max} = V_{max} < \frac{2 \times f_0 \times \cos\theta}{c} \quad \text{and} \quad fd_{max} < \frac{c}{4\,R}$$

[fd_{max} : maximum frequency shift; f_0: transmitted frequency; V_{max}: maximum blood flow velocity; cos θ: cosine of the angle θ between beam and blood flow; c: mean velocity in soft tissues (c = 1,540 m/s); R: depth]

76

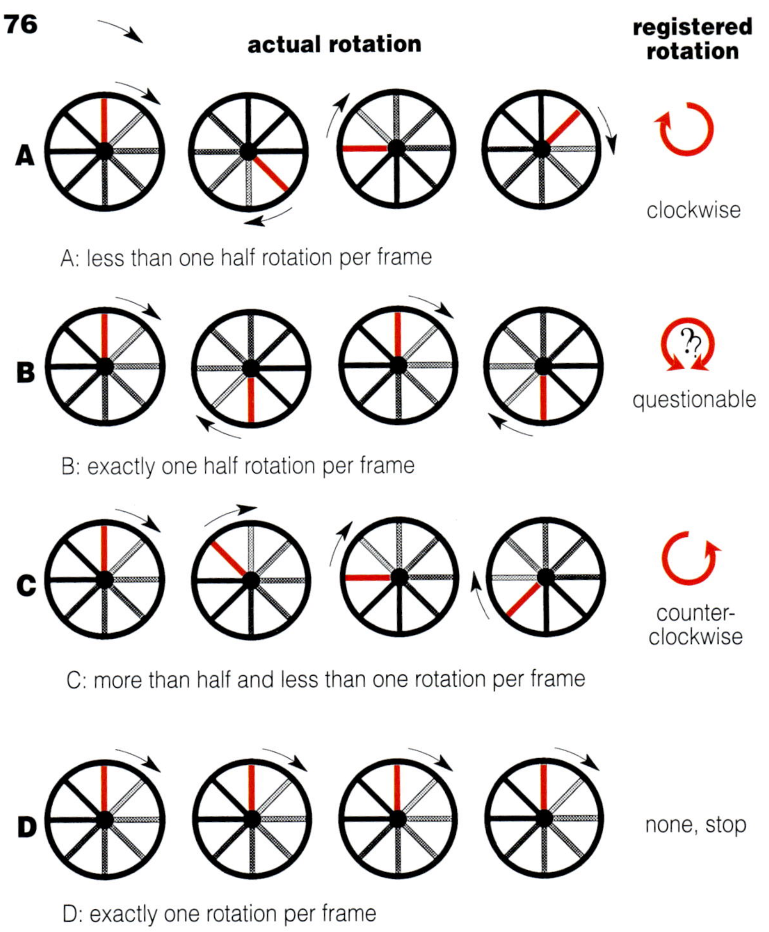

76 Schematic drawings of the stroboscope effect or aliasing, exemplified by a rotating stagecoach wheel. (According to Hatle and Anglessen (1985)[5] and Fehske (1988)[3]).

77

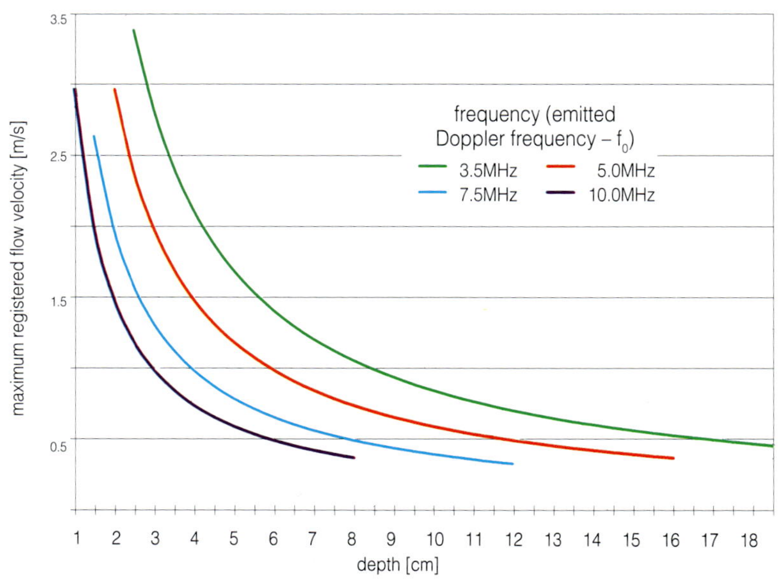

77 Maximum measured blood flow velocities depending on depth or the distance between the transducer and the sample volume. The frequencies are commonly used in veterinary medicine.

By combining these two equations, it is possible to calculate the maximum blood flow velocity (V_{max}), depending on depth (R), or the sample volume, and transmitted frequency (f_0). This is done with the sound beam parallel to blood flow ($\theta = 0$ and $\cos\theta = 1$).

$$V_{max} = \frac{2 \times f_0 \times \cos \Theta}{c} < \frac{c}{4R} \quad \text{this results in}$$

$$V_{max} < \frac{c}{8R \times f_0}$$

The Doppler shift may be registered above the Nyquist limit, although the frequency and flow velocity will be underestimated because of aliasing.

The maximum flow velocities at different frequencies dependent on depth are recorded in **77**.

When the Doppler shift is greater than half the pulse repetition frequency and less than the maximum pulse repetition rate, blood flow is reversed while the flow direction is the same (aliasing). Although flow is directed towards the transducer, it is not recorded above the baseline or in red colours, but below the baseline and in shades of blue. This is comparable to the wheels rotating backwards (**79, 82**).

When the Doppler shift frequency spectrum is great, PW Doppler mode displays a wide pattern above and below the baseline (**80**) and colour-flow Doppler tracings record a colourful mosaic-like image (**83**). Flow direction and velocity are not discernible. Earlier, this aliasing spectrum was falsely described as turbulences (see Laminar and Turbulent Flows, page 64) which may also generate wide frequency spectra.

Aliasing can be avoided by applying the following methods:

Depth (R) Reduction

Depth can be reduced by changing the transducer position and thereby utilizing more effectively the highest pulse repetition rate. This method is not realistically possible, since the distance between the transducer and the heart or vessel is determined individually. The acoustic windows are usually too small to allow the transducer to be repositioned.

Zero Baseline Shift

By moving the zero baseline, the measuring range can be doubled. Flow tracings are then only registered in one direction (**85**).

Transducer with Lower Doppler Frequency (f_0)

Higher flow velocities can be measured by reducing the Doppler frequency. This in turn leads to a decrease in image quality (**86**).

Increasing the Pulse Repetition Frequency (HPRF Doppler)

High pulse repetition frequency (HPRF) Doppler transmits multiple short pulses and receives an echo from a determined depth. In addition, a second or third echo can be registered during an allotted time frame. The Nyquist limit is therefore doubled or tripled, but at the same time a second or third sample volume is recorded along one half or one third of the distance (**87**). Depth discrimination and sample definition are lost.

The most common and easiest methods to correct aliasing and increase the Nyquist limit are shifting the baseline and increasing the pulse repetition frequency. Both methods can be set in preprocessing.

Doppler Controls

Gain

The Doppler signal can be amplified in a linear or overall fashion, comparable to that in one- or two-dimensional sonography. The overall gain control uniformly amplifies all echoes regardless of their origin (**143, 144**).

The gain setting should allow good recognition of the flow tracing without any background artefacts. The overall gain control must be set at the maximum level in patients which are hard to image or do not have a clipped hair coat. Mirror image artefacts occur along the baseline because of high gain settings (see Doppler Artefacts, page 72; **139, 140**).

Wall Filter (High Pass Filter, Low Velocity Reject)

An unwanted Doppler shift can be registered from moving heart and vessel walls and valves. The wall filter eliminates these echoes (see Doppler Artefacts, page 72; **141, 142**). Since the heart and vessel structures are slow moving compared to cardiac and arterial blood flow, only the lower velocities up to 400 Hz have to be filtered. 400 Hz correspond to 0.12 m/s velocity at a frequency of 5 MHz. Slower venous blood flows can be registered by removing or decreasing the wall filter. Higher flow velocities may require a wall filter of up to 1,200 Hz. This leads to a loss of velocity tracings up to 0.2 m/s at a frequency of 5 MHz.

Threshold (Reject)

The signal filter to reduce background noise with CW and PW Doppler modes is called threshold. At the same time, low-intensity signals may be eliminated. If the filter is set too high, it will not register low intensities from maximum velocities. For this reason, the threshold setting should not be too high.

Velocity Range

The velocity range or maximum velocity can be allotted in all Doppler modes. In PW and colour-flow Doppler sonography this is only possible up to the registered maximum velocity mentioned above. The velocity range should be set as low as possible in PW and colour mode, so that the entire scale is used without aliasing.

Sample Volume Position and Size

The sample volume or gate in PW Doppler should be placed in the centre of the vessel or area to be examined. Blood flow should not be perpendicular to the sound beam in this area. The sample volume size should be small enough to allow for good axial resolu-

78

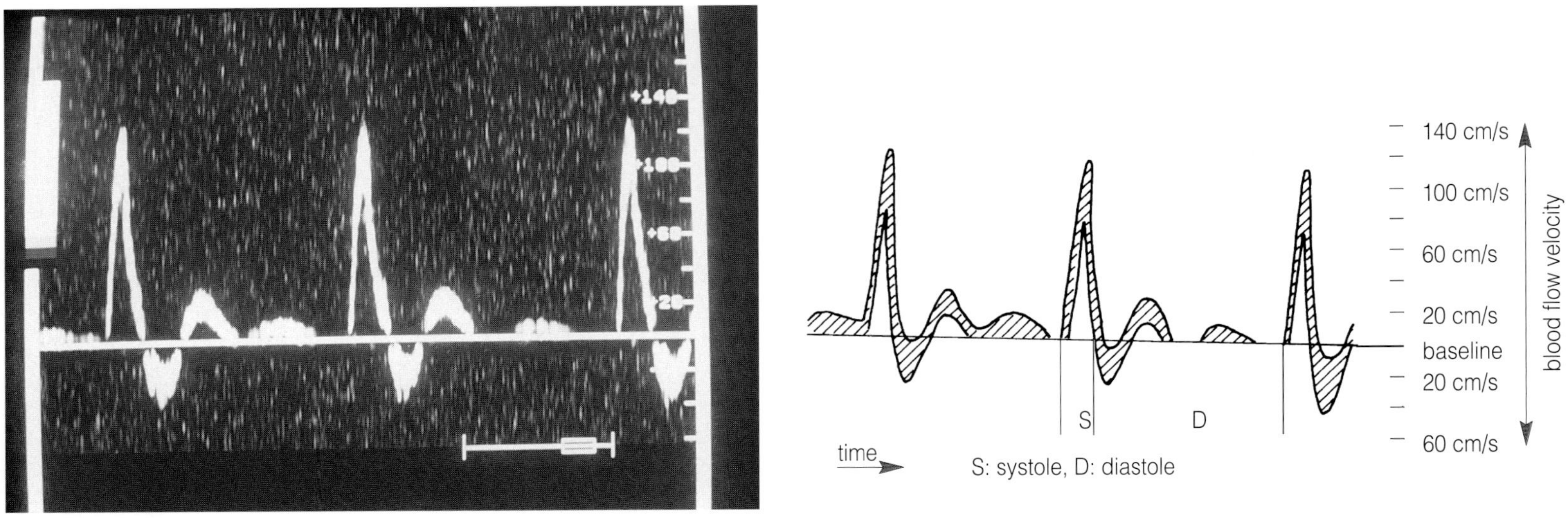

79

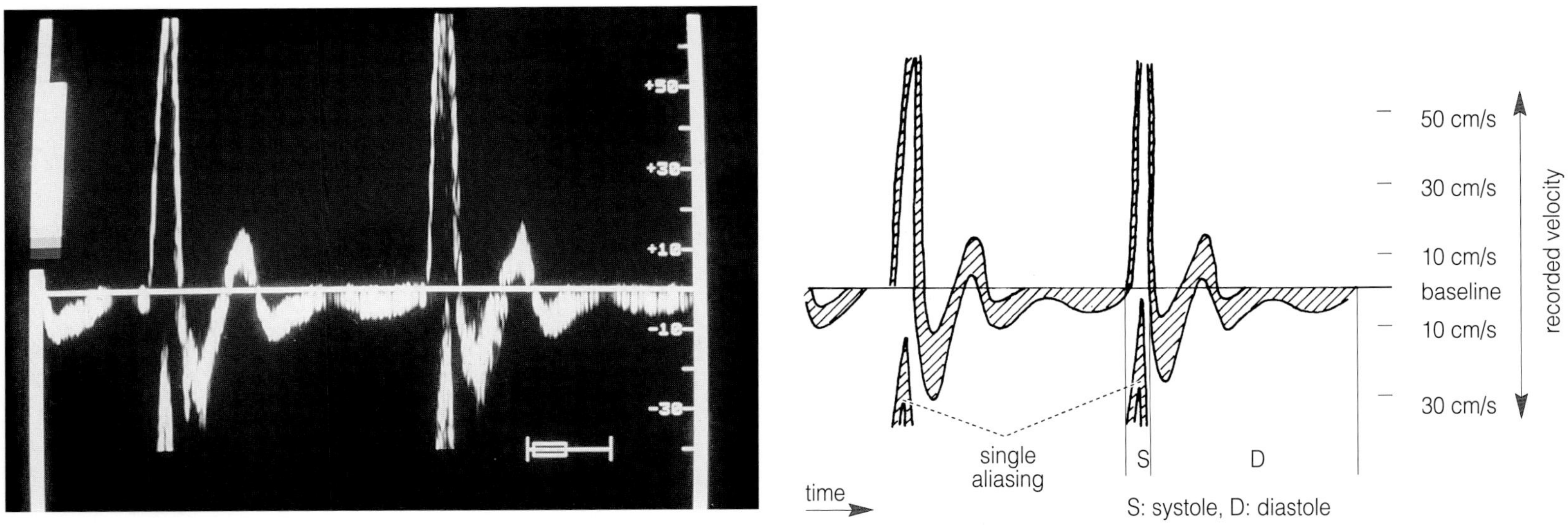

80

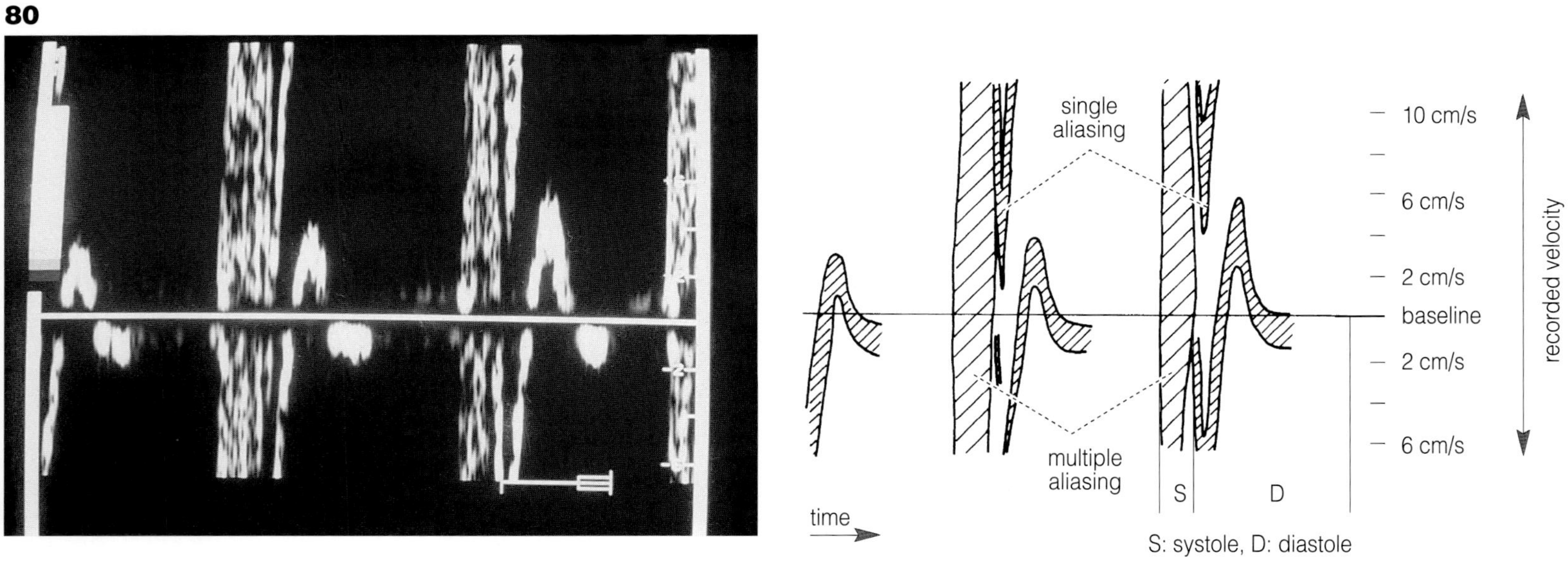

78–83 Blood flow display in the femoral artery of a dog with PW (**78–80**) and colour-flow (**81–83**) Doppler sonography. The maximum velocity is 120 m/s (normal tracing without aliasing (**78, 81**)). Since the recorded velocity is lower than the actual maximum velocity, single (**79, 82**) or multiple (**80, 83**) aliasing occurs.

tion and a small frequency spectrum with exact topographical association. A bigger sample volume is more sensitive and can detect lower velocities. In colour-flow Doppler the sampling region should be as small as possible and be restricted to the area of interest. This creates a higher frame rate and improved axial resolution.

Time Gain Compensation (TGC)

In colour-flow Doppler mode, a time compensated gain can be set much the same as in one- and two-dimensional sonography. The TGC control compensates for weaker echoes from deeper structures.

81

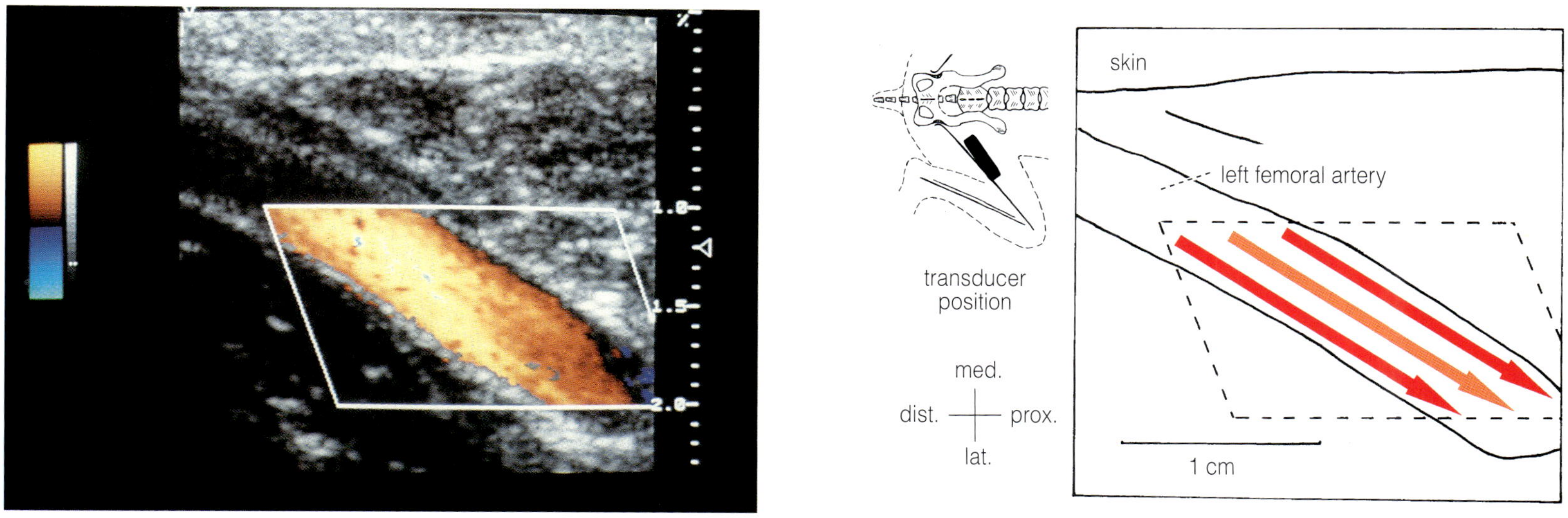

82

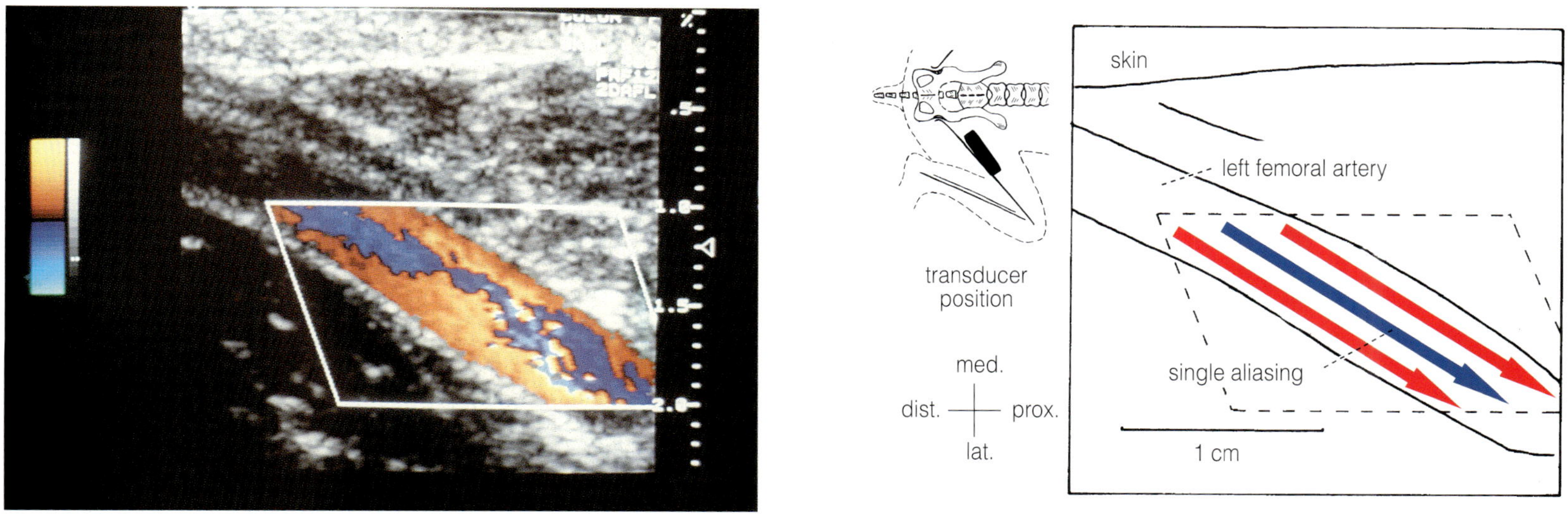

83

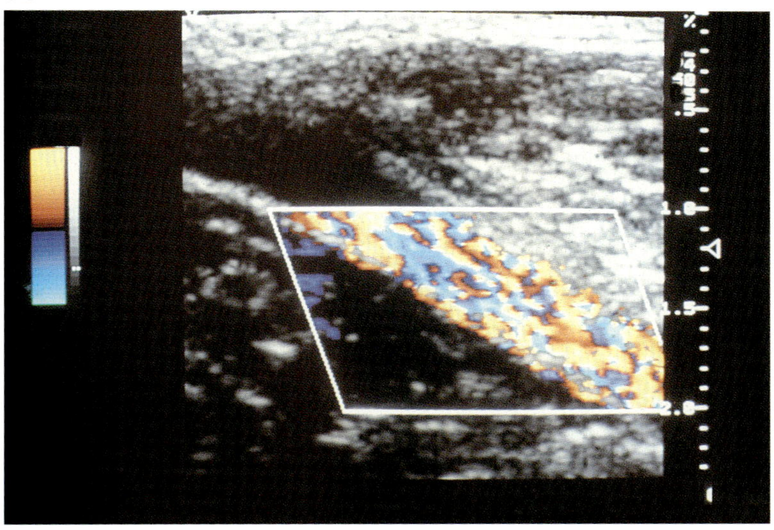

Instrumentation and Documentation

Ultrasound Units

Many of the commercial two-dimensional ultrasound units vary in cost depending on their capacity and power. The difference in quality is determined by resolution, grey scale, controls and versatility, as well as the number of transducers. Most of the units can be switched to M-mode and are capable of cardiac diagnostics. This depends on whether sector transducers are adaptable. Conventional and colour-flow Doppler can be added to some units.

Colour-coded sytems not older than 3–5 years have a high resolution one- and two-dimensional display as well as a conventional Doppler mode. These units are still more expensive than the ‘simpler’ two-dimensional systems described above.

There are three types of sonographic units, differing in size and mobility: portable machines, transportable machines and stationary machines.

The smallest portable ultrasound units weigh about 10 kg and can be carried anywhere (**88**). They are especially practical for veterinarians making house calls or working in a large animal practice. Because of the limited space in these units, quality and controls are somewhat reduced. Many of these systems cannot switch between sector and linear scanners. A cardiac examination is not possible with only linear transducers.

Transportable units up to 40 kg are heavier than portable systems and are usually installed on trolleys in the practice or clinic (**89**). These units can be transported in a passenger car and can be carried by one or two persons. Most of the two-dimensional sonography and conventional Doppler systems belong to this category. These high resolution and versatile systems are recommended for small animal practitioners working in practice or in a clinic.

84

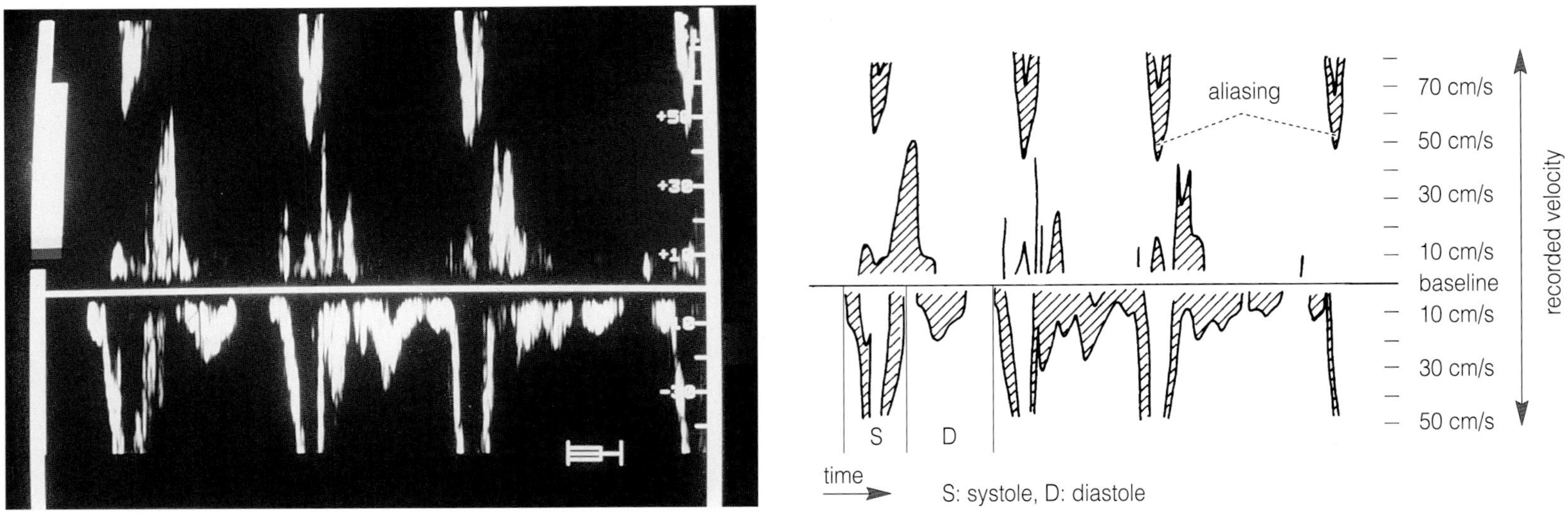

85

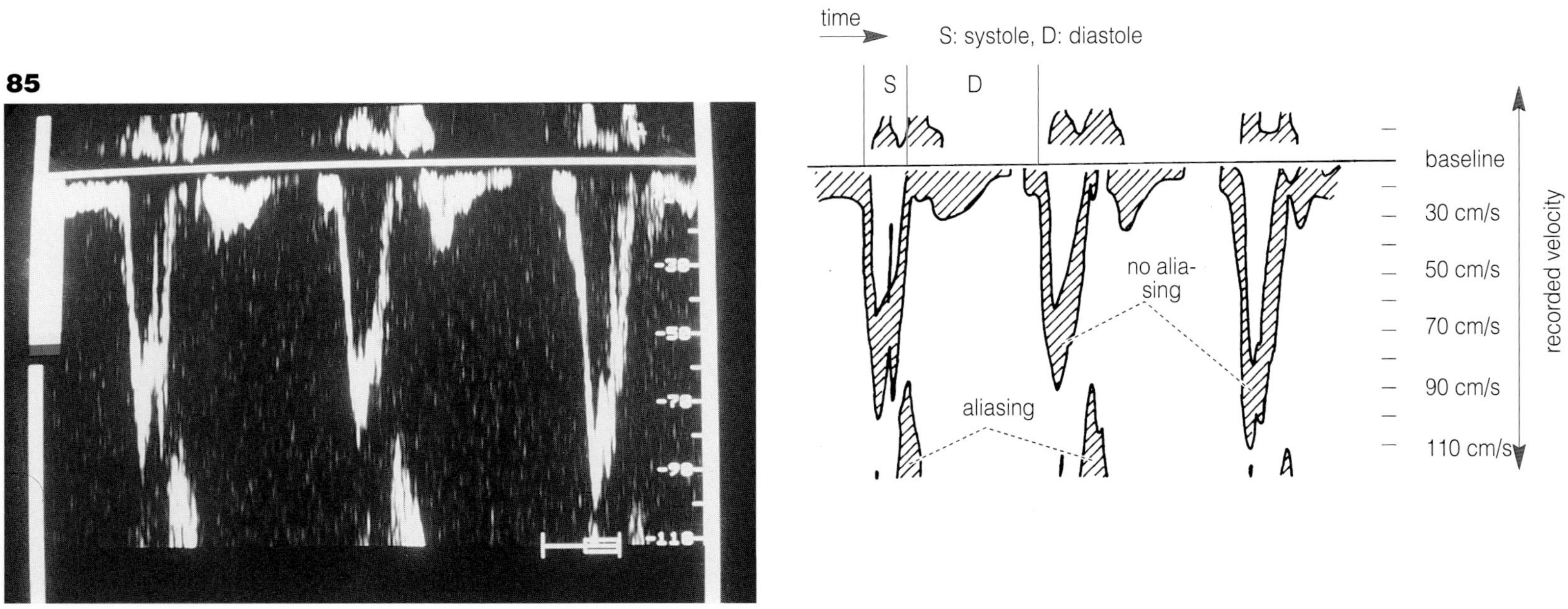

86

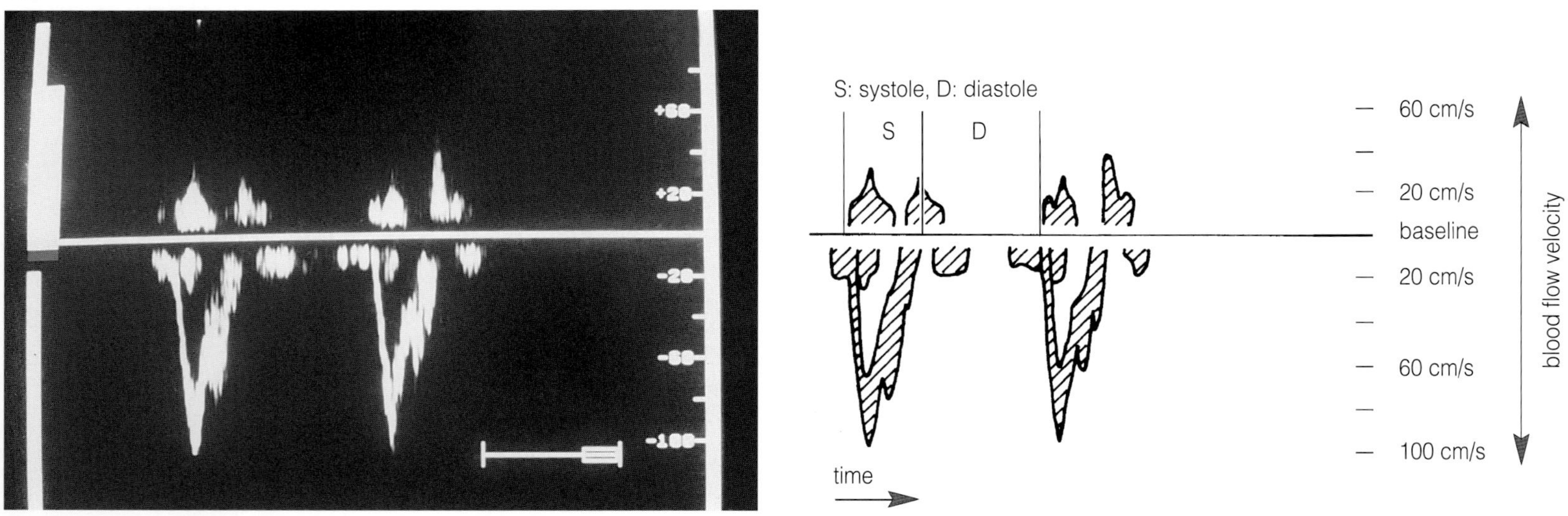

84–86 PW Doppler blood flow tracings in the pulmonary trunk before its division (**84, 85**) and at the pulmonic valve (**86**). Aliasing phenomenon at a Doppler frequency of 6 MHz (**84**); aliasing correction by shifting the baseline (**85**); and using a lower Doppler frequency of 3.0 MHz (**86**).

Stationary ultrasound units are installed permanently on a moveable trolley (90). Most of these units have colour-flow Doppler and are stationary due to their size and weight. They can only be used inside a practice or clinic.

Most veterinarians intending to buy an ultrasound machine are confronted with offers of used human medical systems. These two-dimensional ultrasound systems are not recommended for veterinary practice, since the quality of most systems has greatly improved during the past years, while the cost has been greatly reduced. Small animal practitioners need small transducers with at least 5 MHz and a near-field focus. In human ultrasonography these transducers are only used in pediatrics or in thyroid and vessel diagnostics.

87

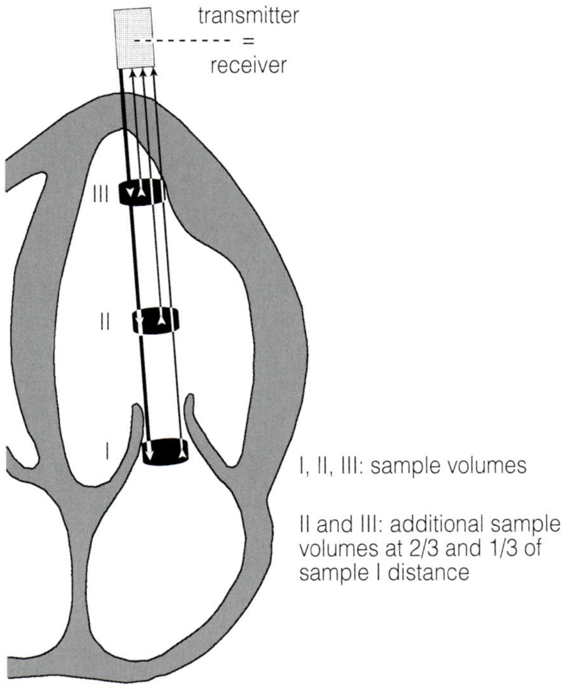

87 Schematic drawing of HPRF Doppler mode.

Ultrasound systems less than five years old, and with colour-flow Doppler, can be bought from human medical practitioners. Buying an additional new transducer may be recommended.

Documentation

Ultrasound images should be recorded with a video recorder and reproduced by additional documentation.

Video Recording

Video recordings of the entire sonographic examination are important for a routine work-up. They are essential for later evaluation of the scanning procedure. Reproductions of frozen images may be incomplete, not typical or false. Some structures or organs in the frozen image may be mistaken for another (**91, 92**).

VHS video recorders are usually used to record black-and-white ultrasound images and are sufficient for documentation. For sonographic examinations outside of the practice it is better to use lightweight recorders. Professional U-matic video systems are higher in quality than VHS recorders, but they are also more expensive. Colour-flow Doppler images should be recorded on S-VHS video recorders.

A sonographic beginner can learn a great deal by reviewing video recordings of sonographic examinations and by studying and evaluating them in slow motion. Questionable findings can then be discussed with a more advanced sonographer.

Frozen images from a video film can be reproduced later with acceptable quality. Digitalized reproductions from video recordings are also possible.

88

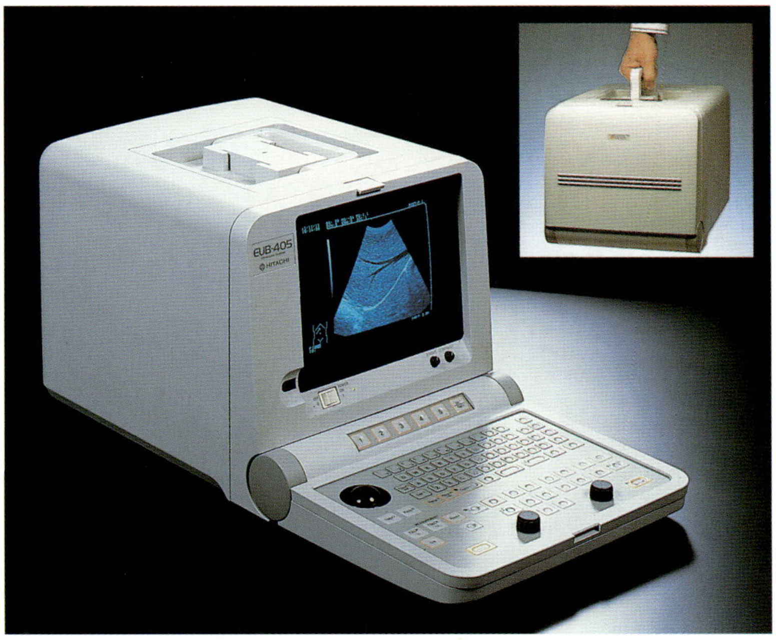

89

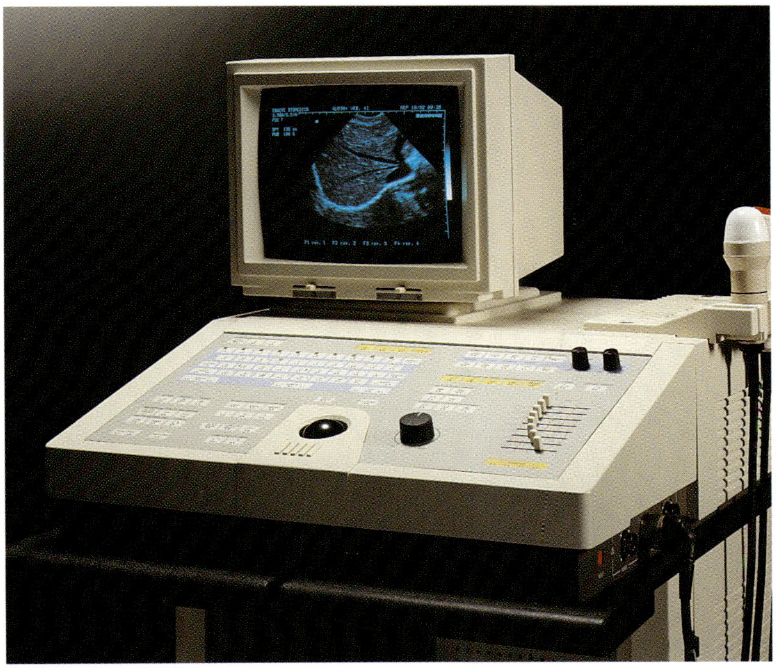

90

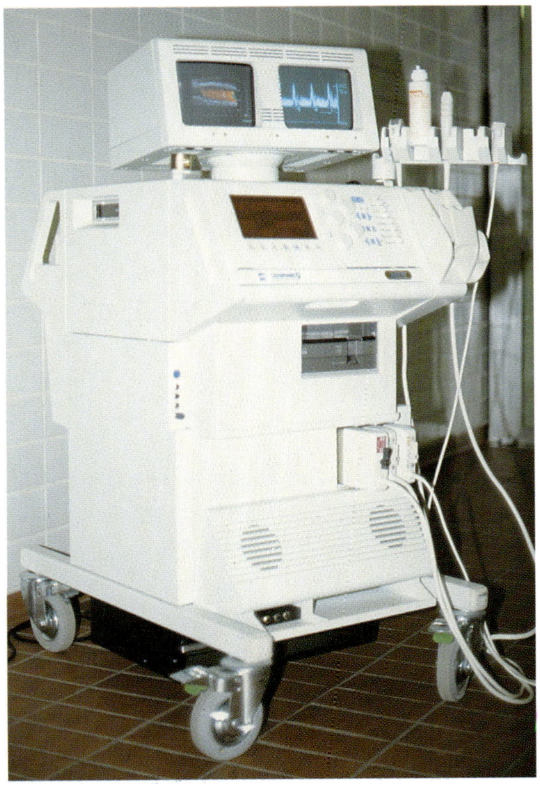

88–90 Portable (**88**), transportable (**89**) and stationary (**90**) ultrasound units.

91

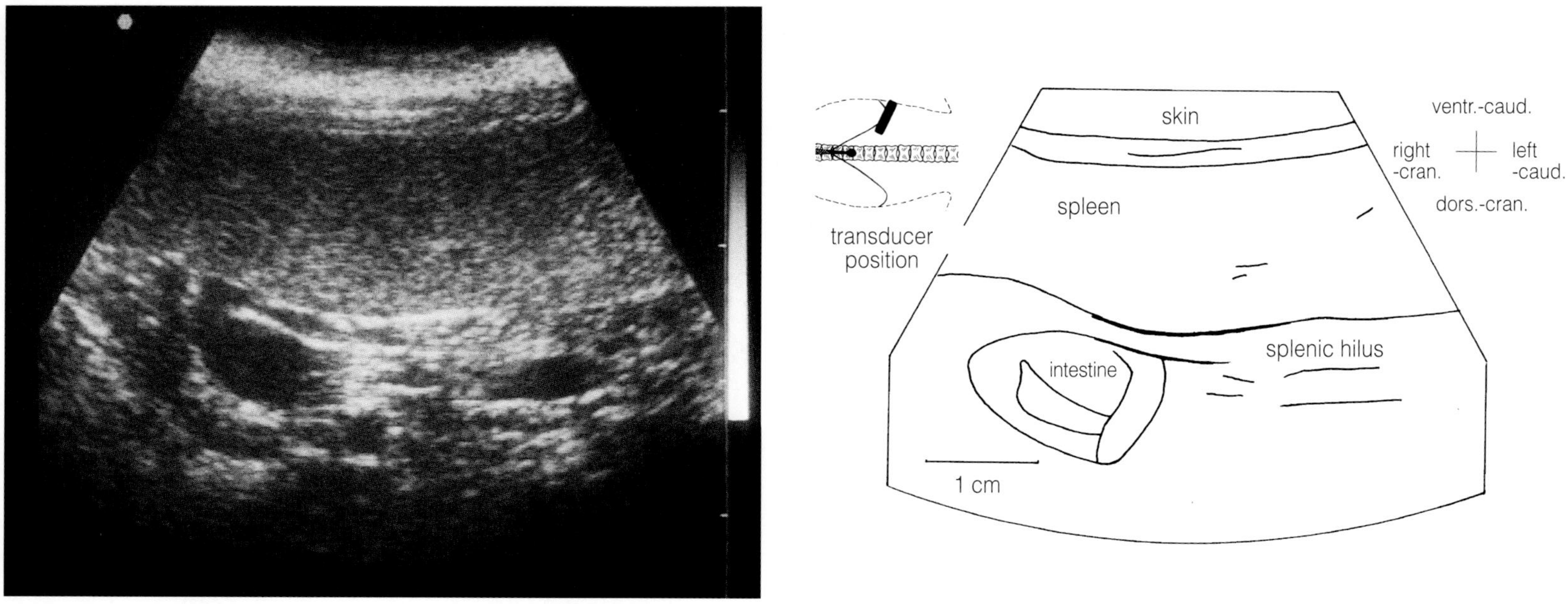

92

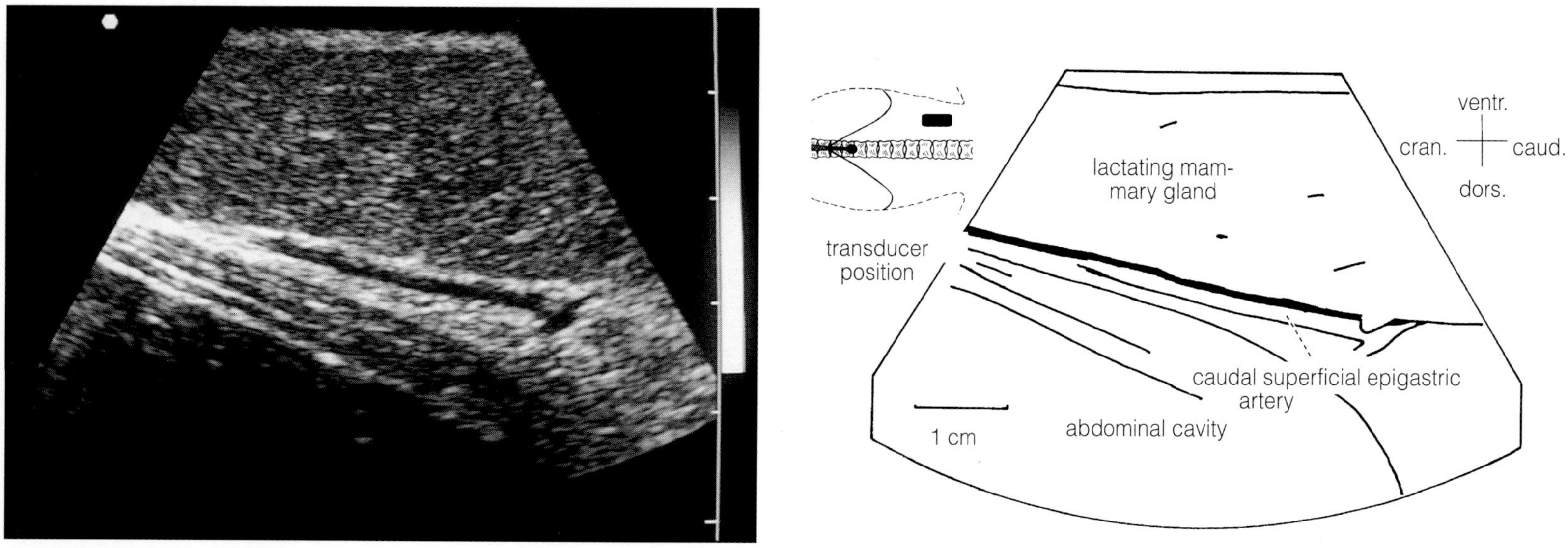

91, 92 Ultrasonographic images of the spleen (**91**) and the lactating mammary gland (**92**) of a dog. The displayed organs may be mistaken for each other, although they have typical sonographic structures.

Frozen Image Documentation

Images should be documented for patient charts and for owners. The simplest and least expensive image documentation method with adequate quality is a video printer (93).

Multiformat cameras or polaroid cameras (95) offer good quality reproductions. These methods are more expensive and the images, usually slides (96), are not immediately available. Another method is to photograph the image from the screen with a camera on a tripod in a darkened room (94).

> Images should initially be recorded on video and additionally reproduced using a video printer and/or camera (97). The system of choice depends on quality and cost expectations of the sonographer.

Acoustic Coupling Gel

Ultrasound examinations require a stable surface and good transducer–skin contact. Air trapped between the transducer and the body surface prevents ultrasonographic imaging or causes artefacts (see Reverberation and Mirror-Image Artefacts, page 70; **135**). Good skin contact is achieved by using an ultrasonographic coupling medium, otherwise called acoustic gel or coupling gel. This acoustic coupling gel should be applied liberally when examining animals, since contact is more difficult to achieve with the skin of dogs and cats than of humans (see Patient Preparation, page 77). Besides commercially available gels (e.g. Sonogel® – distributed in Germany by Fa. Anne Wiebke Linde, Bad Camberg; or Aquasonic® Parker Laboratories Inc., Orange, New York), useful coupling gels can be produced in every pharmacy using the following prescription[6] (98):

Ingredient	Parts	
Glycerol 85%	1,500.0	
Distilled water	8,360.0	
Euxyl K 100	10.0	(preservative)
Carbopol 940	40.0	
Sodium hydroxide solution 15%	90.0	

[Euxyl K 100®, Fa. Schuelke & Mayr, Hamburg, distributed by Fa. Synopharm, 22885 Barsbuettel-Hamburg; Carbopol 940®, distributed by Fa. Synopharm, 22885 Barsbuettel-Hamburg]

93

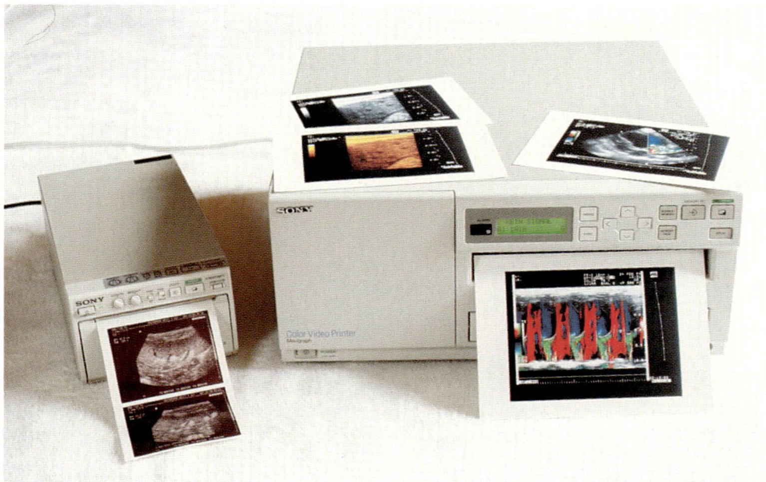

94

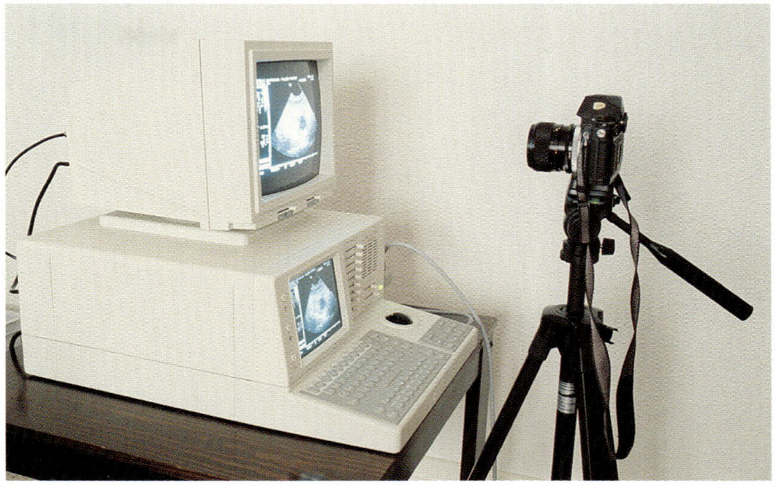

95

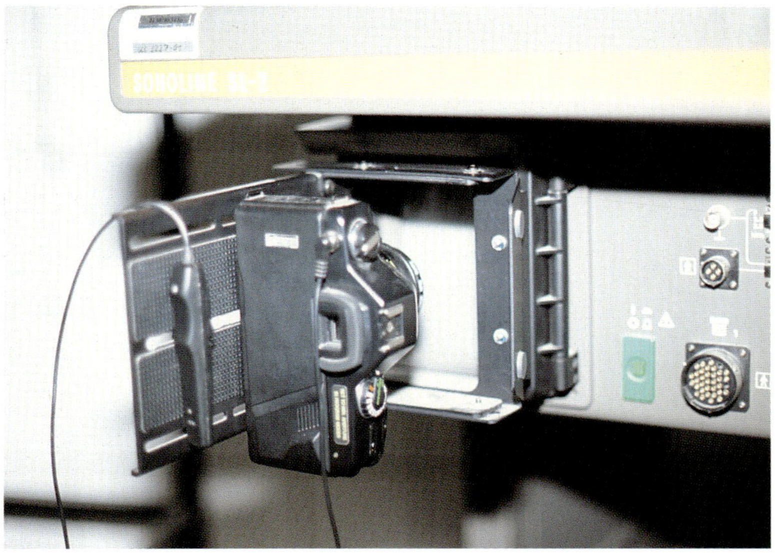

96

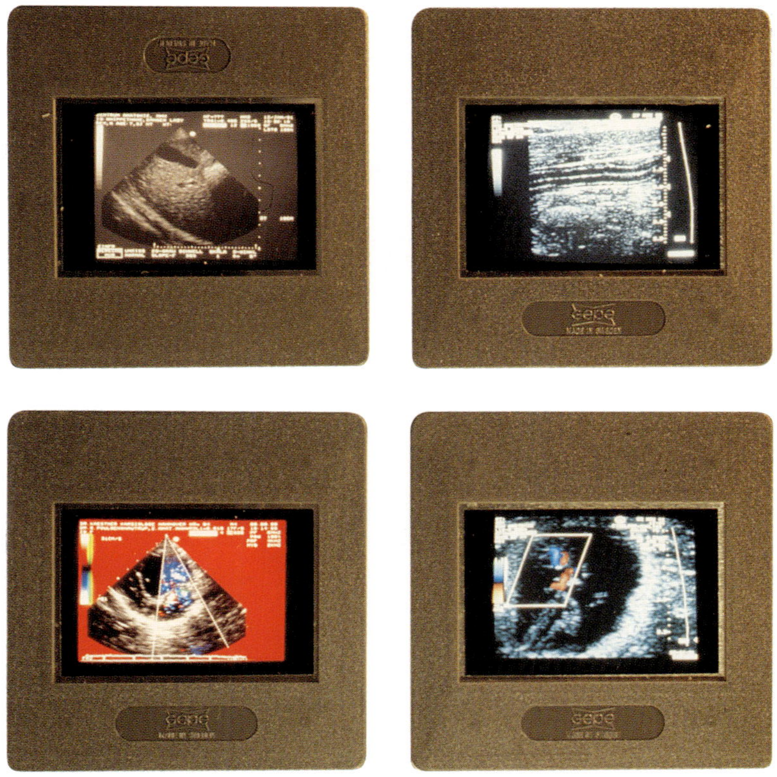

93–96 Various documentation systems for frozen images. Commercial black-and-white and colour video printer with prints (**93**); camera set up in front of the main monitor (**94**); polaroid camera installed on an additional monitor (**95**); slides (**96**).

97

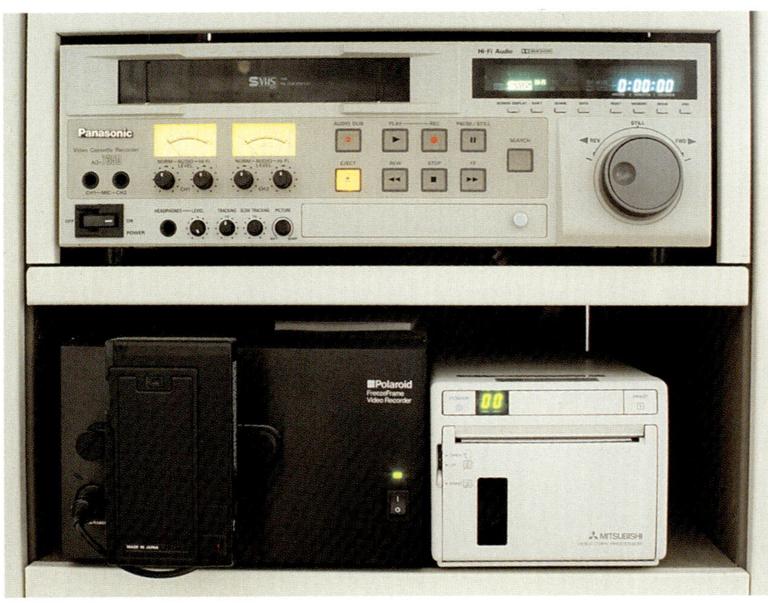

97 Ideal documentation system with a video recorder (top), polaroid camera (bottom left) and video printer (bottom right).

98

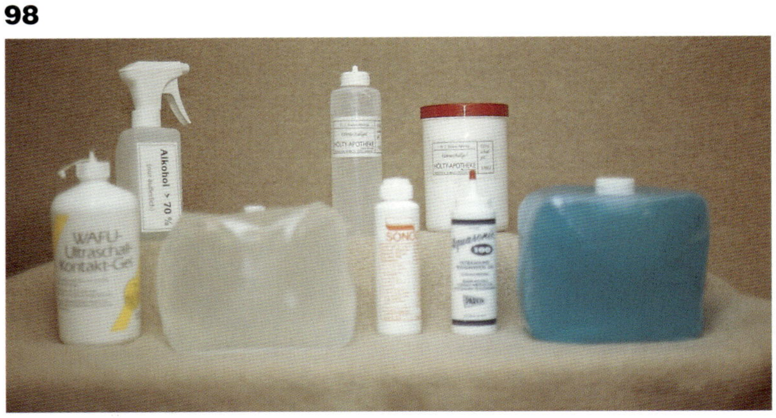

98 High-percentage alcohol (back left), self-made acoustic gel (back middle and right) and various commercial gels (front).

99

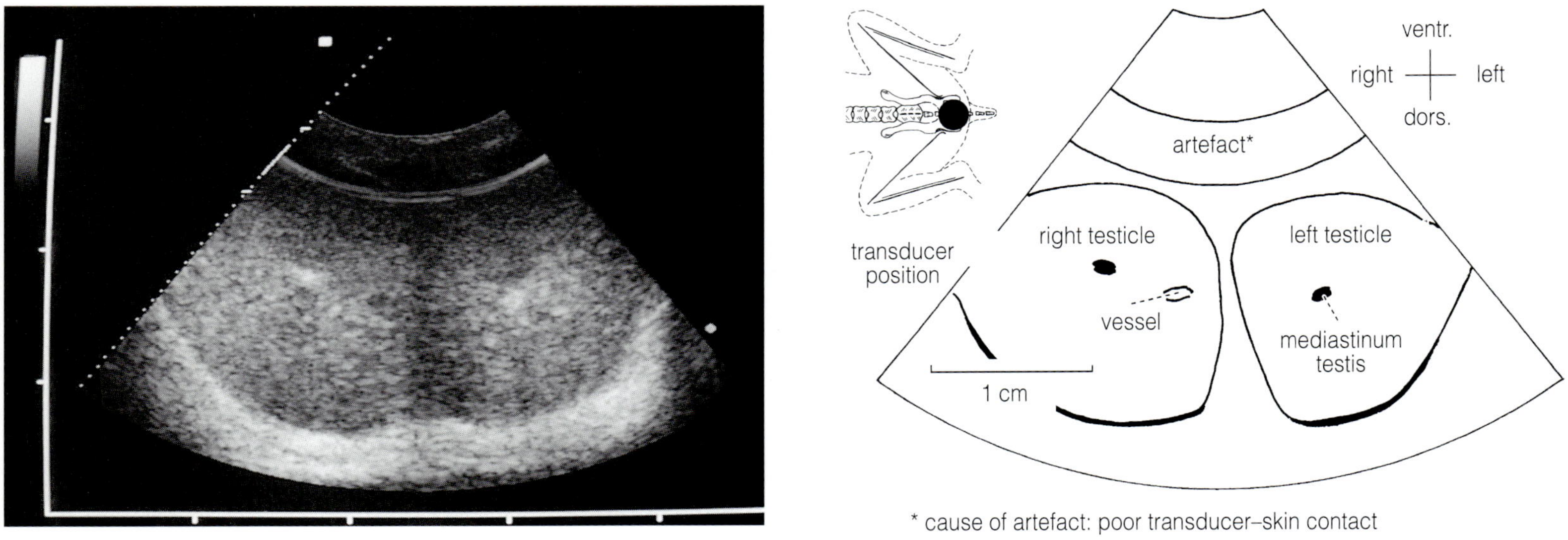

100

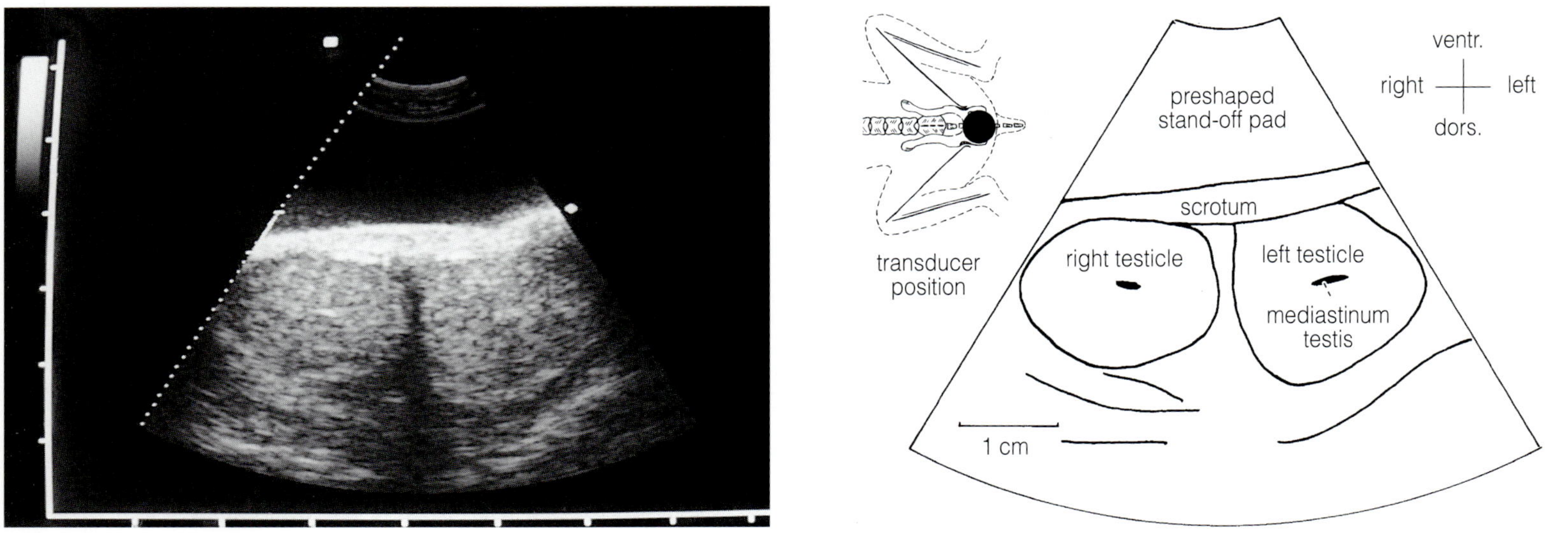

99–102 Transverse (**99, 100**) and longitudinal (**101, 102**) views of the testes of a male dog. Without stand-off pad (**99**); with preshaped stand-off pad (**100**); with built-in stand-off pad (**101**, opposite); with second testicle as a 'natural' stand-off pad (**102**, opposite).

Some contact gels may spoil when stored for too long. Large supplies should be stored in a cool, dark place. Daily or weekly requirements can be kept at room temperature.

Although most dogs and cats try to lick off the gel during or after the examination, the author has not encountered any digestive problems with examined adult animals during the last eight years. In one case, kittens ingesting acoustic gel from the mammary glands of their mother developed a mild diarrhoea. Generally, all gel residue should be wiped or washed off the animal following an examination. The transducers should be cleaned after use, since dried gel may damage the probe surface.

103

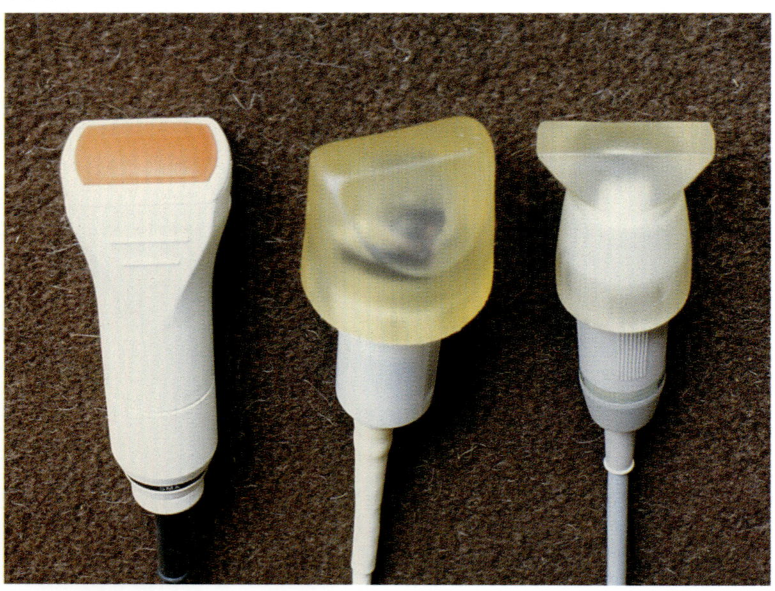

103 Built-in (left) and preshaped (middle, right) stand-off pads.

Commercial acoustic gels are available in large quantity containers (0.85 litre, 5 litres and 10 litres) and in smaller bottles of 0.25 litre. Sterile gel packages are commercially available for intraoperative use.

Stand-Off Pads

Stand-off pads lengthen the distance between the transducer and skin as well as other superficial structures (99–102). At the same time, these stand-off pads adjust to uneven contours and surfaces such as the neck, groin or mammary glands.

Sector transducers have poor resolution in the near field. Low frequency linear transducers with a deeper focal zone also show poor detail in the near field.

'Homemade' stand-off pads are not recommended. They usually consist of a thin plastic bag, such as a condom, containing boiled water to remove air bubbles. Small air bubbles in the water distort the image distal to the stand-off device. The user may also find it difficult to hold the fluid-filled device with one hand while

101

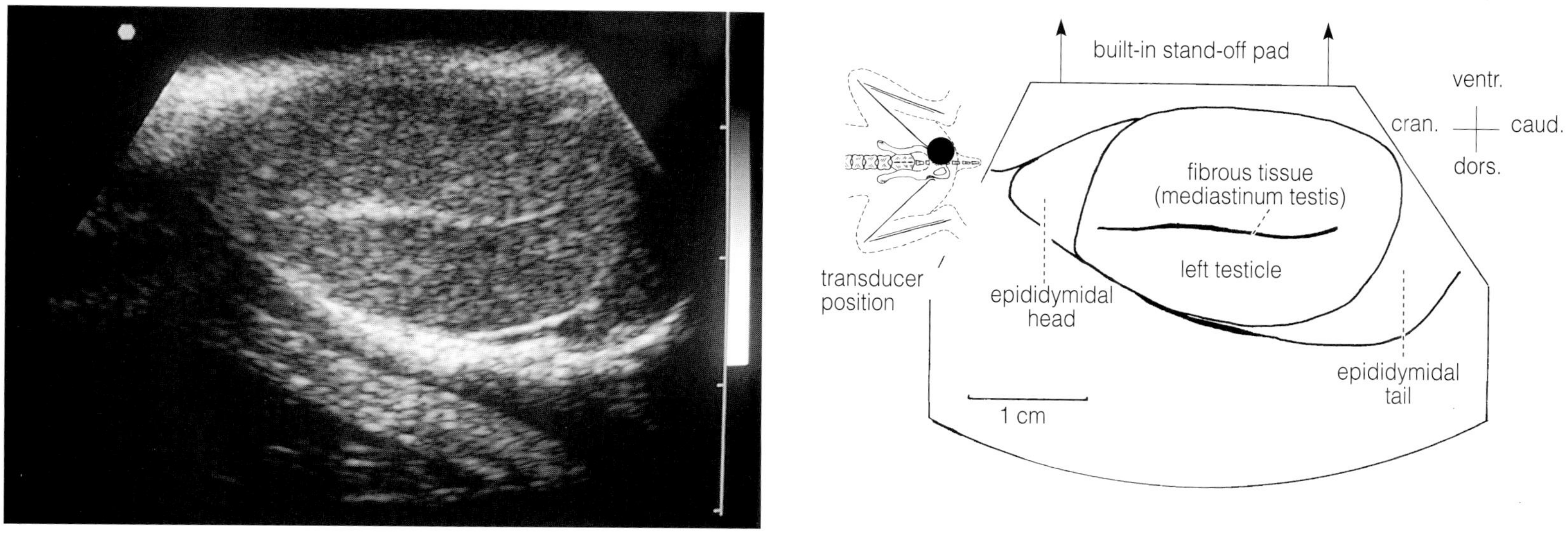

102

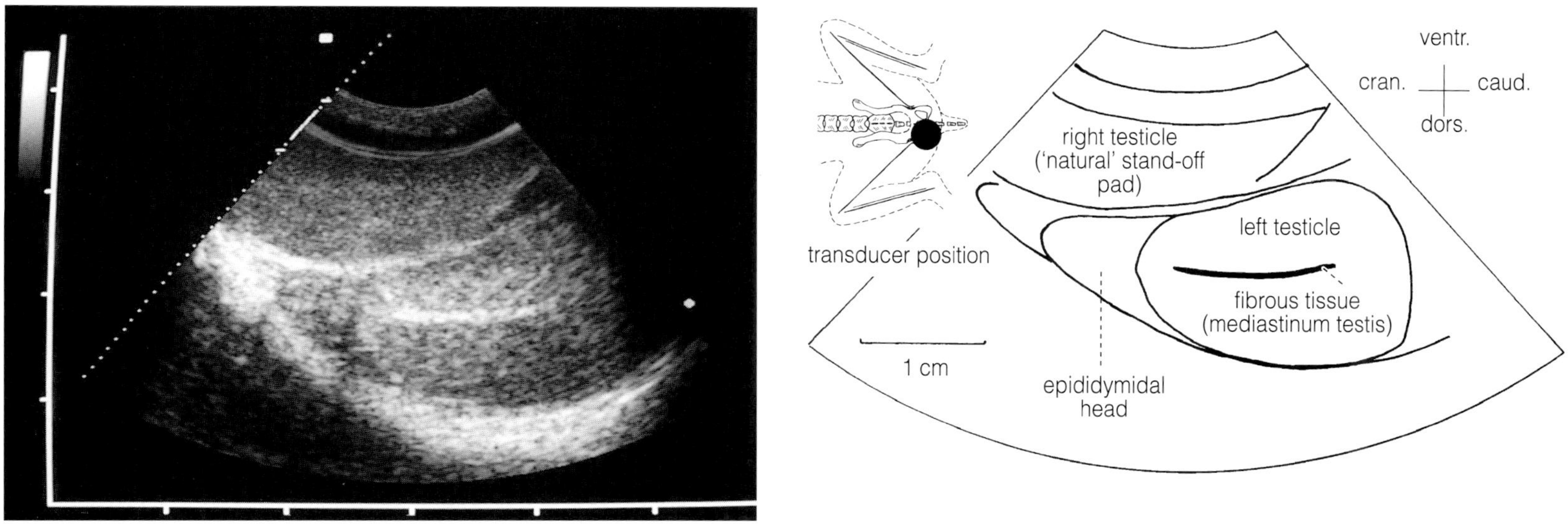

guiding the transducer with the other hand, and at the same time adjusting the power controls and maybe even holding the animal.

Commercially available synthethic stand-off pads (Somnokit®) are composed of softened polyvinyl chloride. Their gel-like substance comes in various shapes and sizes. Apart from pads, preshaped stand-off devices for sector, curved-array and linear transducers are available (**103**). The size of the stand-offs must be compatible with the transducers to allow for good contact between the probe and the pad. The width of the stand-off pad depends on the transducer frequency. Lower frequencies need a wider stand-off pad than higher frequencies.

Sterile, single use stand-off devices are available for intraoperative use. High frequency 10 or 15 MHz sector transducers often have a built-in stand-off device.

The main disadvantage of all stand-off pads is the varying acoustic impedance between the stand-off (relatively low impedance of 1.52×10^6 to 1.56×10^6 [Ns/m^3]) and the skin (relatively high impedance of 2.15×10^6 [Ns/m^3]). This may lead to sound reflections at the interface and may cause reverberation artefacts (**104**) (see Reverberation and Mirror-Image Artefacts, page 70).

104

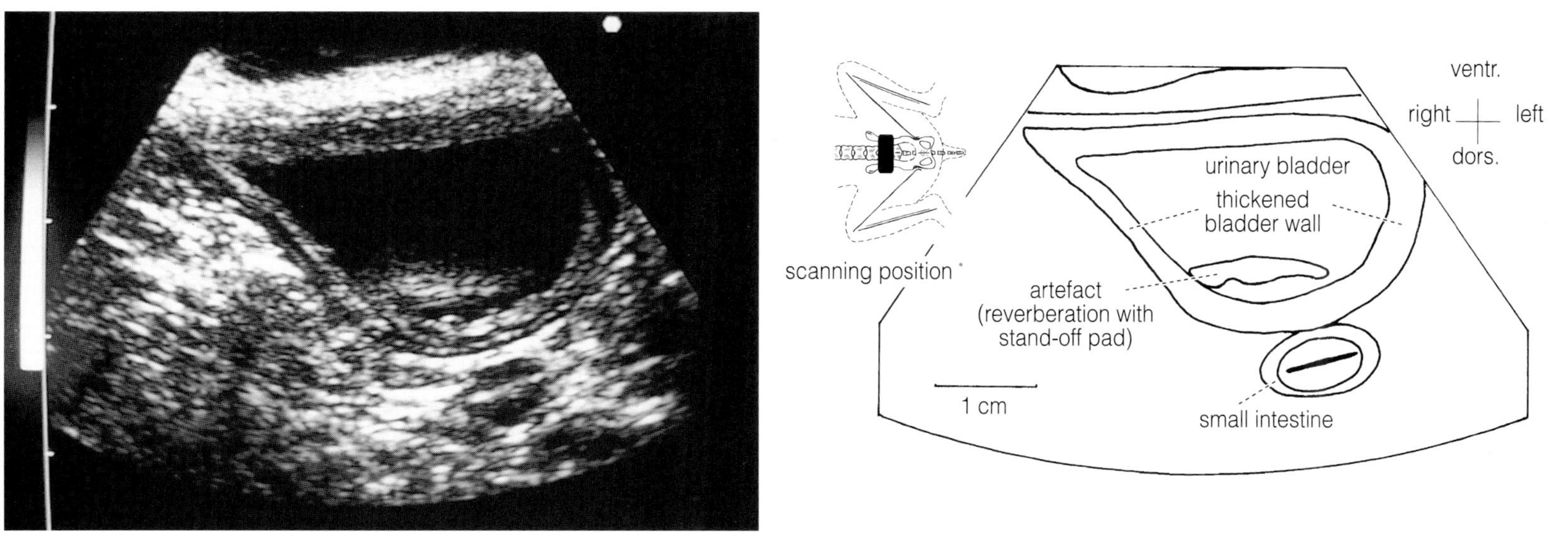

104 Typical artefact (reverberation) in the urinary bladder of a dog when using a built-in stand-off pad.

Contrast Agents

Contrast agents can be used to display certain cavities not detected sonographically (e.g. salpinx) or to display blood flow without Doppler. These agents contain gaseous substances, distributed as microbubbles[4]. Strong ultrasonographic reflections appear at the interfaces between blood and bubbles, due to the different impedances of blood or fluids and gas or air. These interactions make blood flow visible in the two-dimensional sonogram.

'Homemade' contrast mediums utilize bubbles entrapped in an agitated liquid, such as a sterile saline solution, patient blood or carbon dioxide. In Germany, commercial ultrasonographic contrast mediums (used mainly in human medicine) are available (105).

In echocardiography the contrast agents displayed in 105 are injected intravenously and are visible in the veins from the injection site to the right atrium, right heart chamber and pulmonary arteries. The microbubbles are then distributed, diluted and

105

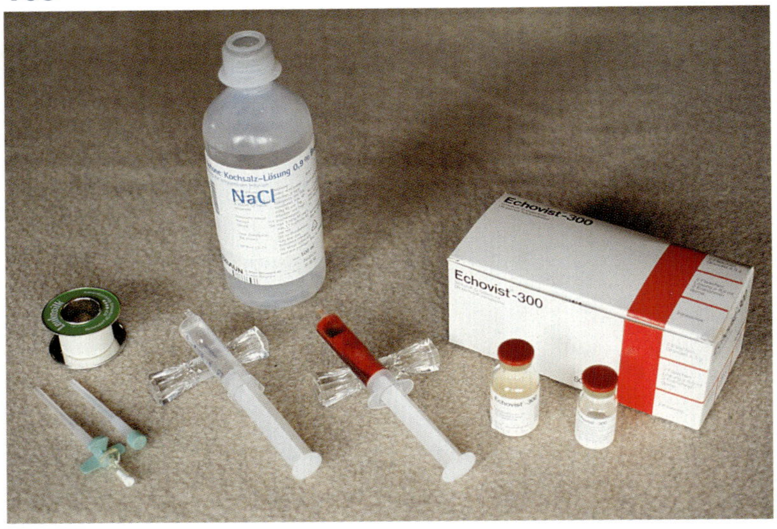

105 Agitated saline solution (left) and patient blood (middle) as well as a commercial contrast agent (right [Echovist®-300, Fa. Schering, Berlin]) for ultrasonography.

106

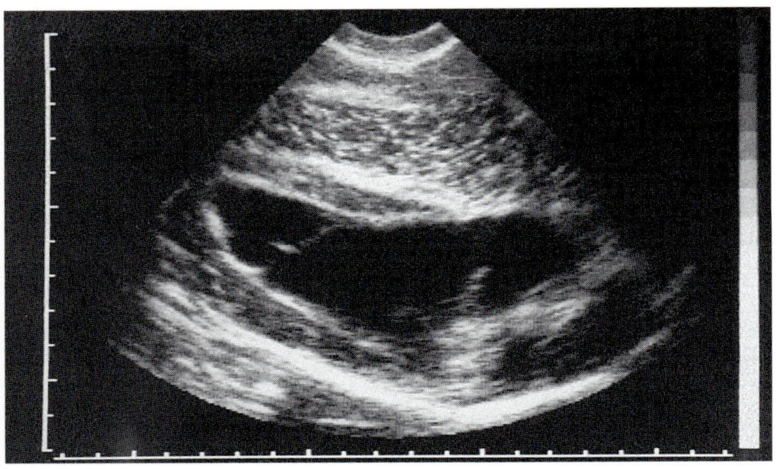

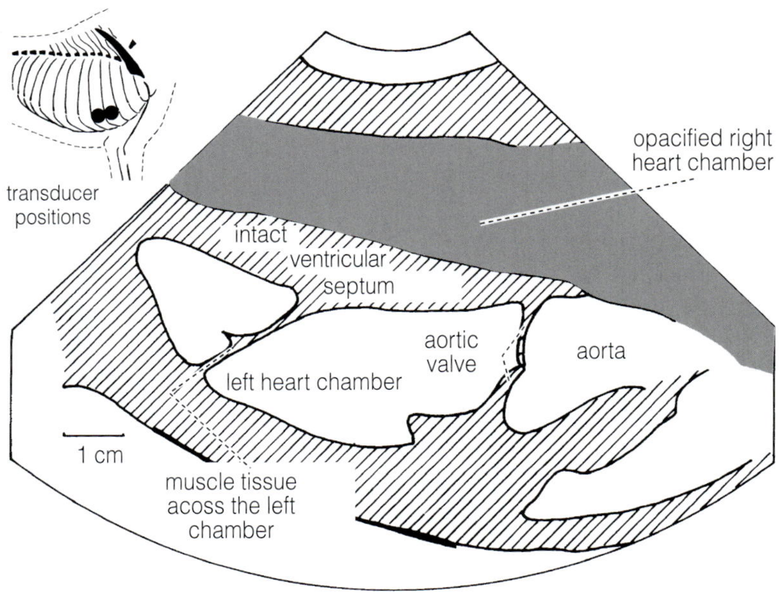

107

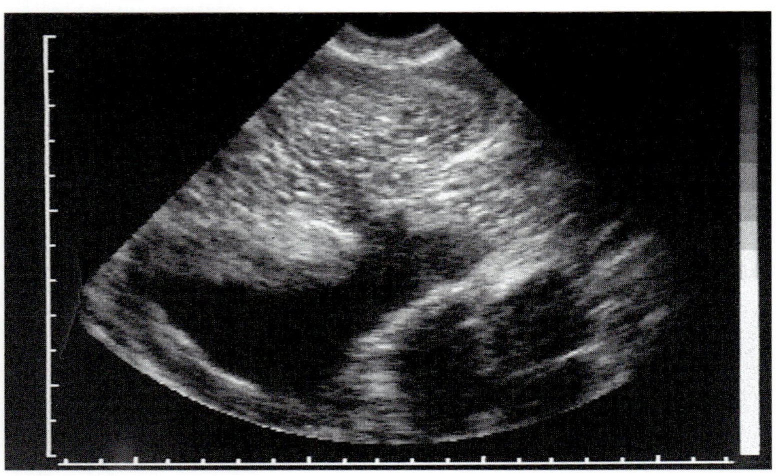

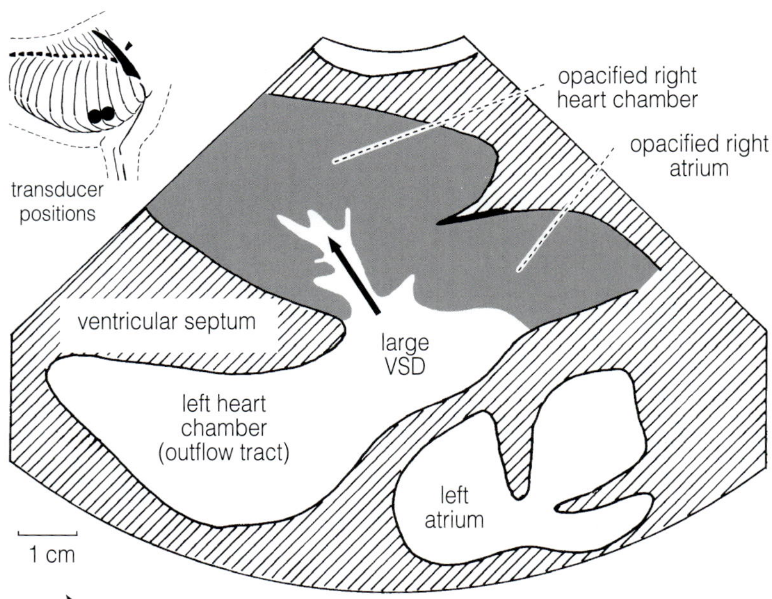

↖: negative contrast effect with a left-to-right shunt
VSD: ventricular septal defect

106, 107 Parasternal long-axis view of a normal heart (**106**) and a heart with a ventricular septal defect (**107**) after contrast application in the jugular vein. A negative contrast effect (**107** – arrow) in the opacified right heart chamber identifies the ventricular septal defect (VSD), which would not have been recognized in a two-dimensional sonogram.

removed within the pulmonary capillaries. This prevents imaging of the pulmonary veins, left atrium, left heart chamber and arteries. Contrast studies are helpful in detecting congenital heart diseases such as atrial and ventricular septal defects[1] (**106, 107**). They are also useful to determine tricuspid and pulmonary insufficiencies.

Since late 1995, a contrast medium (Levovist®, Fa. Schering, Berlin) has become available which passes through the pulmonary circulation. It can also be seen in the left atrium, left ventricle, aorta and other arteries.

References

1 Bonagura JD and Pipers FS (1983) Diagnosis of cardiac lesions by contrast echocardiography. *J. Am. Vet. Med. Assoc.* **4**, 396–402.

2 Bubenheimer P and Kneisel GD (1989) *Dopplerechokardiographie*. Verlag Edition Medizin, Weinheim.

3 Fehske W (1988) *Praxis der Konventionellen und Farbkodierten Doppler-Echokardiographie*. Verlag Hans Huber, Bern, Stuttgart, Toronto.

4 Fritzsch T, Mützel W and Lange L (1985) Aktueller Stand der Entwicklung von Kontrastmitteln für die Echokardiographie. In: Erbel R, Meyer J and Brennecke R (Eds.) *Fortschritte der Echokardiographie*. Springer Verlag, Berlin, Heidelberg, pp. 117–125.

5 Hatle L and Angelsen B (1985) *Doppler Ultrasound in Cardiology: Physical Principles and Clinical Applications*. 2nd Edn. Lea & Febiger, Philadelphia.

6 Johannigmann J, Ried A and Detter A (1984) Ein verbessertes Ultraschallgel. *Gynäkol. Praxis* **8**, 413–414.

7 Kaarmann H and Wessels G (1991) II–1 Physikalische Grandlagen. 10. Ergänzungslieferung. In: Braun B, Günther R and Schwerk W (Eds.) *Ultraschalldiagnostik. Lehrbuch und Atlas. Vol I*. Verlag Ecomed. Landsberg, München, Zürich.

8 Kruck I and Biamino G (1988) *Quantitative Methoden der M-Mode-, 2D- and Doppler-Echokardiographie*. Boehringer Mannheim GmbH, Galenus Mannheim GmbH, Mannheim.

9 Laubenberger (1990) *Technik der medizinischen Radiologie*. 5th Edn. Deutscher Ärzte Verlag, Köln

4 Sonographic Phenomenons and Artefacts

Cordula Poulsen Nautrup

Sonographic Imaging of Tissue

The two-dimensional sonogram is a cross-sectional image (**108–111, 115**), displaying large acoustic interfaces in their actual size and smaller structures with a diverging design (see Interaction of Ultrasound Beams with Tissues, page 21; Scattering, Absorption and Divergence, page 22). Sonographic tissue images are different than radiographs (shadow or sumation image [**113, 114**]) and computed tomograms (digital radiographic cross-sections [**112**]). Conventional radiographs and computed tomographs show different structures depending on the amount of x-rays absorbed, while sonography uses the reflection off tissue interfaces to produce an image[7, 8]. Because of these imaging differences, radiological terms such as opaque, hyperdense, hypodense and isodense, opacity and translucence should not be used to describe ultrasonographic images.

Sonographic images are produced by echoes or reflections.

Table 7 Synonyms for echo-free, echo-poor and echo-rich. (*The author's preferred terms are printed in italics.* Terms such as cystic or cystoid for echo-free and solid for echo-rich should be avoided because of overinterpretation.)

Echo-free	Echo-poor	Echo-rich
reflex-free	*reflex-poor*	*reflex-rich*
		echogenic
		reflexogenic
	low echo intensity	high echo intensity
		highly reflective
	poorly echodense	*echodense*
	low echodensity	*high echodensity*
anechogenic	*poorly echogenic*	*highly echogenic*
anechoic	*hypoechoic*	*hyperechoic*
sonolucent		
translucent		
transonic		sonodense
		white

108

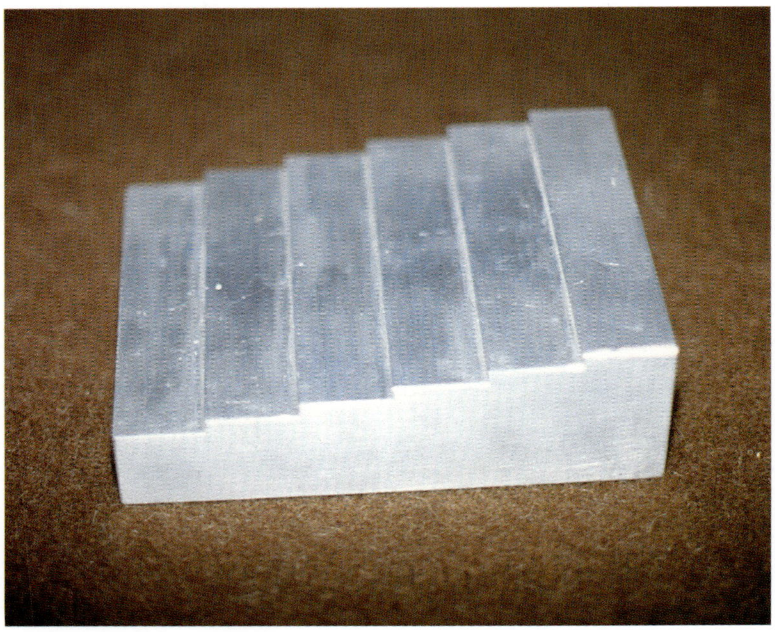

109

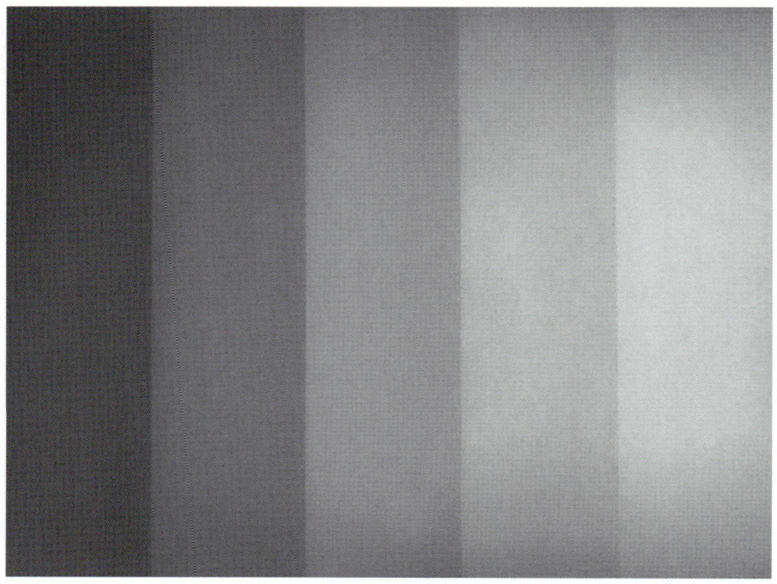

110

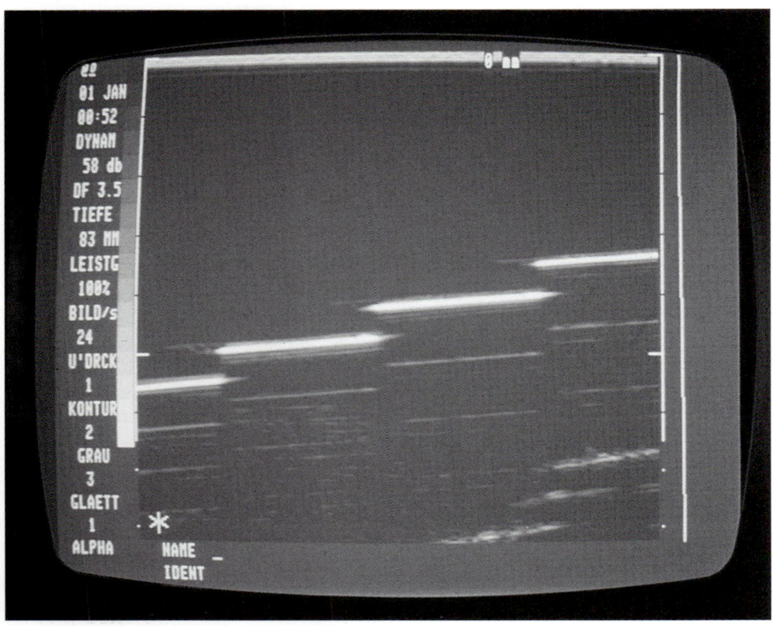

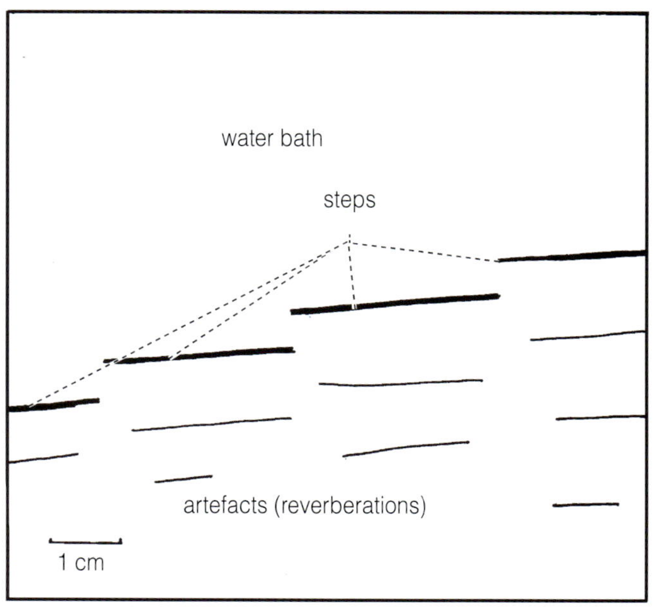

Echogenicity is the ability of each tissue or interface to reflect and scatter ultrasound waves and to produce an image on the screen. The sonographic images of tissues are evaluated for texture, surface, margins, size and topographic location.

In sonography each tissue structure can be well demarcated or not defined and can have a rough or smooth surface. The length, width or area of a structure can be measured. These measurements are available in all ultrasound units. Movement of structures, organs or a fetus should be monitored by the real-time examination. This motion is usually caused by breathing or movement of the organ itself. The topographical location should always be evaluated. This is done by imaging adjacent structures.

> Echogenicity, echo determined size and echo intensity, as well as echo distribution, characterize sonographic textures, surfaces and margins.

Echo Intensity, Echo Size, Echo Density

The three echo parameters, intensity, size and density, describe the appearance of ultrasound images and differentiate between anechoic (echo-free), hypoechoic (echo-poor) and hyperechoic (echogenic, echo-rich) areas. Tissue quality is often described differently. Commonly used terms are listed in *Table 7*.

111

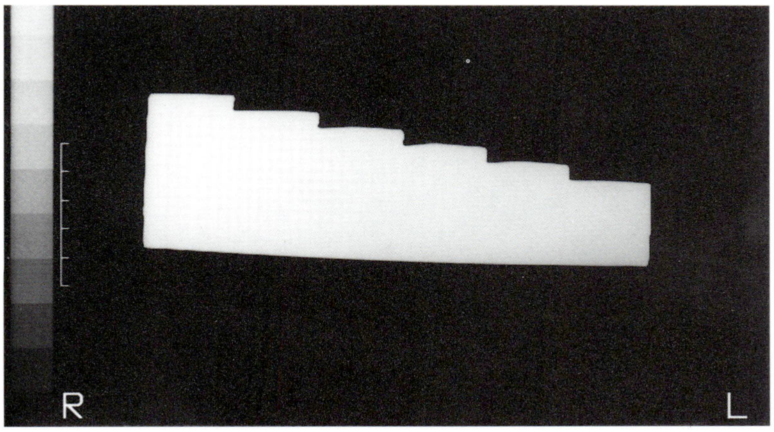

112

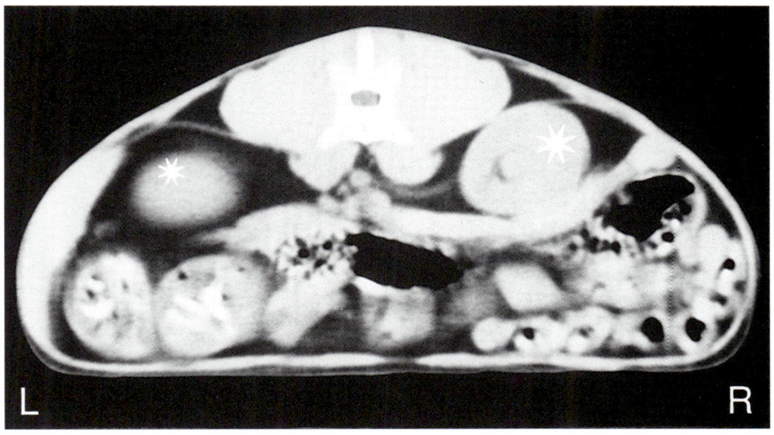

113

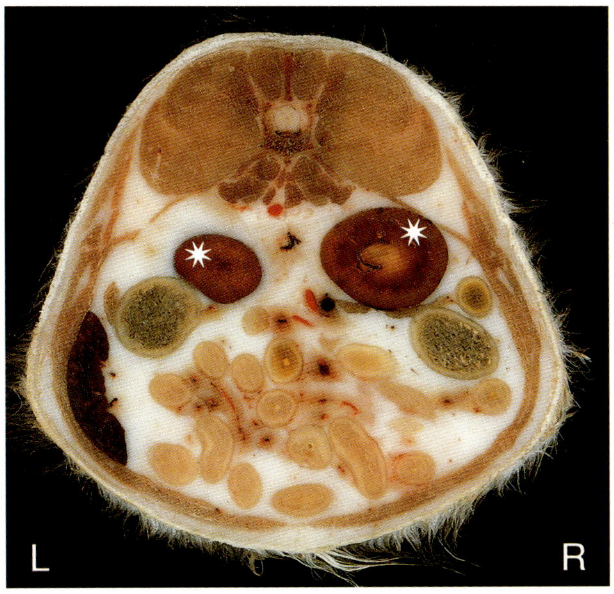

114

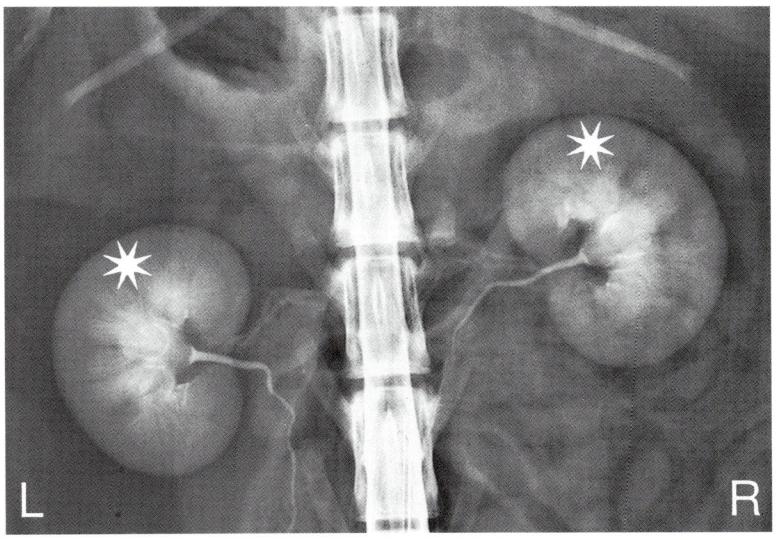

115

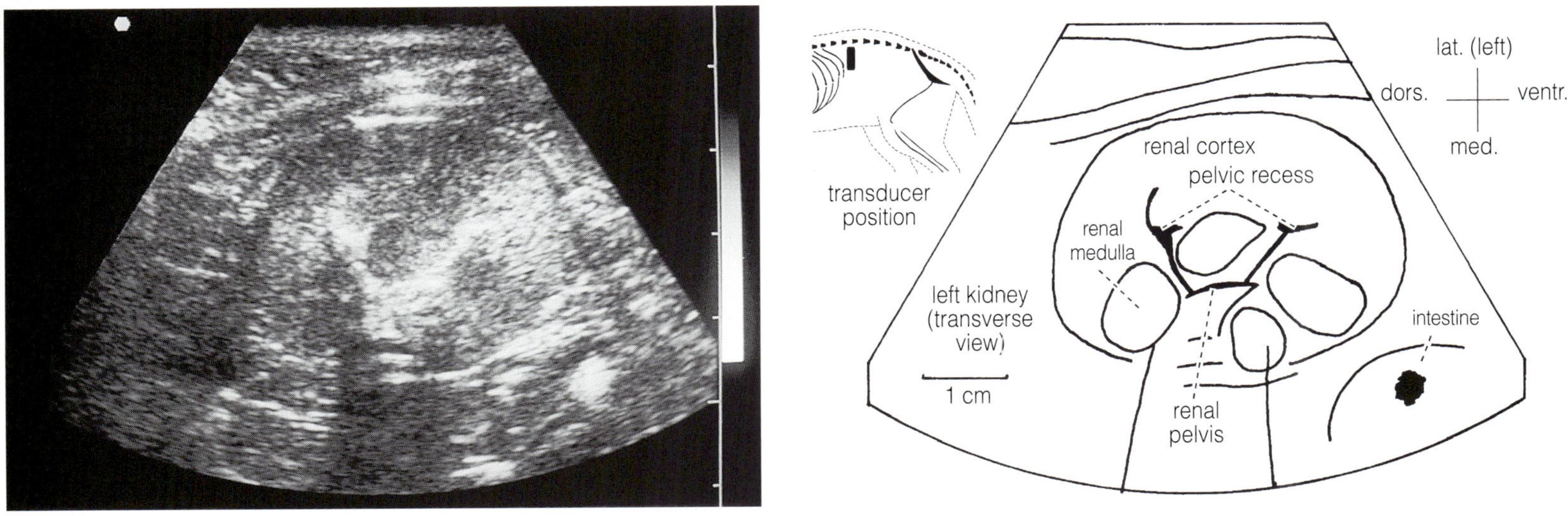

108–115 Comparative display of various imaging methods using aluminum stairs (**108–111**) and feline kidneys (**112** – star; **113** – star; **114** – star). Photographs (**108, 113**), radiographs (**109, 114**), two-dimensional ultrasonography (**110, 115**) and computed tomography (**111, 112**).

116

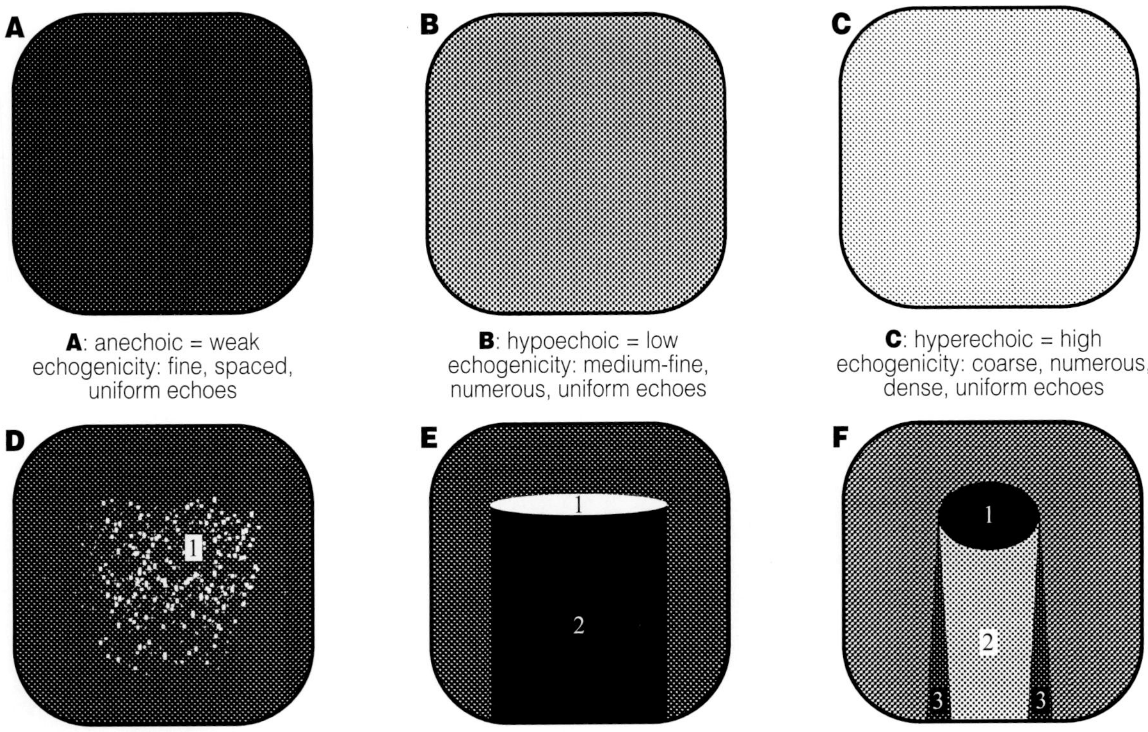

A: anechoic = weak echogenicity: fine, spaced, uniform echoes

B: hypoechoic = low echogenicity: medium-fine, numerous, uniform echoes

C: hyperechoic = high echogenicity: coarse, numerous, dense, uniform echoes

D: non-uniform, distributed, echogenic echoes in an echo-poor area

E: echogenic area (1) with complete acoustic shadowing (2) through total reflection

F: anechoic area (1) with acoustic enhancement (2) and edge-shadowing (3)

116 Schematic drawings of echo intensity, size, density and distribution (**A, B, C, D**) as well as a hyperechoic (**E**) and an anechoic (**F**) area with distal shadowing (**E**) and enhancement (**F**).

Echo-free

Tissues without acoustic interfaces, such as fluids, bile (**117**), urine, blood, ingesta and amniotic fluid, are echo-free. They are displayed as black areas on the screen and paper (**116F**). Pathological fluid accumulations, such as ascites, pleural effusion, pericardial effusion, hydro-, haemo- or pyometra, abscesses, haematomas or cysts, may also have an anechoic appearance.

> An area without echoes is anechoic. Registered echoes may have a fine or coarse texture (referring to dot size), low or high intensity, and low or high homogeneity[2] (**116A–F**).

Low Echogenicity

Structures low in echogenicity are displayed as fine, dispersed, weak or medium to dark grey echoes (**116A**). The renal medulla (**118**), intestinal musculature and some striated muscles are normally echo-poor. Tumours (hepatomas: see **50, 51**) may be hypoechoic. Hypoechoic parenchymal texture may be found with acute liver congestion or oedematous pancreatitis.

Medium Echogenicity

A number of parenchymal organs, such as liver (**117**), spleen, pancreas, salivary glands, thyroid gland, adrenals, renal cortex

117

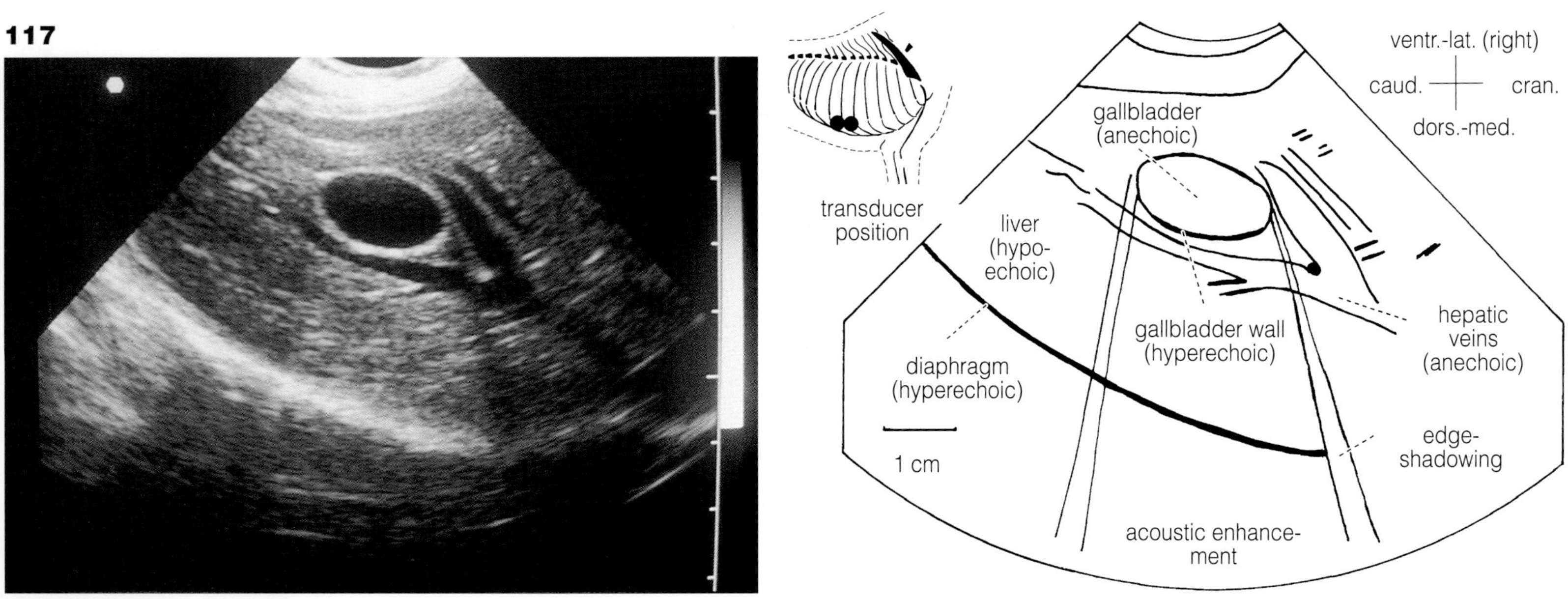

117 Ultrasound image of a canine liver with liver parenchyma (texture with low to medium echogenicity), gallbladder, vessel (anechoic structures), vessel wall and diaphragm (echogenic structures).

118

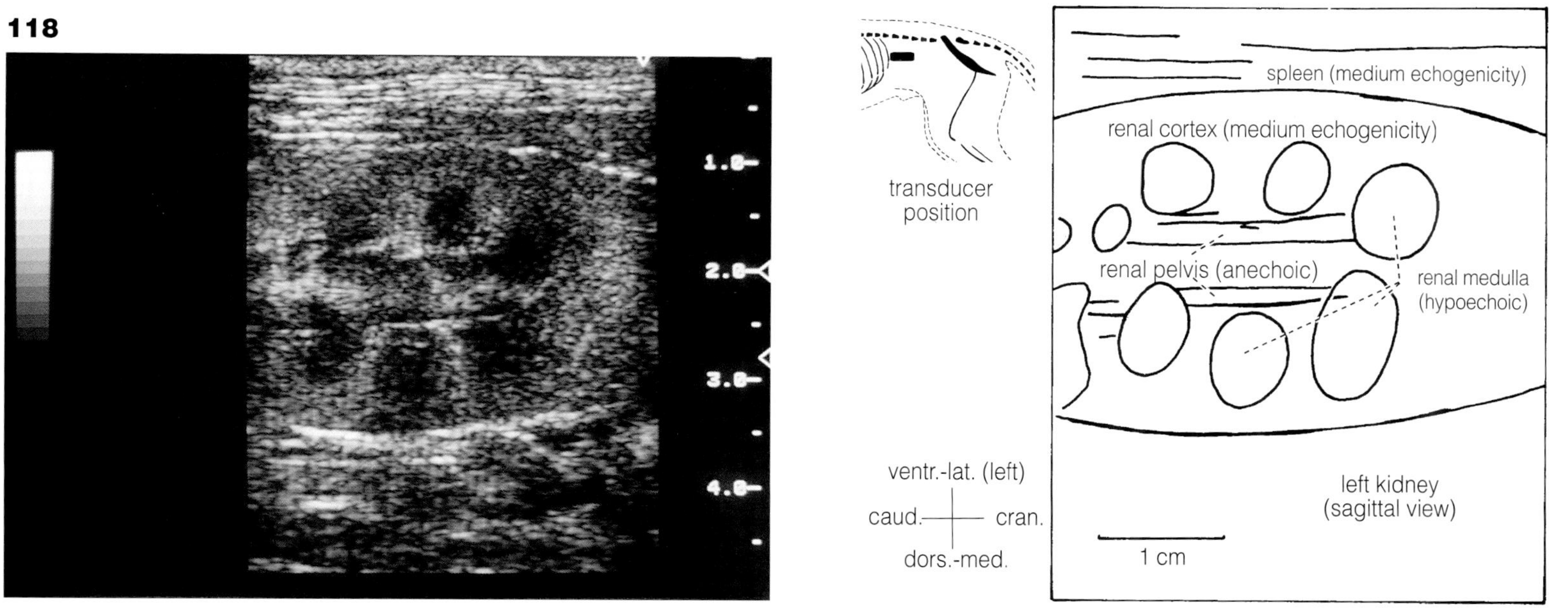

118 Ultrasound image of a canine kidney (sagittal view) with renal cortex (medium echogenicity) and renal medulla (low echogenicity).

119

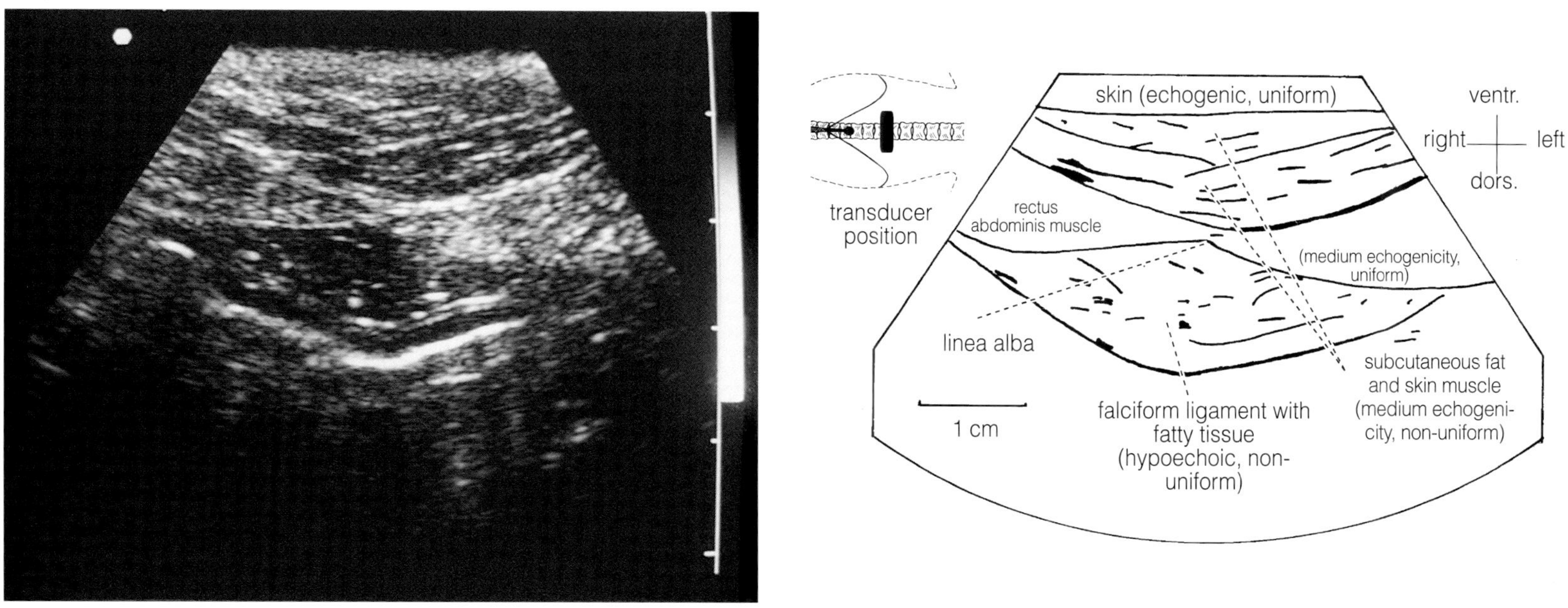

119 Ultrasound image of the ventral abdominal wall in the area of the linea alba. The muscles and fatty tissue show a non-uniform texture with low, medium and high echogenicity.

(**118**), testis and prostate, normally show medium echogenicity. Images of these tissues consist of numerous, uniform, fine to medium-fine, high to medium-intense, or light to medium-grey echoes with medium density (**116B**).

High Echogenicity

Tissue interfaces with markedly differing acoustic impedances cause high intensity reflections, seen as white or light grey images on the screen or paper (**116C**). These structures are termed hyperechoic (*Table 7*). Arterial walls (**117**), fibrous organ margins, interstitial fibrous tissue, the diaphragm (**117**) and pericardium are usually echogenic. Interfaces with calcifications, bony tissue or gas and air-filled organs, e.g. trachea, oesophagus, stomach and intestine, are also hyperechoic. Total reflection at these interfaces causes distal acoustic shadowing (see Acoustic Shadowing and Enhancement, page 70).

Textures with numerous large acoustic interfaces are uniformly echogenic. These tissues appear as homogenous, coarse to fine, high to medium-intense echoes, or as white to medium-grey echoes with a high density on the screen. They include, for example, the normal lactating mammary gland or a pathological fatty degeneration of the liver as well as a number of tumours.

Echo Density or Homogeneity

> Echo distribution may be uniform (homogenous) or non-uniform (non-homogenous) (**116A–F**).

Normal parenchymal organs, such as the liver, spleen, pancreas, salivary glands, thyroid glands, prostate or testis, have uniform echoes consisting of multiple echoes with medium echogenicity. Striated muscles and fatty tissue normally have a non-uniform echo texture (**119**). Pathological lesions with a non-homogenous echo distribution and structural defects include metastases, tumours (**120**) and liver cirrhosis, as well as various types of pancreatitis.

120

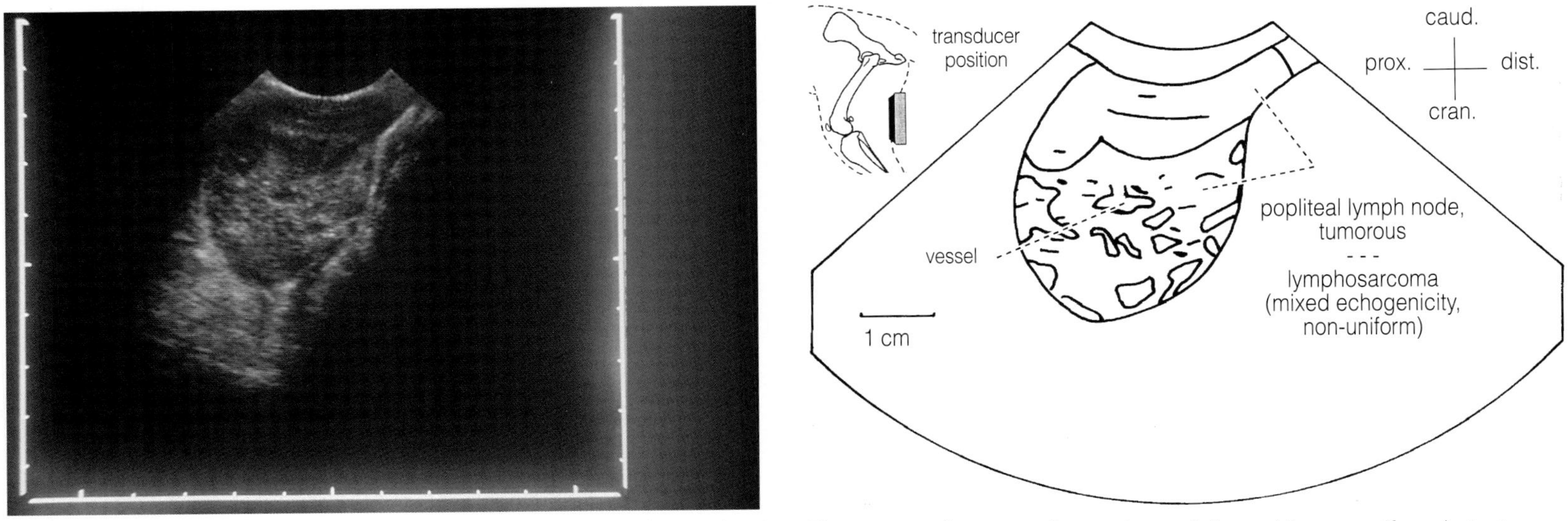

120 Ultrasound image of a lymphosarcoma in the popliteal fossa of a dog. The tumour shows medium echogenicity and is non-uniform in texture.

Dopplersonographic Rheology

Dopplersonographic blood flow follows the physical principles of basic rheology (Greek *rhein* = to flow; rheology = flow principles, field of mechanics).

Flow Profiles

Blood flows at a constant velocity, showing a laminar parabolic flow profile with the lowest velocity near the vessel wall and the highest in the centre of the vessel[5] (**121A, 122**).

When blood accelerates or the vessel diameter is enlarged, a flat flow profile is obtained. The velocities are nearly uniform over the vessel diameter, except for a narrow area near the wall (**121B, 123**).

Blood flow in the cardiovascular system is slightly more complicated due to pulsations of the beating heart, elastic vessel walls, vessel branching and pressure drop in the arterioles and capillaries[3, 4].

> Flow profiles are variable. The highest velocity of cells is always found in the centre of the vessel (**122–124**).

In pulsed Doppler sonography the sample volume should always be placed in the centre of a three-dimensional vessel to measure maximum blood flow velocities (**124**). For frequency spectrum tracings (see Doppler Frequency Spectrum, page 28) of all flow velocities, the gate should cover the entire vessel diameter (**125**).

Laminar and Turbulent Flows

In laminar flows the fluid layers with different velocities move ahead without producing whirlpools. Non-laminar flows are turbulences that disrupt centre flow.

Laminar flow may become non-laminar, when wall lesions (i.e. plaques), higher flow velocities or smaller vessel diameters cause turbulences.

The spectral display of laminar blood flow is above and below the baseline in conventional CW and PW Doppler, and red and blue in colour Doppler (see Doppler Effect, page 24; Colour-Flow Doppler, page 48).

In conventional Doppler modes, turbulent blood flows are displayed as non-uniform velocity tracings above and below the baseline. When velocities are too high, PW Doppler tracings of turbulences may be confused with aliasing (see Aliasing and

121

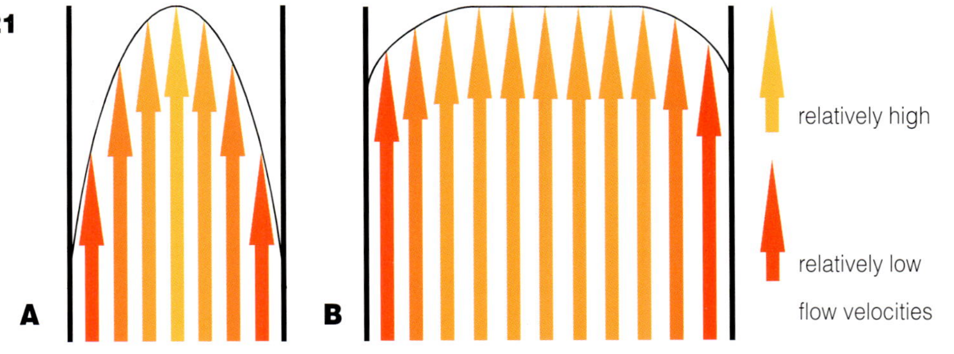

122

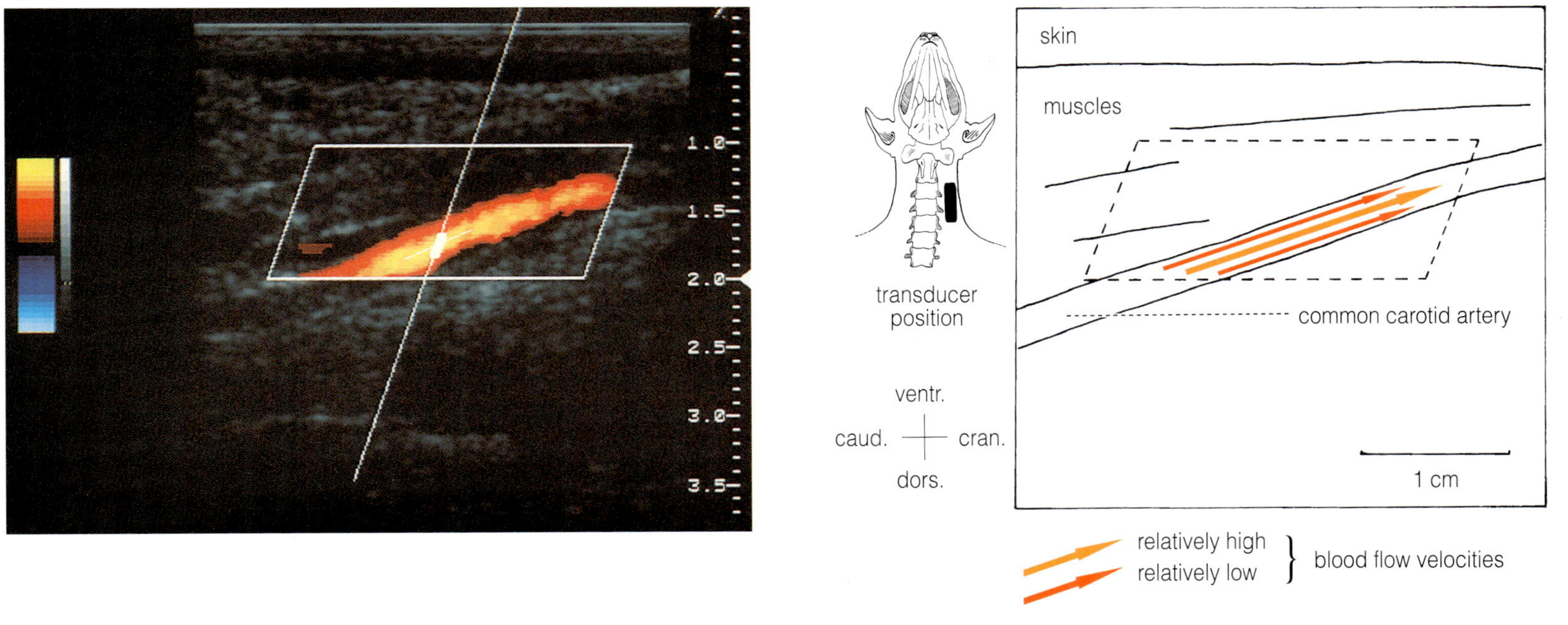

123

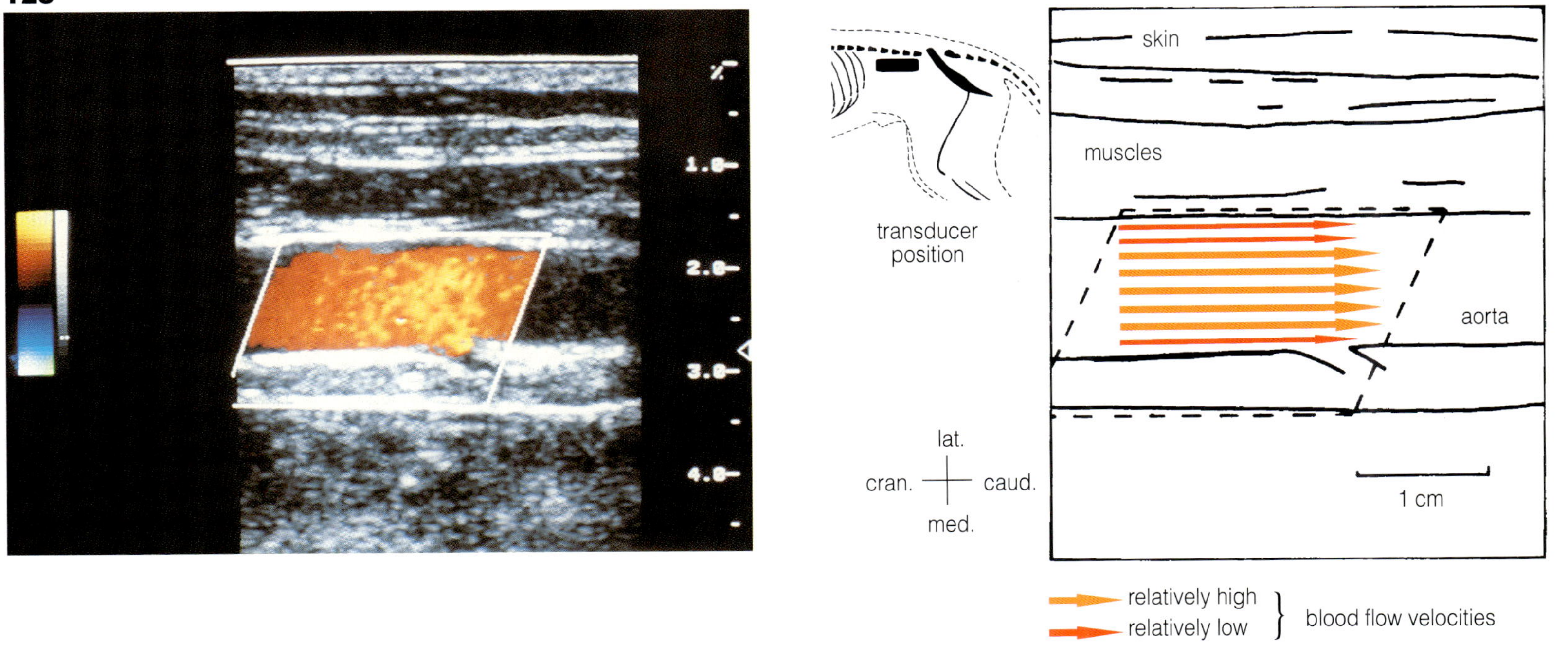

121–123 Schematic drawings of laminar blood flow velocity profiles in a vessel with a small (**121A**) and large (**121B**) diameter. Colour-coded Doppler studies in a small (common carotid artery – **122**) and a large vessel (aorta – **123**) during systole. The maximum velocity is found in the centre of both vessels.

124

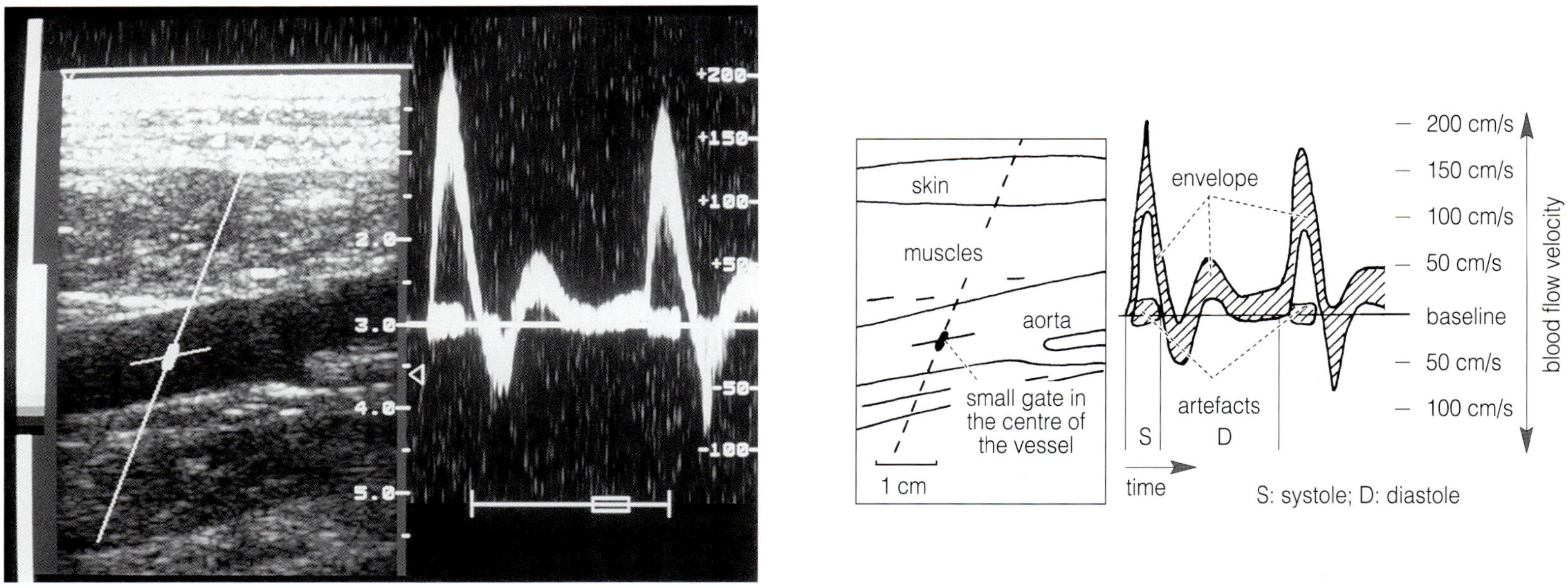

125

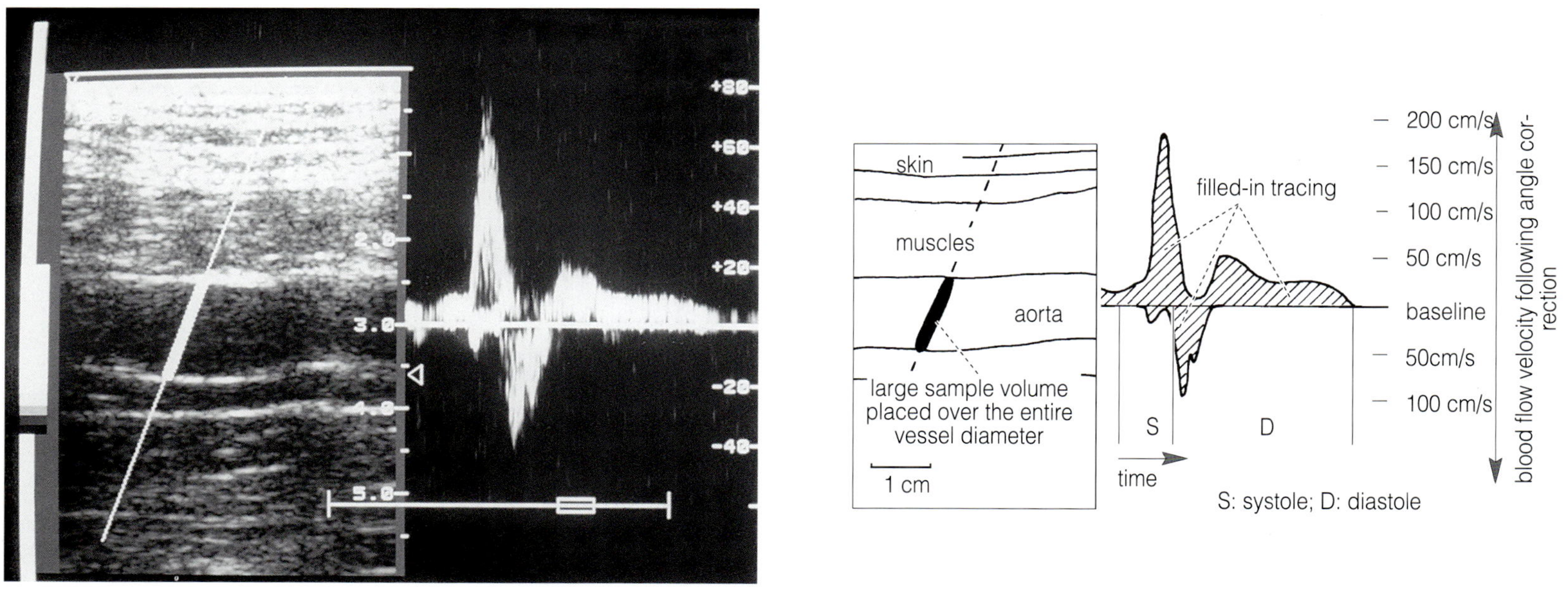

124, 125 PW Doppler echography of the aorta. Display of an envelope or recording maximum velocity by placing a small gate in the centre of the vessel (**124**); display of a filled-in curve or tracing of multiple velocities by placing a large sample volume over the entire vessel diameter (**125**).

Nyquist Limit, page 48). Turbulences are yellow or green in colour flow Doppler (**128, 129**).

Turbulences distal to a stenotic lesion appear as whirlpools (**126**). The stenosis causes an increase in flow velocity distal to the obstruction – called a jet. The maximum velocity and distribution of this jet help to assess the stenotic lesion. Turbulences are seen at the margins of the jet. These turbulences vary and do not indicate the severity of a stenosis[4]. Turbulences are also associated with valvular regurgitation (**127–129**). In this case, two blood flows meet head-on: a retrograde regurgitant jet and a regular ventricular or atrial flow. Additionally, turbulences can be found with atrial or ventricular septal defects (**130**), aorto-pulmonary shunts or patent ductus arteriosus.

126

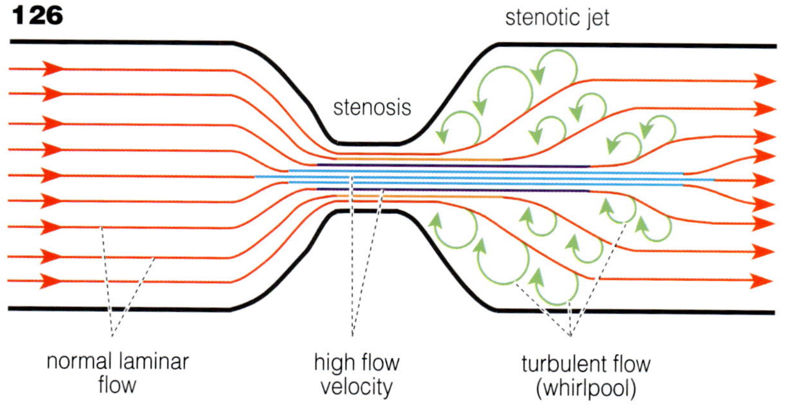

126 Schematic drawing of turbulent flow in a stenotic lesion.

127

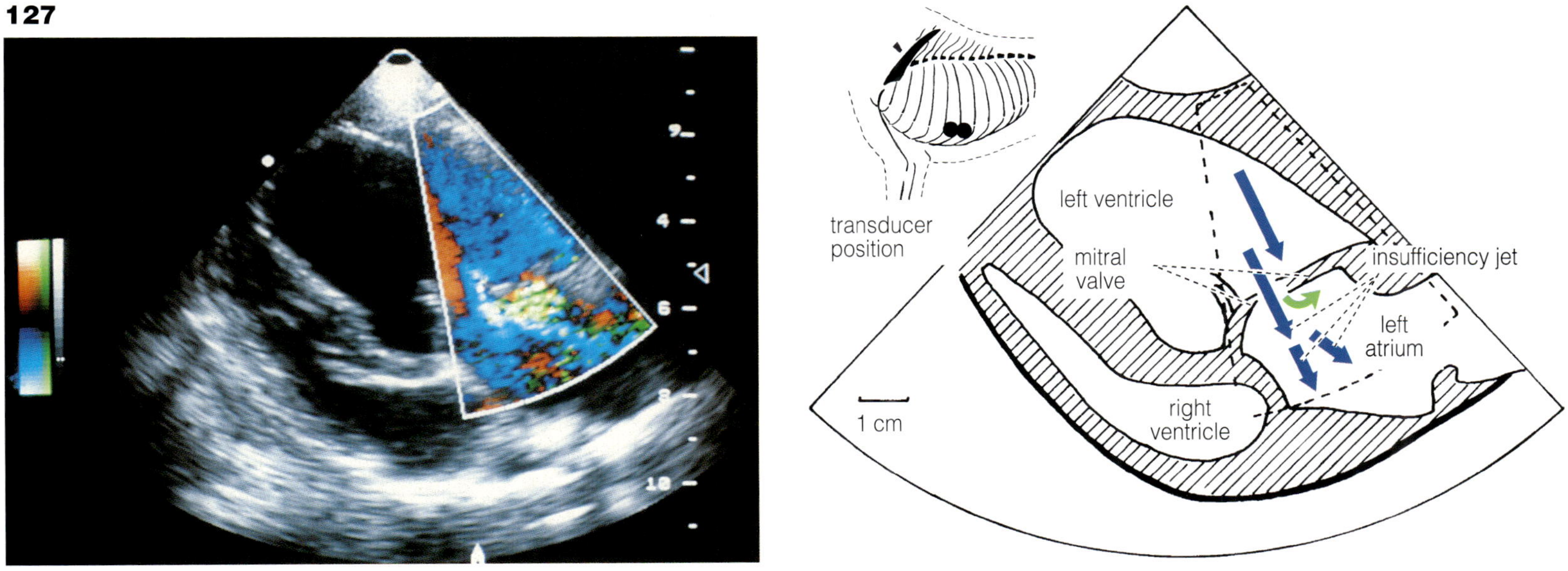

128

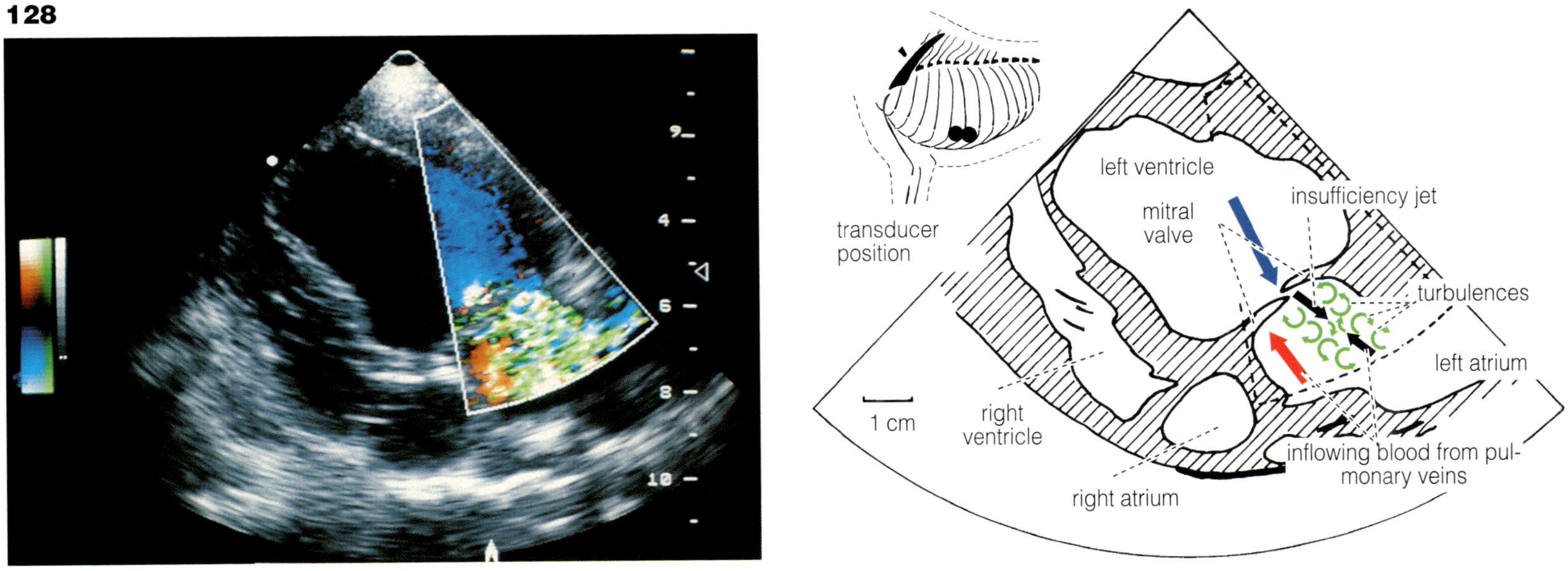

129

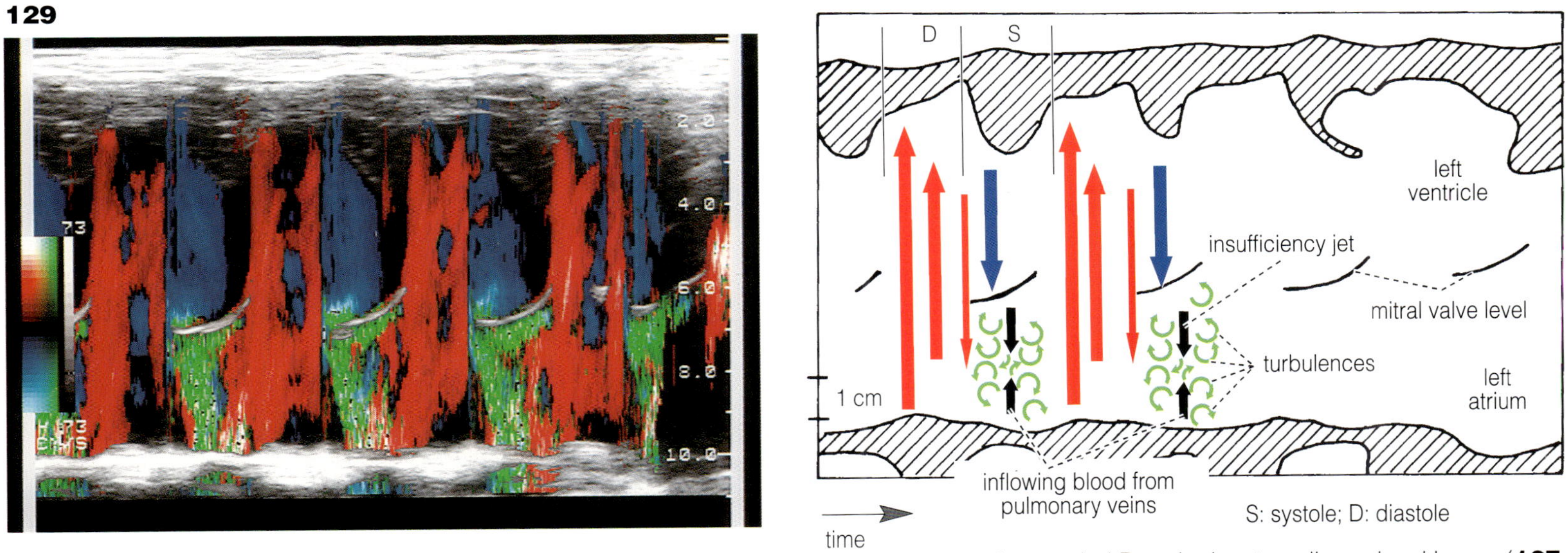

127–129 Laminar and turbulent flow with mitral regurgitation in a dog, demonstrated with colour-coded Doppler in a two-dimensional image (**127, 128**) and M-mode (**129**). Blood flowing back into the atrium (insufficiency jet) does not produce turbulences (**127** – blue colour). Turbulences are caused by regurgitated blood meeting inflowing blood from pulmonary veins (**128, 129** – yellow and green colour).

130

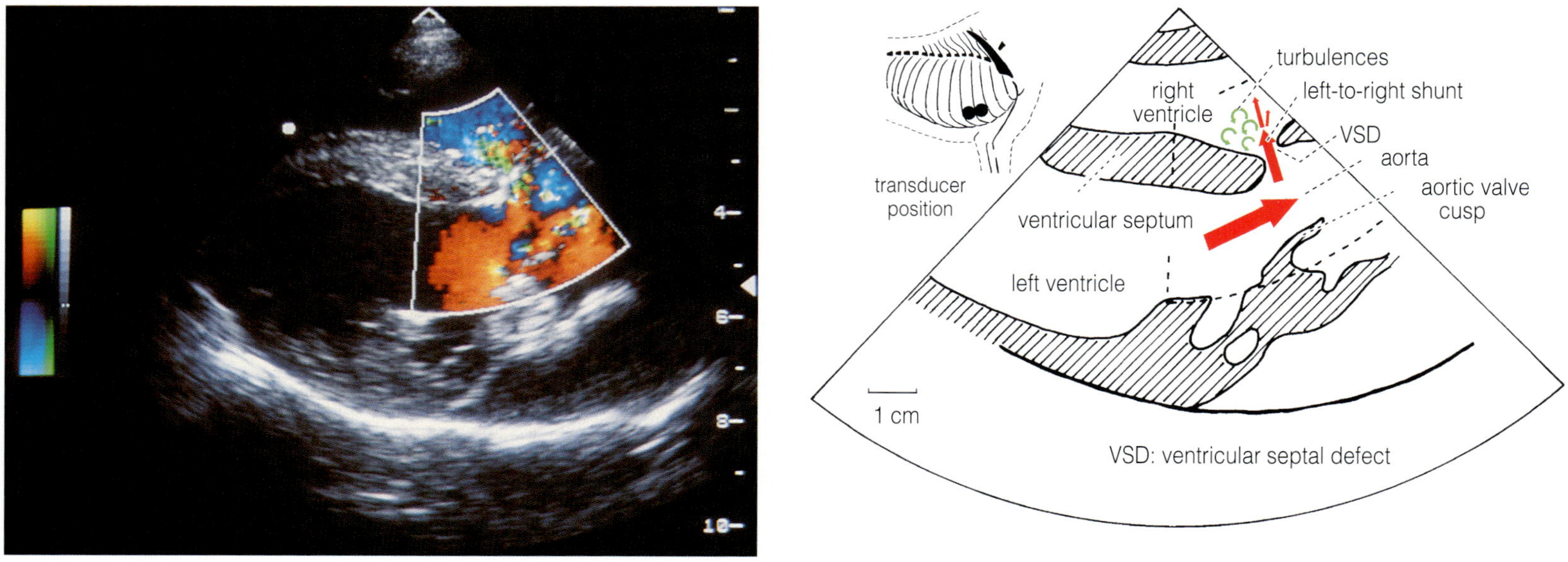

130 Colour-coded Doppler echocardiography of a ventricular septal defect (VSD) with turbulences in a dog.

131

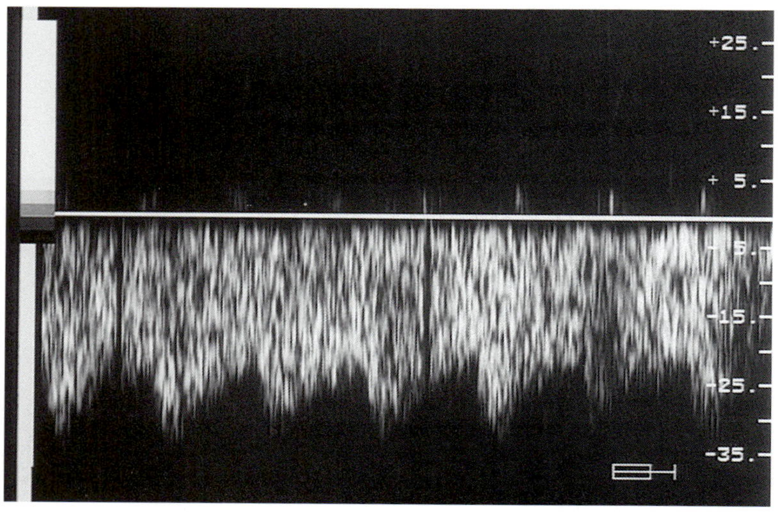

131, 132 Two vascular spectral tracings. Low peripheral resistance – placental vessel of a pregnant cat (**131**); high peripheral resistance – femoral artery in a dog (**132**).

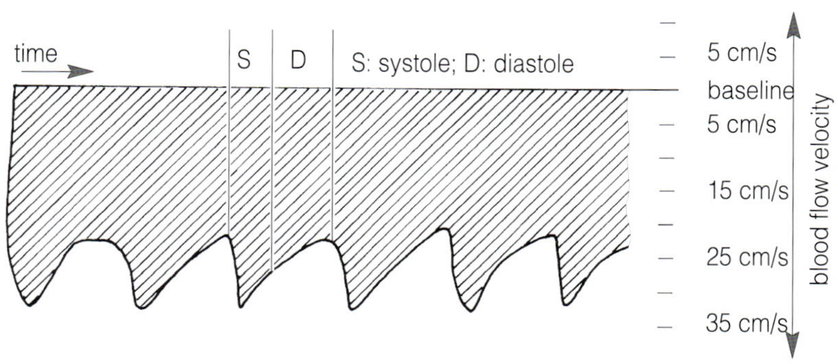

132

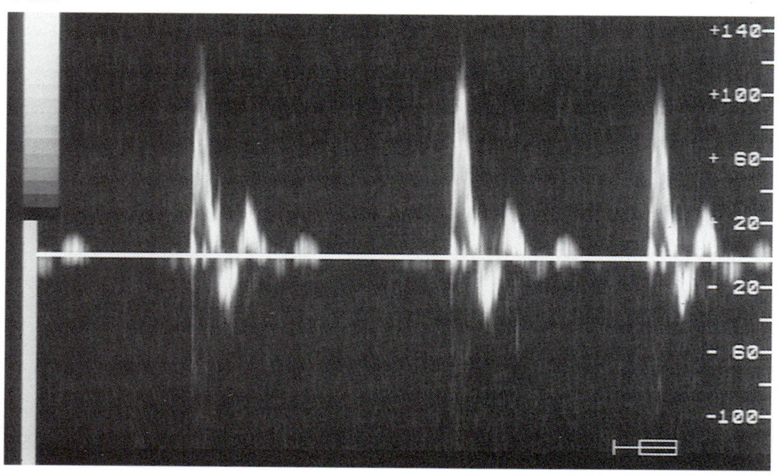

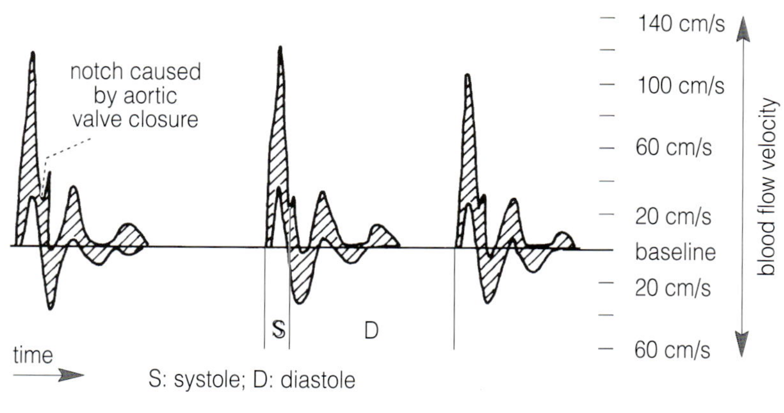

Dopplersonographic Spectral Tracings

In conventional CW and PW Doppler, every part of the heart or vessel has a characteristic normal spectral tracing and flow profile [6].

Peripheral resistance influences flow direction and velocity during systole and diastole in the vessels.

Vessels with low peripheral resistance, such as the uterine vessels of pregnant dogs or the common carotid arteries in cats and small dogs, record more or less high flow velocities during systole as well as diastole (131). Vessels in high resistance areas show a triphase or multiphase blood flow reading with high systolic forward motion, early diastolic backflow and absent end-diastolic flow (132).

Some velocity tracings have additional flow profiles; these will be discussed in the sections on cardiovascular physiology.

Most of the vascular flow profiles known from human medicine[6] apply, with some exceptions, to the dog and cat. Further studies are needed to determine these differences.

133

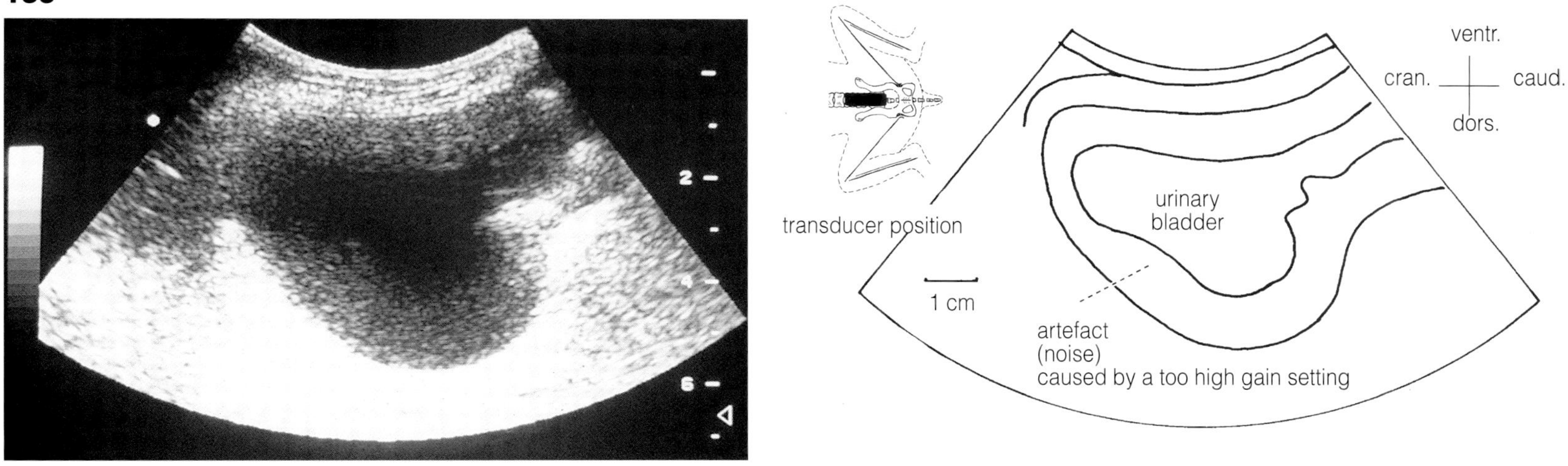

134

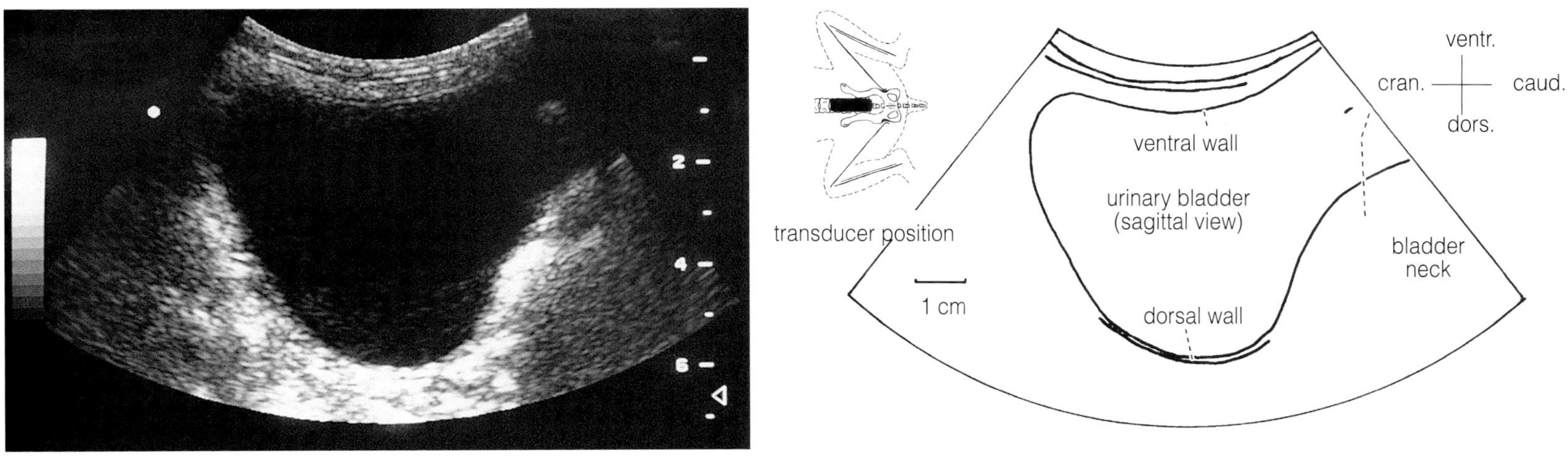

133, 134 Noise artefact in a canine urinary bladder caused by a too high gain setting (**133**), compared with a normal sonographic gain setting (**134**).

135

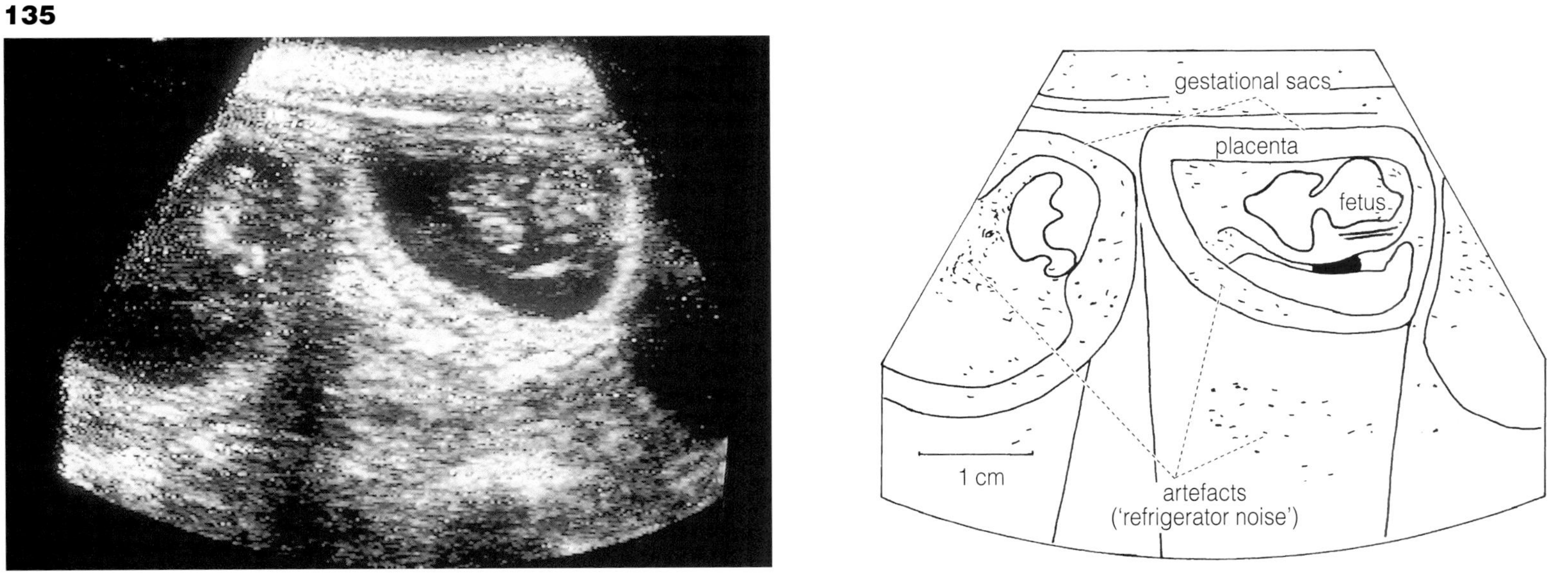

135 Noise artefact over the entire image caused by refrigerator interference. The image shows three gestational sacs in a cat 28 days post breeding.

Imaging Artefacts

Numerous physical and technical sonographic artefacts can prevent adequate assessment of an image (Latin: *ars, artis* = art; *facere* = to do). Some of these 'artificial' phenomenons, such as shadowing or enhancement, may lead to additional findings.

Noise Artefacts

Noise artefacts are displayed as small to medium-sized, more or less non-uniform echoes on the image. They are ususally caused by the gain control being set too high and, in most cases, appear in anechoic areas (**133, 134**). These artefacts can be suppressed by reducing the time gain compensation (TGC) at this depth.

136

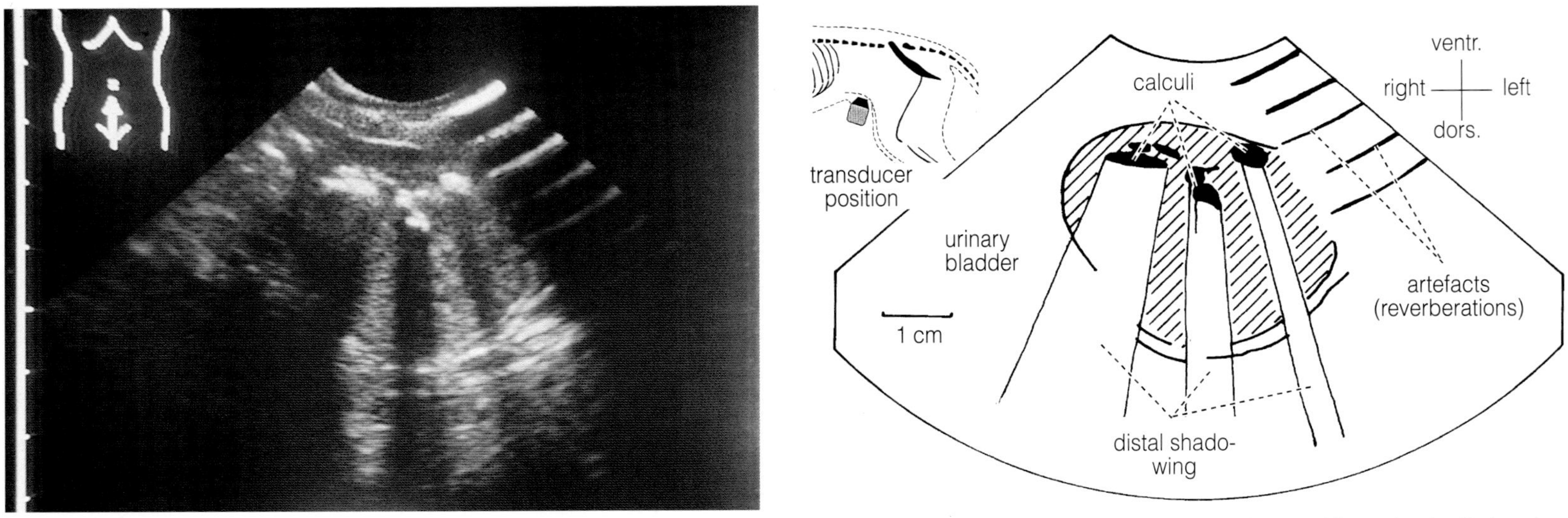

136 Reverberations due to incomplete transducer–skin contact. The ultrasound image is of a canine urinary bladder with cystitis and calculi showing uniform distal shadowing.

137

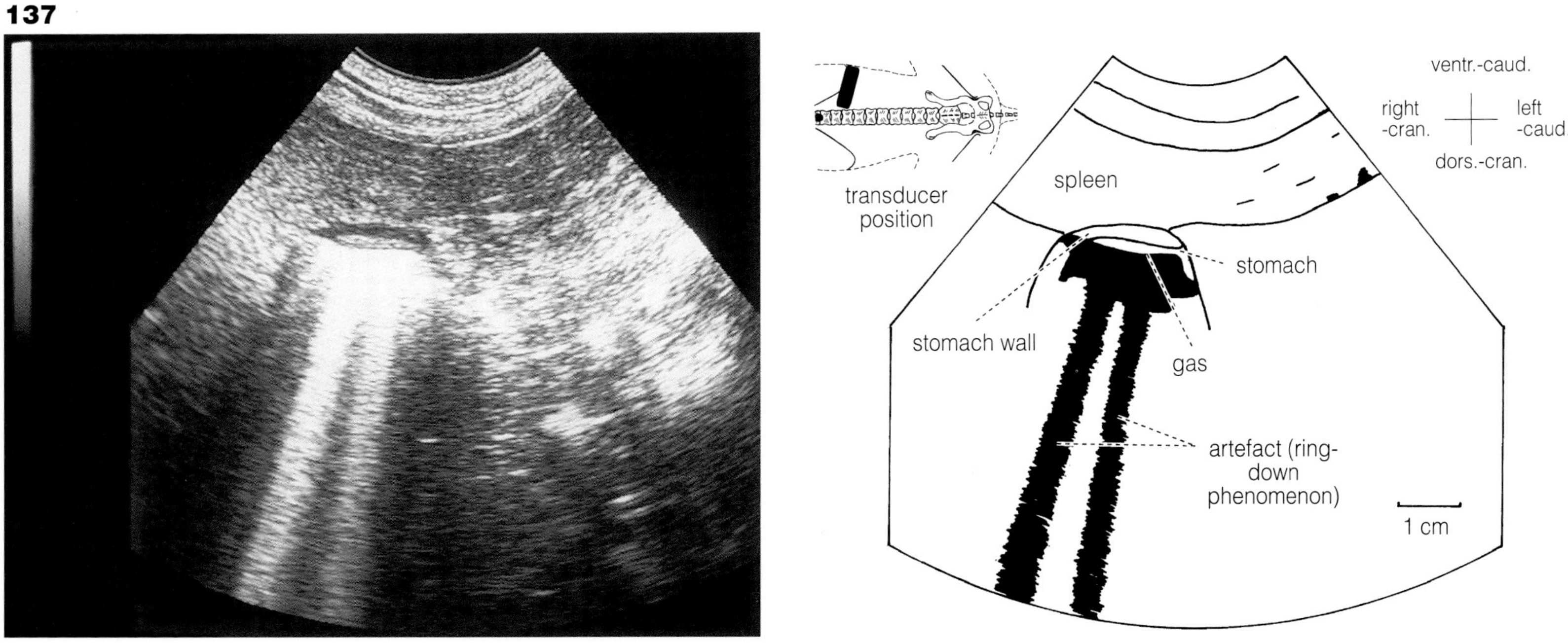

137 Reverberations (ring-down artefact) distal to gas in the stomach of a dog.

Interfering echoes that lead to noise artefacts in the entire image, or at least in part of the image, may be caused by the simultaneous use of additional ultrasound units in a room or other electrical devices. Older ultrasound systems are often very sensitive to interferences by electrical units (refrigerator, heating system, fans, steriliser, etc.). Electrical interference, such as a refrigerator being turned on, reduces image quality and produces 'refrigerator noise artefacts' in some areas of the image (**135**).

Reverberation and Mirror-Image Artefacts

Interfaces with high acoustic impedance differences produce multiple reflections, which are seen as numerous parallel lines to the original echo with decreasing echo intensity. These repetitious echoes are called reverberations. Reverberations are usually caused by insufficient transducer contact with the skin, by air entrapped between the probe and the patient, or if the area does not allow contact with the entire transducer (**136**).

Gas-filled bowel or stomach can also create reverberations. Instead of shadowing, numerous linear reverberations are produced distal to the gas-filled intestine. This is also called ring-down artefact[1] (**137**).

Another form of reverberation is the mirror-image artefact. These artefacts appear at the diaphragmatic interface and concern mainly the heart and liver (**138**). To remove these artefacts the overall gain and TGC must be decreased.

Acoustic Shadowing and Enhancement

Acoustic shadowing appears distal to tissue interfaces with impedance differences. Total reflection of sound waves occurs at these interfaces. The area distal to the reflector cannot be imaged sonographically. Shadowing is displayed as a uniform black area on the screen and is seen distal to bone, calcifications and gas-filled structures (**116E, 135, 139**). Incomplete shadowing may appear distal to stones and calculi (**140**). The area distal to these structures produces weak echoes.

138

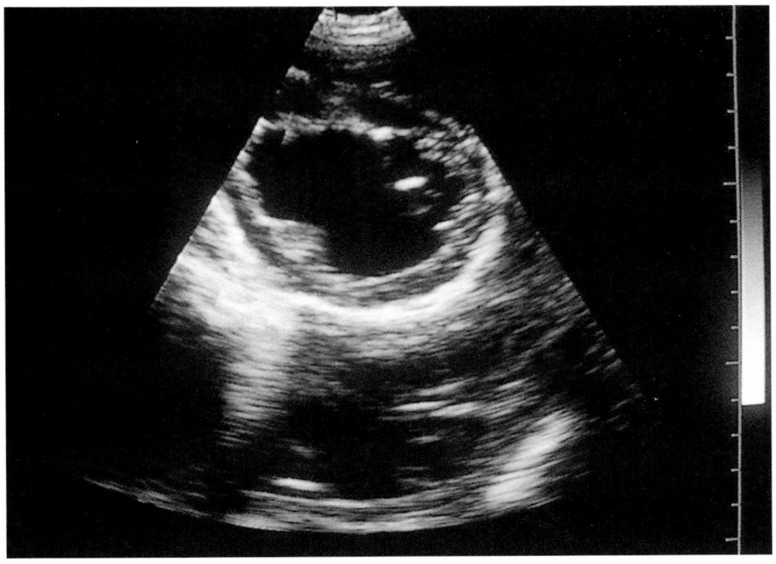

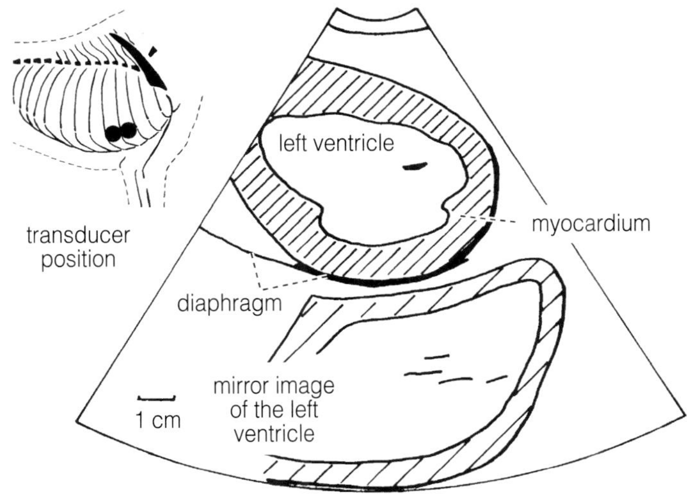

138 Mirror-image artefact of a canine heart at the diaphragm.

139

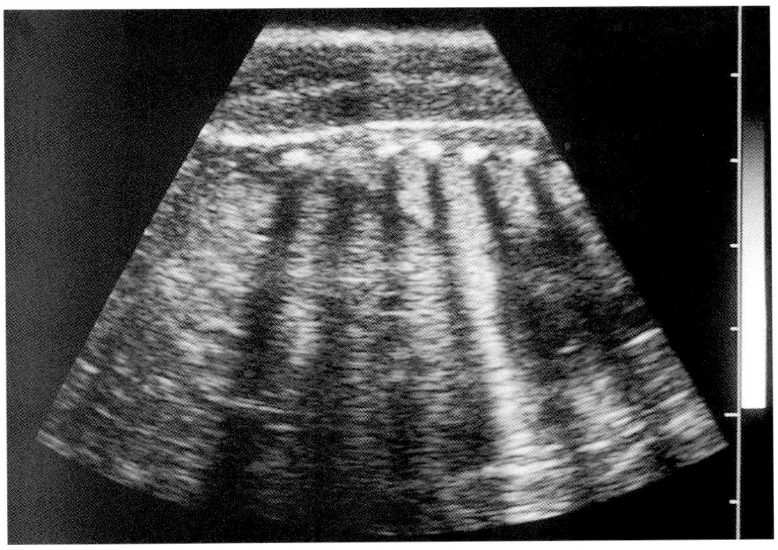

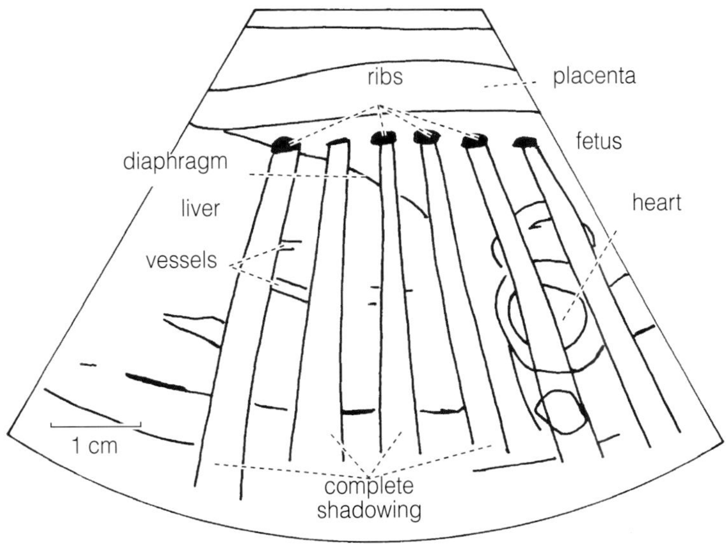

140

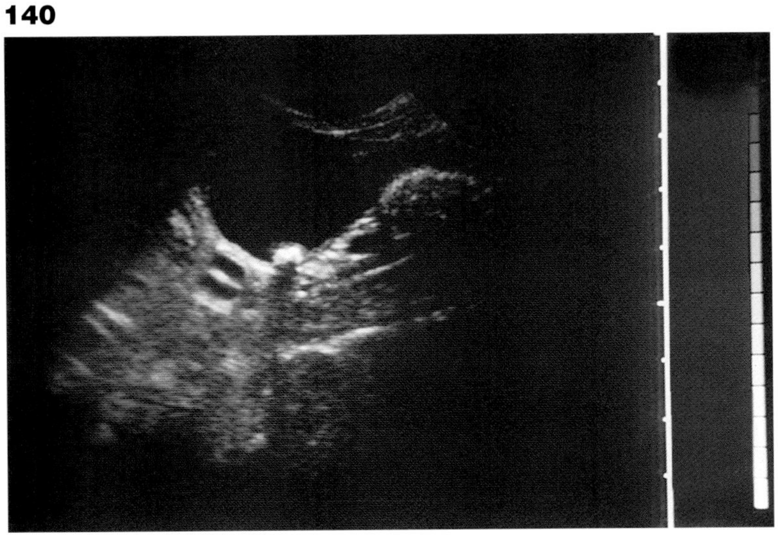

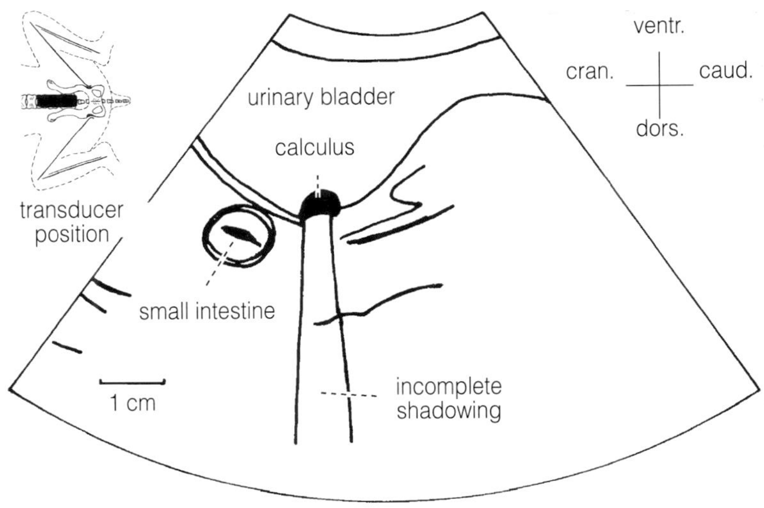

139, 140 Complete shadowing distal to ribs with total reflection of a canine fetus (**139**) (see also **135**) and incomplete shadowing distal to reflecting urinary calculi in a dog (**140**).

141

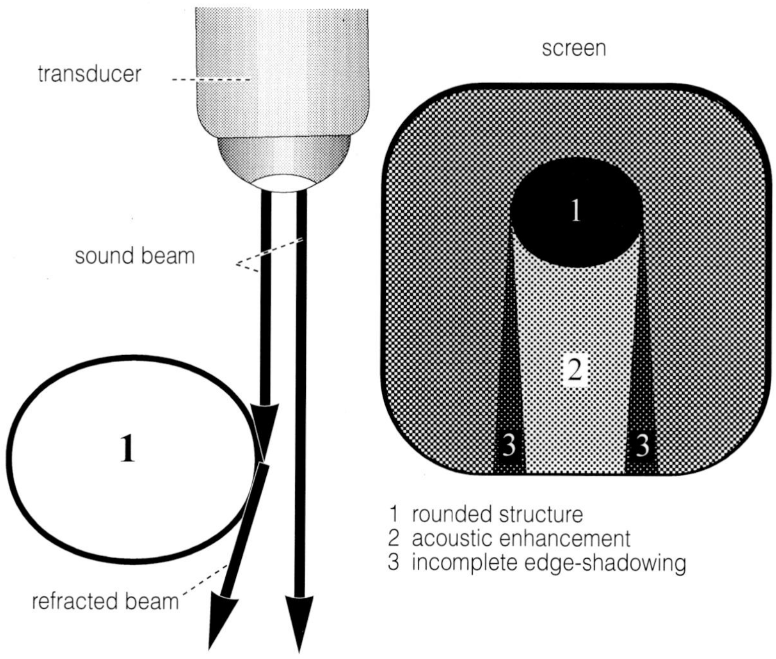

142

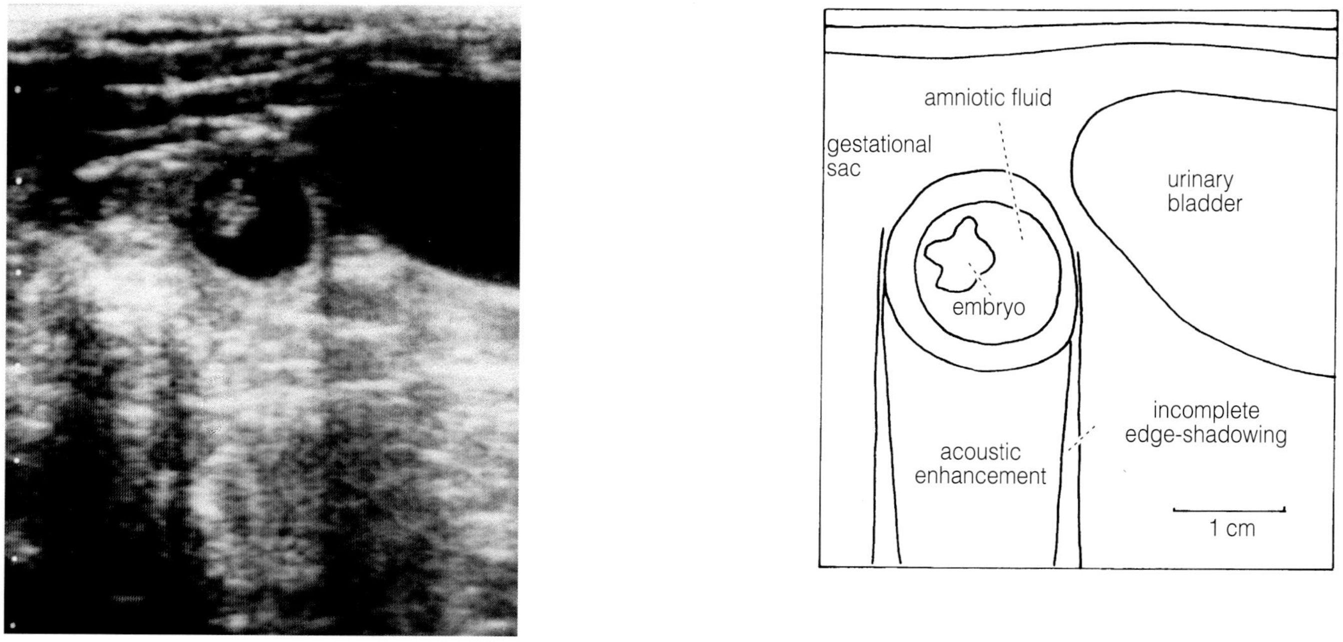

141, 142 Schematic drawing (**141**) and ultrasound image (**142**) of incomplete edge-shadowing due to refraction at the rounded margins of a gestational sac. Acoustic enhancement is also seen distal to the gestational sac.

Refraction causes the soundbeam to diverge distal to the lateral margins of cystic or rounded structures. Edge-shadowing shows a thin anechoic line distal to the rounded margin (see Reflection, Transmission and Refraction, page 21) (**116F, 117, 141, 142**).

Acoustic enhancement occurs distal to fluid-filled organs and structures. Structures in this area are displayed more clearly (**116F, 117, 141, 142**). Low attenuation of the sound beam produces a higher echo amplitude distal to fluids than behind soft tissues. Distal enhancement is useful for diagnosis. Enhancement distal to a filled urinary bladder helps to image the uterus, including gestational sacs in early pregnancy.

Slice-Thickness Artefacts

Slice-thickness artefacts are seen along the margins of cystic structures as fine lines of irregular echoes (**143, 144**). When a wide ultrasound beam, often seen in the near or far field (Resolution, page 32), meets an interface at an oblique angle, the echoes on the screen are weak in intensity and have an irregular contour (**143, 144**). This echogenic edge is seen in the urinary bladder or gallbladder and may be mistaken for cystitis or sludge. A slice-thickness artefact can be corrected by adjusting the focal zone and/or changing the transducer angulation. This allows the sound beam to travel perpendicular to the edge and displays the actual wall structure.

Doppler Artefacts

The most common PW Doppler artefact is a mirror image of the spectral display along the baseline. The 'mirror' signal intensity may be as strong or weaker than the actual intensity. This 'double' spectral display appears when flow direction is not apparent, which means that blood flow is perpendicular to the sound beam (**23**).

Muscle contractions or heart and vessel valve motion may produce false and unwanted signals. The signals will mask flow information in CW and PW Doppler. These artefacts can be avoided or at least decreased by adjusting the wall filter or changing the location of the measuring range (CW Doppler), or by adjusting the sample volume (PW Doppler) (**145**).

143

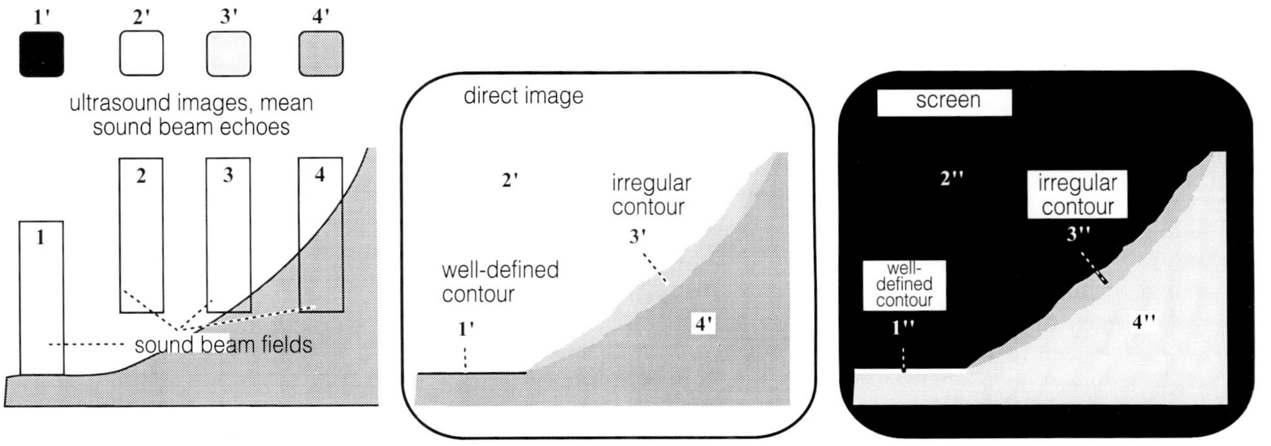

144

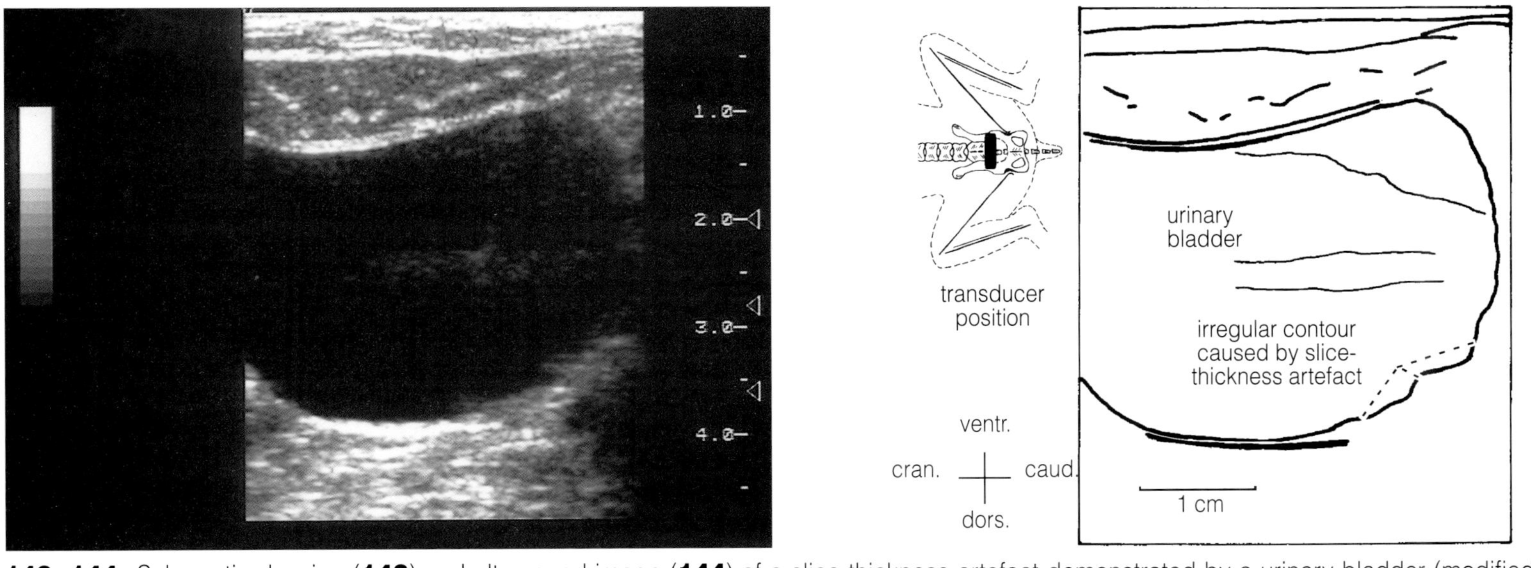

143, 144 Schematic drawing (**143**) and ultrasound image (**144**) of a slice-thickness artefact demonstrated by a urinary bladder (modified from Kaarmann and Wessells, 1991[7]).

145

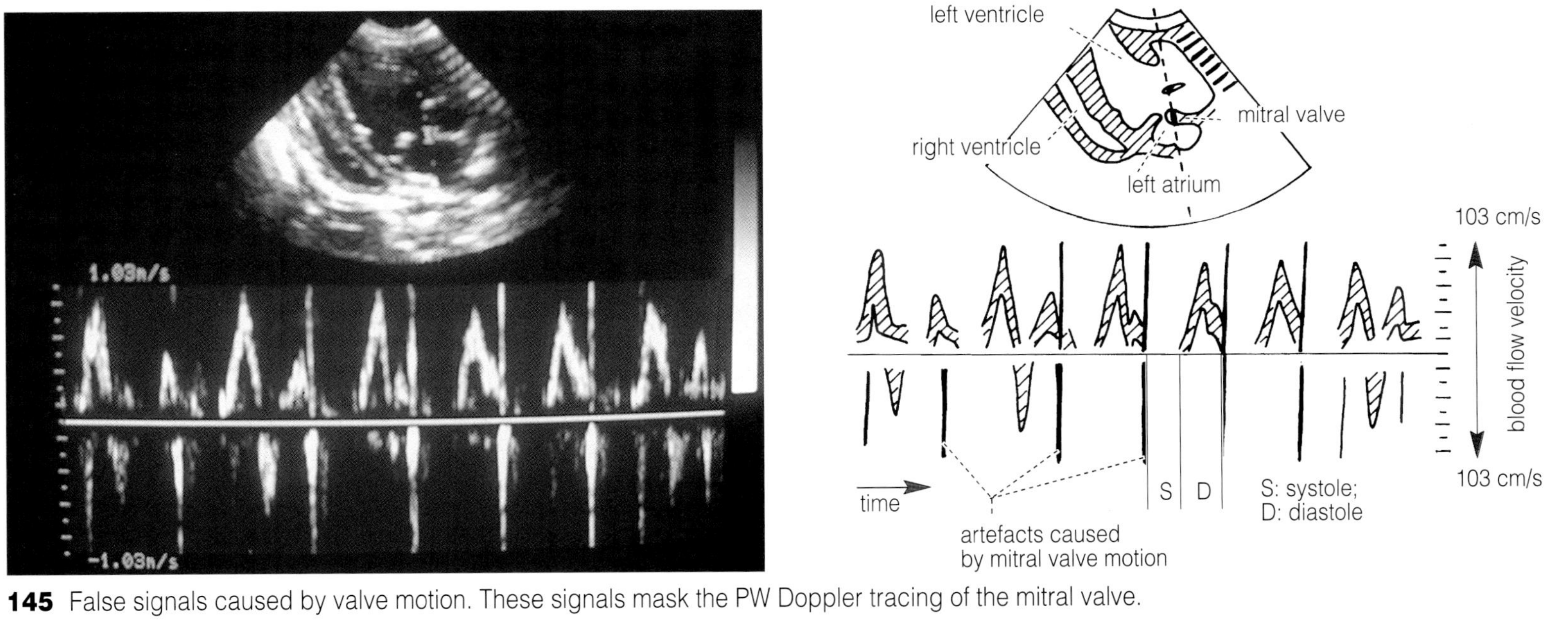

145 False signals caused by valve motion. These signals mask the PW Doppler tracing of the mitral valve.

146

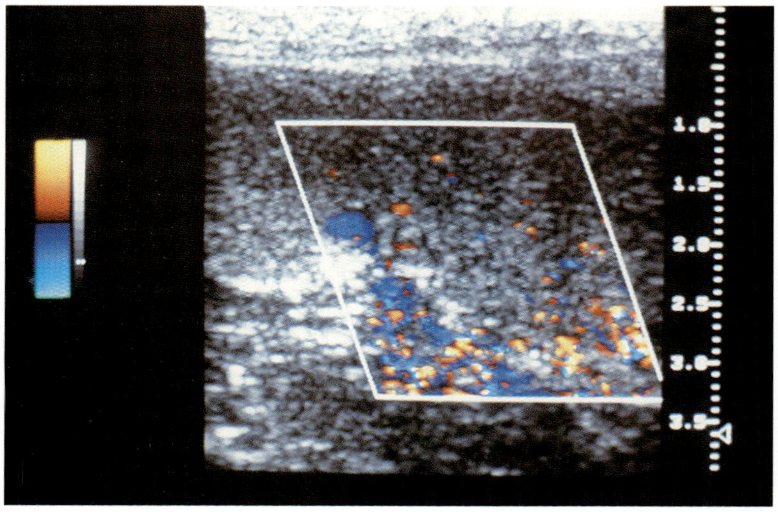

147

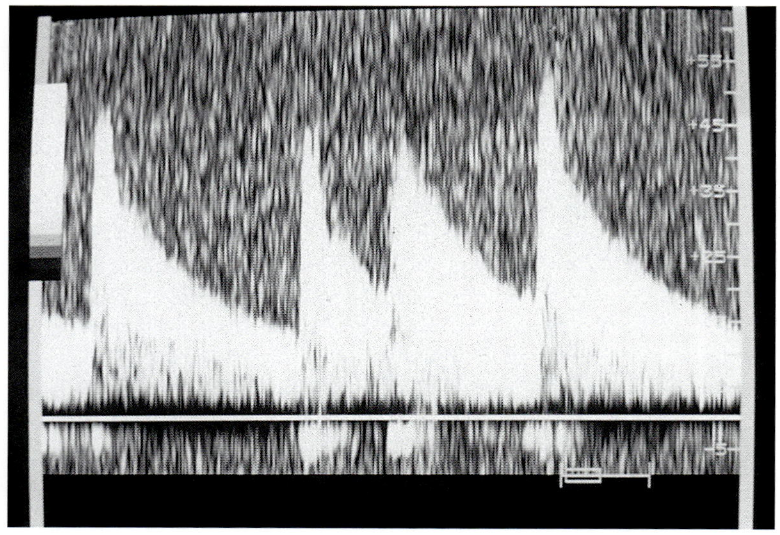

148

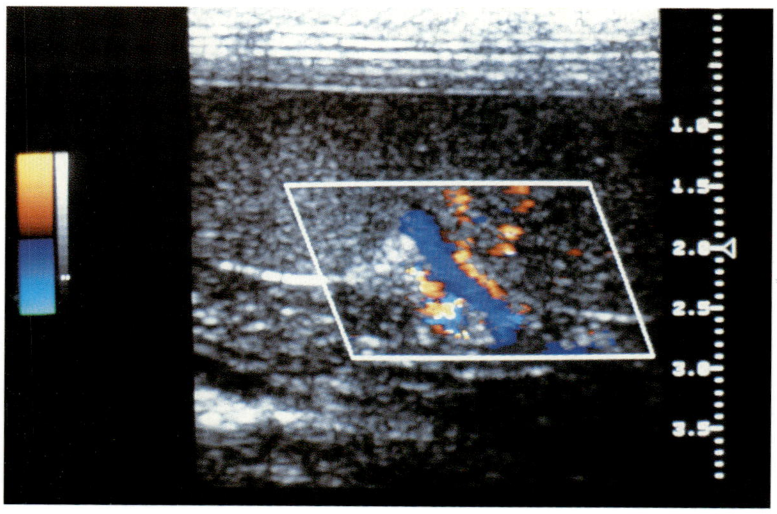

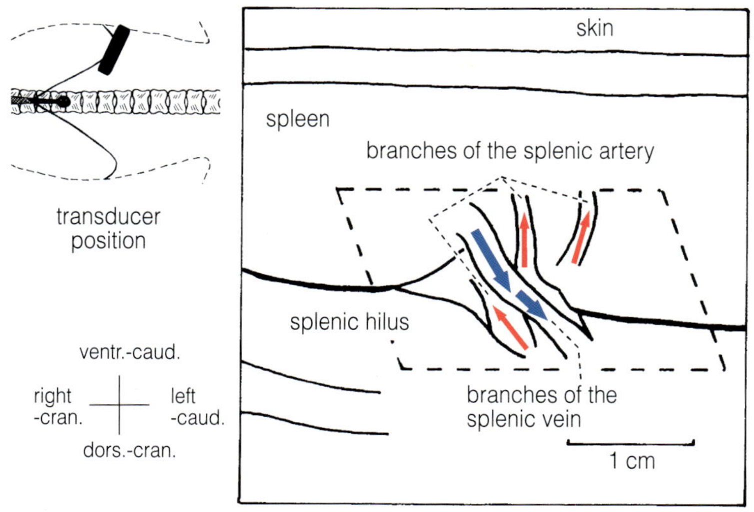

149

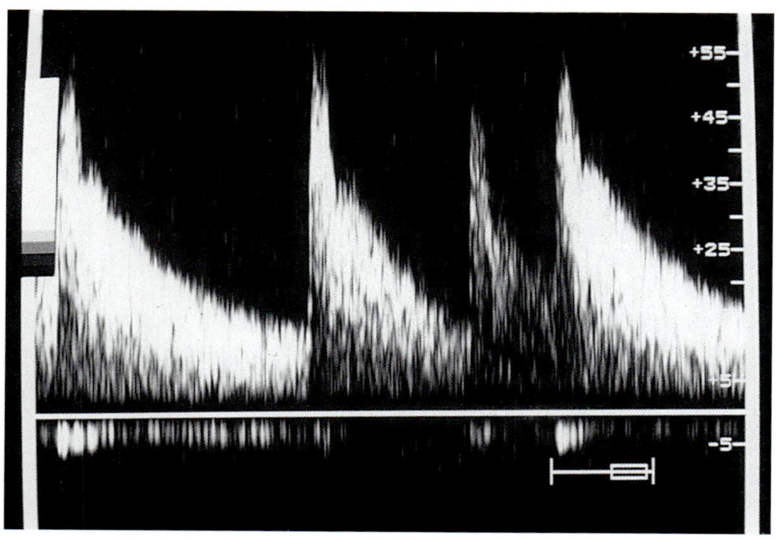

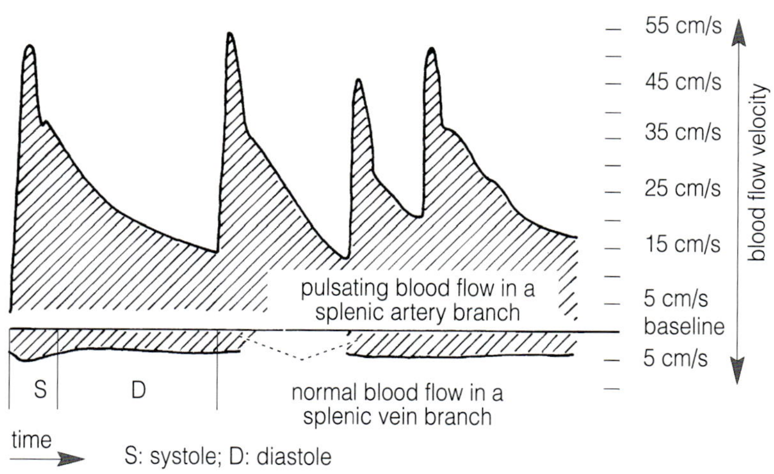

146–149 High gain setting with low noise reduction in a colour-flow Doppler (**146**) and PW Doppler (**147**) display of the splenic artery, compared to the normal display (**148, 149**).

150

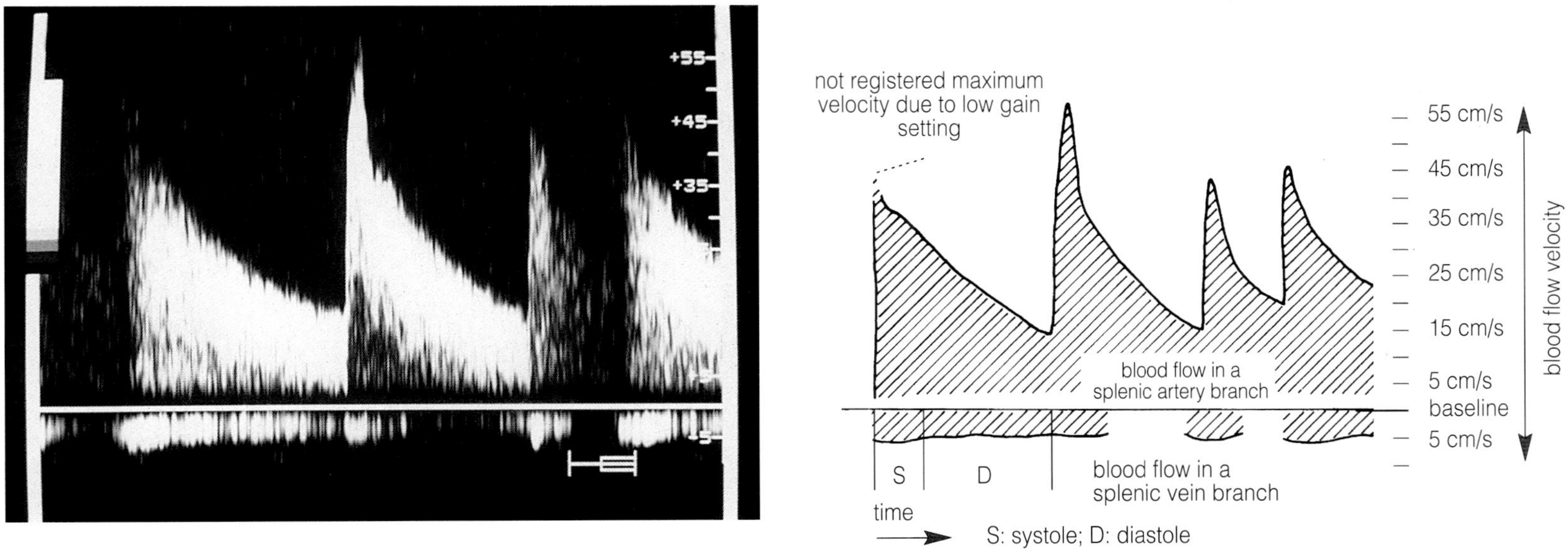

150 Low systolic maximum velocity tracing of the splenic artery in the first signal caused by a low overall gain setting.

Too high a gain setting in colour flow Doppler examinations may produce colour signals in areas without blood flow. In conventional CW and PW Doppler echography these artefacts, as well as any background noise, can be eliminated by reducing the gain and increasing the reject control (**146–149**). Maximum velocities in colour-coded and PW Doppler will not be displayed and are therefore underestimated when the gain is set too low (**150**).

Delayed colour-coded spectrums are caused by technical difficulties. Colour-coded images of blood flow are superimposed on existing two-dimensional sonographic images. These two images may not appear simultaneously when the examined structures move very fast. This problem can be solved by increasing the pulse-repetition rate or the frame rate.

References

Cited References

1 Avruch L and Cooperberg PL (1985) The ring-down artefact. *J. Ultrasound Med.* 4, 21–28.

2 Bönhof JA (1987) Richtig benennen – besser erkennen. Ein Beitrag zur Terminologie der Sonogrammbeschreibung. *Ultraschall Klin. Prax.* 2, 178–184.

3 Bubenheimer P and Kneisel GD (1989) *Doppler-Echokardiographie*. Verlag Edition Medizin, Weinheim.

4 Fehske W (1988) *Praxis der Konventionellen und Farbkodierten Doppler-Echokardiographie*. Verlag Hans Huber, Bern, Stuttgart, Toronto.

5 Gobrecht H (1990) Mechanik der Flüssigkeiten und Gase. In: Gobrecht H: *Mechanik, Akustik, Wärme. Vol. I.* Bergmann, Schaeffer (Eds) *Lehrbuch der Experimentalphysik*. 10th Edn. Verlag Walter de Gruyter, Berlin, New York, pp. 302–392.

6 Grant EG and White EM (Eds.) (1988) *Duplex Sonography*. Springer Verlag, New York, Berlin, Heidelberg.

7 Kaarmann H and Wessels G (1991) II–1 Physikalische Grandlagen. 10. Ergänzungslieferung. In: Braun B, Günther R and Schwerk W (Eds.) *Ultraschalldiagnostik. Lehrbuch und Atlas. Vol I.* Verlag Ecomed. Landsberg, München, Zürich.

8 Poulsen Nautrup C (1991) Einführung in die physikalisch-technischen Grandlagen der Röntgen- and Ultraschalldiagnostik. In: Budras KD and Fricke W: *Atlas der Anatomie des Handes. Lehrbuch für Tierärzte und Studierende*. 3rd Edn. Schlütersche Verlagsanstalt and Druckerei, Hannover, pp. 68–77.

Additional Reading

Goldstein A and Madrazo BL (1981) Slice thickness artefacts in gray-scale ultrasound. *J. Clin. Ultrasound* 9, 365–375.

Kremkau FW and Taylor KJ (1986) Artefacts in ultrasound imaging. *J. Ultrasound Med.* 5, 227–237.

Robinson DE, Wilson LS and Kossof G (1981) Shadowing and enhancement in ultrasonic echograms by reflection and refraction. *J. Clin. Ultrasound* 9, 181–188.

Sommer FG and Taylor KJW (1980) Differentiation of acoustic shadowing due to calculi and gas collections. *Radiol.* 135, 399–403.

Ziskin MC, LaFollette P, Radecki PD and Villafana T (1986) The retrolenticular afterglow: an echo enhancement artefact. *J. Ultrasound Med.* 5, 385–389.

Ziskin MC, Thickman DI, Goldberg NJ, Lapayowker MS and Becker JM (1982) The comet tail artefact. *J. Ultrasound Med.* 1, 1–7.

5 Examination Techniques

Cordula Poulsen Nautrup

Indications and Requirements

Every sonographic examination requires a specific indication. Ultrasonography is one of many examination methods. It is not meant to replace, but rather to supplement other diagnostic methods such as clinical, laboratory or radiological examinations.

Two-dimensional ultrasonography displays macroscopic, anatomical and pathological structures (see Interaction of Ultrasound Beams with Tissues, page 21; Scattering, Absorption and Divergence, page 22; Sonographic Imaging of Tissue, page 60). Histological or functional diagnostics are not possible with ultrasonography. Because the examination is in real-time, motion and organ displacement may be displayed.

Follow-up examinations are helpful and are recommended when imaging embryonal and fetal development and monitoring and assessing diseases, as well as when evaluating therapy results. These follow-up examinations are easy to reproduce because they are painless, harmless and without any adverse effects on the patient.

Specific sonographic indications depend on the organ system involved and these are described in Part II (Chapters 6–12) of this textbook. Two-dimensional ultrasonography is useful for most soft tissue diseases. Gynaecological and obstetrical sonographic examinations are particularly valuable before, during and after pregnancy, as well as during parturition. Palpation and hormone analysis should not be overlooked. A cardiological diagnosis and prognosis should always encompass one- and two-dimensional ultrasonography in addition to primary auscultation, electrocardiogram assessment and thoracic radiography.

Sonographic imaging of the respiratory system, such as the larynx, trachea and lungs, is not possible. Ultrasonography of the brain is difficult in adult dogs and cats with ossified fontanelles (see Brain, page 88). Skeletal ultrasonographic imaging is basically possible (see Monitoring Bone Healing with B-Mode Ultrasonography, page 371; Ultrasonographic Usefulness and Limitations in Monitoring Secondary Fracture Healing, page 377), although bone imaging will always be a radiological domain.

Additional Doppler imaging gives information on blood flow and organ blood supply. Changes in blood supply usually appear sooner than clinical and morphological lesions and are displayed in varying blood flow patterns (see Gestational Age Estimation, page 304). If technically possible, each two-dimensional sonographic examination should be followed by Doppler imaging. This is especially true for most cardiological diseases, which are often only recognized through Doppler imaging (see Doppler Echocardiography, page 137; Echography of Heart Disease, page 142).

(*Table* 5 [page 44] gives an overview of the applications and indications of the different ultrasonographic methods.)

In addition to technical equipment, skill and indications, ultrasonography requires a suitable room for a relaxed examination, plenty of time and, of course, appropriate patient preparation (see Patient Preparation, page 77).

151

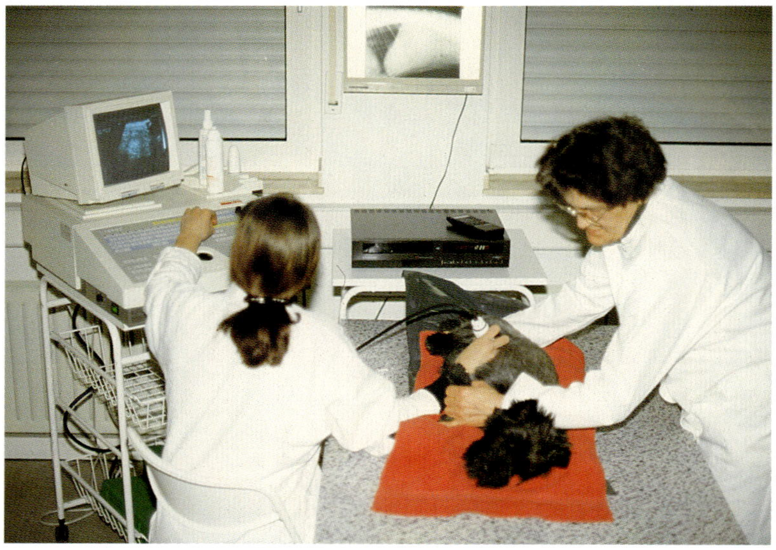

151 Example of a simple but practical sonographic workplace.

Examination Room

The examination room should be darkened, since bright daylight or artificial light will blind the sonographer and reflect on the screen. However, an indirect dim light facilitates handling of the ultrasound unit.

An x-ray viewer should be set up for the sonographer to compare the radiographic and sonographic results.

The sonographer should sit comfortably on a rollable chair or stool. A right-handed person should hold the transducer in his right hand, while the left hand adjusts the unit, holds the animal or assists the right hand. Transducer positioning and movement should be slow and calm. Erratic and inconsistent transducer motion produces poor images. For this reason the scanning arm should rest on the table or, better still, on the animal. It is helpful if another person adjusts the unit and the sonographer only freezes the images with a foot pedal. The ultrasound machine should be placed to the near left, diagonally to the line of vision of the (right-handed) sonographer.

The monitor should be seen not only by the sonographer, but also by the patient's owner, who can hold the animal's head (**151**).

Instrument Settings

Every ultrasound machine has basic settings, modified from human medicine for veterinary practice. In most cases, preset programmes for abdominal and cardiological examinations are installed. Preprocessing settings can be tested on ultrasound phantoms or body organs and should be adjusted for the individual patient.

The following points should assist the sonographic beginner with the daily routine setting of an ultrasound unit (modified from Pickuth *et al.*, 1993[2]):

- The machine settings should always be adjusted carefully when one or more sonographers use the unit for different purposes.
- Any electrical appliances which may cause noise artefacts (so-called 'refrigerator noise'; see Noise Artefacts, page 69) should be turned off before the examination
- The ultrasound unit, monitor and documentation (video recorder and/or video printer) should be turned on with either a joint or individual switch.
- Before starting any examination, the unit should be warmed up for about five minutes.
- The monitor settings are adjusted first and should not be altered. The contrast knob is turned up to the maximum setting and then turned back until the text on the image is legible and white without any blurring. Image brightness is adjusted with a dark grey to black monitor background. The grey scale should display multiple grey levels.
- The power output should be set as low as possible, but also as high as neccessary. Examinations in dogs and cats usually need 100% of the maximum allowed 100 mW/cm^2. For cervical, abdominal and pelvic sonographic diagnostics, as well as for sonographic pregnancy monitoring, the maximum dynamic range with image integration should be used. Echocardiography needs a lower dynamic setting (30 or 40 dB) without image integration. These configurations are preset in some ultrasound machines and are available for echocardiography as well as for abdominal ultrasonography (see Preprocessing, page 33).
- Transducer and frequency are chosen according to the examination (see Scattering, Absorption and Divergence, page 22; Resolution, page 32; and Real-Time Ultrasonography, page 42).
- Time gain compensation (TGC) and gain settings are adjusted at the area in question with the help of the urinary bladder, liver and gallbladder or heart of the patient. The TGC controls are set at a medium position. The overall gain settings are adjusted so that the image is easily recognizable in the darkened room. The TGC settings are then fine tuned until the echoes are even throughout the field. Fluid-filled organs should be anechoic (black). Some animals require maximum TGC and gain settings (see Preprocessing, page 33).
- The region of interest is then displayed and the focal zone moved to this depth. If possible, additional focal zones should be added with non-moving organs.
- Adjustments of postprocessing settings are usually not necessary (see Postprocessing, page 37).

Time Frame

An often overlooked requirement for an ultrasound examination is a sufficient time frame. A quick and sloppy scan produces unsatisfactory results and usually leads to a misdiagnosis or incorrect prognosis. The time needed for an examination depends on the skill and experience of the sonographer. The German Society for Ultrasound in (Human) Medicine (DEGUM) offers guidelines for a useful time frame, which represents the absolute minimum for a veterinarian working with less cooperative patients. DEGUM proposes a time frame of 15 minutes for the sonographic examination of an abdominal organ. Each additional organ takes another five minutes, while other examination techniques such as photography, measurements or calculations need an additional 15 minutes[1].

Successful ultrasonography is based on a problem-orientated, systematic examination of the organ or organ system in question. The examination must be extended to other organs or organ systems if the area being examined does not provide diagnostic findings.

Patient Preparation

Examination Time

If possible, ultrasound examinations should be scheduled in the mornings or evenings. Any distracting or painful manipulations of the animal before sonography should be avoided to assure the animal's cooperation or tolerance of the relatively lengthy examination.

Fasting

For best results in abdominal ultrasonography and sonographic pregnancy diagnosis, animals should be fasted for 12–24 hours. Gas-filled intestines in cats, because they may have caught a mouse or rat, will compromise the quality of the ultrasound examination. These animals should be fasted and re-examined. Fasting should not exceed 24 hours, since additional intestinal gas may be produced after this time. Oral gas-reducing agents (Dimeticon, Lefax®; Asche or Sab Simplex®, Parke-Davis) administered after feeding the previous day and again 2–3 hours prior to the sonographic examination will produce better results. Animals should have a full urinary bladder for abdominal and pregnancy examinations. Animals should be allowed to drink *ad libitum* before the examination. A slight decrease in cutaneous turgor will greatly degrade the image quality.

Clipping and Shaving

Clipping and shaving depends primarily on the animal's hair coat. In addition, the scanning area, the size and frequency of the transducer, individual breed differences and, at times, the wishes of the owner must also be taken into consideration.

Animals with wiry hair and/or a thick undercoat must be clipped to produce good images. Long-haired dogs and cats do not have to be clipped when using a mid-frequency transducer. In these cases the hair can be parted after wetting it with alcohol. Most owners will accept hair coat removal when the importance of the examination is understood. Some animals, especially cats, do not like to be clipped. They may not tolerate the following sonographic examination, although it usually has a calming effect on most dogs and cats. Some animals even fall asleep during a longer sonographic examination.

The clipped area should be kept as small as possible, but must also be big enough to image any adjacent organs (**152, 153**). In pregnant animals, especially cats, hair on the ventral abdomen should not be removed around the nipples, since kittens prefer hairy nipples. Clipping of this area may also lead to milk retention and mastitis. Breed characteristics should also be considered before hair coat removal. Chow Chows and Birman cats, for example, have very slow or no hair growth, or it may regrow in a different colouring.

For echocardiographic examinations, the right and left parasternal areas on the thoracic wall and caudal to the olecranon do not have to be clipped, since the hair coat is sparse, except in cats. Pelvic organs can ususally be scanned from the caudoventral abdominal wall without clipping. The neck area, however, always requires hair coat removal.

Sector transducers with a small contact area can be used without hair clipping, as opposed to sector scanners with stand-off pads and linear-array and curved-array transducers. Near-focused, high frequency transducers with 7.5 MHz or more always require complete hair removal in the scanning area.

Acoustic Coupling Gel

When clipping or shaving is not possible, the hair coat and skin should be soaked with 70–98% alcohol before applying the acoustic coupling gel.

To ensure good skin contact and images the coupling gel should not be used sparingly. The gel is usually reapplied frequently during the examination.

> For a good sonographic diagnosis with optimal image quality, the scanning site must be clipped or shaved and liberal amounts of acoustic coupling gel applied to this area.

At the beginning of the examination, the images may sometimes be dark and of poor quality, even though the scanning area has been prepared properly. When the gel is massaged into the skin by tranducer movement, the images improve after a while.

Basically it is wrong to assume that increased transducer pressure can compensate for incomplete scanning area preparation. This increased pressure is not tolerated by animals and their resistance makes the examination more difficult without improving skin contact. Slight transducer pressure may even compress superficial vessels and deform other superficial structures. All sonographic examinations can and should be performed with the transducer placed lightly on the skin, except when scanning the pancreas and adrenal glands.

Sedation

Sedation is usually not necessary for routine evaluation of cephalic, cervical, cardiac and abdominal areas, including pregnancy diagnosis. In the interest of the sonographer and the owner of the patient, it may be necessary to sedate very aggressive animals before a long sonographic examination. For special procedures, such as transoesophageal echocardiography or intravascular sonography, the animal must be sedated or anaesthetized.

152

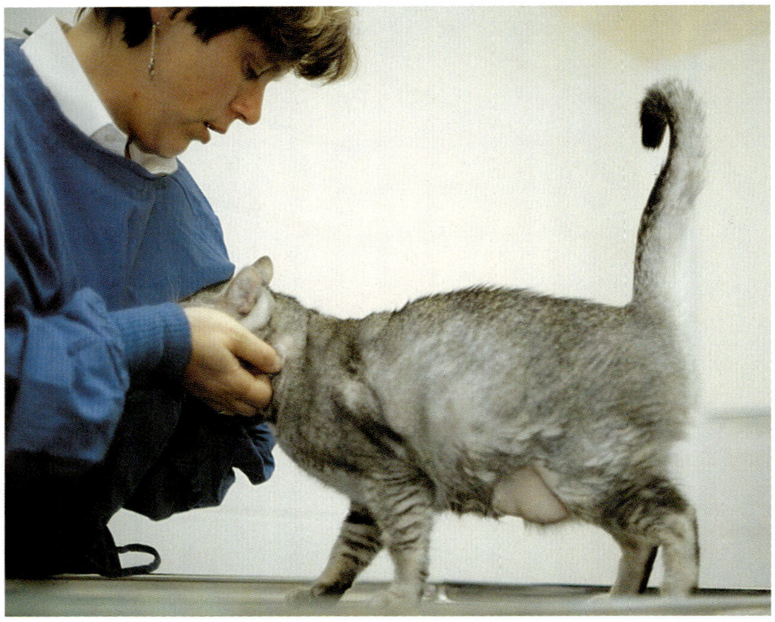

153

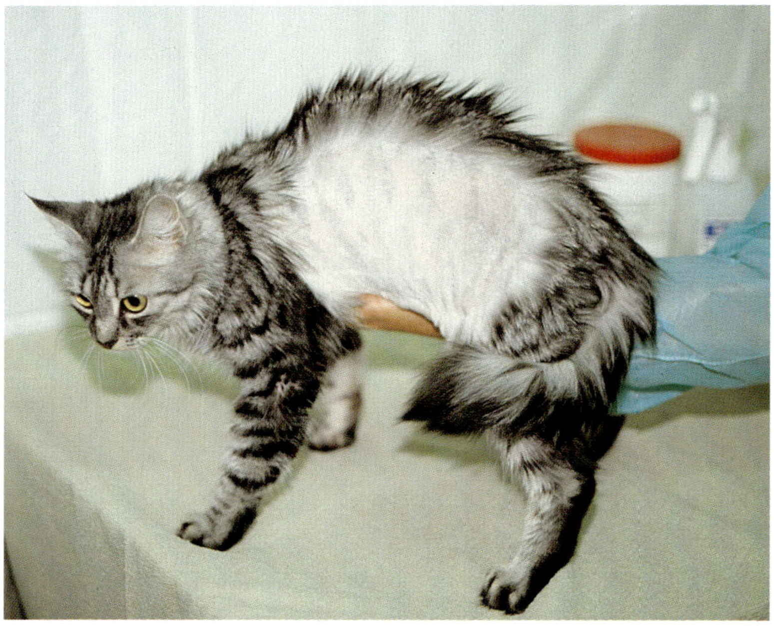

152, 153 Sufficient hair coat removal from the dorsolateral abdominal wall for displaying the kidneys in a cat with gas-filled intestines (**152**). Excessive hair coat removal for an abdominal scan in a cat (**153**).

Patient Positioning

Patient positioning is adapted to the examination in question. The animal should be positioned comfortably for the sonographic examination in order to avoid using excessive restraint. For speedier examinations and better results, the sonographer should always place the patient in the positions he or she most prefers.

Various position changes with different acoustic windows during the examination are helpful in gaining new sonographic perspectives and completing the findings. Echocardiography, for example, can be performed on a standing, sitting or laterally recumbent animal (**154–156**).

A table with a round or oval hole of variable size is extremely helpful for cardiological and abdominal ultrasonography (**157**). For echocardiography the patient is positioned in lateral recumbency over the oval hole with the transducer placed on the thoracic wall from underneath (**158**). The advantage of this method is that the heart moves towards the thoracic wall and lung interference is minimized.

154

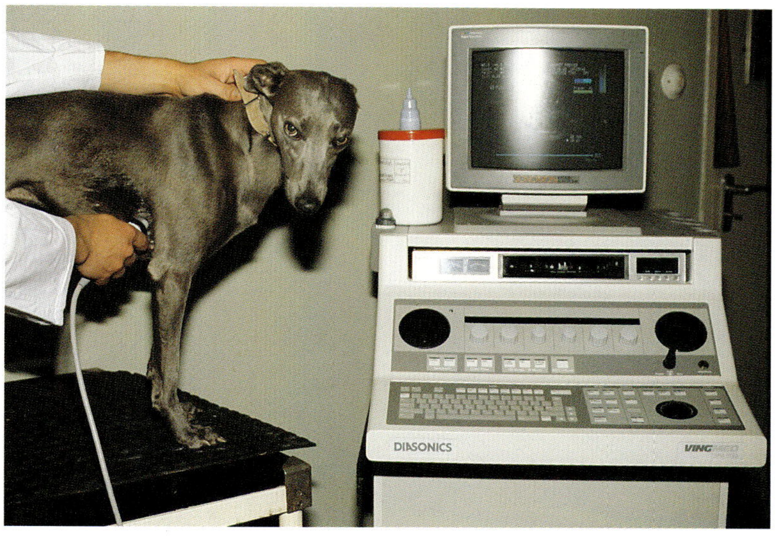

155

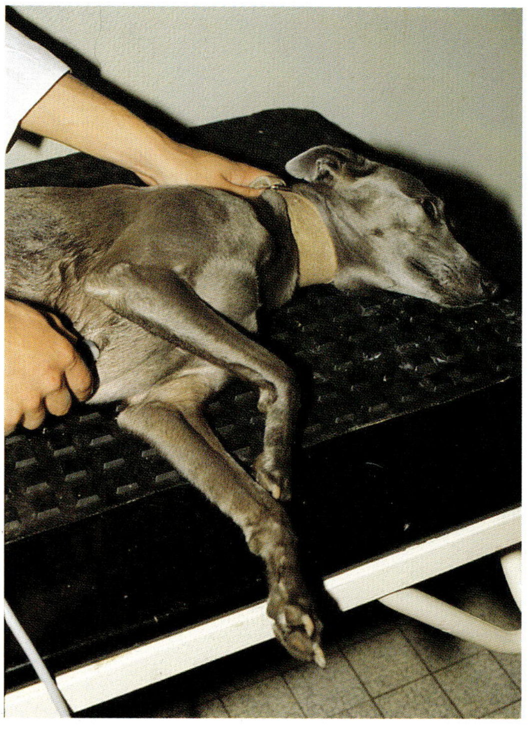

156

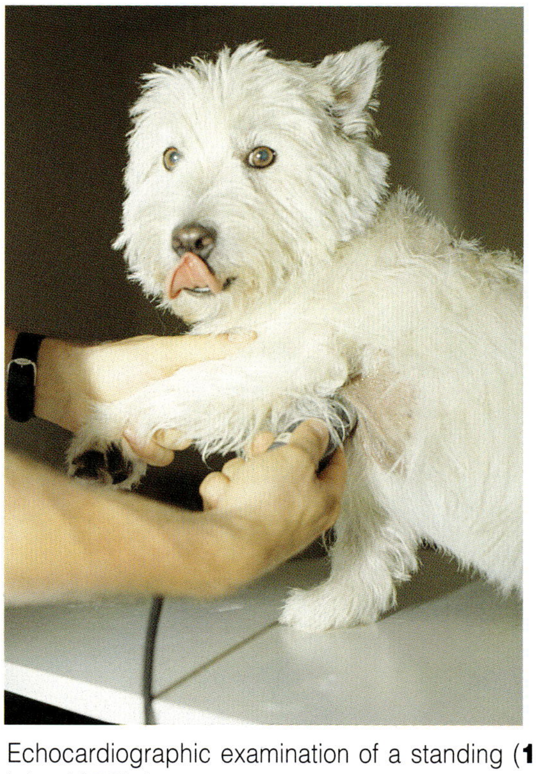

154–156 Echocardiographic examination of a standing (**154**), lying (**155**) and sitting (**156**) dog.

157

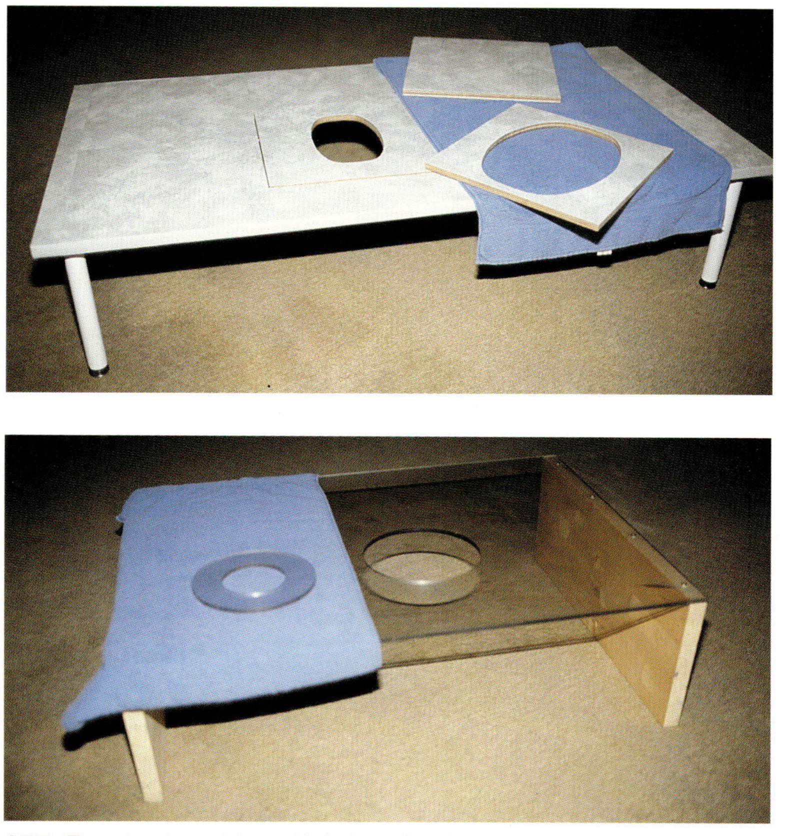

157 Examination tables with holes of various shapes and sizes.

158

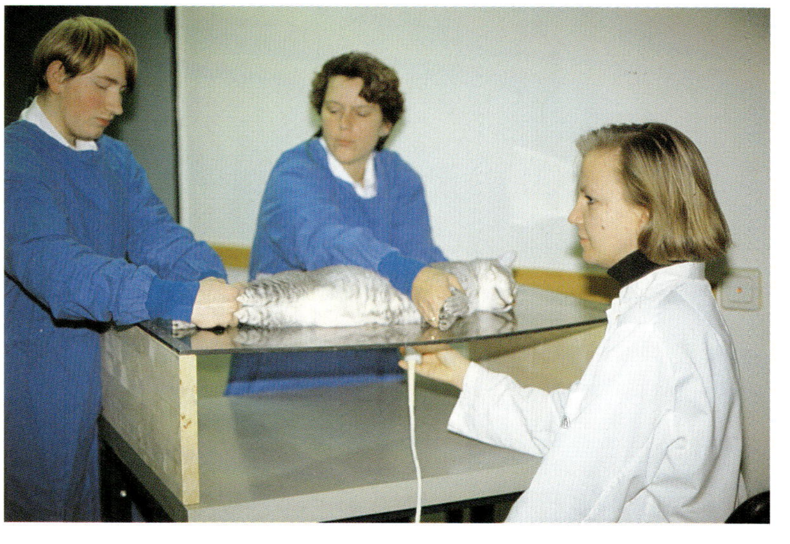

159

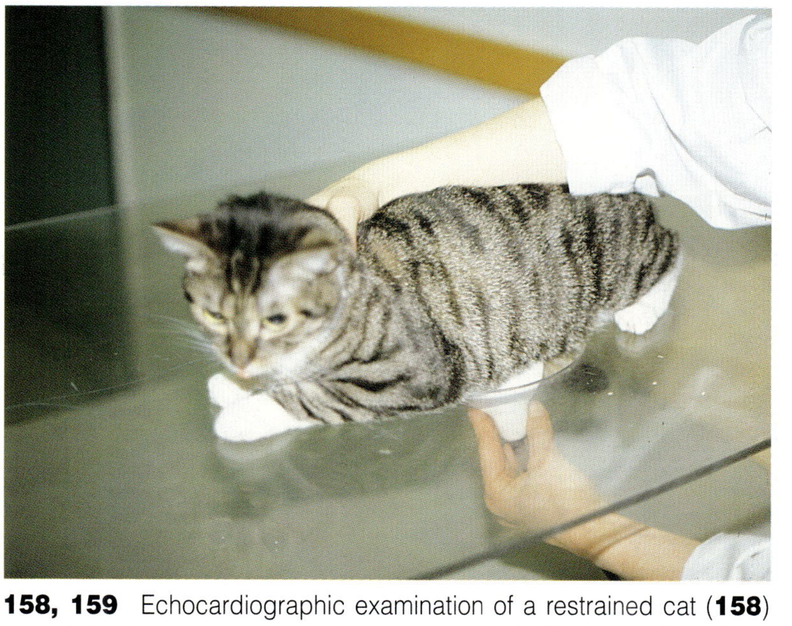

158, 159 Echocardiographic examination of a restrained cat (**158**) and abdominal examination of a relaxed cat (**159**) on a table with a round opening.

160

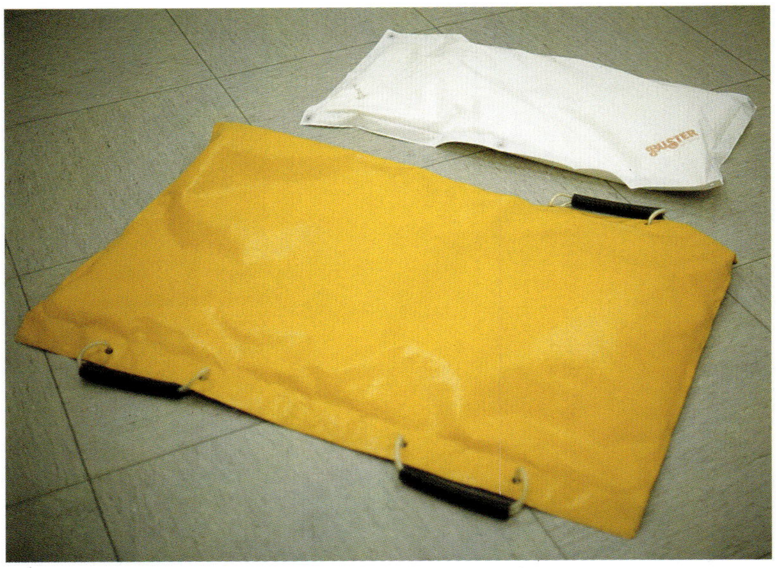

160 Padded surgical mats.

161

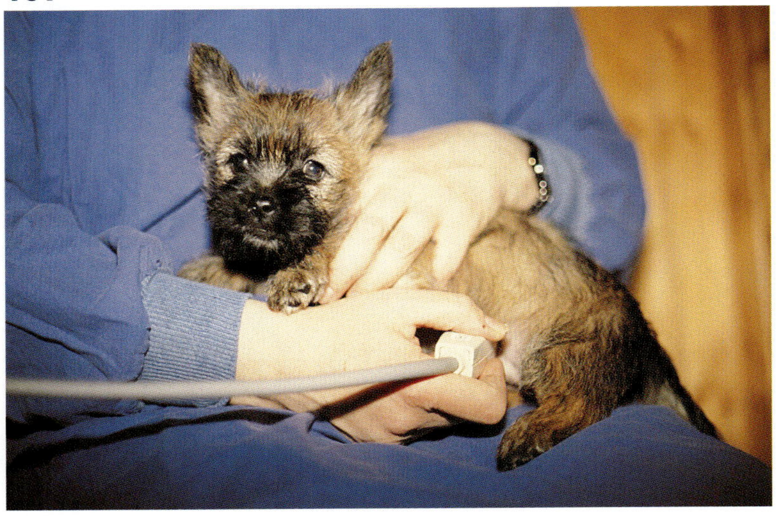

161 Abdominal ultrasonography of a puppy sitting on the sonographer's lap.

162

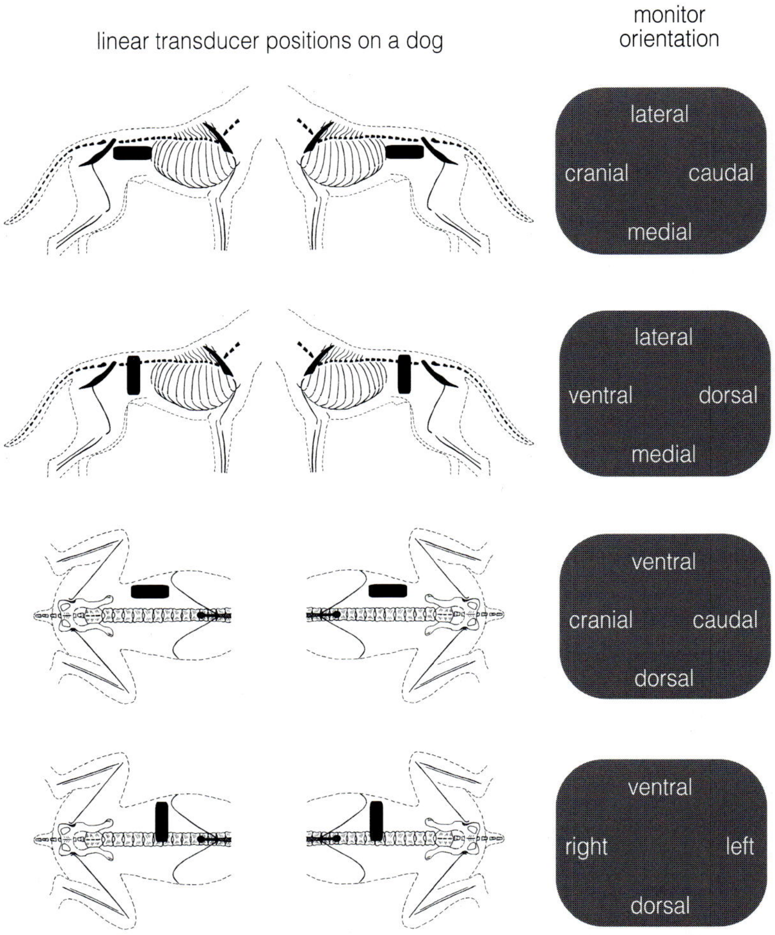

162 Orientation of the patient and of the monitor display in abdominal ultrasonography.

163

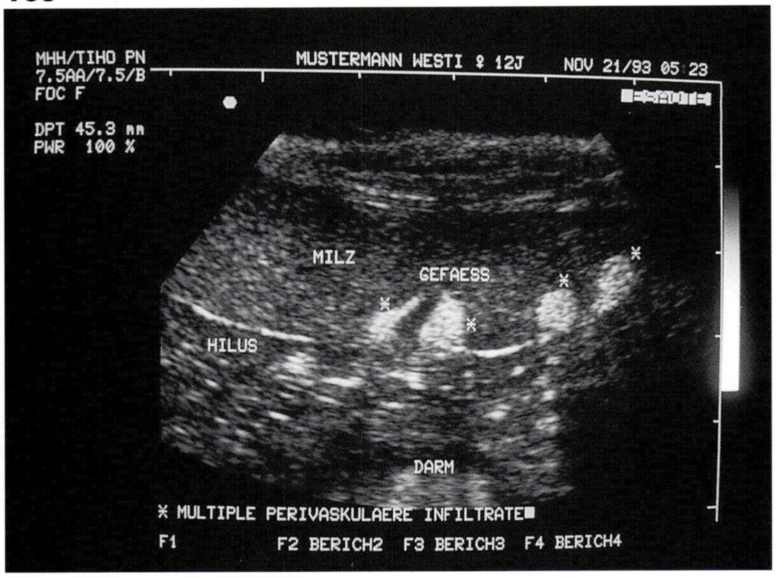

163 Urasound image: hilus = splenic hilus; milz = spleen; gefaess = vessel; multiple perivaskulaere infiltrate = multiple perivascular infiltrates.

164

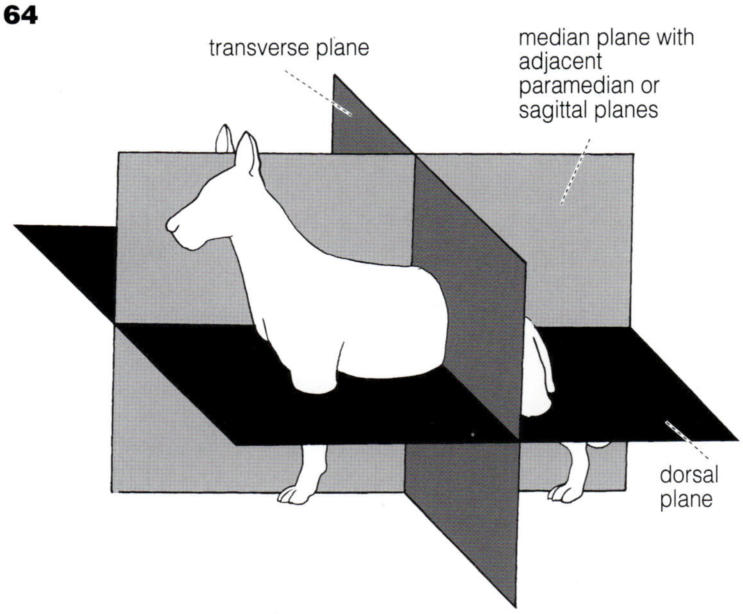

164 Schematic drawing of canine anatomical sections.

Abdominal ultrasonography in cats can also be performed on a table with a round or oval hole. The animals are placed in sternal recumbency over the hole with the transducer applied from beneath the animal through the small opening (**159**).

The animal can also be placed in dorsal recumbency on a padded mat or in a V-shaped trough for sonography of the abdomen and pelvis (**160**).

Longer sonographic examinations of puppies, kittens or docile cats can be done with the sonographer holding the animal on his lap. A right-handed person holds the animal with his left hand

165

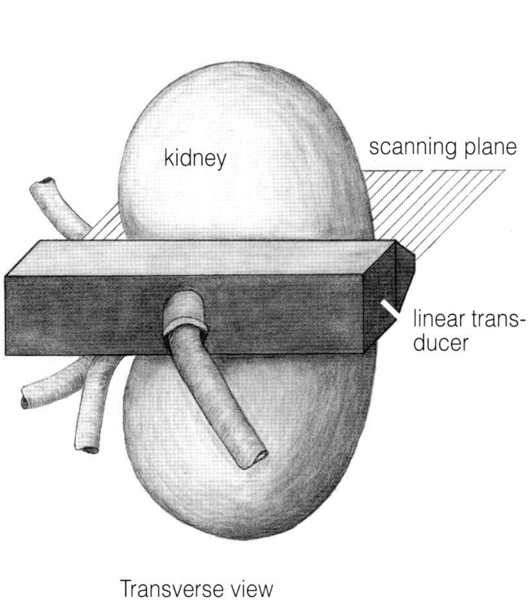

166

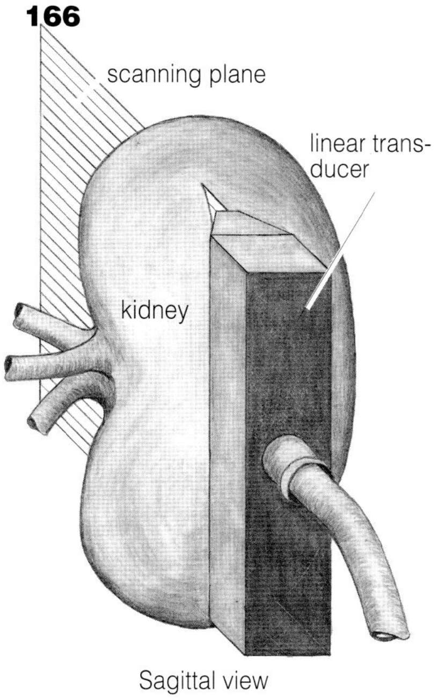

167

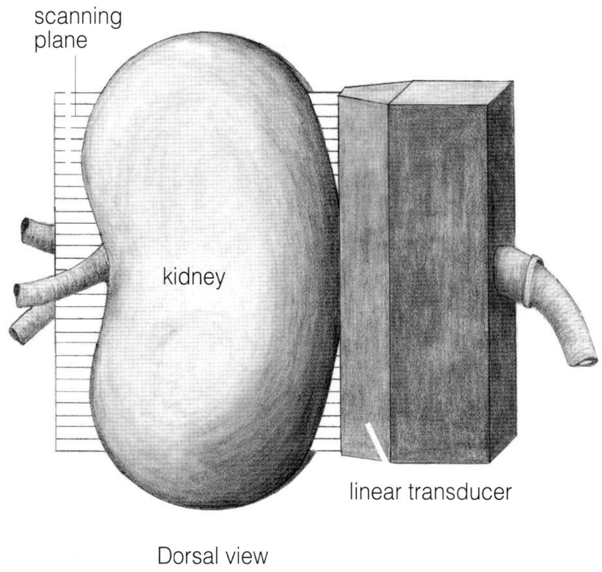

168

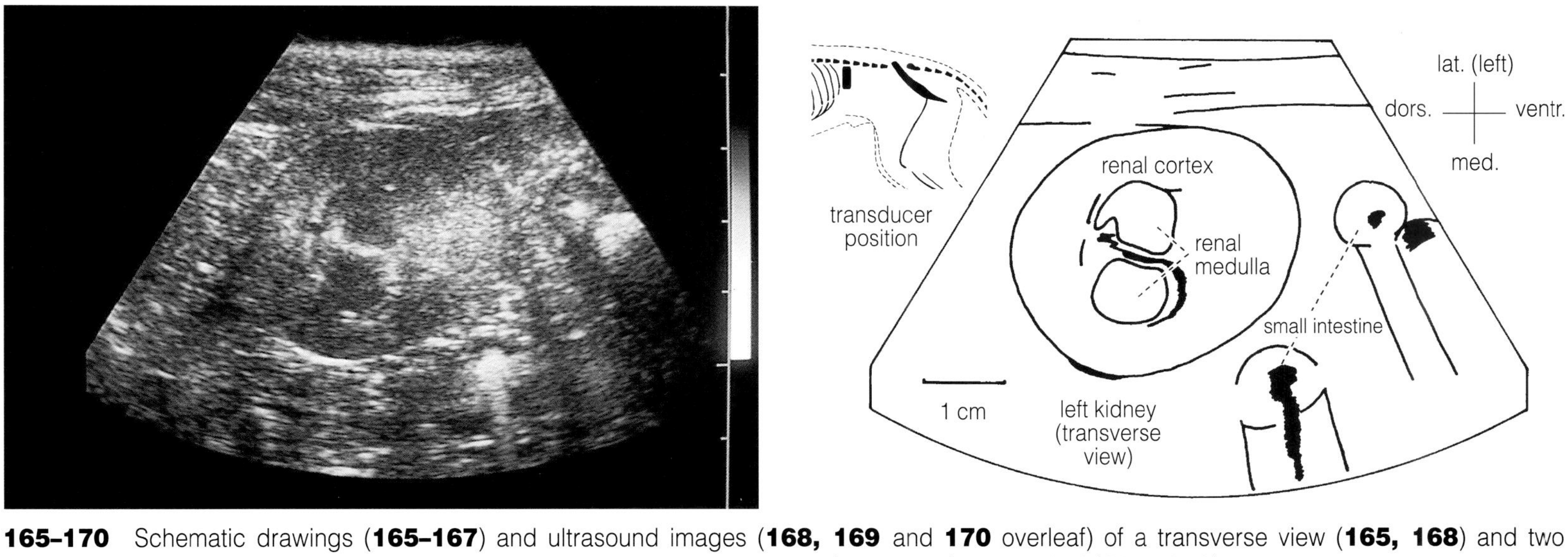

165–170 Schematic drawings (**165–167**) and ultrasound images (**168, 169** and **170** overleaf) of a transverse view (**165, 168**) and two perpendicular longitudinal views of a kidney. The longitudinal views are dorsal (**166, 169**) and sagittal (**167, 170**).

and applies the transducer to the ventral abdominal wall from below with his right hand. The animals are usually very relaxed during this procedure (161).

Image Orientation and Documentation

A uniform image orientation has not been achieved at the present time, even in human medicine. In most cases of cervical, abdominal and pelvic ultrasonography, the right side of the patient corresponds with the left side of the monitor display. Structures cranial to the animal are also displayed on the left side of the screen (162). Images of the heart usually show the heart base on the right side of the display and the apex to the left. The left heart is on the right side and the right heart is to the left of the image (see Echography of the Normal Heart, page 127). Although these image orientations are most commonly used, some sonographers prefer to orientate the displayed image on the opposite side. The labelling in this book is not uniform either. A satisfactory compromise for this inconsistency in publications is to mark the direction on the ultrasound image or the attached sketch with a 'compass-card' (165–167). A uniform orientation of curled fetuses lying in all directions is not plausible. Special image orientations of the eye or extremities are described in the various chapters.

Labelling of ultrasound images and video tapes should always include patient data. It is useful to label all visible structures on the images for clinical use (163). Pathological findings should, if possible, be marked with reference to the affected organ. Multiple views of the individual structures are necessary.

A written report of the sonographic findings should always follow the examination. *Table 7* lists the terminology used to describe an ultrasound image.

To evaluate the findings further, the written report should also include how effectively the animal could be scanned. Gas-filled intestines interfere with sonographic pregnancy monitoring and pulmonary oedema interferes with echocardiography. Some animals may just be difficult to scan without there being any reason.

Imaging planes are described following topographical anatomical nomenclature. Images are displayed in cross-sections or transverse planes and in sagittal, median, paramedian, dorsal and horizontal planes or longitudinal sections. These planes refer to the entire body (164). Organs are usually scanned in transverse views and two perpendicular longitudinal views (165–170). A transverse section of the heart is called a short-axis view; the longitudinal sections are referred to as long-axis views and apical two- or four-chamber views.

169

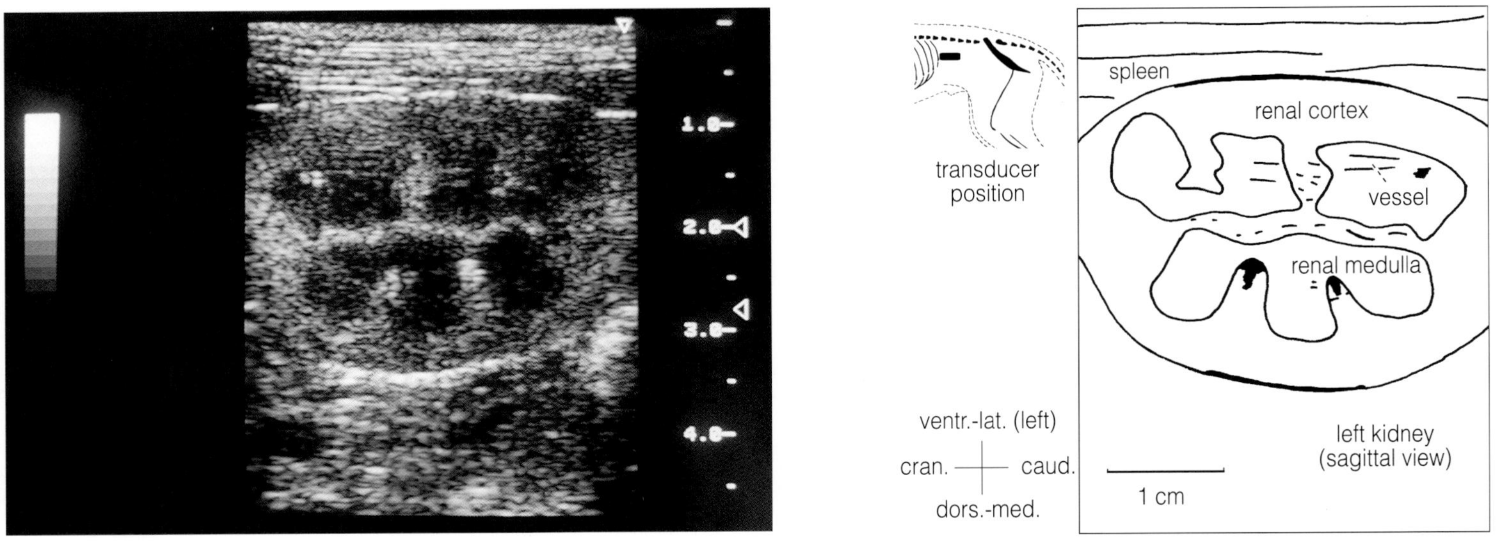

170

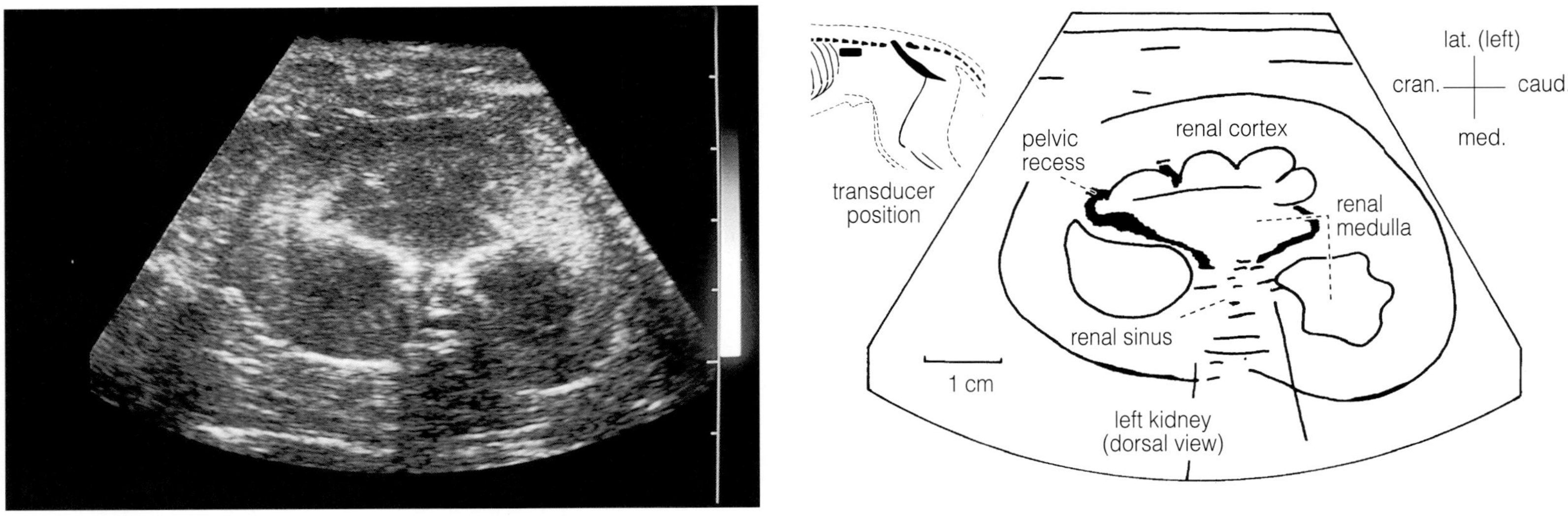

169, 170 Ultrasound images of a kidney (see also **165–168**).

References

1 Lorenz R (1991) *Dynamische Ultraschallanatomie des Abdomens. Leitfaden für Klinik und Praxis*. Hippokrates Verlag, Stuttgart.

2 Pickuth D, Grover CA and Bossi MC (1993) *Sonographie-systematisch*. BON-MED Verlag, Lorch.

PART II CLINICAL ULTRASONOGRAPHIC DIAGNOSIS

6 The Head

To date (1996), ultrasonography of the cranial region in dogs and cats has been limited to soft tissue structures such as muscles, the tongue, the salivary glands, the brain and the eye.

Sonography of the paranasal sinus using A-mode and/or two-dimensional imaging has been employed in human medicine since the late 1960s[7, 8, 10]. This technique is not relevant in veterinary medicine. Compared to humans, adult dogs and cats have thicker skulls and facial bones, which makes the examination more difficult. The same is true for the examination of the canine and feline temperomandibular joint, which is often examined sonographically in humans[6, 16]. In veterinary medicine, radiography is still the method of choice for diagnosing lesions in these areas.

Tongue

Cordula Poulsen Nautrup

High-frequency and high-resolution transducers with small contact areas can easily image cranial soft tissues including muscles and the tongue. The tongue has a characteristic sonographic appearance and should not be mistaken for other structures such as the salivary glands.

Anatomy and Normal Sonographic Findings

With the jaws closed, the tongue (*lingua*) fills almost the entire oral cavity (*cavum oris proprium*). It lies on the bottom of the oral cavity between the mandibular rami. The dorsal and lateral free tip (*apex linguae*) is fastened to the bottom of the oral cavity by the frenulum of the tongue (*frenulum linguae*). The caudal retrolingual region (*radix linguae*) is attached to the hyoid bone (*basihyoideum*) and is flanked on the sides by the paired horns of the hyoid bone (*ceratohyoideum*). The retrolingual region is supplied by various muscles from the bottom of the oral cavity. The lingual muscle (*M. lingualis proprius*) is covered by a mucous membrane. The course of the lingual muscle fibres follows through all three planes. The lyssa is located rostroventrally in the lingual apex and consists of fatty tissue, striated muscles and cartilage.

The scanning positions for the tongue are situated ventrally between the mandibular rami and reach as far as the ventral neck area. Because of the small scanning area, it is best to use sector transducers for the examination.

The tongue has a characteristic shape and a typical arrangement of the lingual muscles. The sonographic image, especially the transverse view, is therefore distinctive.

In the dog the shape of the tongue varies from trapezoid (rostral) to square (caudal). The ventral muscles and the frenulum divide the tongue into two rounded sections of equal size. The dorsal median groove is without sonograpic findings. The tongue itself varies in echogenicity from hyperechoic (ventral) to hypoechoic (dorsal). Echo distribution is homogenous. The tongue is demarcated by a fine anechoic inner margin and a hyperechoic outer margin. Large lingual vessels are displayed as anechoic, round structures. The muscles and/or the frenulum reach into the tongue at a ventromedian angle. A hyperechoic line displays the dorsal margin to the oral cavity.

The transverse view of the tongue in a cat is trapezoid to oval. An oval, hypoechoic area from the centre to the dorsal surface of the tongue is surrounded ventrally and laterally by tissue of moderate echogenicity (**171, 172–175**). The finely granulated echoes are arranged homogenously. The outer margin is displayed as both an anechoic and a hyperechoic double line. The dorsal surface of the tongue is hyperechoic because of the acoustic interface with the air in the oral cavity. The lyssa cannot be visualized in either dogs or cats.

In a longitudinal plane the tongue is uniformly hypoechoic. The ventral longitudinal vessels can be seen as straight, anechoic structures in the dog.

In real-time ultrasonography the tongue retractions can be displayed during swallowing. Dynamic two-dimensional ultrasonography is used to assess lingual function and the act of swallowing in human medicine[5].

171

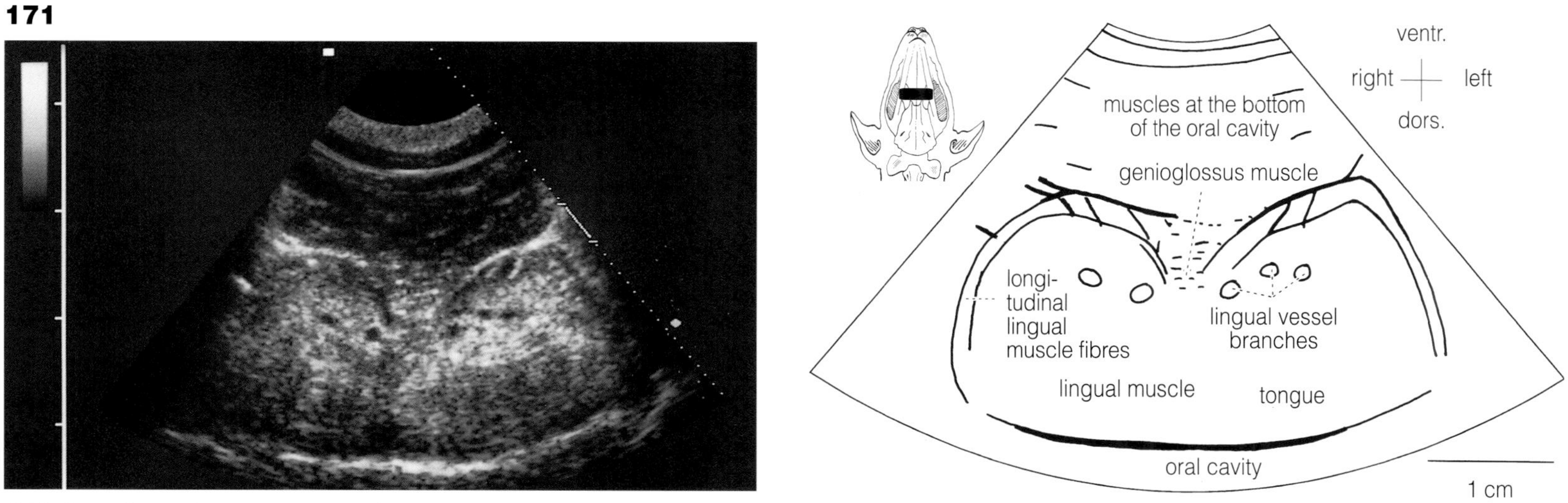

171 Two-dimensional sonogram of a dog. Transverse view of a normal tongue directly rostral to the mandibular rami.

172

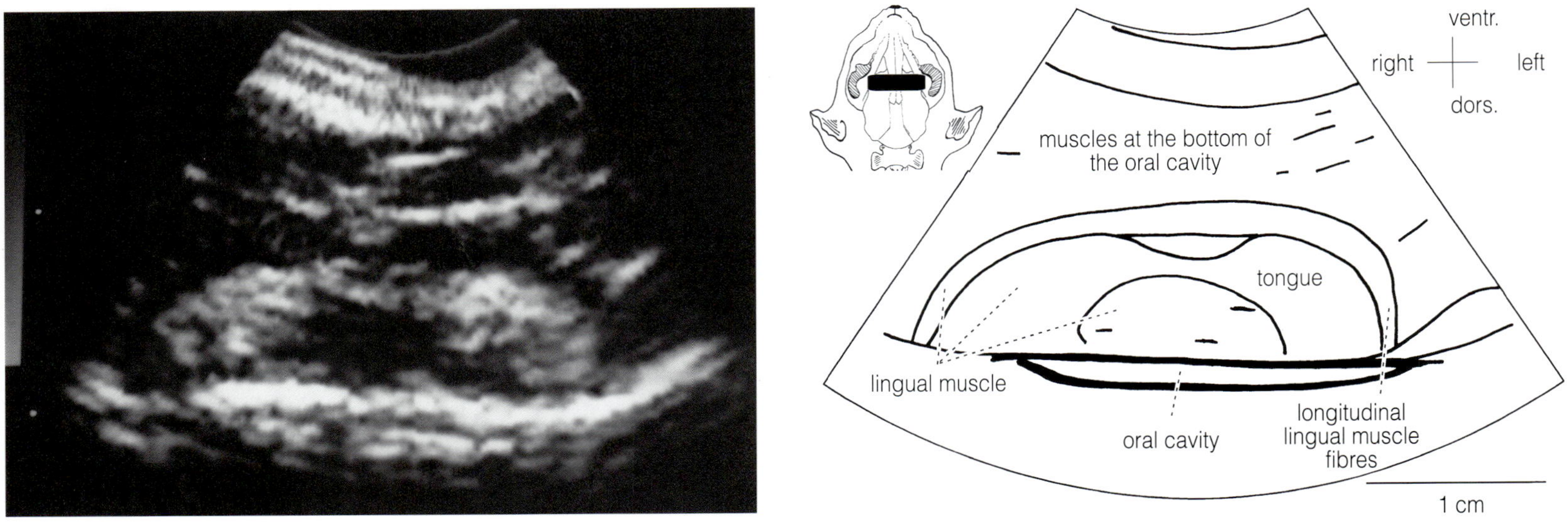

173

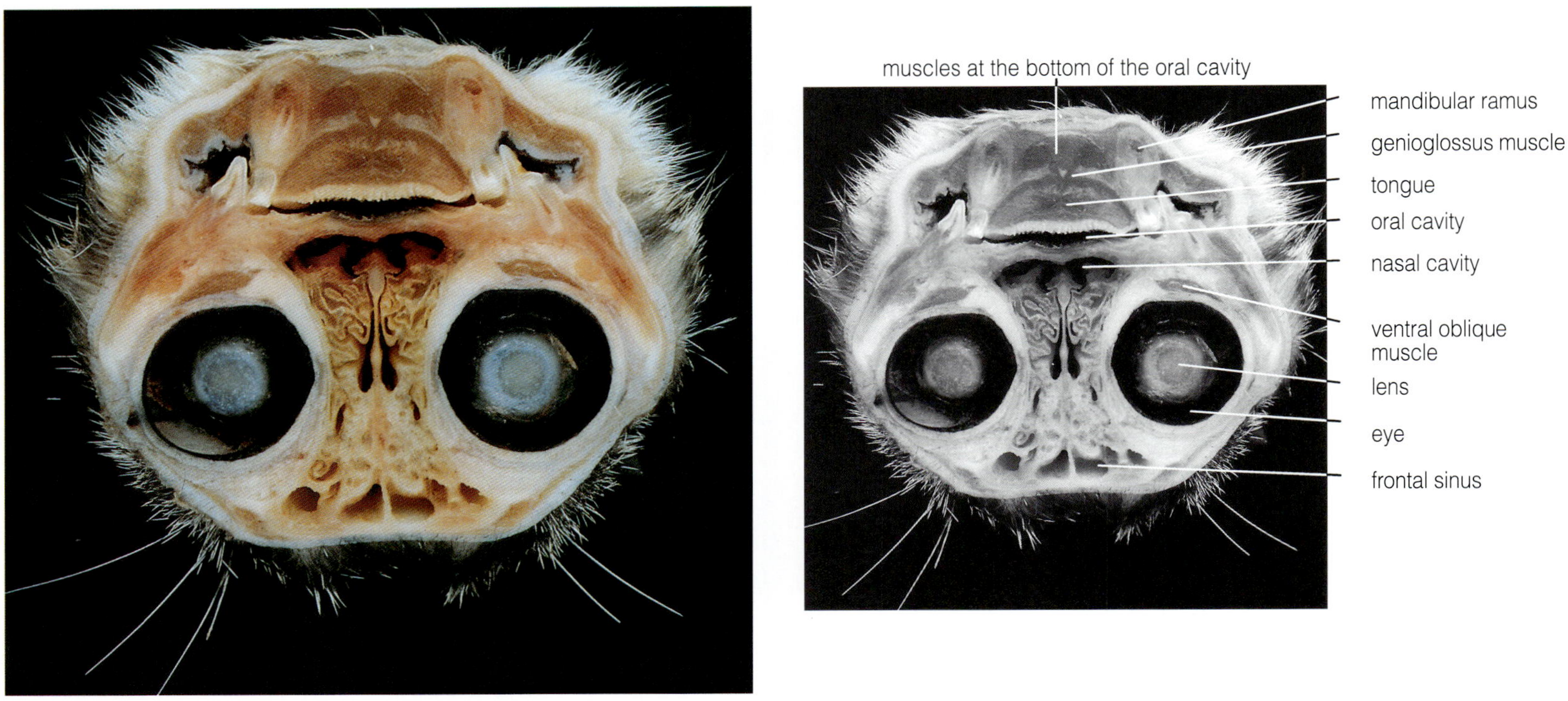

172, 173 Two-dimensional sonogram (**172**) and anatomical section (**173**) of cats. Transverse views of a normal tongue. (See also **174, 175**.)

Sonography of Tongue Disease

Sonographic findings in tongue disease include foreign bodies and neoplasia. A non-metallic foreign body deep in the retrolingual region is better seen sonographically than radiographically[18]. In principle, visual and radiographic examinations should always precede ultrasonography. Inflammatory and neoplastic lesions of the tongue are displayed as non-uniform areas of mixed echogenicity. Inflammation of the mucous membranes should be limited to a visual examination.

Salivary Glands

Cordula Poulsen Nautrup and Hans-Josef Heider

The canine and feline salivary glands (*Gll. salivariae*) include the parotid, mandibular, sublingual and zygomatic salivary glands. Of these, the normal mandibular salivary gland is most easily accessible for ultrasonography.

Instrumentation and Examination Technique

High-resolution transducers with frequencies of 7.5 MHz or, preferably, 10 MHz and higher are used for examination of the salivary glands. Since the skin contact area in the caudal head and cranial neck region is small and uneven, sector transducers should be employed. The salivary glands are located superficially, only a few millimetres under the skin. For this reason, a stand-off pad can help to smooth the uneven surface. Small 10 MHz linear transducers do not need a stand-off pad, although they are usually too long and too wide to examine the head of small to medium-sized dogs or cats. Transbulbar imaging of the zygomatic salivary gland follows the same requirements as ocular ultrasonography.

Anatomy and Normal Sonographic Findings

The parotid salivary gland (*Gl. parotis*) is small, thin and triangular. It is situated directly under the skin and the thin parotideoauricular muscle. The pre- and postauricular ends surround the auricular cartilage. The superficial parotid duct (*Ductus parotideus*) courses across the masseter muscle and opens into the oral cavity at the upper canine tooth. The mandibular salivary gland (*Gl. mandibularis*) is a relatively large, round, globoid structure located ventral to the parotid gland and partially covered by the gland (**176**). It is

174

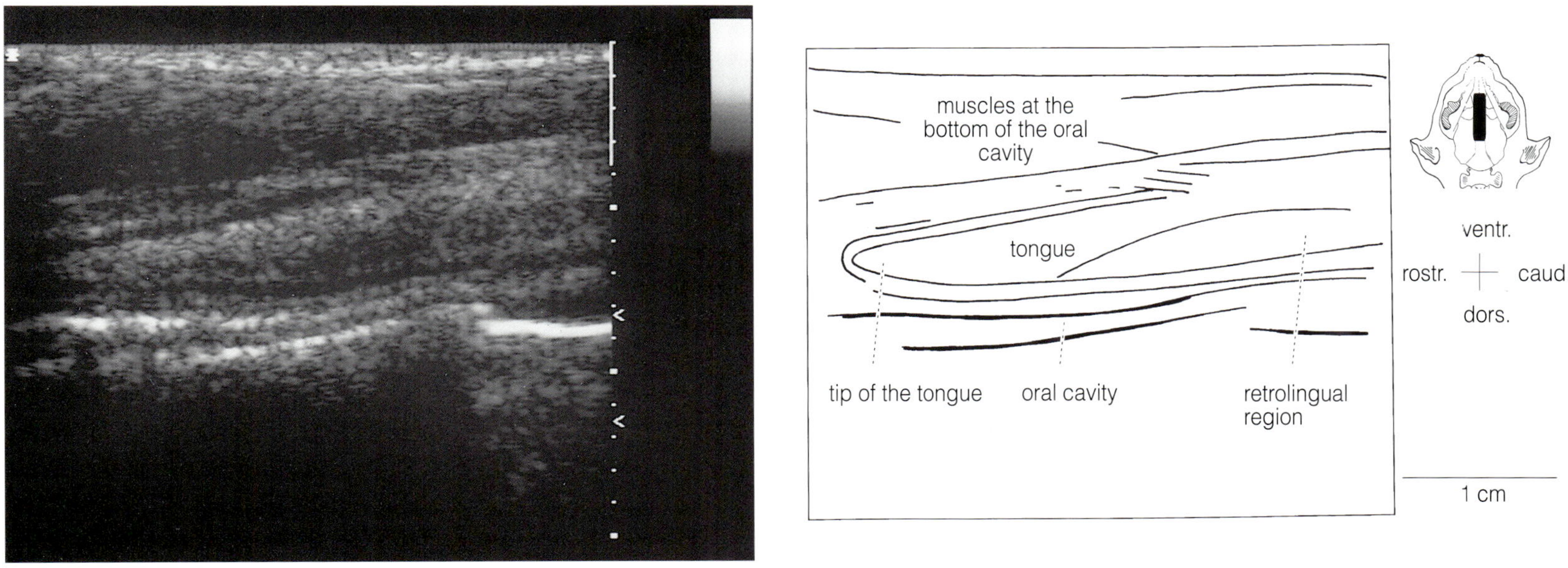

175

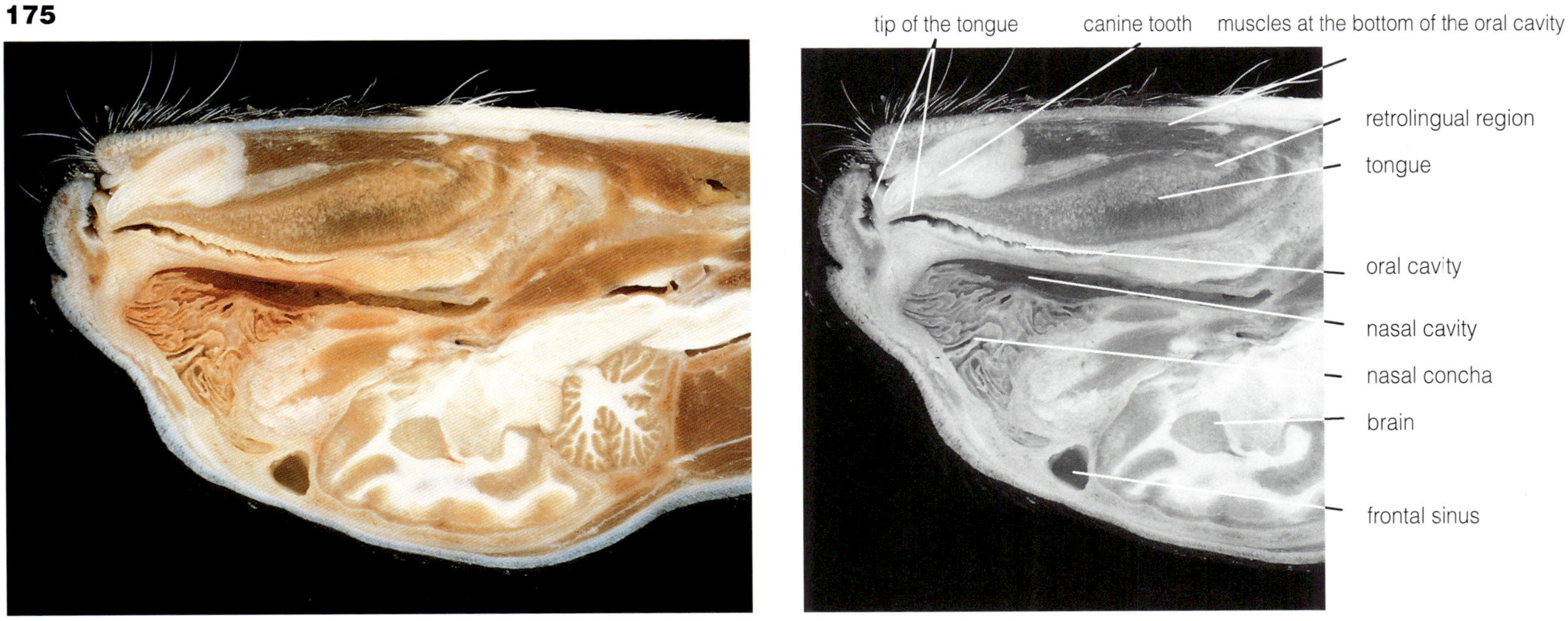

174, 175 Two-dimensional sonogram (**174**) and anatomical section (**175**) of cats. Sagittal views of a normal tongue. (See also **172, 173**.)

176

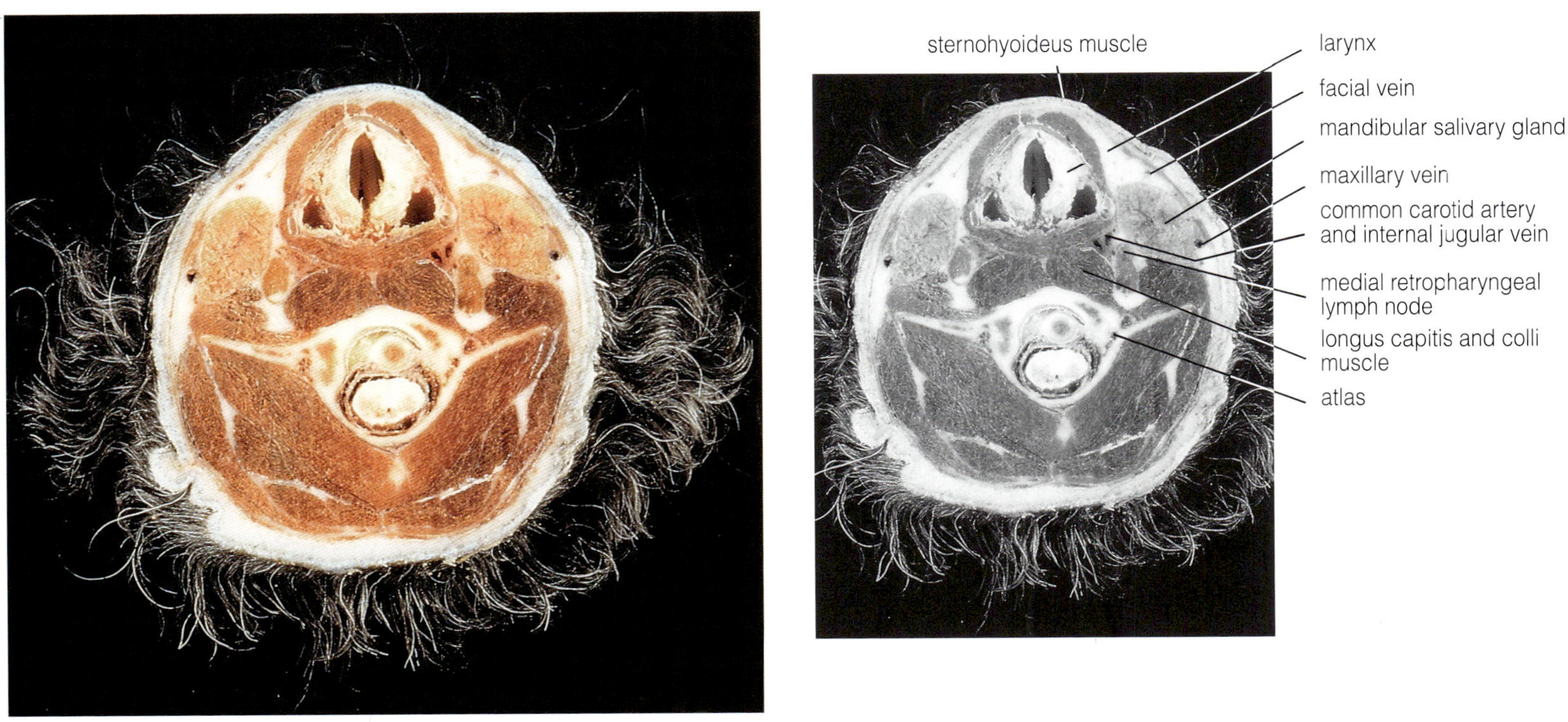

176 Anatomical cross-section of the canine mandibular salivary gland.

177

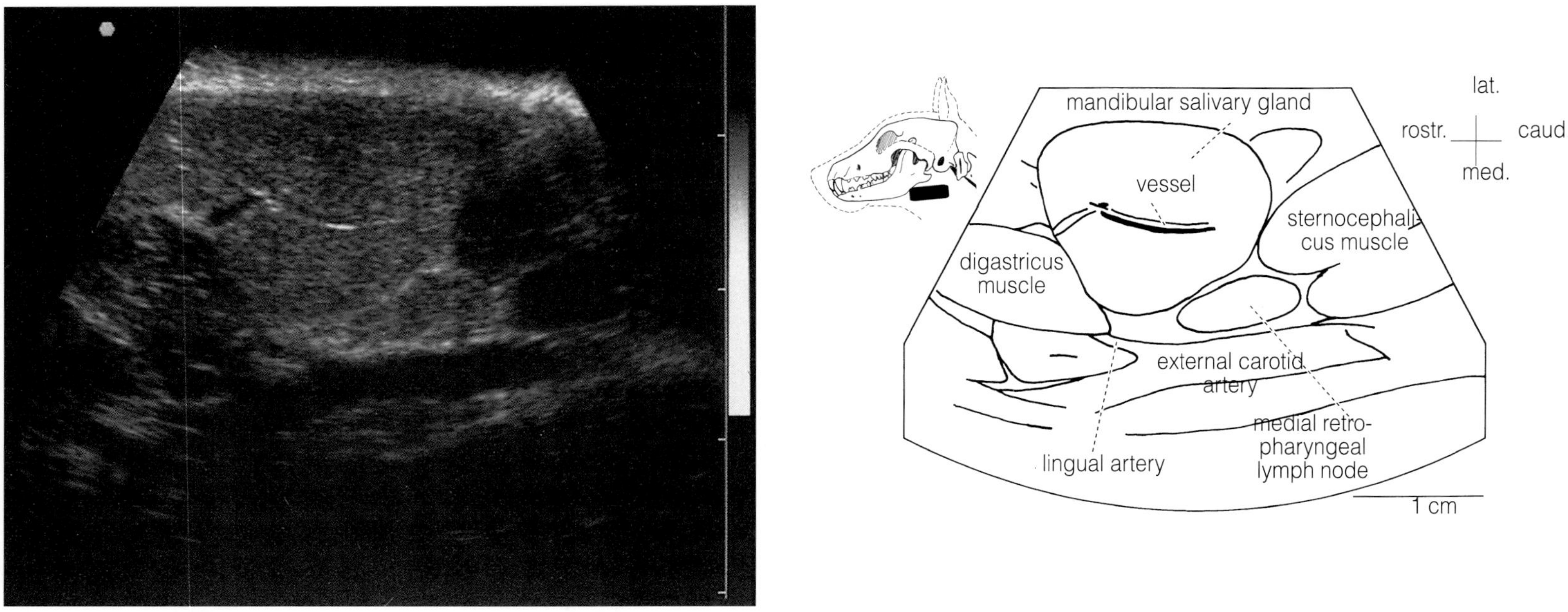

177 Two-dimensional sonogram of a dog. Normal mandibular salivary gland in a dorsal long-axis view.

178

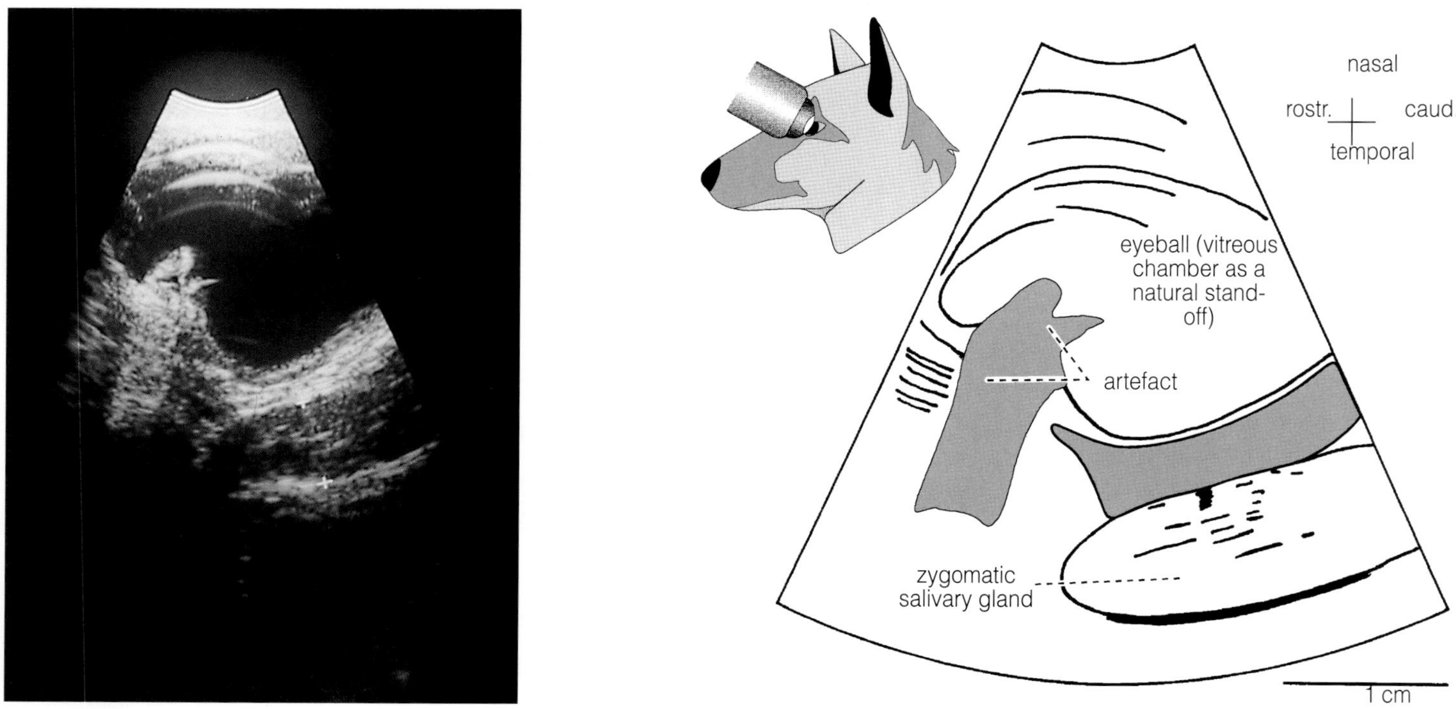

178 Two-dimensional transocular sonogram of a dog. Normal zygomatic salivary gland in a longitudinal plane.

situated caudal to the angle of the mandible and caudoventral to the bifurcation of the maxillary and linguofacial veins. The mandibular lymph nodes are ventral and cranial to the mandibular salivary gland. The monostomatic sublingual salivary gland (*Gl. sublinguialis monostomatica*) is located rostral to the mandibular salivary gland and medial to the mandibular ramus. The mandibular and sublingual salivary ducts run parallel within the muscles at the bottom of the oral cavity.

The parotid salivary gland is scanned directly ventral, cranial and caudal to the cartilage of the ear canal. The image of the normal, thin gland varies. The parenchyma shows low to moderate echogenicity with uniform echoes.

The scanning position for the mandibular salivary gland is caudoventral to the auricular region and caudal to the mandibular ramus. The mandibular salivary gland is large and round to oval in shape (**177**). The parenchyma is moderately echogenic and relatively homogenous, surrounded by a hyperechoic capsule. The interstitial fibrous tissue and vessel walls are seen as central hyperechoic echoes in a long-axis view of the gland. The mandibular salivary gland should not be mistaken for the small, uniformly hypoechoic mandibular lymph nodes located ventral and rostral to the gland. The well-demarcated, uniformly hypoechoic medial retropharyngeal lymph node is seen medial to the mandibular salivary gland. The maxillary and linguofacial veins located lateral to the mandibular salivary gland are compressed by transducer application and should not be used as sonographic landmarks. The external carotid artery, lingual artery and facial artery are easily visualized deep to the mandibular salivary gland.

The monostomatic sublingual salivary gland is sometimes difficult to separate from the mandibular salivary gland. It is positioned more rostral and is smaller and more hypoechoic.

The zygomatic salivary gland (*Gl. zygomatica*) is located ventral to the orbital fibrous tissue and rostromedial to the zygomatic arch. Imaging of this gland is accomplished through ocular sonography.

179

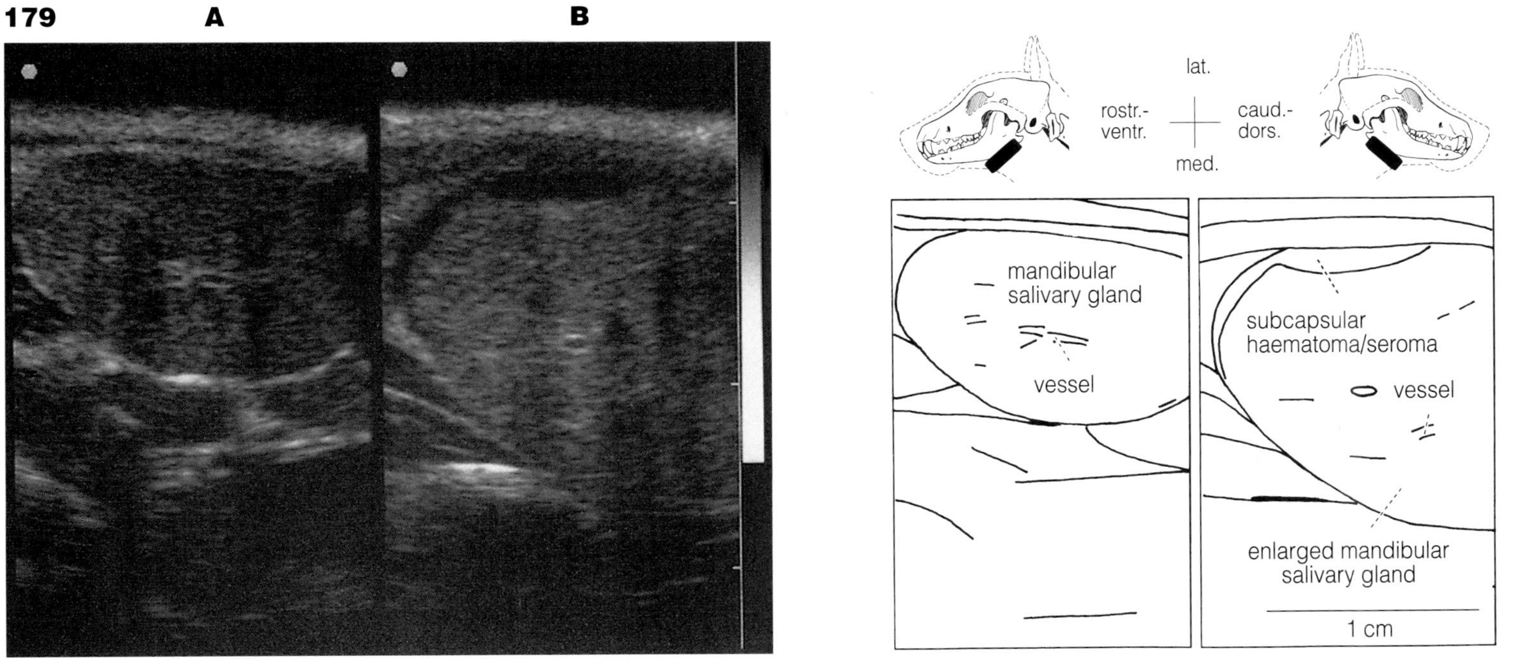

180

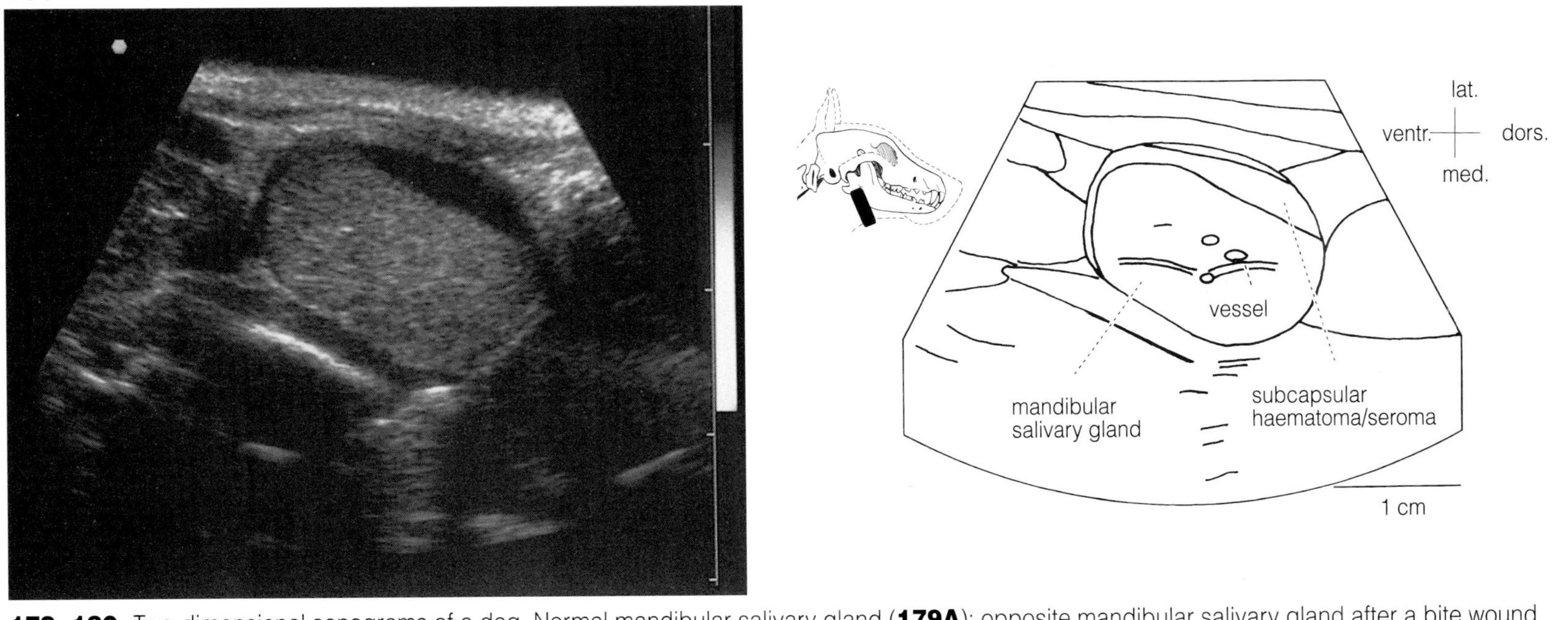

179, 180 Two-dimensional sonograms of a dog. Normal mandibular salivary gland (**179A**); opposite mandibular salivary gland after a bite wound with inflammatory enlargement (**179B**); distinct subcapsular haematoma and seroma (**180**).

The scanning positions are on the eyeball, dorsal to the nasal canthus. The zygomatic salivary gland is oval in a long-axis view and round in a transverse plane. The hypoechoic gland contains various vessels and is surrounded by a hyperechoic margin (178).

Normal salivary ducts cannot be differentiated sonographically.

Sonography of Salivary Gland Abnormalities

Indications for ultrasonography of the salivary glands include all masses on the cheek ventral to the ear and/or caudal to the mandibular ramus, as well as masses under the tongue. Differential diagnosis for an exophthalmus should always consider abnormalities of the zygomatic salivary gland.

Cystic lesions of the mandibular and sublingual salivary glands or their ducts (*meliceris* – neck cyst; *ranula* – sublingual cyst) appear as well-demarcated, anechoic structures with echogenic particles floating within the fluid or attached to the wall. Echogenic septa can reach into the anechoic area. Cystic lesions cannot always be connected to the right salivary gland or duct[1].

Sialitis produces enlargement of the salivary gland without altering the echogenicity. Abscesses are usually non-uniform, ranging from anechoic to hyperechoic. In some cases they are anechoic and cannot be differentiated from cysts. Traumatic haematomas close to the gland capsule also produce masses in the head and neck region. This may lead to enlargement of the adjacent salivary gland. Acute to subacute haematomas are anechoic in the ultrasound image (179, 180).

While the normal salivary ducts are not visualized sonographically, obstruction of these ducts will produce dilated, anechoic structures. An obstruction near the orifice cannot be visualized sonographically. An obstructed parotid duct appears as a large, anechoic structure coursing over the cheek or masseter muscle (181). The dilated salivary duct is displayed with an extremely thin wall. Threadlike, floating echoes within the duct suggest inflammatory debris.

181

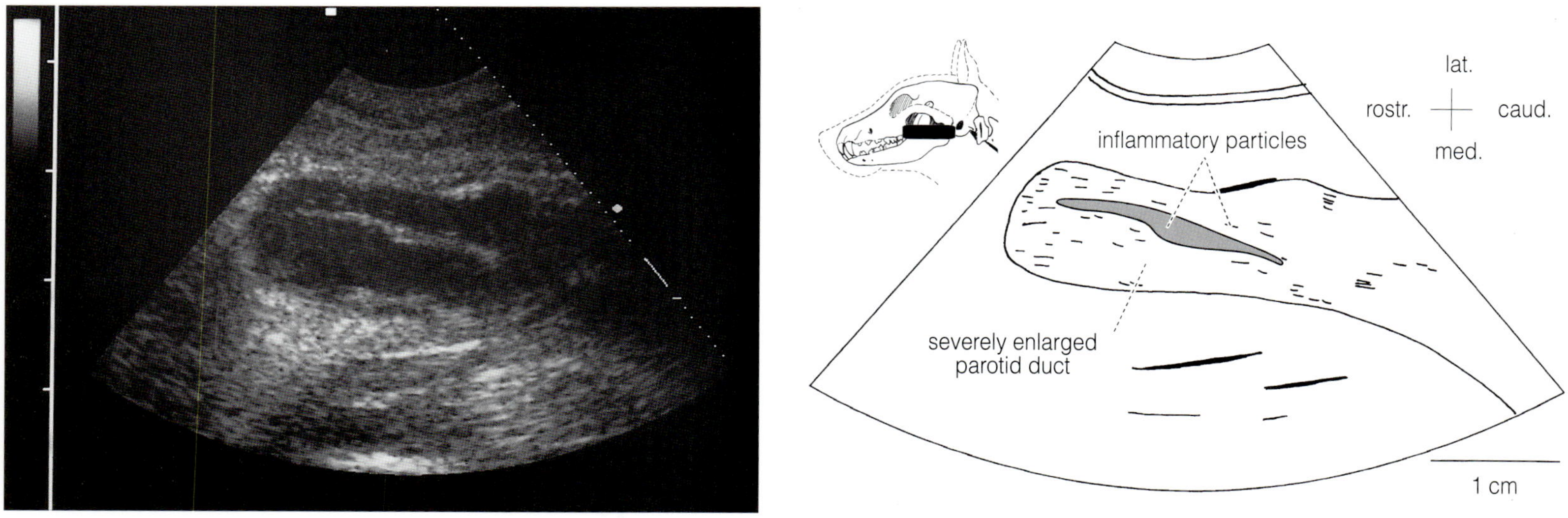

181 Two-dimensional sonogram of a dog. Congested and inflamed parotid duct caused by an obstruction.

Brain

Cordula Poulsen Nautrup

Instrumentation and Examination Technique

Ultrasonography of the brain, especially in puppies and kittens, requires high-resolution transducers (7.5 to 10 MHz) with a near-field focus. Since the contact area is small and uneven, sector probes and very small linear transducers are required.

Young animals are placed on the sonographer's lap for the examination. Hair coat clipping is not necessary if enough coupling gel is used. Transverse and sagittal images of the brain are obtained through the palpable, open rostral fontanelle. Transcutaneous sonography of the canine and feline brain is not possible

182

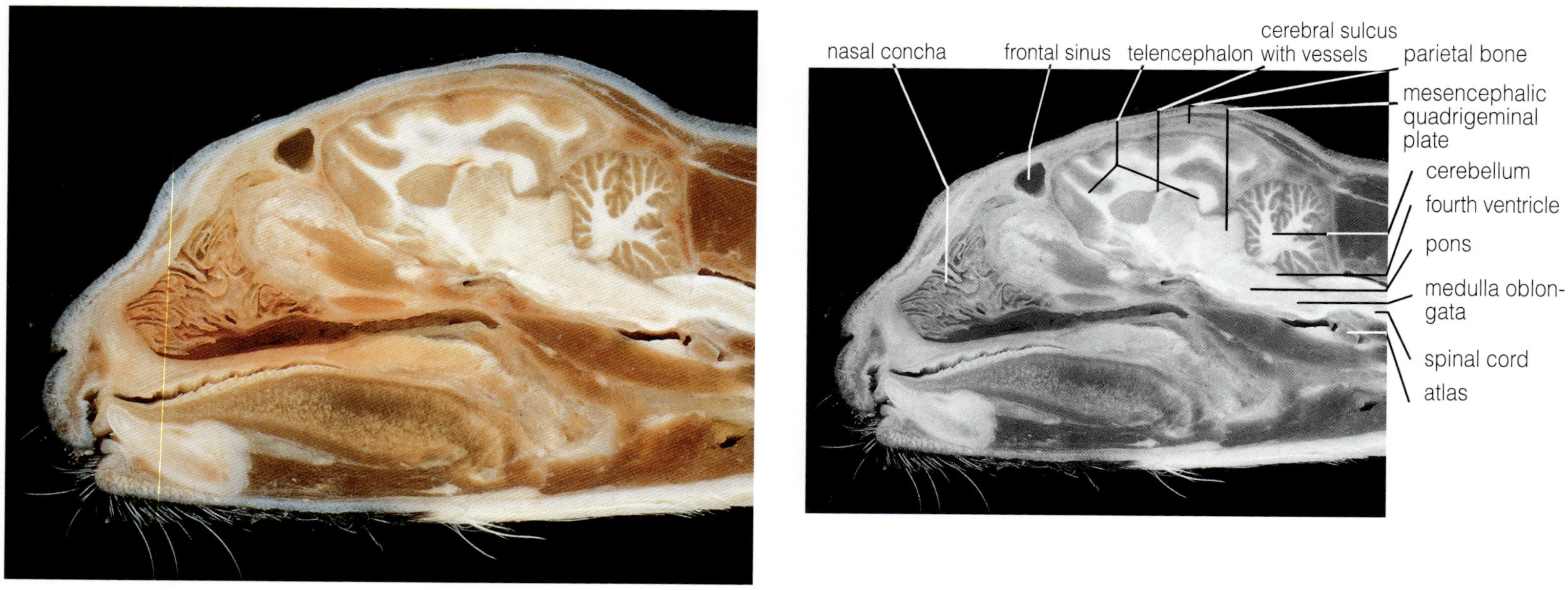

183

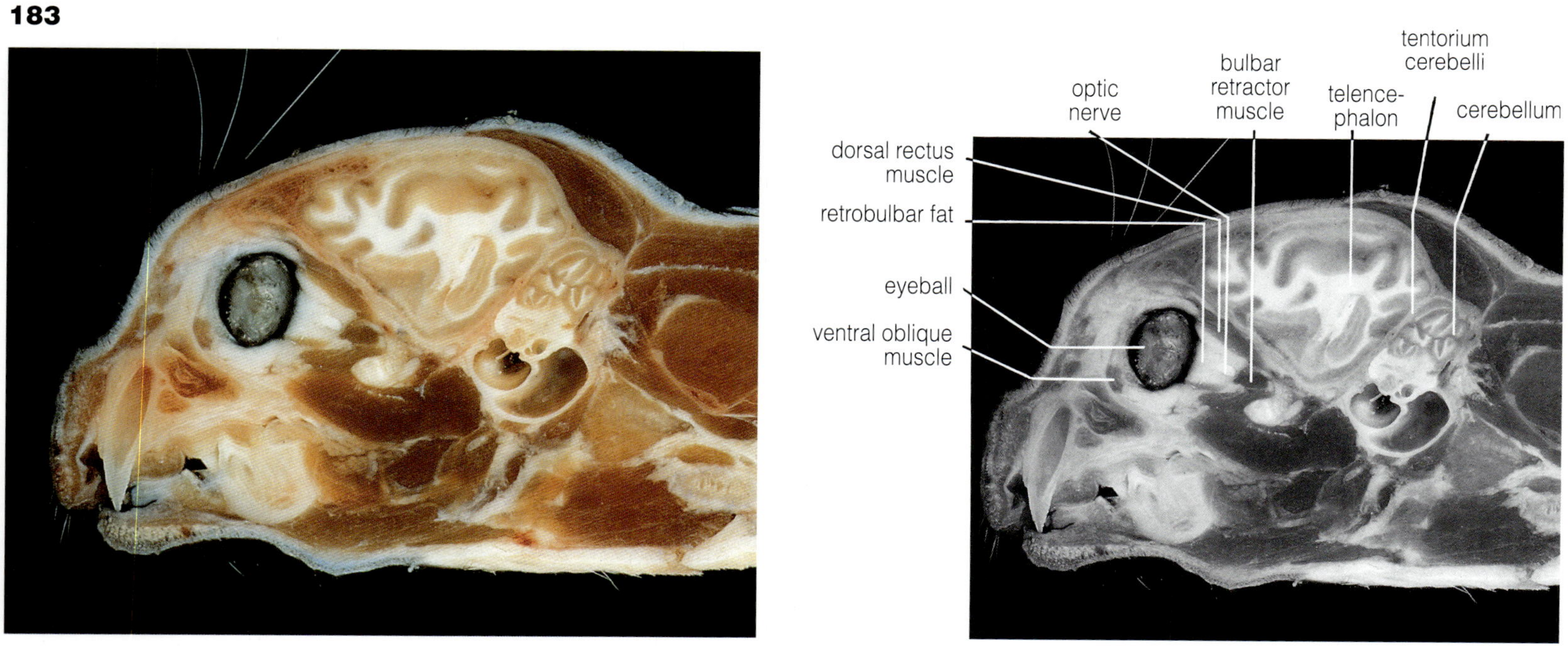

184

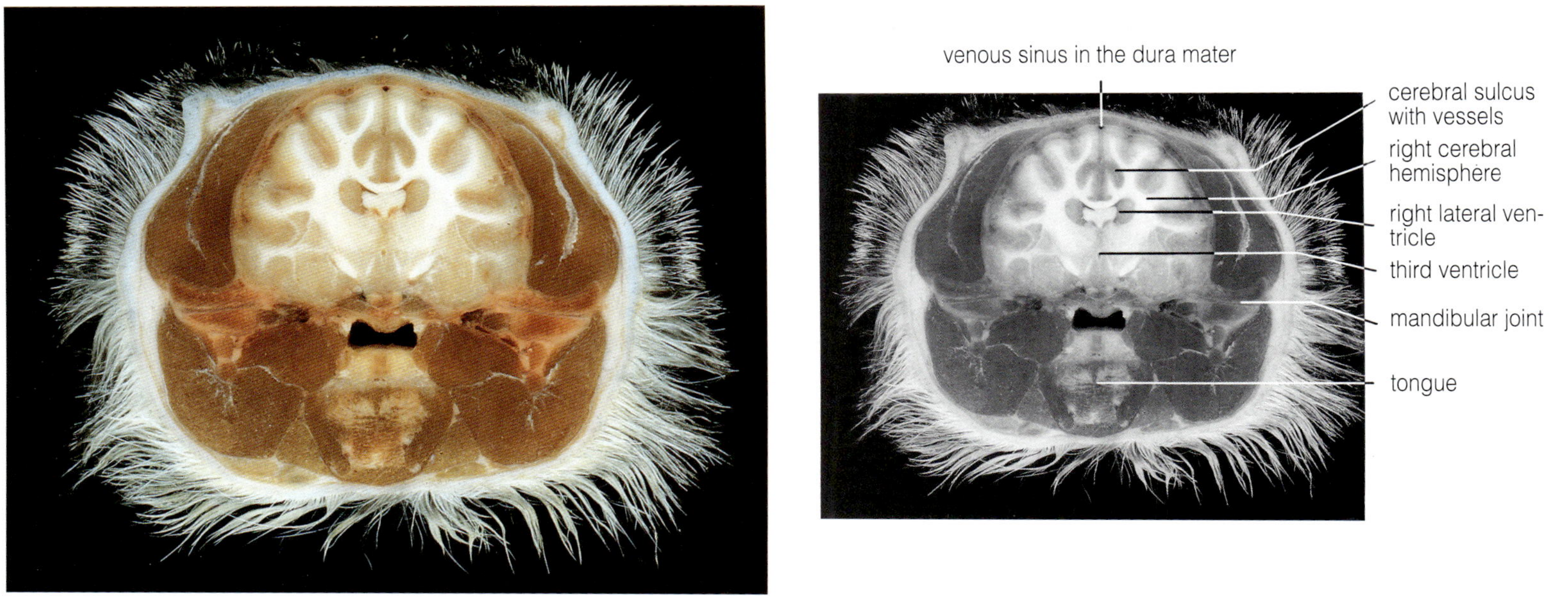

185

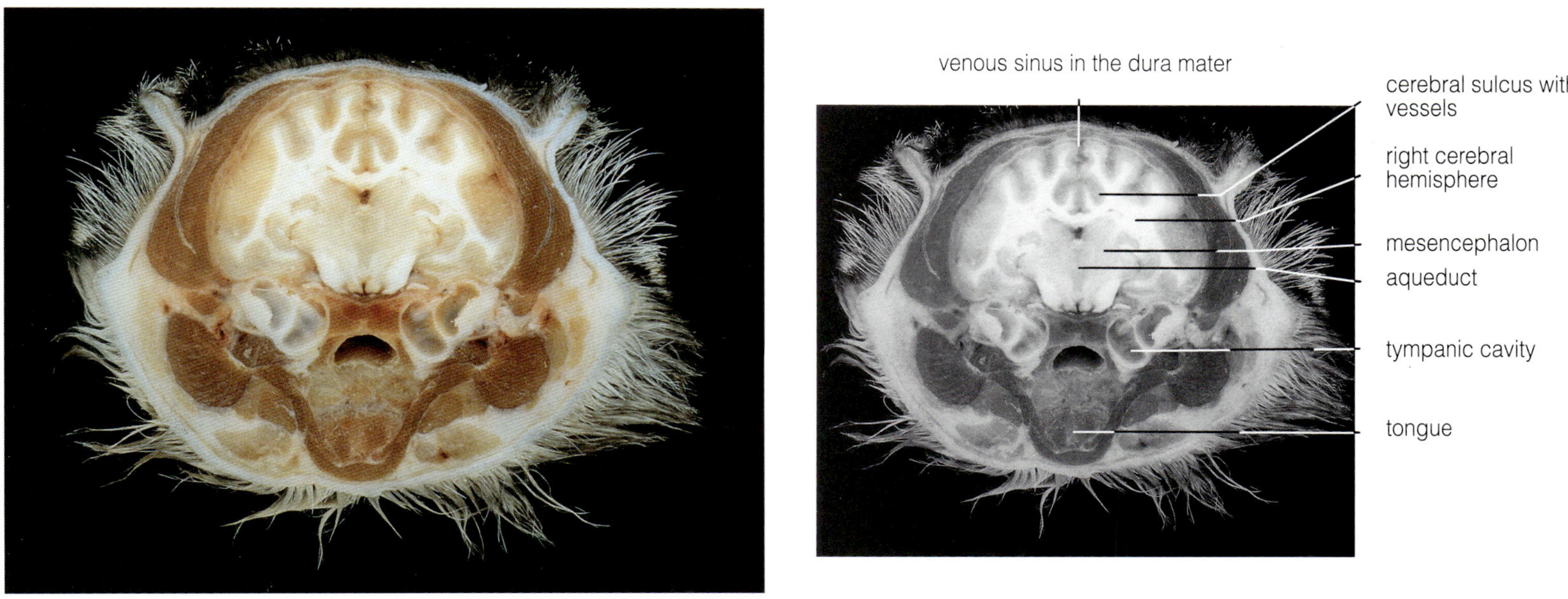

186

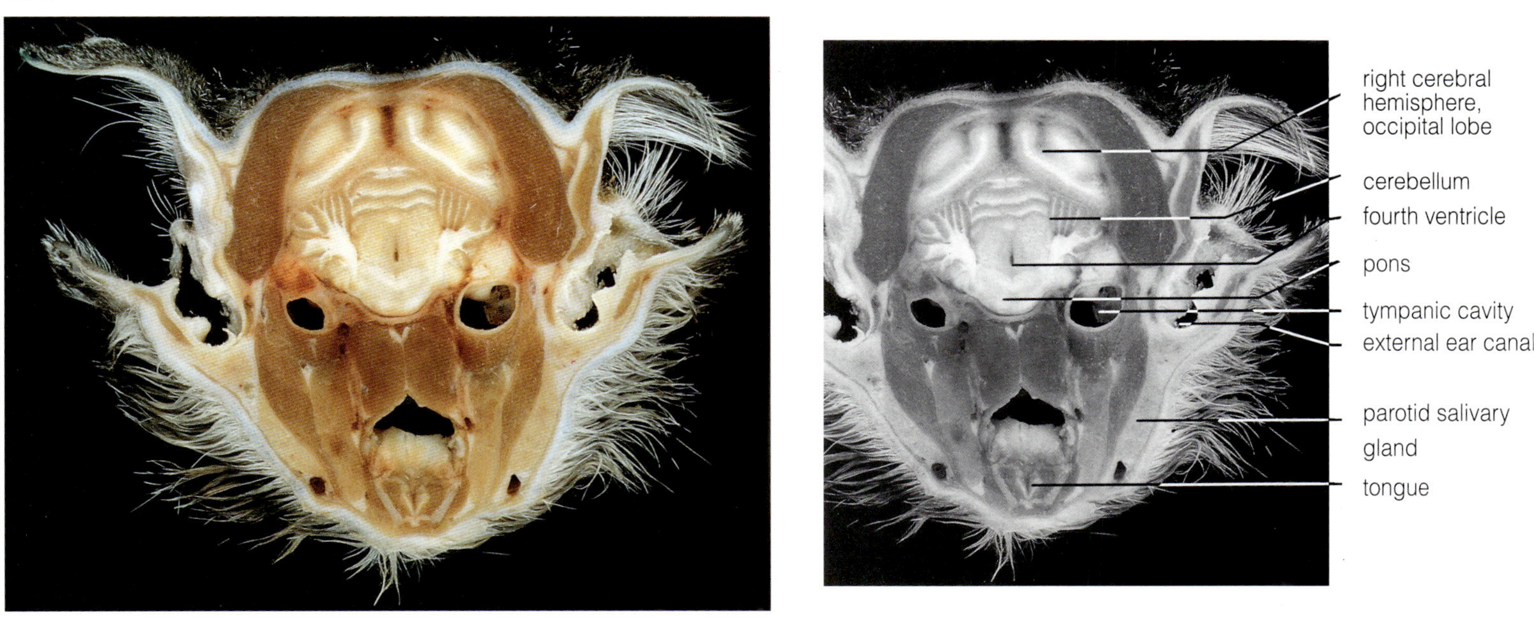

182–186 Anatomical sagittal sections, directly paramedian (**182**) and more lateral at the middle ear (**183**). Anatomical cross-sections at the mandibular joint (**184**), the middle ear (**185**) and the cerebellum (**186**) of an adult cat.

187

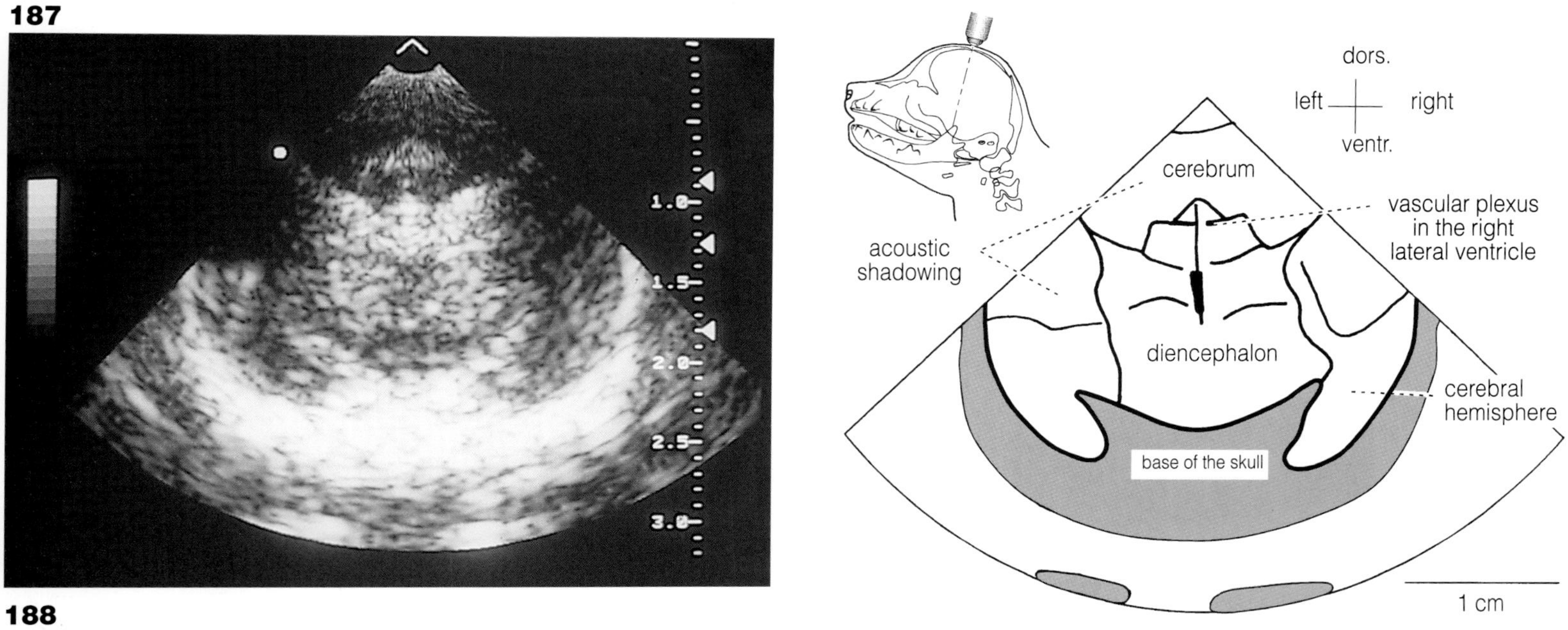

188

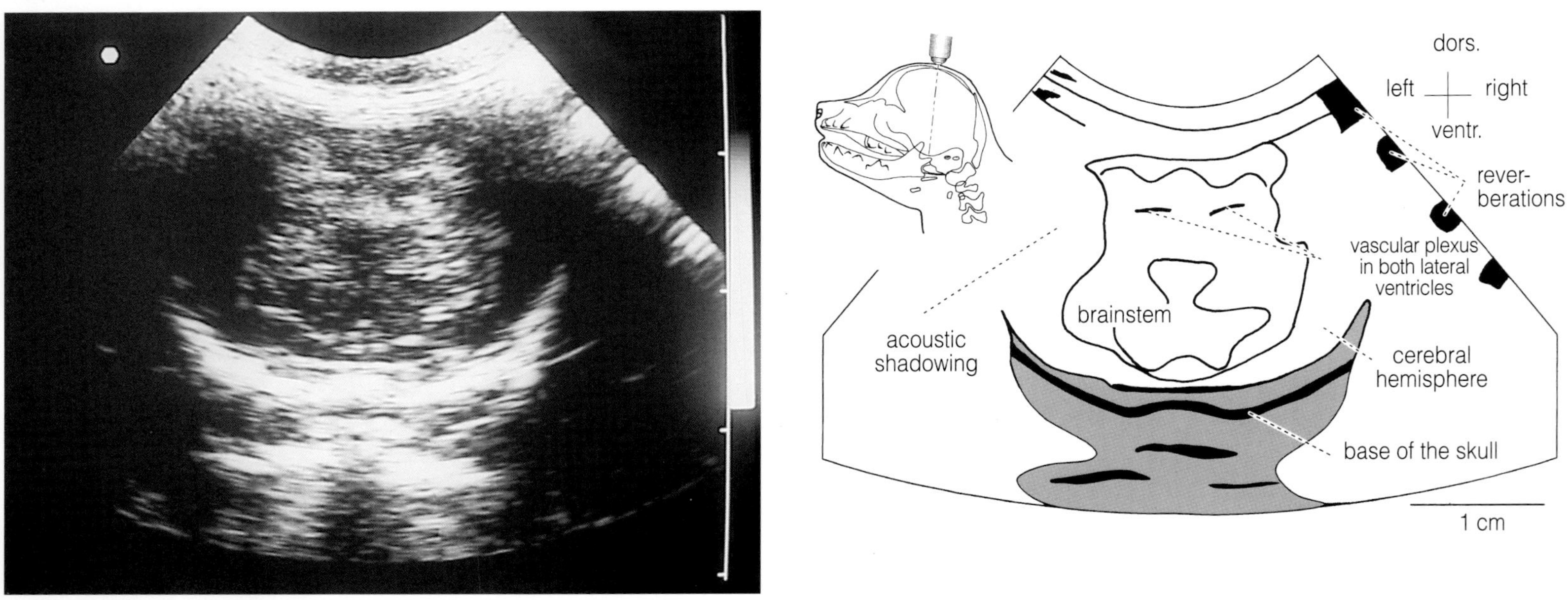

187, 188 Two-dimensional sonogram of a healthy, newborn, medium-sized puppy. Transverse view at the diencephalon (**187**) and the mesencephalon (**188**).

after complete ossification of the cranium, which is usually shortly after birth. The only method of imaging the brain in adult animals is during surgery after trepanation of the skull[12] (see Anatomy and Normal Sonographic Findings, below).

Anatomy and Normal Sonographic Findings

The brain is surrounded on all sides by the bones of the cranium. The roof of the skull or skull cap is dorsal and the base of the skull is ventral. During fetal development, wide fibrous sutures are found between the skull bones. These sutures distend at intersections into the so-called fontanelles. Compared with human fontanelles, most canine and feline fontanelles are already very small at birth (0.5–3 mm) or completely ossified. Chondrodystrophic toy breeds are an exception. In these breeds the frontal fontanelle between the frontal and parietal bone (*fonticulus frontoparietalis*) is relatively large and may remain open for life[17]. The meninges surrounding the brain are called dura mater, arachnoid membrane and pia mater. Wide blood sinuses are found within the dura mater (*sinus durae matris*).

The brain is divided into the following sections from rostral to caudal (182–186):

189

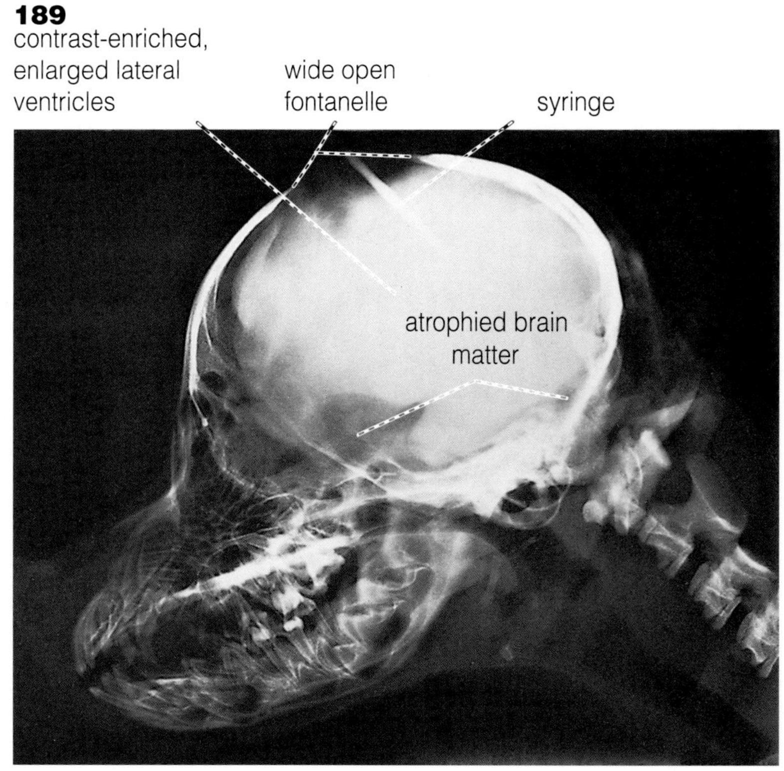

189 Lateral radiograph of a nine-week-old medium-sized puppy with postmortem ventriculography. Severe congenital hydrocephalus with a wide open fontanelle and enlarged opaque lateral ventricles reaching to the base of the skull.

190

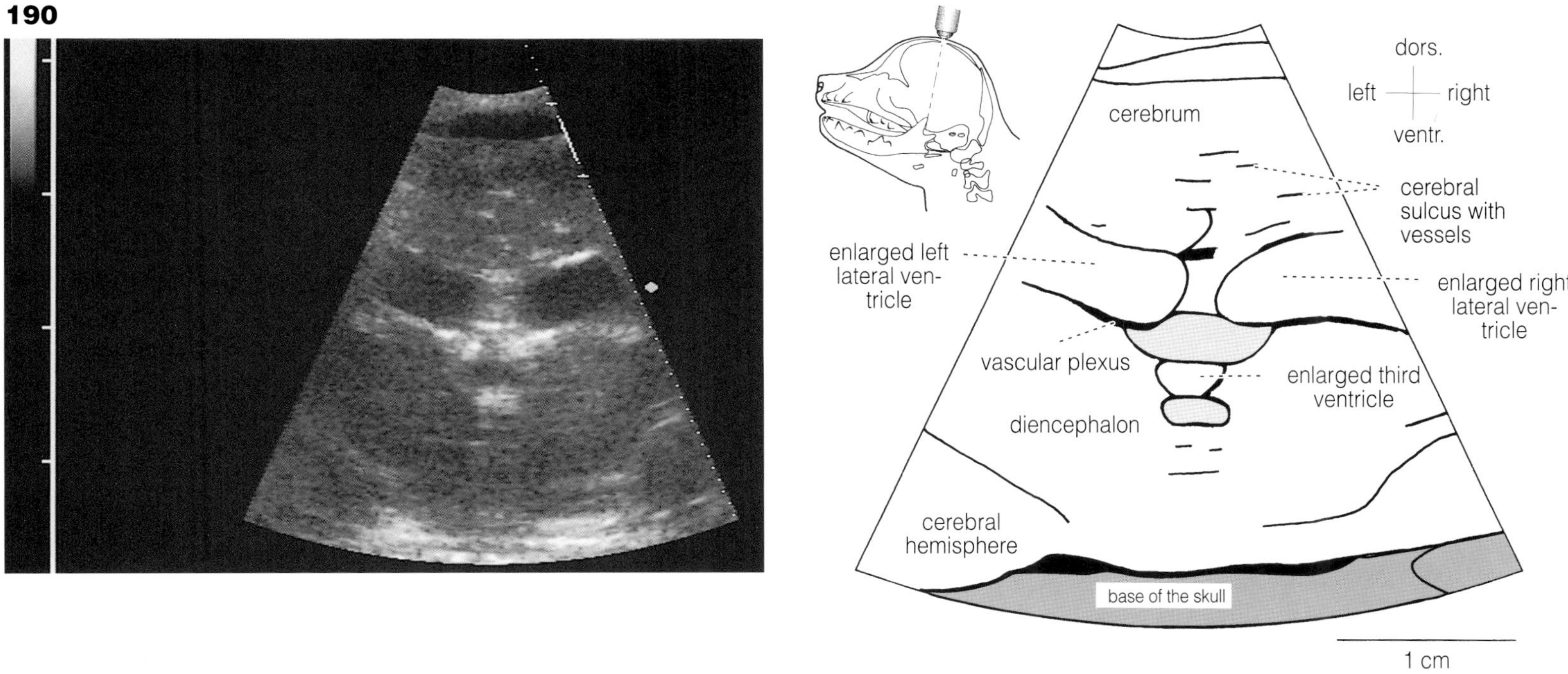

191

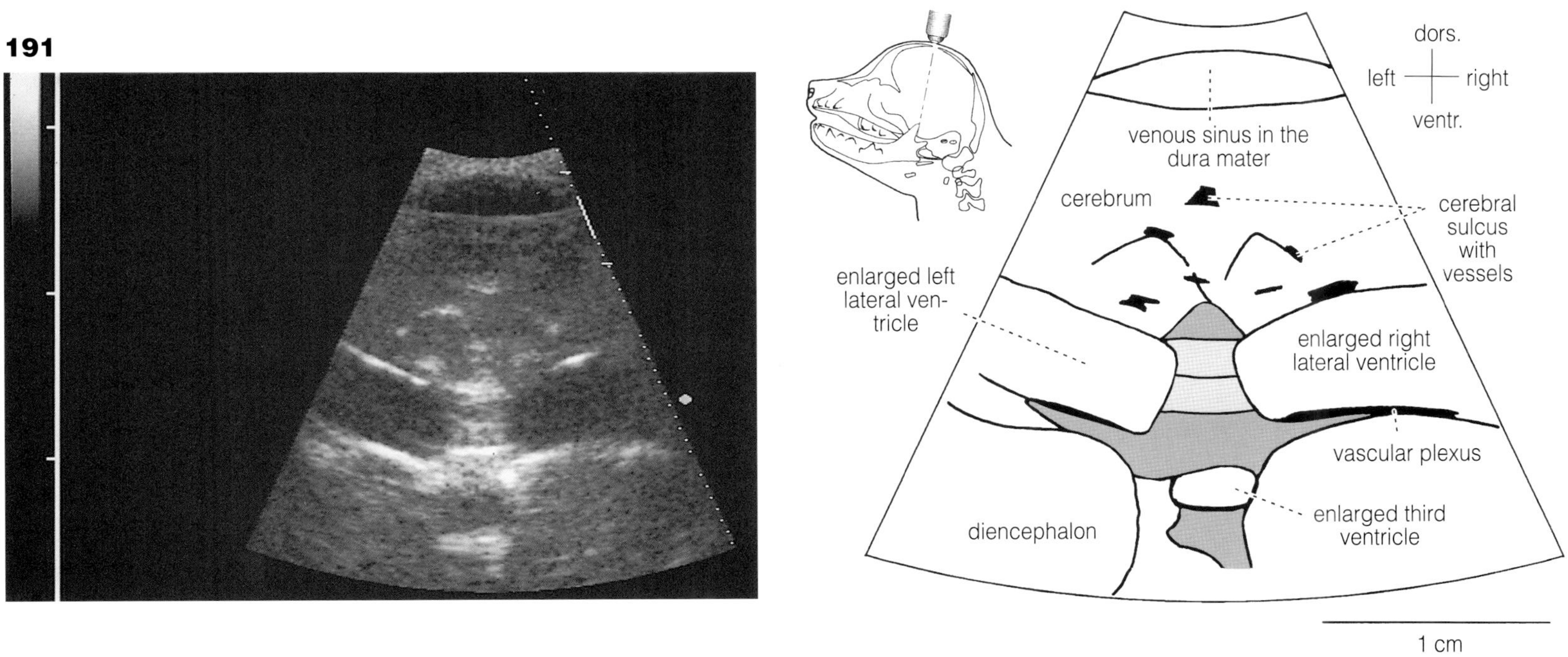

192

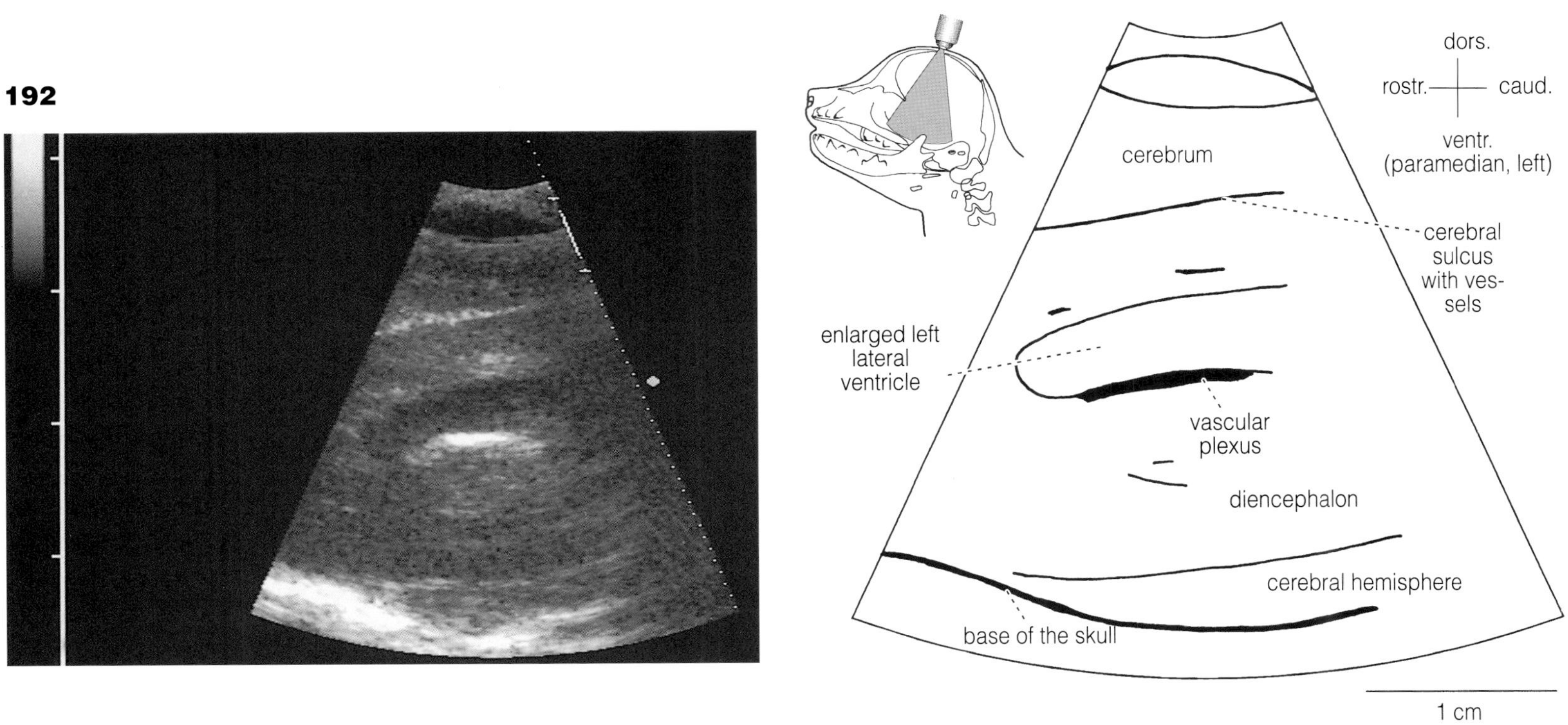

190–192 Two-dimensional sonograms of a three-week-old, medium-sized puppy. Moderate congenital hydrocephalus with wide lateral ventricles and an enlarged third ventricle. Cerebral matter is is still apparent in the transverse (**190, 191**) and sagittal (**192**) views.

- Telencepalon (endbrain) with two hemispheres.
- Diencepalon (interbrain) with the thalamus as well as the epithalamus, metathalamus, subthalamus and hypothalamus.
- Mesencepalon (midbrain) with the quadrigeminal plate (*lamina tecti*) and the cerebral crus (*pedunculi cerebri*).
- Metencephalon (hindbrain) with the cerebellum and the pons.
- Myeloncephalon (marrow brain) with the medulla oblongata.

The ventricles of the brain are important for sonographic diagnostics and they contain clear cerebrospinal fluid (liquor cerebrospinal). Cerebrospinal fluid is produced by the choroid plexus in the ventricles. It flows into the central canal of the spinal chord and through three openings in the fourth ventricle into the subarachnoid space. The first and second ventricles are located paramedian in the cerebral hemispheres as lateral ventricles. The third ventricle is situated within the diencephalon and leads into the narrow mesencephalic aqueduct. The fourth ventricle lies within the rhombencephalon and communicates with the outer cerebral fluid spaces. The ventricles of the dog and cat are usually too small to image sonographically or with computed tomography.

Transcutaneous sonography in normal dogs and cats, except toy breeds, is only possible in the first few days of life. Even then the acoustic window in puppies and kittens is extremely small. The image of the normal brain in newborn puppies and kittens is unremarkable. The displayed section of the brain can be determined by the scanning position and different contours of the hyperechoic base of the brain[13]. The grey and white cerebral matter appears hypoechoic to moderately echogenic. An association to the various brain centres or other structures is not possible. The lateral ventricles and the third ventricle are not fluid-filled spaces. They appear hyperechoic, due to the vascular plexus (**187**). The mesencephalic aqueduct and the fourth ventricle cannot be displayed[13]. Artefacts (reverberations) may appear at the sides of the ultrasound image (**188**).

Ultrasonography of Hydrocephalus

Transcutaneous ultrasonography of the brain is indicated with an open fontanelle in week-old puppies and kittens. Clinical and radiological signs include a larger head than that of littermates and a palpable, open fontanelle (**189**). Sensomotor and psychological dysfunctions are often not apparent. Central nervous disorders generally do not correlate with the enlarged ventricles and brain matter atrophy.

Since most cases of hydrocephalus are congenital, they primarily present with enlarged ventricles. Two-dimensional sonography of the lateral ventricles shows anechoic or fluid-filled spaces. In mild to moderate hydrocephalus, the lateral ventricles are still surrounded by hypoechoic brain matter (**190–192**). Severe hydrocephalus leads to complete atrophy of the cerebral hemispheres (**193, 194, 197, 198, 201**). The brainstem can be recognized ventrocaudally. Ultrasonography is comparable to computed tomographic imaging (**195, 196, 199, 200**). The cause of hydrocephalus, for example obstruction of the mesencephalic aqueduct or a closed fourth ventricle, cannot be determined sonographically. Computed tomography is more reliable in finding these lesions.

193

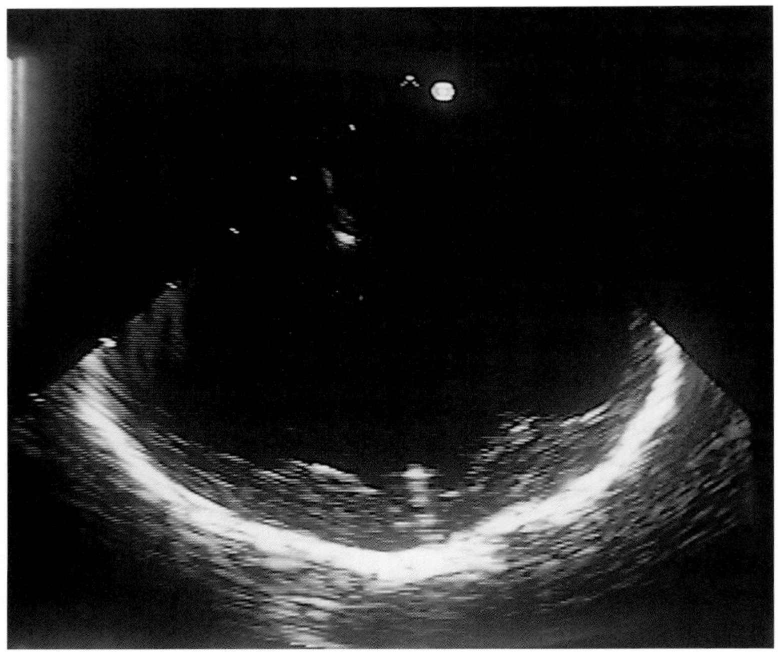

194

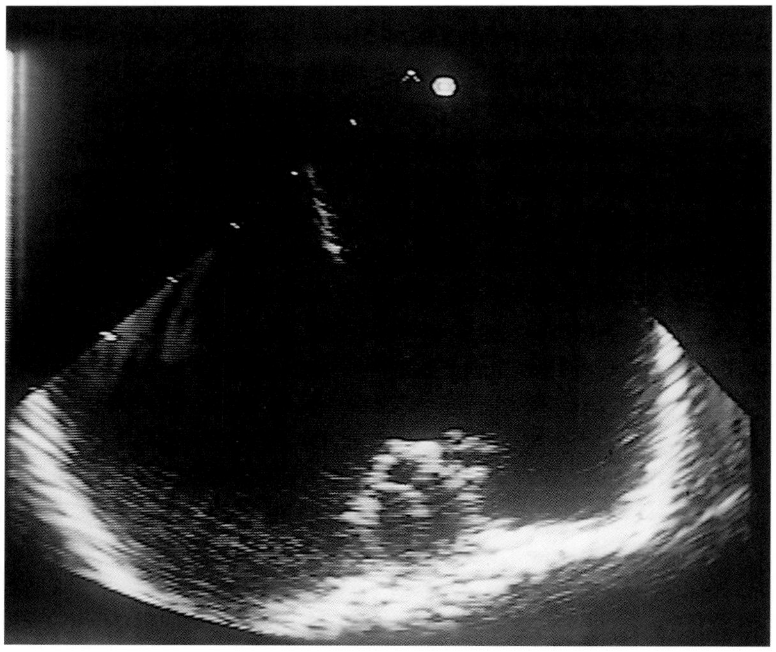

193–196 Two-dimensional sonography (**193, 194**) as well as computed tomography (**195, 196**) in the nine-week-old puppy from **282–284, 289** and **290**. Severe congenital hydrocephalus with almost complete atrophy of the cerebrum and some of the brainstem in various transverse views. (See also **197–200**.)

Eye

Ocular ultrasonography in dogs and cats includes the examination of the eyeball and the orbit.

Instrumentation and Examination Technique

Cordula Poulsen Nautrup and Hans-Josef Heider

Special ophthalmological high-frequency (10 MHz) sonographic units are used to examine the eye. These systems are able to

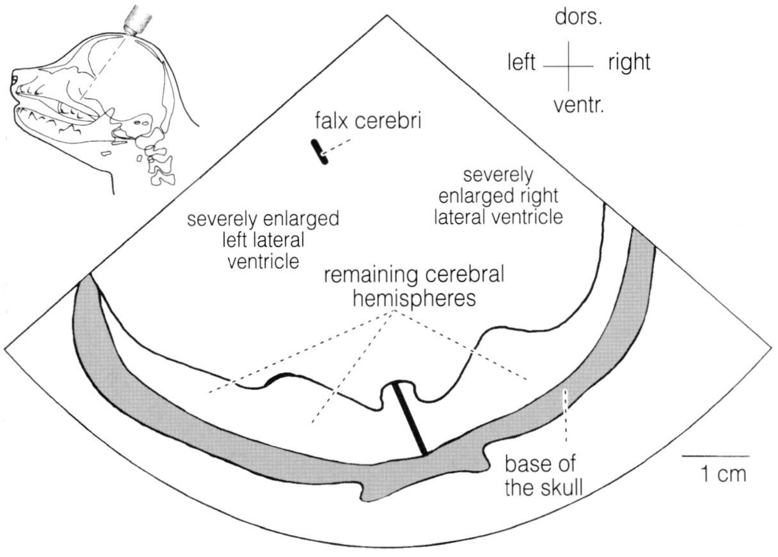

195

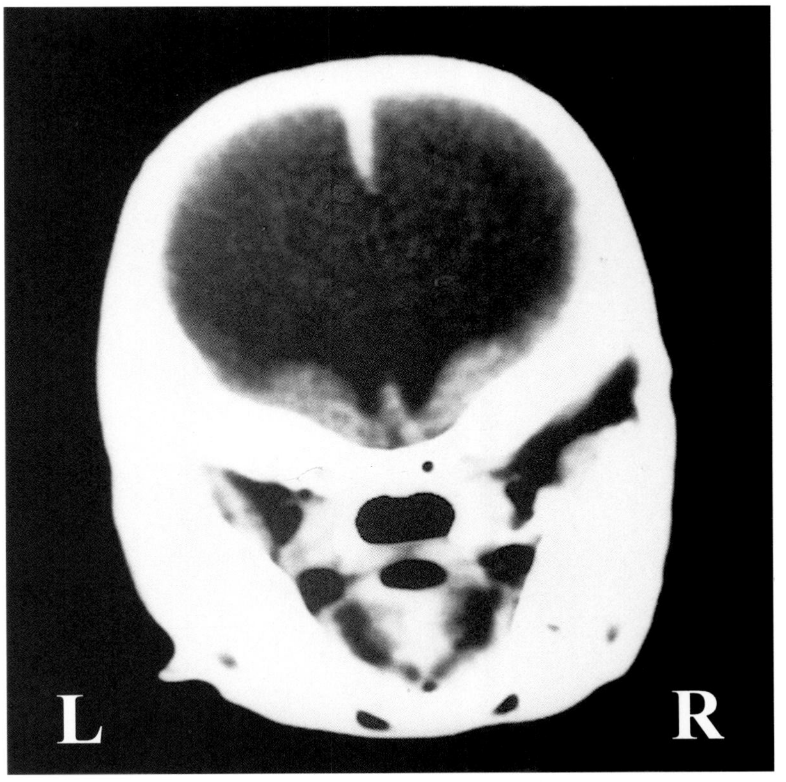

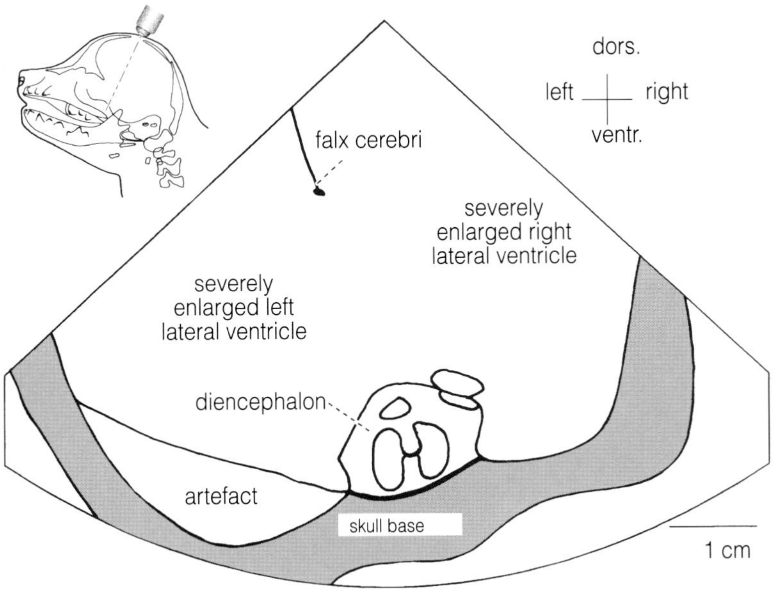

196

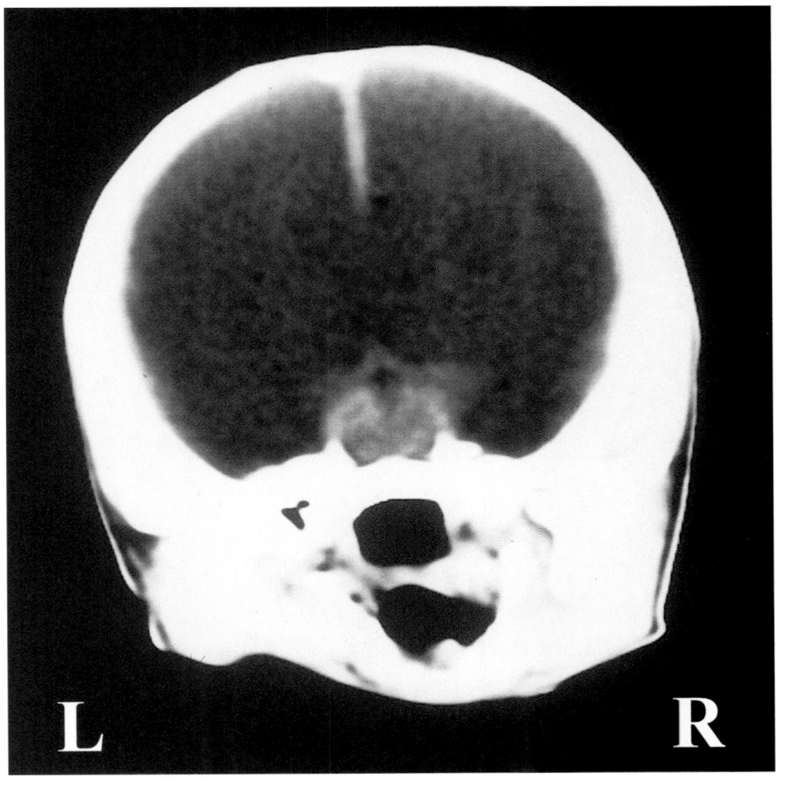

record conventional two-dimensional B-mode images as well as A-mode (see A-Mode; B-Mode, page 39). Cardiac and abdominal ultrasound units can also be used for ocular ultrasonography, as long as they employ high-frequency transducers of 7.5 MHz or 10–12 MHz. Sector scanners or small linear probes can be used. When scanning the anterior chamber with sector transducers, it is advisable to use a soft stand-off pad (see Stand-Off Pads, page 56). Some ophthalmological systems have special concave transducer surfaces that may cause reverberations in the near field (**222, 224, 225**). Methyl cellulose or commercial ocular coupling gel allows good contact. The eyes should always be rinsed thoroughly with saline solution after each examination.

Most dogs and cats can be scanned without the use of sedation. Topical ocular anaesthesia of the conjunctiva and cornea with proxymetacaine (Proparakain-POS® 0.5%, Ursapharm) is mandatory. Aggressive animals may need general anaesthesia. However, this may cause third eyelid protrusion, which can complicate the examination. General anaesthesia also causes nasal and inferior rotation of the eyeball. This can be avoided in small animals by using neuroleptic analgesia with ketamine and xylazine.

197

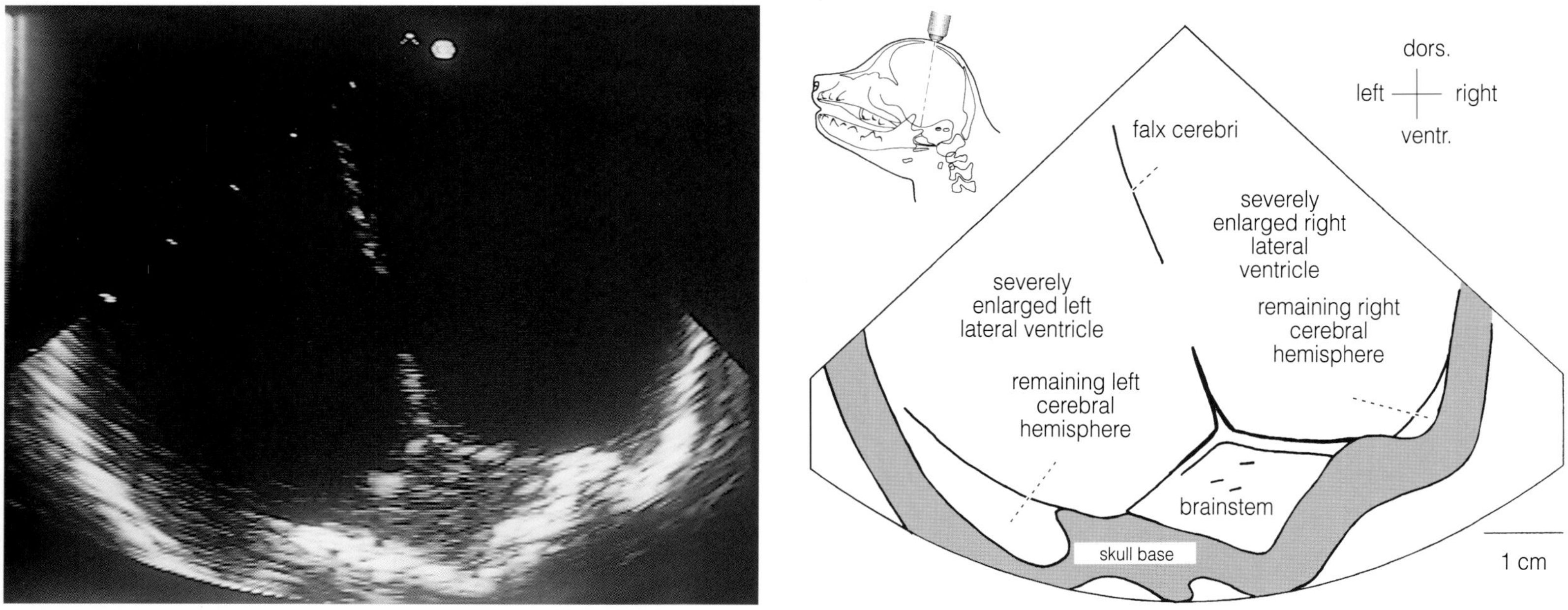

198

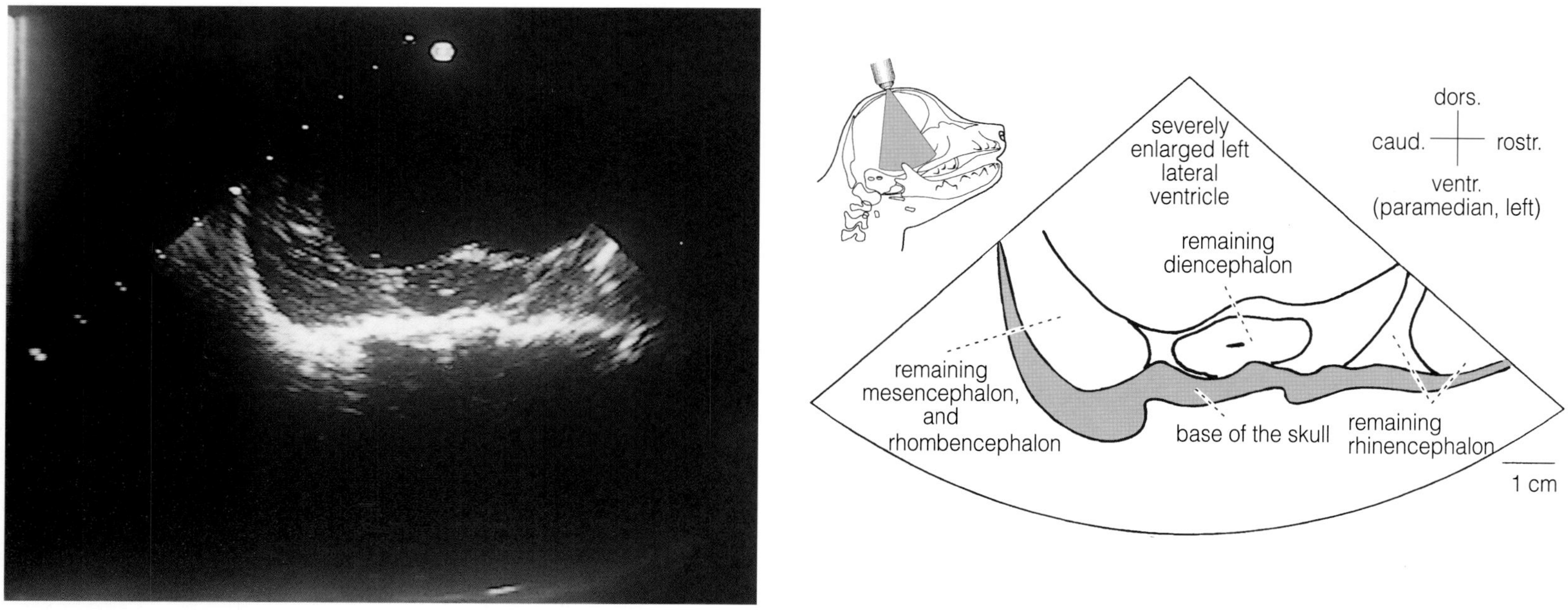

197–200 Two-dimensional sonography (**197, 198**) as well as computed tomography (**199, 200**) in the nine-week-old puppy from **282–284, 289** and **290**. Severe congenital hydrocephalus with almost complete atrophy of the cerebrum and some of the brainstem in various transverse views (**197, 199**) and a paramedian view (**198, 200**). (See also **193–196**.)

Animals are placed in sternal recumbency (202) or in a sitting position for the examination. A second person holds the head of the animal in a normal and comfortable position (203). For routine examinations the transducer is placed directly onto the cornea with or without an offset. In this way, sagittal and dorsal views are obtained (204). Transverse views of a non-sedated animal can only be made when the eyeball is not too deep inside the orbit. Enophthalmos is seen in some breeds or in sick animals. The transducer is placed directly onto the eyeball, or with a stand-off pad, near the temporal canthus (205). The animal can be anaesthetized when a transverse view of the eye is difficult to obtain. Spontaneous ventronasal rotation of the eyeball can be useful for obtaining a diagnosis. The eyeball can also be retracted with sutures.

Anatomy and Normal Sonographic Findings

Cordula Poulsen Nautrup, Hans-Josef Heider and Sabine Eggers

The sonographically relevant parts of the eye are the eyeball and the orbit.

The eyeball is nearly spherical (206). The external fibrous tunic is composed of the transparant cornea and the opaque white sclera. The middle vascular tunic or choroid lies inside the sclera. The thicker portion around the lens is called the ciliary body,

199

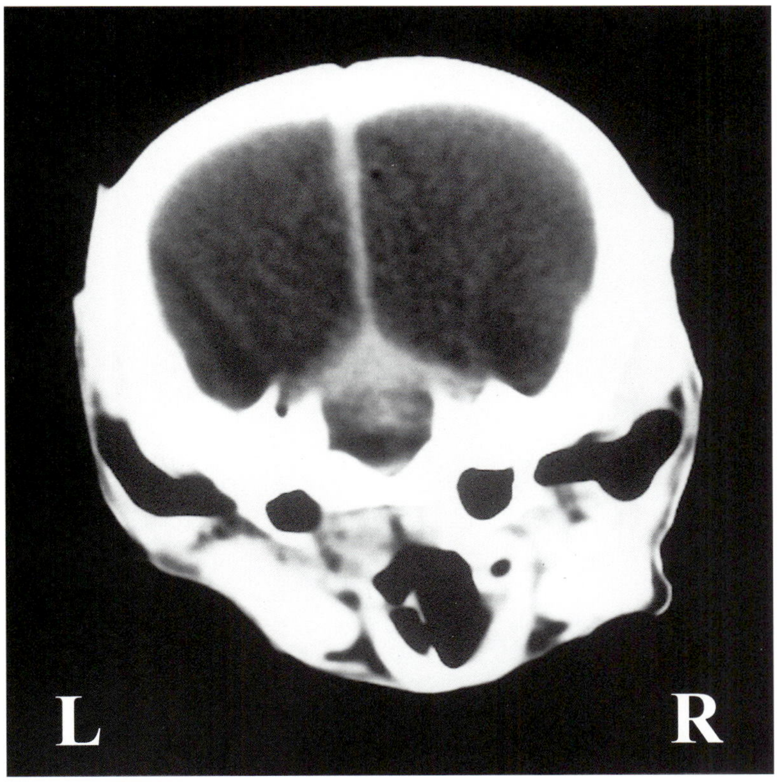

200

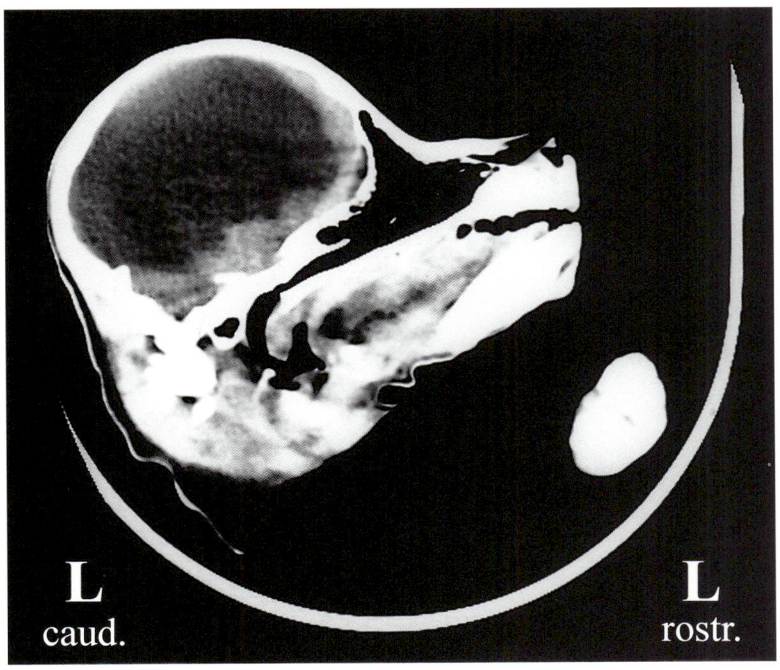

201

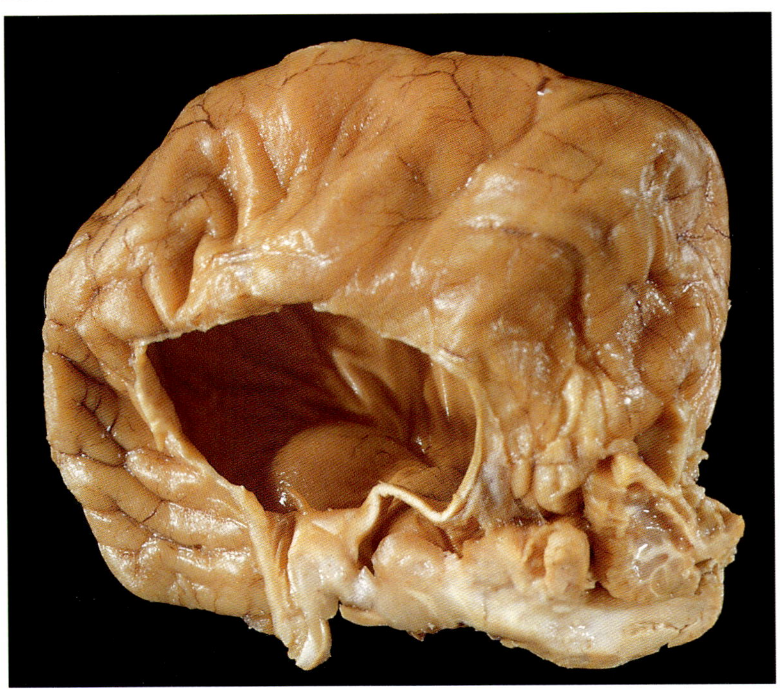

202

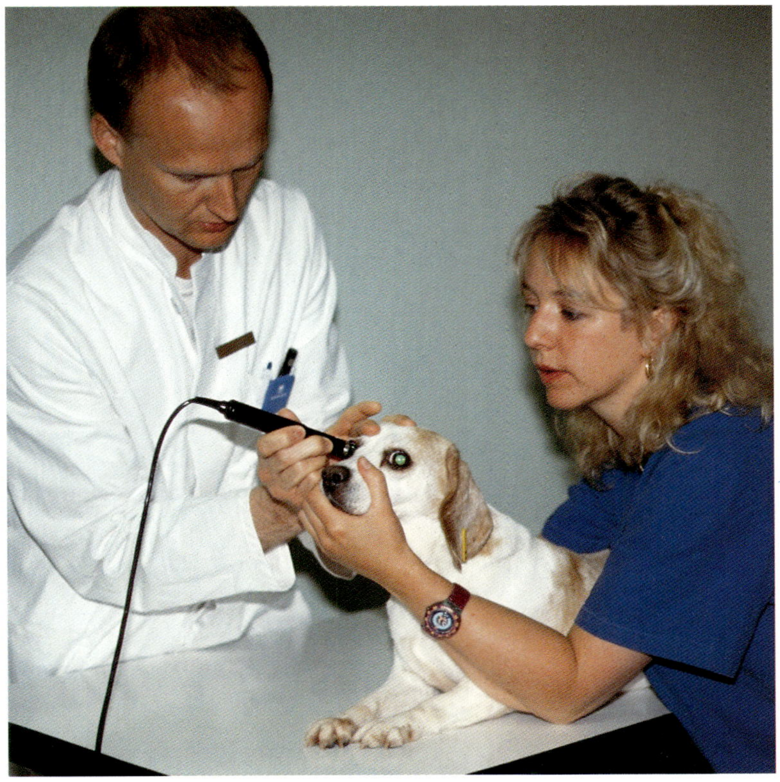

203

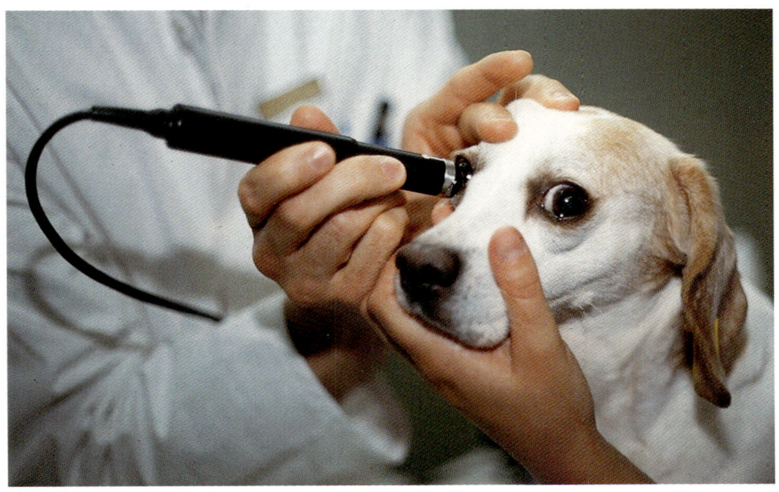

202, 203 Sternal recumbency in a dog with light, almost horizontal fixation of the head (**202**); scanning position for dorsal and sagittal views of a non-sedated dog (**203**).

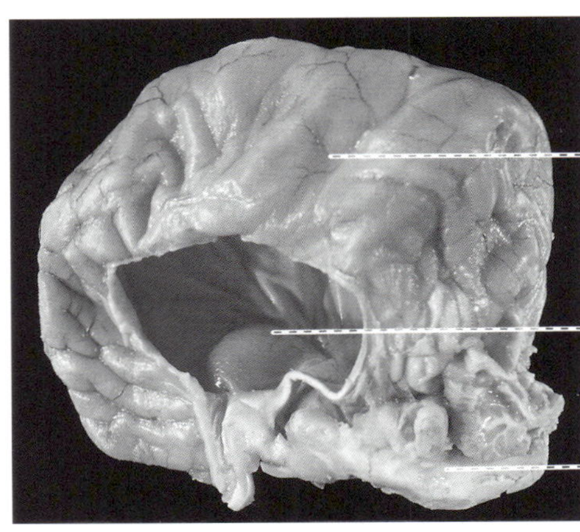

201 Pathological specimen of the right side of the brain of the puppy from **282–284, 287** and **288**. The cerebrum is atrophied to a thin capsule; parts of the brainstem are preserved. The puppy showed few cerebral dysfunctions.

204

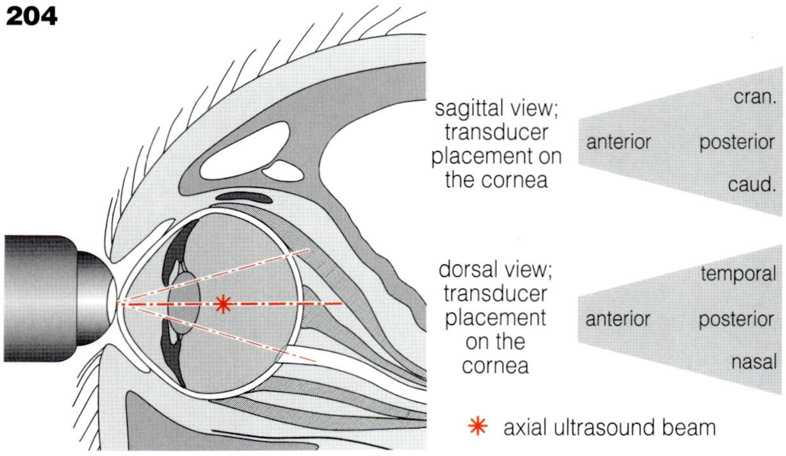

205

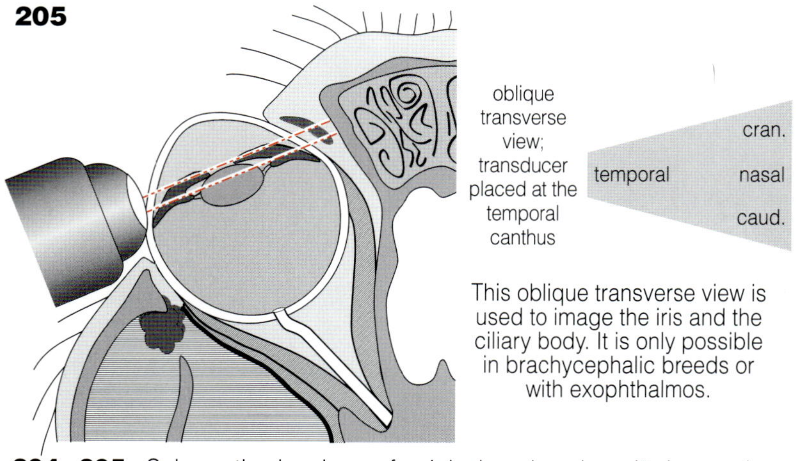

204, 205 Schematic drawings of axial, dorsal and sagittal scanning positions (**204**) as well as a transverse view (**205**), with image orientation.

206

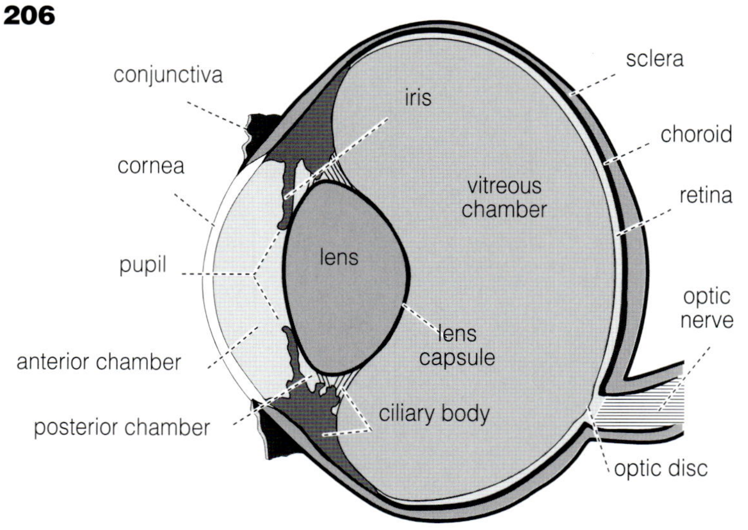

206 Schematic drawing of the eyeball in a sagittal view.

207

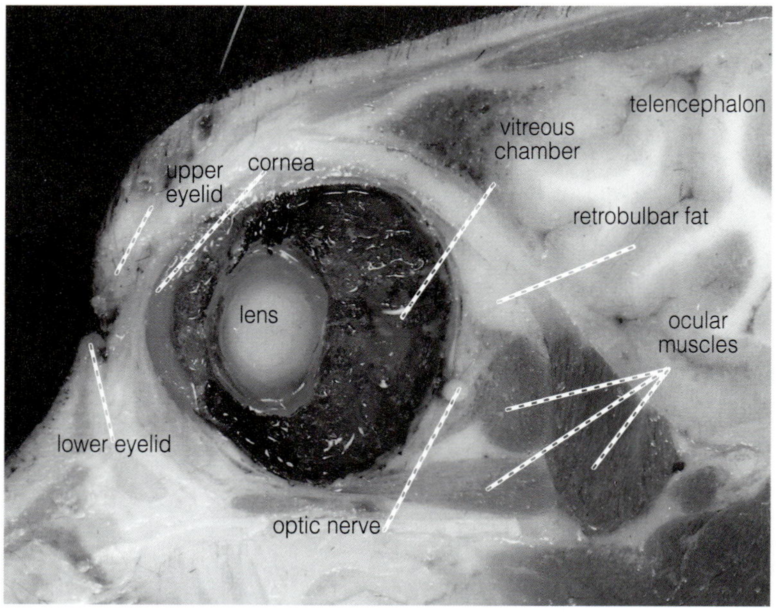

208

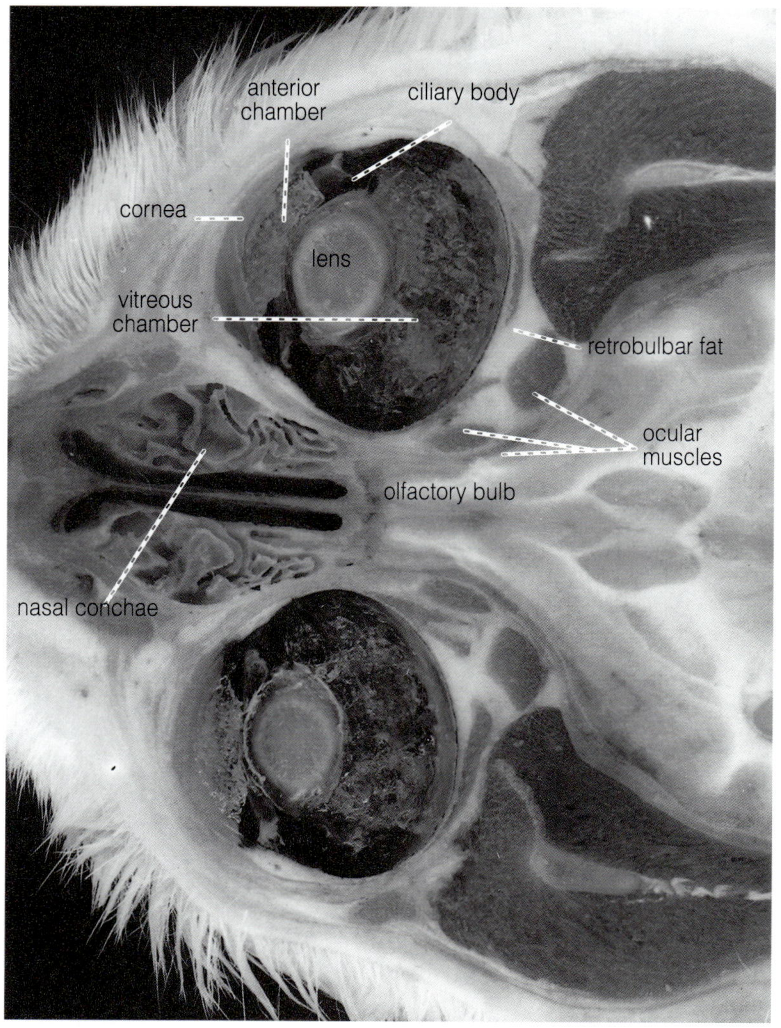

207, 208 Anatomical sagittal (**207**) and dorsal (**208**) sections of a feline orbit.

which suspends the lens. The anterior region is the iris. The iris surrounds the pupil similar to an aperture. The inner sensory layer of the eye is the retina. The lens of the eye is a biconvex clear structure, which is located posterior to the iris. The anterior lens capsule borders the posterior chamber, while the posterior lens capsule is adjacent to the vitreous chamber. The lens is suspended by the ciliary body. The vitreous chamber is bounded by the lens and the retina. Both chambers of the eyeball contain aqueous humour and they communicate through the pupil. The anterior chamber is bounded by the cornea and the iris. The posterior chamber is bounded by the iris, the ciliary body and the lens (206). The optic nerve (II. cerebral nerve) enters the eyeball temporal to the posterior pole of the eye and forms the optic disc on the retina. The external ophthalmic artery and vein accompany the optic nerve near the eyeball.

The orbit is a pyramid-shaped cavity with an open anterior base. The canine and feline orbit is not completely surrounded by bones. The entrance to the orbit is closed by the eyelids. The orbit contains the eyeball and the S-shaped optic nerve, as well as branches of the third to seventh cerebral nerves and sympathetic

209

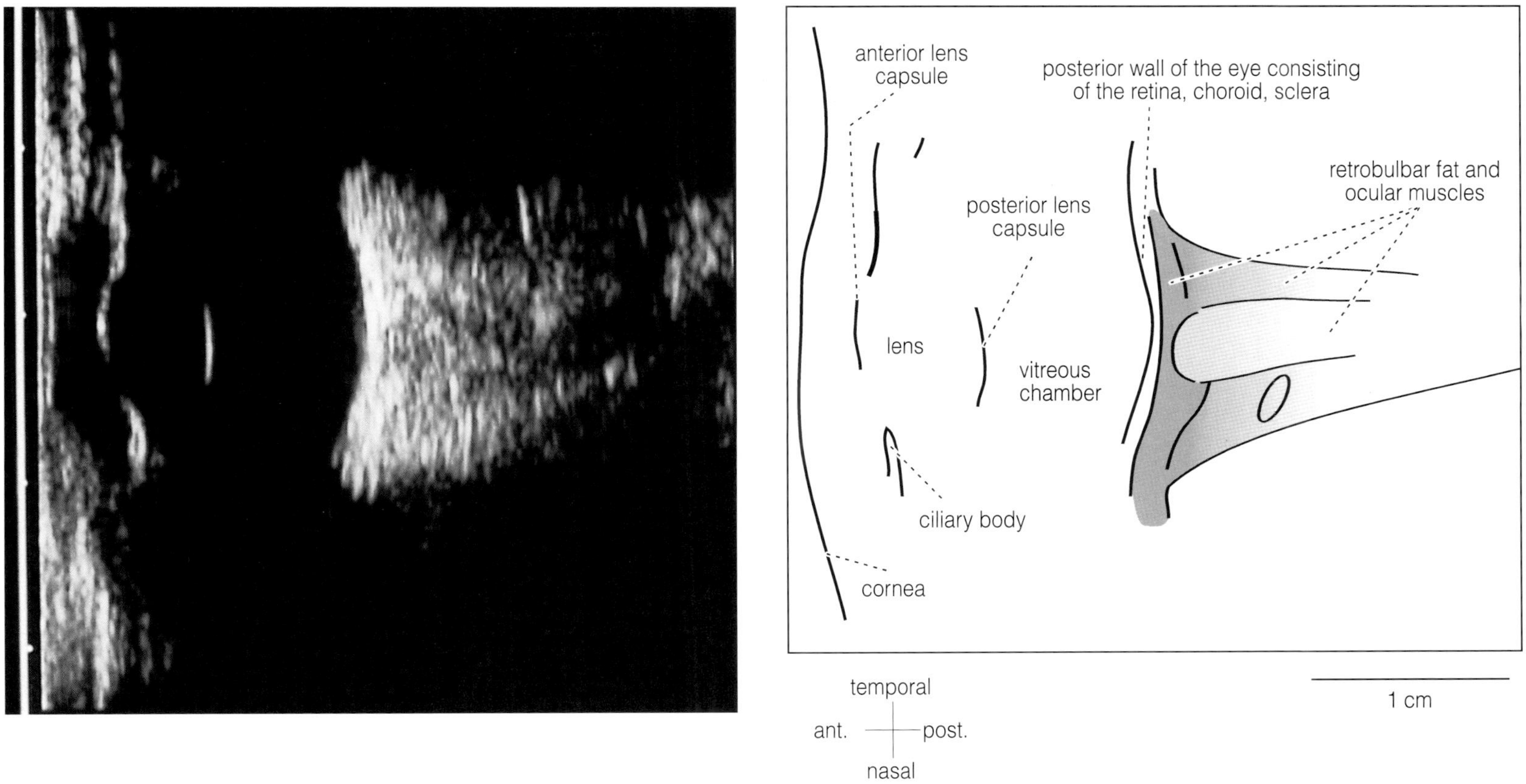

210

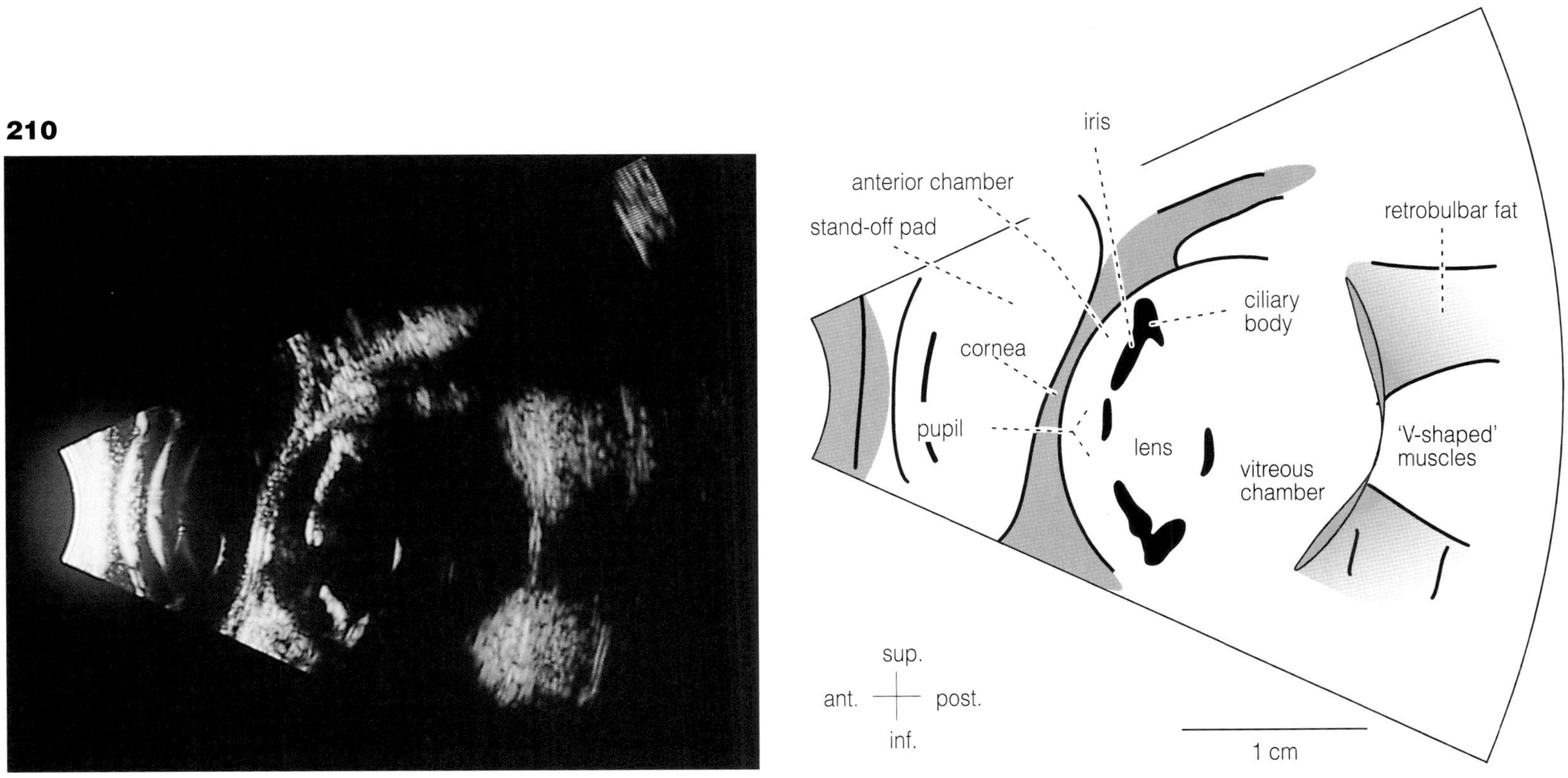

209, 210 Two-dimensional sonographic images of a dog with a small 7.5 MHz linear transducer (**209**) and a 10 MHz sector transducer (**210**). A conventional ultrasound machine was used for **209**, while **210** was imaged with a stand-off pad and a special ultrasound system used in human ophthalmology. Dorsal (**209**) and sagittal (**210**) views of normal eyes.

nervous system, blood vessels, the lacrimal gland and the ocular muscles (four rectus muscles, two oblique muscles and the retractor bulbi muscle). These orbital structures are surrounded by periorbital fibrous tissue. The fibrous tissue is embedded in a fat pad (207, 208). The zygomatic salivary gland is located lateral to the periorbita (178).

Two-dimensional ultrasonography allows evaluation of bulbar structures such as the cornea, the anterior chamber, the iris, the ciliary body, the lens and the vitreous chamber. The posterior section of the bulbar wall can also be visualized (209–213).

The cornea is hyperechoic and can be easily differentiated from the deeper, anechoic, curved anterior chamber. The iris and ciliary body are difficult to separate and they are seen as a V-shaped, echogenic structure behind the anterior chamber near the lens (209–211). The iris is a solid, radial echogenic aperture and is best imaged in a transverse view (212, 213). The elliptical shape of the clear lens is difficult to image in an axial view (sagittal and dorsal). Unless very high frequency probes are used (12 MHz and above), only the middle or perpendicular sound beam is able to visualize the lens capsule. The peripheral portions of the lens are

211

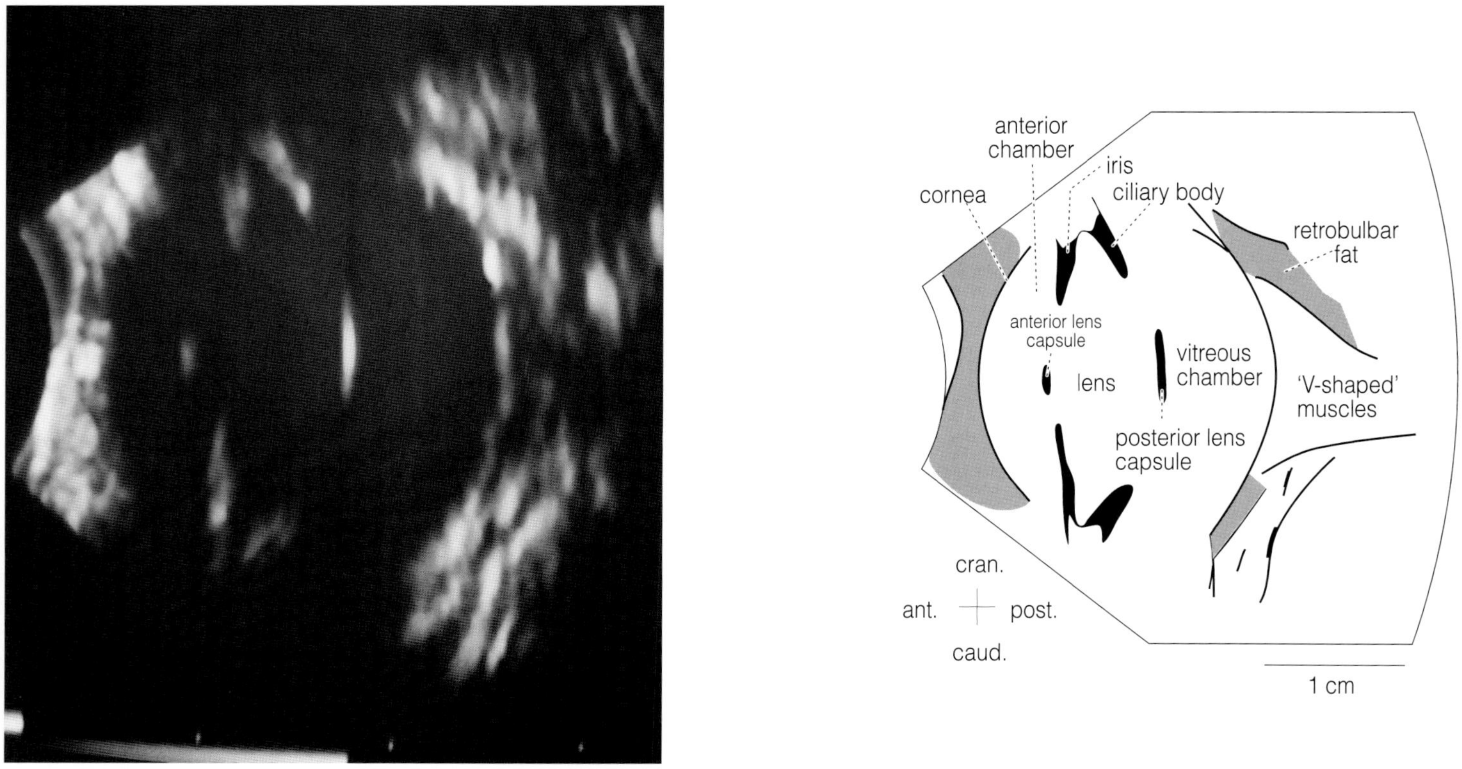

211 Two-dimensional sonogram of a cat using a 10 MHz sector transducer with a conventional ultrasound unit. Sagittal view of the normal eye.

rarely seen in the axial sonogram. The interior of the lens is anechoic. The ultrasound beam travels faster through the lens, which may lead to artefacts deeper to the structure. The posterior wall of the eye may appear protruded behind the lens because of distal enhancement. The vitreous body contains 99% water and is anechoic. The posterior wall of the eye is highly reflective. The three layers of the posterior wall (retina, choroid, sclera) cannot be resolved individually with conventional ultrasound systems (**209–213**).

The retrobulbar area contains hyperechoic fatty tissue. The hypoechoic optic nerve and slightly more echogenic ocular muscles can be differentiated within this echogenic tissue. In a longitudinal view the ocular muscles have a typical V-shape.

A stand-off pad should be used to image the cornea, anterior chamber and iris. Special ultrasound systems with frequencies of 40–100 MHz have been created to give detailed images of the cornea, the anterior and posterior chambers, the lens, the iris and the ciliary body[19].

It is important to avoid any pressure on the eyeball when evaluating the depth of the anterior chamber. Transducer placement on the cornea may already decrease the distance between the cornea echo and that of the anterior lens capsule.

A-mode ultrasonography is still used to measure ocular structures (see A-Mode, page 39). The spikes are equivalent to the acoustic interfaces along the sound beam path (**214**). After the initial echo and the echo-free stand-off echo, the spikes correspond to the cornea, the anterior and posterior lens capsule, the vitreous chamber baseline and the posterior ocular wall (**215–217**). Reproducible sonographic measurements of the eye must be made exactly in the axis of the eye without indenting the cornea (**214**). Biometric values of the dog eye are listed in *Table 8* [4, 20].

Table 8 Direct and sonographic biometric measurements of intraocular lengths in dolichocephalic and mesocephalic dog breeds from Cotrill *et al.*, 1989*[4] and A-mode measurements of intraocular lengths in various non-brachycephalic breeds from Schiffer *et al.*, 1985**[20].

	Dolichocephalic breeds*			**Mesocephalic breeds**			**Non-brachycephalic breeds****
	Direct measurement [mm]	B-mode measurement [mm]	A-mode measurement [mm]	Direct measurement [mm]	B-mode measurement [mm]	A-mode measurement [mm]	A-mode measurement [mm]
Anterior chamber D1	4.0–6.0	2.0–5.5	2.0–5.0	3.0–5.5	2.0–5.0	2.0–5.0	4.26–5.94
Lens D2	5.0–8.0	6.7–8.9	6.7–7.8	5.0–8.0	6.7–8.9	3.3–10.0	6.64–7.84
Vitreous chamber D3	8.5–12.0	9.0–10.0	6.0–11.0	8.0–12.0	7.5–10.0	5.5–10.5	8.87–10.19
Total eye length D4	19.5–22.0	18.3–23.4	16.8–22.8	18.0–20.0	17.8–22.8	15.7–23.3	20.26–23.30

212

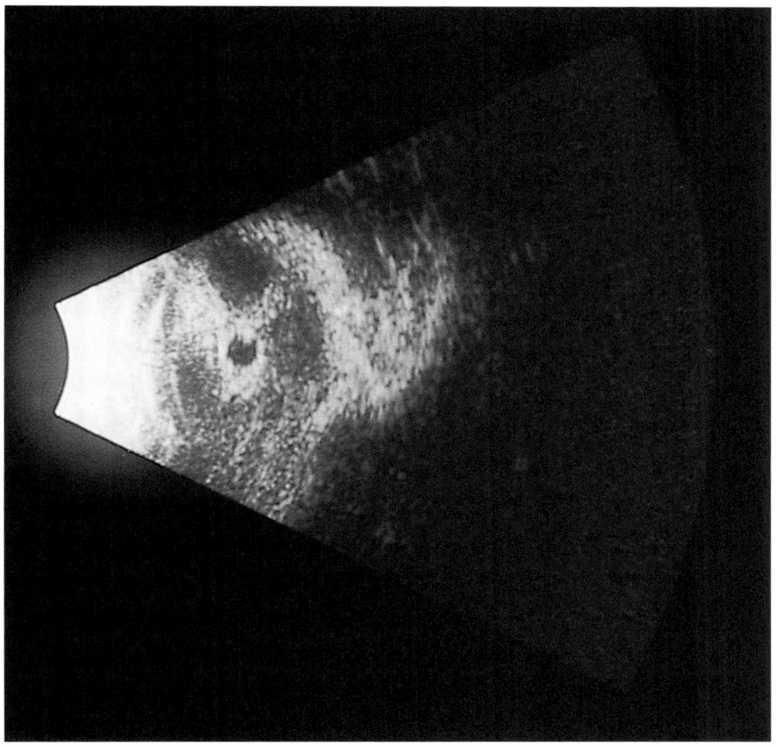

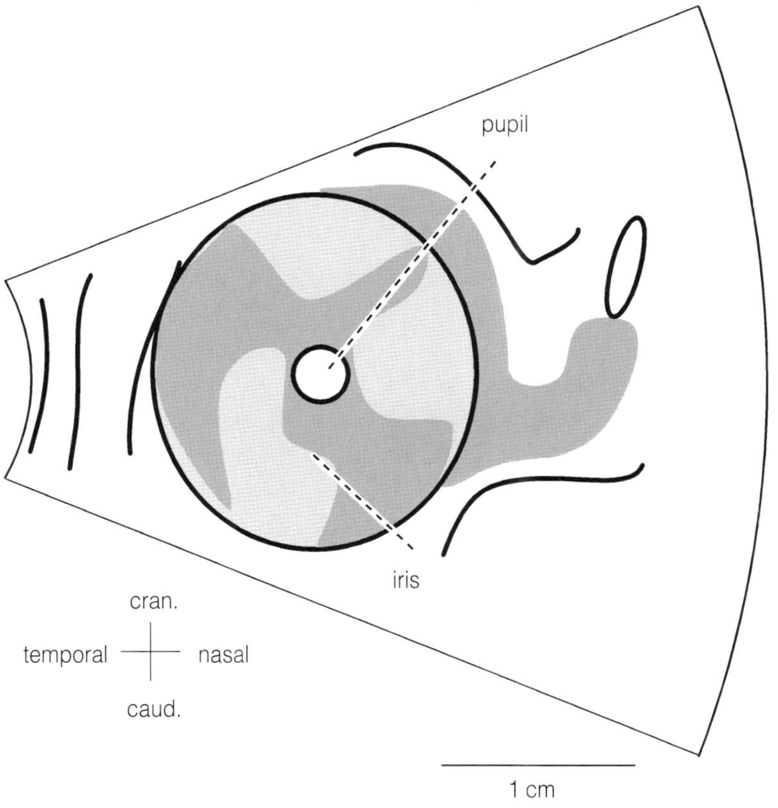

213

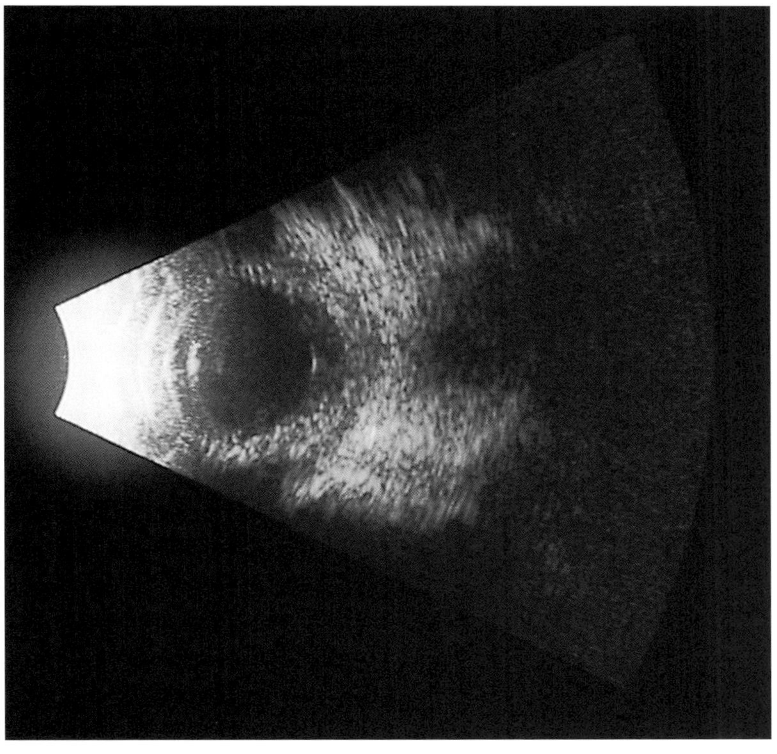

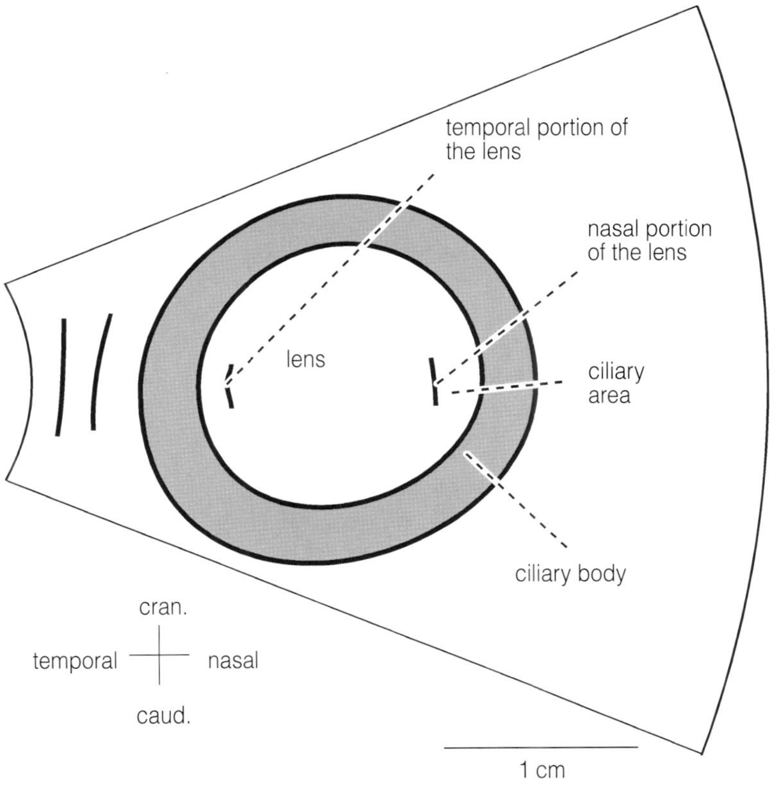

212, 213 Two-dimensional sonograms of a brachycephalic dog using a sector transducer (10 MHz). Tranverse view of a normal eye at the pupil (**212**) and at the lens (**213**).

Ultrasonography of Ocular Disease

Hans-Josef Heider

The indications for ocular ultrasonography include all eyeball lesions of unknown origin with concurrent opacification of the cornea, anterior chamber, posterior chamber, lens or vitreous chamber. Ocular ultrasonography should also be performed when neoplasia, intraocular foreign bodies or retinal and choroidal lesions such as detachments are suspected.

Orbital ultrasonography is indicated for each non-breed related exophthalmos or enophthalmos, especially if it is unilateral.

Ultrasonography of Intraocular Disease

Cornea

Ultrasonographic examination of the cornea is of limited clinical value.

An increase in corneal thickness can be imaged sonographically. This is usually caused by a chronic dysfunction of the epithelium or endothelium of the cornea followed by oedema. These lesions are seen in conjunction with glaucoma.

Precise measurements of corneal thickness in the normal eye are only possible with special A-mode units used in human ophthalmology for refractive surgery preparation. Extensive thick-

214

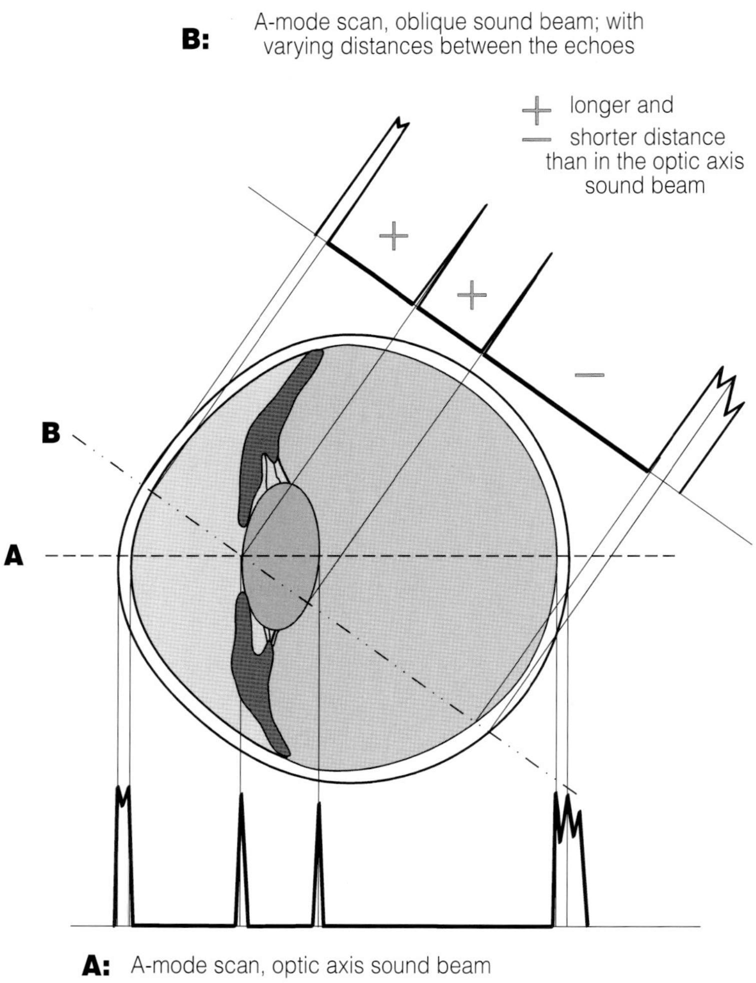

214 Schematic drawing of the acoustic interfaces of the eyeball with the equivalent A-mode scan in an axial (**A**) and oblique (**B**) sound beam.

215

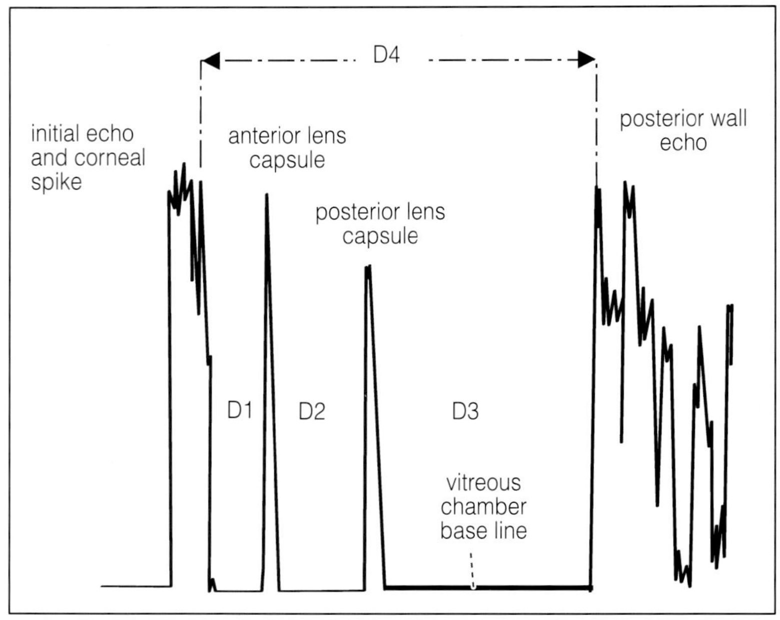

216

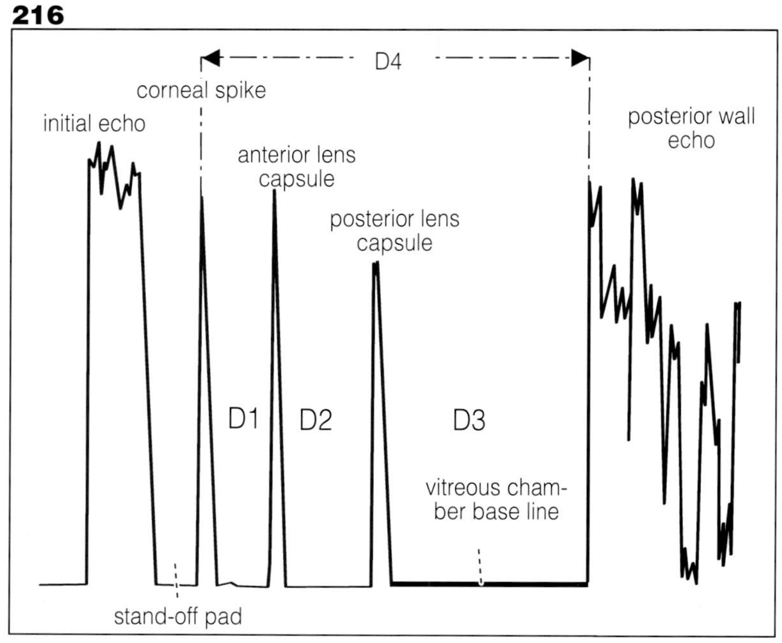

217

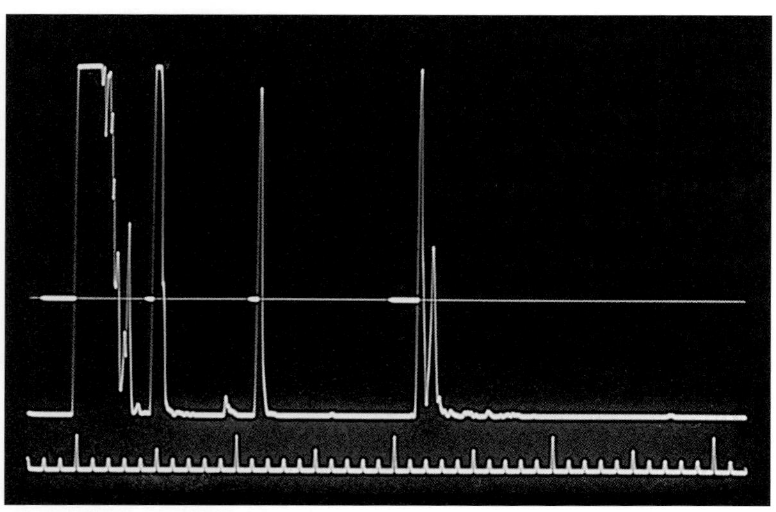

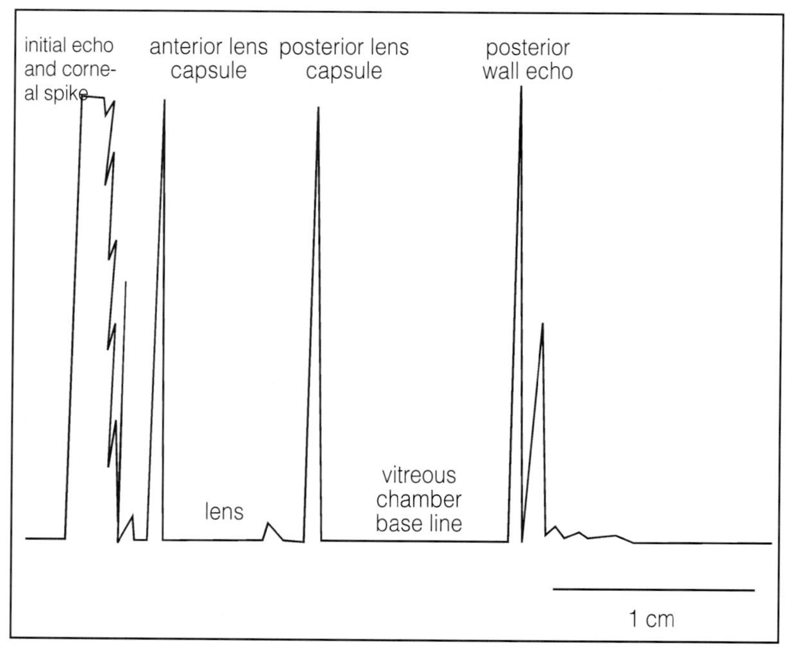

215–217 Schematic drawings (**215, 216**) and a photo (**217**) of a normal canine A-mode scan in the optic axis.

218

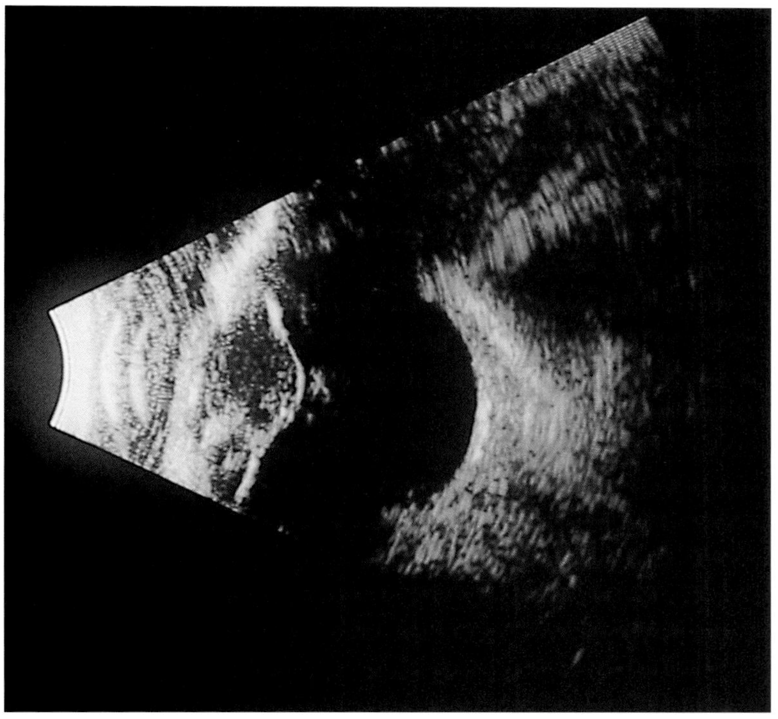

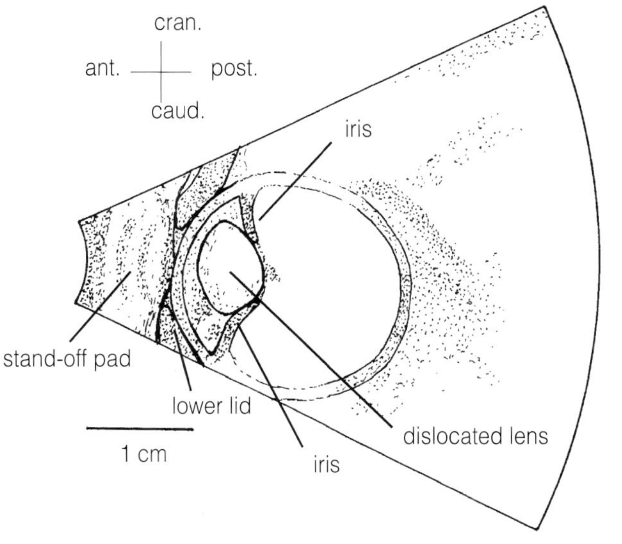

218 Anterior lens dislocation in a dog. The luxated lens is posterior to the cornea and obstructs the pupil. The iris diaphragm is displaced posteriorly.

219

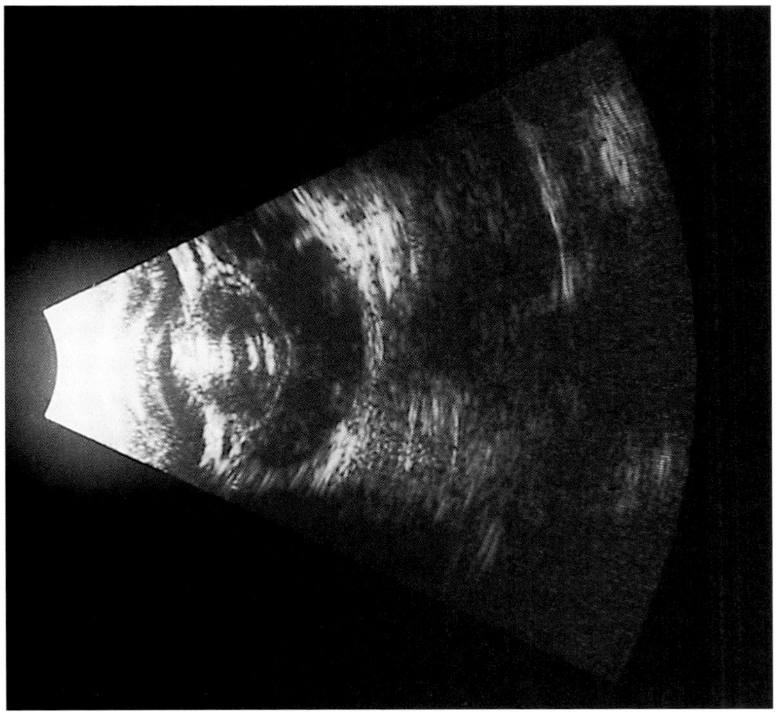

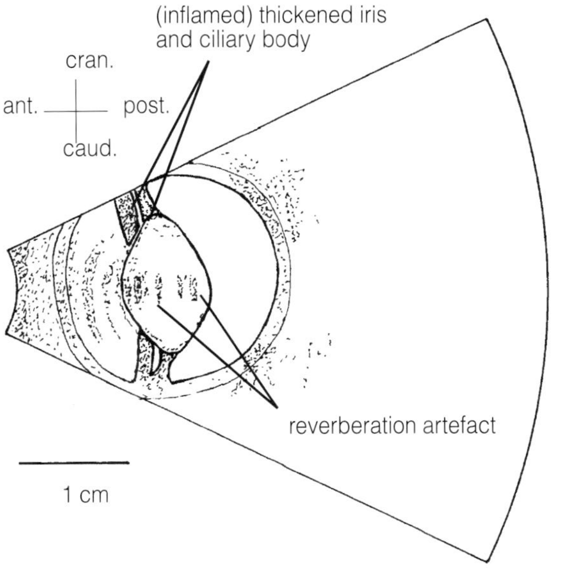

219 Chronic idiopathic uveitis in a cat. Inflammation of the iris and ciliary body leads to thickening and increased echogenicity of these structures. They are more easily recognizable and differentiated than in a normal eye. The lens capsule is diffusely covered with precipitate, which displays the entire lens contour better than in a normal image.

ening can be measured with conventional systems for A-mode biometry. In some cases, measurements can be made with two-dimensional ultrasonography. A stand-off pad places the cornea within the focal zone to image the anterior and posterior portion.

Anterior Chamber

Ultrasonography of the anterior chamber helps to display lesions that result in varying chamber diameters (corneal-to-anterior lens capsule distance) or to visualize pathological contents.

A stand-off pad should always be used to measure the anterior chamber distance in two-dimensional B-mode ultrasonography. The distances are usually easier to measure with A-mode biometry (**214–217**). The anterior chamber is measured from the anterior corneal surface to the anterior lens capsule. The normal measurements for the canine anterior chamber are between 4.26 and 5.94 mm[20].

The anterior chamber distance is decreased with swelling of the lens during cataract formation (intumescent cataract)[14]. This condition should not be confused with indentation of the chamber due to excessive transducer pressure.

The anterior chamber may appear enlarged with glaucoma[14] or with microphakia or aphakia.

Anterior chamber haemorrhage is seen as increased echogen-

220

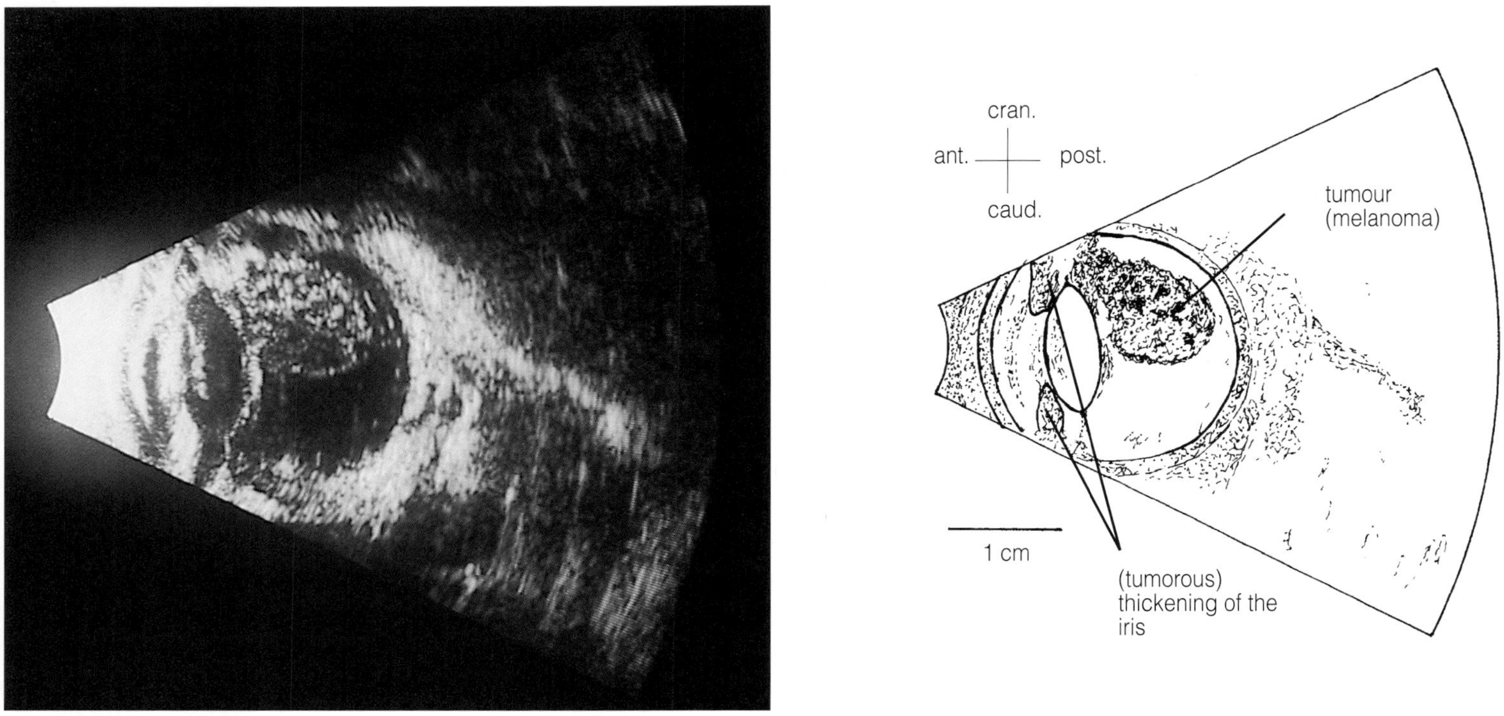

220 Malignant melanoma of the superior portion of the ciliary body in a cat. The extent of the tumour is visible in the upper part of the vitreous chamber. The echogenicity of the mass does not allow differentiation from vitreous chamber haemorrhage.

221

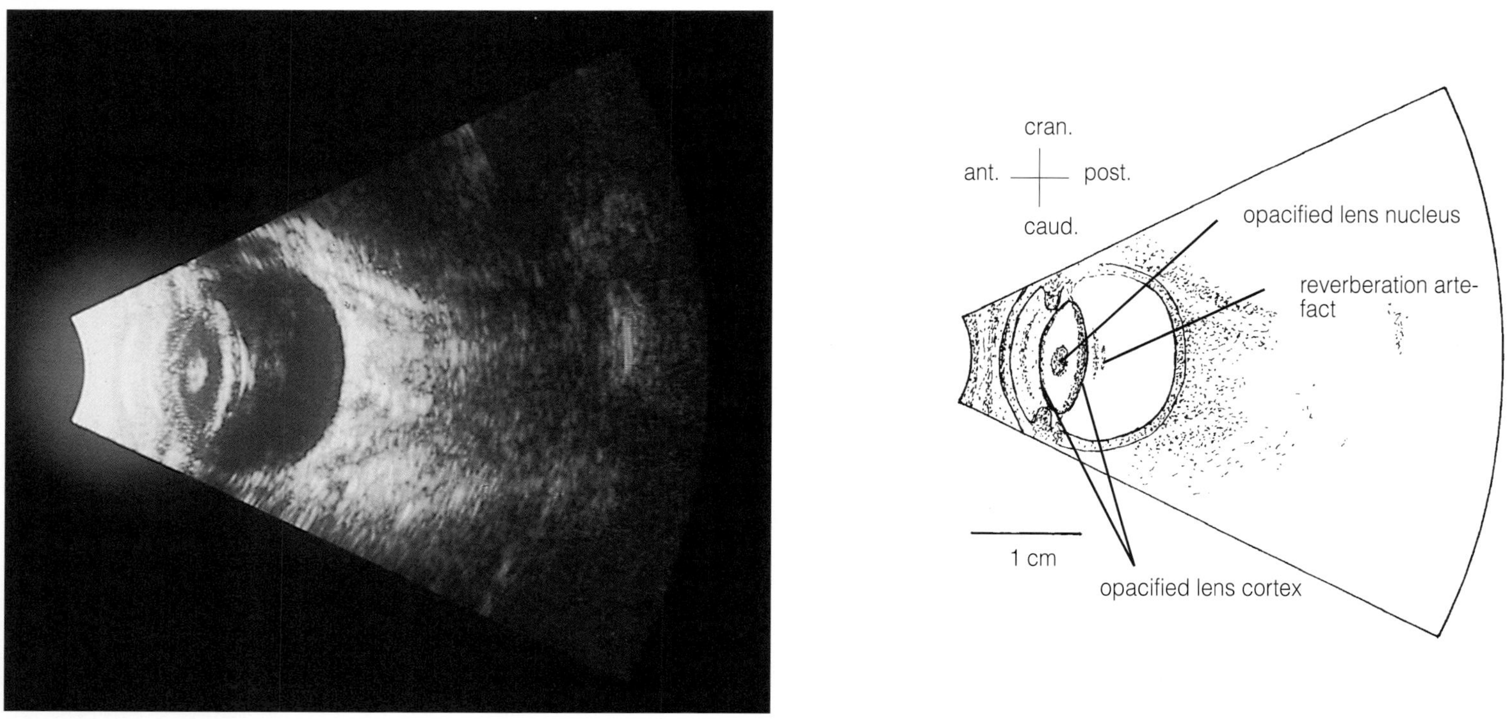

221 Nuclear and cortical cataract in a dog. The nucleus and cortex of the lens body are opacified. The echogenic posterior lens cortex causes reverberation artefacts in the vitreous chamber.

icity of the normally clear aqueous humour. In some cases the echogenic particles move with the flow of the aqueous fluid[21]. Blood clots have moderate echogenicity and are usually more or less attached to the iris or ciliary body. They may appear similar to tumorous masses.

An anteriorly dislocated lens is easier to recognize if it has cataract formation since it is then hyperechoic. A clear dislocated lens is more difficult to find, because the sound beam is never exactly perpendicular to the tilted lens and cannot produce an echo. An anterior lens dislocation is usually accompanied by posterior dislocation of the iris (**218**).

Iris and Ciliary Body

An increase in iris and ciliary body size may be caused by trauma, inflammation (**219**) or neoplasia (**220**). Chronic iridocyclitis results in better sonographic visualization and differentiation of these structures than in the normal eye (**219**).

The size and motility of the pupil is important in assessing prognosis and therapy in eye diseases where there is an opacified cornea. In the human eye the iris diaphragm, pupillary size and pupillary reaction are evaluated ultrasonographically in a transverse view with a maximal converging eyeball[9]. This view is basi-

222

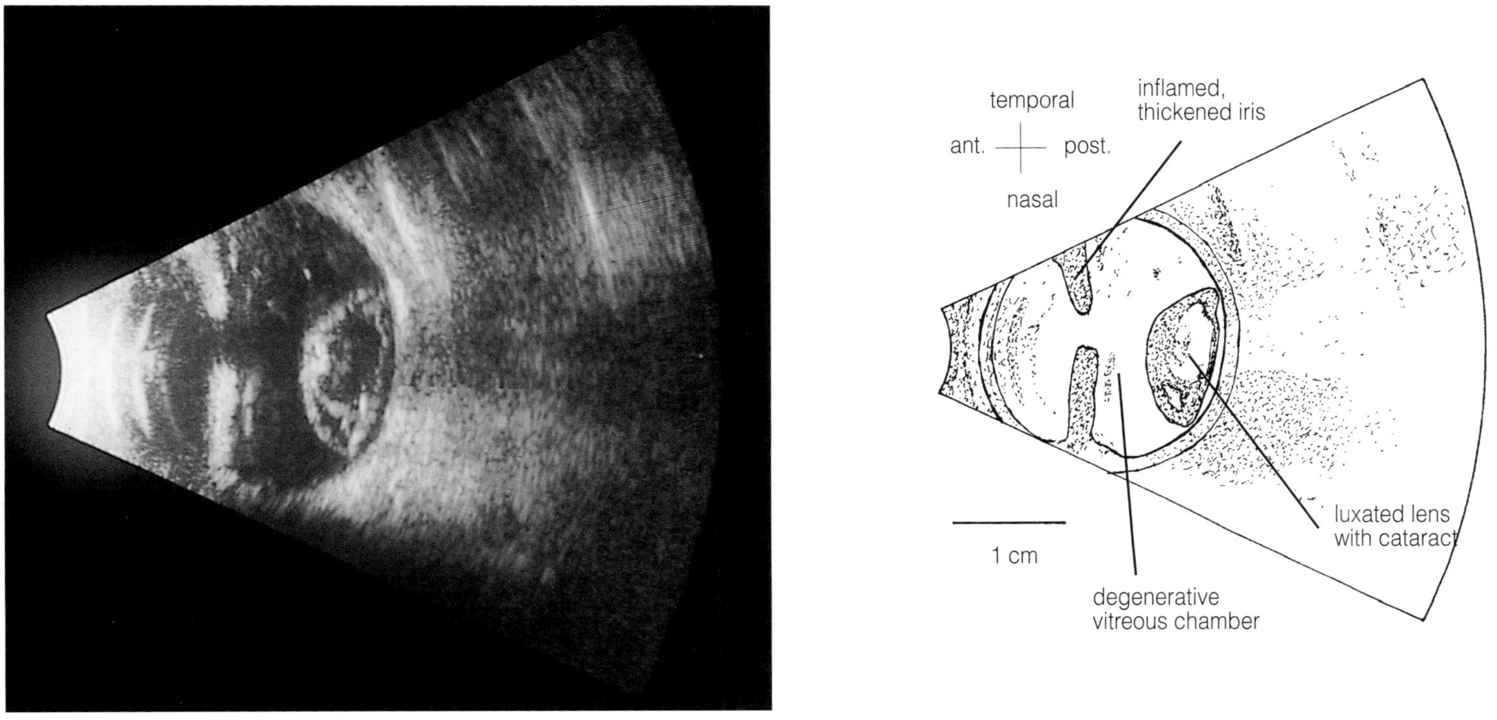

222 Posterior lens dislocation in a cat caused by chronic idiopathic uveitis. The inflamed iris is thickened and hyperechoic, and the iris diaphragm is displaced posteriorly. The lens is deformed and shows opacification of the cortex and around the nucleus. The parallel opacities in the vitreous chamber are degenerative or infiltrative.

cally possible in dogs and cats (**212, 213**). The eyeball must be adducted under general anaesthesia, especially in animals with deep-set eyes. Assessment of pupillary reaction is not possible under these circumstances.

Lens

Ultrasonographic axial measurements of lens diameters in the adult dog are between 6.64 and 7.84 mm[20]. The lens size can be larger during the immature stage of cataract formation due to water retention (see above). A reduction in lens size is found in hypermature cataracts and congenital hypoplastic lenses (microphakia). The lens has a higher sound beam velocity than the aqueous humour and the vitreous chamber, and this should be considered when evaluating and measuring lens thickness in A-mode and B-mode. The lens seems more flattened, and this is more apparent with cataracts.

Ocular lens non-homogenicities are also acoustic interfaces. The lens capsule may be covered with inflammatory particles or red blood cells, or the capsule and subcapsular lens cortex may be opacified. This allows the lens to be visualized in its entirety as opposed to the normal image (**219, 221**). The same is true for a pathologically small lens.

Complete opacification of the lens (*Cataracta incipiens*) may only result in slightly increased echogenicity. Isolated cataract formations within the body of the lens are easier to differentiate (**221**).

Ruptured ligaments of the lens near their attachments, accompanied by water retention during cataract formation, can be visualized peripherally at their attachments in a transverse view[21]. A Morgagni cataract shows an opacified, displaced nucleus in the lens body[21].

Dislocation of the lens can be displayed sonographically. Subluxation of the lens occurs when the ligamentous attachments are loose and the lens tilts away from its normal position. A small gap can sometimes be seen between the posterior portion of the iris and the anterior lens capsule. The iris may also be displaced caudally, which makes the iris diaphragm appear slightly funnel-shaped. This effect is more apparent with complete lens luxation. Anterior lens dislocation results in posterior displacement of the iris (**218**) (see above). Posterior lens dislocation is more easily identified with cataract formation (**222**).

Glaucoma

An increase in size of the eyeball associated with increased intraocular pressure can be visualized in the A-mode and B-mode image. The axial length of the eyeball is greater, as are separate sections such as an enlarged anterior chamber or a longer distance between the posterior lens capsule and the retina[14].

Pathologically reduced posterior wall thickness and optic disc cupping associated with glaucoma are not easily detected with conventional ultraound systems.

Vitreous Chamber

Diseases of the normally anechoic vitreous chamber can be detected early with ultrasonography. Ultrasonographic lesions of the vitreous chamber are seen with the following diseases (modified from Guthoff, 1988[9]):

- Bulbar deformities.
- Vitreous chamber infiltrates.
- Asteroid hyalosis.
- Synchysis scintillans.
- Posterior vitreal detachment.

223

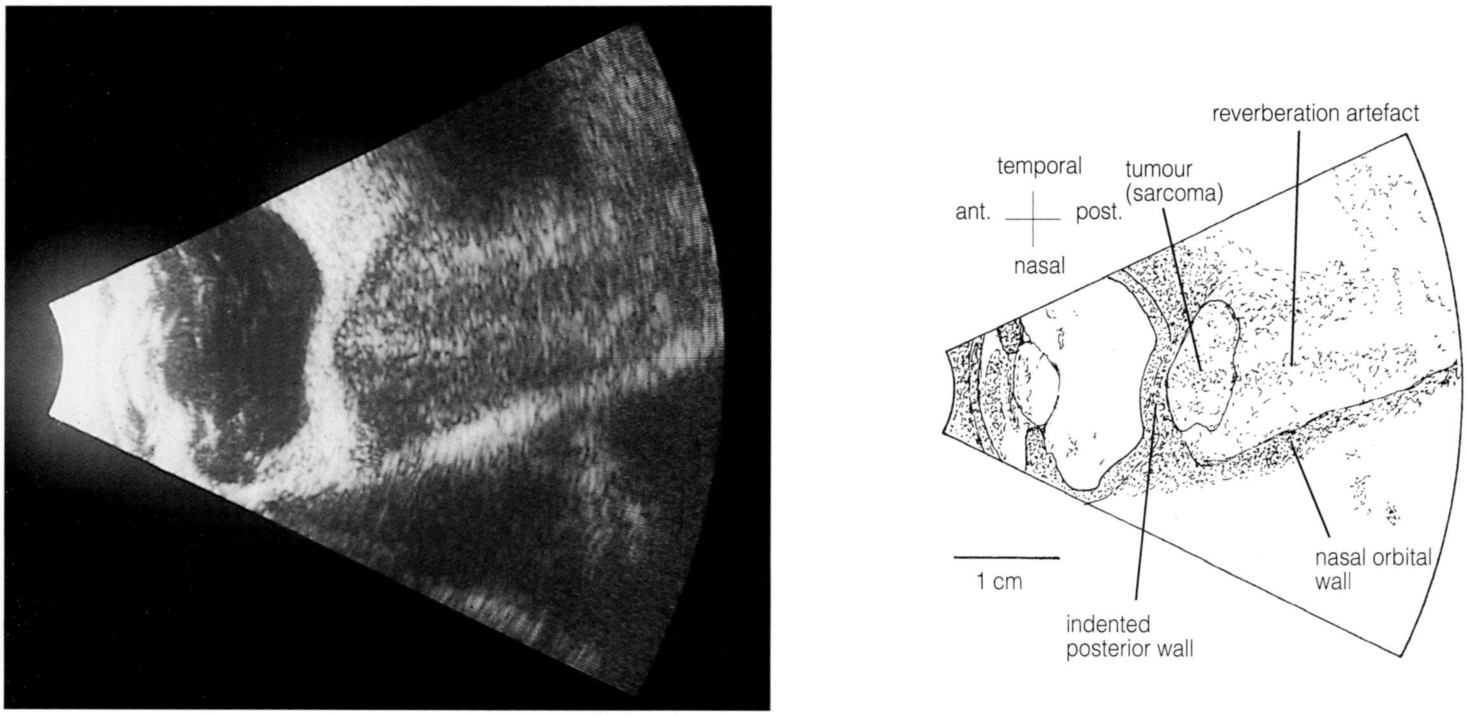

223 Retrobulbar tumour (sarcoma) in a dog with indentation of the posterior wall and associated deformity of the vitreous chamber.

- Vitreal haemorrhage.
- Uveitis.
- Intraocular foreign bodies.
- Persistent hyperplastic primary vitreous (PHPV).
- Retinal detachment.
- Neoplasia of surrounding tissues.

Bulbar deformities. Bulbar deformities are caused by space-occupying lesions, such as tumours, in the retrobulbar area (**223**). These 'real' lesions must be differentiated from artefacts produced near the posterior wall.

Large colobomas and staphylomas on the posterior wall are visualized sonographically as vitreal chamber attachments. The cystic structure and size of these colobomas can often be identified behind the posterior wall.

A pathologically small eyeball and vitreous chamber is seen with congenital disorders (microphthalmia) or shrinkage of the eyeball (phthisis bulbi). In both cases, sonography is helpful in differentiating the diagnosis from other disorders such as collie microphthalmia or simulated micophthalmia in deep-set eyes. In the dog and cat, bulbar phthisis in conjunction with posterior wall thickening cannot be accurately differentiated from micophthalmia.

Vitreous chamber infiltrates, vitreous chamber degeneration. Infiltrates of the vitreous chamber are seen as multiple point-like echoes, usually after increasing the gain setting. They are often found in older dogs in conjunction with cataracts and are considered a form of vitreal degeneration. Vitreous chamber degeneration is sonographically detected in 23–42% of all cases of cataract (in a study with 147[22] and 1,638[3] dogs). The incidence of vitreal degeneration increases with each stage of cataract maturation. These lesions are not known to cause complications in cataract surgery.

Synchysis scintillans. Both asteroid hyalosis and synchysis scintillans have distinct sonographic images without causing vision impairment.

Asteroid hyalosis shows hyperechoic calcium lipid complexes suspended within the vitreous body. Eyeball movement causes marked vitreal aftermotion. Associated vitreal detachment is seen by an anechoic retrovitreal zone (**224, 225**).

Synchysis scintillans, however, is caused by crystaline cholesterol complexes that are not suspended in the vitreous body. These crystals settle in the lower part of the vitreous chamber. Bulbar motion leads to swirling particles within the vitreous followed by infiltrate deposits. This phenomenon can be observed ultrasonographically.

224

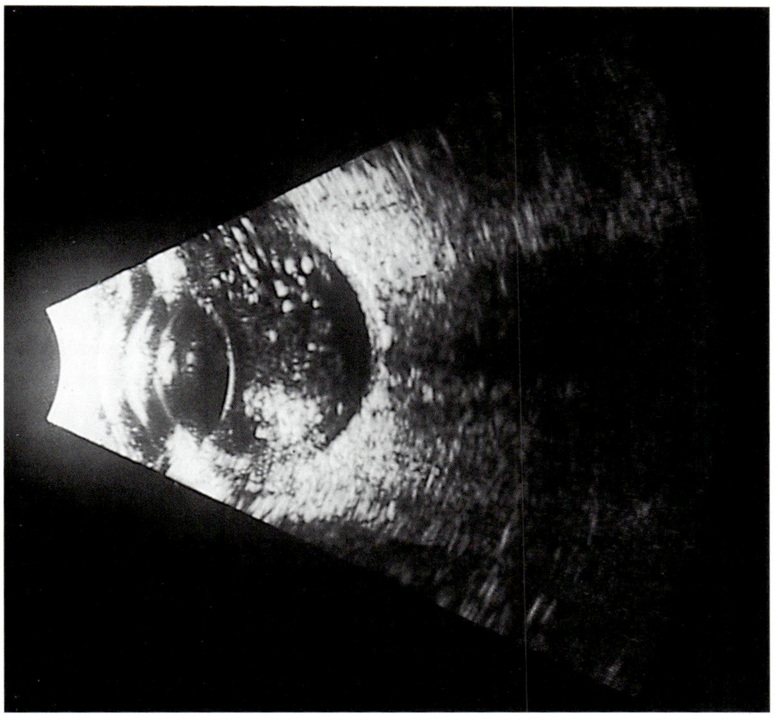

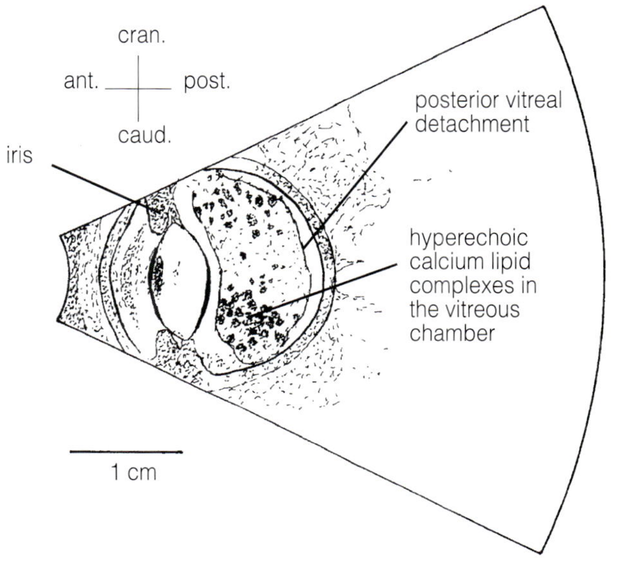

225

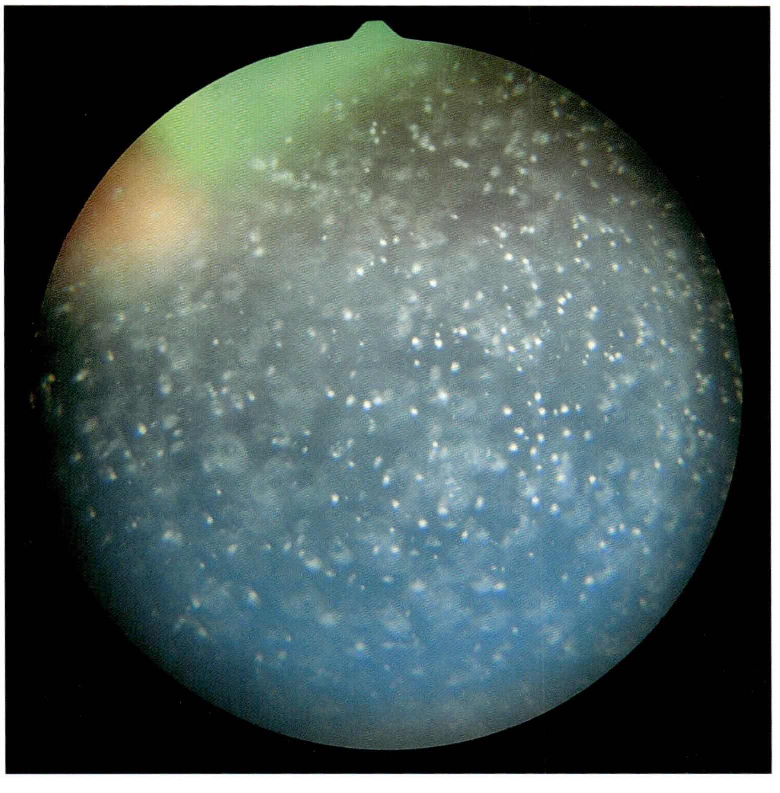

224, 225 Two-dimensional sonogram (**224**) and photograph (**225**) of the vitreous chamber in a dog. Asteroid hyalosis. The calcium lipid complexes in the vitreous body are hyperechoic and appear very large in the sonographic image (**224**), although they are actually small dots (**225**). The posterior portion of the vitreous chamber is detached from the retina (**224**).

Posterior vitreal detachment. Asteroid hyalosis and posterior vitreal detachment are usually associated with cataract formation in the dog. Posterior vitreal detachment is easily identified sonographically when the posterior portion of the vitreous chamber is echogenic due to haemorrhage.

The vitreous chamber may also appear to be more hyperechoic than the anechoic space between it and the retina. Differentiation from retinal detachment is difficult or impossible when the detached part of the vitreal membrane has a V-shaped attachment to the optic disc and the retina.

In one study, posterior vitreal detachment occurred in 7.69% of all canine cataracts; 2.32% of these cases also showed vitreal membrane formation[3]. The authors occasionally found vitreal detachments in dogs following intracapsular extraction of dislocated lenses with partial vitreal resection. Posterior vitreal detachment with trauma to the posterior lens capsule following cataract surgery may result in retinal detachment[2].

Vitreal haemorrhage. Ultrasonography is valuable in assessing possible causes of vitreal haemorrhage, such as neoplasia of the iris and ciliary body or retinal detachment (**226**). It is also useful in establishing a prognosis and therapy.

The sonographic image varies with age, degree and extent of haemorrhage. Mild haemorrhage may appear only as a more hyperechoic posterior vitreous chamber or as echogenic fibrous strands with red blood cells[9]. Blood clots within a degenerated vitreous chamber may appear similar to a solid mass and they are difficult to differentiate from neoplasia. Vitreal haemorrhage shows distinct aftermovement of the red blood cells. In some cases the entire vitreous chamber may be filled with floating blood cells and it have a higher echogenicity.

In humans, haemorrhage with posterior vitreal detachment usually fills the space between the vitreous body and the retina. Severe haemorrhage results in diffusion into the vitreous body structure with a subsequent increase in the number of acoustic interfaces. Haemorrhage in the retrovitreal space will resolve within days or weeks due to good fluid supply. Blood within the vitreous body is resorbed more slowly and can be identified sonographically for a longer period[9]. Comparable findings are seen in the dog.

Uveitis. Sonographic lesions of the vitreous chamber associated with uveitis resemble haemorrhage. Differentiation is only possible with the help of a case history and an ophthalmoscopic examination.

226

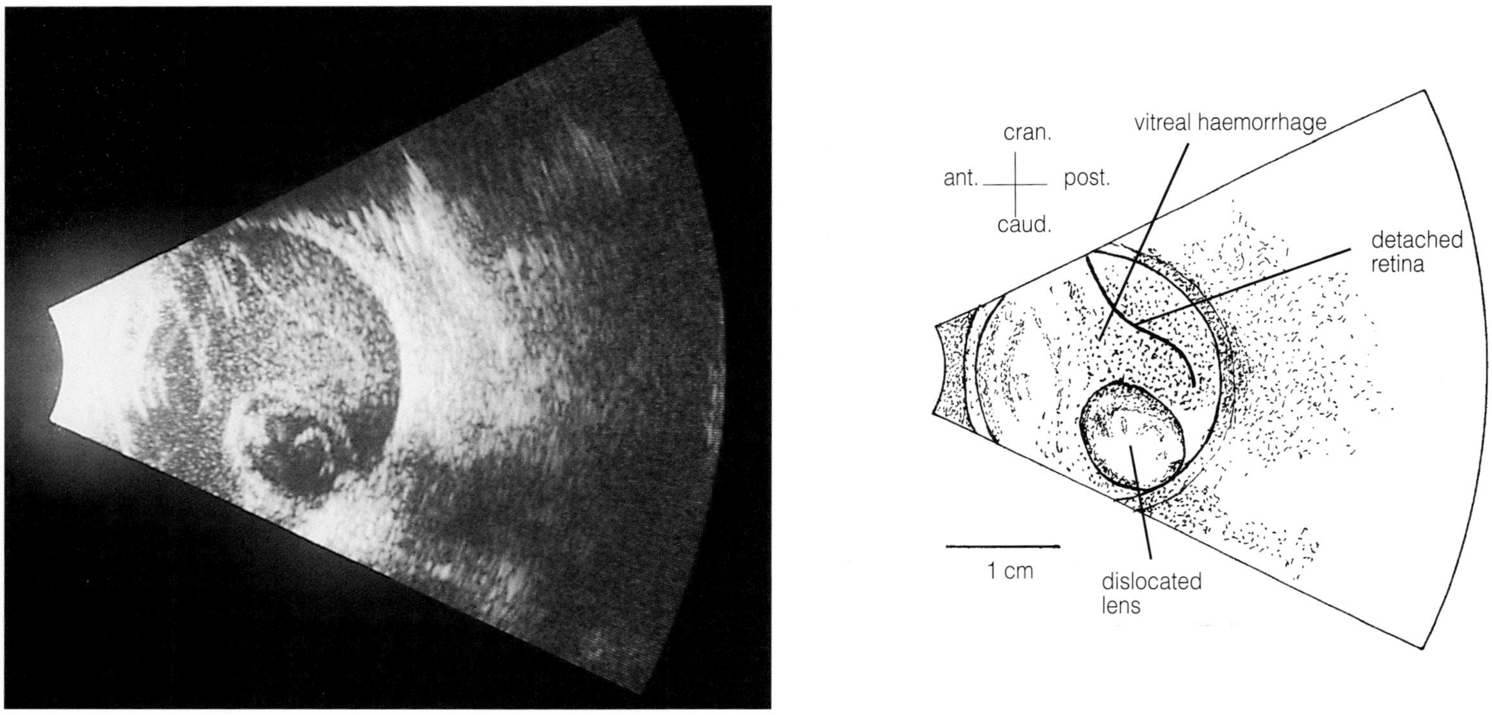

226 Hydrophthalmos, hyphaema, vitreal haemorrhage, posterior lens dislocation and retinal detachment in a dog. Glaucoma was obvious during the clinical/ophthalmological examination. Blood in the anterior chamber prevented evaluation of the posterior portions of the eye. The floating blood particles are dispersed within the vitreous chamber.

227

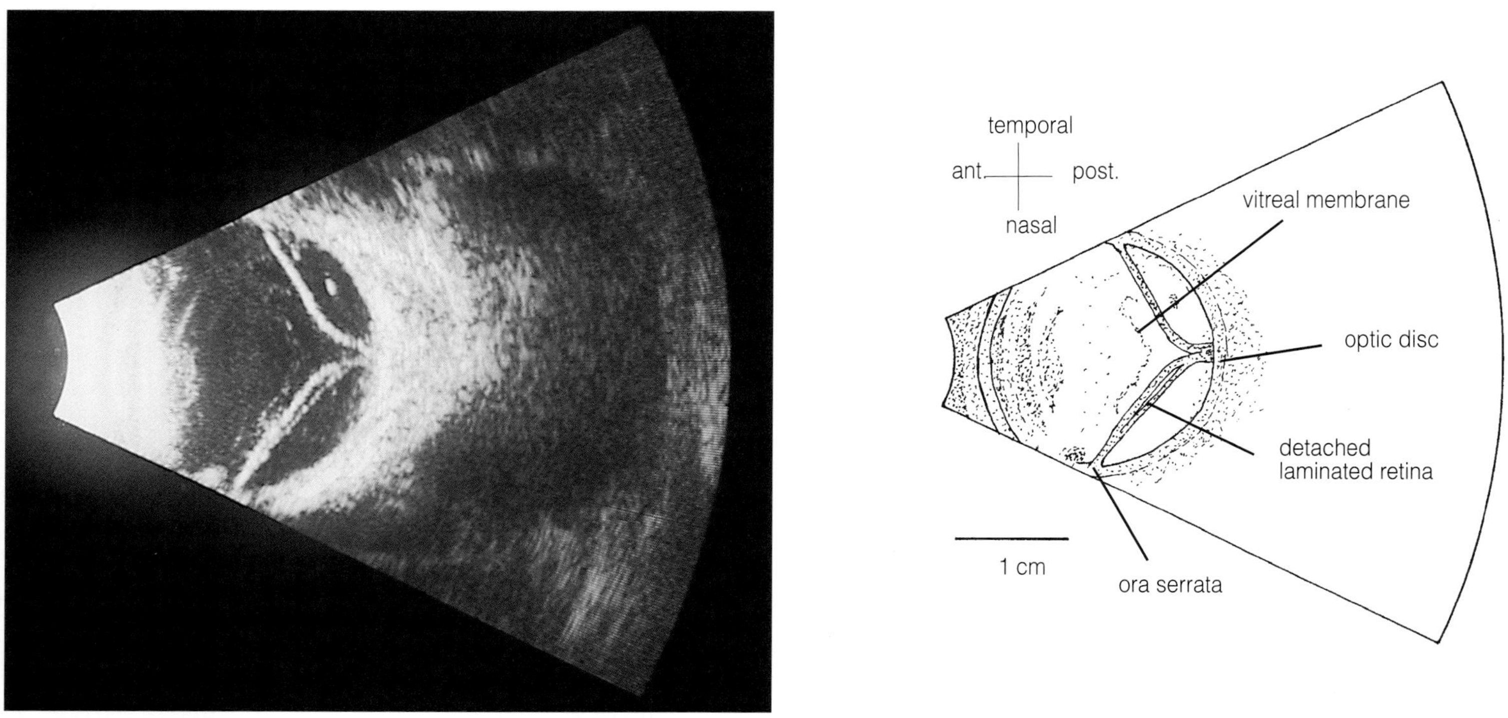

227 Total retinal detachment in a dog. The retina is attached to the wall near the optic disc and the ora serrata and has a V-shaped echo. The lower part appears laminated. Undulating aftermovements of the detached retina were seen after spontaneous bulbar motion.

Intraocular foreign bodies. Ocular foreign bodies are usually echogenic and they are easily detected with ultrasonography. Various factors limit the ability to image these foreign objects. Metallic foreign bodies are detected at a minimum size of 0.3 mm in diameter[9]. An uneven surface produces poor echoes. A slanted surface of the foreign body to the sound beam angle may prevent proper imaging of objects such as glass splinters that usually have strong echoes[9].

Persistent hyperplastic primary vitreous (PHPV). PHPV is a congenital condition with different sonographic images displayed depending on the degree of the lesion. Persistent retrolenticular hyaloid vasculature produces a hyperechoic posterior lens capsule. In severe cases of PHPV the findings include cataracts, a retrolenticular funnel-shaped mass and persistent portions of the hyaloid artery displayed as an echogenic stalk between the posterior lens capsule and the optic disc.

228

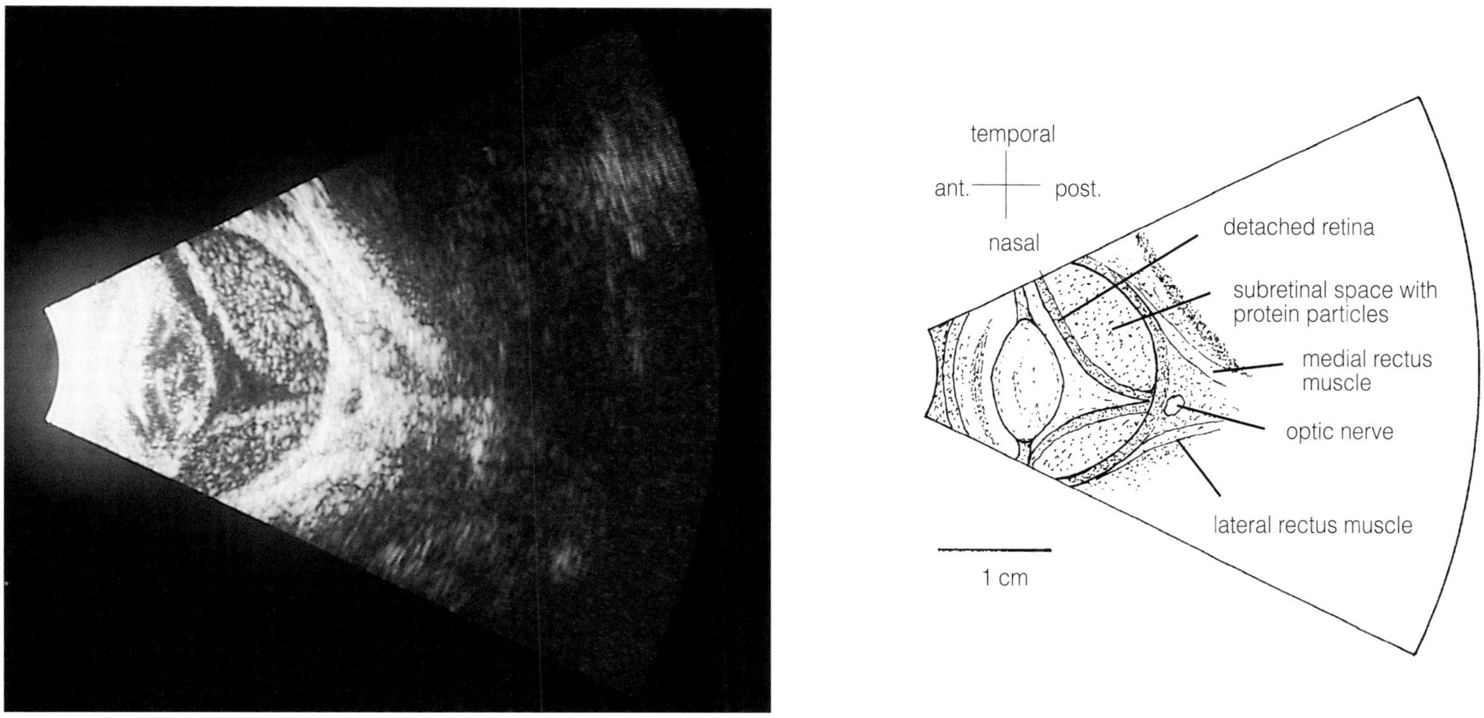

228 Total retinal detachment in a cat. The attachments of the retina at the optic disc and the ora serrata are distinctly visible. The vitreous chamber is compressed. Diffuse echogenicity between the retina and posterior wall is caused by increased protein content in the subretinal fluid. Differential diagnosis includes diffuse subretinal haemorrhage.

229

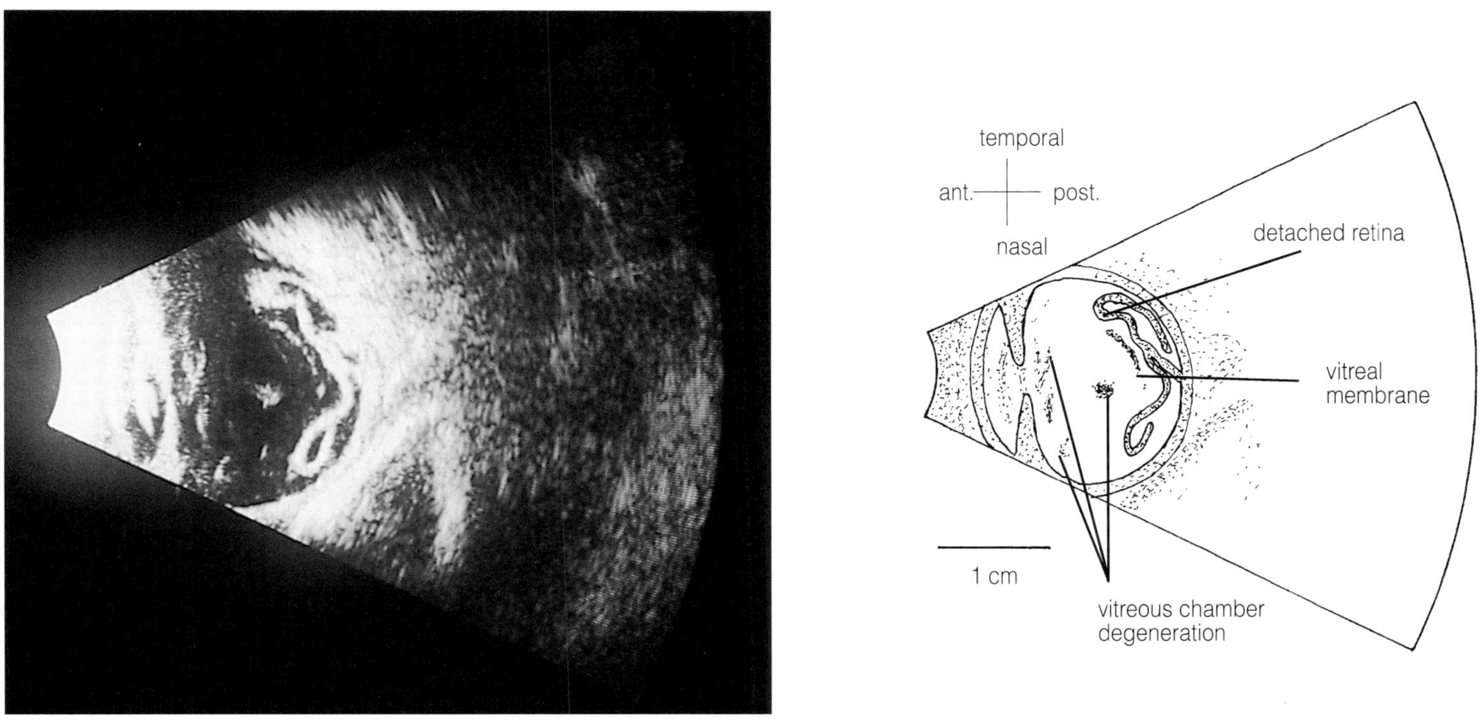

229 Total retinal detachment in a dog as a complication after intracapsular lens extraction. In this case the retina is also detached at the ora serrata and is folded in the posterior portion of the vitreous chamber near its optic disc attachment. Spontaneous bulbar movement resulted in whip-like movements of the retina.

Retinal detachment. Retinal detachment is one of the most important indications for ocular ultrasonography. Ultrasonography is the only method for providing a definitive diagnosis when direct ophthalmoscopy is not possible.

The sonographic image of a detached retina can vary. The typical sonogram of total retinal detachment shows two membranes attached at the optic disc and the ora serrata of each side (**227, 228**). The shape is that of a V or a triangle. Differential diagnosis includes posterior vitreal detachment, which can appear similar to a detached retina. Retinal detachment can be differentiated from posterior vitreal detachment by the fact that there is no attachment to the optic disc. Additional vitreal membrane formation within the vitreous chamber can complicate the diagnosis.

Following abrupt bulbar movements, a ruptured detached retina will move in a whip-like fashion starting at the wall attachment (**229**).

When the attachments at the ora serrata are severed, the detached retina sinks to the posterior portion of the vitreous chamber. The retina can be visualized as a double membrane, attached to the optic disc, near the lower bulbar wall.

The sonographic image of retinal detachment also depends on the duration of detachment. Periretinal proliferation results in thickening of the retina, which is sonographically obvious. The aftermovements show lower amplitudes with trembling instead of floating movements. Older detachments lead to degeneration of the vitreous chamber. The vitreous body shrinks and the vitreous appears more echogenic. This process is accompanied by a narrowing of the funnel-shaped retina and vitreal membrane formation, starting near the optic disc. The end-stage shows the detached retinal portions so close together that the sonographic appearance is T-shaped. Older detachments also result in protein concentration and sedimentation in the subretinal space. These echogenic particles in the sonographic image may be confused with subretinal haemorrhage (**228**).

Ultrasonography of Orbital Disease

Sonographic examinations of the orbit are primarily indicated to differentiate space-occupying lesions in the retrobulbar area. In most cases these lesions are associated with an exophthalmos.

Ultrasonography assists in locating lesions that are either diffuse and non-demarcated or well-defined and focal and also indent the eyeball[15]. Ultrasound alone cannot always differentiate inflammatory diseases from neoplastic lesions in the retrobulbar area.

Inflammation and tumours in the retrobulbar area result in changes of the normal sonographic image. Phlegmonous inflammation appears sonographically similar to a disseminated, invasive tumour. Abscesses are characterized by a well-defined wall and are no different to a well-demarcated mass. Both a tumour and inflammation can have varying sonographic appearances, ranging from diffusely hyperechoic to focal and hypoechoic.

Indentation of the bulbar wall is usually indicative of neoplasia. However, inflammation of retrobulbar structures such as the zygomatic salivary gland can also have the same appearance[15].

Fine-needle biopsy and aspiration cytology of retrobulbar lesions should always be done under ultrasound guidance. The needle can be placed safely into the biopsy area without injuring the optic nerve. The sound beam should always be as perpendicular to the metal biopsy needle as possible to allow for good visualization. The same procedure is used for ultrasound-guided biopsy and aspiration of well-defined retrobulbar abscesses.

References

1 Barr FJ (1990) *Diagnostic Ultrasound in the Dog and Cat*. Blackwell Scientific Publications, Oxford.

2 Boydell P (1992) The significance of posterior vitreous detachment in dogs undergoing cataract surgery. *Paper Synopses BSAVA Congress 1992*, 165.

3 Boydell P and Pike R (1993) Ultrasonographic findings in 1,638 canine eyes with cataract. *Proc. 24th Annual Meeting, Am. Coll. Vet. Ophthalmol.* 152.

4 Cottrill NB, Banks WJ and Pechman RD (1989) Ultrasonographic and biometric evaluation of the eye and orbit of dogs. *Am. J. Vet. Res.* **50**, 898–903.

5 Fuhrmann R and Diedrich P (1993) Videogestützte dynamische B-Mode-Sonographie der Zungenfunktion während des Schluckens. *Fortschr. Kieferorthop.* **54**, 17–26.

6 Gateno J, Miloro M, Hendler BH and Horrow M (1993) The use of ultrasound to determine the position of the mandibular condyle. *J. Oral. Maxillofacial Surg.* **51**, 1081–1086.

7 Gianoli GJ, Mann WJ and Miller RH (1992) B-mode ultrasonography of the paranasal sinuses compared with CT findings. *Otolaryngol. Head Neck Surg.* **107**, 713–720.

8 Gilbricht E and Heidelbach JG (1969) Über diagnostische Möglichkeiten mit dem Ultraschall-Echolot-Verfahren bei Erkrankungen der Kieferhöhlen. *Z. Laryng. Rhinol. Otol.* **48**, 363–373.

9 Guthoff R (1988) *Ultraschall in der Ophthalmologischen Praxis*. Enke Verlag, Stuttgart.

10 Heidelbach JG and Gilbricht E (1969) Über die Anwendung des Ultraschallecholotverfahrens in der Stirnhöhlendiagnostik. *Z. Laryng. Rhinol. Otol.* **48**, 699–706.

11 Hudson JA, Cartee RE, Buxton DF, Simpson ST and Steiss JE (1990) Ultrasonographic diagnosis of canine hydrocephalus *Vet. Radiol.* **31**, 50–58.

12 Hudson JA, Simpson ST, Cartee RE and Buxton DF (1989) Ultrasonographic anatomy of the canine brain. *Vet. Radiol.* **30**, 13–21.

13 Hudson JA, Simpson ST, Cox NR and Buxton DF (1991) Ultrasonographic examination of the normal canine neonatal brain. *Vet. Radiol.* **32**, 50–59.

14 Lohmann B (1994) *Biometrie am Handeauge mit Hilfe des A-Modus Ultraschallverfahrens*. Gießen, Justus-Liebig-Univ., Veterinärmed. Fak., Diss.

15 Morgan R (1989) Ultrasonography of retrobulbar diseases of the dog and cat. *J. Am. Anim. Hosp. Assoc.* **25**, 393–399.

16 Nabeih YB and Speculand B (1991) Ultrasonography as a diagnostic aid in temporomandibular joint dysfunction: a preliminary investigation. *Int. J. Oral. Maxillofacial. Surg.* **20**, 182–186.

17 Nickel R, Schummer A, Wille K-H and Wilkens H (1992) Passiver Bewegungsapparat, Skelettsystem. Herkunft des Kopfskelettes. In: Nickel R, Schummer A and Seiferle E (Eds.) *Lehrbuch der Anatomie der Haustiere. Vol. I.* 6th Edn. Verlag Paul Parey, Berlin, Hamburg, pp. 131–133.

18 Orikarinen KS, Nieminen TM, Makarainen H and Pyhtinen J (1993) Visibility of foreign bodies in soft tissue in plain radiographs, computed tomography, magnetic resonance imaging, and ultrasound. An *in vitro* study. *Int. J. Oral. Maxillofacial. Surg.* **22**, 119–124.

19 Pavlin CJ and Foster FS (1994) *Ultrasound Biomicroscopy of the Eye*. Springer Verlag, New York, Berlin, Heidelberg.

20 Schiffer SP, Rantanen NW, Leary GA and Bryan GM (1982) Biometric study of the canine eye using A-mode ultrasonography. *Am. J. Vet. Res.* **43**, 826–830.

21 Spaulding KA (1994) Ocular sonography. Vortrag, gehalten auf dem 1. *Basic Science Course in Veterinary and Comparative Ophthalmology*. Raleigh, North Carolina, USA.

22 Van der Woerdt A, Wilkie DA and Myer CW (1993) Ultrasonographic abnormalities in the eyes of dogs with cataracts: 147 cases (1986–1992). *J. Am. Vet. Med. Assoc.* **203**, 838–841.

7 The Neck

Cordula Poulsen Nautrup, Wolfgang Kästner, Bettina Denkewitz and Sven Reese

Ultrasonography of neck organs and large vessels has been routinely applied in human medicine for the last 25 years[2, 6, 8, 9, 10, 11]. Anatomical and technical problems restrict ultrasonography of the neck in the dog and cat. There are fewer indications for cervical examinations in small animals than in humans.

Neck structures identified sonographically include the oesophagus, trachea, thyroid gland, muscles and superficial cervical lymph nodes, as well as large arteries and veins. Normal parathyroid glands cannot be differentiated sonographically because of their small size and similar echotexture with the thyroid gland. Normal deep cervical lymph nodes are also not always visible. Large cervical nerves and the brachial plexus produce similar echos to the surrounding fat and fibrous tissue and are difficult to visualize.

Instrumentation and Examination Technique

Sonographic evaluation of the small and superficial cervical structures requires a high-resolution transducer with a frequency of at least 7.5 MHz or, preferably, 10–13 MHz. The neck structures are located in the near field and should be scanned using a linear transducer or a stand-off pad with sector-array or curved-array probes. A soft, flexible stand-off pad is useful for good skin contact in the uneven neck area and one should also be used with linear transducers. The small neck area in dogs and cats allows only short and narrow transducers with a small contact surface.

The use of high-frequency transducers requires proper clipping of the ventral and lateral neck area in dogs and cats. Dogs with a short, fine and thin hair coat, such as Whippets, Boxers or Dobermanns, do not have to be clipped. In some cases, close clipping and the use of commercial gels with preservatives can lead to skin irritations.

The examination is performed on a standing or laterally or dorsally recumbent animal with the neck extended. Some animals do not tolerate this position or the slight pressure on the neck. Because of this, the examination should be done quickly. Ultrasonography of the neck in non-sedated dogs and cats is possible only for quick examinations and/or in calm and well-behaved animals. Ultrasonography of the neck is indicated in clinically apparent cases such as masses. It may also be used for individual organs, such as an enlarged thyroid gland, or large arteries in patients with uncertain central nervous dysfunctions.

The sonographic area should be scanned in several transverse and longitudinal planes. Oblique longitudinal views (**230**) should be scanned in addition to the normal sagittal and dorsal views (**231**). A comparison of both sides of the body is helpful in finding small lesions.

Patient and image orientation is not uniform in human medicine. It is advisable to use the same orientation principles as in the abdominal scan (**232**) (see Image Orientation and Documentation, page 81).

Muscles, Fibrous Tissue and Fat

Anatomy and Normal Sonographic Findings

The paired sternocephalicus muscle is seen regularly on cervical ultrasound examinations and is located ventrally and laterally. It arises from the sternum and inserts on the temporal and occipital bones. These muscle form the ventral margin of the superficial jugular furrow. The cleidocephalicus and omotranversarius muscles are located dorsally. The sternohyoideus and sternothyroideus muscles are identified along the length of the ventral neck.

230

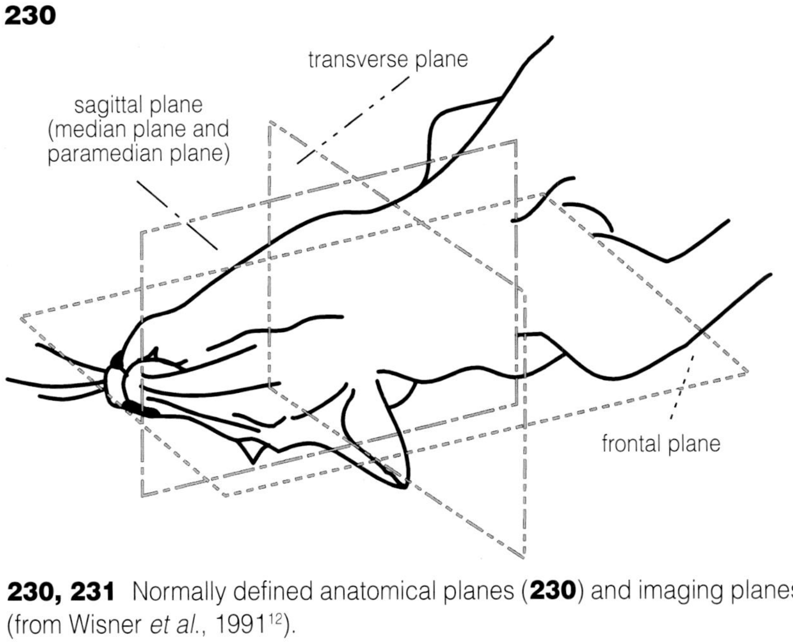

231

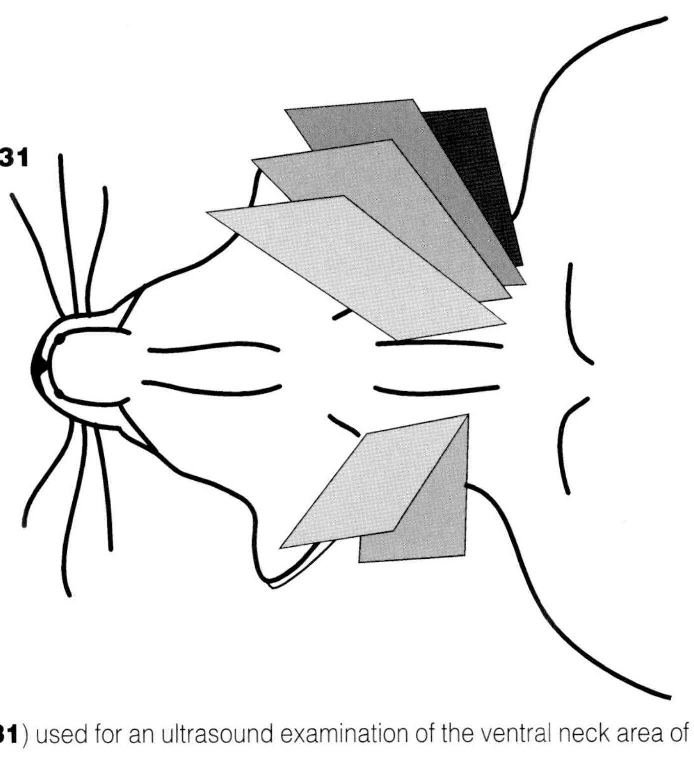

230, 231 Normally defined anatomical planes (**230**) and imaging planes (**231**) used for an ultrasound examination of the ventral neck area of a cat (from Wisner *et al.*, 1991[12]).

232

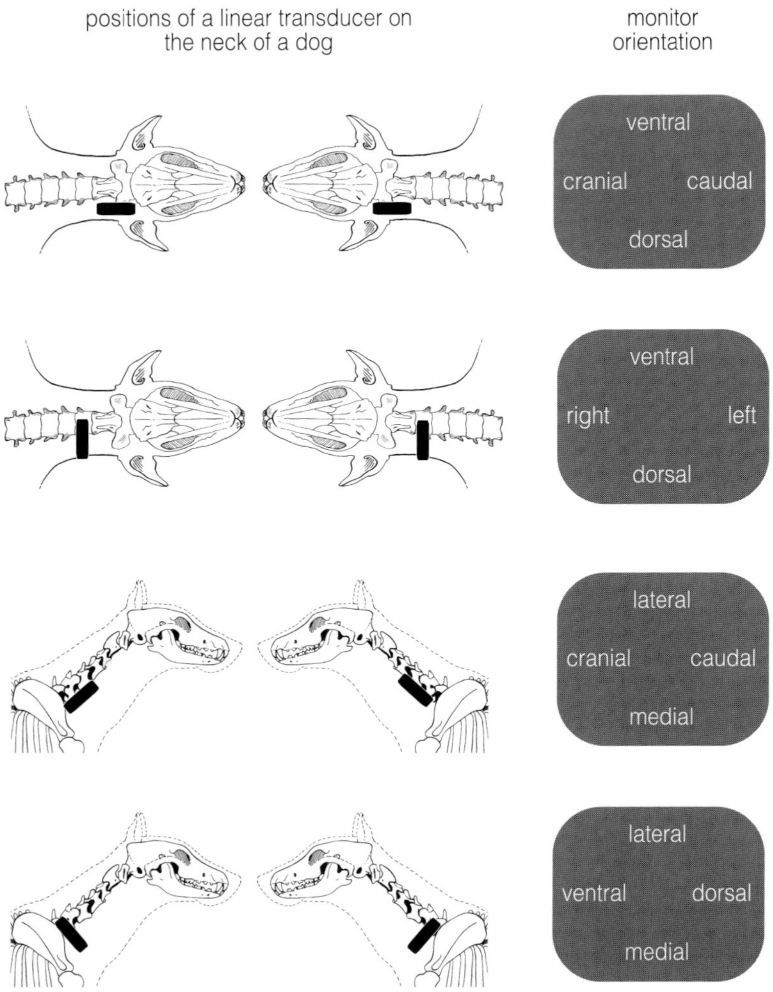

232 Patient and monitor orientation in cervical ultrasonography. (In some of the following images of the thyroid gland and common carotid artery (**243, 247, 248, 255, 256, 258**) the right monitor side is cranial and the left side of the patient is caudal.)

Cervical muscles appear more or less hypoechoic to hyperechoic and non-uniform (**238–240, 243, 255, 256, 258**). The echogenicity depends on the angle of the scan and the amount and distribution of fibrous tissue within and around the muscles. The muscles are followed along their path in transverse (**238, 239**), sagittal, dorsal and oblique views (**240, 243, 255, 256, 258**).

Fibrous tissue, including fascia and fat, is distributed between the muscles and neck structures. These tissues, as well as the nerves and deep cervical lymph nodes, appear moderately to highly echogenic. The individual structures are difficult to differentiate, although they delineate the muscles and other cervical organs (**236, 254**). In transverse views the vagus nerve is seen as a round, hypoechoic structure, well demarcated from the surrounding hyperechoic tissue.

Ultrasonography of Muscle and Connective Tissue Lesions

One of the most frequent indications for ultrasonography of the neck is undifferentiated masses. The sonographic diagnosis follows a complete history and clinical examination and should determine the extent of the lesion as well as the involvement of muscles or other neck structures.

Large, demarcated or diffuse masses following trauma are usually acute haematomas or inflammatory disease including oedema, phlegmons and abscesses. Acute haematomas are sonographically homogenous and hypoechoic to moderately echogenic. As the haematoma matures and organizes, it becomes more echogenic and more non-uniform. Inflammatory lesions have a completely different image and show hyperechoic areas with anechoic pockets of different sizes (**233, 234**). Depending on the type of lesion, there is a more or less clearly defined margin. It is not always possible to determine the involvement of neck musculature or other structures.

Pieces of wood[7] or large inorganic foreign bodies made of glass, plastic or metal are easily visualized[4, 5]. Small organic foreign bodies such as foxtails are almost impossible to find[1].

A tentative diagnosis can only be made on ultrasonography after a clinical examination. Histopathological examination produces a definitive diagnosis. Sonographically uniform and non-uniform masses should always include neoplasia in the differential diagnosis.

Thyroid and lymph node disease can also produce lesions on the ventral and lateral neck area (see Thyroid Gland and Parathyroid Glands, page 113; Lymph Nodes, page 117).

Larynx, Trachea and Oesophagus

Anatomy and Normal Sonographic Findings

The palpable larynx is located ventromedian to the head–neck border and joins the palpable trachea caudally. Both structures are covered ventrally by the long sternohyoideus muscles.

Sonography of air-filled structures can only assess the surface. The sound beam is completely reflected at the interface between the larynx or trachea wall and intraluminal air, which produces distal shadowing and/or reverberation artefacts. The reverberations are more distinct on a transverse plane (**236, 239**). In a sagittal view the trachea, especially in young and middle-aged animals, has a characteristic striped appearance due to alternating cartilage and connective tissue (**235**).

The cervical oesophagus is located dorsal to the trachea and it courses caudally, where it shifts to the left of the trachea. The oesophagus can be imaged from the left jugular furrow in a longitudinal plane with a slightly dorsomedian or horizontal scanning direction. Transverse views are made from the left or right cranially and ventrally in the caudal portion. The oesophagus shows a hyperechoic centre associated with intraluminal mucus and air. The mucosa and submucosa are moderately echogenic and difficult to differentiate. The thicker muscle layer is hypoechoic and is surrounded by a hyperechoic margin (**236**). The function of the oesophagus can be evaluated in the conscious patient by oral application of shaken (hyperechoic) or boiled water (anechoic).

Ultrasonography of Laryngeal, Tracheal and Oesophageal Lesions

Diseases of the larynx and trachea are usually diagnosed using radiology and computed tomography. An involvement of these

233

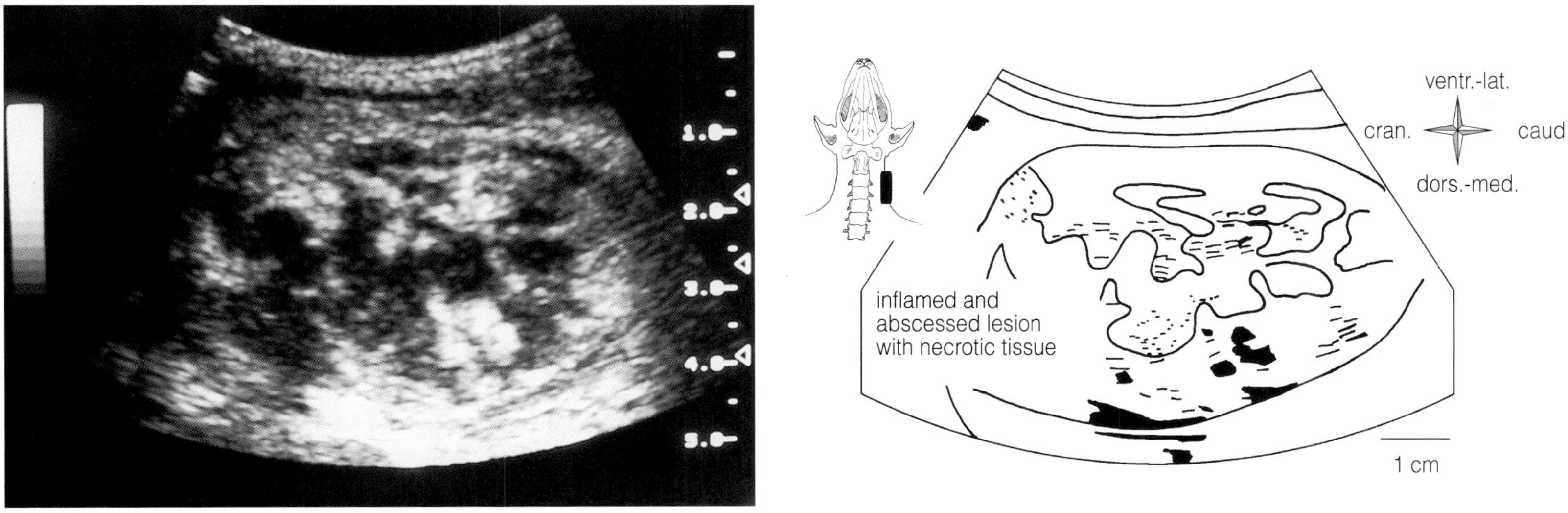

234

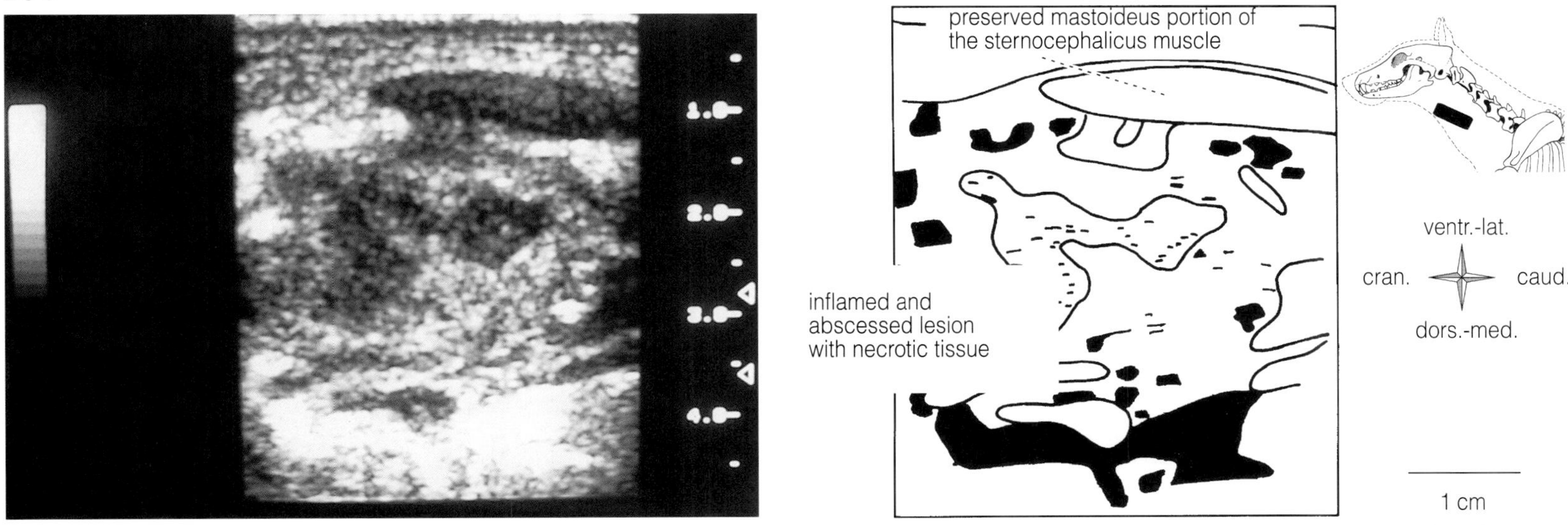

233, 234 Two-dimensional sonography in a dog. Large, traumatic inflammatory lesions ventrolaterally (**233**) and laterally (left side) (**234**) on the neck. Non-homogenicity and poor definition is characteristic of these lesions.

235

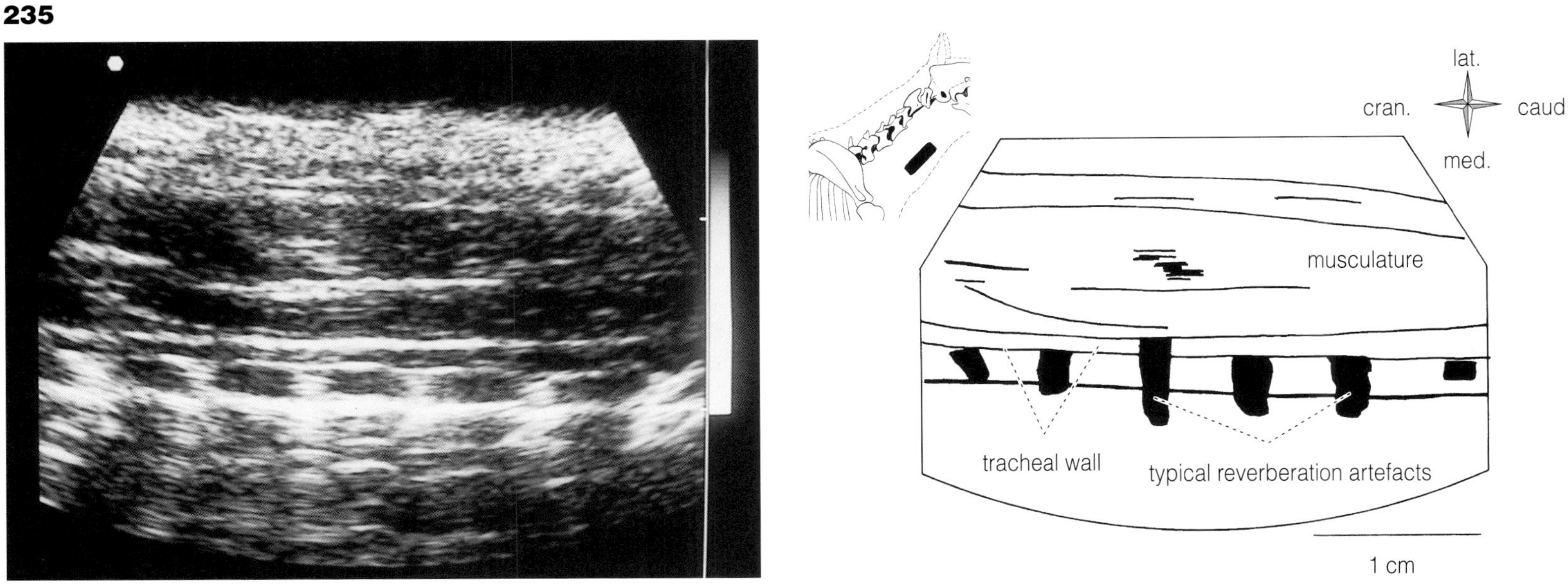

235 Two-dimensional sonography in a two-year-old dog. Longitudinal view of the normal trachea.

236

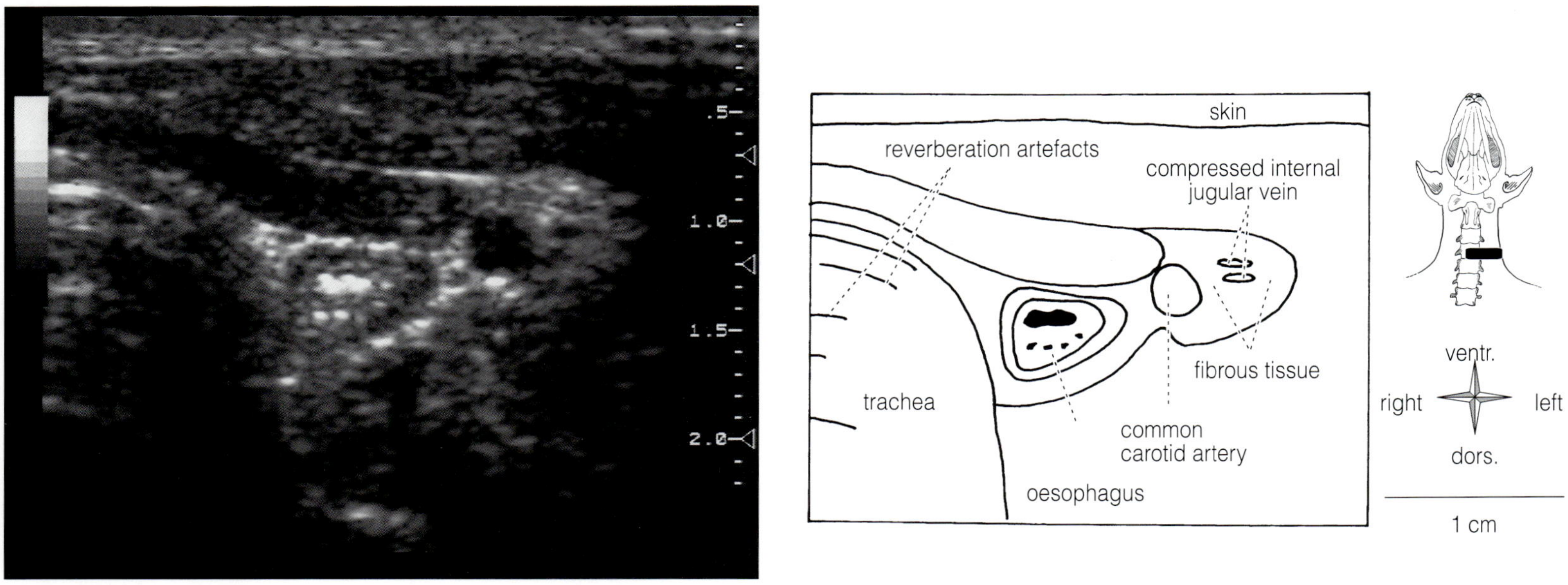

236 Two-dimensional sonography in a dog. Transverse view of the normal oesophagus.

237

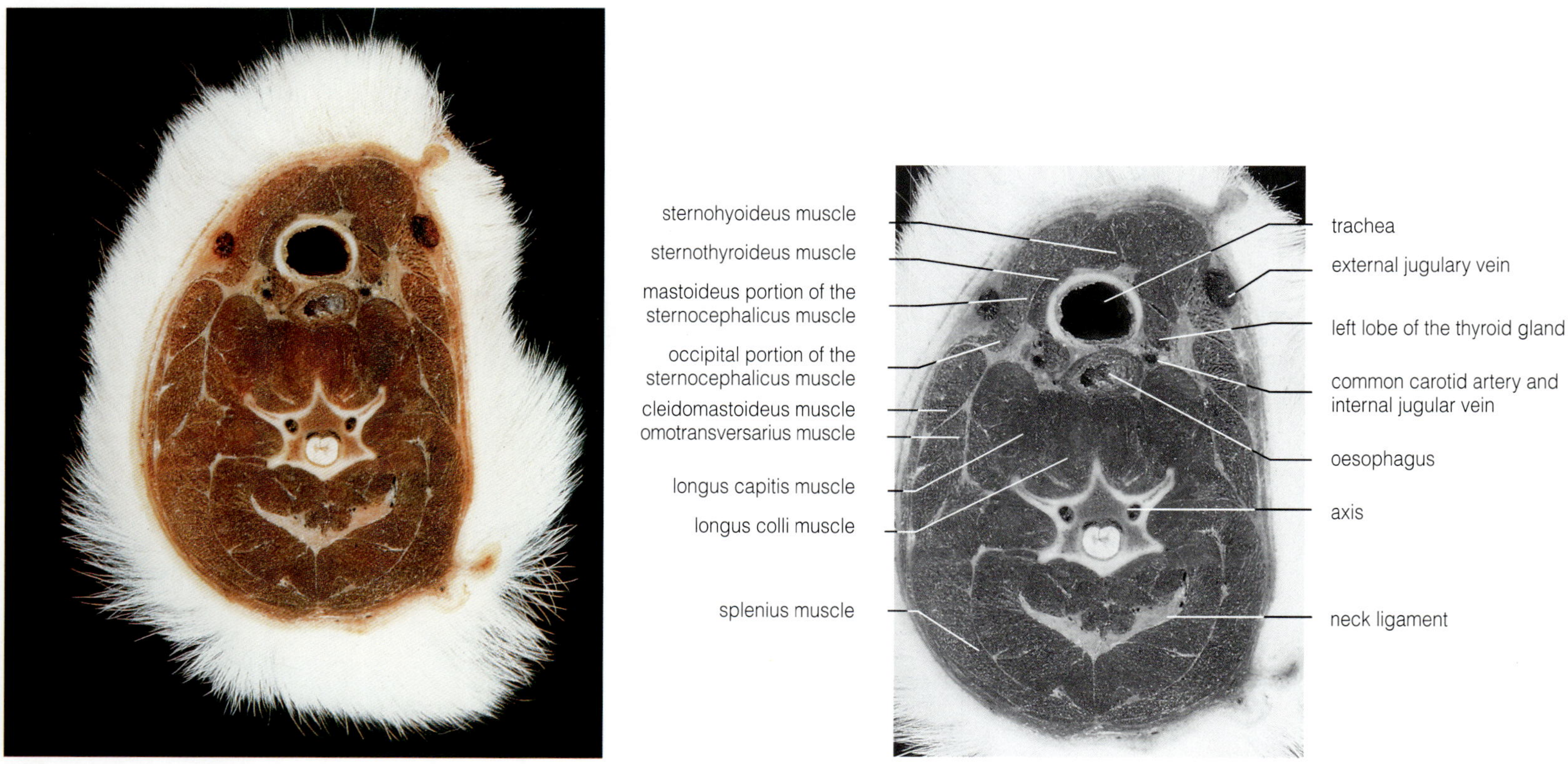

237 Anatomical cross-section directly caudal to the larynx at the thyroid gland of a dog.

238

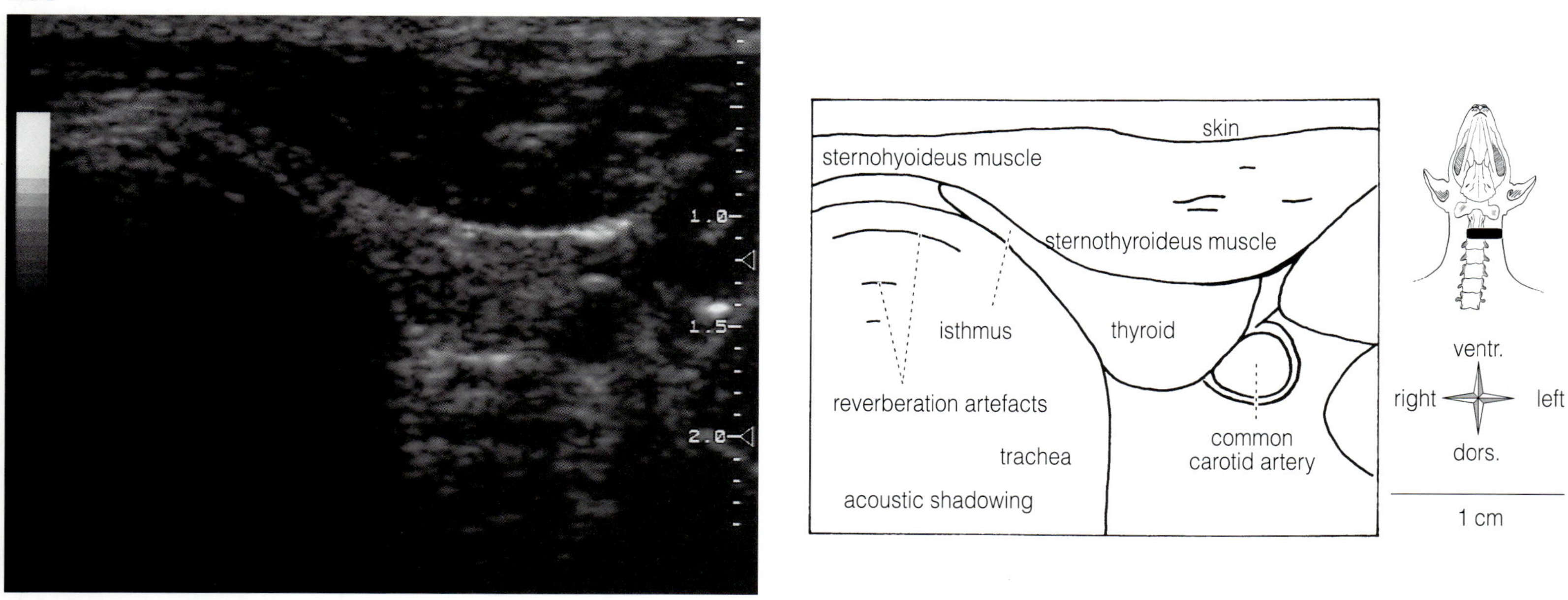

238 Two-dimensional sonogram of a dog. Normal left thyroid lobe in a transverse view. A thin line of glandular tissue (isthmus) is seen next to the trachea.

239

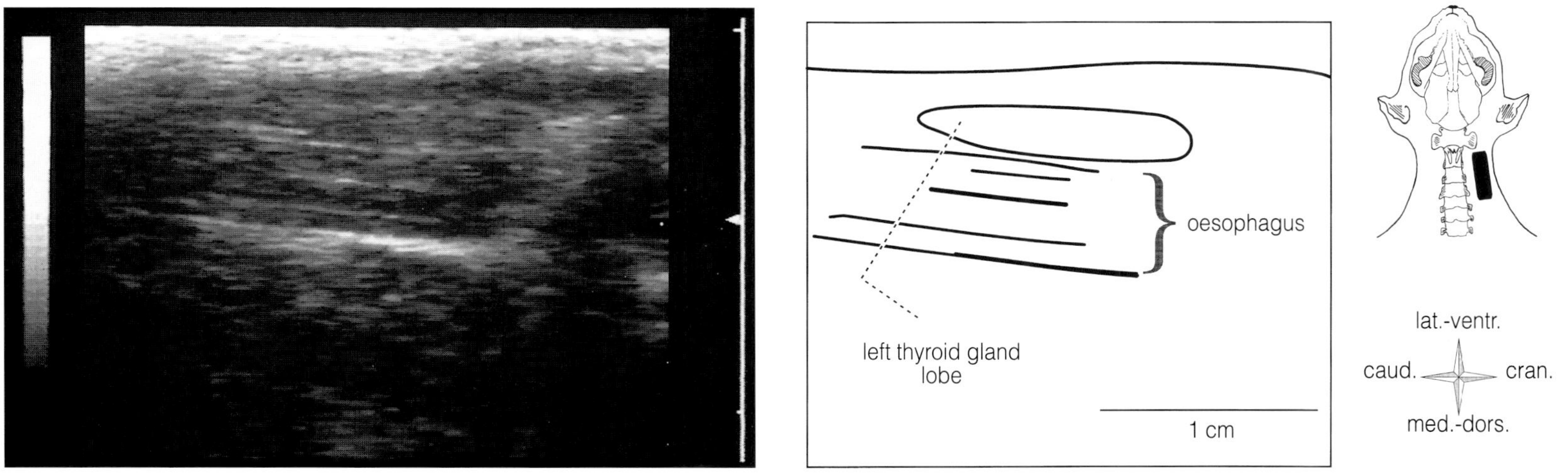

239 Two-dimensional sonography of a cat. Normal left thyroid lobe (and oesophagus) in a paramedian longitudinal view.

240

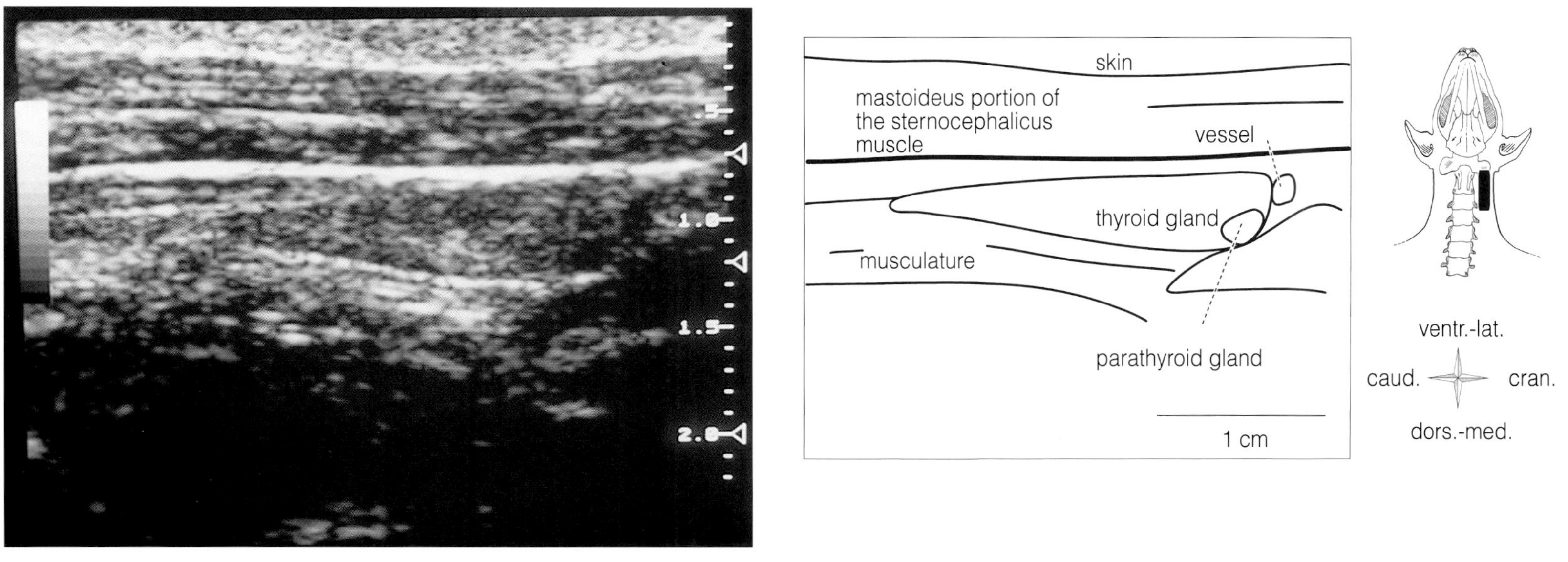

240 Two-dimensional sonogram of a dog. Normal left thyroid lobe and parathyroid gland in a paramedian longitudinal view.

structures with lesions in the neck area can be ruled out using ultrasonography by evaluating the surface or the width of the lumen. These ultrasound examinations are time consuming and do not always bring helpful results.

The same is true for lesions of the oesophagus. Wall lesions, obstructions and dilations are easier to diagnose in the neck area than in the thorax (see Oesophagus, page 25). Functional sonography of the oesophagus may determine the location and cause of decreased oesophageal movement or disorders in fluid and food passage.

Thyroid Gland and Parathyroid Glands

Anatomy and Normal Sonographic Findings

The thyroid gland consists of two lobes that are round in the transverse plane and flattened, oval-shaped in the longitudinal view. The lobes are situated to the left and right of the ventral trachea, directly caudal to the larynx (**237**). The lobes are occasionally connected by a thin glandular isthmus over the ventral aspect of the trachea in large dogs. The thyroid lobes are approximately the size of a pea to a large walnut in dogs, depending on the breed, and pea-size in adult cats.

Cross-sections of the thyroid gland are achieved by multiple transverse planes directly caudal to the palpable larynx. The thyroid gland is imaged in its long axis by rotating the transducer to a sagittal and dorsal plane. The transducer is positioned in the jugular furrow for these longitudinal views.

Normal thyroid glands image similar to other parenchymal organs, with uniform echos of moderate echogenicity and density surrounded by a fine echogenic demarcation. In the transverse plane the thyroid gland is round to oval, trapezoid or rectangular (**238, 239**). Ventrolateral to the trachea, a thin glandular isthmus can be imaged in some dogs (**238**). The thyroid gland is oval with a rounded cranial and a pointed caudal end in the longitudinal view (**240**). In some large dogs, fine anechoic areas are located around the thyroid lobes. These vessels and their blood flow can be verified using colour-coded Doppler sonography (**243**). With the help of colour-coded Doppler sonography, even small vessels in small or medium-sized dogs or cats can be identified by their blood flow (**243**).

The thyroid gland is located lateral to the trachea and medial to the common carotid artery (**238, 239**).

241

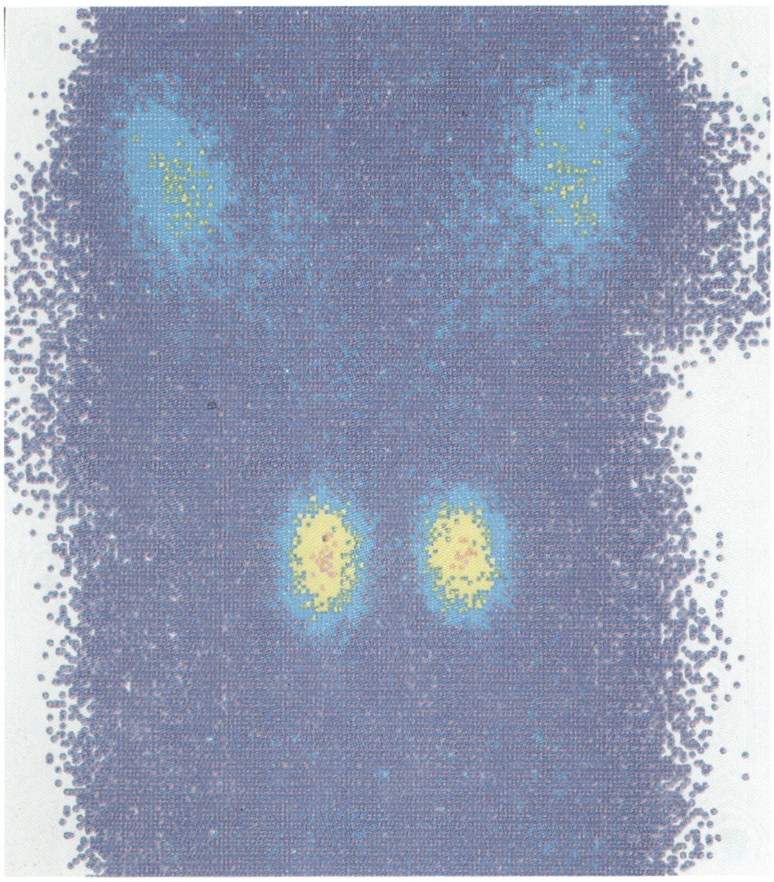

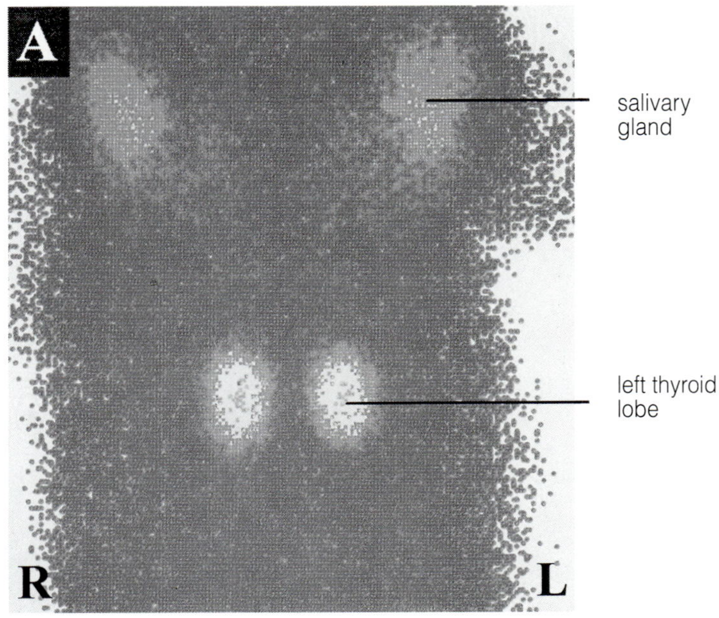

242

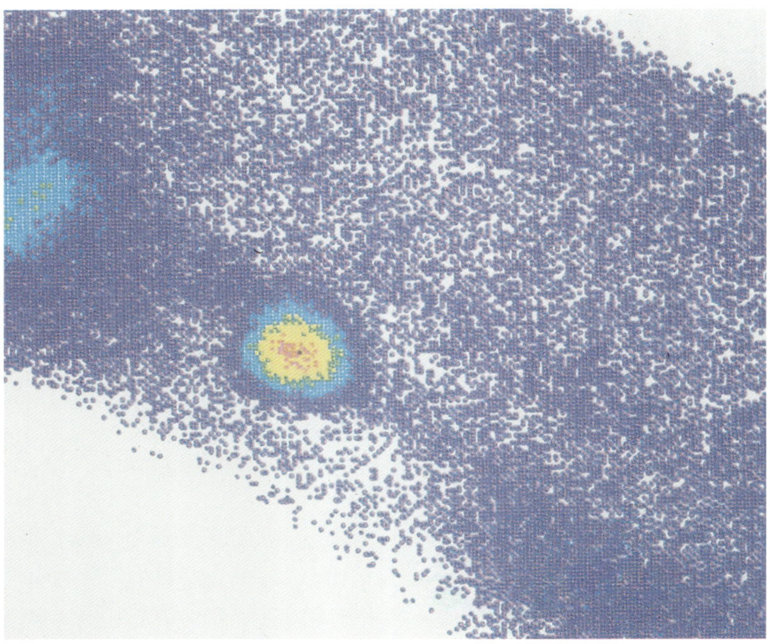

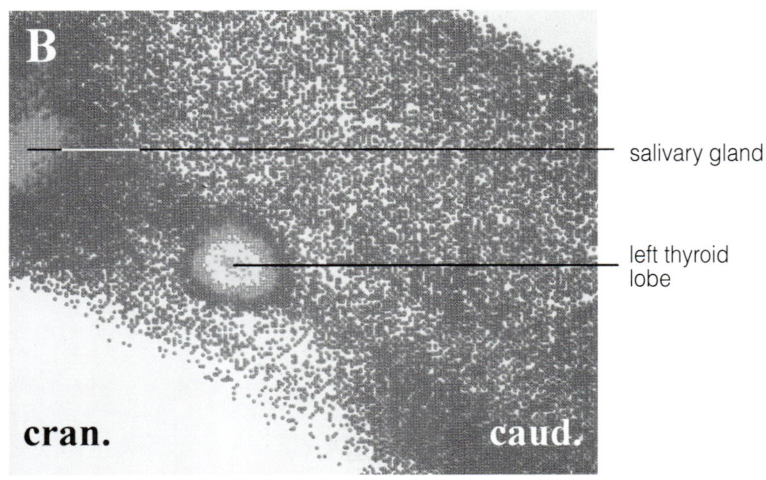

241, 242 Scintigraphy in a dog. Normal thyroid gland from a ventral view (**241**) and a left view (**242**). (Copied with permission from Anne Westhoff, Hannover.)

243

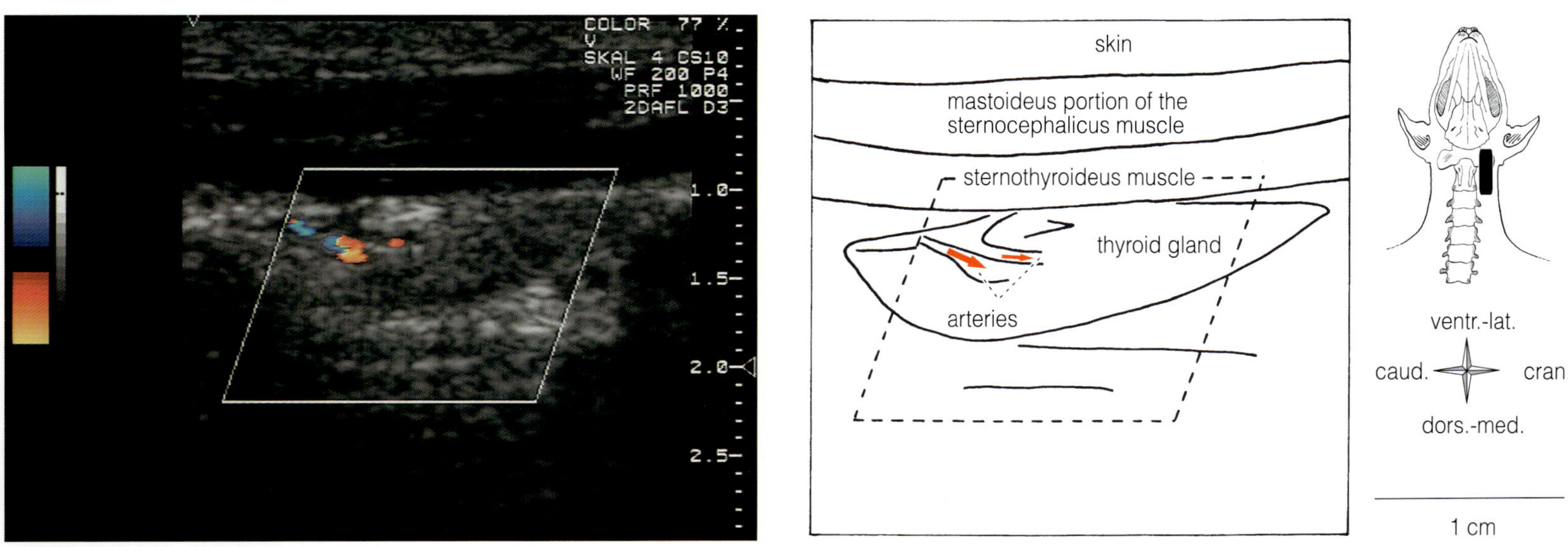

243 Colour-coded Doppler sonography in a dog. Normal left thyroid lobe in a longitudinal plane with arterial vessels.

244

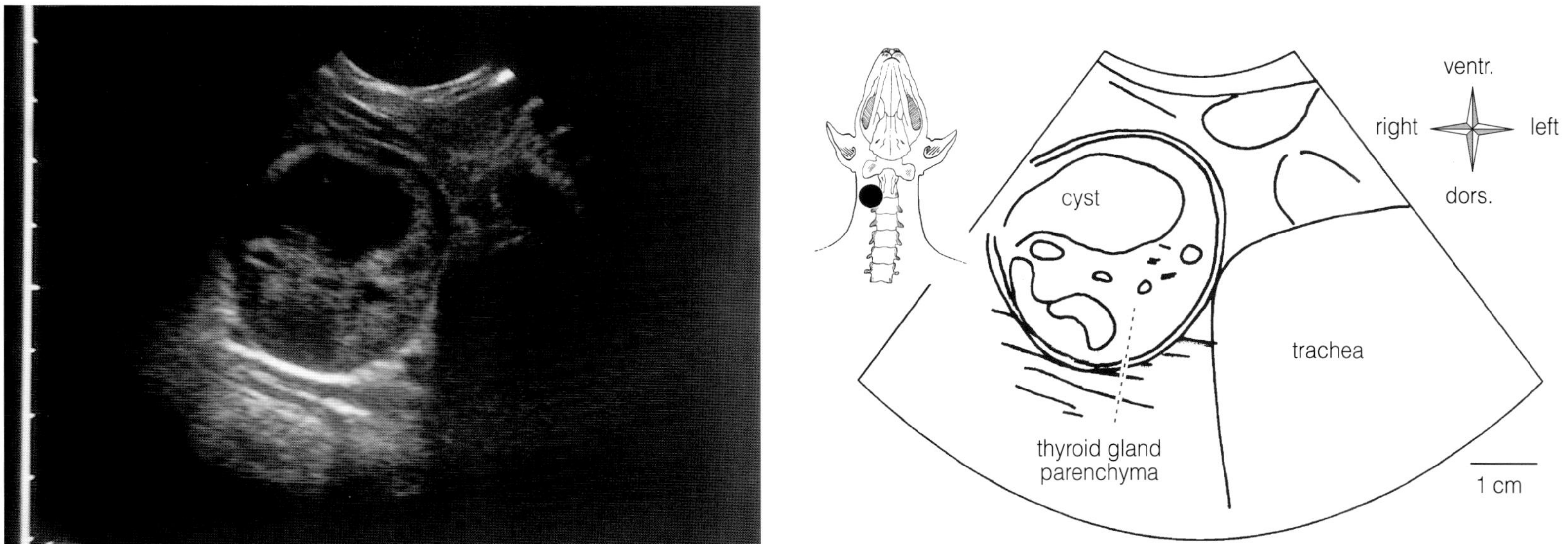

244 Two-dimensional sonogram of a dog. Cystic lesion in the right thyroid lobe.

245

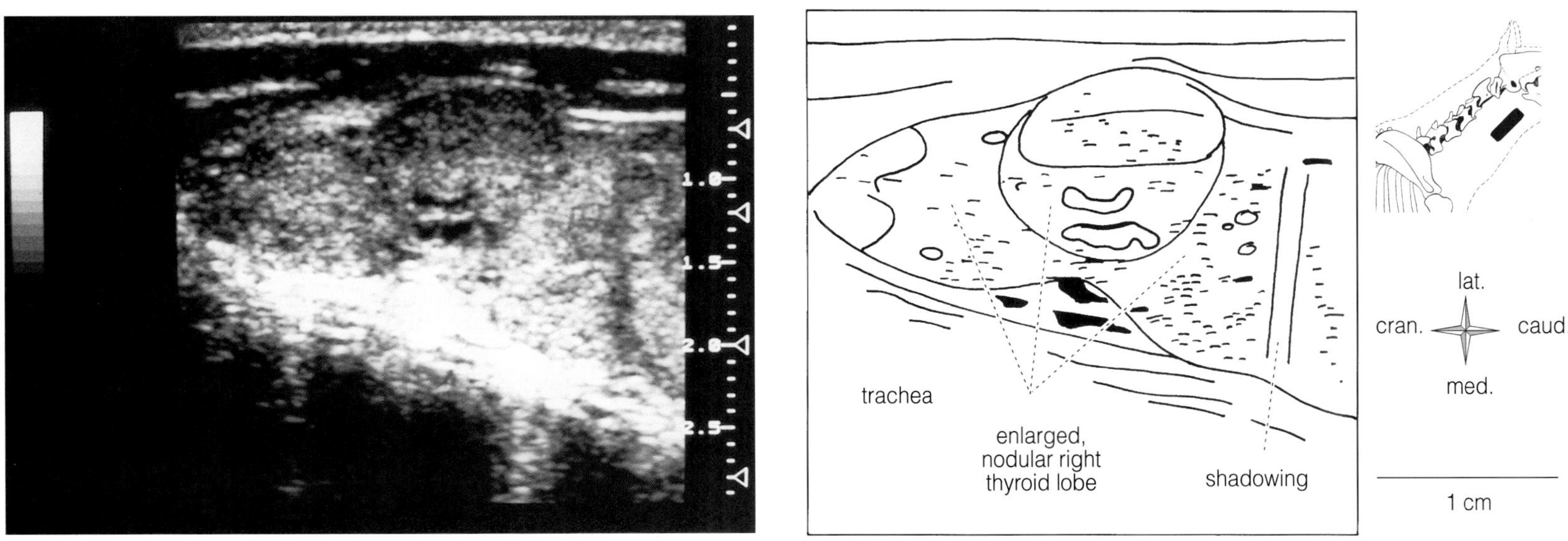

246

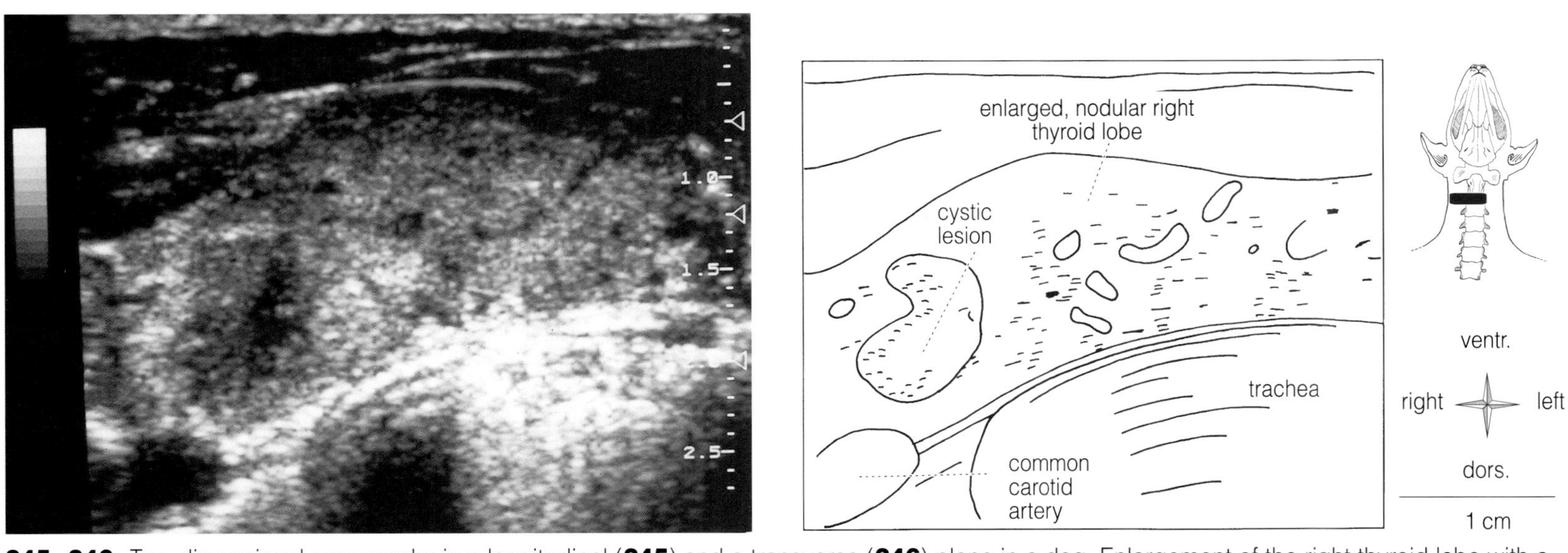

245, 246 Two-dimensional sonography in a longitudinal (**245**) and a transverse (**246**) plane in a dog. Enlargement of the right thyroid lobe with a two-year euthyroid condition. Nodular and cystic lesions are found within the glandular parenchyma. The benign nodules protrude over the surface of the thyroid capsule without spreading to the capsule itself. The left thyroid lobe is normal.

247

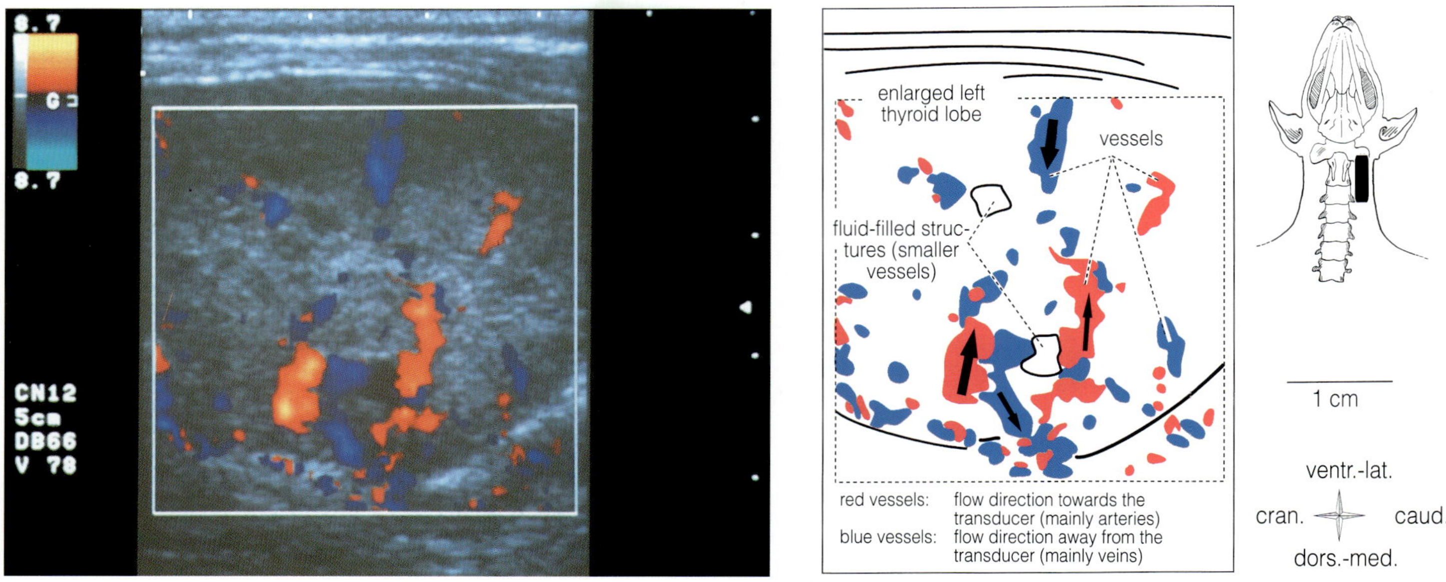

248

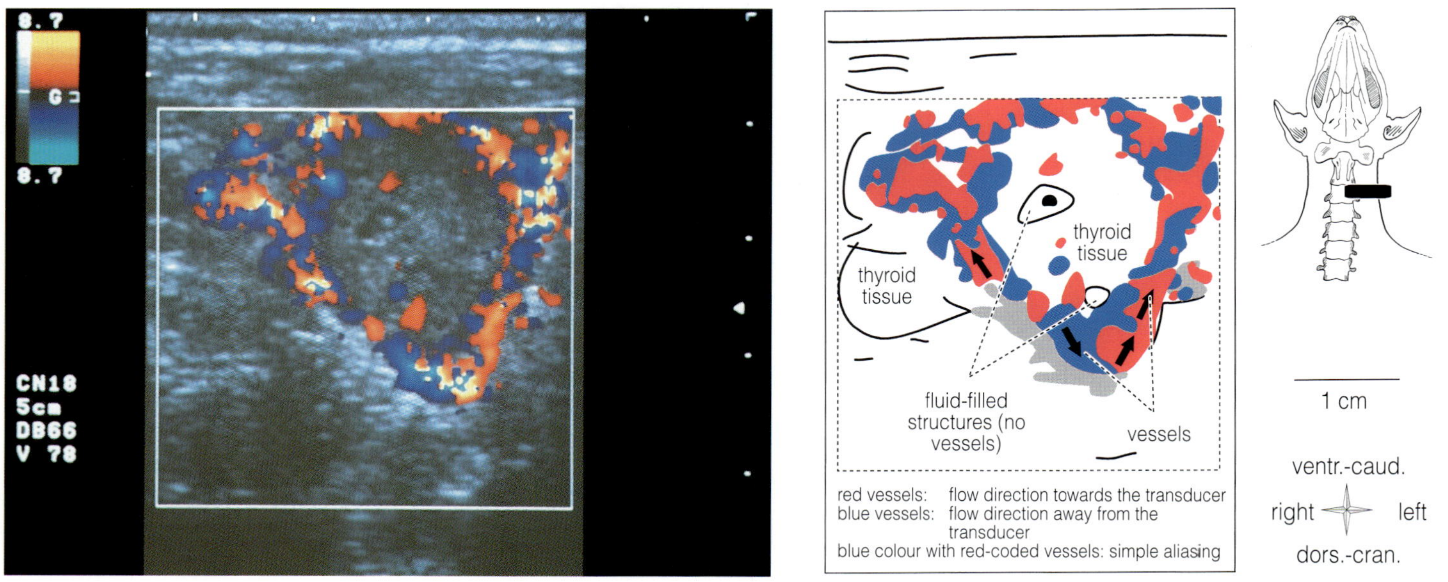

247, 248 Colour-coded Doppler sonogram of a dog. The enlarged thyroid lobe shows colour enhancement due to dilated vessels and additional blood supply.

The parathyroid glands are found embedded medially and laterally in the parenchyma of each thyroid lobe. Normal parathyroid glands are seen as hypoechoic to anechoic rounded structures in high-resolution sonograms. The more cranially located, outer parathyroid gland is visible in dogs (**240**).

Ultrasonography of Thyroid Lesions

Ultrasonography of the thyroid is indicated when there are mass lesions in the glandular area as well as with hyperthyroid or hypothyroid conditions. Ultrasonographic examinations should be accompanied by determinination of serum levels of triiodothyronine (T3) and thyroxine (T4) as well as thyroid-stimulating hormone (TSH) levels. These values usually determine therapy. Ultrasonography should be followed by scintigraphy, if possible (**241, 242, 249, 250**), and a fine-needle aspirate or biopsy.

Masses associated with euthyroid conditions are due to goitre. The thyroid gland is usually diffusely enlarged without any inflammation or nodular lesion. Both thyroid lobes are equally enlarged with normal echogenicity and texture.

Thyroid enlargements are more frequently associated with more or less demarcated nodules, cysts or calcifications. These lesions may be caused by euthyroid, hypothyroid or hyperthyroid conditions. The sonographic image is always irregular (**244**).

Cystic lesions are round to oval, anechoic, well-demarcated structures with distal acoustic enhancement (**245, 246**). Calcifications are recognized as strong hyperechoic structures with distal shadowing (**245**). Nodules may be echogenic with hypoechoic margins (**245**), hypoechoic and well-defined (**246**), or hypoechoic with irregular margins. The contours of the thyroid gland may appear cauliflower-like due to these nodules (**245**). A nodular thyroid gland may appear brighter and more colourful in colour Doppler sonography due to the number of large vessels and the blood supply (**247, 248**).

Two-dimensional and Doppler sonography cannot distinguish between benign and malignant mass lesions (**245, 246, 252**). Malignancies are suspected if there is poor definition and invasive tumour growth.

Acute and chronic thyroiditis, with or without abcessation, cannot be differentiated from cystic or nodular lesions.

249

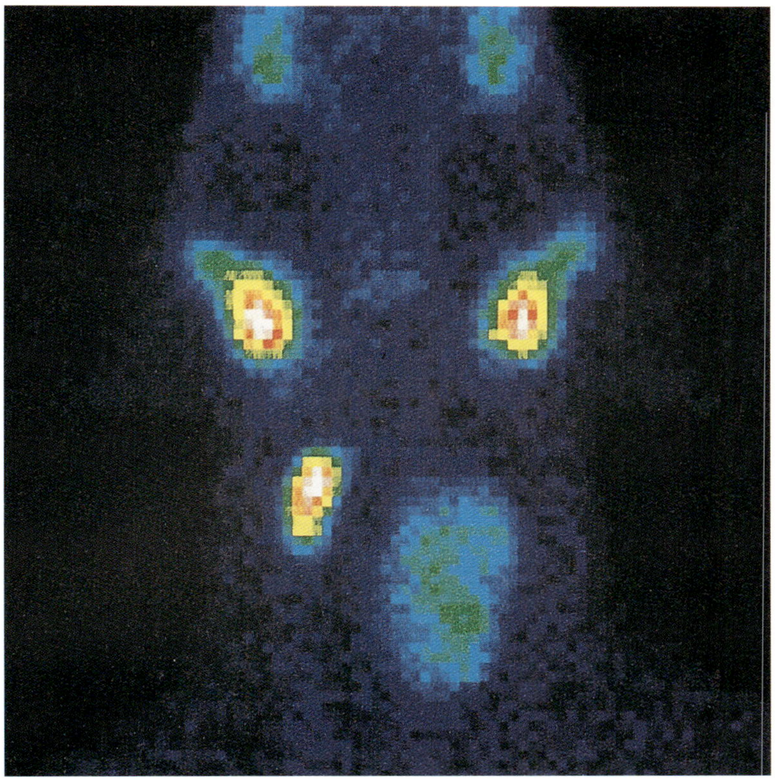

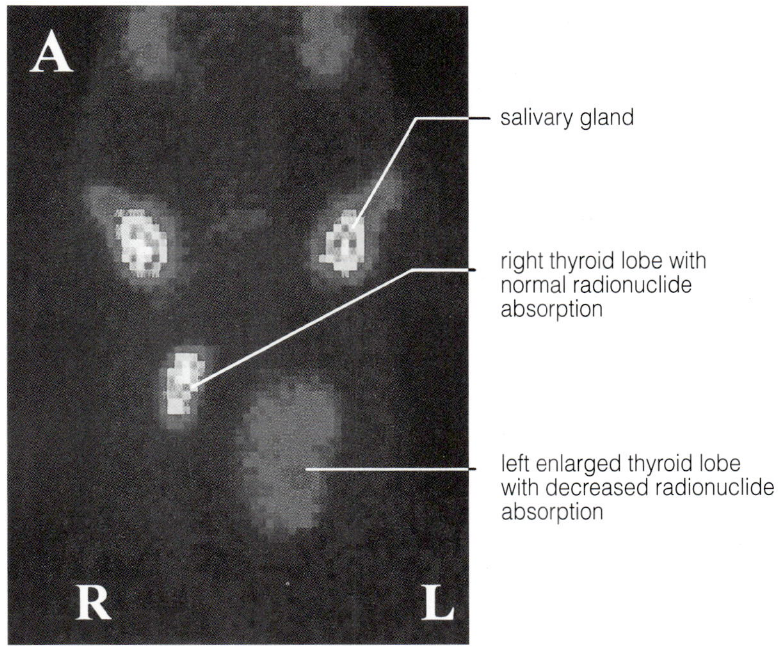

250

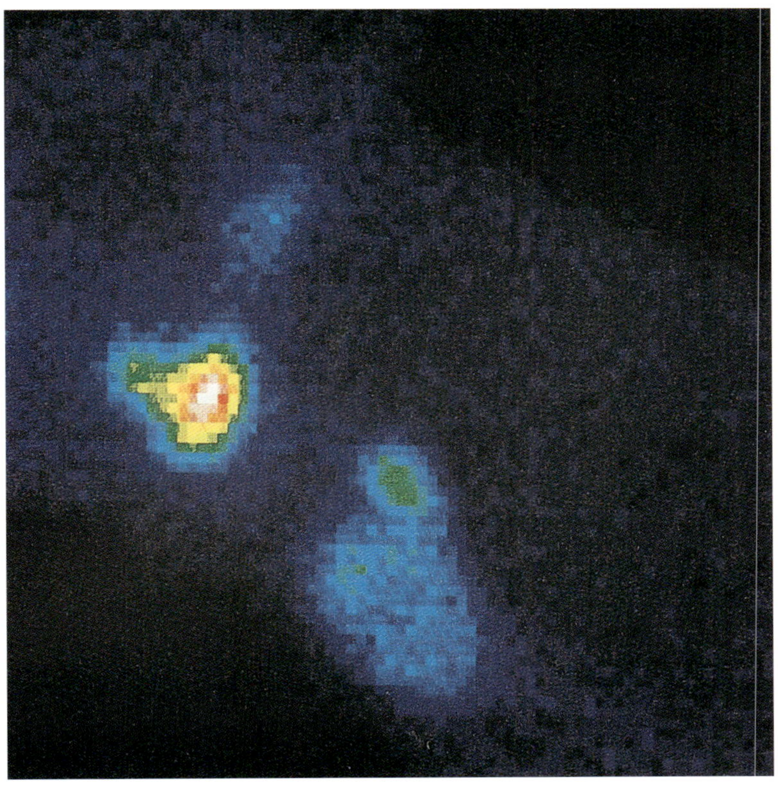

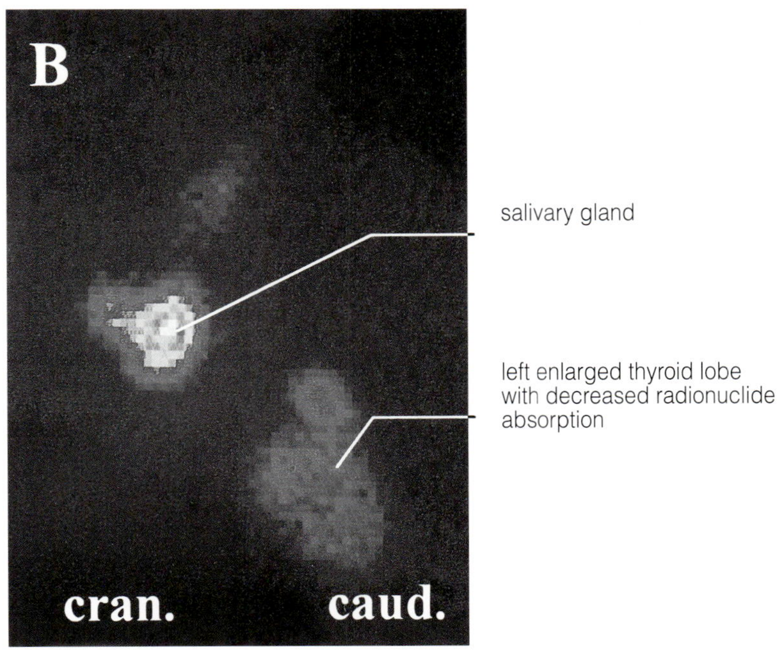

249, 250 Scintigrams from a ventral (**249**) and a left (**250**) view in a dog. Nodular left-sided struma with decreased radionuclide absorption. (Copied with permission from Anne Westhoff, Hannover.)

Lymph Nodes

Anatomy and Normal Sonographic Findings

One to three palpable superficial cervical lymph nodes are located cranial to the scapula beneath the omotransversarius muscle. The superficial cervical lymph nodes are visualized in a transverse plane by placing the transducer directly in front of the scapula and directing it towards the cranial edge. A long-axis view is achieved by rotating the transducer 90 degrees. The lymph nodes are uniformly hypoechoic with a hyperechoic demarcation (253).

The deep cervical lymph nodes are located near the thyroid gland and the trachea. They are small and not consistently visualized ultrasonographically.

Ultrasonography of Lymph Node Disease

Lymph node ultrasonography is indicated with blood profile irregularities such as leucocytosis and/or lymphocytosis as well as palpable enlarged deep cervical lymph nodes.

Lymphoma allows sonographic visualization of the deep cervical lymph nodes. They are seen adjacent to the trachea as round to oval, hypoechoic, well-demarcated structures. Differentiation

251

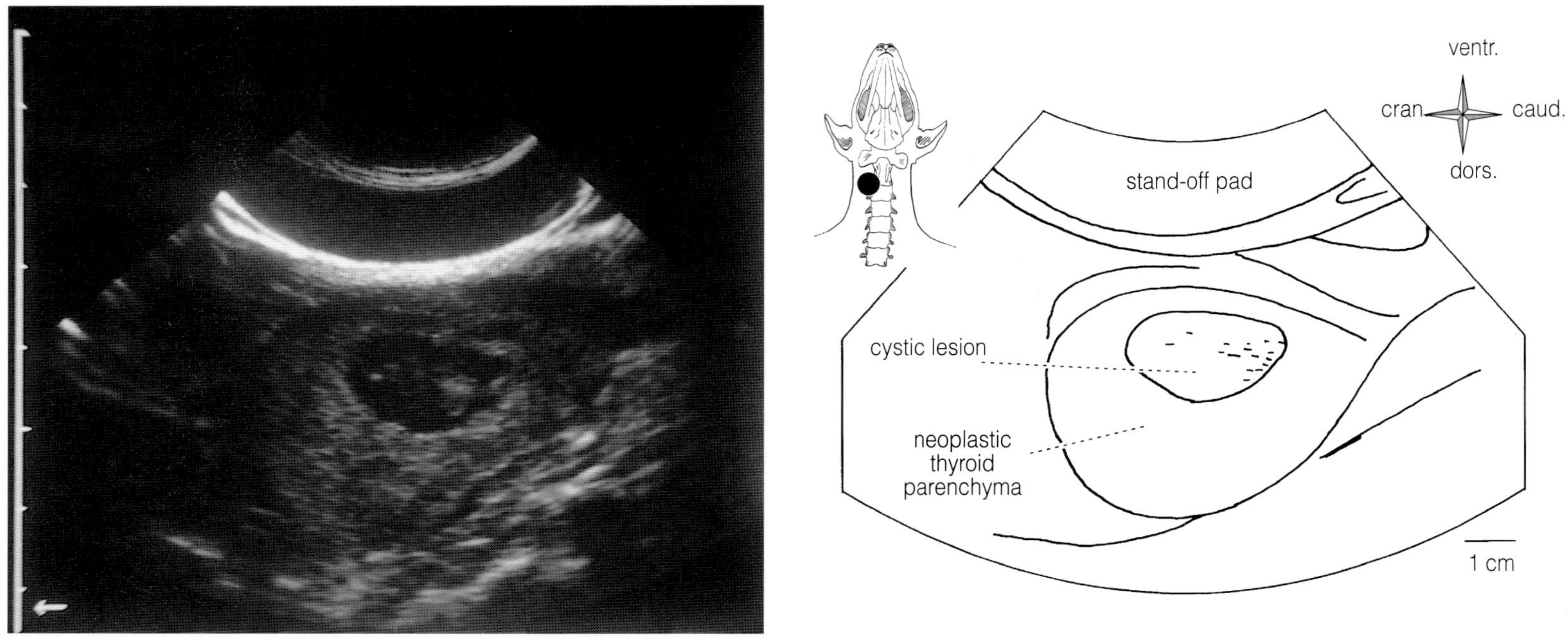

251 Two-dimensional sonogram of a dog. Carcinoma of the right thyroid lobe. The mass is well-demarcated but non-uniform in texture with fluid-filled lesions.

252

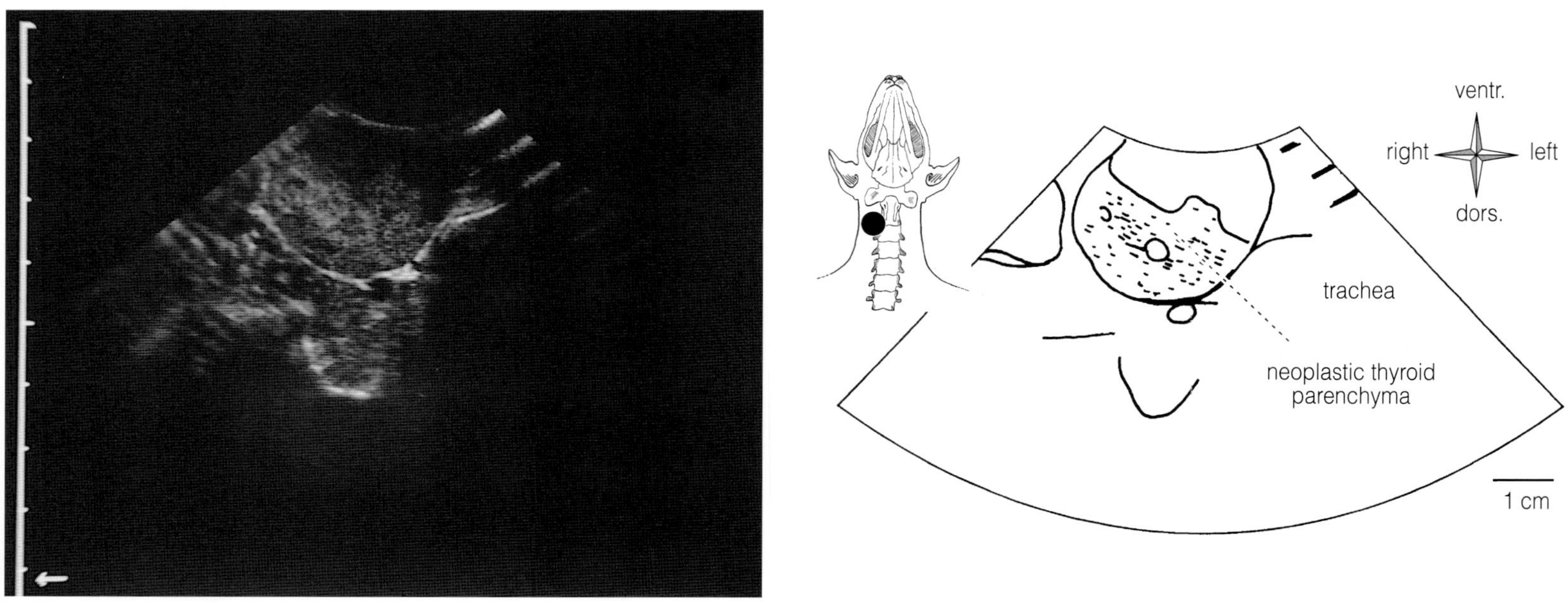

252 Two-dimensional sonography in a dog. Solid carcinoma of the right thyroid lobe. This mass is also well-demarcated. It appears more homogenous than the benign nodule in **245** and **246**.

253

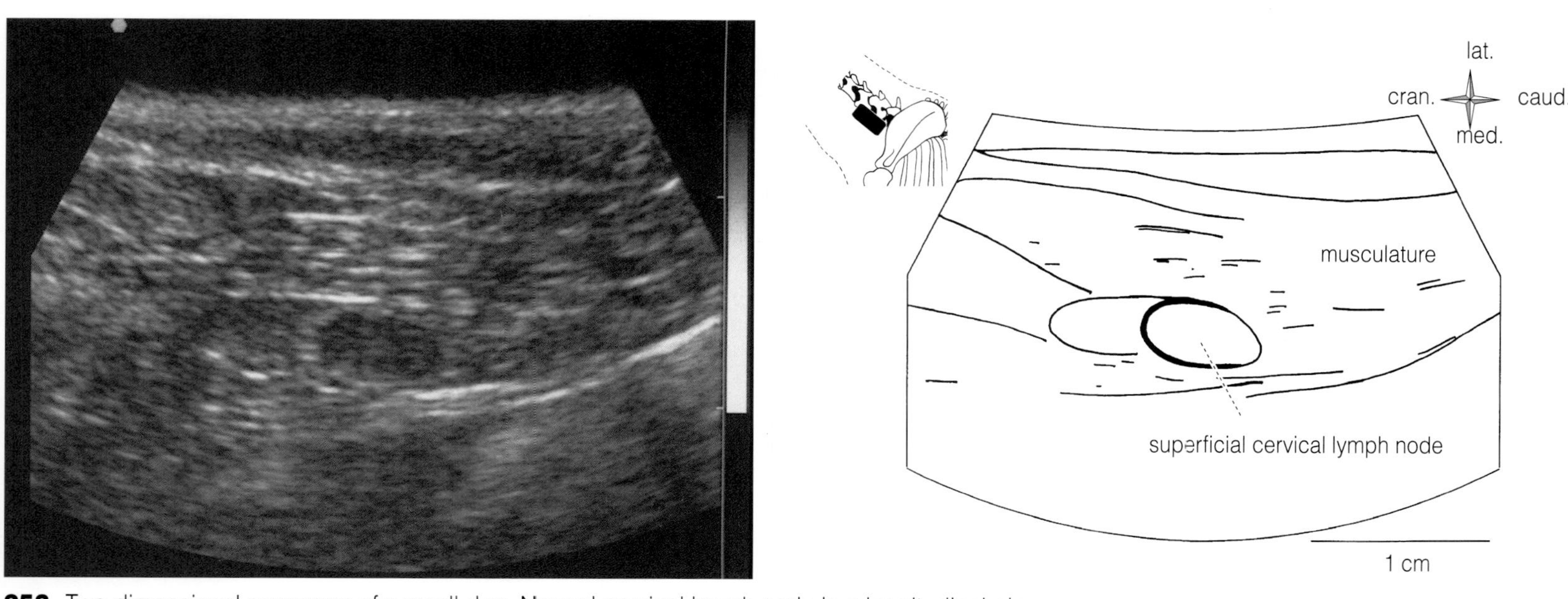

253 Two-dimensional sonogram of a small dog. Normal cervical lymph node in a longitudinal plane.

254

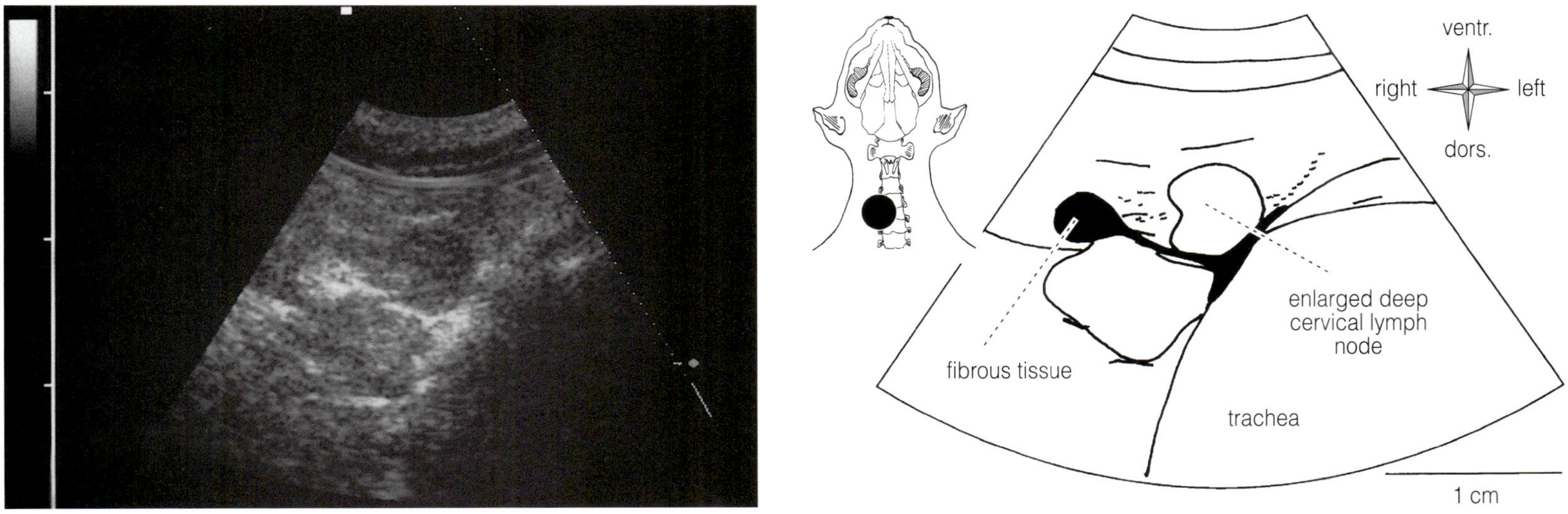

254 Two-dimensional sonogram of a cat. Solitary, enlarged deep cervical lymph node lateral to the trachea.

255

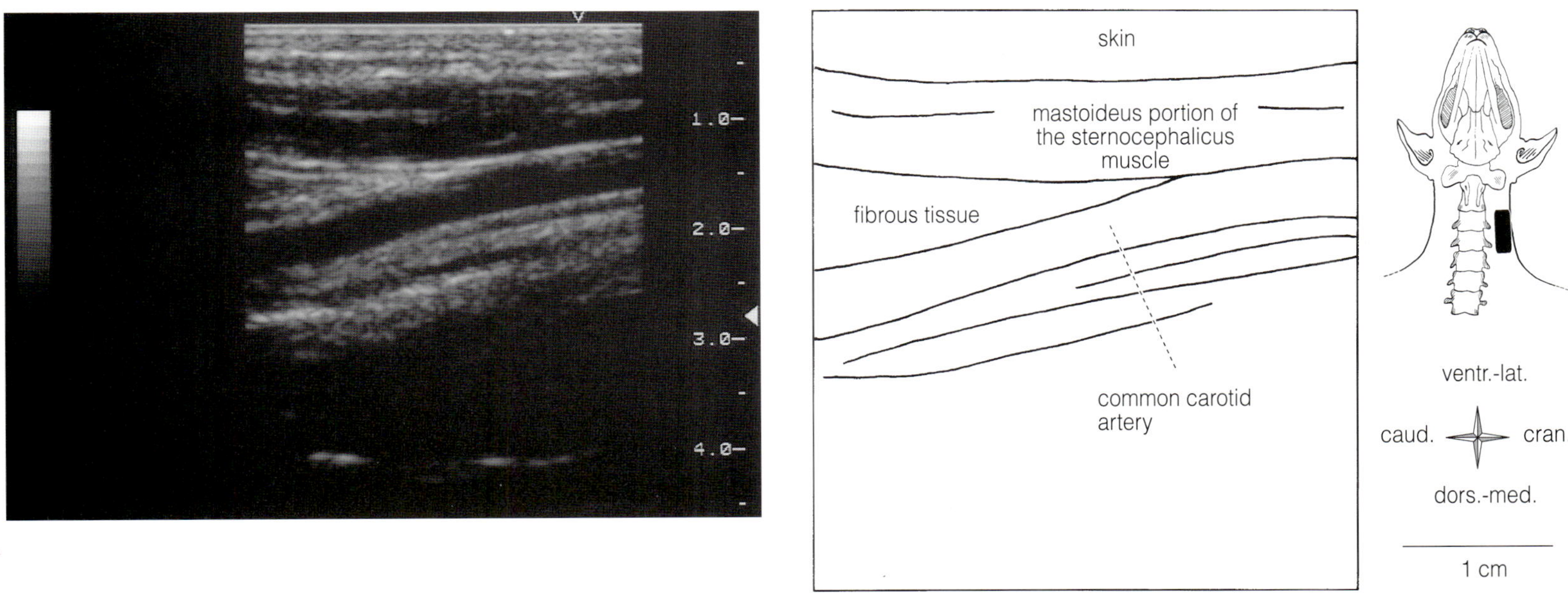

256

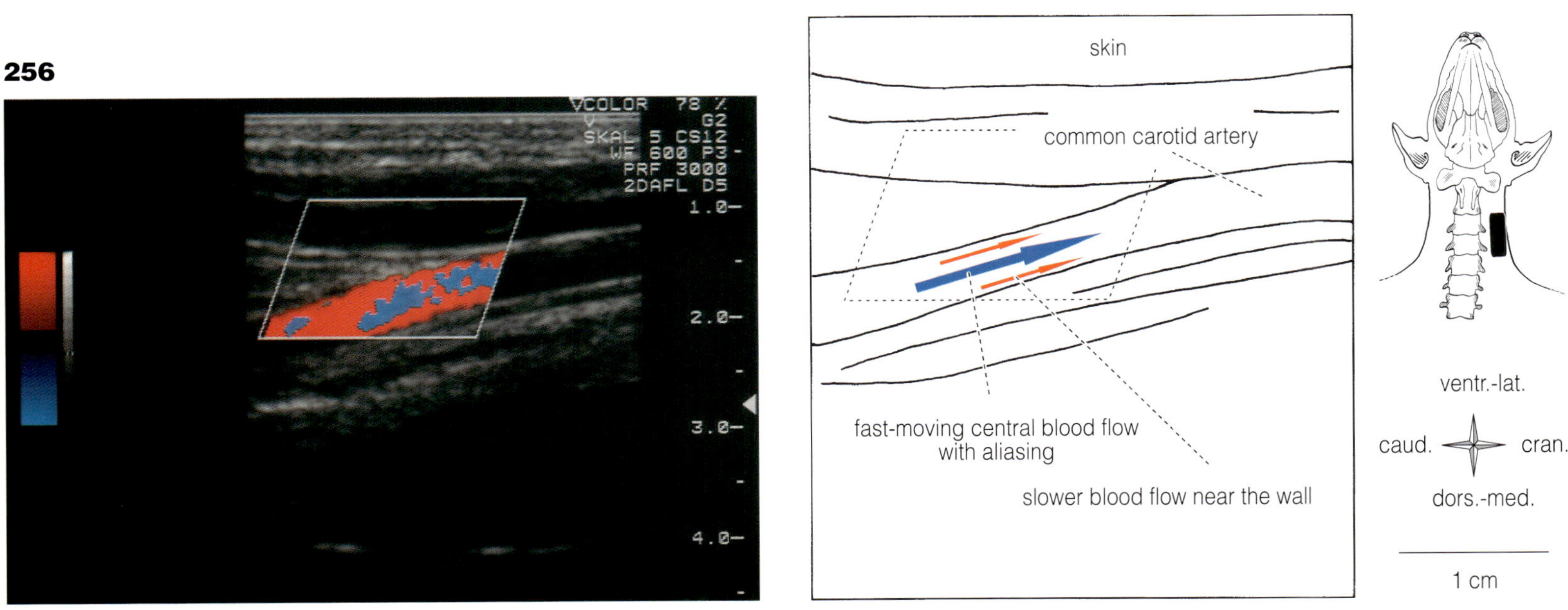

255, 256 Two-dimensional sonogram (**255**) and colour-coded Doppler echogram (**256**) of a dog. Normal left common carotid artery with normal blood flow in a longitudinal view. Colour-coded sonography (**256**) shows simple aliasing.

257

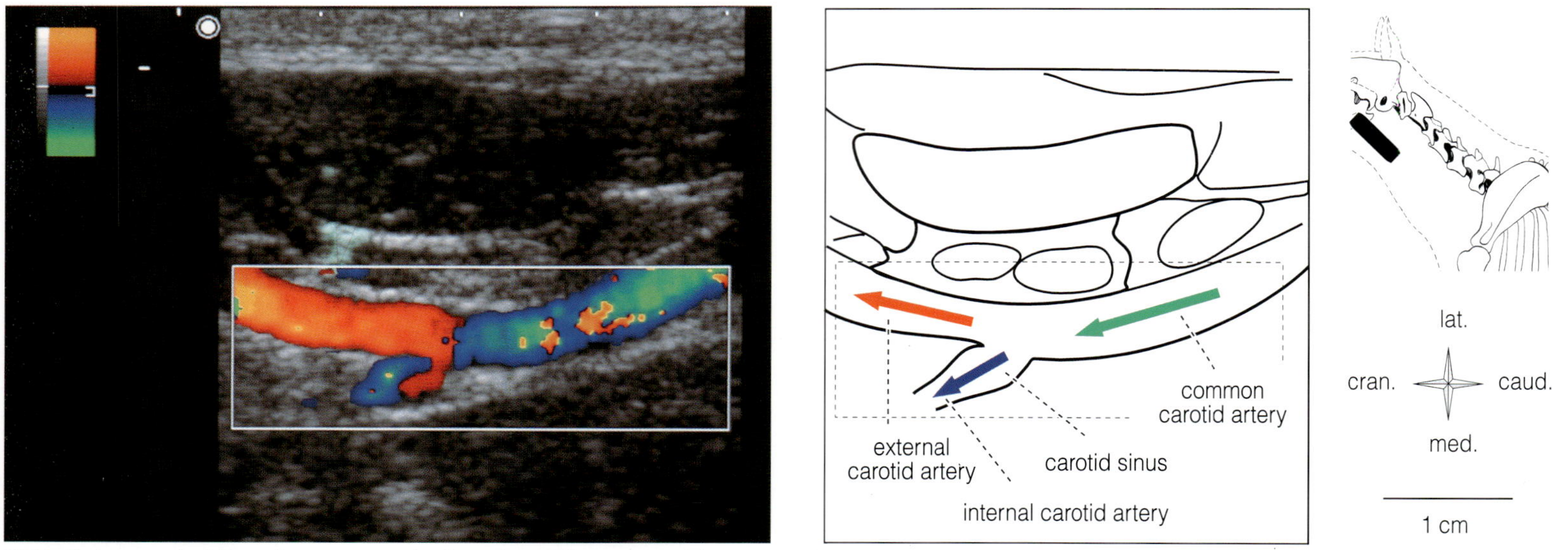

257 Colour-coded Doppler sonography in a dog. Bifurcation of the external and internal carotid arteries.

258

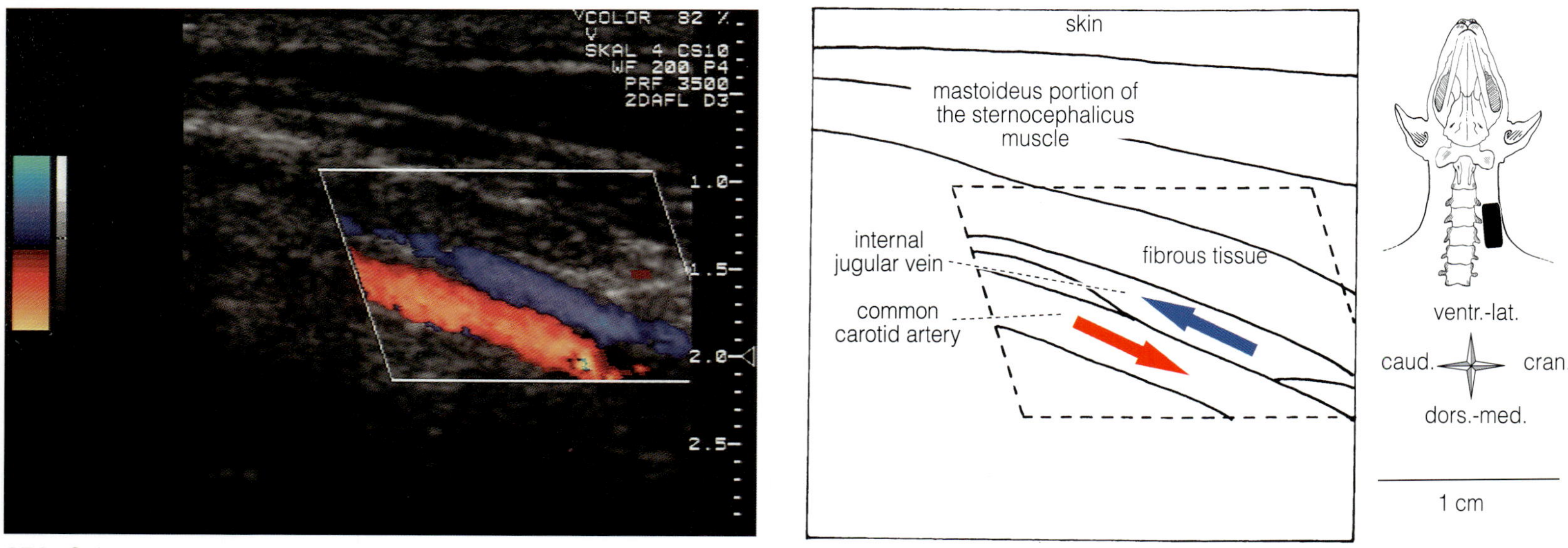

258 Colour-coded Doppler sonography in a dog. Normal common carotid artery and internal jugular vein.

259

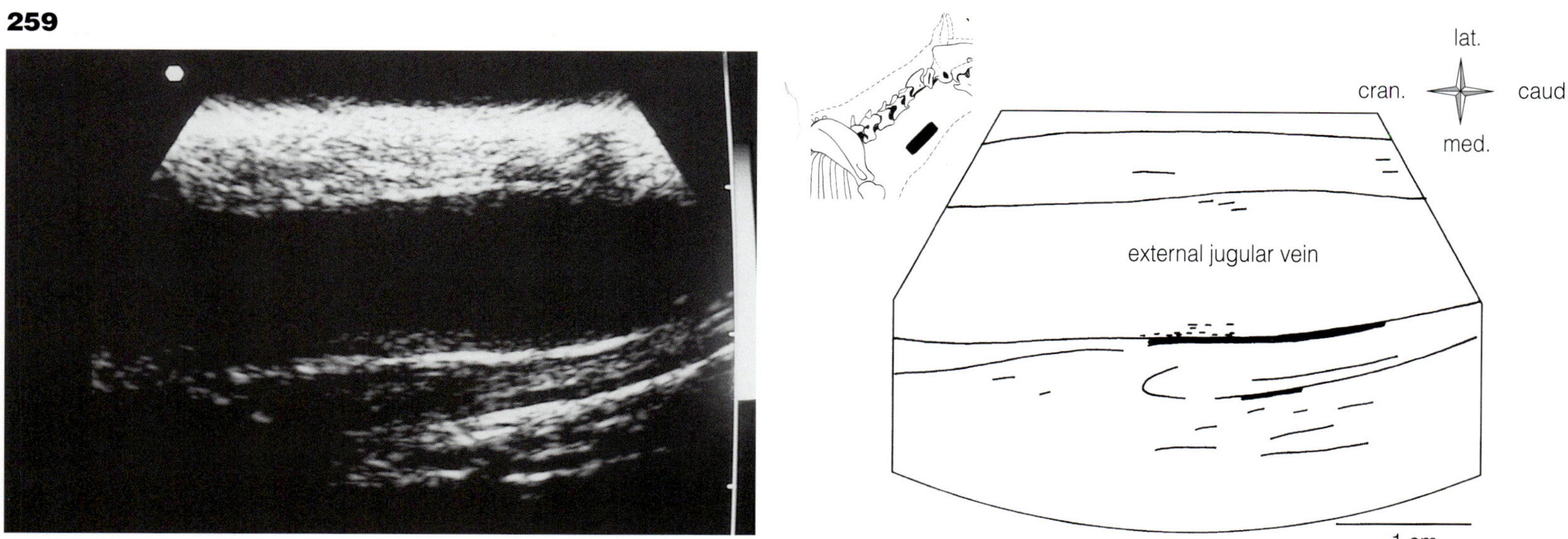

259 Two-dimensional sonogram of a dog. Normal large external jugular vein.

260

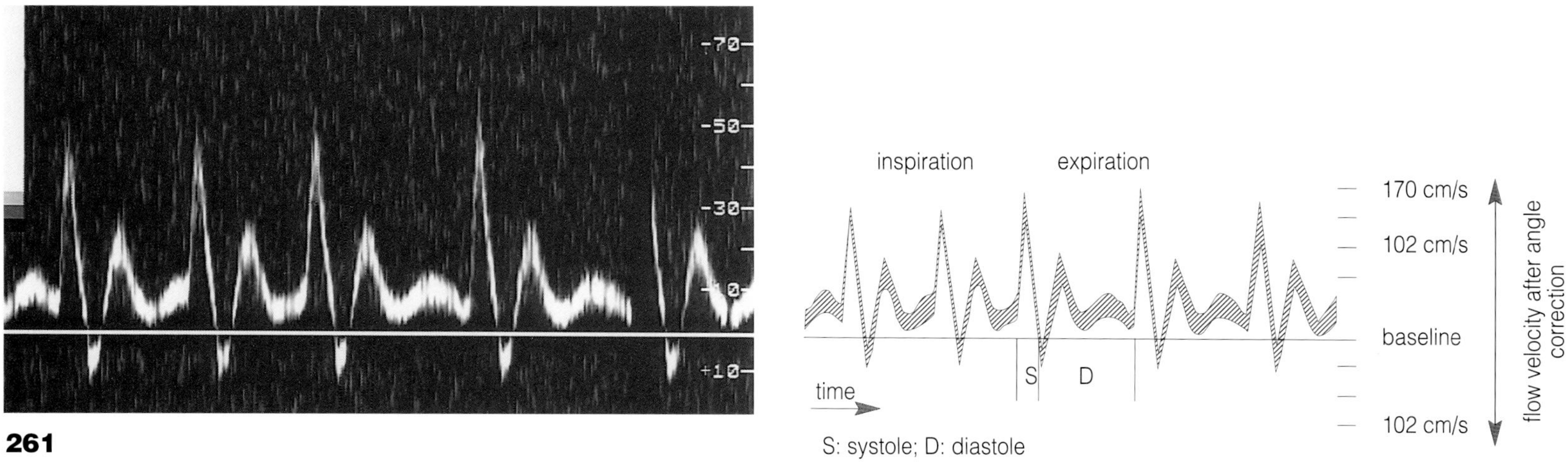

261

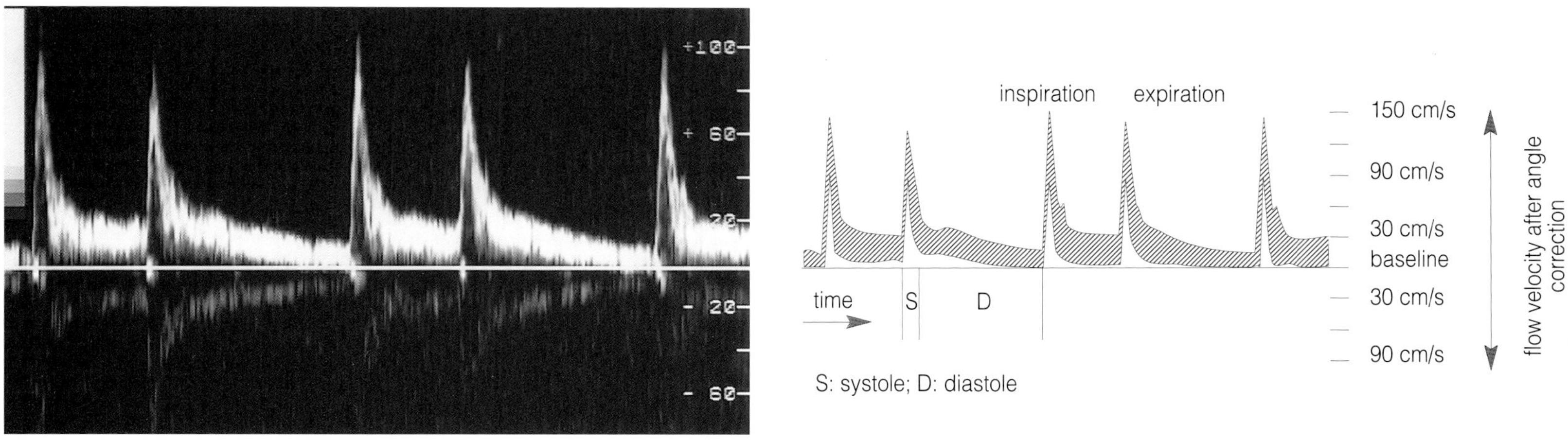

262

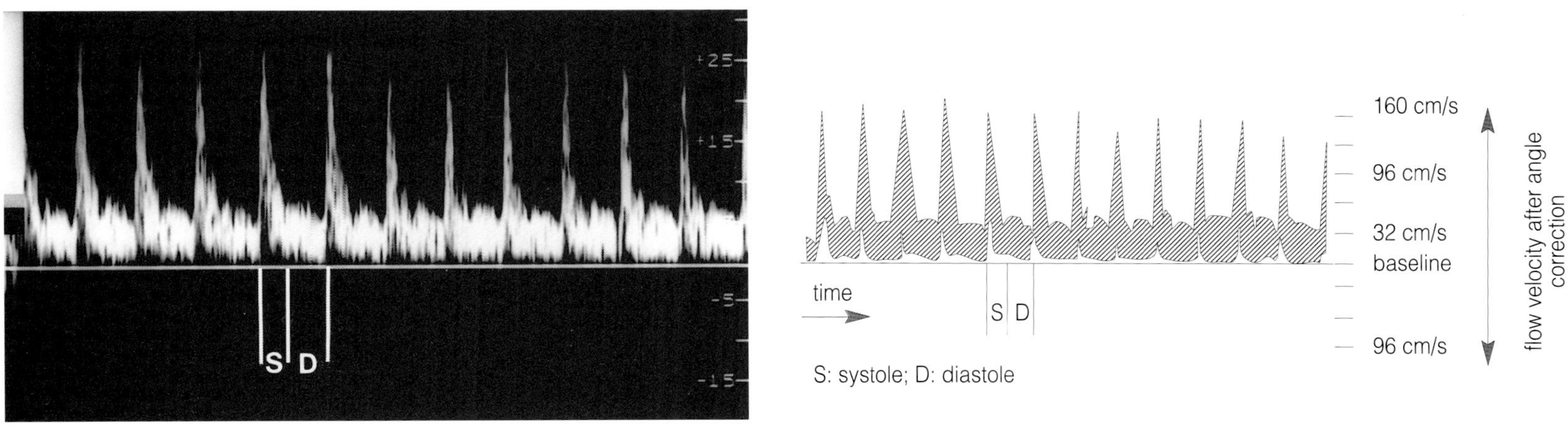

263

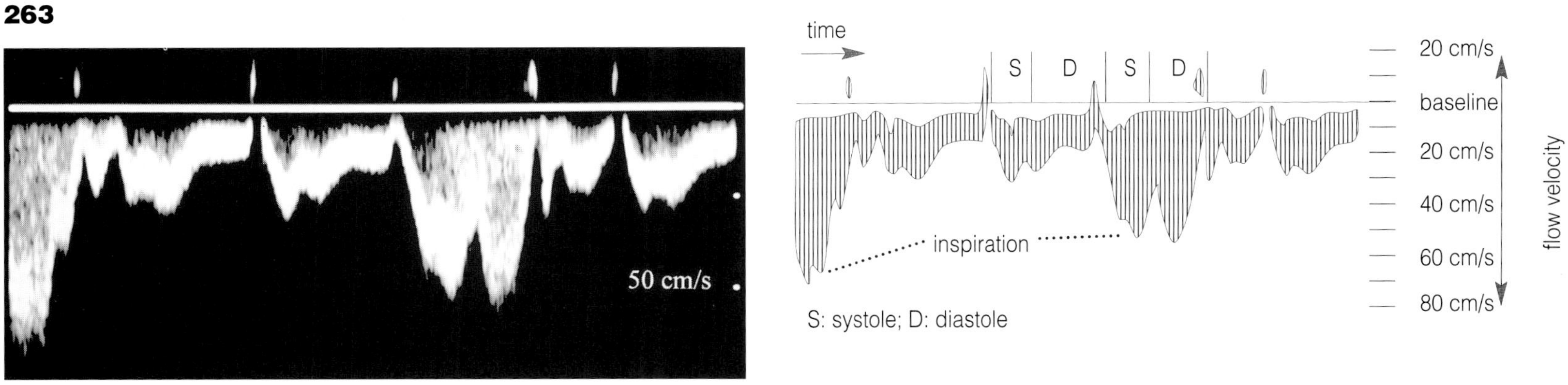

260–263 Pulsed-wave (PW) Doppler of the common carotid artery of a large (**260**) and a small (**261**) dog, and of a cat (**262**). PW Doppler echogram of the internal jugular vein (**263**) with characteristic pulsating blood flow, dependent on heart beats and inspiration.

from normal lymph nodes is possible only by comparing their size and enlargement. The echogenicity, density and texture of lymphomatous lymph nodes is not conclusive of tissue transformations. Ultrasonographic imaging cannot distinguish between benign and malignant disease. Superficial lipomas in the neck area are also hypoechoic, well-defined and homogenous and they should not be confused with diseased lymph nodes. Inflammatory lymph node enlargement cannot be differentiated sonographically from neoplastic lymph nodes.

Ultrasonography may be helpful in determining the extent of compression of the trachea, osophagus or larynx caused by enlarged lymph nodes.

Large Vessels

Anatomy and Normal Sonographic and Doppler Findings

Large vessels in the neck area include the paired common carotid arteries (internal and external) and the paired internal and external jugular veins. The common carotid artery and the internal jugular vein are located to the right and left of the trachea and larynx. The common carotid artery bifurcates at the junction of the head and neck into the larger external carotid artery and the thinner internal carotid artery. The large external jugular vein lies in the jugular furrow directly beneath the skin muscle.

Two-dimensional sonographic cross-sections of the left and right common carotid artery are easy to produce and should be made first. The transducer is placed in the middle to the left and right of the trachea in a transverse plane and moved from caudal to cranial. Long-axis views are made by rotating the probe 90 degrees. The transducer is then tilted in the jugular furrow from a sagittal to a dorsal plane to visualize the entire vessel. The characteristic anechoic lumen is surrounded by an hyperechoic arterial wall (**255, 256**). It is difficult to image the cranial bifurcation into the internal and external carotid artery (**257**). The internal jugular vein runs parallel to the common carotid artery and is not visible due to transducer compression (**236, 258**). The superficial large external jugular vein is even more likely to collapse than the deeper jugular vein (**259**).

Normal blood flows in the common carotid artery vary greatly (**260–263**). Large dogs have a bidirectional blood flow (**260**), while small dogs and cats have a unidirectional flow (**261, 262**). The bidirectional blood flow causes an early diastolic regurgitation to the heart. Unidirectional blood flow allows the blood to move in a cranial direction during the entire systole and diastole with slower diastolic motion. Maximum flow velocity is 50–110 cm/s in cats and 80–150 cm/s in dogs. Velocities are higher caudally than cranially. Venous blood flow in the external and internal jugular vein is constant and pulsating and is dependent on heart contractions and respiration (**263**). Flow velocity increases during atrial filling (ventricular systole) and inspiration.

Ultrasonography of Cervical Vessel Lesions

Two-dimensional and Doppler ultrasonography of large cervical vessels is indicated with all cerebral deficiencies.

Both the arteries and the veins should be examined carefully for wall lesions, with or without stenosis, as well as for thrombosis. Plaques and mural thrombosis are visualized only with exact long-axis views of the vessel. By manually compressing the left or right external jugular vein caudally, the vein will not collapse with transducer pressure and it can be assessed for wall lesions and thrombosis.

Stenosis is recognized by higher flow velocities with pulsed-wave Doppler and local aliasing in colour Doppler sonography. Blood flow changes behind the stenosis [3].

References

Cited References

1 Barr FJ (1990) *Diagnostic Ultrasound in the Dog and Cat*. Blackwell Scientific Publications, Oxford.

2 Brinker RA, Landiess DJ and Croley RF (1968) Detection of carotid artery bifurcation stenosis by Doppler ultrasound. *J. Neurosurg.* **29**, 143–148.

3 Von Büdingen HJ and Von Reutern G-M (1993) *Ultraschalldiagnostik der Hirnversorgenden Arterien. Dopplersonographie der Extra- und Intrakraniellen Arterien, Duplexsonographie*. Georg Thieme Verlag, Stuttgart, New York.

4 Fornage BD, Nasca S and Durville A (1987) Sonographic detection and three-dimensional localization of a metallic foreign body in soft-tissue in a dog. *Br. Vet. J.* **143**, 278–281.

5 Fritsch R and Gerwing M (1991) *Sonographie bei Hand und Katze*. Enke Verlag, Stuttgart.

6 Fujmoto Y, Oka A, Omoto R and Hirose M (1967) Ultrasound scanning of the thyroid gland as a new diagnostic approach. *Ultrasonics* **5**, 177–180.

7 Little CM, Parker MG, Callowich MC and Sartori JC (1986) The ultrasonic detection of soft tissue foreign bodies. *Invest. Radiol.* **21**, 275–277.

8 Miyazaki M and Kato K (1965) Measurement of cerebral blood flow by ultrasonic Doppler technique, hemodynamic comparisons of right and left carotid artery in patients with hemiplegia. *Jpn. Circ. J.* **29**, 383–386.

9 Rutherford RB, Hiatt WR and Kreutzer EW (1977) The use of velocity wave form analysis in the diagnosis of carotid artery occlusive disease. *Surgery* **82**, 695–702.

10 Spencer MP, Reid JM, Davis DL and Paulson PS (1974) Cervical carotid imaging with a continous wave doppler flowmeter. *Stroke* **5**, 145–154.

11 Thijs LG, Roos P and Wiener JD (1972) Use of ultrasound and digital scintiphoto analysis in the evaluation of solitary thyroid nodules. *J. Nucl. Med.* **13**, 504–509.

12 Wisner ER, Mattoon JS, Nyland TG and Baker TW (1991) Normal ultrasonographic anatomy of the canine neck. *Vet. Radiol.* **32**, 185–190.

Additional Reading

Brunetton J-N. (1987) *Ultrasonography of the Neck*. Springer Verlag, Berlin, Heidelberg, New York.

Föhn J (1992) *Sonographische und Duplexsonographische Untersuchungen an der Ventralen Halsregion des Rindes*. Zürich, Univ., Veterinärmed. Fak., Diss.

Fruehwald F and Blackwell DE (1992) (Eds) *Atlas of Color-coded Doppler Sonography: Vascular and Soft Tissue Structures of the Upper Extremity, Thoracic Outlet and Neck*. Springer Verlag, Wien, New York.

Hell B and Norer B (1990) *Atlas der Ultraschalldiagnostik im Kopf-Hals-Bereich*. Georg Thieme Verlag, Stuttgart, New York.

Klima G (1993) *Schilddrüsen-Sonographie*. Verlag Urban and Schwarzenberg, München, Wien, Baltimore.

Koischwitz D (1993) *Sonographie der Kopf-Hals-Region*. Springer Verlag, Berlin, Heidelberg, New York.

8 Thoracic Cavity without the Heart

Ralf Tobias

Ultrasonographic examinations of the thoracic cavity and its organs are limited by anatomical considerations and by basic acoustic physics. Bones surrounding the thorax, such as vertebrae, ribs and the sternum, allow only a small acoustic window. The air-filled lungs pose another sonographic obstacle, since the sound beams are reflected from their surface. Normal lung tissue and structures covered by the lungs are not sonographically accessible. Because of the small acoustic window, sector scanners or micro-convex transducers should be used. Conventional linear-array and curved-array transducers have a large contact area and are useless for these examinations.

Indications for thoracic ultrasonography (see *Table* 9) are usually found as a result of previous radiographic examination. Ultrasonography is helpful in locating diffuse or defined radiographic opacities and associating them with organs or tumours. The consistency of a diffuse precardial thoracic shadow can also be determined with ultrasonography. Pleural effusion can, for example, be differentiated from a solid tumour. Lung lesions can only be scanned near the surface or when air-filled tissue is displaced. Furthermore, lesions of the oesophagus can be found. Examination of the diaphragm for hernias should be made from the thorax as well as from the abdomen.

Table 9 Indications for thoracic ultrasonography without the heart.

Indications for thoracic ultrasonography:
• Areas dampened with percussion.
• Radiographic thoracic opacities indicating a lesion.
• Superficial lung lesions.
• Lung lesions with displacement of air-filled tissue.
• Oesophageal lesions.
• Diaphragmatic lesions, hernias.

264

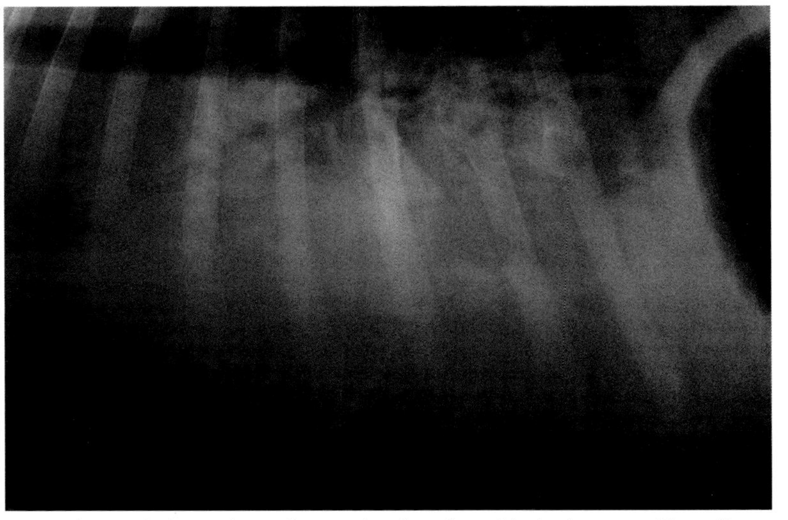

264 Lateral thoracic radiograph of a dog. Hydrothorax with uniform shadowing of the pleural cavity and an indistinguishable heart.

Hydrothorax, Haemothorax, Chylothorax, Pyothorax

Radiography of pleural effusion shows a partial or complete, homogenous opacification with organ detail loss (**264**). Ultrasonography, on the other hand, can diagnose the presence of fluid and assess thoracic organs such as the heart, pericardium, mediastinum and diaphragm. Free fluid in the pleural cavity, similar to ascites, improves the image quality of thoracic structures (**265**; see Gastrointestinal Tract, page 165; Liver and Gallbladder, page 181). Atelectatic lung tissue can also be visualized within the pleural effusion.

Ultrasonography of anechoic or slightly echogenic fluid does not allow differentiation of its quality, e.g. transudate, exudate, blood, lymph or pus. A definitive diagnosis of the effusion must be made by tapping the thoracic cavity. Percutaneous thoracentesis should be ultrasound-guided to ensure safe needle passage and to minimize injuries to other thoracic organs such as the heart and pericardium. A summary of sonographic abnormalities is given in *Table 10*, page 125.

265

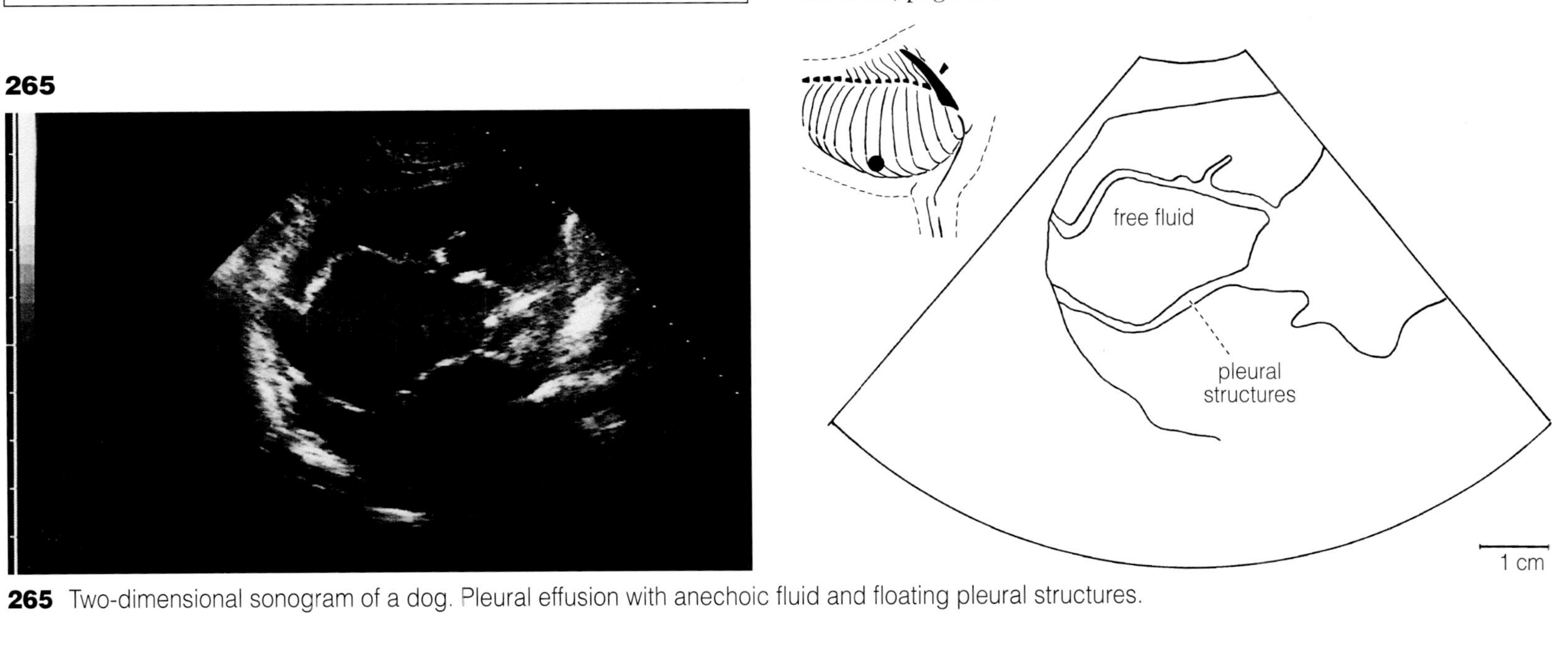

265 Two-dimensional sonogram of a dog. Pleural effusion with anechoic fluid and floating pleural structures.

266

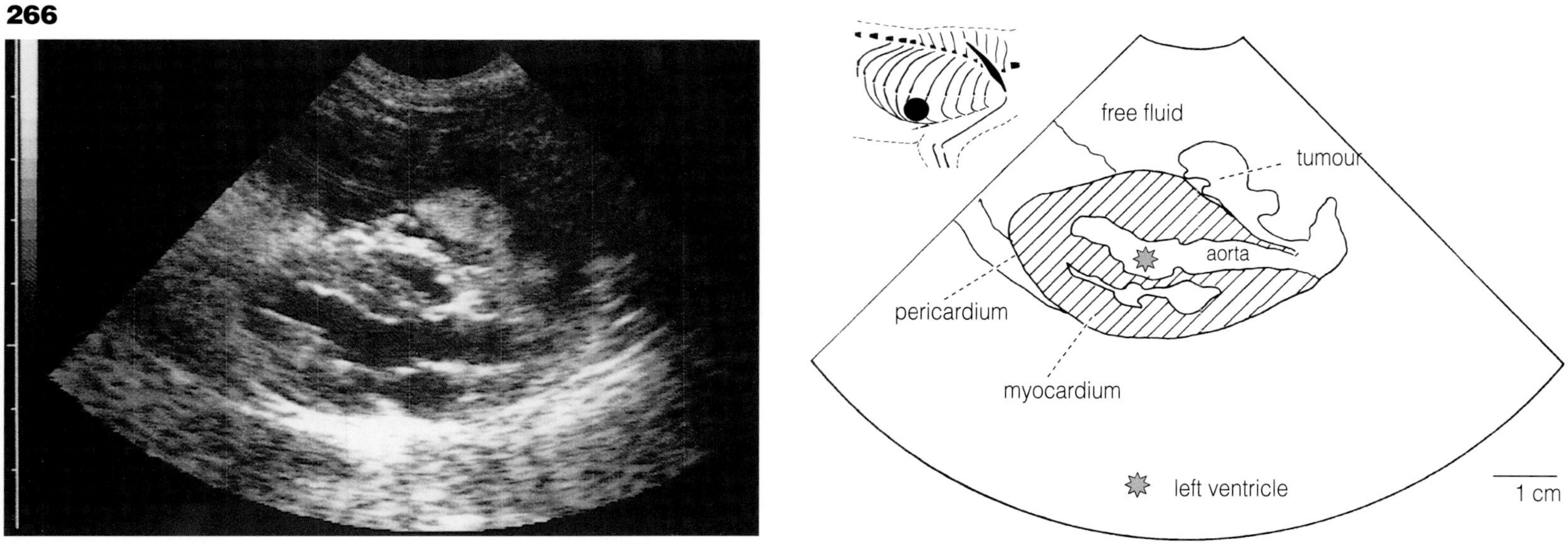

266 Two-dimensional sonogram – cat. Thymic leukemia with neoplasia near the heart. The non-uniformly echogenic tumour tissue is surrounded by anechoic fluid.

267

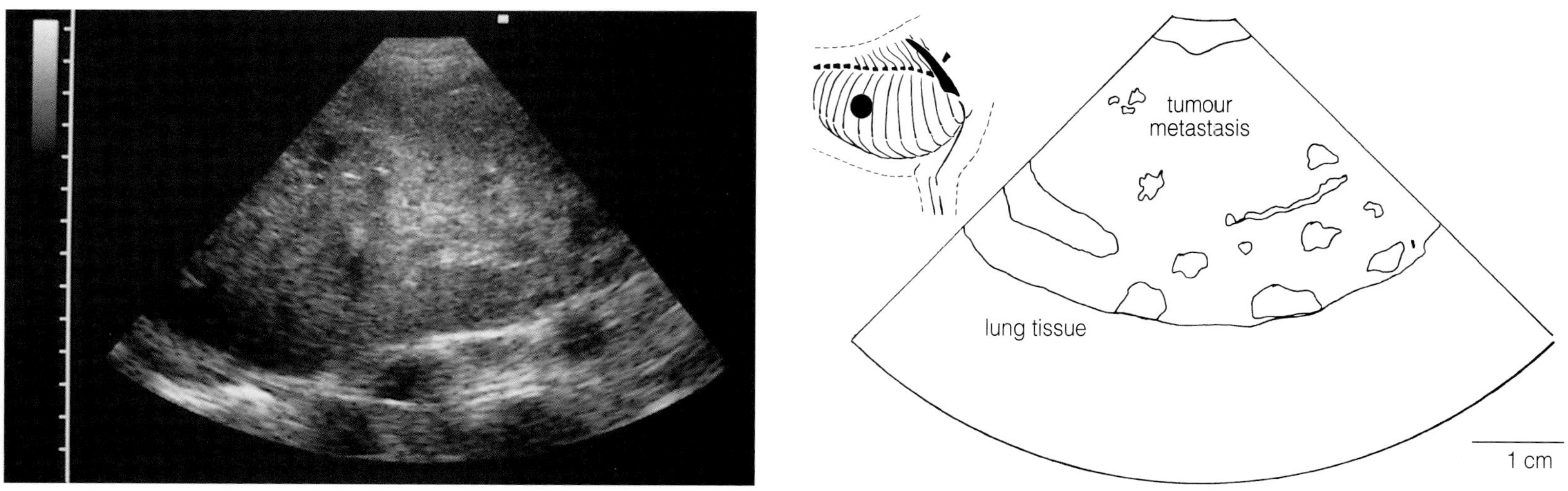

267 Two-dimensional sonogram – dog. Large tumour metastasis of mixed echogenicity in the lung, secondary to mammary tumours.

268

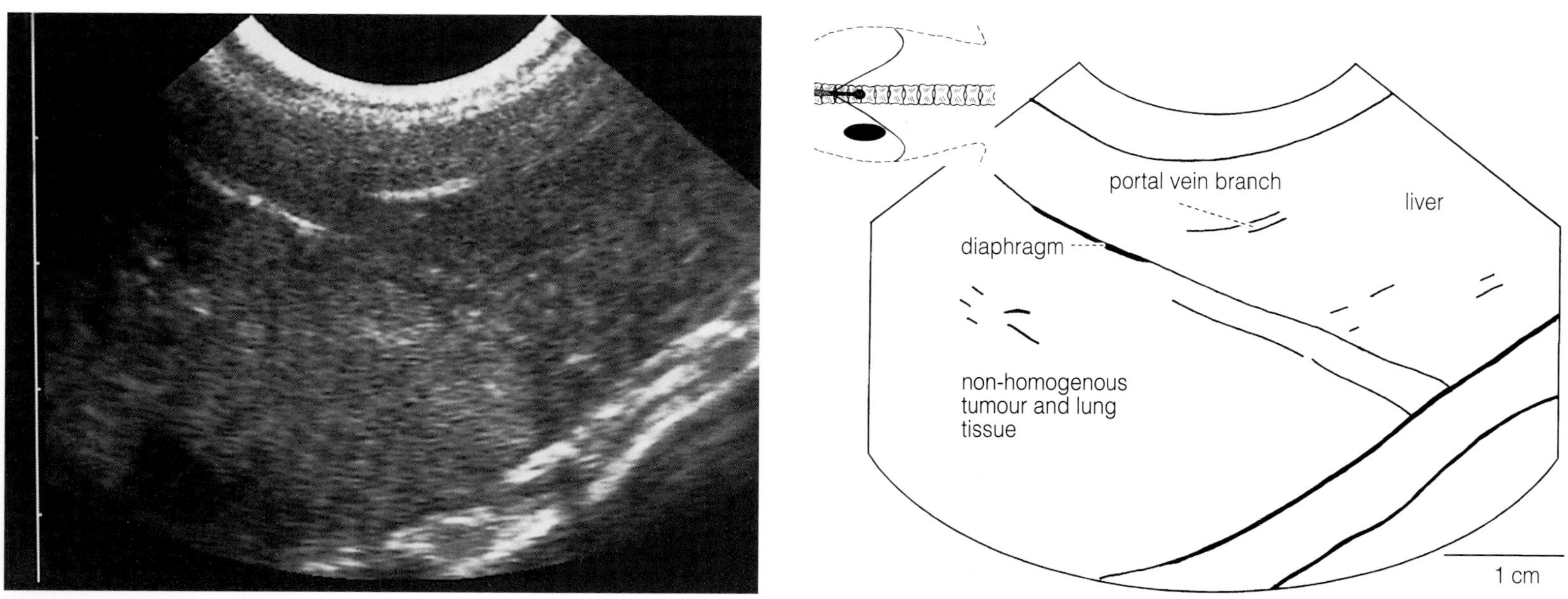

268 Two-dimensional sonogram – cat. Mixed echogenic lung tissue with bronchial carcinoma. Because this cat has been scanned from the ventral abdomen, this image should not be mistaken for a mirror image artefact of the lung at the diaphragm. A mirror image artefact will show identical structures in front of and behind the diaphragm, which is not demonstrated in this sonogram. (Copied with permission from K. Weber, Puettlingen.)

269

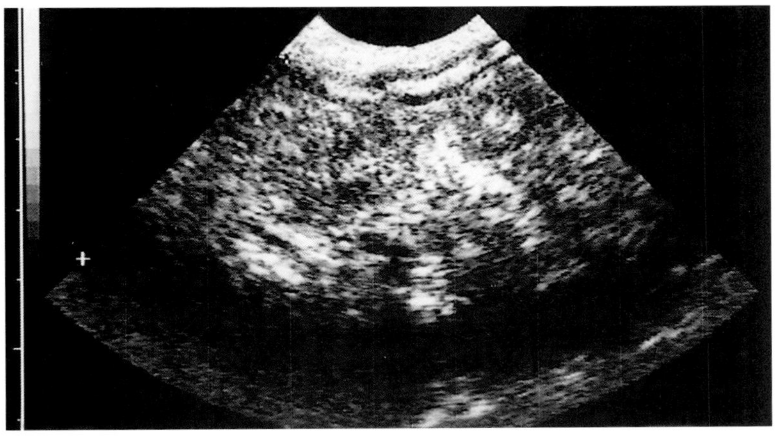

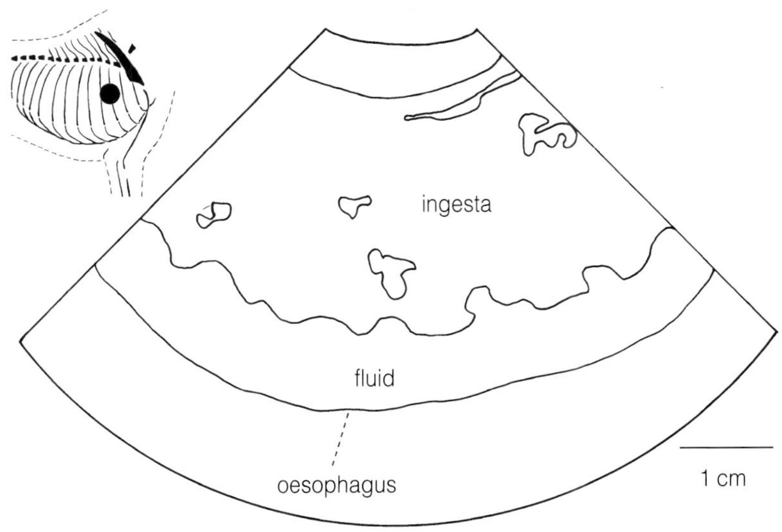

269 Two-dimensional sonogram – dog. Megaoesophagus with large amounts of ingesta. Real-time imaging showed no movement of the oesophagus.

270

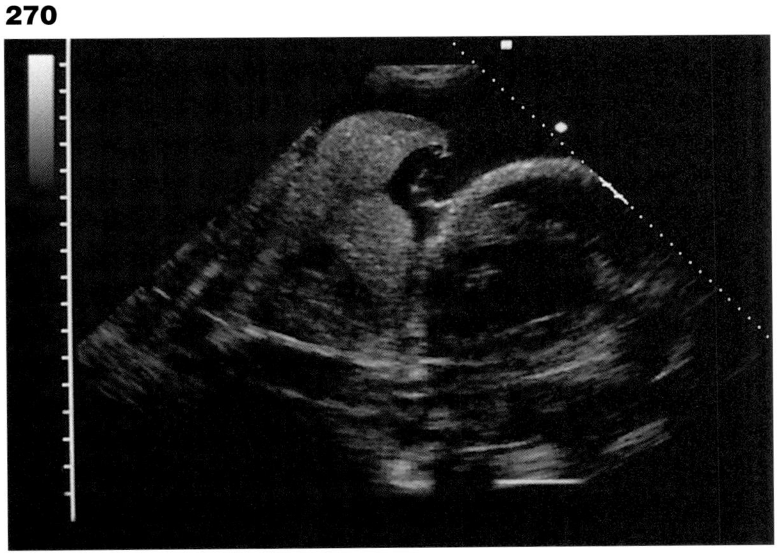

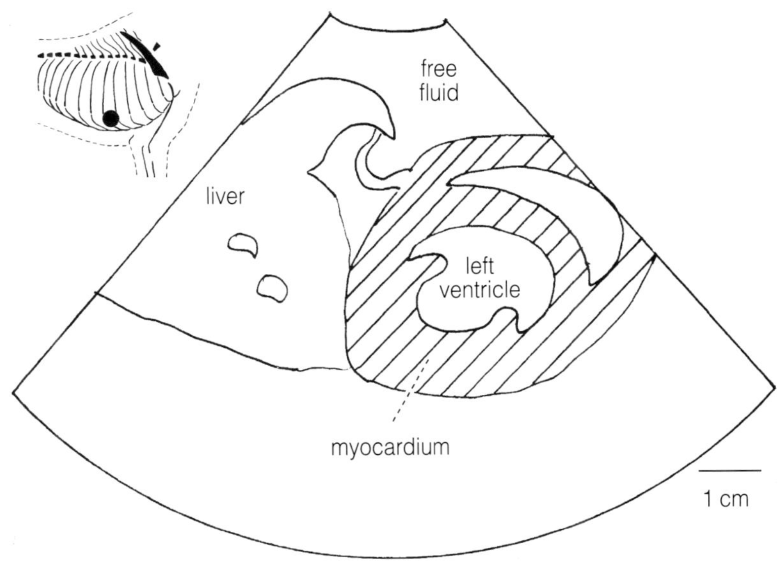

270 Two-dimensional sonogram – dog. Diaphragmatic rupture with displaced liver lobes in the thoracic cavity and pleural effusion.

Table 10 Two-dimensional ultrasonography with hydrothorax, haemothorax, chylothorax and pyothorax.

Sonographic abnormalities:
• Anechoic or slightly echogenic free pleural fluid.
• Good thoracic organ definition including atelectatic lung tissue.
• Floating pleural structures.

Table 11 Two-dimensional ultrasonography with pleural neoplasia. (*Secondary abnormalities are shown in italics.*)

Sonographic abnormalities:
• Non-homogenous, well-defined nodules with mixed echogenicity.
• Hypoechoic to anechoic demarcated structures with abscesses or cysts.
• *Pleural effusion.*

Neoplasia

Neoplastic lesions in the thoracic cavity are often accompanied by pleural effusion (see *Table 11*). Pleural fluid allows tumours to be detected more easily by improving the acoustic window (**266**).

Radiography is the imaging method of choice when looking for pleural tumours and metastases, especially within the lungs. The size of intrapulmonary tumours is more easily visualized on lateral and dorsoventral radiographs. The consistency of pleural tumours can be determined with ultrasonography when they are near the lung surface and/or air-filled lung tissue is displaced. Solid lung tumours have a mixed echogenicity (**267, 268**), while cysts or abscesses are hypoechoic to anechoic.

Oesophagus

Transthoracic sonography of the normal oesophagus is difficult, because it is surrounded by air-filled lung tissue. The wall of a megaoesophagus filled with ingesta can sometimes be distinguished as an echogenic line (**269**). The ingesta shows mixed echogenicity with shadowing. When water is mixed with food in the oesophagus, acoustic contrasts are improved. Ultrasonography can be used to evaluate oesophageal motion.

Table 12 Two-dimensional ultrasonography with diaphragmatic hernias or ruptures. (*Secondary abnormalities are shown in italics.*)

Sonographic abnormalities:
• *Abdominal organs in the pleural cavity.* • *Pleural effusion.*

Diaphragm

The diaphragm is seen as an echogenic line from the lateral thoracic wall and the ventral abdominal wall. Pleural or peritoneal fluid facilitates diaphragmatic imaging. A stomach filled with ingesta or barium makes visualization of the diaphragm more difficult. Ultrasonography of the diaphragm is indicated with suspected hernias or ruptures (see *Table 12*).

Sonographic diagnosis of diaphragmatic hernias is made indirectly by imaging abdominal organs within the thoracic cavity, e.g. liver, liver lobes, stomach or small intestines (**270**). The diaphragmatic defect is usually not detected. A definitive diagnosis should be made radiographically with a contrast study.

Congenital defects of the diaphragm and pericardium such as peritoneopericardial diaphragmatic hernias are often found by chance during echocardiographic examinations (see Peritoneopericardial Diaphragmatic Hernia, page 143; **313–315**).

References

Barr FJ (1990) *Diagnostic Ultrasound in the Dog and Cat*. Blackwell Scientific Publications, Oxford.

Carothers M and Guillermo Couto C (1989) Respiratory neoplasia. In: Kirk RW (Ed.) *Current Veterinary Therapy X. Small Animal Practice*. WB Saunders, Philadelphia, London, Toronto.

Fritsch F and Gerwin M (1993) *Sonographie bei Hand und Katze*. Enke Verlag, Stuttgart.

Schwerk WB and Görtz C (1993) III.2 Pleura and Lunge. 12. Ergänzungslieferung. In: Braun B, Günther R and Schwerk W (Eds.) *Ultraschalldiagnostik. Lehrbuch und Atlas. Vol 2*. Verlag Ecomed. Landsberg, München, Zürich.

9 The Heart

Ralf Tobias and Cordula Poulsen Nautrup

Echography of the Normal Heart

Ultrasonography of the heart (echocardiography) is an imaging method accepted worldwide in cardiac diagnostics. Echocardiography should only be considered in conjunction with clinical, electrocardiographic and radiological examinations.

While one- and two-dimensional echocardiography has been routinely employed in human medicine since the late 1960s, its use in veterinary medicine began in the late 1970s (see History of Diagnostic Ultrasonography, page 18).

Transthoracic echocardiography is commonly used in veterinary medicine (**271**). Transoesophageal echocardiography uses a special probe to image the heart from the oesophagus and it has an experimental status in veterinary medicine (see Interventional Ultrasonography, page 390).

Several echocardiograms in this chapter are produced transthoracically. Ultrasonographic contrast studies with intravenous application of agitated saline solution or Echovist® (Firma Shering, Berlin) can be added to each procedure (see Contrast Agents, page 58; **105–107**).

Transthoracic echocardiography is performed on the recumbent, or preferably on the sitting or standing animal, from the left and/or right thoracic wall (**271**). The use of a table with an opening is useful for echocardiographic examinations. The dog or cat is placed in lateral recumbency over the opening with the transducer applied from beneath the animal (see Patient Positioning, page 78; **157, 158**). Patients with dyspnoea should be examined in an upright position to allow easier respiratory movements.

The transducer is placed into the third to fifth or sixth intercostal space, ventrolaterally on the thoracic wall. The size of the acoustic window is limited by the surrounding lungs and ribs.

Good transducer–skin contact is achieved by applying high-percentage alcohol and liberal amounts of coupling gel. Hair clipping is only necessary in thick-coated animals (see Patient Preparation, page 77).

One-Dimensional Echocardiography

Time-motion mode, also referred to as TM-mode or M-mode, is considered a one-dimensional technique, although it displays two dimensions: depth (superimposed interfaces or structures) and time (motion of structures during systole and diastole).

M-mode echocardiography traces the motion of cardiac structures, e.g. ventricular wall, septum or heart and vessel valves, along a horizontal axis as dots of varying brightness. This type of tracing produces an unusual anatomical image (**272**).

M-mode ultrasonography is still the method of choice for cardiac measurements, e.g. wall thickness and chamber diameters. It is also useful in recording cardiac motion patterns such as valve movements. For M-mode evaluation the sound beam must be perpendicular to these structures. A combination of one- and two-dimensional echocardiography is easiest and most practical. The region of interest is imaged in the two-dimensional echocardiogram, the selected 'sound beam' is placed into this region, and the unit switched to M-mode (see One-dimensional B-Mode, page 39;

271

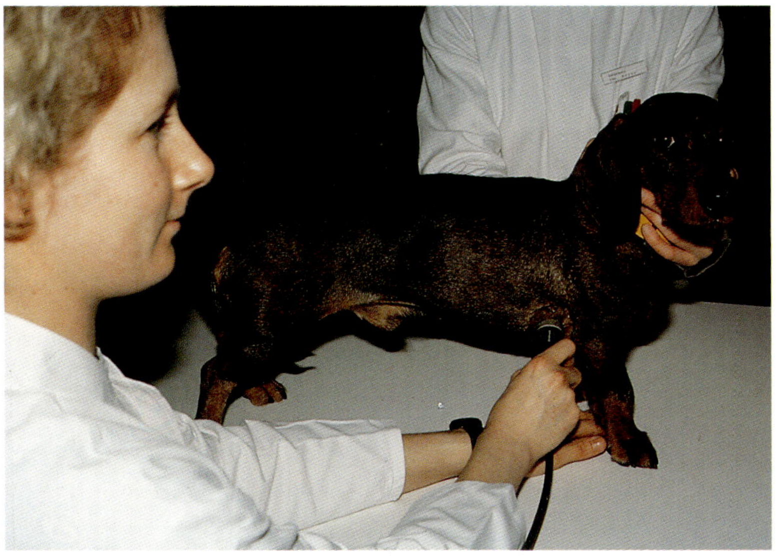

271 Transthoracic echocardiography of a standing patient (Wire-haired Dachshund).

272

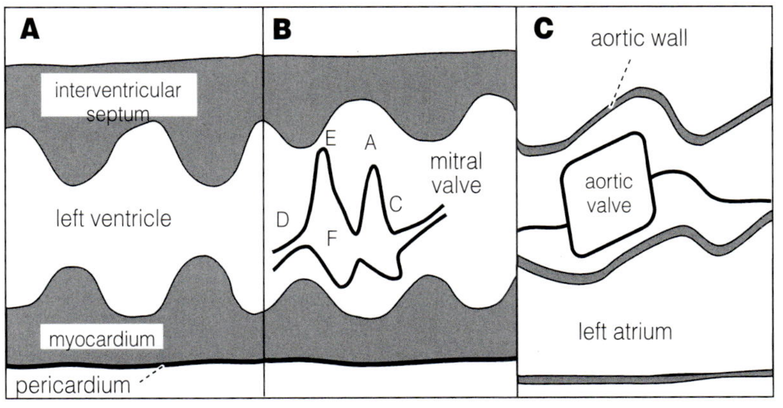

272 Schematic drawing of a M-mode echocardiogram of a left canine heart at various levels: **A:** at the papillary muscles; **B:** at the mitral valve; **C**: at the aortic valve.

55–61). By angulating and moving the transducer slightly, numerous regions can be traced in M-mode (**272–275**). *Table 13* (page 132) summarizes the cardiac structures visualized with M-mode.

The scanning positions for M-mode echocardiography are almost exclusively on the right thoracic wall. Two-dimensional images produced in a parasternal long-axis and short-axis view are the basis for M-mode echocardiography. Three areas, normally obtained in a parasternal long-axis view, are important for M-mode tracings:

- M-mode directly below the mitral valve with visualization of the right ventricular wall and chamber, the interventricular septum and the left ventricle, as well as the pericardium, chordae tendinae and the left ventricular wall (**273**).
- M-mode of the mitral valve leaflets with visualization of the right ventricular wall and chamber, the tricuspid valve, the interventricular septum, the anterior (septal) and/or posterior (parietal) mitral leaflets, the left chamber and ventricular wall, and the pericardium (**274**).
- M-mode at the level of the aortic root with visualization of the right atrium and ventricle, the tricuspid valve, the aortic root with the aortic valve, the left atrium and the left pulmonary artery (**275**).

273

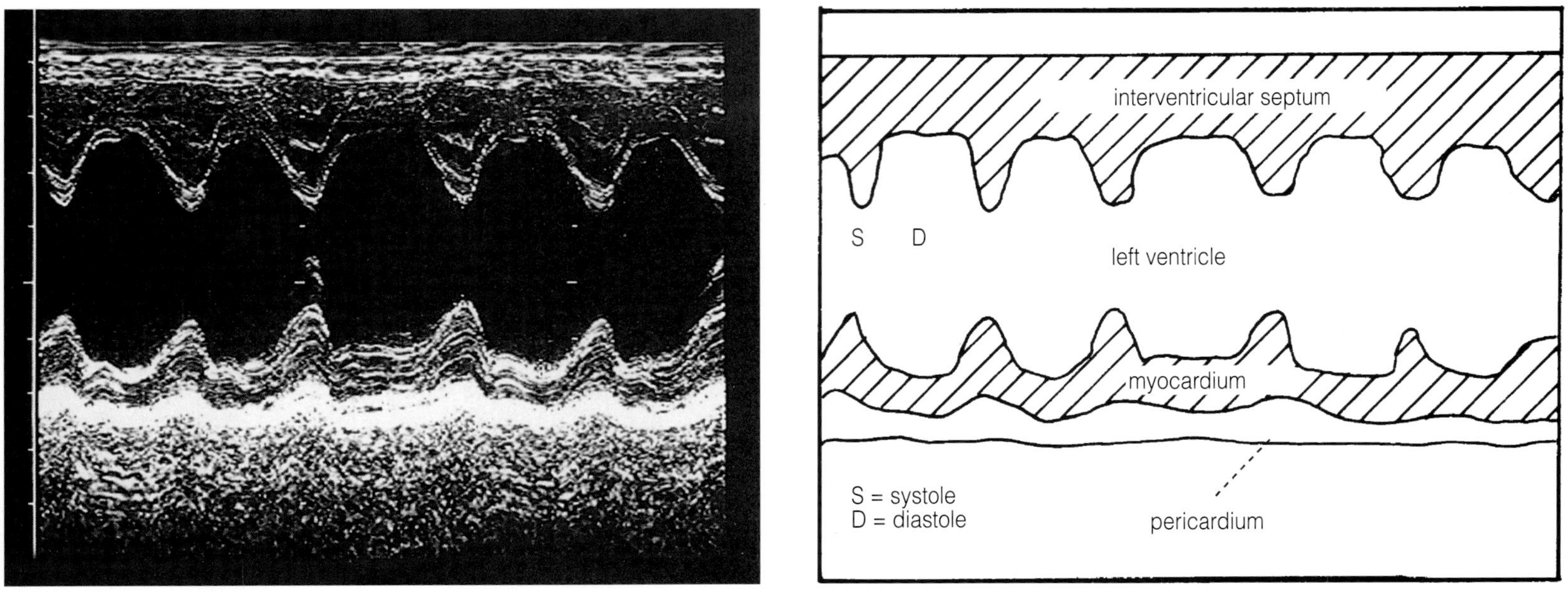

273 M-mode – dog. View of the interventricular septum, left ventricle and left ventricular wall directly below the mitral valve.

274

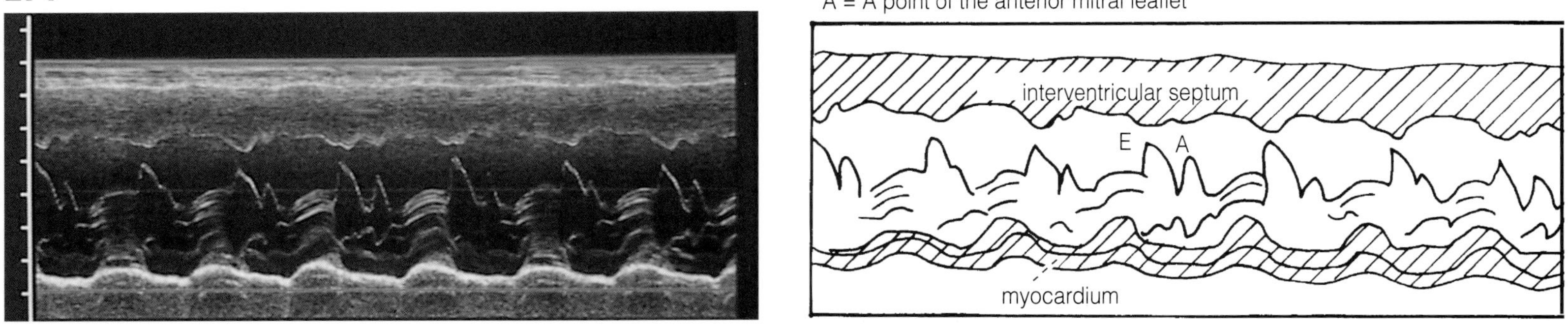

274 M-mode – dog. Image of the interventricular septum, left ventricle, anterior and posterior mitral leaflets, left ventricular wall and pericardium.

275

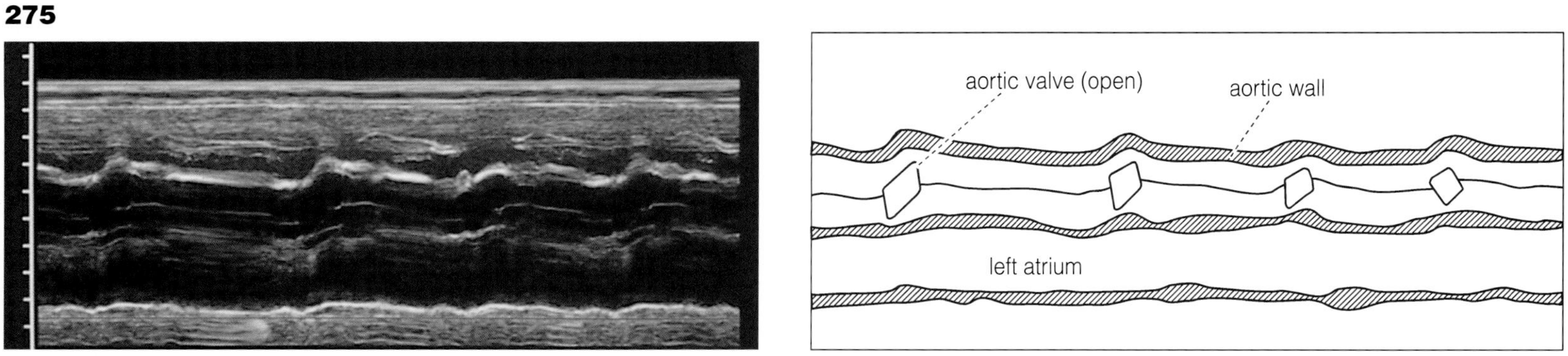

275 M-mode – dog. Image of the aortic valve, aortic root and left atrium. The LA/aortic root ratio is used to evaluate left atrial enlargement. They are normally of equal size.

Imaging and measurements of ventricular walls and chambers, as well as evaluation of the mitral valve, are especially easy in the two-dimensional short-axis view (90 degrees to the long-axis view). Ventricular wall thickness and internal dimensions are measured by placing the scan line between the papillary muscles. Mitral valve motion is displayed by placing the sound beam through the opening and closing leaflets.

Echocardiographic measurements are discussed in One- and Two-dimensional Echocardiographic Measurements, page 136.

Two-Dimensional Echocardiography

The two-dimensional echocardiogram (2DE) offers a more anatomically 'correct' image of the heart than the M-mode echocardiogram. The structures are imaged within the pie-shaped area of a sector transducer. The 90 degree scanning area is traced about 30 times per second, which produces a real-time image. The two-dimensional technique shows loss of detail compared to M-mode imaging.

Evaluation of cardiac and valvular motion is similar to M-mode.

276

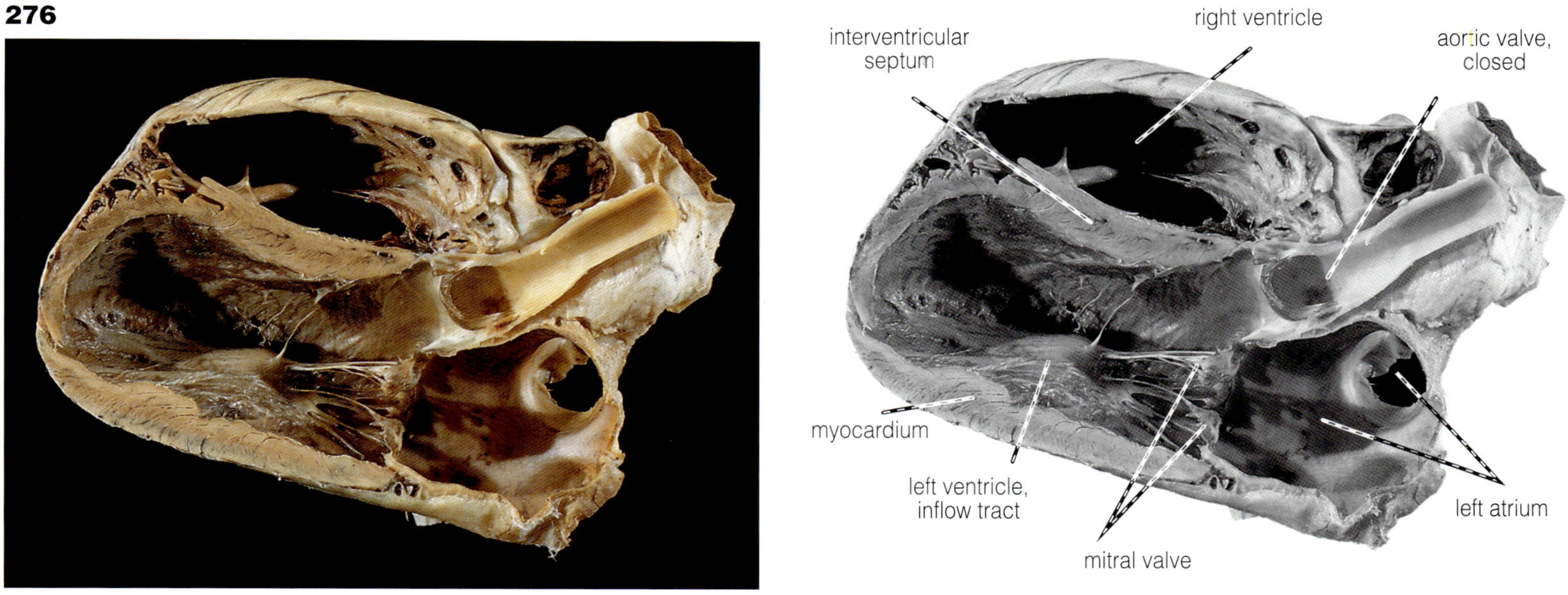

276 Anatomical specimen of a canine heart with the left ventricular inflow tract, comparable to the sonographic long-axis view in **277, 288**.

277

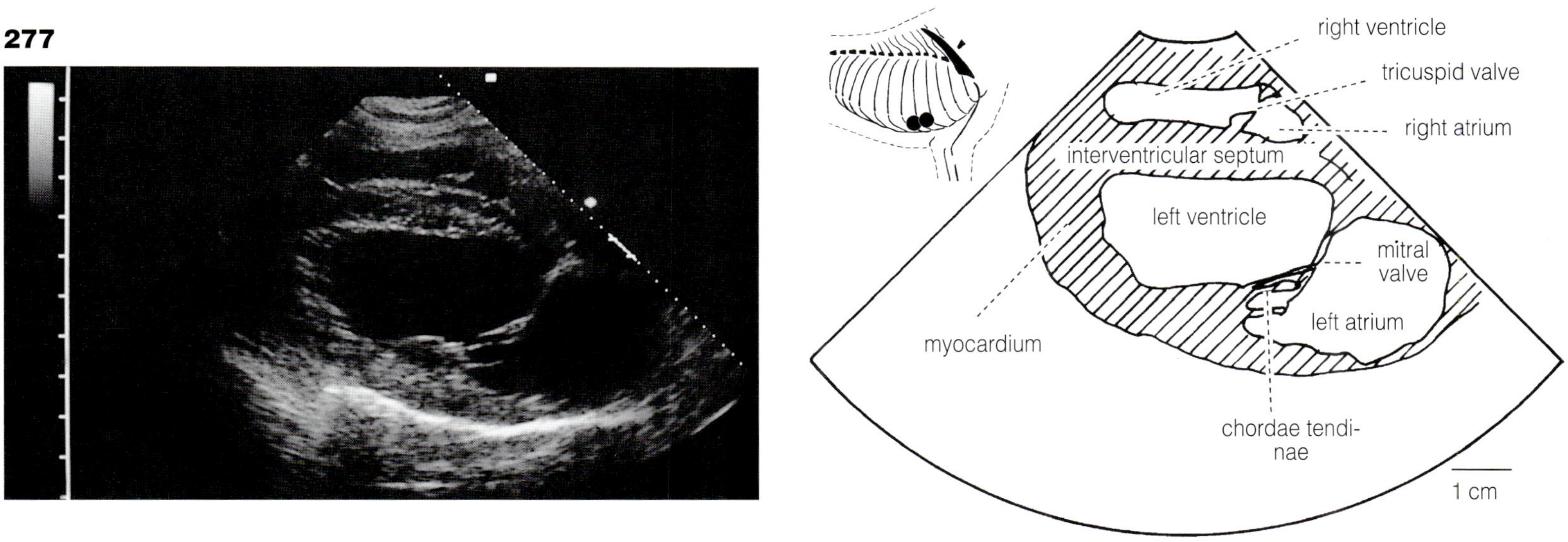

278

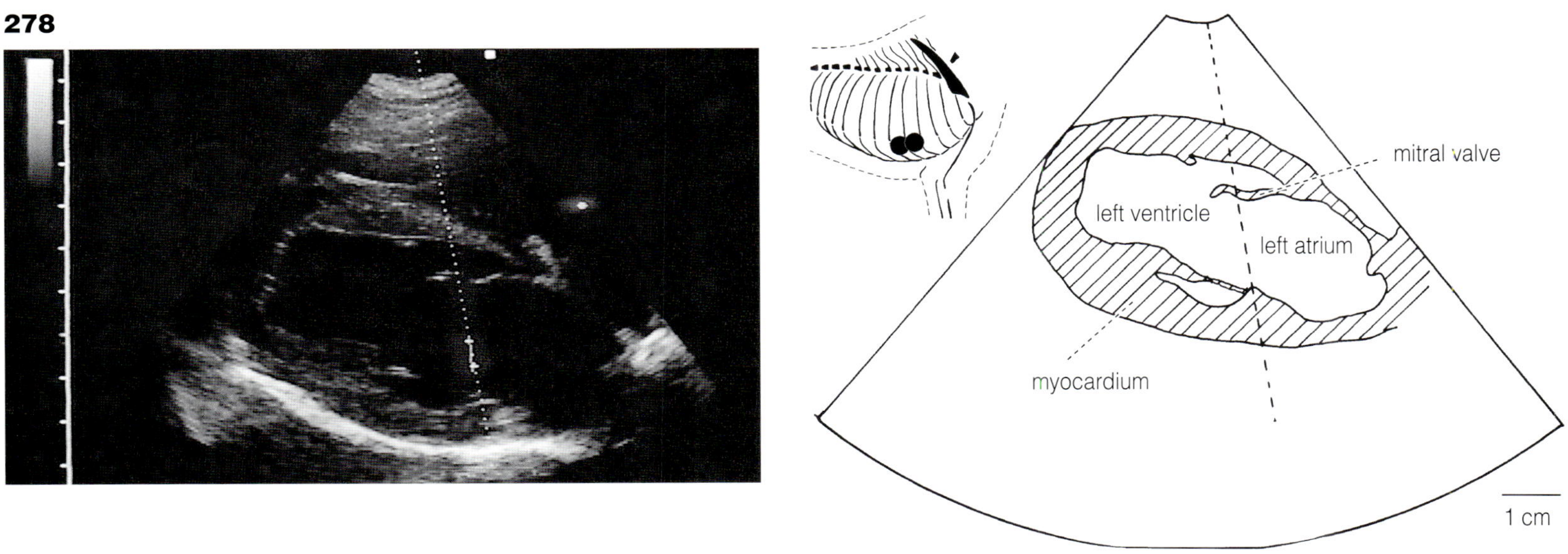

277, 278 Two-dimensional echocardiograms – dog. The long-axis views show the left ventricle, left atrium, myocardium and the mitral valve in different phases. Systolic closed (**277**) and diastolic open (**278**) mitral valve with an aligned M-mode scan .

Morphological and functional evaluation of each heart structure is a clear advantage of echocardiography over conventional radiography, in which the heart silhouette is seen only as an opacity.

Basically there are numerous imaging planes. The standard imaging planes are long-axis and short-axis views as well as apical two-chamber and four-chamber views (*Tables 14–16*, pages 132, 133)[25, 26, 31, 33].

For a long-axis view, the transducer is placed in the third to fifth intercostal space at a right parasternal location. This allows parallel imaging of the left ventricle, mitral valve and left inflow

279

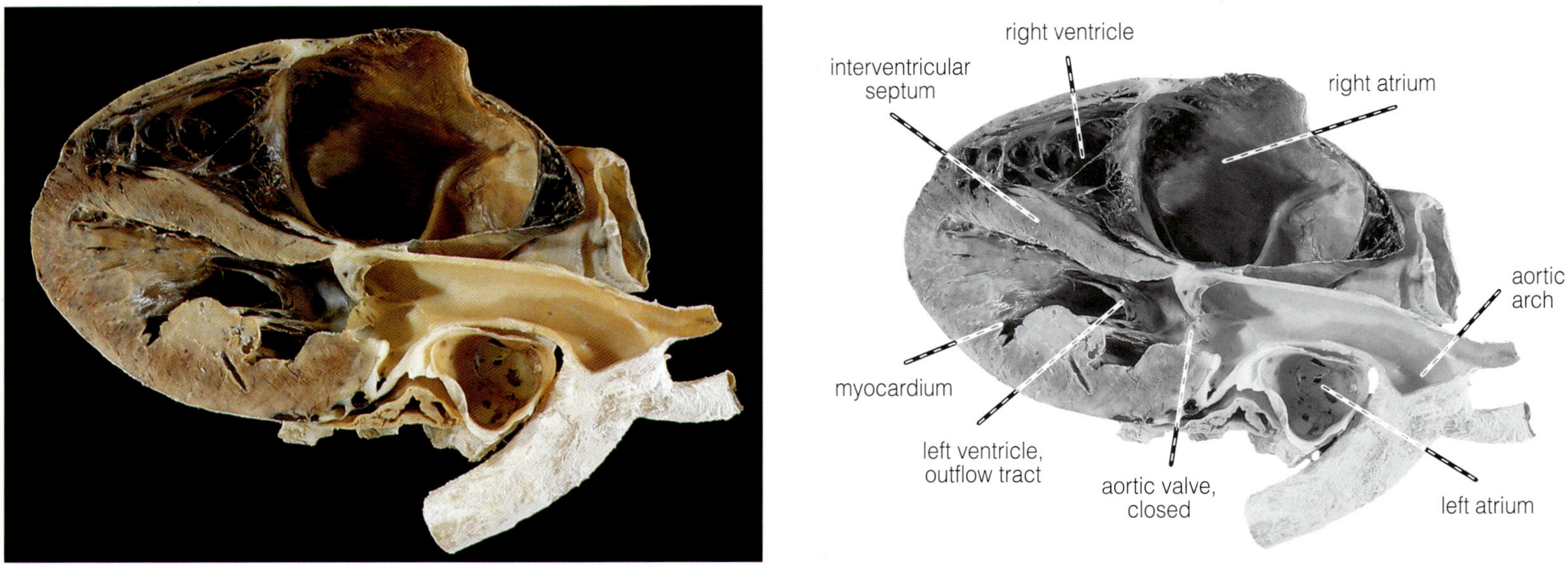

279 Anatomical specimen of the left ventricular outflow tract.

280

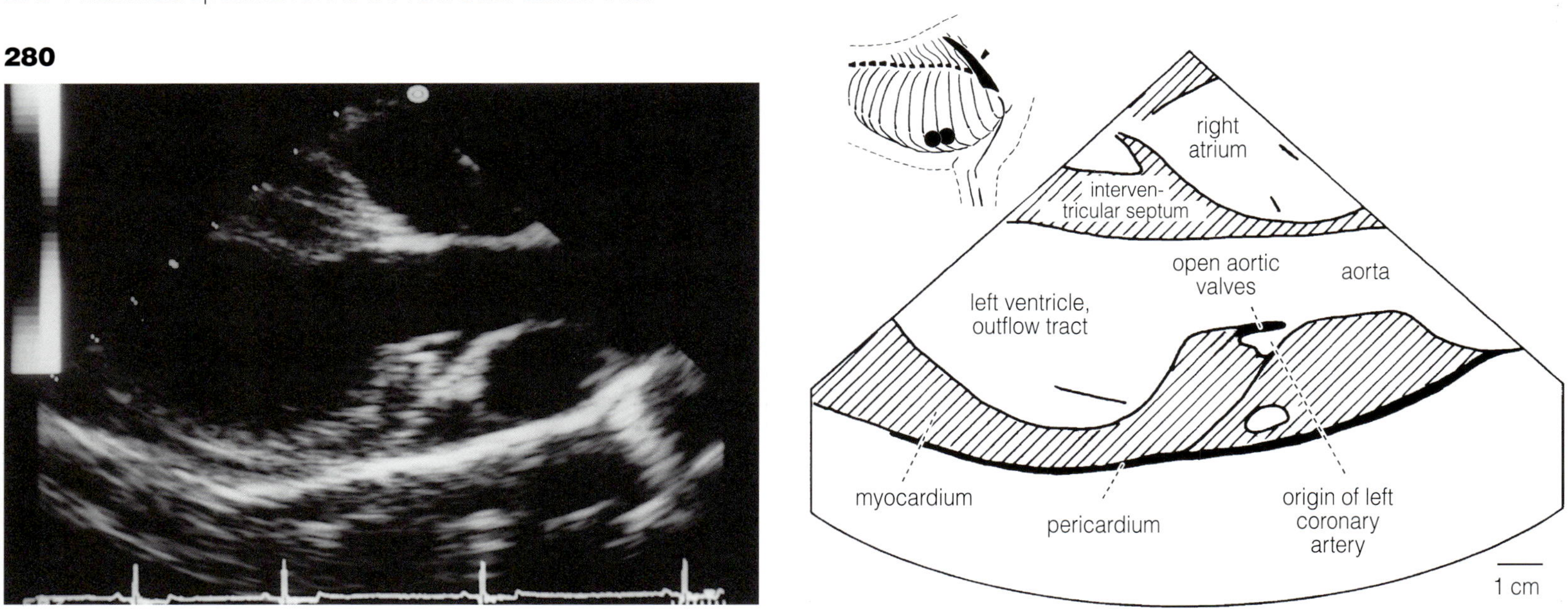

281

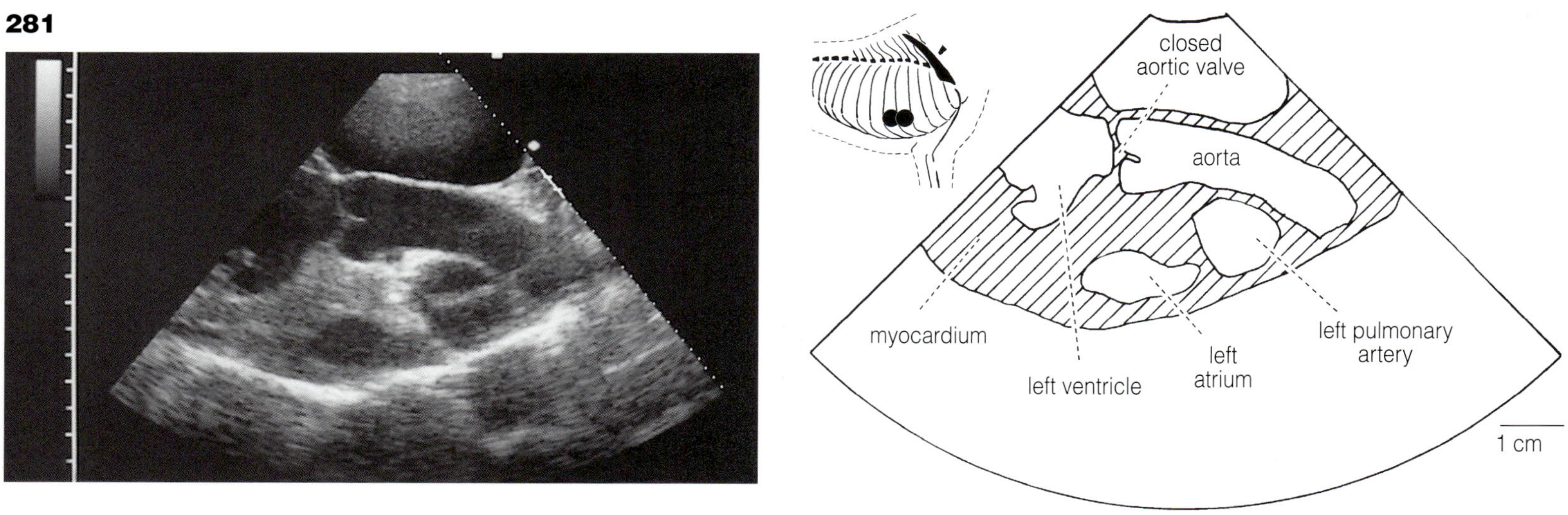

280, 281 Two-dimensional echocardiograms – dog. The long-axis views show the left ventricular outflow tract, the aortic valve, the aortic root and the aorta in different phases. Systolic open (**280**) and diastolic closed (**281**) aortic valve. Instead of the usual echo with two closed aortic valve leaflets, a middle echo is commonly seen, displaying the contact area of the leaflets.

tract (276–278). The left ventricular outflow tract is displayed by angulating the transducer caudally about 20 degrees (279–281). The right heart is not clearly visualized, apart from the interventricular septum.

Short-axis views are obtained by rotating the transducer 90 degrees. The four standard planes are located at the levels of the cardiac apex, the papillary muscles, the mitral valve and the aortic valve. Short-axis planes should always be evaluated from the apex to the heart base.

While the left ventricle is nearly round with a uniform thickness of the myocardium and septum, the right ventricle is sickle-shaped with a thinner myocardium (282–288).

282

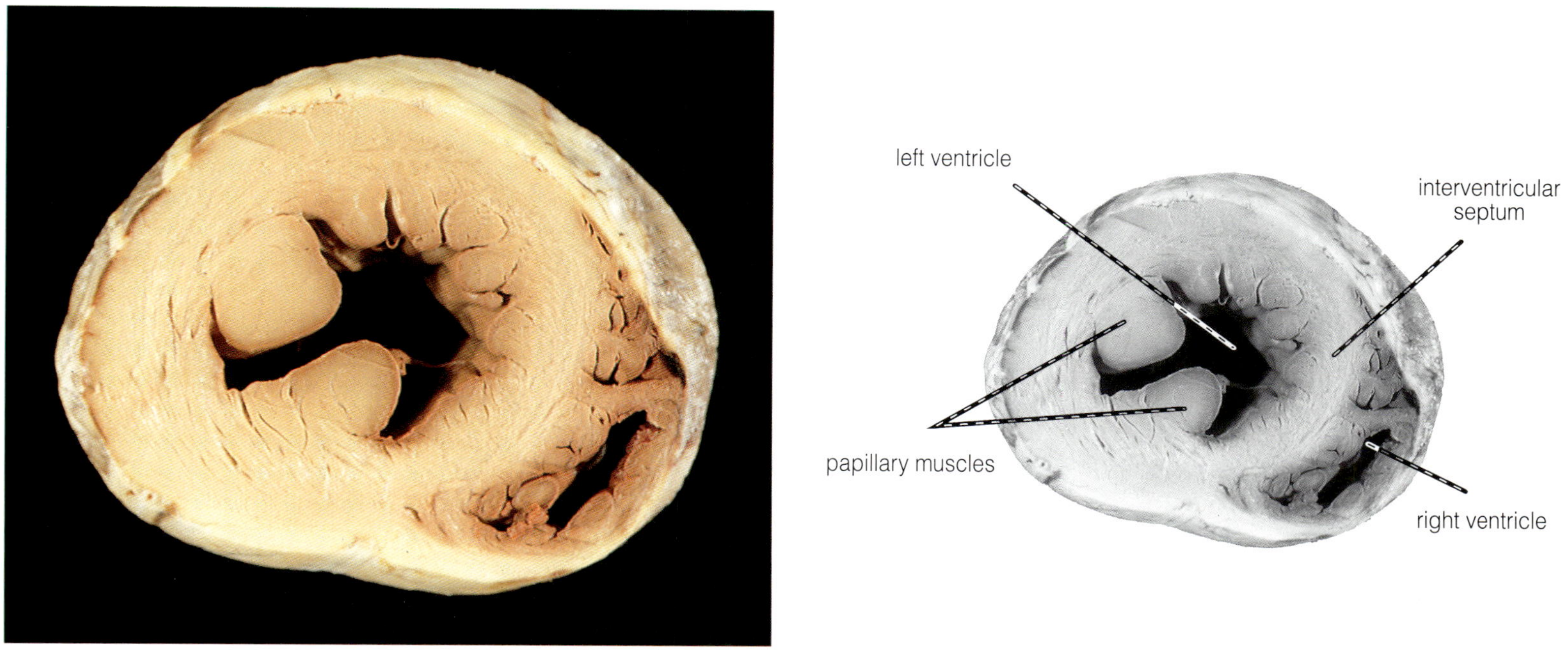

283

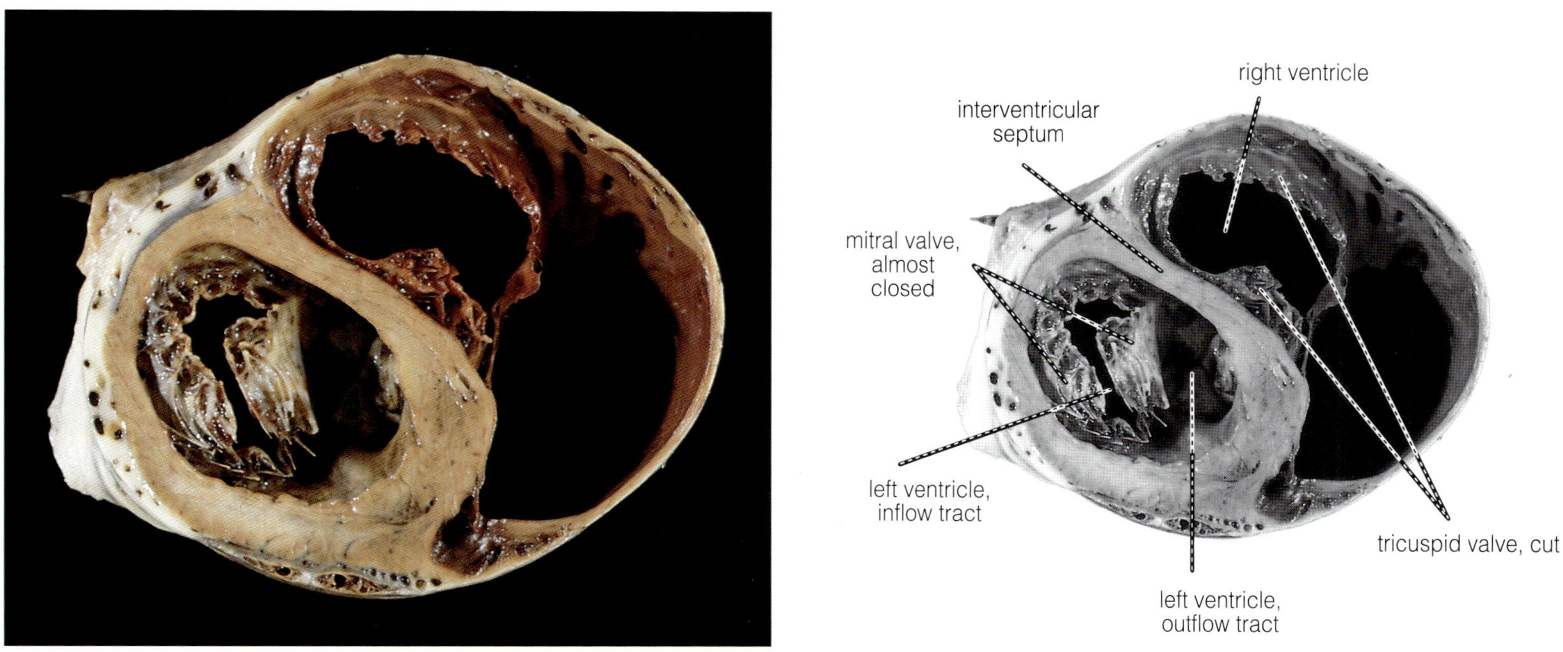

284

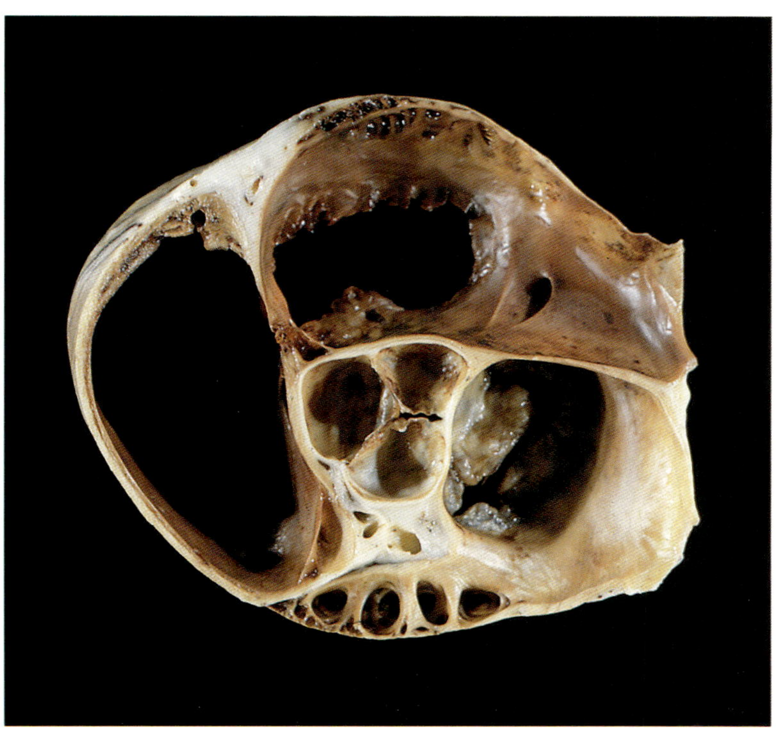

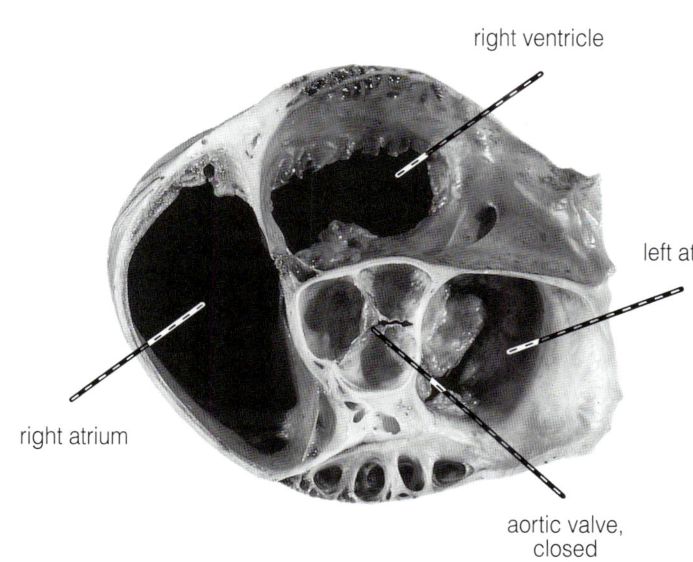

282–284 Anatomical cross-sections at various levels of a canine heart, comparable to sonographic short-axis views. Cross-section at the level of the papillary muscles (**282**); the atrioventricular valves (**283**); and the aortic valve (**284**).

285

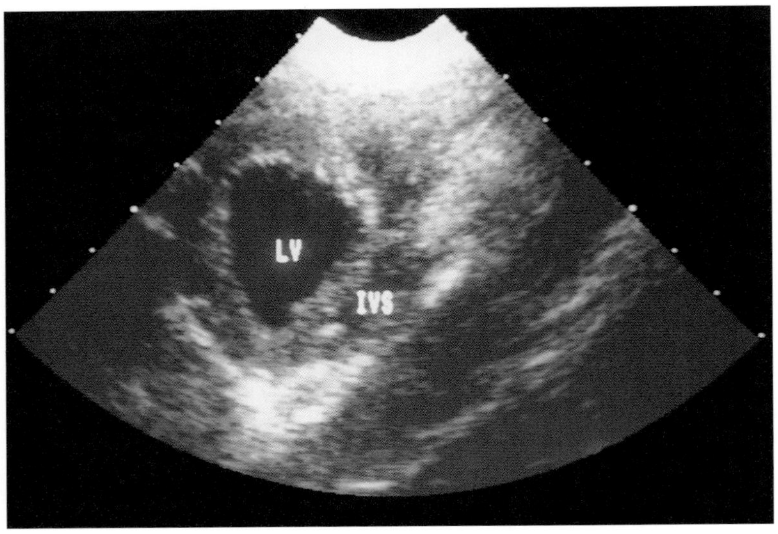

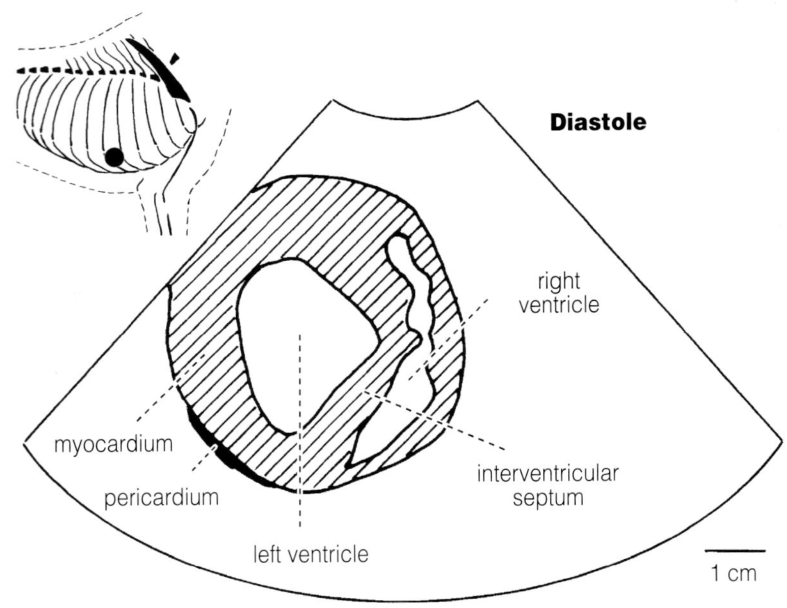

286

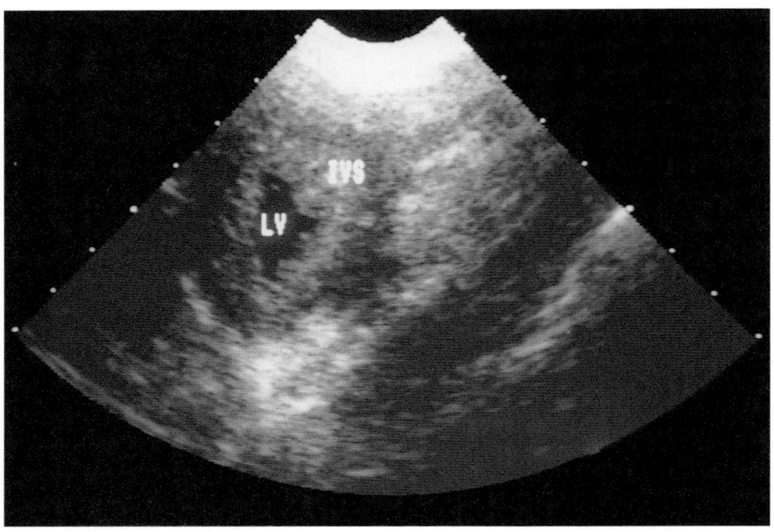

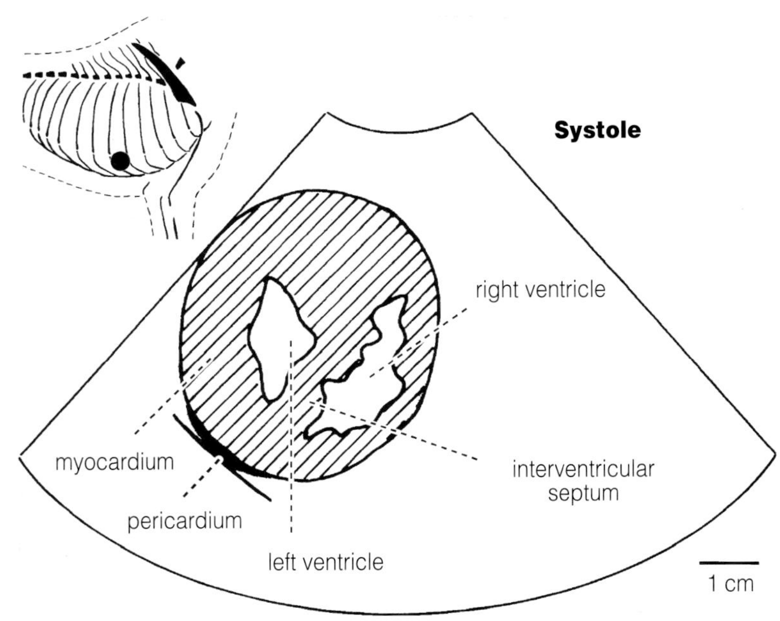

285, 286 Two-dimensional echocardiograms – dog. End-diastolic (**285**) and end-systolic (**286**) short-axis views at the apex.

Table 13 Summary of the cardiac structures displayed with M-mode echocardiography.

Anatomical structures visualized with M-mode:
• Anechoic or slightly echogenic free pleural fluid. • Ventricular walls. • Myocardium. • Interventricular septum. • Atria. • Ventricles. • Atrioventricular valves. • Chordae tendinae. • Papillary muscles. • Aortic root and valve. • Pericardium and pericardial cavity.

Table 14 Summary of the anatomical structures visualized by two-dimensional echocardiography in the left ventricular long-axis view.

Anatomical structures in the left ventricular long-axis view with two-dimensional echocardiography:
• Myocardium. • Interventricular septum. • Atrial septum. • Atria. • Ventricles. • Atrioventricular valves. • Chordae tendinae. • Papillary muscles. • Aortic root and valve. • Pulmonary valve (limited). • Origin of left and right coronary artery (limited). • Pericardium and pericardial cavity.

287

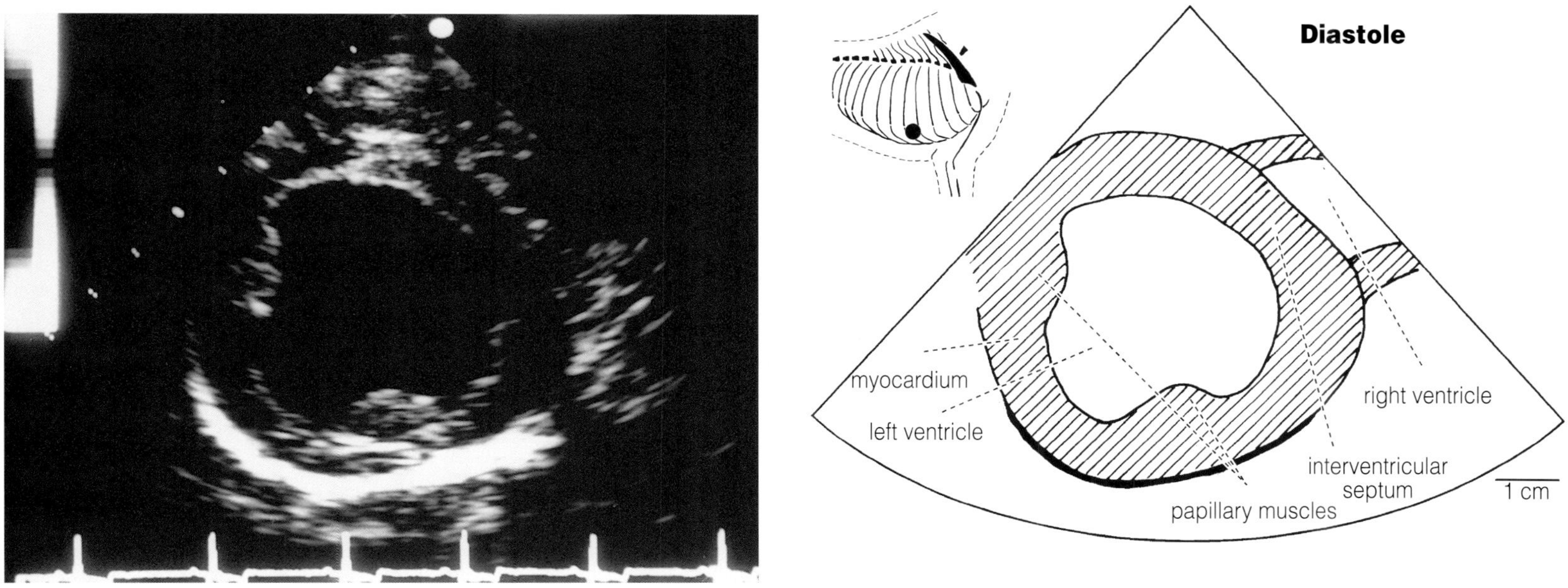

288

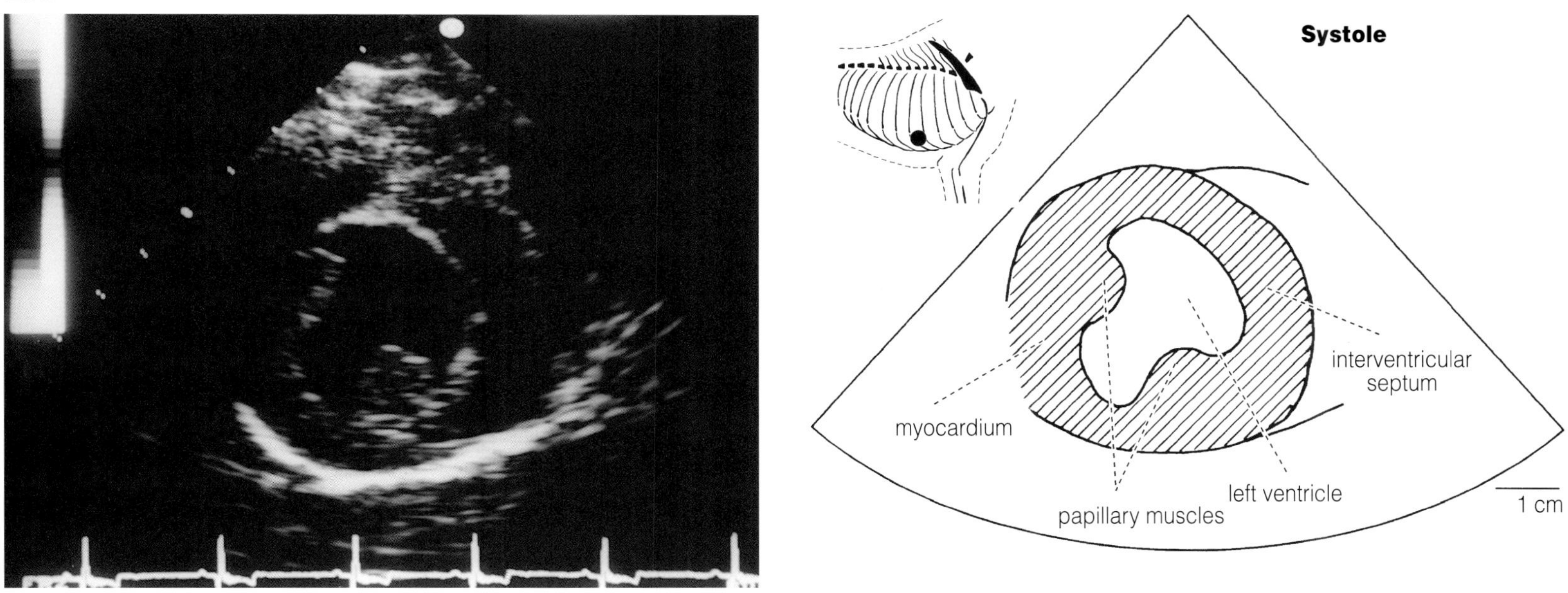

287, 288 Two-dimensional echocardiograms – dog. End-diastolic (**287**) and end-systolic (**288**) short-axis views at the papillary muscles.

Table 15 Summary of the anatomical structures visualized by two-dimensional echocardiography in the left ventricular short-axis view.

Anatomical structures in the left ventricular short-axis view with two-dimensional echocardiography:
• Myocardium. • Interventricular septum. • Ventricles. • Mitral valve and partial tricuspid valve. • Chordae tendinae. • Papillary muscles. • Aortic valve. • Pulmonary valve (limited). • Pericardium and pericardial cavity.

Table 16 Summary of the anatomical structures visualized by two-dimensional echocardiography in the four-chamber and five-chamber views.

Anatomical structures in the four-chamber and five-chamber views with two-dimensional echocardiography:
• Myocardium (limited, parallel to sound beam). • Interventricular septum (limited, parallel to sound beam). • Atrial septum (limited, parallel to sound beam). • Atria (partially). • Ventricles. • Atrioventricular valves. • Aortic root and valve (only in five-chamber view). • Pericardium and pericardial cavity.

289

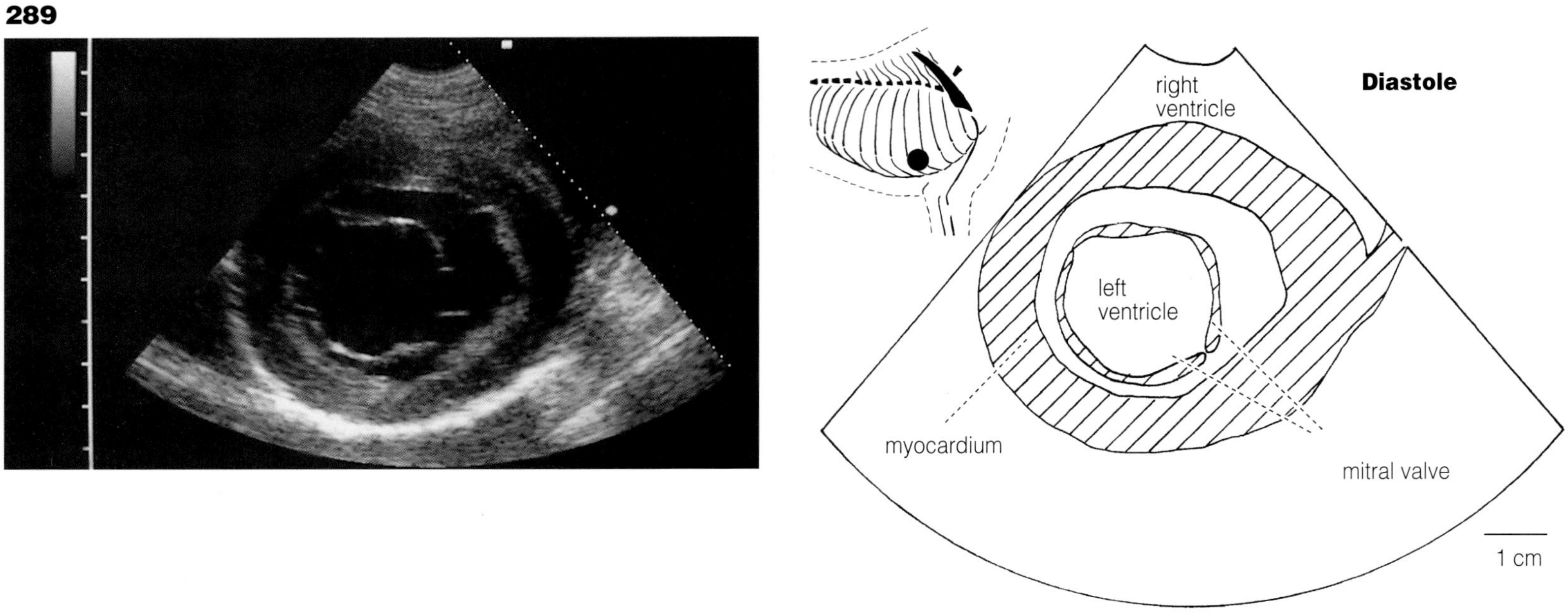

290

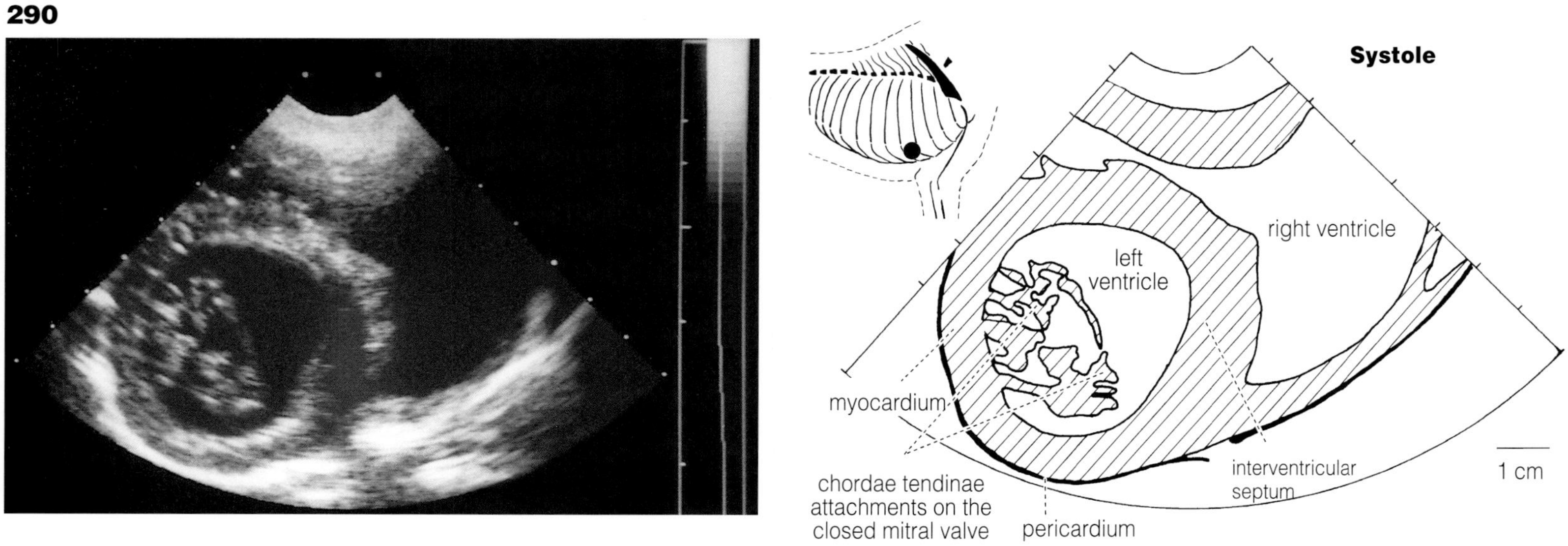

289, 290 Two-dimensional echocardiograms – dog. Short-axis view of the heart at the level of the open (**289**) and closed (**290**) mitral valve. **290:** Because of systolic heart motion, the tips of the mitral leaflets are not seen, although the transducer position is unchanged. The image shows the attachment of the chordae tendinae closer to the apex (see **55–61**; One-dimensional B-Mode, page 39).

In diastole the wide open septal and parietal mitral leaflets have an oval to round, so-called 'fish-mouth', appearance. Complete closure of the mitral valve during systole is usually missed. During systole, cardiac motion moves the scanning plane towards the apex and displays the chordae tendinae as numerous echogenic dots (282–284, 289, 290) (see One-dimensional B-Mode, page 39; 55–61). The left ventricular outflow tract is registered between the septal mitral leaflet and the interventricular septum.

A transverse view of the closed aortic valve during diastole shows a Y-shape of the right, left and septal coronary cusps. Completely open cusps cannot be separated from the aortic wall (282–284, 291, 292).

The main pulmonary artery or pulmonary trunk is difficult to image from the right thoracic side. The right ventricular outflow tract can be displayed by angulating the transducer slightly from the aortic short-axis view. Evaluation of the pulmonary valve is easier from the left third to fourth intercostal space. The sound beam is directed caudodorsally. With an almost transverse view of the aorta at the valve level, the main pulmonary artery is located above the aorta and nearer to the transducer. In this image the pulmonary trunk and pulmonary valve are seen in a longitudinal plane and they can be followed to the bifurcation into the pulmonary arteries (305).

For complete cardiac evaluation the heart must be imaged in a left apical four-chamber view (293). The four-chamber view displays the ventricles and atria, as well as portions of the septa. Systolic and diastolic atrioventricular valve motion can also be evaluated.

In the apical four-chamber view, the heart appears to be upside down with the atria more distal. The left atrium and left ventricle are usually on the right hand side of the image or monitor. Slight

291

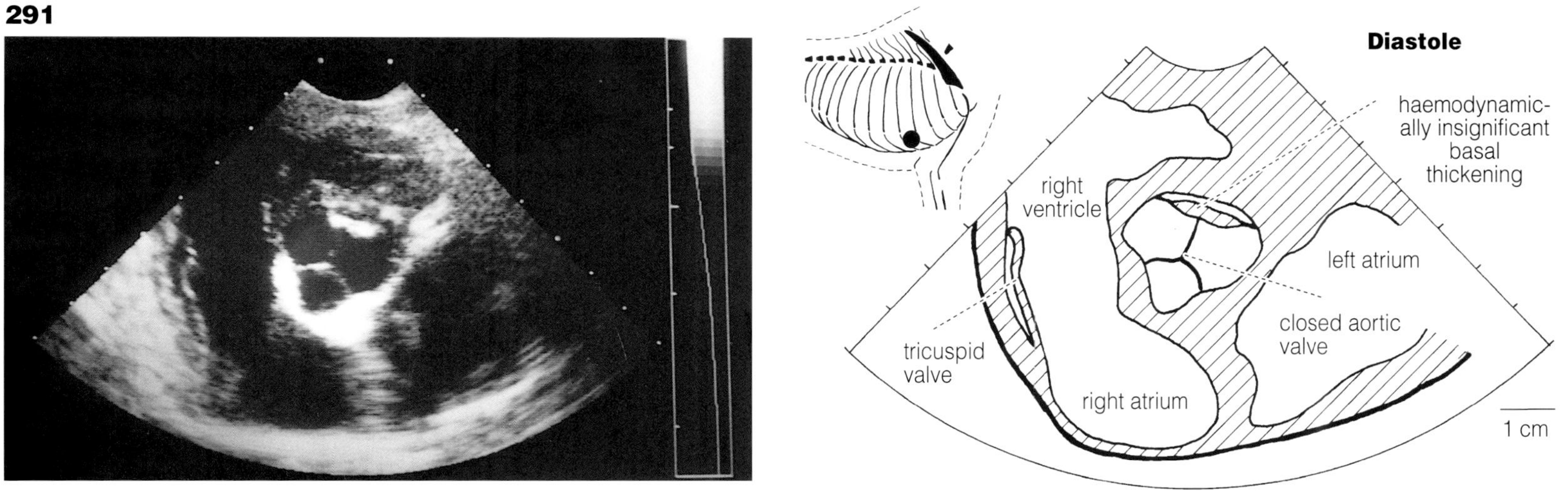

292

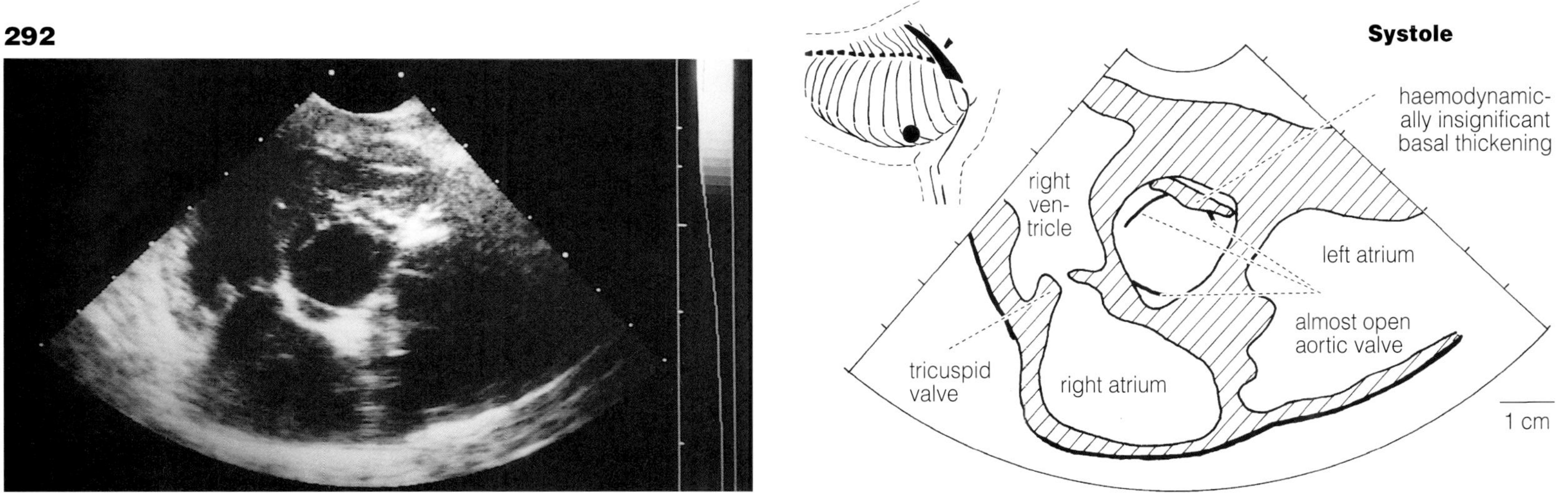

291, 292 Two-dimensional echocardiograms – dog. Short-axis view at the end-diastolic closed (**291**) and early-systolic almost open (**292**) aortic valve.

293

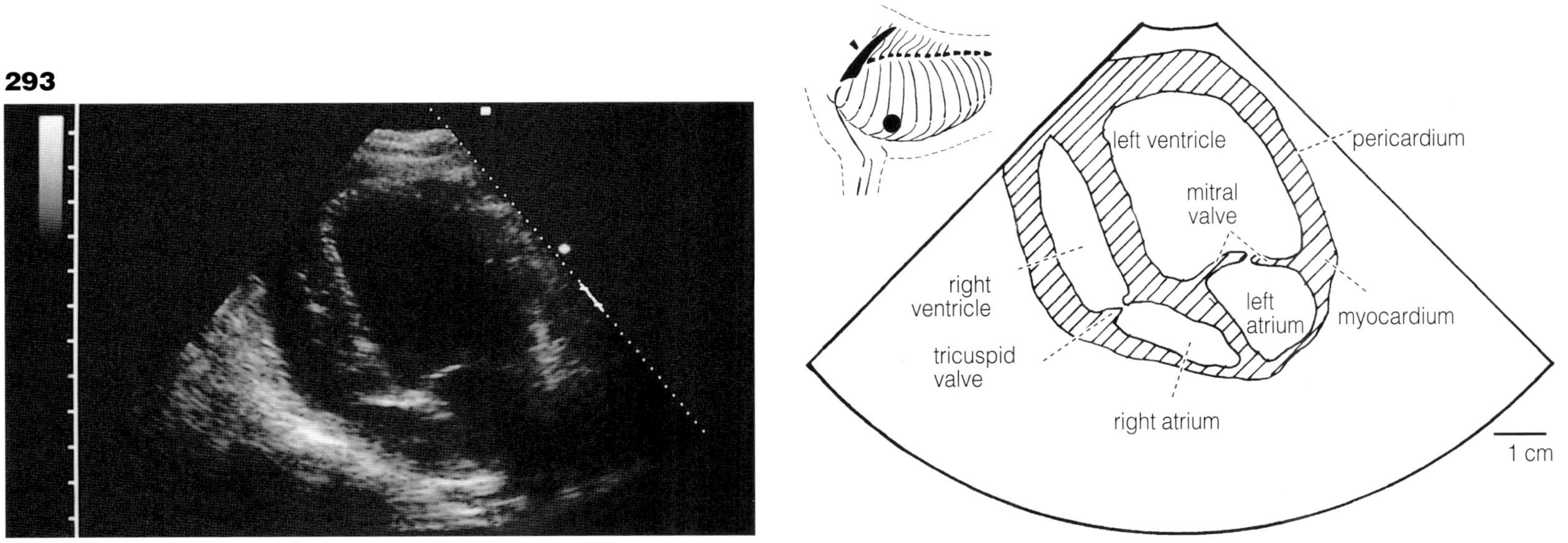

293 Two-dimensional echocardiogram – dog. Four-chamber view. In this 'upside-down' view of the heart, it is possible to evaluate the four chambers (left and right atrium, left and right ventricle), the myocardium and the atrioventricular valves.

294

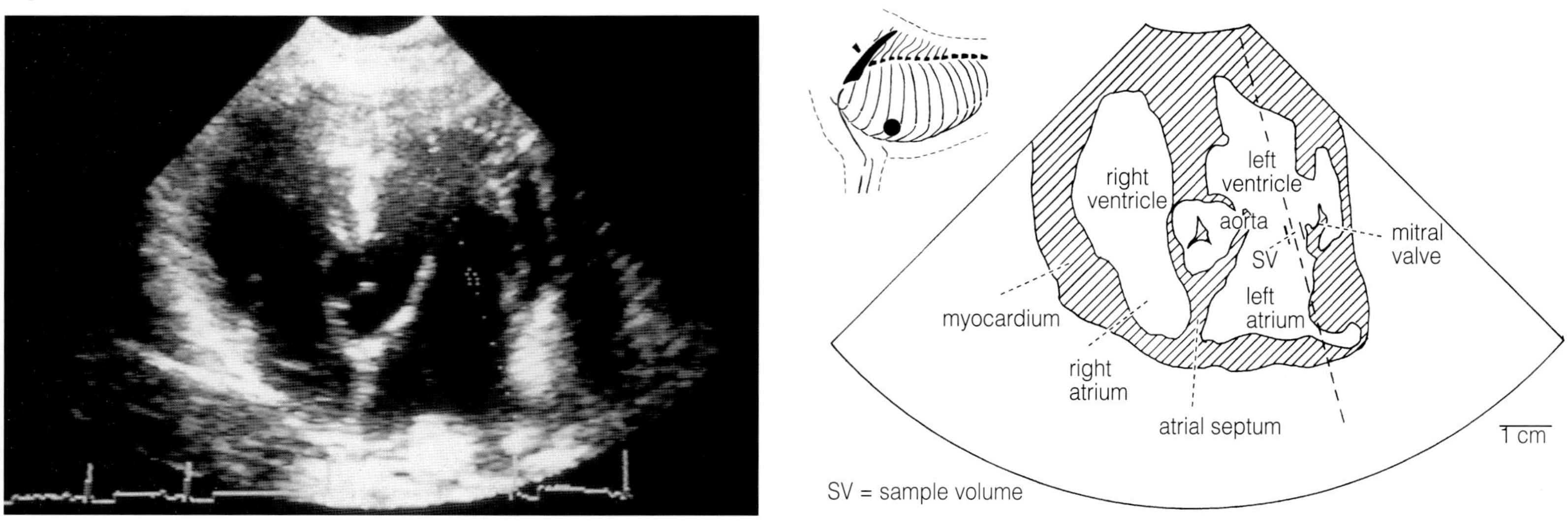

294 Two-dimensional echocardiogram – dog. Five-chamber view. Besides the atria and the ventricles, the closed aortic valve, i.e. its middle echo, and the aortic root are visualized.

rotation of the transducer produces an image with the aortic valve and ascending aorta medial to the mitral valve or atrial septum. This view is also called a five-chamber view (**294**)[31, 33].

295

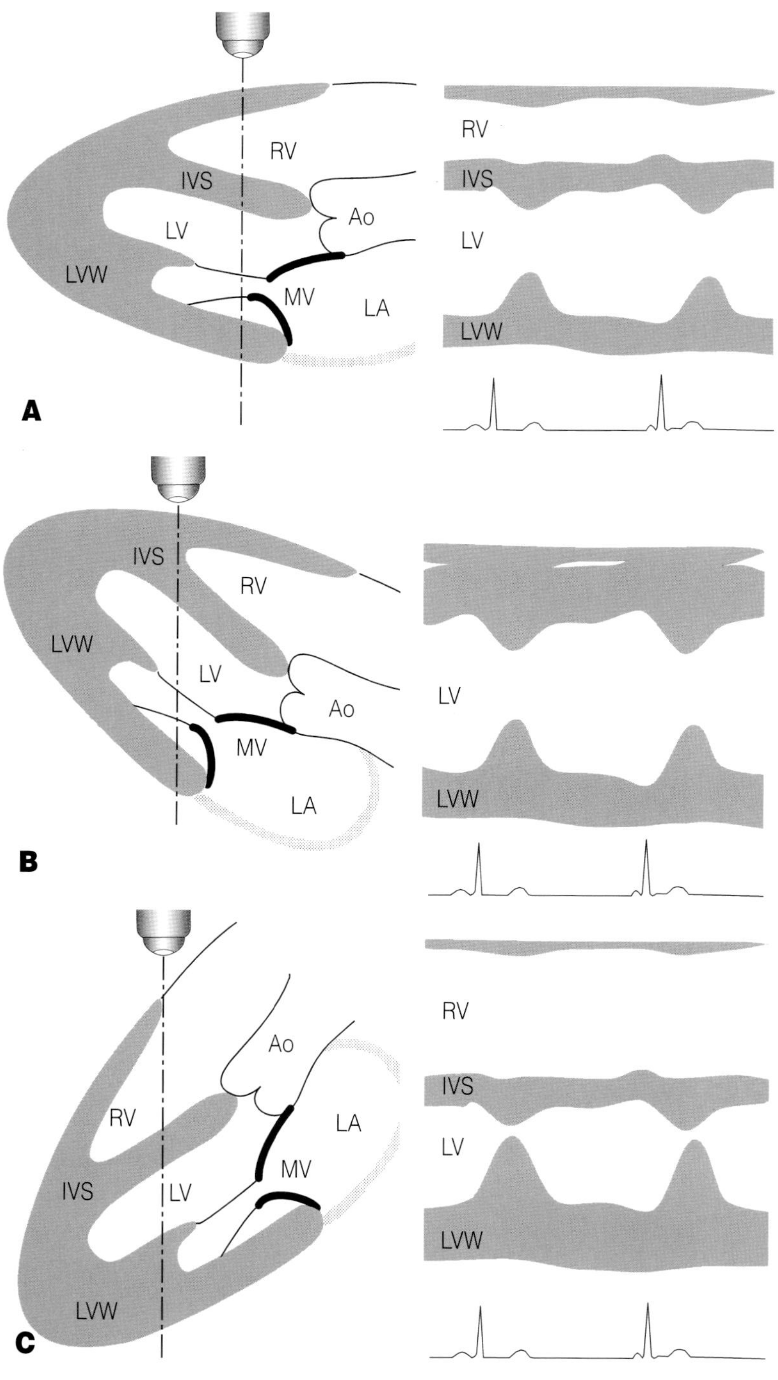

One- and Two-Dimensional Echocardiographic Measurements (Tables 17, 18)

Quantification of separate structures leads to an objective evaluation of pathological lesions. Many authors have given normal echocardiographic reference values in various dog breeds and cats. These values are derived from calculations using the body weight, body surface or age of individual breeds[22, 27, 28]. Body weight is the reference variable of choice for routine measurements of ventricular diameters and ventricular and septal wall thickness.

M-mode measurements are indicated when recording a structure over time and receiving clearer detail. The sound beam must be perpendicular to the cardiac structure to receive an accurate, reproducible and comparable image. Any deviation from a perpendicular image will lead to values with normal ratios but too high measurement values (**295A**).

A clinically relevant measurement is the left ventricular fractional shortening (FS). The relative systolic dimension change of the left ventricle is given in per cent, expressing myocardial contractility (**296**).

$$FS = \frac{LVDd - LVDs}{LVDd} \times 100$$

[FS: fractional shortening; LVDd: left ventricular end-diastolic dimension; LVDs: left ventricular end-systolic dimension]

The systolic shortening fraction measures chamber dimensions from the ventricular wall endocardium to the interventricular septum. The measurements are made from the third or fourth intercostal space. The scanning planes are described above (One-dimensional Echocardiography).

295 Schematic drawing of the sound beam's influence on measuring parameters. Compared to an exact perpendicular sound beam (**A**), an oblique scan will overestimate ventricular dimensions, although FS is the same (**B**). When the sound beam also passes through a papillary muscle, FS will be too high (**C**). [Ao = aorta; IVS = interventricular septum; LA = left atrium; LV = left ventricle; LVW = left ventricular wall; MV = mitral valve; RV = right ventricle.]

Reproducible shortening fraction measurements are received by exact placement of the scan line in the M-mode. The authors find that the best and most practical site is between the papillary muscles in the short-axis view. Inclusion of contracting papillary muscles in the measurement results in a too high shortening fraction (**295A**). Values greater than 30% are considered normal. A hypercontractile heart will show shortening fractions greater than 40%. Some dogs with severely dilated hearts will have similarly high FS values, although haemodynamic function is reduced (see Hypertrophic Cardiomyopathy, page 148). Dog breeds such as Greyhounds, hunting dogs and other dogs in training have normal FS values of less than 30%. Excessive movement or stress will increase these values – 'athlete's heart' (author's note). Statistical interpretation of these values will have to be examined.

> The systolic shortening fraction is an important index in diagnosing and evaluating cardiomyopathies. When measuring FS, it is imperative to consider the history and clinical symptoms of the animal, as well as ensuring an exact scanning plane.

This statement states that all M-mode measurements require an exact placement of the sound beam in the two-dimensional echocardiogram.

The same is true when determining the mitral valve opening area. An M-mode tracing at the level of the mitral valve shows the M-shaped echo of the anterior leaflet and the low amplitude W-shape of the posterior leaflet between the interventricular septum and the left chamber wall (**273**)[22]. It is not always possible to display both leaflets at the same time in the M-mode tracing.

Table 17 Useful and recommended measurements in one- or two-dimensional echocardiography.

Anatomical measurements in one-dimensional (M-mode) or two-dimensional echocardiography (2DE):	
• Right ventricular wall (RVW)	M-mode
• Right ventricular end-diastolic dimension (RVDd)	M-mode
• Right ventricular end-systolic dimension (RVDs)	M-mode
• End-diastolic and end-systolic interventricular septum (IVSd and IVSs)	M-mode
• End-diastolic and end-systolic left ventricular wall (LVWd and LVWs)	M-mode
• Left ventricular end-diastolic dimension (LVDd)	M-mode
• Left ventricular end-systolic dimension (LVDs)	M-mode
• Fractional shortening (FS)	Calculated automatically
• End-systolic left atrial dimension (LA)	2DE – parasternal long-axis view
• End-diastolic aortic diameter (AoD)	2DE – parasternal long-axis view
• End-diastolic aortic bulbus diameter (AoB)	2DE – parasternal long-axis view
• Mitral valve opening (DE-slope)	M-mode

Mitral valve opening in one-dimensional M-mode begins at point 'D'. The maximum valve opening point is at 'E. The slope from 'D' to 'E' signifies early-diastolic opening of the anterior (septal) mitral leaflet (**272**). The opening excursion is given in millimetres and may be higher with a prolapsed valve or ruptured chordae tendinae. The 'EF' slope, given in mm/s, represents the mid-diastolic closure rate of the anterior mitral leaflet. This last parameter has little significance in dogs and cats because of their relatively high heart rates and short diastoles. A decrease in the 'EF' slope is seen with mitral stenosis in humans[30, 10]. The distance between the 'E' point (maximal early diastolic opening point) and the ventricular septum serves as a useful diagnostic index. Left ventricular hypertrophy decreases the 'E' point to septal separation (EPSS)[2, 4, 29], while dilated cardiomyopythy shows an increase of this distance. The 'A' point indicates initial closure of the mitral valve and 'C' represents complete closure (**272**).

The size of the left atrium (LA) is determined by comparing it with the diameter of the aortic root (Ao). This end-diastolic measurement is made in a left ventricular long-axis view in two-dimensional echocardiography. The LA/aortic root ratio should be 1.0 in normal dogs[5, 22].

Doppler Echocardiography

The Doppler methods described in Chapter 3 (Doppler Mode, page 45) have become an important part of veterinary cardiac diagnostics. They are used to evaluate normal and pathological blood flows near the heart valves and to diagnose cardiac lesions[9, 10]. These methods include continuous-wave (CW), pulsed-wave (PW) and colour-coded Doppler.

Special ultrasound units record the Doppler signals on a monitor and acoustically. The audible signal is smooth and whistling with laminar flow or noisy and hissing with turbulent flow. Since most patients are disturbed by the Doppler sounds, they should be received over head sets or turned off completely.

Table 18 M-mode measurements of the dog depending on body weight (modified from Lombard, 1984[22]), and of the cat (modified from Soderberg *et al.*, 1984[29]). (n.a. = not available)

Animal Body weight (kg)	Dog 1–10	Dog 11–20	Dog 21–30	Dog 31–40	Dog 41–50	Cat
LVDd [mm]	23–29	30–37	37–44	45–51	52–59	11.16–14.48
LVDs [mm]	13–17	18–22	23–27	28–33	33–38	6.80–9.86
FS [%]	43–41	40–38	38–37	38–36	37–36	21.87–47.13
LVWd [mm]	5–7	7–8	8–10	10–11	11–13	2.05–4.21
LVWs [mm]	n.a.	n.a.	n.a.	n.a.	n.a.	4.67–6.27
IVSd [mm]	5–7	7–8	8–10	10–11	11–13	n.a.
LAs [mm]	14–17	17–21	21–24	25–28	28–32	8.17–11.51
AoB [mm]	15–18	18–21	21–25	25–28	28–32	8.03–10.81
RVDd [mm]	7–9	9–10	11–12	13–14	14–16	n.a.

296

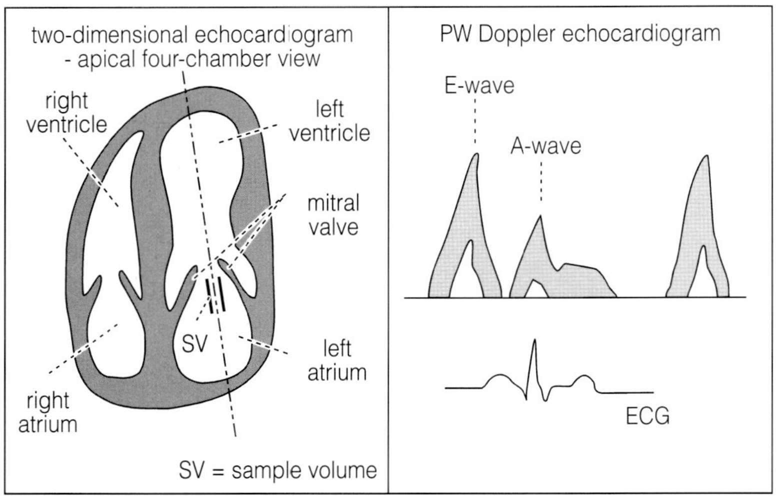

297

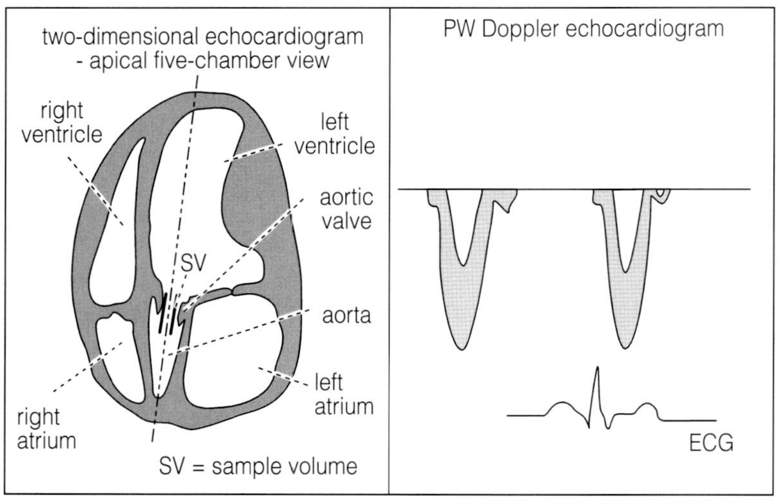

298

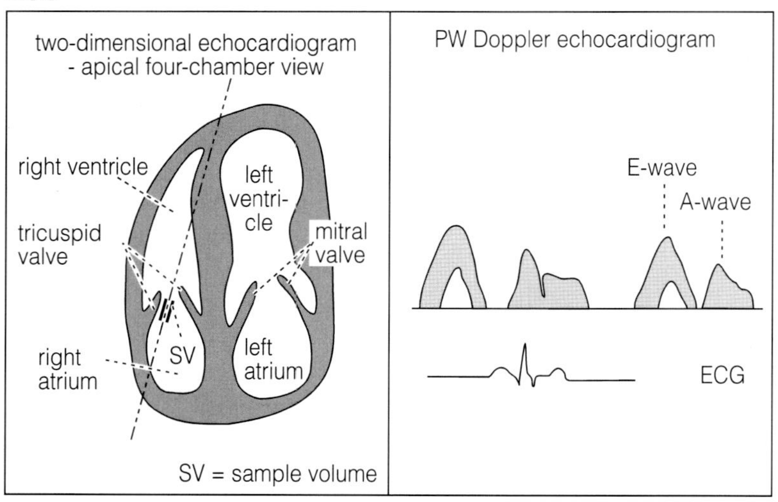

299

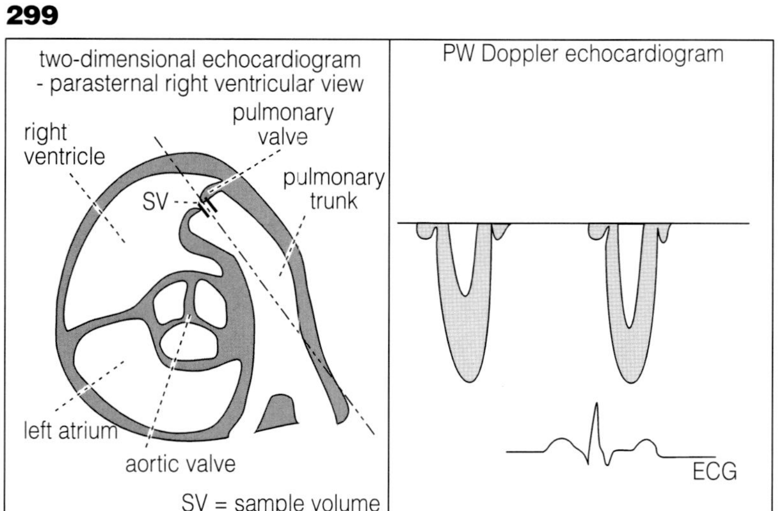

Conventional CW and PW Doppler echocardiograms are displayed by a graph. Spectral Doppler recordings show time (systole and diastole) on the x-axis and flow direction and velocity along the y-axis. The Doppler signal is generally above the baseline when flow is towards the transducer (**296, 298, 302, 303**). Blood flow away from the transducer is traced below the baseline (**297, 299, 300, 301**; see Doppler Effect, page 24, **16–18**).

The grey scale of the Doppler signal is proportional to the number of blood cells moving at the same velocity. The brighter an area in the black-and-white Doppler echocardiogram, the more blood cells are moving at the same velocity. Unwanted, low-frequency Doppler shifts (Doppler shift = difference between transmitted and received frequencies [see Doppler Effect, page 24]), caused by myocardial and vessel wall movement, can be reduced with filters (see Doppler Controls, page 49). Quick valve motion produces thin, vertical Doppler signals that cannot be filtered (artefacts). These artefacts are apparent at early- and end-systole (see Doppler Artefacts, page 72; **145**).

To optimize the Doppler method, it is necessary to direct the transmitted beam parallel to the blood flow. Blood flow measurements are made from a left apical four-chamber view. In this view the atria and ventricles are on top of each other (**293**). When the ultrasound beam cannot be aligned parallel to the blood flow, an angle correction factor is employed in the PW Doppler mode (see Doppler Effect, page 24; **21–23**).

PW Doppler mode, combined with two-dimensional echocardiography, can accurately localize the area to be measured. For an overview of flow velocity distribution or to locate abnormal flows, e.g. insufficiencies, numerous areas have to be traced. This sampling for cardiac abnormalities is also referred to as 'mapping'. The image has to be switched from two-dimensional to a Doppler mode for this procedure. Another limitation of PW Doppler is its inability to measure high flow velocities, seen with abnormal blood flows. High velocities in PW Doppler lead to aliasing (see Aliasing and Nyquist Limit, page 48; **78–83**). CW Doppler is used to measure high flow velocities. It cannot determine the exact location of an abnormal signal or use an angle correction factor. CW Doppler is best for finding small insufficiency jets at the mitral and tricuspid valves (see Continuous-Wave Doppler, page 46; Pulsed-Wave Doppler, page 46).

The flow velocities measured with CW or PW Doppler echography are the basis for semi-quantitative determination of pressure gradients at stenotic heart or vessel valves and for helping to evaluate the severity of a stenosis. The pressure gradient refers to the difference between prestenotic and poststenotic hydrostatic pressure.

The modified Bernoulli equation determines that the sum of hydrostatic pressure (to be measured) and back pressure is the same in all areas, when flow acceleration and viscous friction are

296–299 Schematic drawings of beam/sample volume alignment with CW and PW Doppler and normal tracings in black-and-white Doppler echocardiography. Over the mitral valve (**296**); over the aortic valve (**297**); over the tricuspid valve (**298**); and over the pulmonary valve (**299**).

300

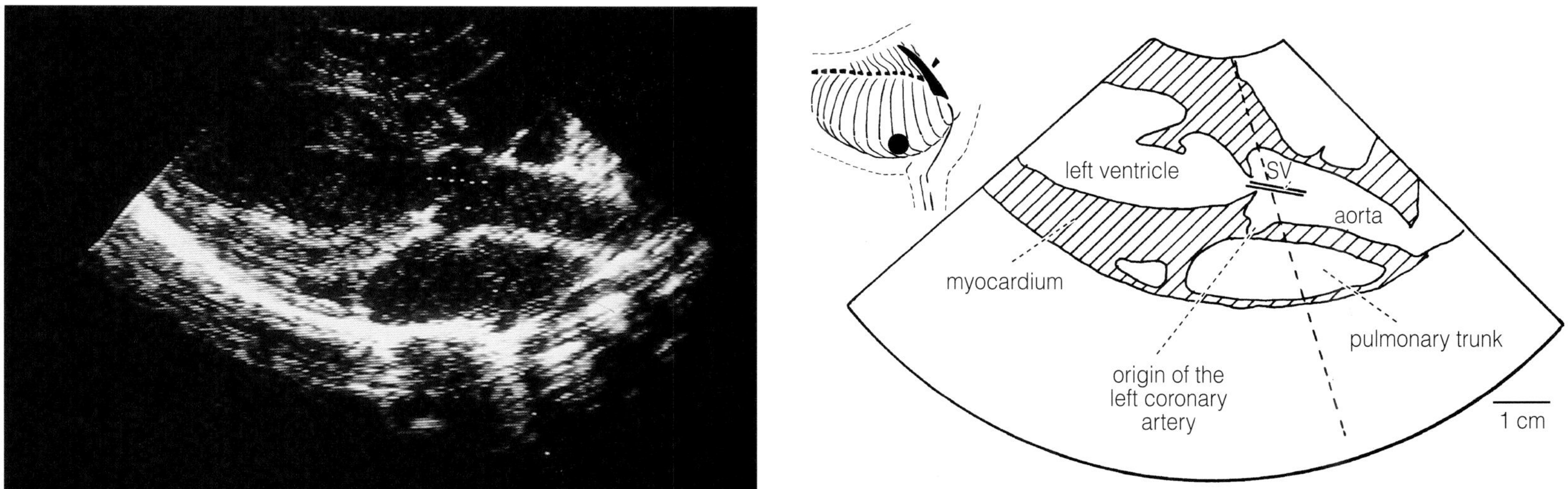

SV = sample volume

301

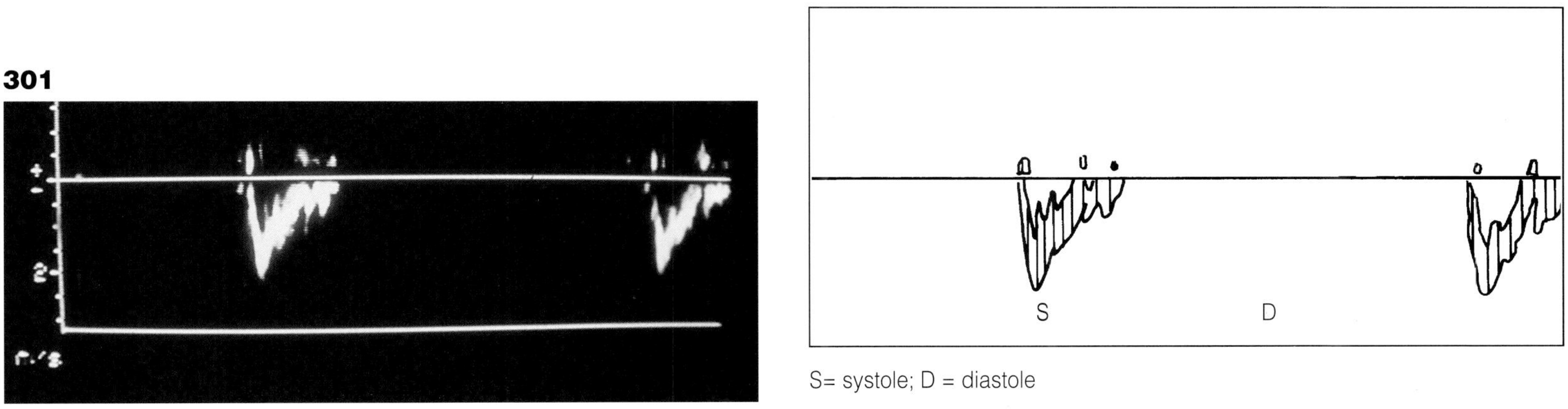

S= systole; D = diastole

300, 301 Two-dimensional echocardiograms – dog. Left ventricular outflow tract with the angle-corrected sample volume placed at the aortic valve level for PW-Doppler (**300**). PW Doppler echocardiogram at the aortic valve level with the characteristic triangular flow profile below the x-axis (**301**).

302

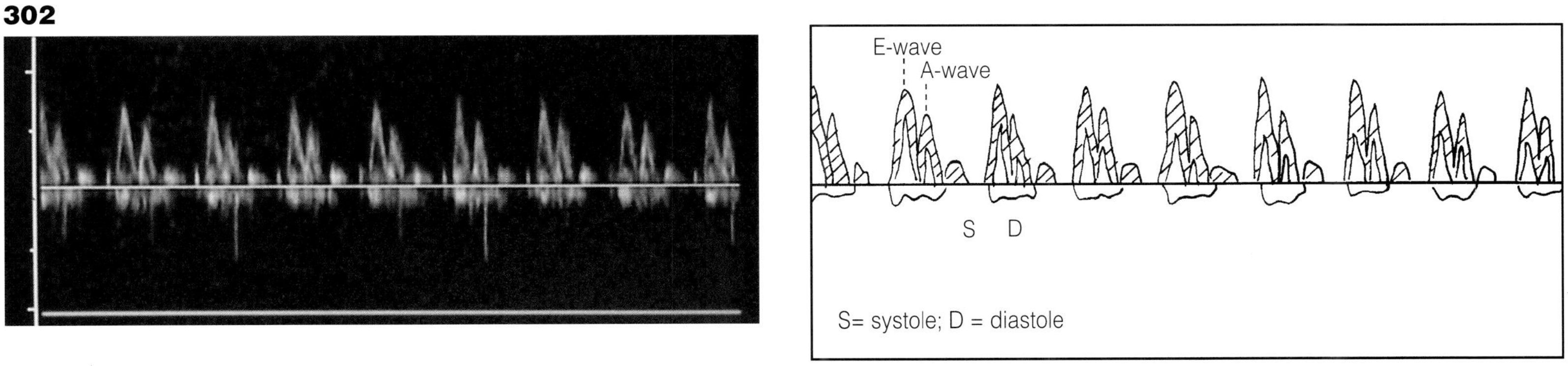

302 PW Doppler echocardiogram – cat. Left ventricular inflow tract at the mitral valve level or slightly towards the atrium with the typical Doppler signal above the x-axis.

ignored. Back pressure is calculated from fluid velocity and density.

$$Pb = \frac{1}{2} \rho \times v$$

[Pb: back pressure; ρ: density; v: blood flow velocity]

Following the modified Bernoulli equation, this becomes:

$$P + Pb = \text{constant} \quad \text{or} \quad P_1 + P_2 = P_2 + Pb_2$$

$$P_1 + \frac{1}{2}\rho v_1^2 = P_2 + \frac{1}{2}\rho v_2^2$$

[P_1: hydrostatic pressure proximal to the obstruction; ρ: blood density proximal and distal to the obstruction; v_1: velocity proximal to the obstruction; P_2: hydrostatic pressure distal to the obstruction; v_2: velocity distal to the obstruction]

$$P_1 - P_2 = \Delta P = \frac{1}{2}\rho v_2^2 - \frac{1}{2}\rho v_1^2$$

$$\Delta P = \frac{1}{2}\rho (v_2^2 - v_1^2)$$

By substituting a value for blood density and converting the hydrostatic pressure to mmHg, $\frac{1}{2} \times \rho$ equals 4.

$$\Delta P = 4 (v_2^2 - v_1^2)$$

[ΔP: pressure gradient $P_1 - P_2$ in mmHg; v_2: velocity distal to the obstruction in m/s; v_1: velocity proximal to the obstruction in m/s]

In the normal heart the velocity v_1 (proximal to the obstruction) is usually much less than 1 m/s, while the postobstructive velocity v_2 is always much more. For this reason, v_1 can be dropped from the equation.

303

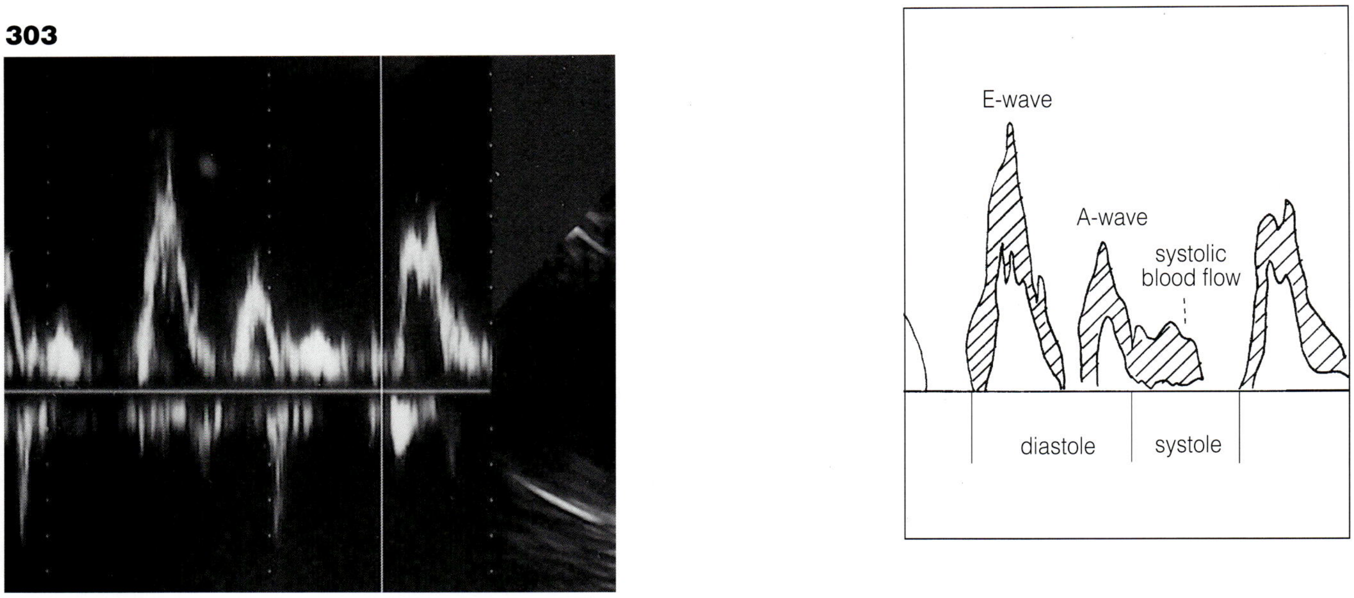

303 PW Doppler echocardiogram – dog. Left ventricular inflow at the mitral valve level. The early-diastolic E-wave normally has a higher peak and longer duration than the following A-wave after atrial contractions. Maximal early-diastolic velocities, immediately after valvular opening, are measured at the E-point. The A-point represents maximal inflow velocities after atrial systole.

304

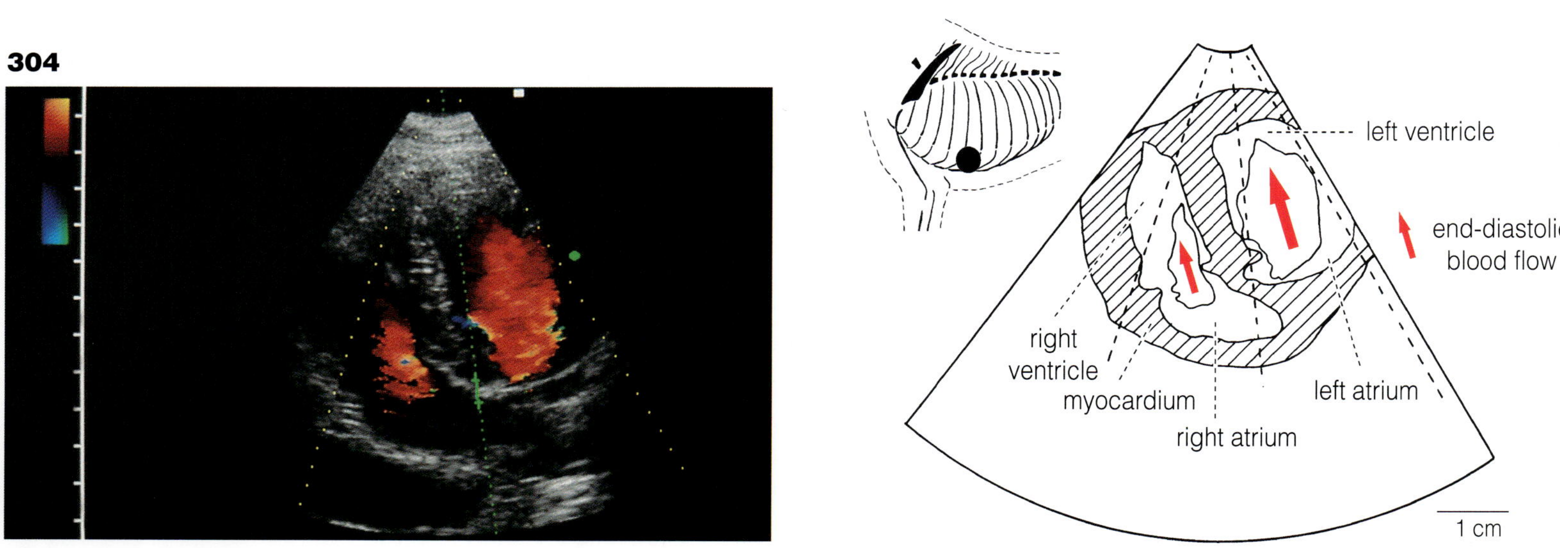

304 Colour-flow Doppler echocardiogram – dog. End-diastolic filling at the AV valves in a four-chamber view. Blood flowing towards the transducer is coded in red.

This results in the simplified but exact 'modified' Bernoulli equation used in clinical diagnostics:

$$\Delta P = 4\, v_2^{2}$$

[DP: pressure gradient $P_1 - P_2$ in mmHg; v_2: velocity distal to the obstruction in m/s]

The modified Bernoulli equation applies only to mild and moderate, small obstructions. Severe, large obstructions produce viscous friction with relatively low poststenotic velocities. In these cases the pressure gradient is underestimated, because the Bernoulli equation does not consider the energy loss caused by friction.

The more obstructed an area, the higher the pressure gradient becomes. In human medicine, pressure gradients over 50 mmHg with aortic stenosis are considered critical. Gradients between 30 and 50 mmHg require further diagnostics. If possible, the aortic opening area should also be examined. Valvular pulmonic stenosis in humans is categorized with gradients between 20 and 30 mmHg as mild, between 30 and 80 mmHg as moderate, and greater than 80 mmHg as severe[7, 13]. Similar values for dogs and cats do not exist and results should be analyzed carefully. The stenosis should be categorized by secondary abnormalities:

- Aortic stenosis: secondary left ventricular hypertrophy or dilatation; secondary mitral insufficiency with or without left atrial enlargement.
- Pulmonic stenosis: secondary right ventricular hypertrophy with abnormal septal movement to the right or dilation; secondary tricuspid insufficiency with or without right atrial enlargement; and hepatic vein congestion.

Colour-flow Doppler imaging identifies turbulences and cardiac abnormalities more rapidly than other Doppler modes (*Table 19*). Laminar blood flow towards the transducer is red; flow away from the transducer is blue (**304**, see Doppler Effect, page 24; Colour-Flow Doppler, page 48). As blood flows at lower velocities, the colours become darker. High flow velocities, seen, for example, with regurgitation, lead to aliasing and a colour shift (see Aliasing and Nyquist Limit, page 48). Turbulences appear in yellow or green colours (see Laminar and Turbulent Flows, page 64).

305

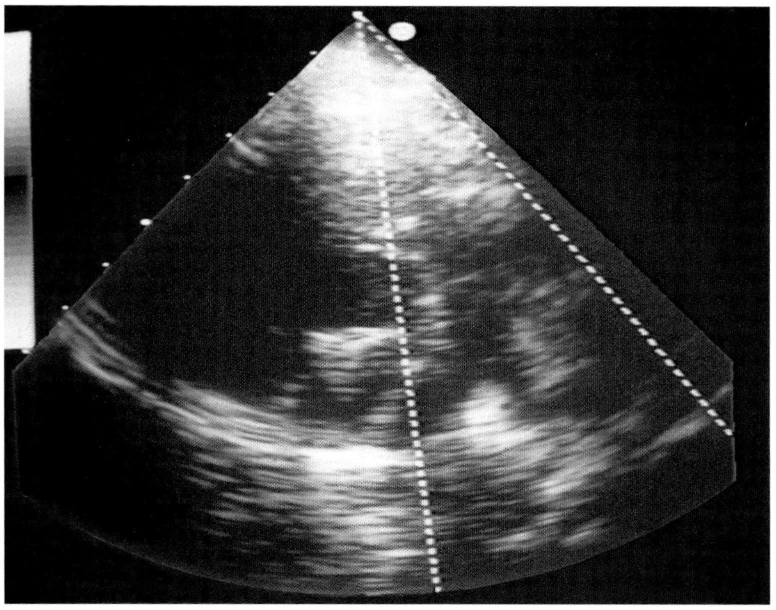

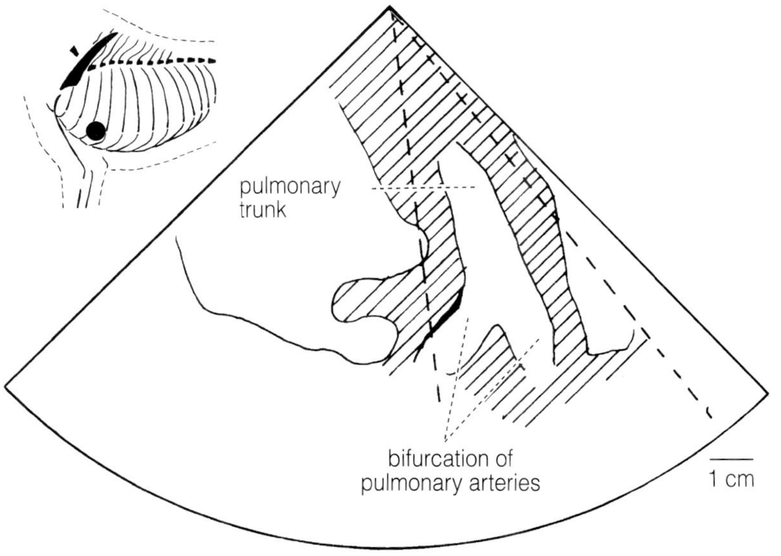

305 Two-dimensional echocardiogram – dog. Normal pulmonary trunk and pulmonary arteries.

Flow Velocities in Doppler Echocardiography

The ideal transducer positions for Doppler examinations are located on the left thoracic wall (see **296–299**). (*Table 20* gives the clinical indications for Doppler examinations.) The mitral, tricuspid and aortic valve areas are displayed in four- or five-chamber views. Blood flow is nearly parallel to the sound beam in these views. The pulmonary valve, including the pulmonary trunk and bifurcating pulmonary arteries, should be scanned from the left third intercostal space. In this plane the aorta and left atrium are in a short-axis.

PW Doppler is able to evaluate relatively low flow velocities in the normal heart. The Doppler signal across the mitral valve resembles its M-mode image of the septal leaflet. The double-peaked, M-shaped signal consists of the E-wave, followed by a smaller A-wave. The E-wave has a higher peak and corresponds to early diastolic blood flow at the beginning of diastole, immediately following valvular opening. The late diastolic A-wave represents atrial contraction. The distance between the E-wave and the A-wave depends on the heart rate. A rapid heart rate causes the two peaks to move closer together. The E- and A-waves cannot be differentiated with tachycardia. Bradycardia produces a mid-diastolic L-wave between the E- and the A-wave. Blood flow is towards the transducer and is therefore displayed above the baseline (**296**). Flow profiles across the tricuspid valve are similar to those across the mitral valve. E- and A-peaks, i.e. maximal early and end-diastolic velocities, are usually somewhat lower than those of the mitral valve (**298**). The height of the peaks of both the mitral and tricuspid valves are influenced by respiratory action. The E-waves appear higher during inspiration.

Table 19 Blood flow displayed in colour-coded Doppler echocardiography.

Colour	Flow direction	Flow velocity	Types of flow
Red colour	Towards the transducer		Laminar flow
Blue colour	Away from the transducer		Laminar flow
Dark colour		Low flow velocity	
Bright colour		High flow velocity	
Colour shift		Very high velocities with aliasing	
Yellow or green colour		Turbulences	

Table 20 Clinical indications for Doppler echocardiography.

Heart disease	Preferred method
Congenital or aquired AV and semilunar valvular insufficiencies	PW Doppler CW Doppler
Congenital or aquired AV and semilunar valvular stenoses	PW Doppler CW Doppler
Evaluation of haemodynamic effects with cardiomyopathies	PW Doppler CW Doppler
Congenital heart abnormalities: (a) atrial and ventricular septal defects (ASD, VSD) (b) patent ductus arteriosus (PDA) (c) aorto-pulmonary shunt (APS) (d) tri-, tetralogy, e.g. tetralogy of Fallot	Colour-flow Doppler
Treatment re-examinations	PW Doppler CW Doppler Colour-flow Doppler

Doppler profiles across the aortic and pulmonary valve are directed away from the transducer and displayed below the baseline. The spectrum resembles an asymmetric, triangular peak with maximal early systolic velocities (**297, 299**). High velocities are registered during inspiration and with low heart rates. These are caused by prolonged diastolic phases and higher right ventricular output. Normal flow velocities in the dog are listed in *Table 21*.

Table 21 Normal flow velocities in the dog (modified from Kirberger *et al.*, 1992[17] and Madron, 1991[24]).

Valve	Velocity in m/s Kirberger *et al.*	Madron
Mitral		
E-wave	0.59–1.18	0.75–1.00
A-wave	0.33–0.93	0.5–0.75
Tricuspid		
E-wave	0.49–1.13	0.80
A-wave	0.32–0.94	0.60
Aortic	1.06–2.29	1.20–1.70
Pulmonary	0.88–1.61	1.05–1.30

Aorto-pulmonary shunts have larger connecting defects near the vessel valves and show the same clinical signs as a PDA. These shunts are more difficult to correct than PDA and require open-heart surgery because of their location within the pericardium. Regurgitating blood from the aorta into the main pulmonary artery causes turbulence, which is seen near the valves. To differentiate aorto-pulmonary shunts from PDA, the direct connection between the aorta and the main pulmonary artery should be found using colour-flow Doppler. This can prove difficult, even with large shunts. The aorta should be examined carefully in all planes (long-axis, short-axis) from the left and right thorax. The length and size of the open communication is usually underestimated sonographically. It is difficult to determine the actual size and volume of a shunt.

Secondary abnormalities, such as pulmonary and tricuspid insufficiencies, may be assessed using CW, PW or colour Doppler. Two-dimensional echography is valuable in determining secondary changes of the left ventricle. The left ventricle may become severely dilated and have low-normal to decreased shortening fractions. A distended fibrous annulus leads to incomplete mitral valve closure with regurgitation in Doppler echography[3, 25, 26].

Secondary abnormalities of these congenital defects are displayed radiographically as cardiomegaly and pulmonary congestion. The ECG shows higher ventricular amplitudes.

Echography of Heart Disease

Ralf Tobias

Echography is an important diagnostic tool for determining congenital and aquired heart diseases in dogs and cats. Other methods include a clinical examination, especially auscultation, electrocardiography and radiography. The following section discusses commonly occuring heart diseases and their sonographic appearance. In describing the cardiac abnormalities, some of the sonographic findings are not complete. *Tables 22–33* list the echocardiographic findings associated with each abnormality.

Congenital Defects

*Patent Ductus Arteriosus (*Ductus botalli*) and Aorto-Pulmonary Shunt (Table 22)*

With a patent ductus arteriosus (PDA), oxygen-enriched blood passes from the aorta through the open ductus arteriosus into the pulmonary trunk or the left pulmonary artery and back into the pulmonary circulation. A right-to-left shunt rarely occurs[11]. The ductus arteriosus is located outside the pericardium.

An auscultatory continuous machine-like murmur is typical for a PDA[16]. Colour Doppler shows strong turbulence with mosaic-like colours within the main pulmonary artery up to its bifurcation and, occasionally, distal to it in the left pulmonary artery. Defects in the wall of the pulmonary trunk may be detected with two-dimensional echocardiography; however, they are not conclusive, because they are parallel to the sound beam (**305**).

Table 22 Echocardiographic findings with patent ductus arteriosus (PDA) and aorto-pulmonary shunts (APS). (*Secondary abnormalities are printed in italics.*)

Echocardiographic findings	Congenital defect	Method
Turbulences in the entire main pulmonary artery	PDA	Colour Doppler
Turbulences in the main pulmonary artery near the valve	APS	Colour Doppler
Patent ductus arteriosus	PDA	Limited 2DE
Aorto-pulmonary shunt	APS	Limited 2DE Colour Doppler
Blood flow in the ductus arteriosus	PDA	Limited colour Doppler
Ventricular and atrial dilation, especially left	*PDA, APS*	*M-mode, 2DE*
Low-normal to decreased systolic shortening fractions	*PDA, APS*	*M-mode*
Increased EPSS	*PDA, APS*	*M-mode*
Pulmonary and tricuspid valve regurgitation	*PDA, APS*	*CW, PW, colour Doppler*
Systolic mitral regurgitation	*PDA, APS*	*CW, PW, colour Doppler*

306

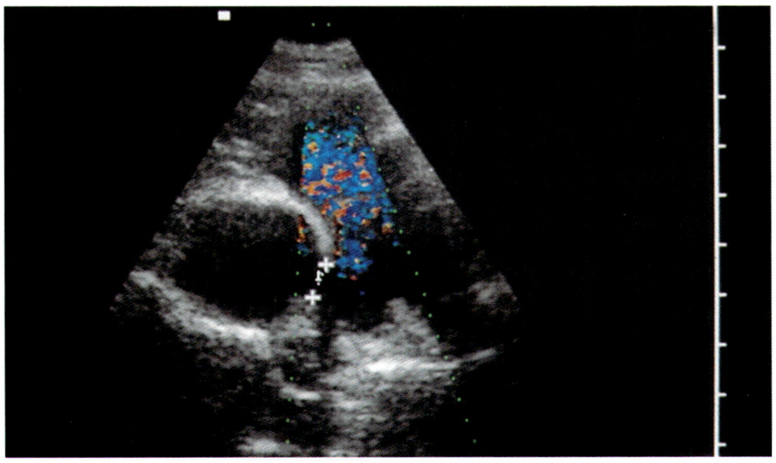

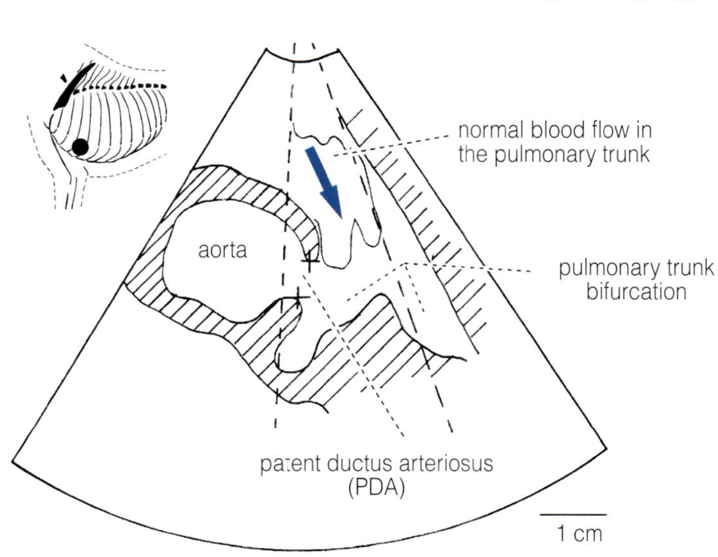

307

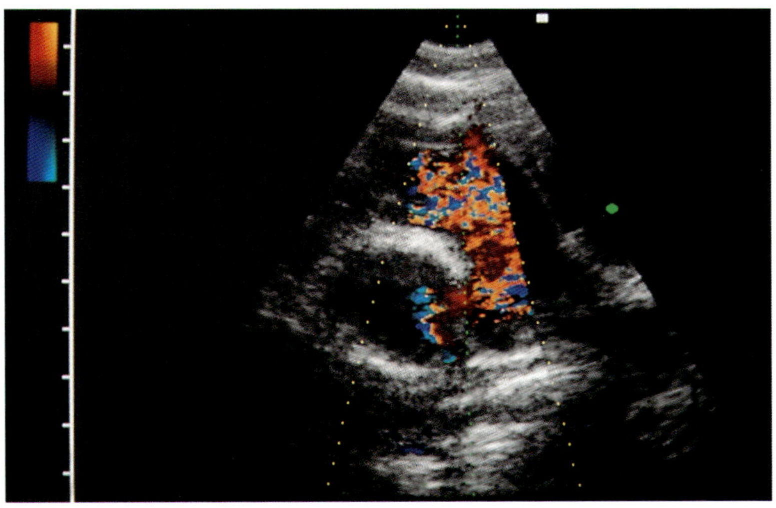

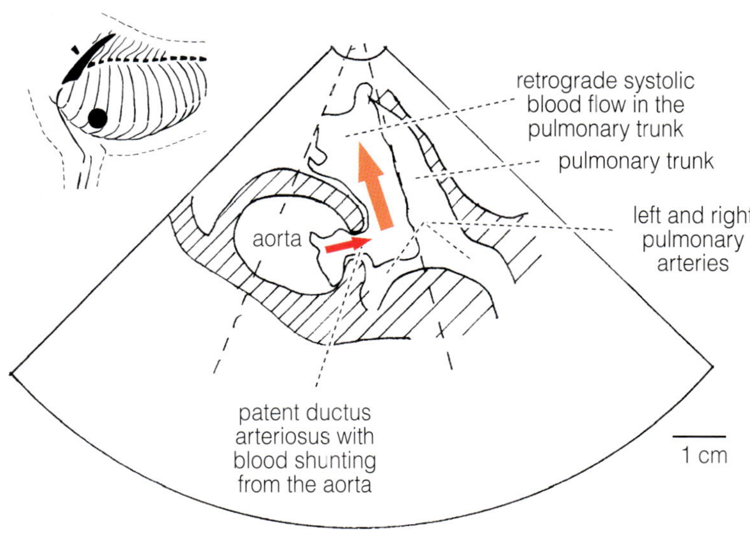

306, 307 Patent ductus arteriosus in a dog. Two-dimensional (**306**) and colour-coded (**307**) Doppler echocardiograms.

Septal Defects (Table 23)

Ventricular septal defects (VSDs) occur as isolated abnormalities or as part of the complex tetrology of Fallot. They are most commonly located in the membranous part of the interventricular septum below the aortic valve. Muscular septal defects are not as common[11].

During auscultation, holosystolic heart murmurs are heard over the left and right hemithorax. Smaller septal defects usually have louder murmurs than larger openings in the interventricular septum. Blood flow is commonly from the left ventricle to the right ventricle during systole[11, 16].

VSDs are imaged from both the left and the right thorax in parasternal long-axis and short-axis views. It is useful to examine the septum from various planes and with different transducer positions, since even large defects may be overlooked and artefacts may lead to a false interpretation. Very large VSDs are recognized as anechoic openings in the septum, using a parasternal ventricular long-axis view (**309**). Movement of the interventricular septum after loss of its membranous portion is characteristic of a VSD. In early diastole the muscular part of the septum pushes into the septal cusp of the closed aortic valve. Large defects result in volume and pressure overload, which causes enlarged, dilated ventricles and atria[3, 23, 26]. Contrast echocardiography recognizes medium-sized to large VSDs without any problems[1]. The contrast-free, anechoic blood of the left ventricle is pressed into the contrast-enriched, echogenic right ventricle during systole. This is displayed as a negative contrast jet within the right ventricle (see Contrast Agents, page 58; **106, 107**).

Blood flowing through the septal defect is called a jet and is easily displayed with colour Doppler. The turbulences are recognized as yellow or green colours (**310, 311**). Large septal defects have slower flow velocities with fewer turbulences and more uniform colours[7].

An atrial septal defect (ASD) is a rare congenital abnormality in the dog and cat. A typical heart murmur is not usually heard. Concurrent pulmonic stenosis may produce a quiet systolic heart

Table 23 Echocardiographic findings with ventricular (VSD) and atrial septal defects (ASD). (*Secondary abnormalities are printed in italics.*)

Echocardiographic findings	Congenital defect	Method
Anechoic septal dropout	Very large VSD, ASD	Limited 2DE
Shunting blood	VSD, ASD	Colour Doppler, limited contrast echocardiography
Strong turbulences around the shunt	VSD	Colour Doppler
Right ventricular hypertrophy	*VSD*	*M-mode, 2DE*
Abnormal septal motion	*VSD*	*M-mode, 2DE*
Ventricular and atrial dilation, especially right sided	*VSD, ASD*	*M-mode, 2DE*

308

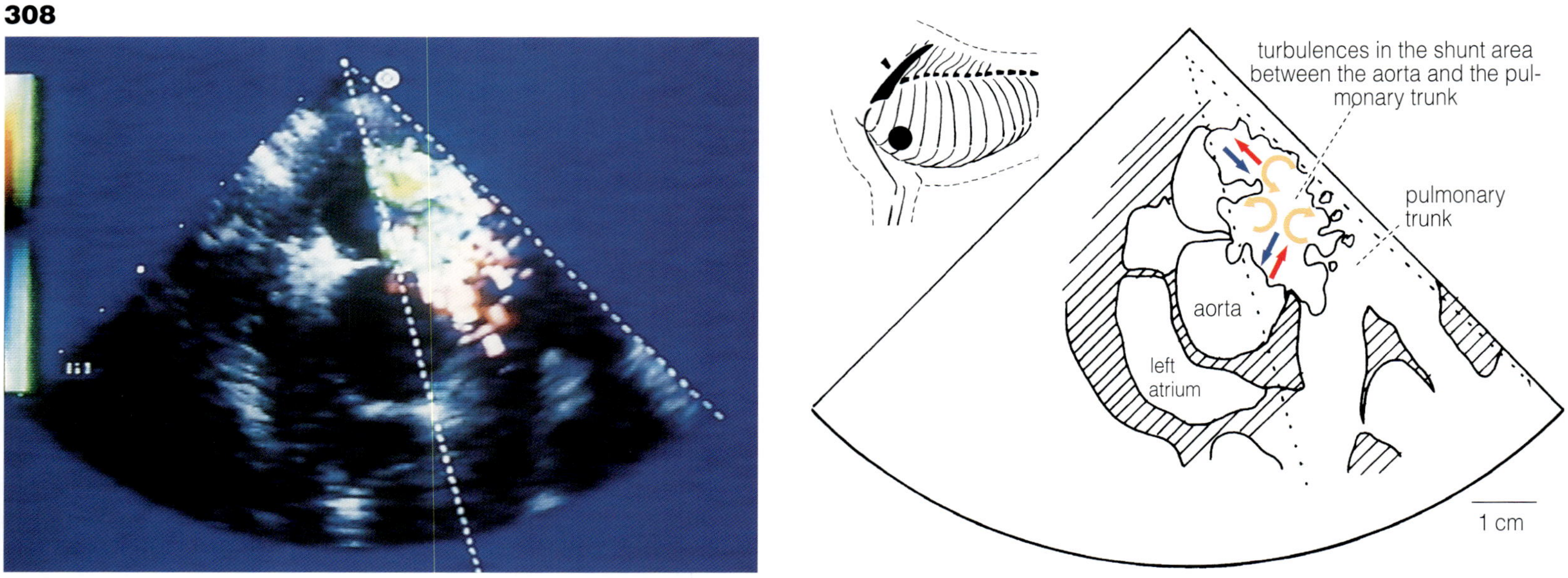

308 Colour-coded Doppler echocardiogram – dog. Aorto-pulmonary shunt with turbulences near the valves.

309

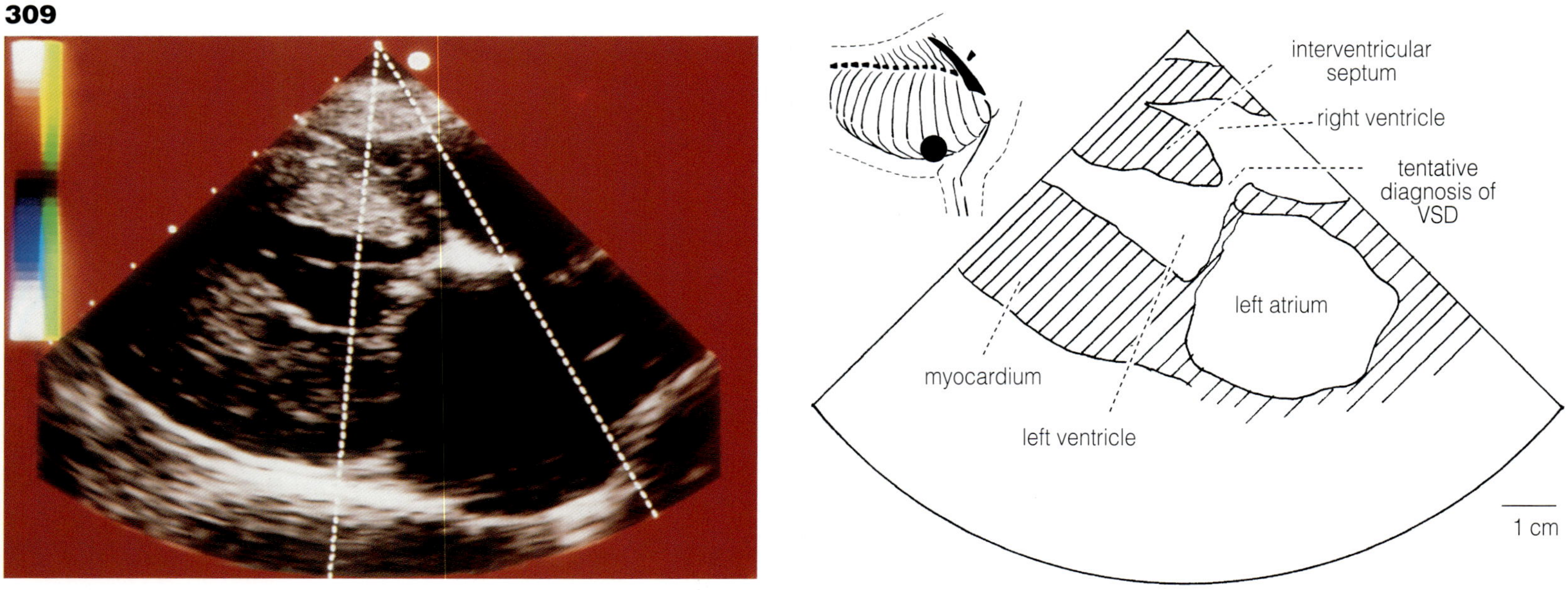

310

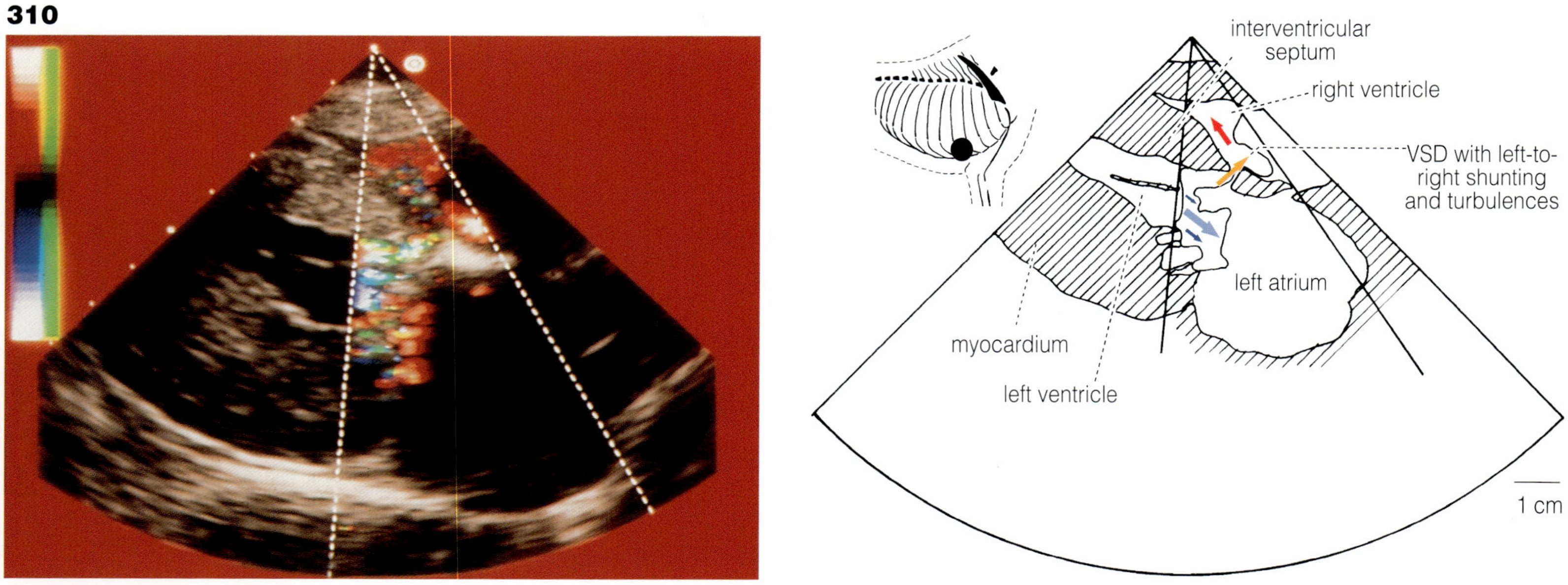

309, 310 Two-dimensional and colour Doppler echocardiograms – dog. VSD with a small anechoic area in the membranous part of the septum in a left ventricular long-axis view (**309**) and left-to-right shunt with colour Doppler (**310**).

murmur in the left third intercostal space.

Very large ASDs may be imaged echocardiographically in right and left parasternal long-axis views. Artefacts may cause septal dropout and simulate an ASD. The area of the fossa ovalis in the atrial septum is thin and produces few echoes, which may appear to be an ASD. Volume and pressure overload may cause RA and LA dilation. Colour-coded Doppler is useful in diagnosing ASDs and evaluating haemodynamic patterns (312)[18, 23, 25]. Non-apparent ASDs may be detected using transoesophageal echocardiography[19].

311

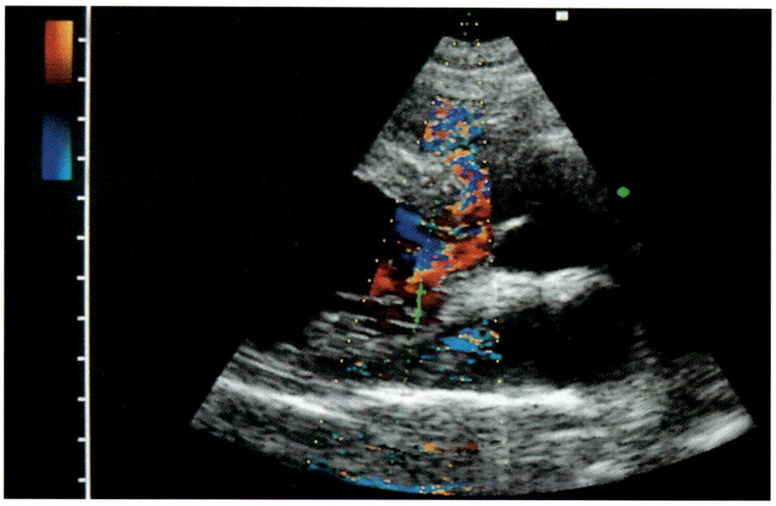

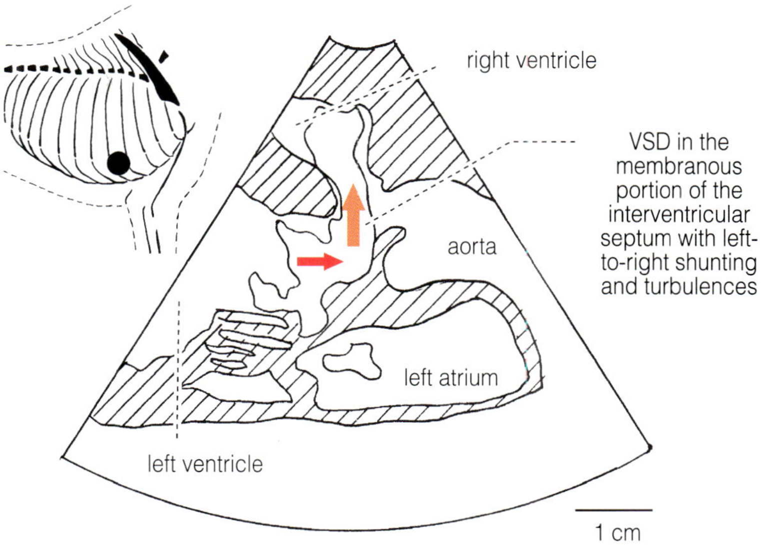

312

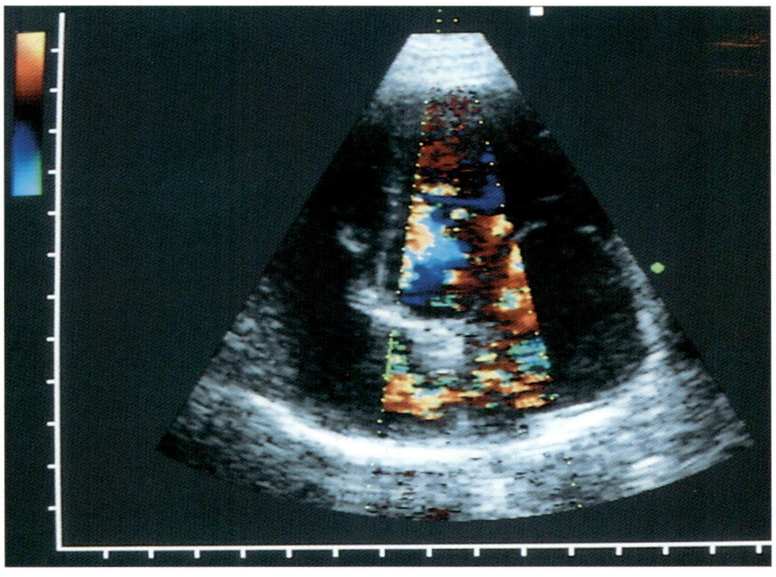

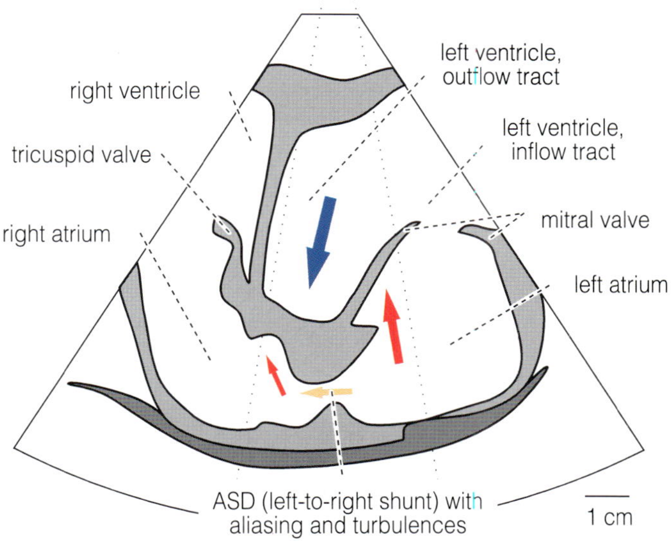

311, 312 Colour-flow Doppler echocardiogram – dog. VSD with left-to-right shunting (**311**) and ASD (**312**).

Peritoneopericardial Diaphragmatic Hernia (PPDH) (Table 24)

The most common congenital defect of the pericardium is the postembryonic persistent communication between the peritoneal and pericardial cavity[11, 12]. Radiographs show an enlarged heart silhouette and diffuse shadowing in the area connecting the thorax and the abdomen (**313**). Two-dimensional echocardiography can occasionally discern herniated abdominal organs within the pericardial sac (**314, 315**). Since the animals are usually without any clinical symptoms, PPDH may be an incidental finding.

Table 24 Echocardiographic findings with peritoneopericardial diaphragmatic hernias.

Echocardiographic findings	Method
Abdominal organs, usually liver, within the pericardial sac	2DE
Normal heart or occasional left ventricular myocardial disease and mitral valve abnormalities	M-mode, 2DE, colour Doppler, PW Doppler, CW Doppler

313

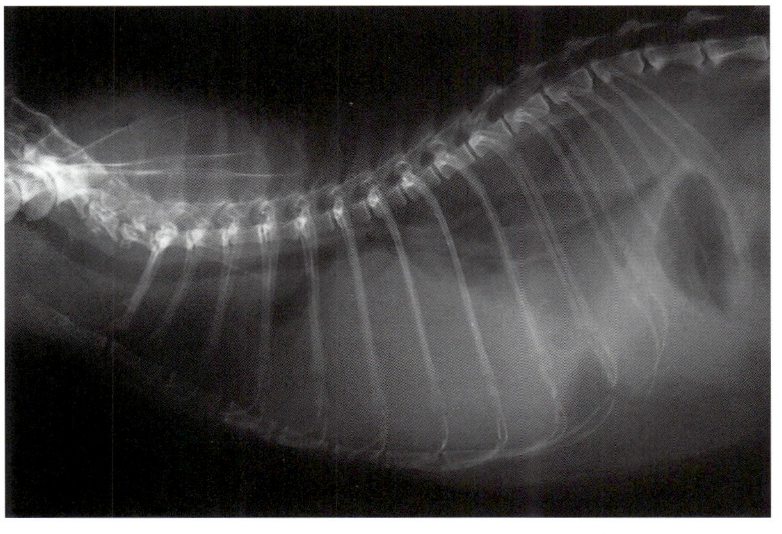

313 Lateral radiograph – cat. Cardiomegaly and diffuse shadowing between the heart silhouette and the diaphragm, indicative of a peritoneopericardial diaphragmatic hernia.

314

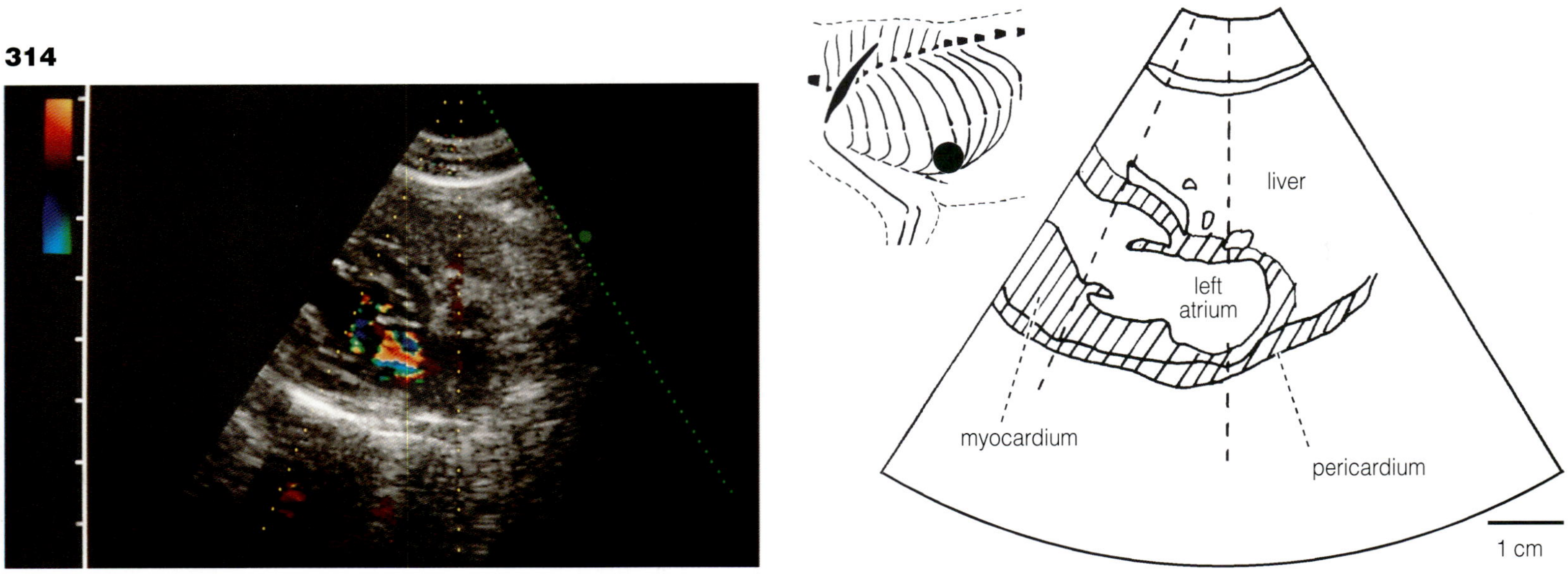

314 Colour-flow Doppler echocardiogram – cat. Portions of the liver are seen within the pericardial sac. Colour Doppler shows additional mitral insufficiency.

315

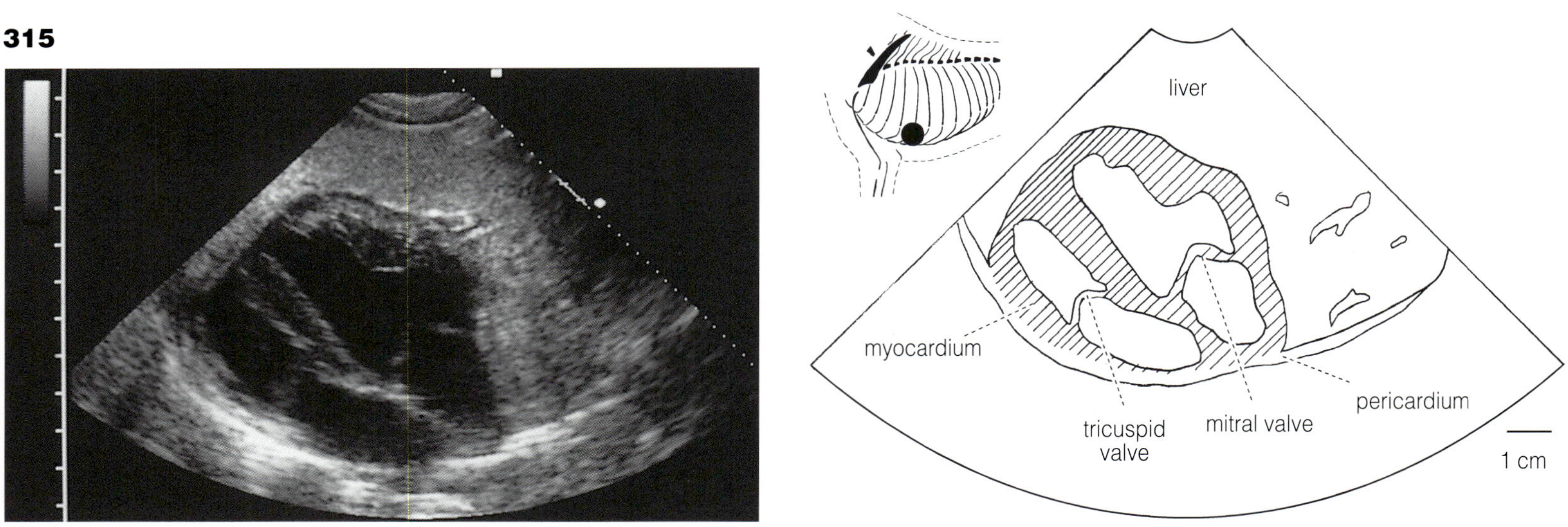

315 Two-dimensional echocardiogram – dog. The liver is seen within the pericardial sac.

Myocardium and Ventricles

While radiography of myocardial and ventricular diseases can only visualize changes in heart size, echocardiography is able to recognize the underlying heart disease. Myocardial disease includes dilated or hypertrophic cardiomyopathy, depending on morphology and heart function. Cardiomyopathies are classified as primary or secondary. Primary cardiomyopathies are idiopathic, while secondary cardiomyopathies have infectious, metabolic, traumatic, dietary, toxic or neoplastic causes[8, 14].

316

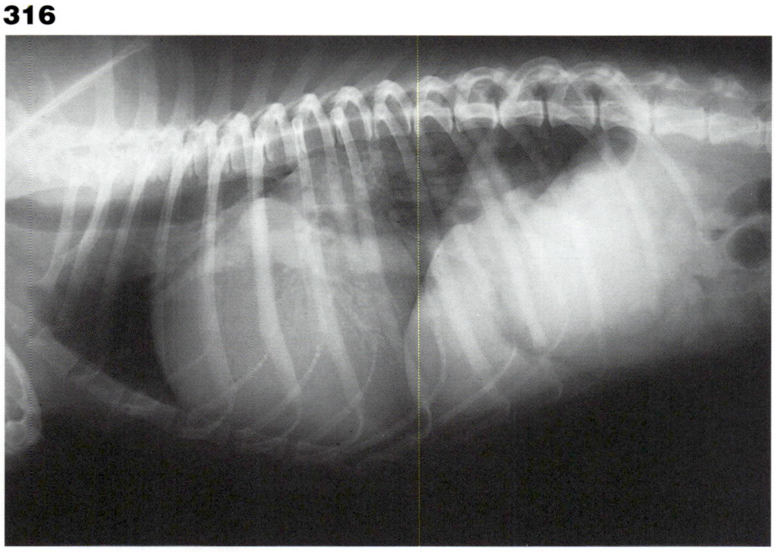

316 Lateral radiograph – dog. This dog, suffering from heart disease, shows severe cardiomegaly with a greatly enlarged left atrium. The enlarged atrium outlines the Y-shaped bifurcation of the trachea, which is usually invisible.

Two-dimensional and M-mode echocardiography is used to examine cardiomyopathies. Doppler echocardiography is used to evaluate blood flow and to document secondary insufficiencies. Scanning positions are located on either side of the thorax. The heart is evaluated in long-axis and short-axis views, as well as the four-chamber view. With the help of two-dimensional echocardiography, myocardial contractility, ventricular to atrial dimensions, and valve motion can be visualized. M-mode sonography then measures septal and wall thickness and calculates the systolic shortening fraction.

Dilated Cardiomyopathy (Table 25)

Dilated cardiomyopathy (DCM), also called congestive cardiomyopathy, is a heart disease seen occasionally in cats and more often in dogs. Feline dilated cardiomyopathy occurs in Oriental shorthaired cats. In dogs this disease affects middle-aged, large breeds.

Patients with DCM have systolic heart murmurs. ECGs record

317

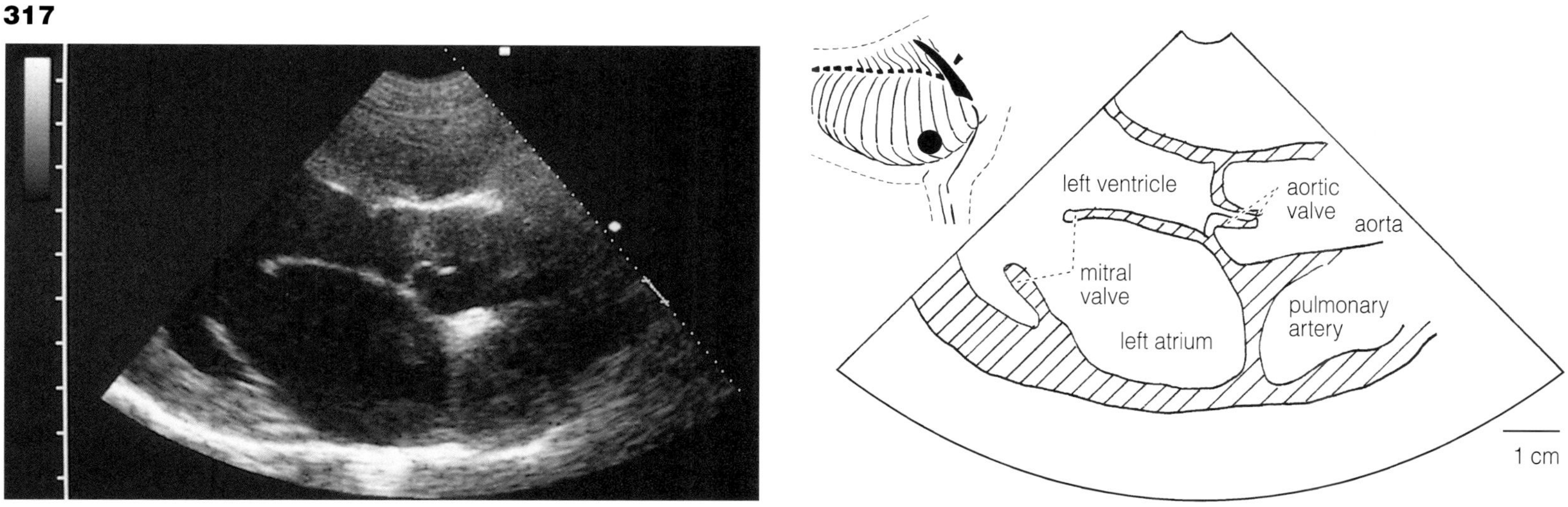

317 Two-dimensional echocardiogram – dog. Dilated cardiomyopathy with simultaneous imaging of the mitral and aortic valve.

318

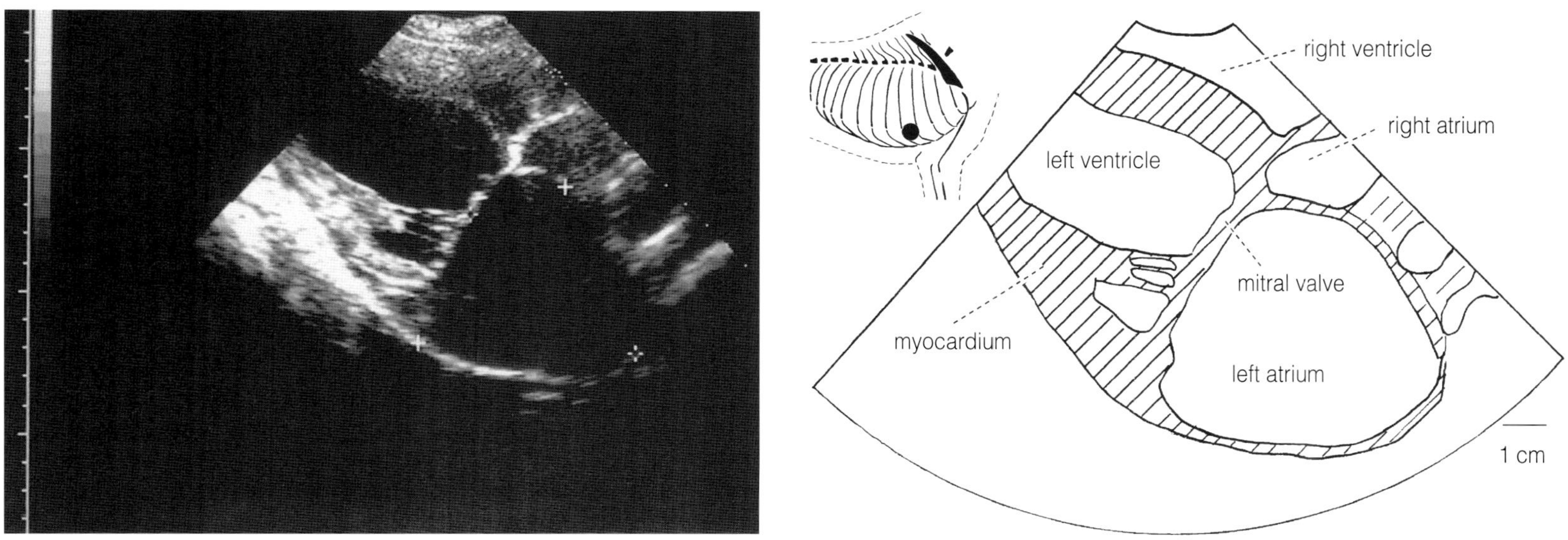

318 Two-dimensional echocardiogram – dog. Dilated cardiomyopathy with greatly decreased myocardial thickness and increased left ventricle dimensions. Mitral regurgitation causes enlargement of the left atrium.

arrhythmias, such as ventricular extrasystoles and/or atrial fibrillation. Radiography shows generalized cardiomegaly and lung congestion (**316**). AV valve insufficiency with regurgitation is caused by a distended fibrous annulus. Wall thickness is reduced and diminished myocardial contractility indicates systolic dysfunction[21].

The 2-D echocardiogram of patients with DCM shows a characteristic hypokinesis of the heart. M-mode tracings record diminished septal and ventricular wall excursions. In severe cases there is little difference between systolic and diastolic wall thickness (**319, 320**). Ventricular internal dimensions also remain unchanged. Shortening fractions are greatly decreased (**320**). Displacement of the heart base, with simultaneous imaging of the mitral and aortic valve in a parasternal left ventricular long-axis view, is characteristic of DCM (**317**). This image cannot be produced in the normal patient. Diminished MV excursions in M-mode are typical for DCM. Some dogs with DCM show increased contractility of the septum and LV wall, which is haemodynamically ineffective because of increased LV internal dimensions (**321**). End-diastolic aortic root dimensions are small, due to reduced cardiac output. Mitral regurgitation is responsible for the greatly enlarged left atria (**318–320**). In some cases, DCM is accompanied by pericardial effusion (see Pericardium, page 161).

Table 25 Echocardiographic findings with dilated cardiomyopathy (DCM). (*Secondary abnormalities are printed in italics.*)

Echocardiographic findings	Method
Simultaneous imaging of the aortic valve and mitral valve in a right parasternal left ventricular long-axis view	2DE
Round ventricles	2DE
Decreased ventricular wall thickness	2DE, M-mode
Increased ventricular internal dimensions	2DE, M-mode
LV hypokinesis (some dogs with ineffective hyperkinesis)	2DE, M-mode
Decreased systolic shortening fraction	M-mode
Increased EPSS	M-mode
Decreased aortic root dimension	*M-mode, 2DE*
Mitral regurgitation	*CW Doppler, PW Doppler, colour Doppler*
Left atrial enlargement	*M-mode, 2DE*
Pericardial effusion	*M-mode, 2DE*

319

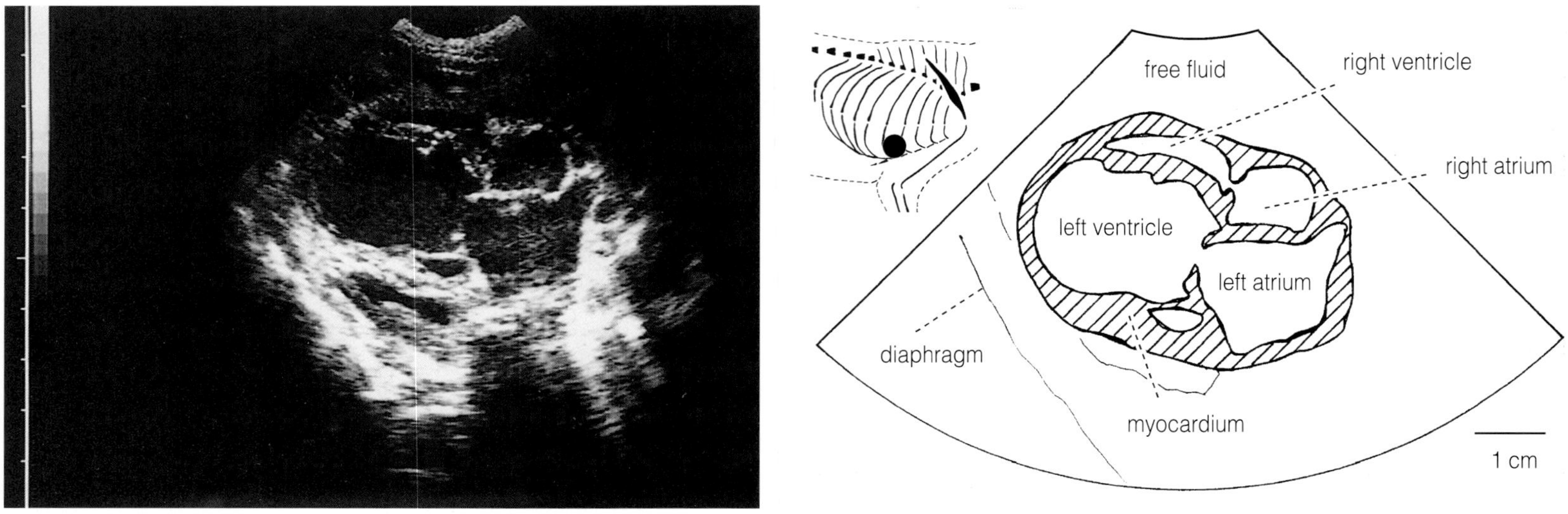

320

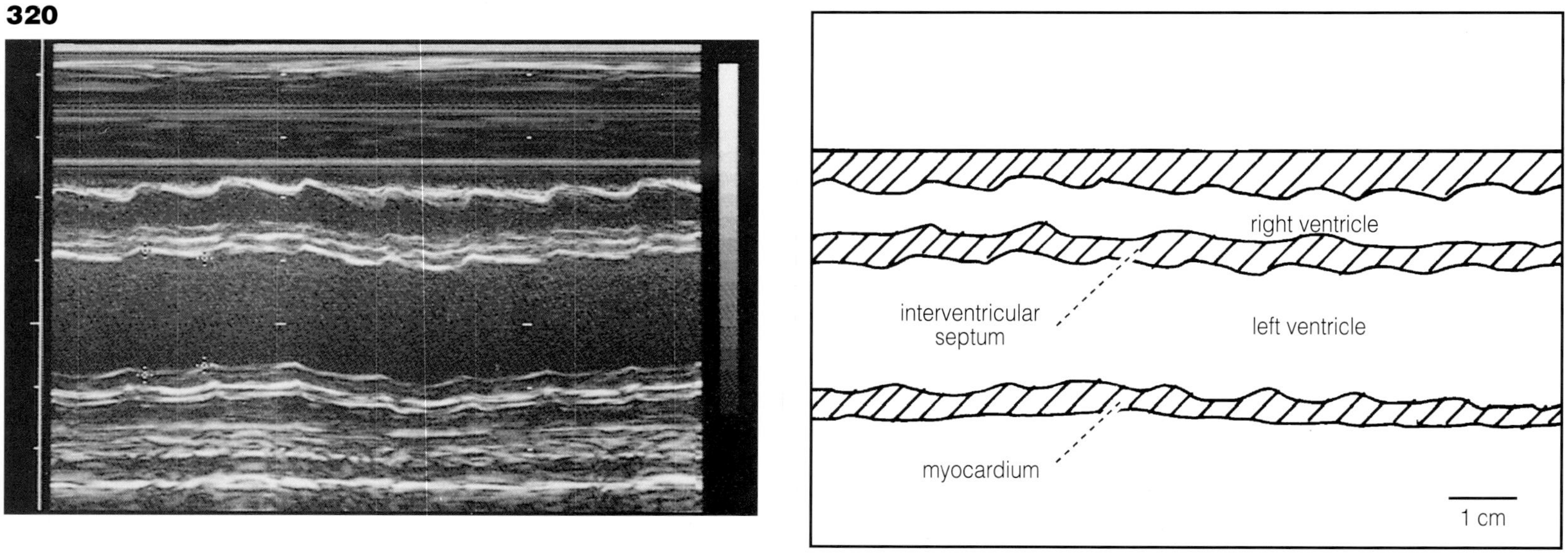

319, 320 Two-dimensional (**319**) and M-mode (**320**) echocardiograms – cat. Severe dilated cardiomyopathy with diminished contractility (FS = 13%).

321

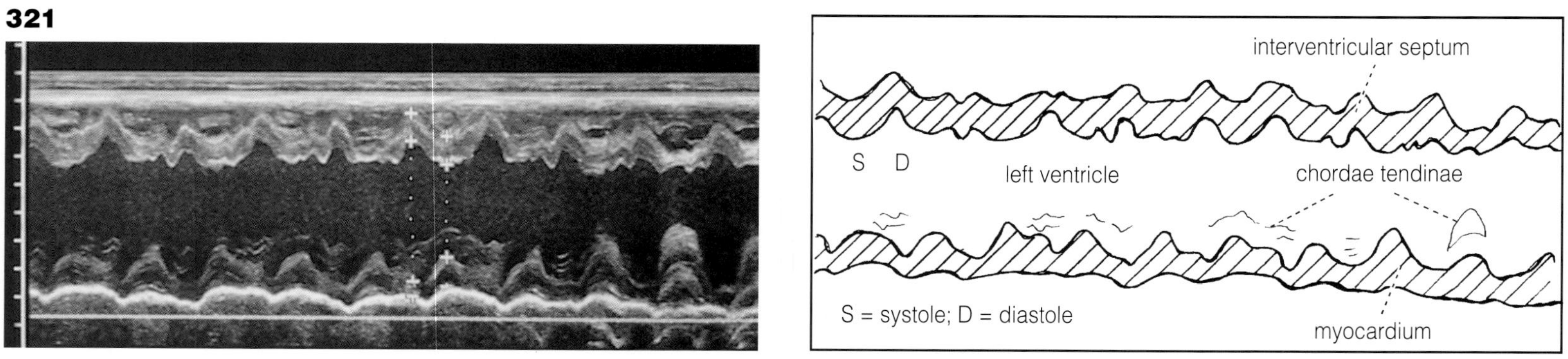

321 M-mode echocardiogram – dog. Severe ventricular dilation with haemodynamically ineffective hypercontractility and end-systolic volume overload (FS = 43%).

Hypertrophic Cardiomyopathy (Table 26)

Hypertrophic cardiomyopathy (HCM) is a common myocardial disorder in cats and is occasionally found in dogs. Hypertrophy of the ventricular walls and/or interventricular septum may be symmetric or asymmetric and is usually concentric. Ventricular hypertrophy is either idiopathic or secondary to aortic stenosis or increased sympathicotonia[14, 30]. The LV outflow tract becomes obstructed when the septum is hypertrophied near the heart base.

Radiography shows moderate cardiomegaly with left atrial enlargement (322).

One- and two-dimensional echocardiography displays septal and LV wall thickening with a greatly reduced ventricular lumen (323, 324, 328). The heart chambers become larger with secondary dilation. Myocardial contractility is normal or increased. Mitral regurgitation can be evaluated using CW, PW or colour Doppler. The left atrium is usually enlarged with moderate to severe regurgitation. Some dogs with HCM show signs of endocardial fibrosis. This is recognized in the echocardiogram by increased echogenicity of the endocardium.

Table 26 Echocardiographic findings with hypertrophic cardiomyopathy (HCM). (*Secondary abnormalities are printed in italics.*)

Echocardiographic findings	Method
Symmetric or asymmetric septal and/ or LV hypertrophy	2DE, M-mode
Reduced internal ventricular dimensions	2DE, M-mode
Normo- or hyperkinesis of the LV (hypokinesis with secondary dilation)	2DE, M-mode
Normal to increased shortening fraction (decreased FS with dilation)	M-mode
Decreased EPSS	M-mode
Left atrial enlargement	*M-mode, 2DE*
Thromboembolism	*2DE, colour Doppler*
Mitral regurgitation (less than with dilation)	*CW Doppler, PW Doppler, colour Doppler*
Pericardial effusion	*M-mode, 2 DE*

322

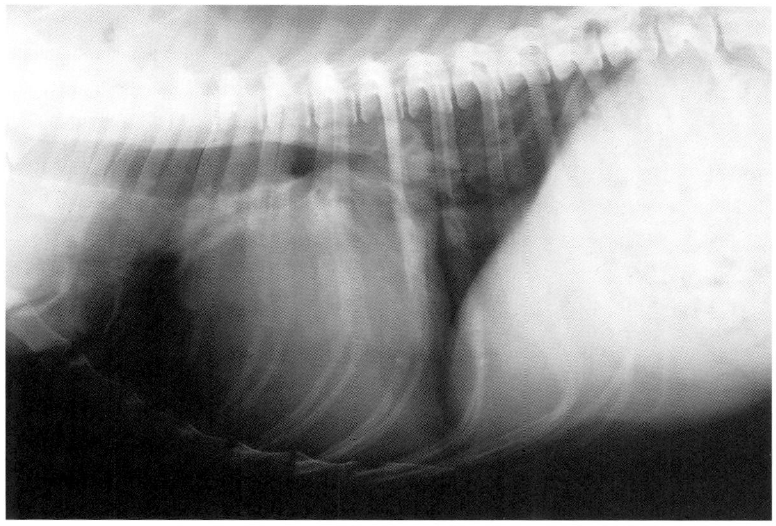

322 Lateral radiograph – dog. Hypertrophic cardiomyopathy with moderate cardiomegaly and left atrial dilation.

323

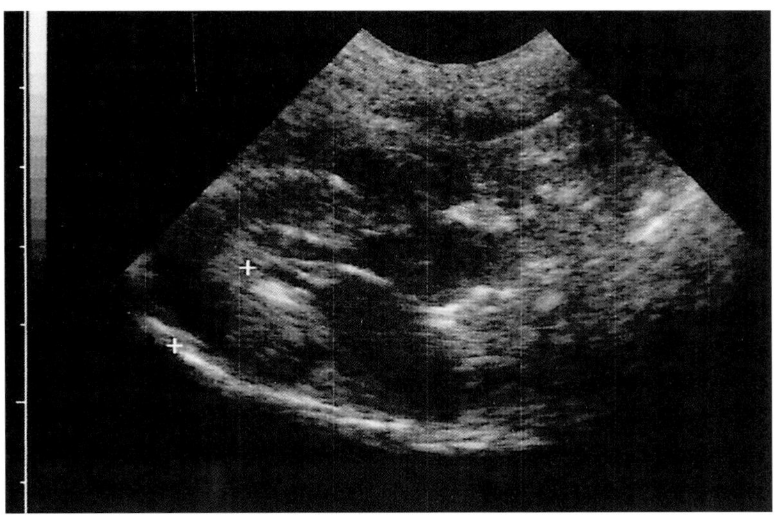

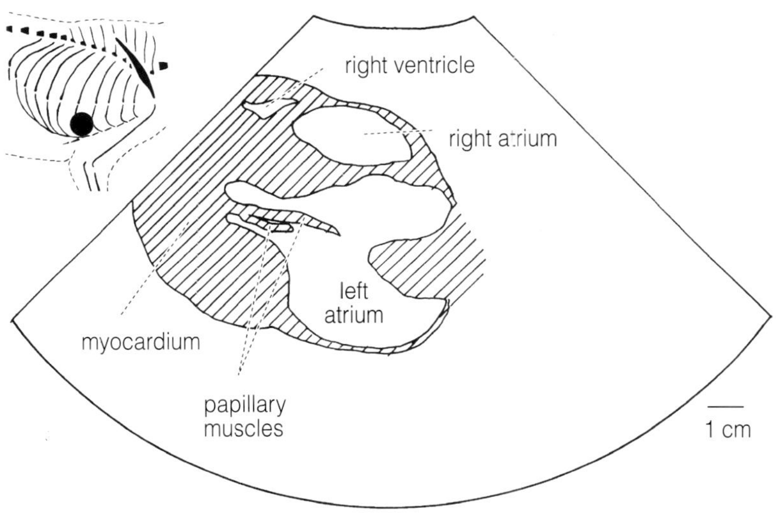

324

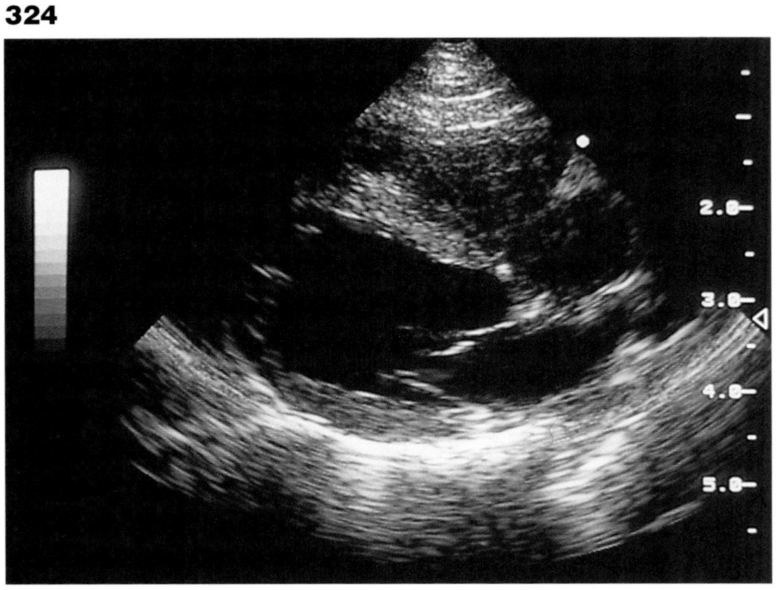

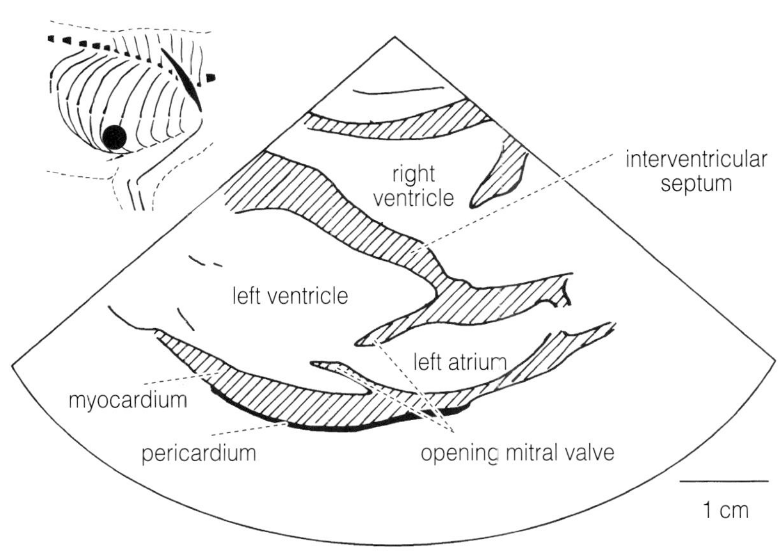

323, 324 Two-dimensional echocardiograms – cat. Hypertrophic cardiomyopathy with thickening of the myocardium, papillary muscles and chordae tendinae. The left atrium shows secondary enlargement, caused by reduced left ventricular load (**323**). A normal heart for comparison (**324**).

325

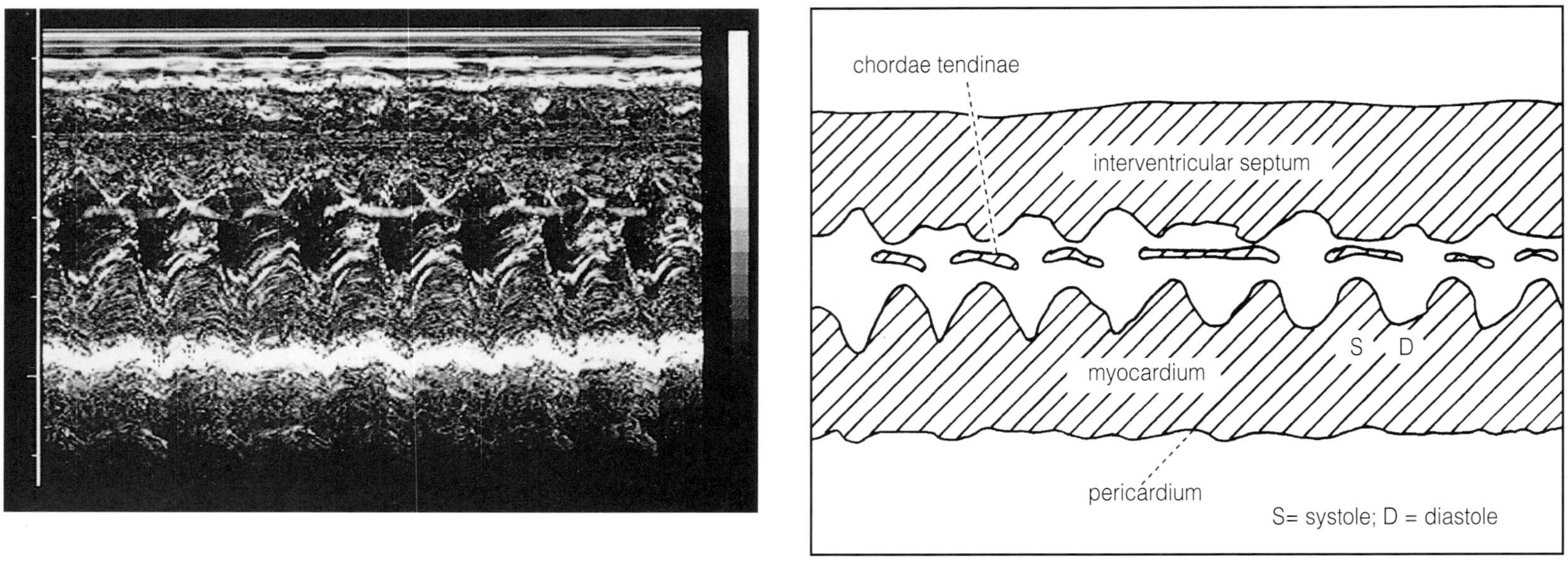

325 M-mode echocardiogram – cat. Hypertrophic cardiomyopathy with hypertrophic septum and ventricular wall and reduced left ventricle lumen. The thickened chordae tendinae are seen as hyperechoic lines within the ventricle.

326

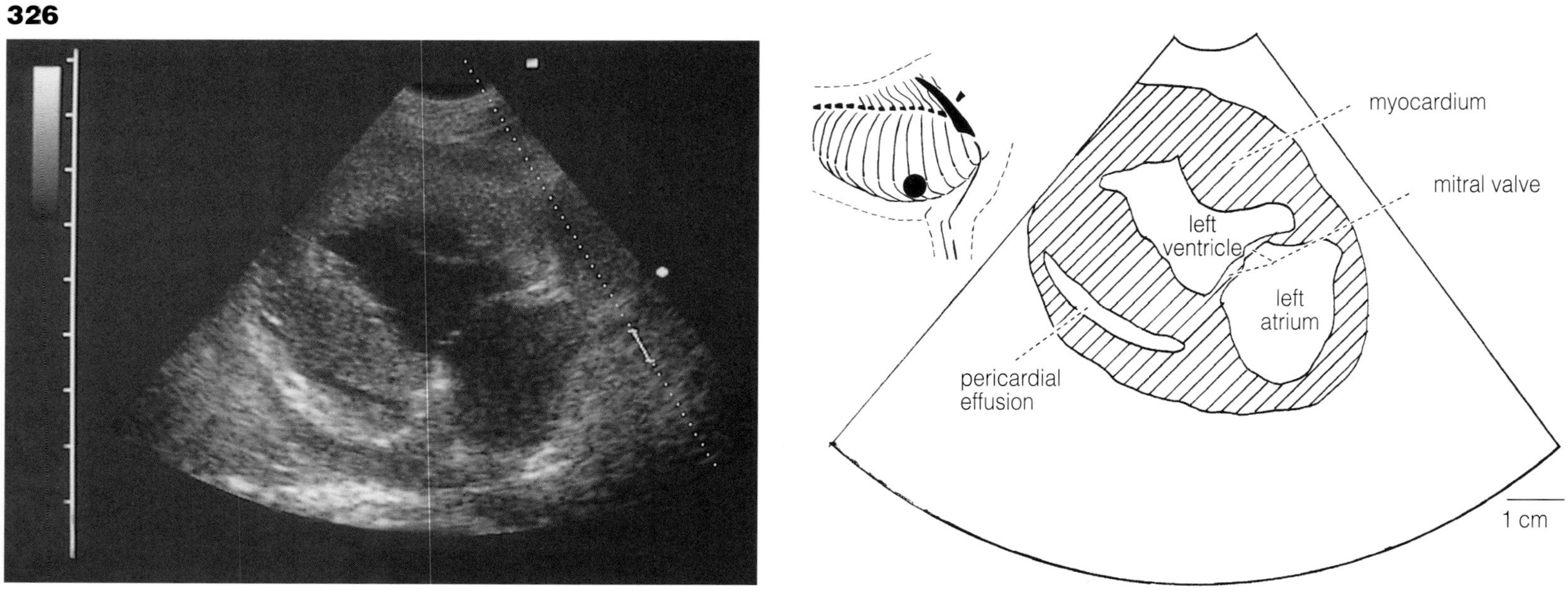

327

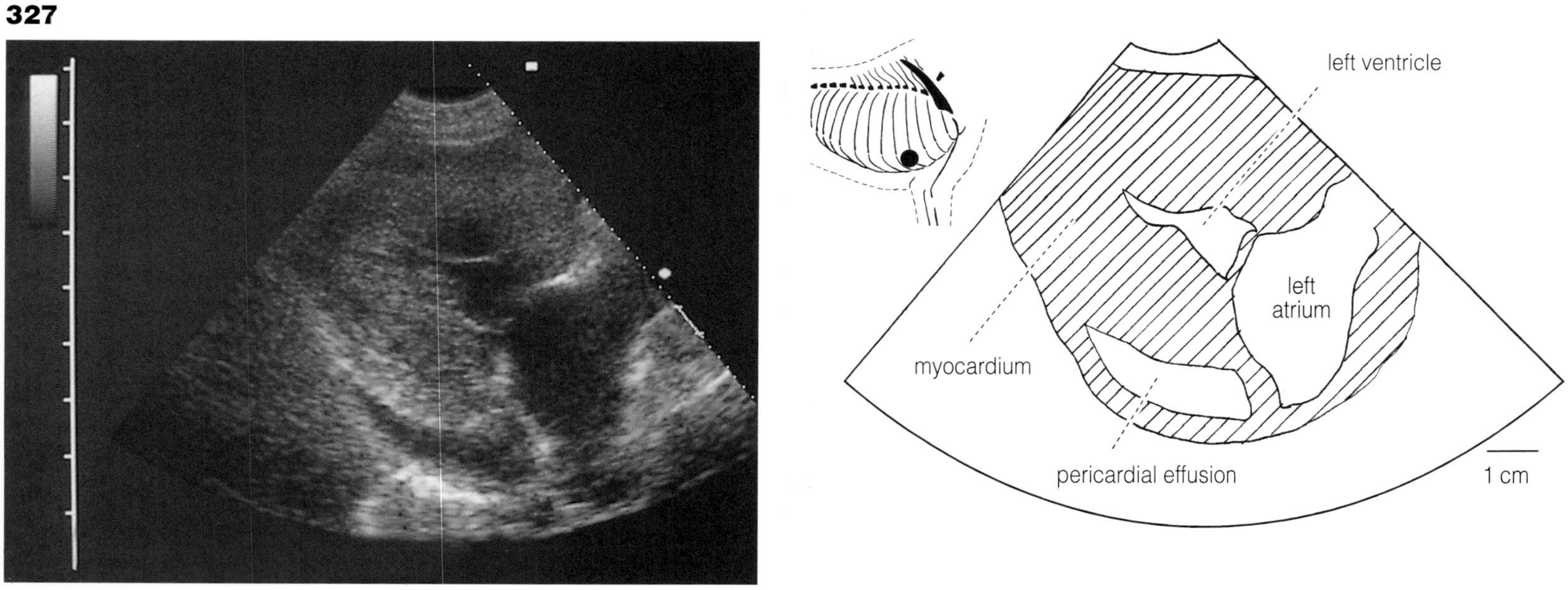

326, 327 Two-dimensional echocardiograms – dog. Hypertrophic cardiomyopathy with thickened septum and ventricular wall during diastole (**326**) and systole (**327**). Ventricular internal dimensions are almost unchanged in diastole (**326**). Mild pericardial effusion can be noticed (**326, 327**).

328

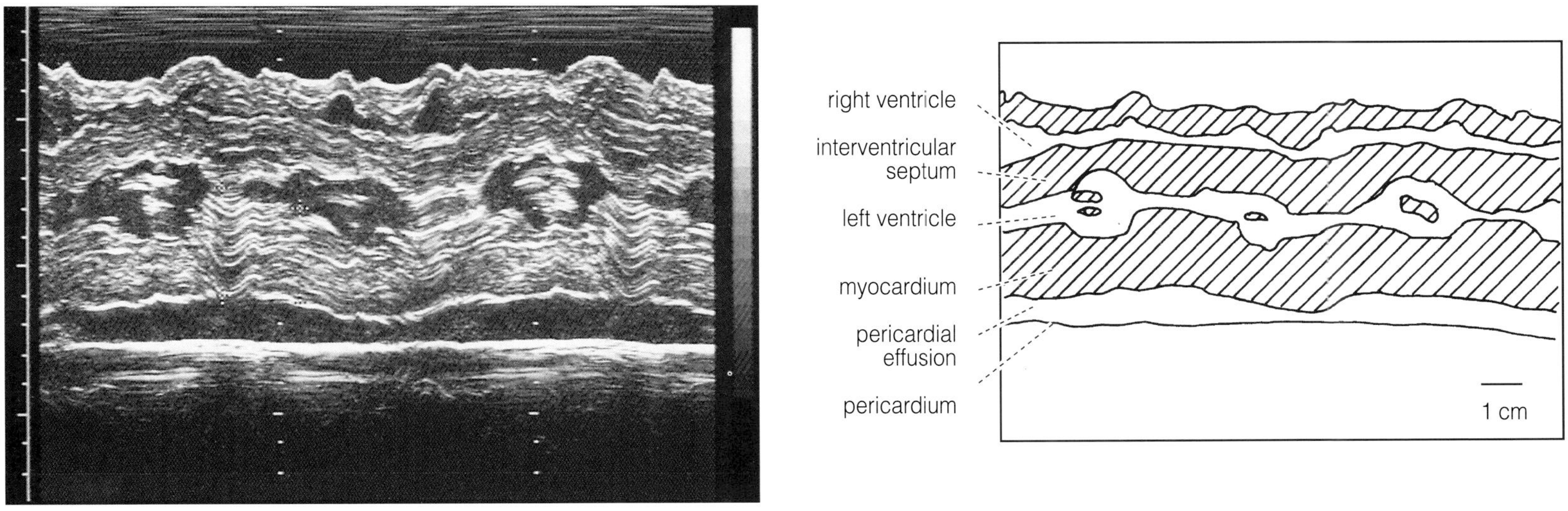

328 M-mode echocardiogram – dog. Hypertrophic cardiomyopathy with pericardial effusion indicating congestive heart failure.

329

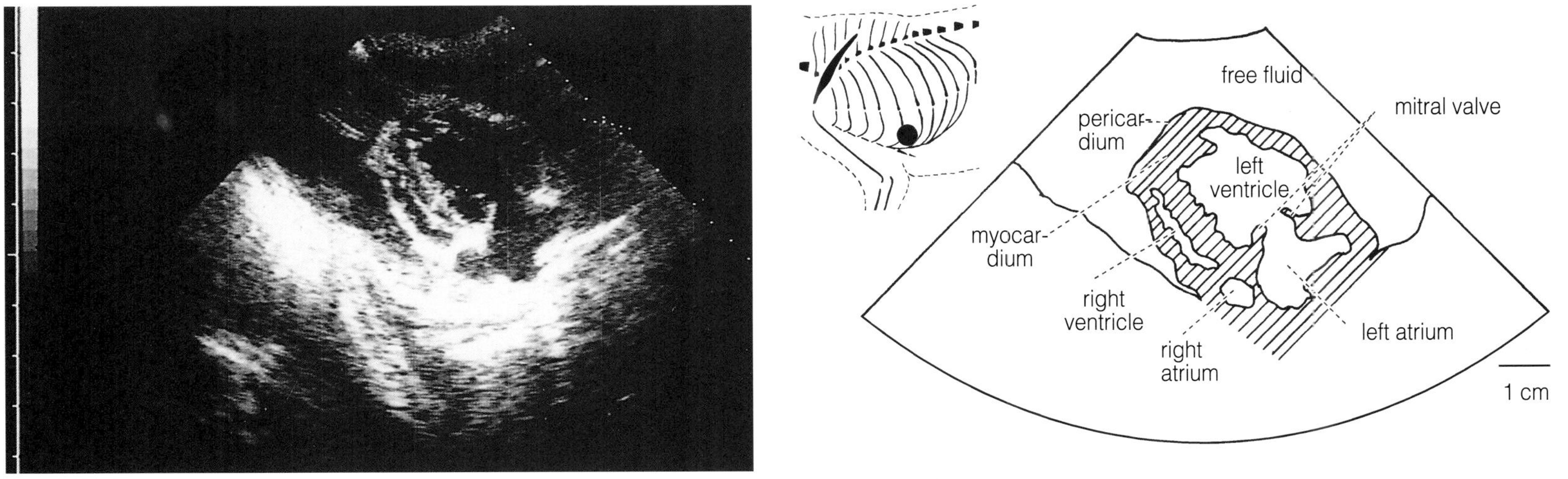

329 Two-dimensional echocardiogram – cat. Endocarditis with pyothorax showing irregular endocardial echoes.

Endocarditis (Table 27)

Infective endocarditis is usually caused by bacteraemia from other organs. Endocarditis affects the AV and semilunar valves, as well as the mural endocardium[15, 16]. The myocardium, epicardium or pericardium are rarely involved, but cases have been reported[6]. The cause of endocarditis is unknown.

In one- and two-dimensional echocardiography, endocarditis is visualized as shaggy, fibrinous, hyperechoic deposits on the endocardium (**329–331**). These vegetations lead to valvular insufficiencies with typical echographic features. Echocardiography cannot determine the duration of the infection. Acute myocarditis does not have a characteristic echographic image. Secondary echocardiographic lesions, such as decreased contractility and AV insufficiencies, seen in conjunction with history and other clinical examinations (ECG and blood profiles), allow a tentative diagnosis. Infection causes myocardial scars, which are seen as hyperechoic lesions in the one- and two-dimensional echocardiogram.

Table 27 Echocardiographic findings with endomyocarditis and myocarditis. (*Secondary abnormalities are printed in italics.*)

Echocardiographic findings	Disease	Method
Shaggy, fibrinous, hyperechoic vegetations on the valves, occasionally on the ventricular endocardium	Endocarditis	2DE, M-mode
Hyperechoic myocardial scars	Myocarditis	2DE, M-mode
Contractility changes, usually hypokinesis	*Myocarditis*	*M-mode, 2DE*
Arrhythmias	*Myocarditis*	*M-mode, 2DE*
AV regurgitation	*Endocarditis*	*CW Doppler, PW Doppler, colour Doppler*

330

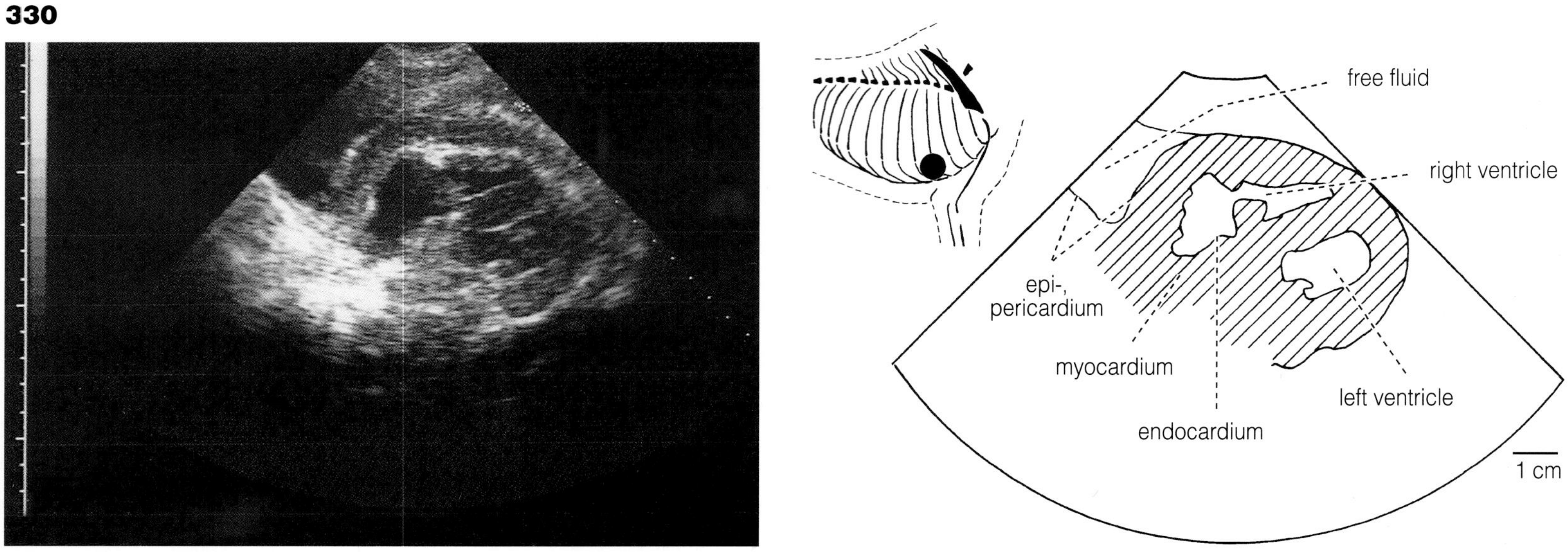

330 Two-dimensional echocardiogram – dog. Endocarditis, myocarditis and pericarditis with a distinctly non-uniform echogenicity, caused by microbiologically and histologically determined, disseminated coccidioidomycosis.

331

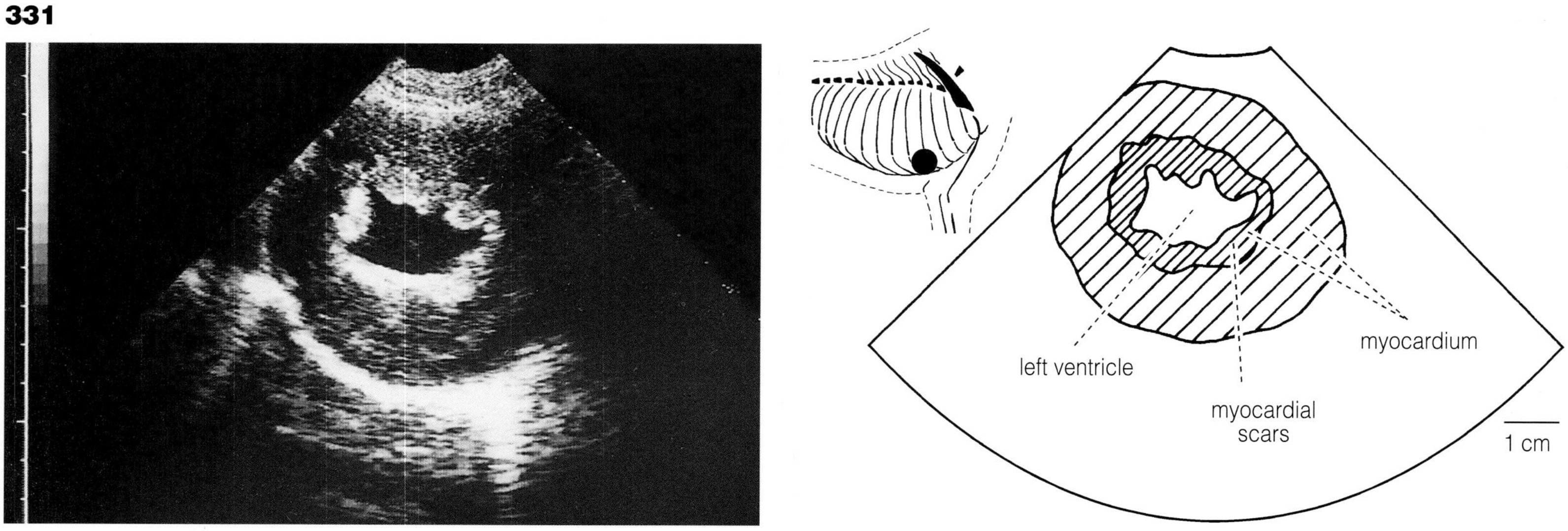

331 Two-dimensional echocardiogram – dog. Echogenic myocardial scars at the papillary muscle level.

Table 28 Echocardiographic findings with tumours and thrombi. (*Secondary abnormalities are printed in italics.*)

Echocardiographic findings	Disease	Method
Structures with mixed echogenicity (anechoic to hyperechoic)	Tumour and thrombus	2DE
Ball-shaped or polymorph, attached to endocardium or projecting into the chambers	Tumour and thrombus	2DE
Turbulences near the masses	Tumour and thrombus	Colour Doppler
Pericardial effusion	*Tumour*	*M-mode, 2DE*

332

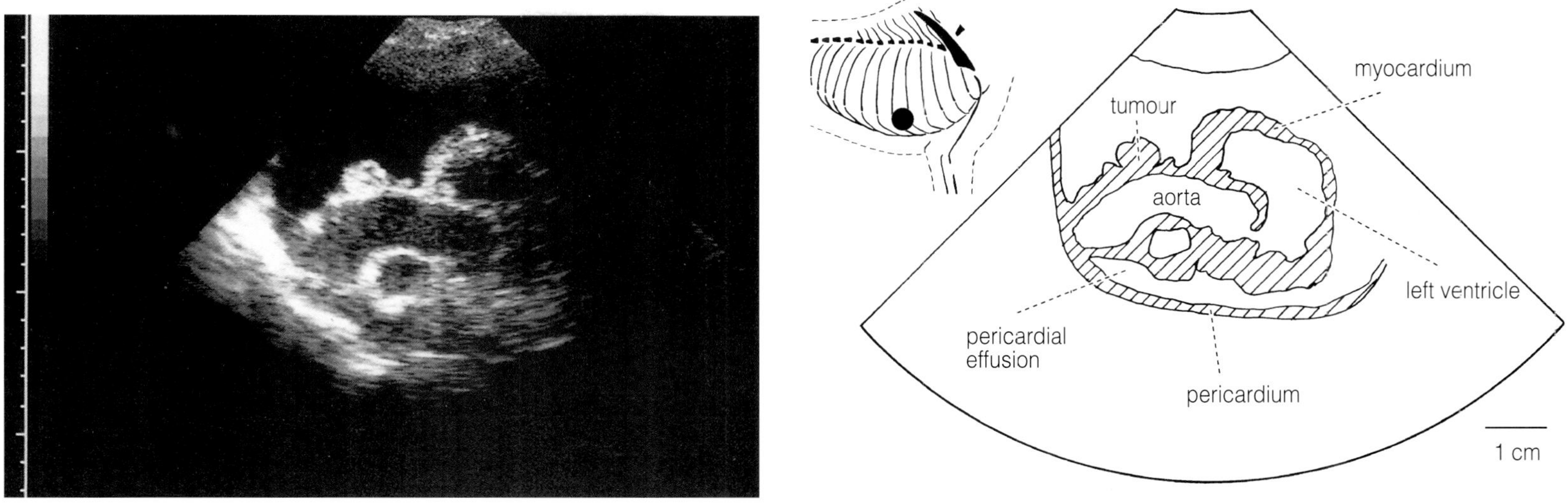

332 Two-dimensional echocardiogram – dog. Echogenic mass at the heart base, causing progressive haemorrhagic pericardial effusion. A chemodectoma was diagnosed pathohistologically.

333

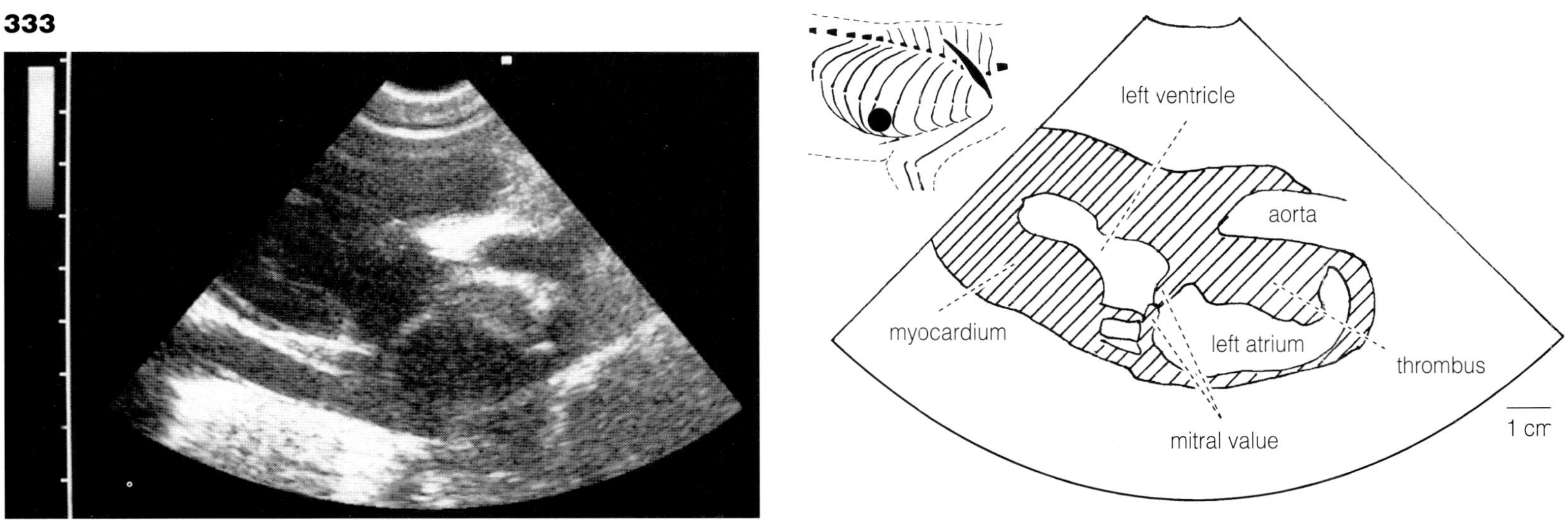

333 Two-dimensional echocardiogram – cat. Echogenic mural mass within the greatly enlarged left atrium, in conjunction with hypertrophic cardiomyopathy. The floating thrombus is seen in the real-time image.

Cardiac Masses (Table 28)

Neoplasia and thrombi in the heart are always associated with severe clinical manifestations, e.g. syncope, arrhythmia or congestion.

Tumours are recognized as masses of variable size in two-dimensional echocardiography. Classification of neoplasia is not possible with echocardiography. Histopathology is required to determine the type of tumour.

Haemangiosarcoma is the most common primary heart tumour in the dog. It is rarely seen with secondary metastasis. With the help of two-dimensional echocardiography, haemangiosarcomas are detected in the right atrium. Chemodectomas are located around the perimeter of the aortic wall and are found mainly in middle-aged to old Boxers. These tumours may also infiltrate arteries and ventricles (**332**). Chemodectomas are usually more echogenic than the more hypoechoic or anechoic haemangiosarcomas[11, 25, 26, 32].

Endocardial masses are usually indicative of a thrombus. These masses may also float within the heart cavities. The mixed echogenicity of a thrombus is similar to that of neoplasia. Thrombi are difficult to differentiate, depending on their localization (**333**). They are often not found with transthoracic echocardiography, especially when they are in the enlarged left atrium (feline hypertrophic cardiomyopathy). Transoesophageal imaging may be helpful. Thrombi and tumours are difficult to differentiate echocardiographically.

Mitral and Aortic Valves

Mitral Valve

Diseases of the septal and parietal mitral valve leaflets are commonly seen in dogs, with a lower incidence in cats. Acquired valvular disease is a cause of clinical disorders in middle-aged and older dogs.

The mildest form of atrioventricular valve disease is mitral valve prolapse. The cause is not known. Two-dimensional echocardiography shows systolic prolapse of a valvular leaflet into the left atri-

334

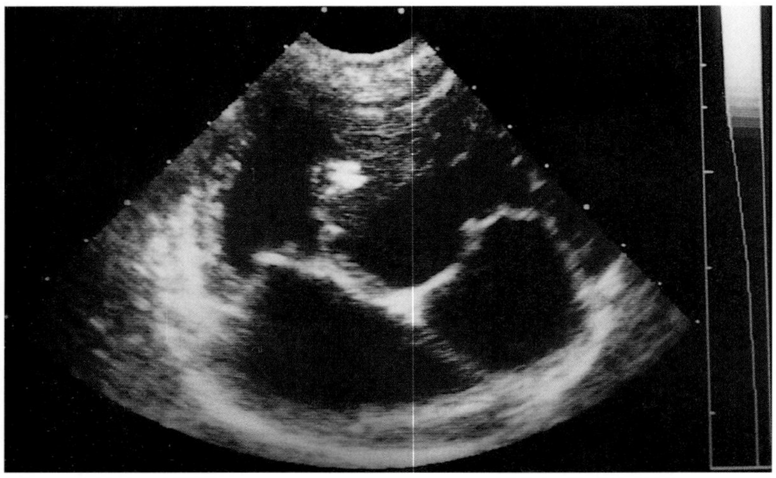

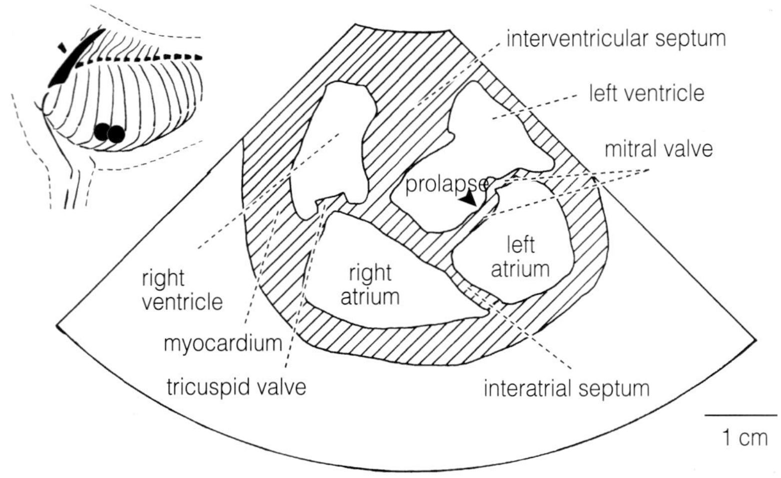

334 Two-dimensional echocardiogram – dog. Mitral valve prolapse of the closed septal leaflet during systole, bulging into the left atrium.

um (**334**). The image is achieved in a parasternal left ventricular long-axis view or a four-chamber view. Concurrent regurgitation must be determined with the help of Doppler methods.

The most common left AV valve disease is mitral valve endocardiosis, causing valvular insufficiency (see *Table 29*, page 156)[15]. Mitral stenosis is not as common. Mitral endocardiosis is diagnosed mainly in smaller breeds, such as Wire-haired Dachshunds and Toy Poodles. Males are more commonly affected. Mitral insufficiency is caused by chronic fibrotic, myomatous, degenerative valvular disease, which leads to shortening and thickening of the leaflets, thinning and shortening of the chordae tendinae, and papillary muscle atrophy or hypertrophy. These lesions are summarized by the term endocardiosis. Mitral regurgitation allows blood to flow from the ventricle back into the left atrium during systole. Systolic heart murmurs of varying grades can be auscultated in the fifth intercostal space over the mitral valve. Radiography shows moderate to severe cardiomegaly with an enlarged left atrium (**335**).

Echocardiographic diagnosis is made on one- and two-dimensional examinations, as well as with Doppler. Two-dimensional images show valvular thickening and 'knobbly' enlargements at the ends of the leaflets, which may be shortened in severe cases

335

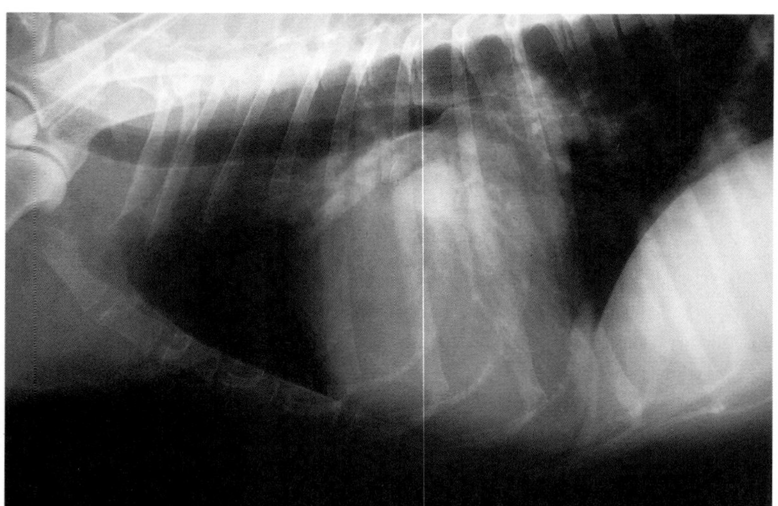

335 Lateral radiograph – dog. Cardiomegaly with left atrial enlargement, caused by regurgitant blood flow with mitral insufficiency.

(**336, 337**). The shortened appearance of the valve does not correlate with haemodynamic function and permits only a tentative diagnosis of mitral insufficiency.

Mitral insufficiency is also caused by widening of the fibrous annulus in dilated cardiomyopathy. Secondary abnormalities in M-mode examinations include left atrial and, in some cases, left ventricular enlargement (**337**). The papillary muscles may be hypertrophied. Ruptured chordae tendinae are recognized by uncoordinated leaflet motion during diastole and a prolapsing leaflet during systole. Ruptured chordal remnants may be seen as fine echoes. Shortening fractions are usually increased. The severity of mitral insufficiency cannot be diagnosed with M-mode or two-dimensional sonography. Estimation of mitral regurgitation is made according to secondary changes, such as left atrial enlargement, which usually signify haemodynamic disorders.

Doppler echocardiography provides semiquantitative evaluation of mitral insufficiency. Colour Doppler is more sensitive than auscultation. The examination is made in a left apical four-chamber view. PW Doppler examinations can detect a regurgitant jet by placing the sample volume in the left atrium above the mitral valve (**337**). Sample volumes placed below the valve in the left ventricle are difficult to evaluate, because of normal blood flow in the left ventricular outflow tract and slight regurgitation in the direction of the mitral valve. Although the sample volume is placed in the left atrium, the heart base may shift during systole, which leads to contamination by flow tracings of the left ventricular outflow tract.

> Normal systolic flow tracings in the aorta should not be misinterpreted as mitral regurgitation!

Spectral Doppler 'mapping' of the area of regurgitant flow includes not only the length of the jet, but all angles within the left atrium. 'Jet-lesions' of the left atrium are caused by regurgitant jets hitting the atrial wall. These pathological findings are not recognized sonographically[11, 15].

Conventional Doppler echocardiography shows mitral insufficiency as a parabolic regurgitant signal below the baseline and between the C and D points (**339**). Since regurgitant jets have high flow velocities, the Nyquist limit is reached quickly with PW Doppler and aliasing occurs (**338**). Peak velocities must be deter-

336

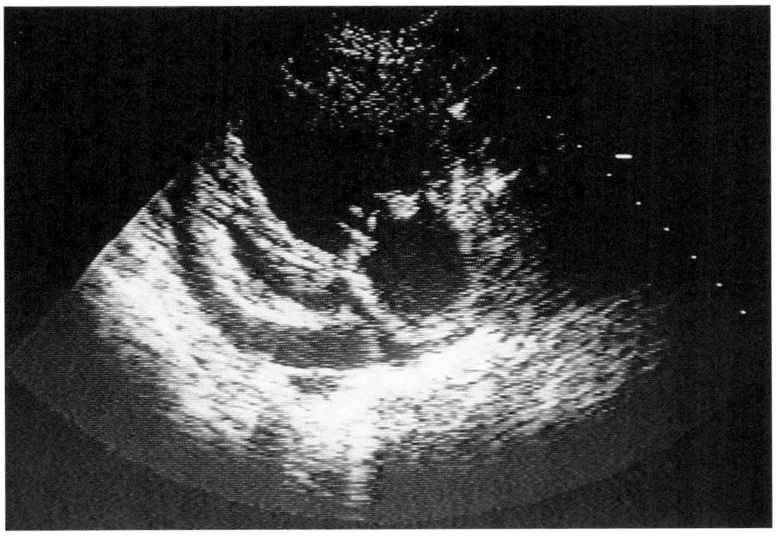

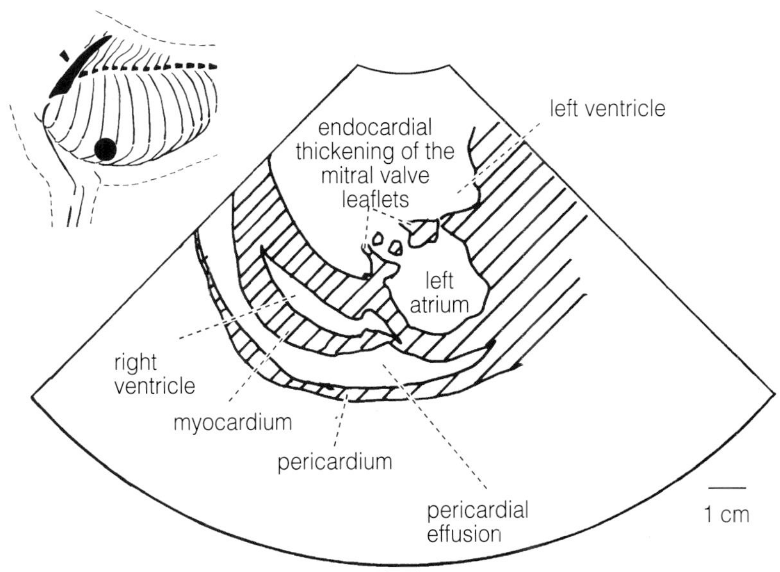

336 Two-dimensional echocardiogram – dog. Endocardiosis with distinctly thickened and shortened mitral leaflets. Additional pericardial effusion is indicative of mitral insufficiency.

337

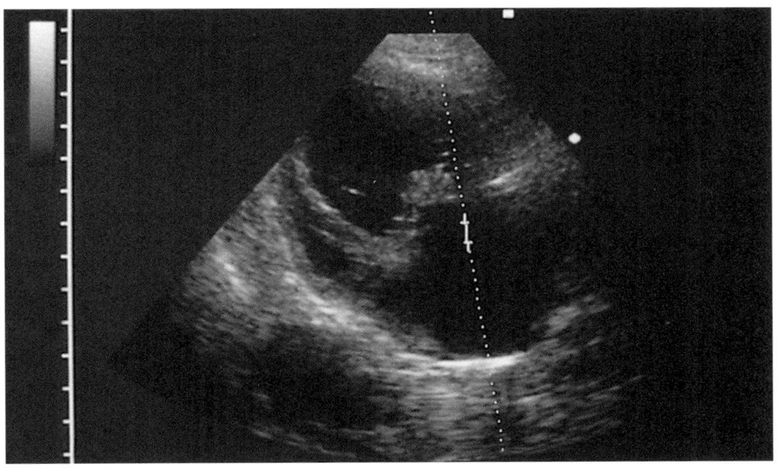

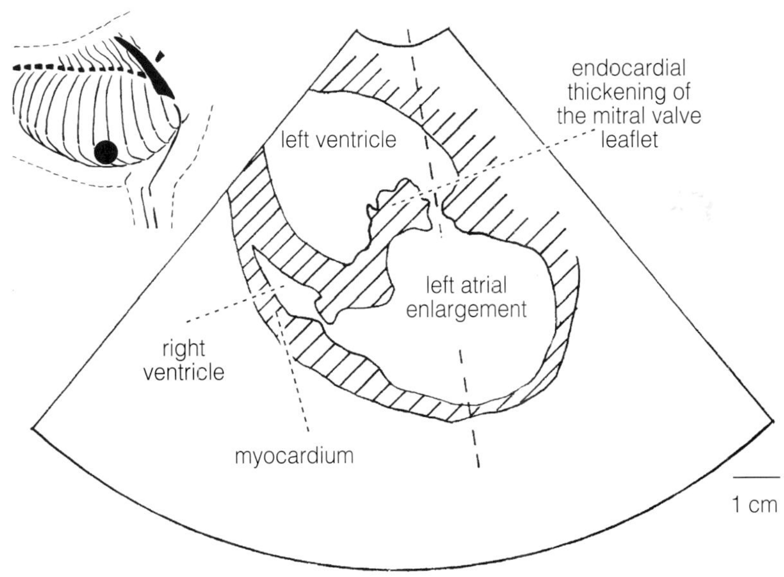

337 Two-dimensional echocardiogram – dog. Endocardiosis with left atrial enlargement. For a definitive diagnosis of insufficiency, the PW Doppler sample volume is placed in the left atrium.

338

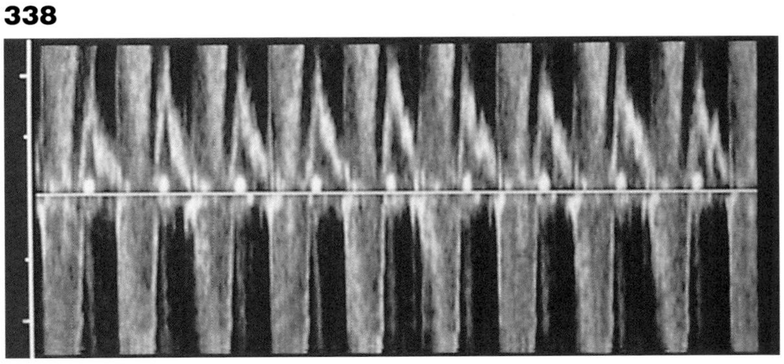

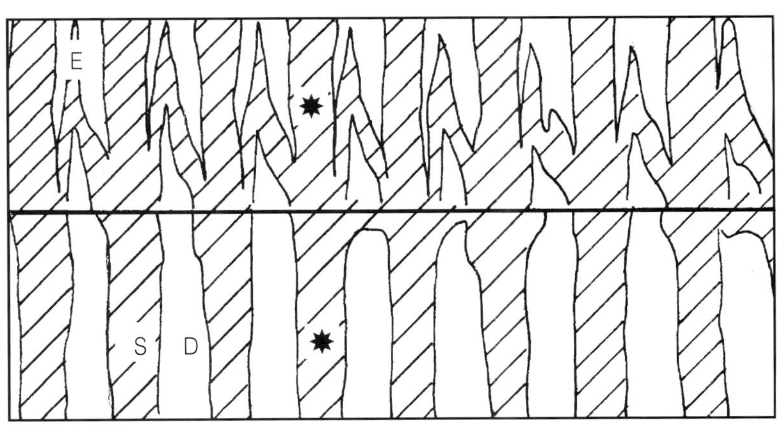

E = E-wave ✸ = systolic regurgitation, aliasing
S = systole; D = diastole

338 PW Doppler – dog. Mitral insufficiency with aliasing. Flow velocities have exceeded the Nyquist limit. Regurgitation is apparent above and below the baseline.

339

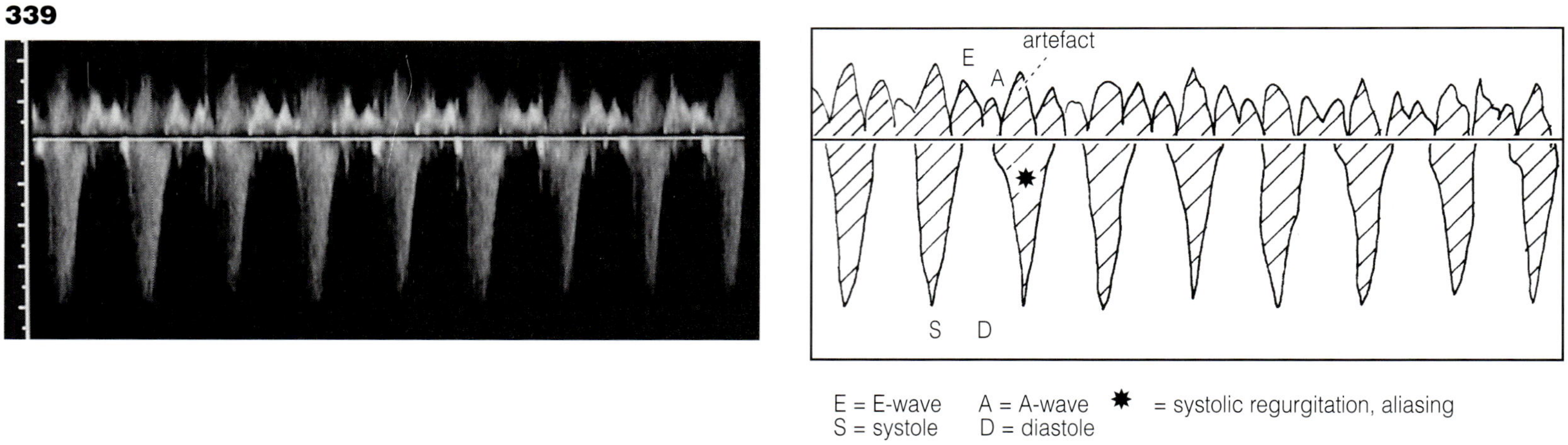

339 CW Doppler – dog. The high regurgitant signal is traced with the sample volume in the centre of the insufficiency. By increasing the Doppler gain, the tracing would have a rounded, parabolic amplitude.

340

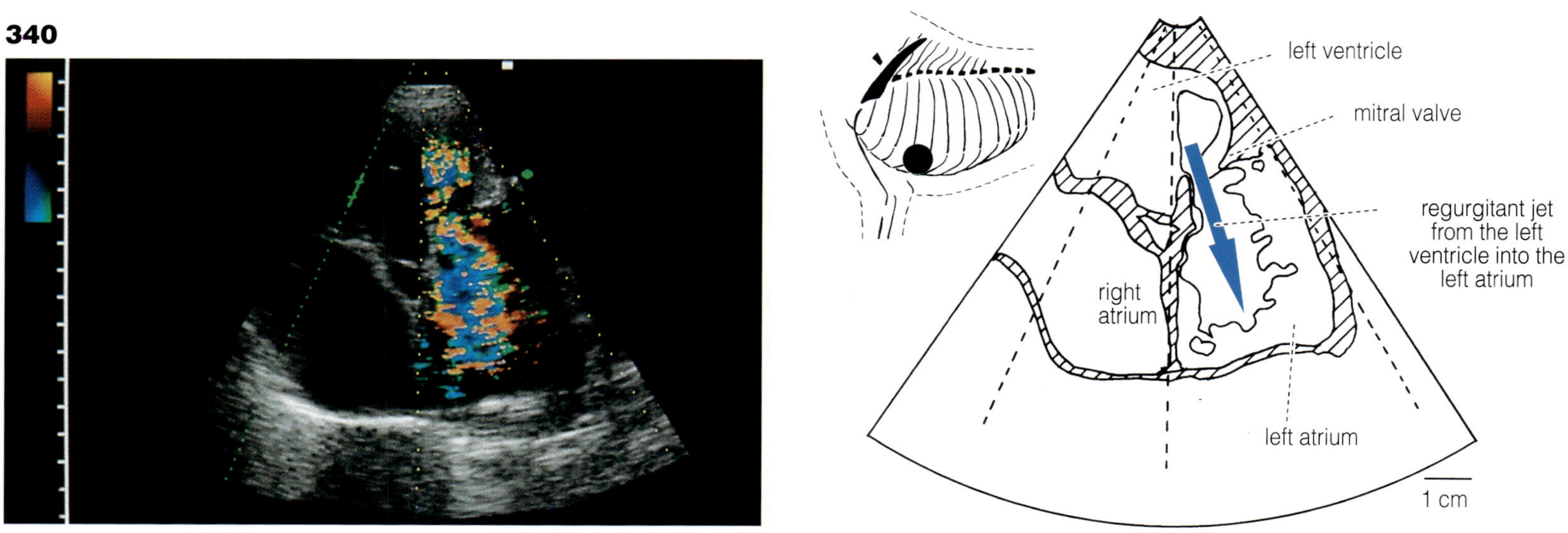

340 Colour-flow Doppler echocardiogram – dog. Mitral insufficiency with a central regurgitant jet from the left ventricle into the left atrium. Severe insufficiency is indicated, because the regurgitant jet almost reaches the atrial roof. Atrial dilation is caused by valvular insufficiency.

mined with CW Doppler (**339**). Regurgitation is found in the whole systole or in early systole, depending on the severity of the mitral insufficiency. Apart from these extremes, there are numerous other forms.

In colour Doppler echocardiography, high velocities will also exceed the Nyquist limit. The regurgitant blood shows a colour shift in the middle of the jet (**340**). Aliasing and turbulences in severe AV valve insufficiencies produce a mosaic-like colour image of the regurgitant jet (**341, 342**). Colour Doppler is superior to PW Doppler in finding small regurgitant jets and determining their angle and width. With a combination of M-mode and colour Doppler, regurgitation can be recorded over time (**342**).

Mitral stenosis occasionally occurs with valvular thickening. In M-mode the usual M-shaped mitral valve shows a flattened E to F slope. Valvular movement is reduced in two-dimensional echocardiography. The left atrium is enlarged, while the left ventricular dimensions are normal. Higher velocities through the narrow mitral valve opening in the direction of the apex are recorded with Doppler sonography[7].

Table 29 Echocardiographic findings with mitral valve endocardiosis and mitral insufficiency. (*Secondary abnormalities are printed in italics.*)

Echocardiographic findings	Disease	Method
Thickened, non-uniform valvular structure	Endocardiosis	M-mode, 2DE
Papillary muscle hypertrophy	Endocardiosis	M-mode, 2DE
Increased DE slope	Endocardiosis	M-mode
Ruptured chordae tendinae	Endocardiosis	2DE
Systolic regurgitation	Insufficiency	PW Doppler, CW Doppler, colour Doppler
Left atrial enlargement	*Insufficiency*	*M-mode, 2DE*
Hyperkinesis	*Endocardiosis, insufficiency*	*M-mode, 2DE*
Ventricular dimensions normal, hypertrophied or dilated	*Endocardiosis, insufficiency*	*M-mode, 2DE*

341

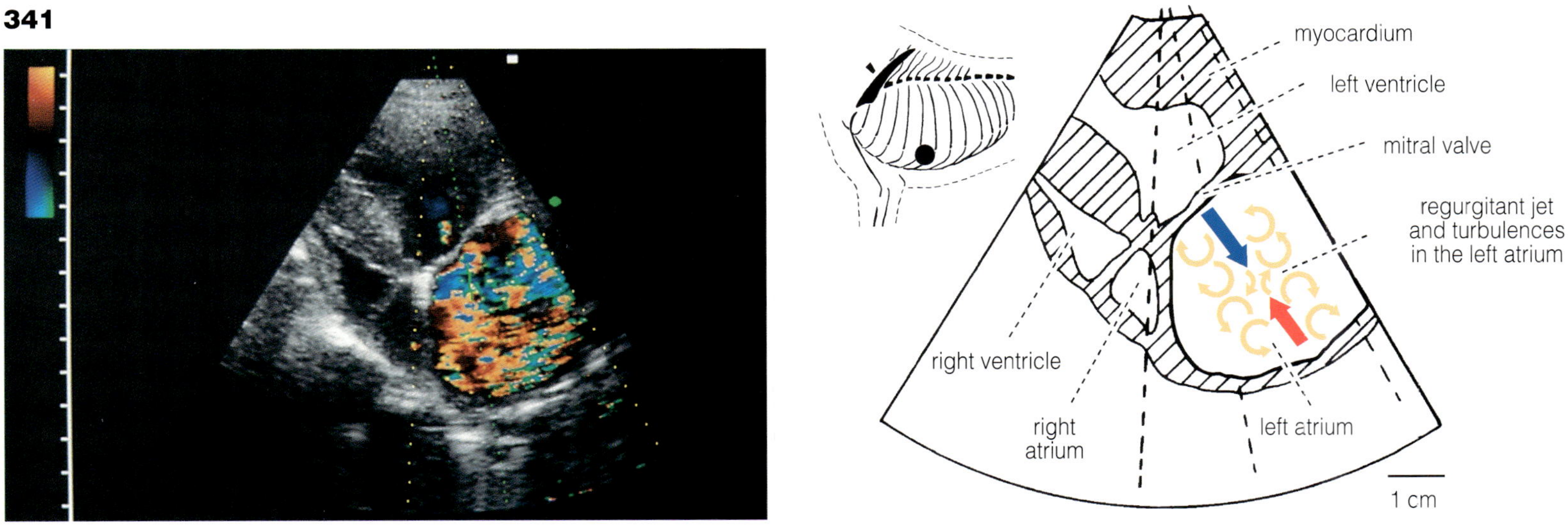

341 Colour-flow Doppler echocardiogram – dog. Mitral insufficiency with characteristic colour mosaic in the left atrium, caused by regurgitant flow meeting inflowing blood from the pulmonary veins. In the real-time image, regurgitation was seen through the insufficient valve. This is proof of mitral insufficiency (see Laminar and Turbulent Flows, page 64; **126–129**).

342

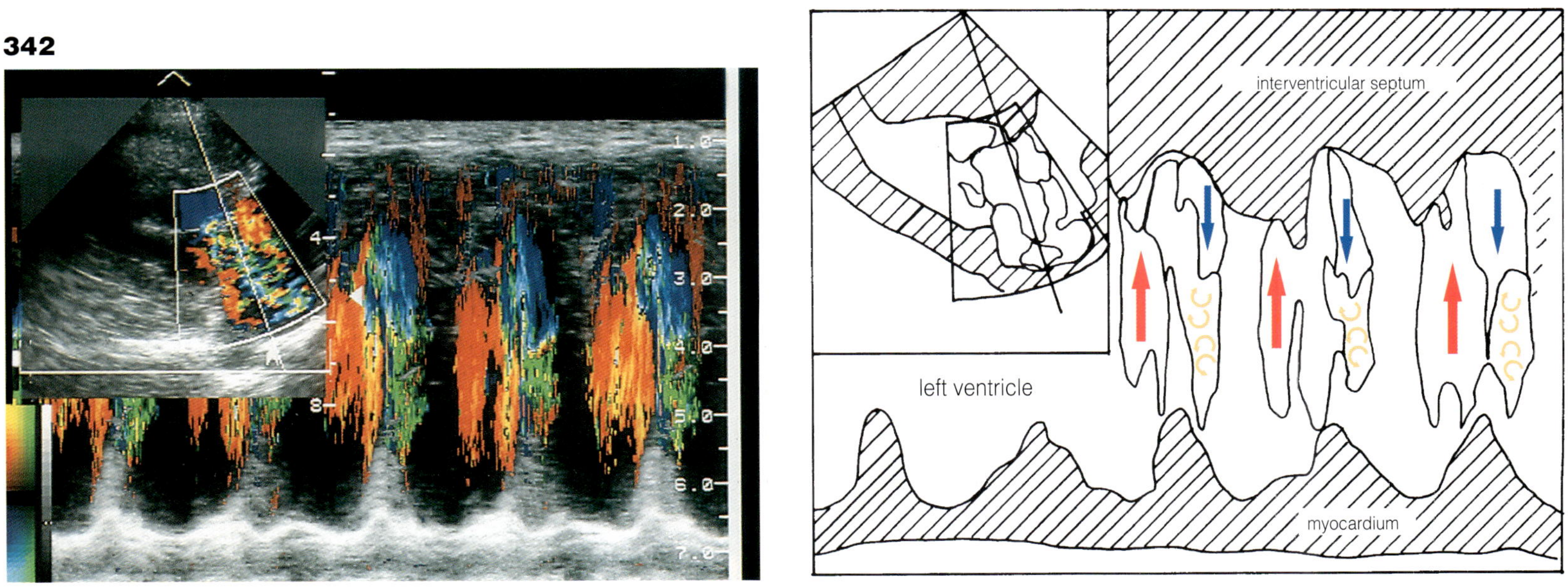

342 M-mode with colour Doppler – dog. Mitral insufficiency with systolic regurgitation (blue colour) and turbulences (yellow/green colour).

Aortic Valve (Table 30)

Aortic stenosis is seen in dogs, especially Boxers, and less frequently in cats. Subvalvular aortic stenosis is caused by a fibrotic ring obstructing the left ventricular outflow tract. Valvular and supravalvular stenoses are occasionally found. A characteristic systolic crescendo–decrescendo heart murmur is heard over the aortic valve[11, 16, 30]. Radiographs show left heart enlargement and, in some cases, poststenotic aortic dilation. Left ventricular systolic pressure overload results in LV hypertrophy and secondary mitral insufficiency. Mitral regurgitation leads to left atrial enlargement. The aorta is imaged from the right thoracic wall in short-axis and long-axis views. A five-chamber view displays the aorta from the left thorax. In this view the aorta runs longitudinally between both atria (**294, 296–299**). Subvalvular fibrous ridges or rings are distinguished as hyperechoic structures (**343**). Valvular aortic stenosis shows thickened, hyperechoic aortic cusps (**344**). Severe stenosis reduces valvular mobility.

PW Doppler has limited use in diagnosing aortic stenosis because of the high velocities involved. CW Doppler should always be used additionally. Flow velocities in the stenotic and

Table 30 Echocardiographic findings with aortic stenosis. (*Secondary abnormalities are printed in italics.*)

Echocardiographic findings	Method
Subvalvular, valvular, or supravalvular hyperechoic obstructions	2DE
Reduced valvular mobiltiy	M-mode, 2DE
Increased poststenotic aortic dimensions	M-moce, 2DE
High flow velocities in the stenotic and poststenotic areas	PW Doppler, CW Doppler, colour Doppler
Hyperkinesis	*M-mode, 2DE*
Ventricular dimensions normal, hypertrophied, or dilated	*M-mode, 2DE*
Mitral insufficiency	*PW Doppler, CW Doppler, colour Doppler*

343

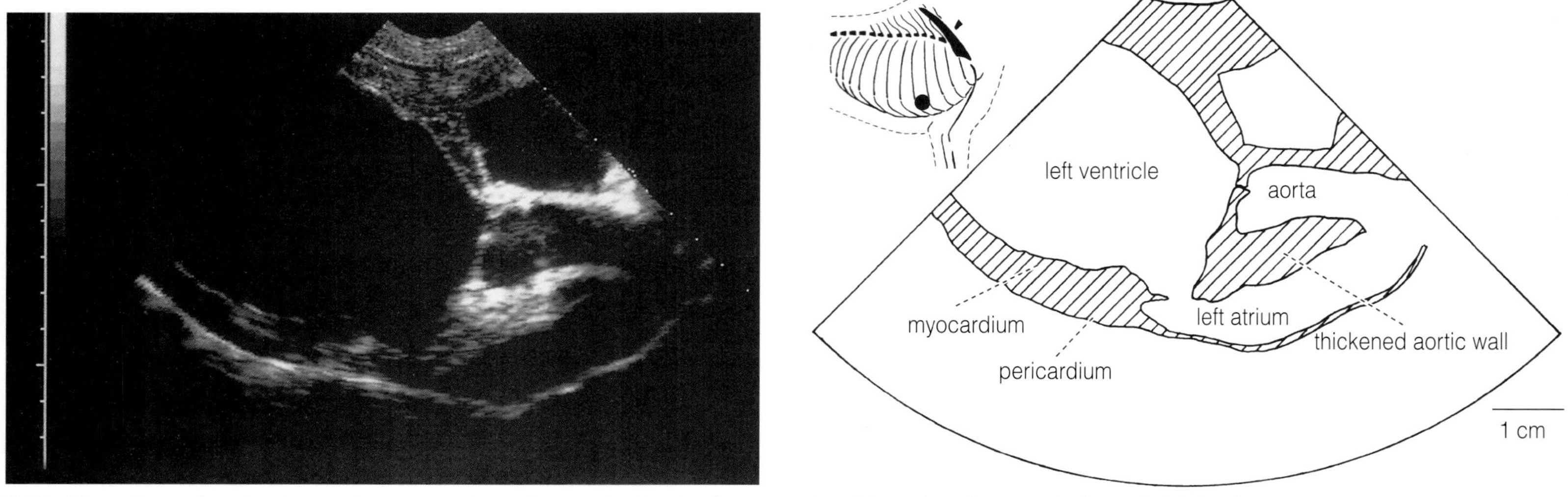

343 Two-dimensional echocardiogram – dog. Supravalvular aortic stenosis with typical hyperechoic wall thickening around the aortic root and echogenic ridges into the lumen. This puppy shows secondary left ventricular dilation, which is indicative of progressive, severe cardiac decompensation.

344

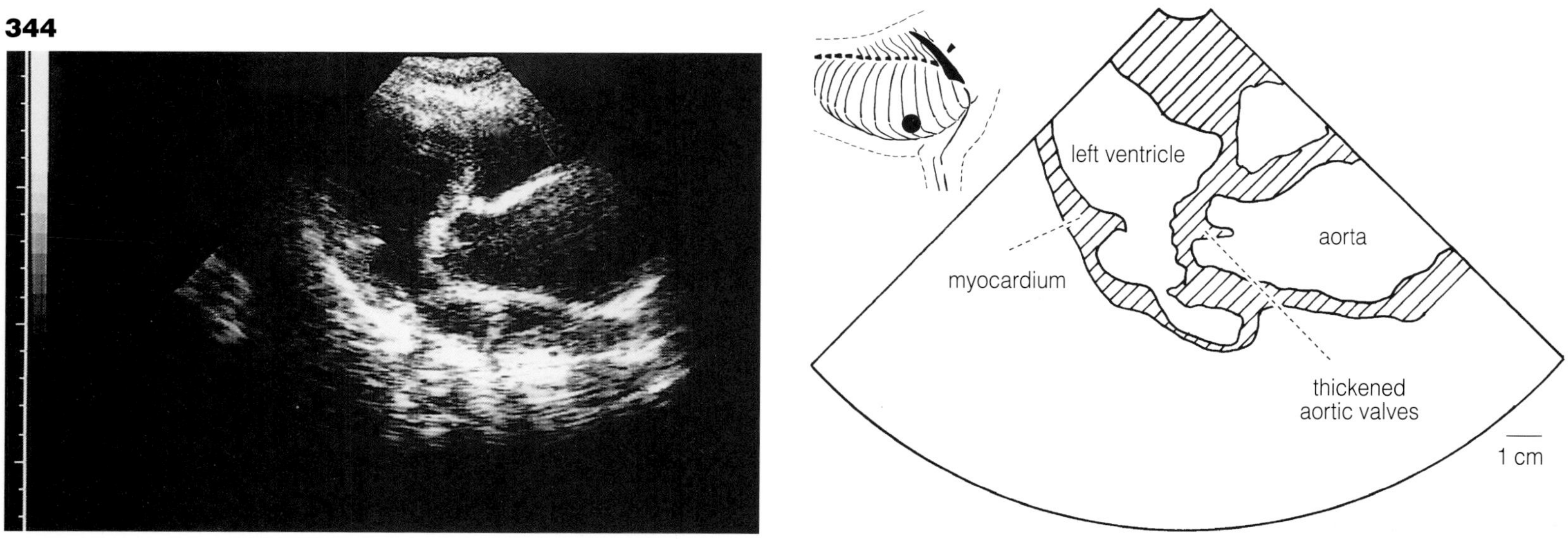

344 Two-dimensional echocardiogram – dog. Valvular aortic stenosis with extremely thick valves and distinctly reduced mobility in real-time imaging. Poststenotic aortic dilation is seen.

345

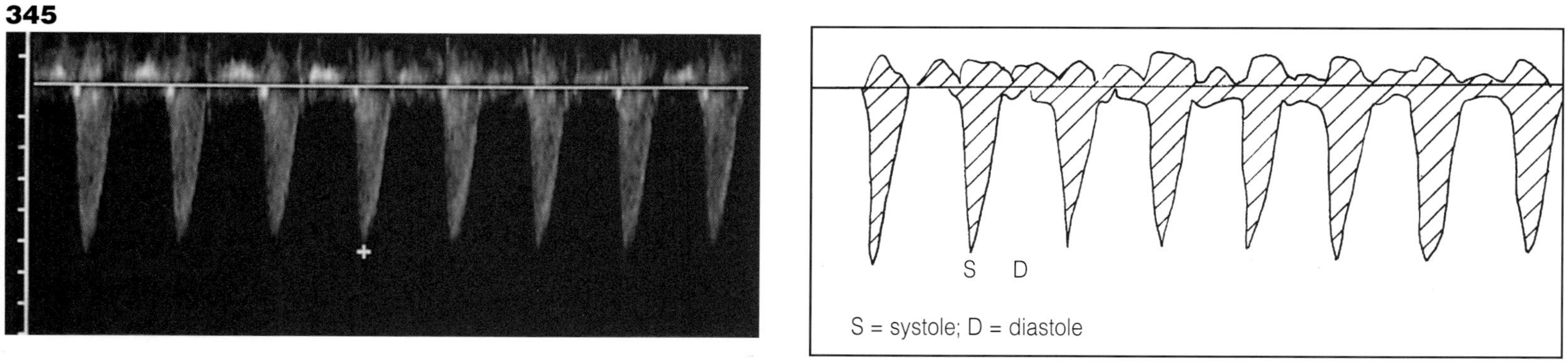

345 CW Doppler – dog. Valvular aortic stenosis with poststenotic flow velocities of 4 m/s (normally up to 1.7 m/s).

poststenotic areas greatly exceed 2 m/s (**345**). Colour Doppler displays high central and turbulent lateral flows as mosaic-like colour combinations in the poststenotic area. Semiquantitative evaluation of flow velocities is possible with colour Doppler. Peak velocities are adjusted to avoid aliasing (**346**).

Aortic insufficiency is recognized in two-dimensional echocardiography by slight fluttering of the septal mitral leaflet, caused by diastolic regurgitation. The aortic valves are sonographically normal[7, 13]. Left ventricular volume overload may lead to hypertrophy or dilation. Doppler echography displays regurgitant jets. Clinically significant aortic insufficiency is rare in both dogs and cats[16]. Colour Doppler may distinguish small, relatively slow regurgitant jets over the aortic valve. Since these jets do not correlate with heart murmurs, they appear to be a normal finding [personal communication, Poulsen Nautrup].

Tricuspid and Pulmonary Valves

Tricuspid Valve

Isolated abnormalities of the tricuspid valve are rare. Tricuspid insufficiency is usually associated with other diseases[15, 16]. Tricuspid valve diseases are similar to those of the mitral valve described above (Mitral Valve). The tricuspid valve is imaged

346

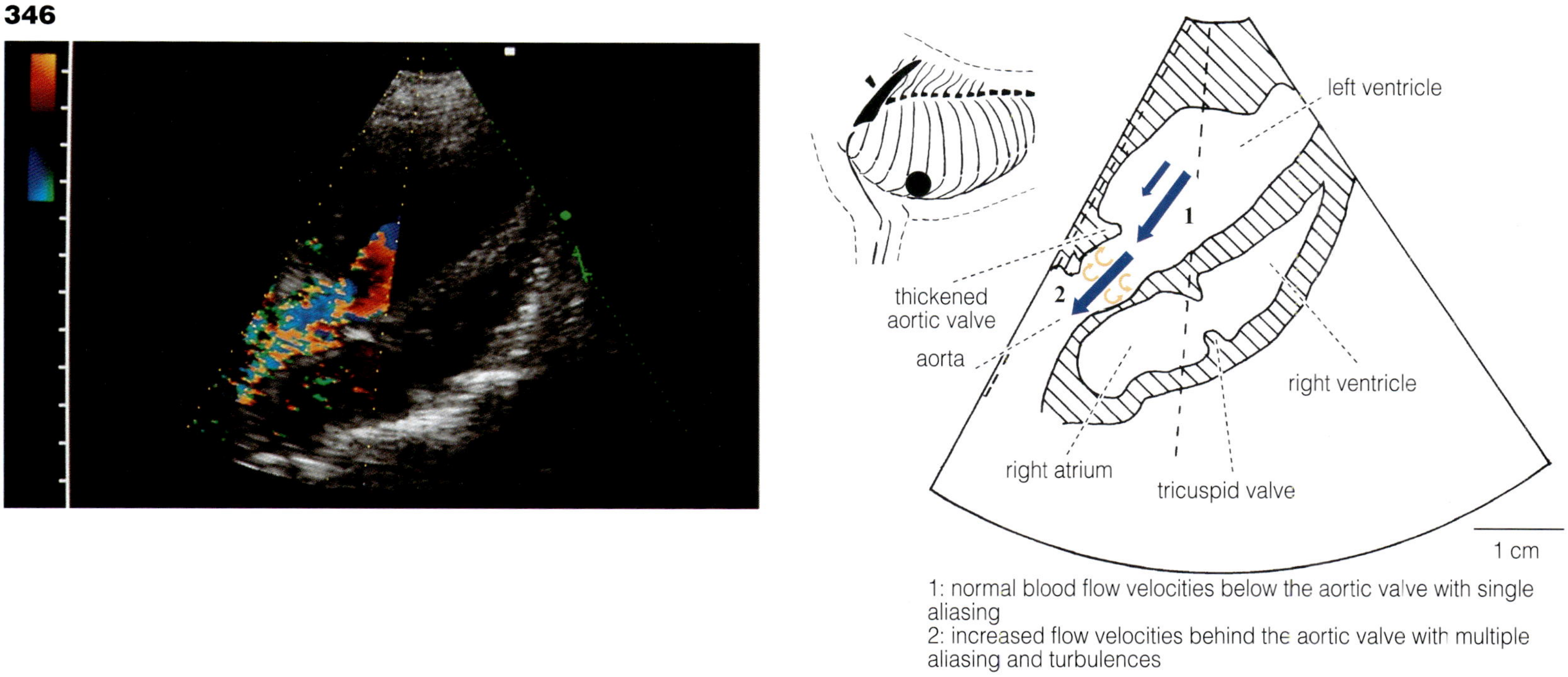

346 Colour Doppler echocardiogram – dog. Long-axis view. Subvalvular aortic stenosis with turbulent flow near the valves (green colour) and aliasing (multicoloured) due to high flow velocities.

347

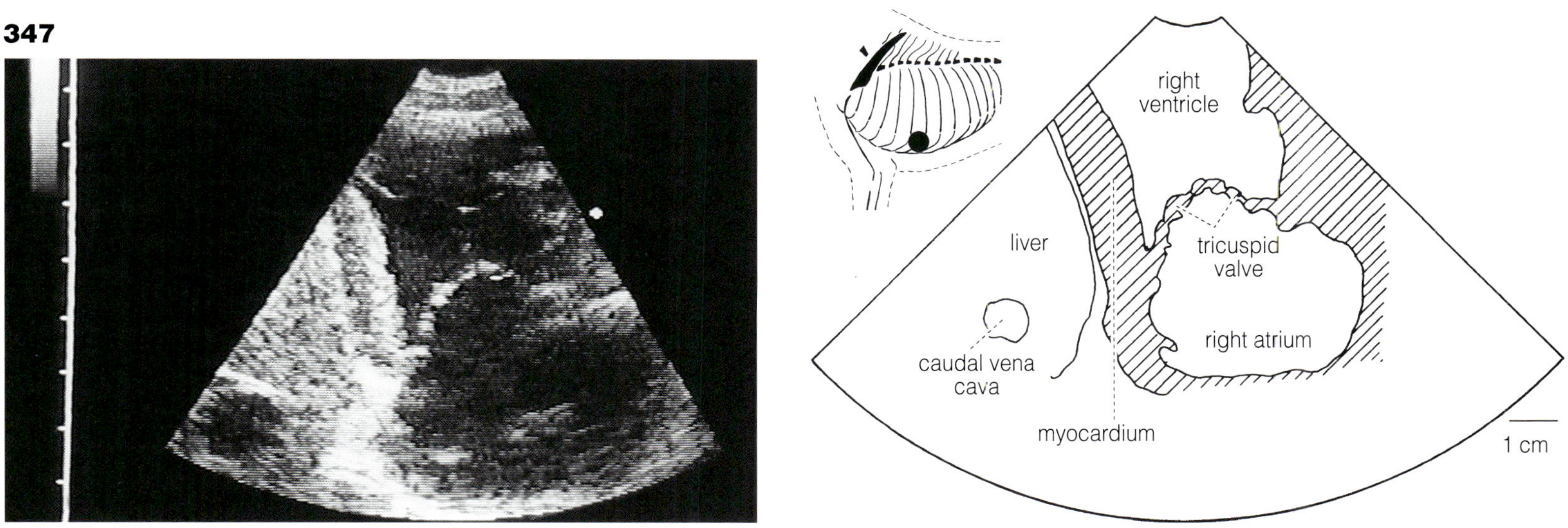

347 Two-dimensional echocardiogram – dog. Tricuspid insufficiency with pulmonic stenosis, showing right atrial enlargement and ventricular dilation. The tricuspid valve is thickened and shows an irregular surface, similar to AV valve endocardiosis.

348

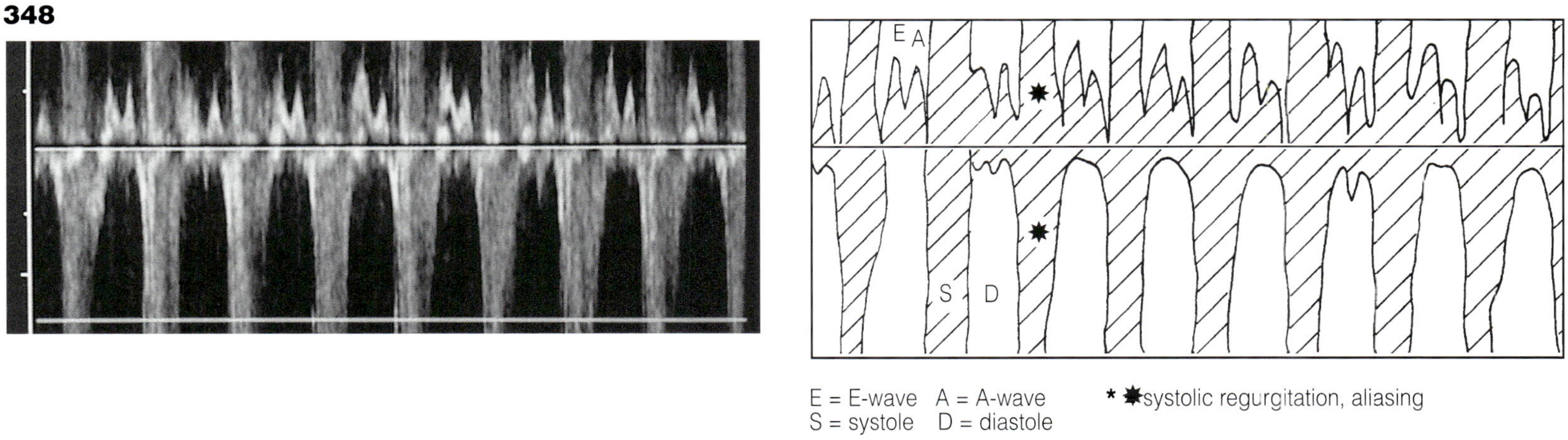

348 PW Doppler – dog. Tricuspid insufficiency with systolic regurgitation. Regurgitant jet velocities exceed the Nyquist limit and lead to aliasing.

from the left thorax in a right ventricular long-axis and a four-chamber view (347). Imaging of the tricuspid valve and the right ventricle is more difficult than the left heart, and is occasionally unsatisfactory. This is partly because of the three valvular leaflets and the half-moon shape of the right ventricle. Doppler signals of tricuspid regurgitation are registered over the entire systole (348). (*Table 31*, page 161, gives echocardiographic findings with tricuspid endocardiosis and insufficiency.)

349

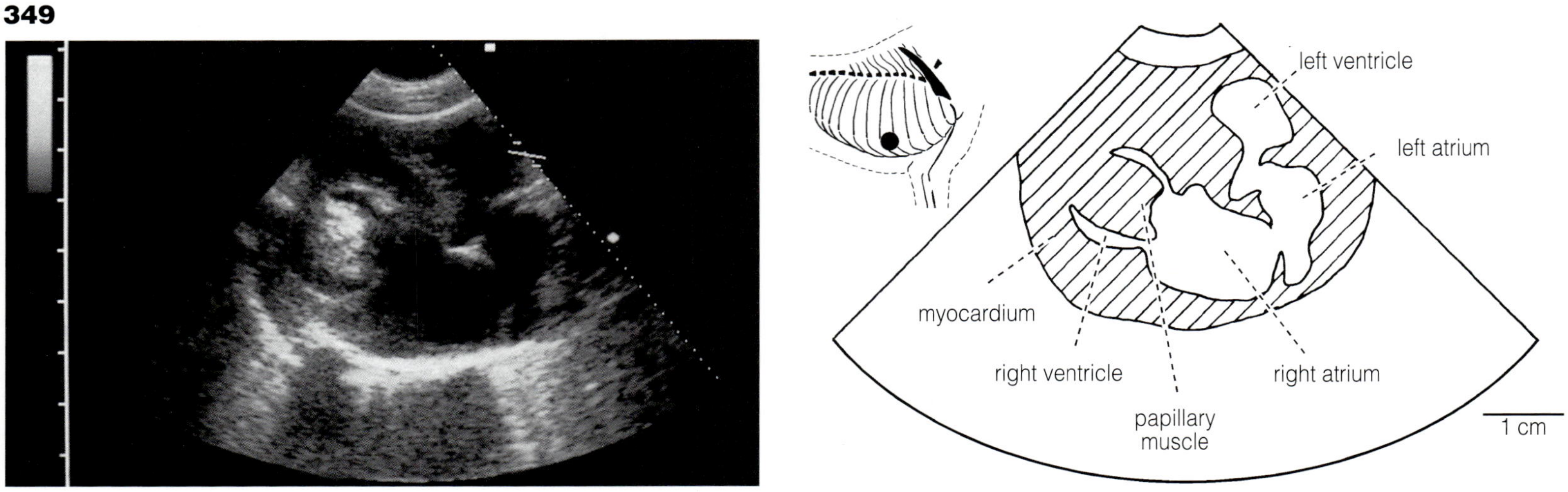

349 Two-dimensional echocardiogram – dog. Pulmonic stenosis with severe right ventricular hypertrophy. The hyperechoic endocardium and myocardium of the hypertrophied papillary muscles may be caused by infection of these layers. Secondary tricuspid insufficiency causes right atrial dilation.

350

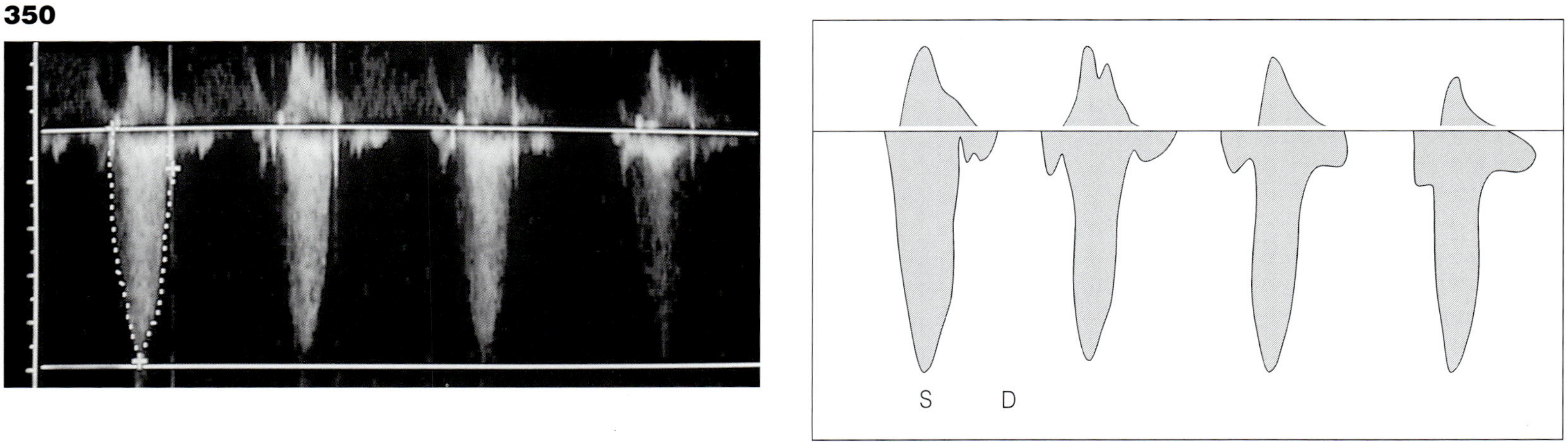

S = systole; D = diastole

350 CW Doppler echocardiogram – dog. Pulmonic stenosis with high stenotic and poststenotic flow velocities of 7 m/s (normally up to 1.3 m/s) and parabolic tracings.

351

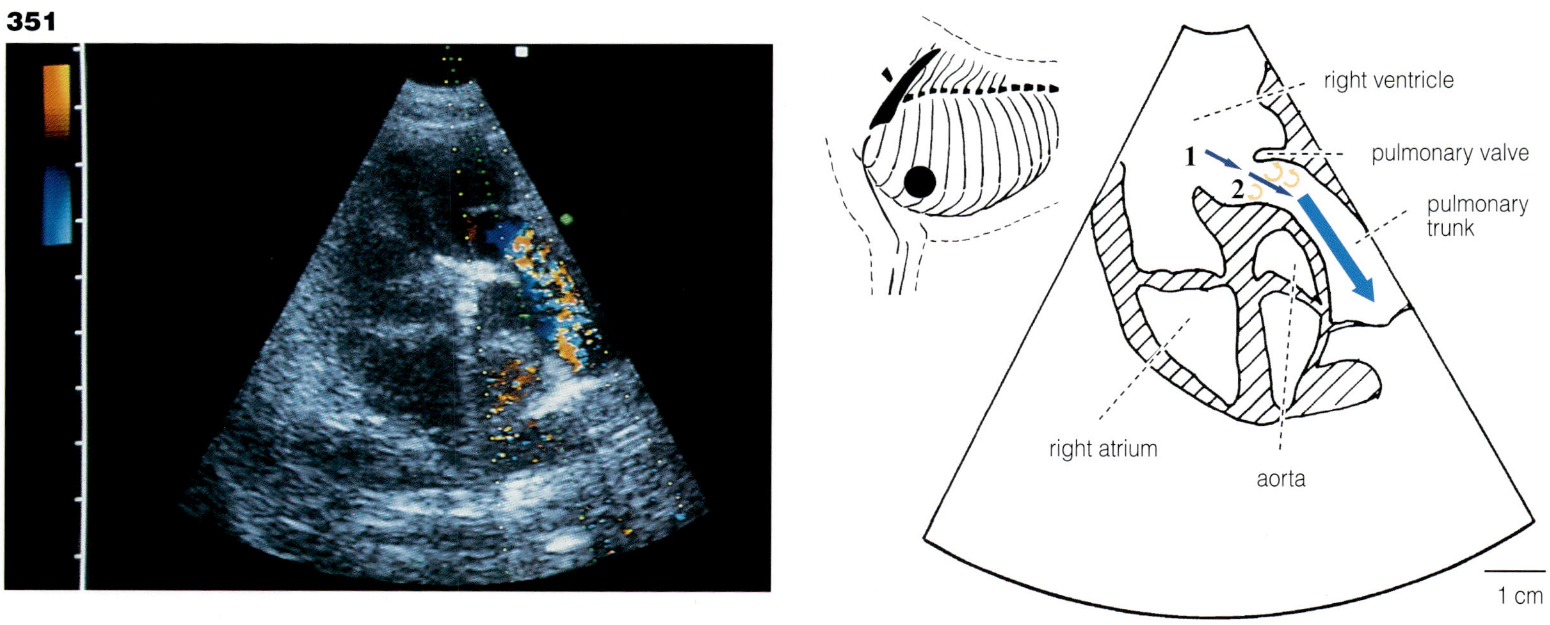

1: normal blood flow velocities below the pulmonary valve
2: increased flow velocities behind the pulmonary valve with aliasing and turbulences

351 Colour-flow Doppler – dog. Pulmonic stenosis with poststenotic aliasing, caused by high flow velocities and turbulences.

352

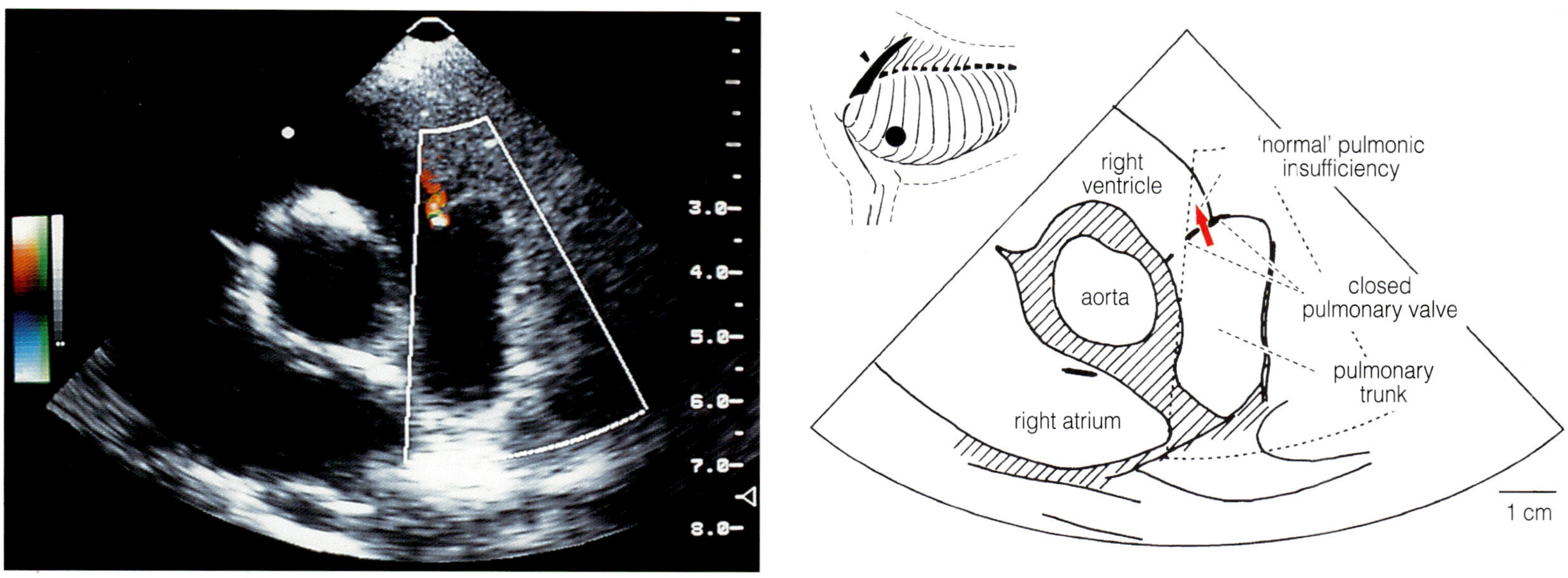

352 Colour-flow Doppler – dog. Mild pulmonic insufficiency with relatively low velocities under 0.78 m/s and without heart murmurs.

Table 31 Echocardiographic findings with tricuspid valve endocardiosis and tricuspid insufficiency. (*Secondary abnormalities are printed in italics.*)

Echocardiographic findings	Disease	Method
Thickened, non-uniform valvular structure	Endocardiosis	M-mode, 2DE
Systolic regurgitation	Insufficiency	PW Doppler, CW Doppler, colour Doppler
Right atrial enlargement	*Insufficiency*	*M-mode, 2DE*
Abnormal septal motion	*Endocardiosis, insufficiency*	*M-mode, 2DE*
Ventricular dimensions normal, hypertrophied or dilated	*Endocardiosis, insufficiency*	*M-mode, 2DE*

353

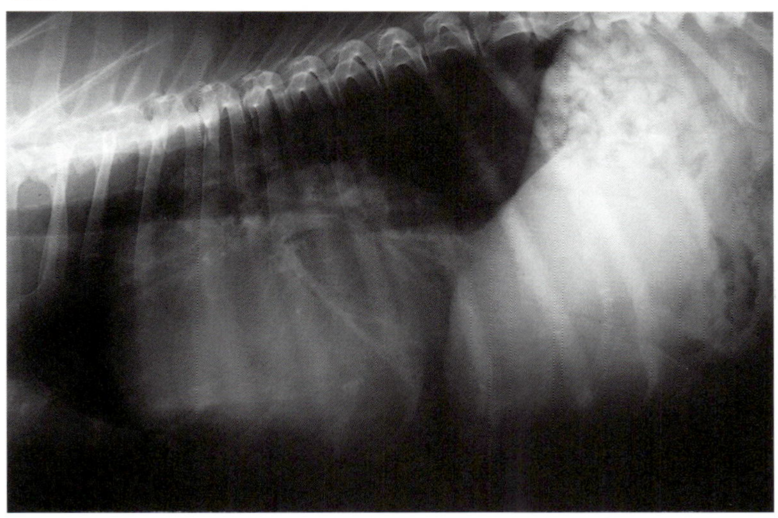

353 Lateral thoracic radiograph – dog. Pericardial effusion with 'pumpkin-shaped' heart.

Pulmonary Valve

Systolic crescendo–decrescendo heart murmurs in the left third intercostal space indicate stenosis in the main pulmonary artery. The ECG shows signs of right axis deviation[11, 16]. The pulmonary valve is imaged longitudinally from the left thorax (**296–299, 305**). Pulmonic stenosis shows thickened hyperechoic valves with reduced mobility (*Table 32*, page 163). Secondary abnormalities include right ventricular hypertrophy and atrial enlargement (**349**). Conventional Doppler echocardiography measures higher flow velocities. The parabolic flow tracings are recorded below the baseline (**350**). High stenotic and poststenotic velocities result in multiple aliasing with colour Doppler. Combined with turbulences, this aliasing produces a colourful poststenotic mosaic (**351**). Insufficiencies seen in colour Doppler without additional heart murmurs appear to be a normal finding (**352**)[13] (personal communication, Poulsen Nautrup).

Pericardium

Congestive heart failure and neoplasia may cause pericardial effusion. Radiographs of severe pericardial effusion show a 'pumpkin-shaped' heart (**353**). Milder pericardial filling results in slight enlargement of the heart silhouette, which is usually overlooked. The ECG shows low voltage and electrical alternans.

> Radiographic enlargement of the heart should be examined echocardiographically for pericardial effusion. Differential diagnosis includes almost all other cardiac diseases.

Sonographic examinations are possible from the left or right thorax in parasternal long-axis and short-axis views. Pericardial effusion is displayed as an anechoic to hypoechoic space between

354

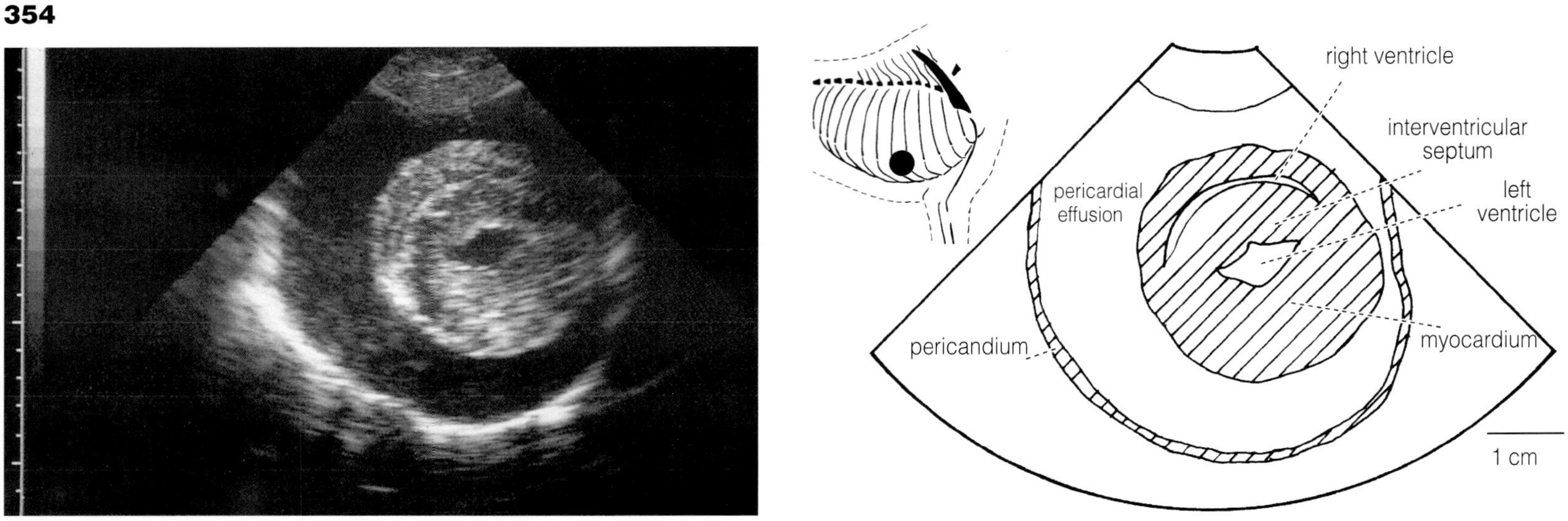

354 Two-dimensional echocardiogram – dog. Pericardial effusion.

355

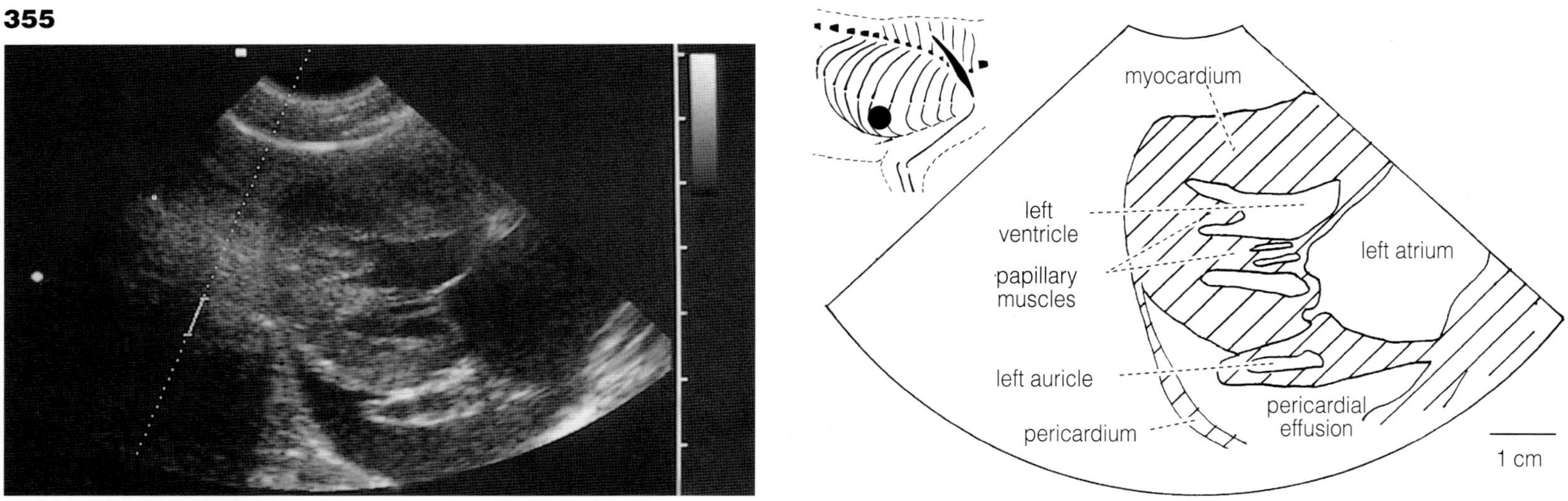

355 Two-dimensional echocardiogram – cat. Pericardial effusion. The irregular myocardium and echos within the fluid are probably inflammatory.

356

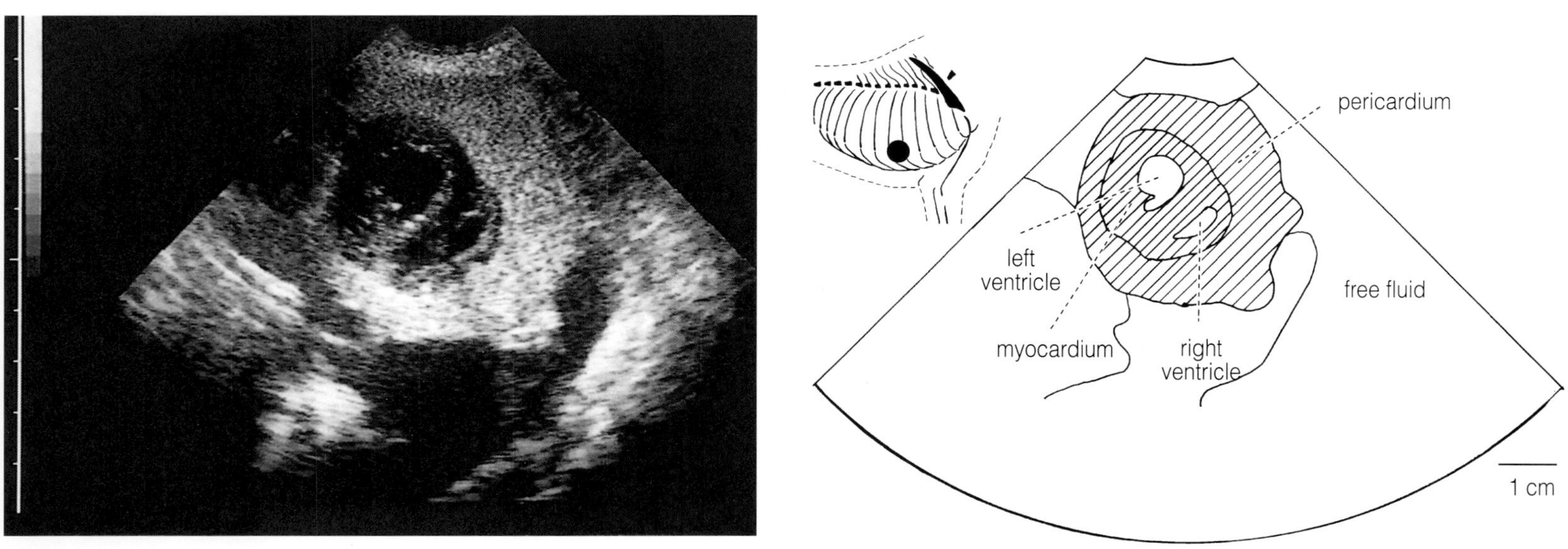

356 Two-dimensional echocardiogram – dog. Pericarditis.

Table 32 Echocardiographic findings with pulmonic stenosis. (*Secondary abnormalities are printed in italics.*)

Echocardiographic findings	Method
Thickened, hyperechoic valves	2 DE
Reduced valvular mobiltiy	M-mode, 2DE
Increased poststenotic pulmonary trunk dimensions	M-mode, 2DE
High flow velocities in stenotic and poststenotic areas	PW Doppler, CW Doppler, colour Doppler
Right ventricular hypertrophy with abnormal septal motion	*M-mode, 2DE*
Occasional right ventricular dilation	*M-mode, 2DE*
Tricuspid insufficiency	*PW Doppler, CW Doppler, colour Doppler*

Table 33 Echocardiographic findings with pericardial effusion.

Echocardiographic findings	Method
Anechoic to hypoecoic fluid-filled space between the epicardium and the pericardial sac	M-mode, 2DE
Hyperechoic pericardial thickening with chronic pericarditis	M-mode, 2DE
Swinging heart	2DE
Neoplasia, fibrin or other signs of inflammation	M-mode, 2DE

the epicardium and the pericardial sac (**354, 355**). Fluid echogenicity does not indicate its quality. The hyperechoic pericardial sac should be traced as far as possible, to differentiate pericardial from pleural effusion (see Hydrothorax, Haemothorax, Chylothorax and Pyothorax, page 123). The effusion becomes more abundant towards the cardiac apex. It is not possible to determine the exact amount of fluid with echocardiography. Severe pericardial effusion results in a swinging motion of the heart, caused by reduced mobility[34]. This swinging motion does not include the pericardial sac. Depending on the amount of pericardial effusion, the heart walls may show diastolic collapse with decreased mobility and reduced filling. Pericardiocentesis is necessary to reduce the pressure and the procedure should be ultrasound guided. Pericarditis causes fibrotic thickening of the pericardium. In two-dimensional echocardiography the pericardium appears as a wide hyperechoic shell around the heart (**356**). *Table 33* gives echocardiographic findings with percardial effusion.

References

Cited References

1 Bonagura JD and Pioers FS (1983) Diagnosis of cardiac lesions by contrast echocardiography. *J. Am. Vet. Med. Assoc.* **182**, 396–402.

2 Bonagura JD, O'Grady MR and Herring DS (1985) Echocardiography: principles of interpretation. *Vet. Clin. North Am.* **15**, 1177–1194.

3 Bonagura JD and Herring DS (1985) Echocardiography: congenital heart disease. *Vet. Clin. North Am.* **15**, 1195–2108.

4 Bonagura JD and Herring DS (1985) Echocardiography: acquired heart disease. *Vet. Clin. North Am.* **15**, 2109–2125.

5 Boon J, Wingfield WE and Miller CW (1983) Echocardiographic indices in the normal dog. *Vet. Radiol.* **24**, 214–221.

6 Brunnberg L, Hart S, Tobias R and Wohlsein P (1993) Disseminierte Kokzidioidomykose bei einem Hand. I: Klinische Befande. *Kleintierpraxis* **38**, 83–88.

7 Bubenheimer P and Kneissl GD (1989) *Doppler-Echokardiographie*. Verlag Edition Medizin, Weinheim, Basel, Cambridge.

8 Cobb MA (1992) Idiopathic dilated cardiomyopathy: advances in aetiology, pathogenesis and management. *J. Small Anim.Pract.* **33**, 113–118.

9 Darke PGG (1990) Dopplerechocardiography in small animals. *Vet. Internat.* **2**, 3–13.

10 Darke PGG (1992) Dopplerechocardiography. *J. Small Anim.Pract.* **33**, 104–112.

11 Ettinger SJ and Suter PF (1970) *Canine Cardiology*. WB Saunders, New York, Philadelphia, London.

12 Evans SM and Biery DN (1980) Congenital peritoneopericardial diaphragma hernia in the dog and cat: a literature review and 17 additional case histories. *Vet. Radiol.* **21**, 108.

13 Fehske W (1988) *Praxis der Konventionellen und Farbkodierten Doppler-Echokardiographie*. Verlag Hans Huber, Bern, Stuttgart, Toronto.

14 Fuentes VL (1992) Feline heart disease: an update. *J. Small Anim.Pract.* **33**, 130–137.

15 Kersten U and Brass W (1973) Untersuchungen zur Ätiologie und Pathogenese der Endokardiose und Endokarditis des Handes. *Dtsch. Tierärztl. Wschr.* **80**, 293–316.

16 Kersten U (1989) Zirkulationsapparat. In: Suter PF and Niemand HG (Eds) *Praktikum der Handeklinik*. Verlag Paul Parey, Hamburg and Berlin, pp. 394–427.

17 Kirberger RM, Van den Berg PB and Darazs B (1992) Doppler echocardiography in the normal dog. Part I: Velocity findings and flow patterns. *Vet. Radiol.* **33**, 370–379.

18 Kirberger RM and Berry WL (1992) Atrial septal defect in a dog: the value of Doppler echocardiography. *J. South Afric. Vet. Assoc.* **63**, 43–48.

19 Köhler E (1990) *Ein- und zweidimensionale Echokardiographie mit Dopplertechnik: Untersuchung, Befandung und Interpretation*. 4th Edn. Enke Verlag, Stuttgart.

20 Kujat C (1986) III 2.1 Echokardiographie im Erwachsenenalter. 4. Ergänzungslieferung. In: Braun B, Günther R and Schwerk W (Eds.) *Ultraschalldiagnostik. Lehrbuch und Atlas. Vol 2*. Verlag Ecomed. Landsberg, München, Zürich.

21 Lombard CW (1984) Echocardiographic and clinical signs of canine dilated cardiomyopathy. *J. Small Anim.Pract.* **25**, 59–70.

22 Lombard CW (1984) Normal values of canine M-mode echocardiogram. *Am. J. Vet. Res.* **45**, 2015–2018.

23 Lombard CW (1986) Klinische Echokardiographie bei Hand und Katze. *Berl. Münch. Tierärztl. Wschr.* **99**, 293–300.

24 Madron E de (1991) Rôle de l'échocardiographie doppler en mode continu et pulsé dans le diagnostic et l'évaluation de la sévérité des cardiopathies des petits animaux. Deuxième partie: caractéristiques Doppler des principales cardiopathies. *Pratique Méd. Chirur. Anim. Compagnie* **26**, 31–42.

25 Moise SN (1989) Echocardiography: therapeutic implications. In: Kirk RW (Ed.) *Current Veterinary Therapy X, Small Animal Practice*. WB Saunders, Philadelphia, London, Toronto, Montreal, Sydney, Tokyo, pp. 201–218.

26 Moise SN (1988) Echocardiography. In: Fox PR (Ed.) *Canine and Feline Cardiology*. Churchill Livingston, New York, Edinburgh, London, pp. 113–156.

27 Pipers FS (1979) Echocardiography in the domestic cat. *Am. J. Vet. Res.* **40**, 882–886.

28 Sisson D and Schaeffer H (1991) Changes in linear dimensions of the heart, relative to body weight, as measured by M-Mode echocardiography in growing dogs. *Am. J. Vet. Res.* **52**, 1591–1594.

29 Soderberg SF, Boon JA, Wingfield WE and Miller CW (1983) M-Mode echocardiography as a diagnostic aid for feline cardiomyopathy. *Vet. Radiol.* **24**, 66–73.

30 Stepien RL and Bonagura JD (1991) Aortic stenosis: clinical findings in six cats. *J. Small Anim.Pract.* **32**, 341–350.

31 Thomas WP (1984) Two-dimensional, real-time echocardiography in the dog: technique and anatomic validation. *Vet. Radiol.* **25**, 50–64.

32 Thomas WP, Sisson D and Bauer TG (1984) Detection of cardiac masses in dogs by two-dimensional echocardiography. *Vet. Radiol.* **25**, 65.

33 Thomas WP, Gaber CE, Jacobs GI, Kaplan PM, Lombard CW, Moise NS and Moses BL (1993) Recommendations for standards in transthoracic two-dimensional echocardiography in the dog and cat. Echocardiography Committee of the Specialty of Cardiology, American College of Veterinary Internal Medicine. *J. Vet. Intern. Med.* **7**, 247–52.

34 Trautvetter E and Bob M (1986) Zur Diagnose des Perikardergusses beim Hand mit Hilfe der zweidimensionalen Echokardiographie. *Berl. Münch. Tierärztl. Wschr.* **99**, 308–310.

Additional Reading

Bommer WJ and Haerten RL (1991) Die wachsende Rolle des Ultraschalls in der kardiovaskulären. *Medizin. Electromedica* **59**, 115–127.

Bonagura JD and Pipers FS (1981) Echocardiographic features of pericardial effusion in dogs. *J. Am. Vet. Med. Assoc.* **179**, 49–56.

Brown DJ, Knight DH and King RR (1991) Use of pulsed-wave Doppler echocardiography to determine aortic and pulmonary velocity and flow variables in clinically normal dogs. *Am. J. Vet. Res.* **52**, 543–550.

Dennis MO, Nealeigh RC, Pyle RL, Glbert SH, Lee AC and Miller C (1978) Echocardiographic assessment of normal and abnormal valvular function in beagle dogs. *Am. J. Vet. Res.* **39**, 1591–1598.

Fioretti M and Maccio S (1991) Interpretation, diagnostischer Wert und Grenzen der Echokardiographie bei Mitralendokardiose des Handes. *Vet. Internat.* **2**, 2–11.

Hagio M and Otsuka H (1987) Pulsed Doppler echocardiography in normal dogs and calves, and three cases of valvular regurgitation. *Jpn. J. Vet. Sci.* **49**, 1113–1125.

Jiang L, Siu SC, Handschuhmacher MD, Luis-Guerrero J, Vazquez-De-Prada JA, King ME, Picard MH, Weymann AE and Levine RA (1994) Three-dimensional echocardiography. *In vivo* validation for right ventricular volume and function. *Circulation* **89(5)**, 2342–2350.

Kirberger RM (1991) Mitral valve E point to ventricular septal separation in the dog. *J. South Afric. Vet. Assoc.* **62**, 163–166.

Kirberger RM, Van den Berg PB and Grimbeek RJ (1992) Doppler echocardiography in the normal dog. Part II: Factors influencing blood flow velocities and a comparison between left and right heart blood flow. *Vet. Radiol.* **33**, 380–386.

Köhler E (1993) *Klinische Echokardiographie*. 3rd Edn. Enke Verlag. Stuttgart.

Lehmkuhl LB and Bonagura JD (1994) Comparison of transducer placement sites for Doppler echocardiography in dogs with subaortic stenosis. *Am. J. Vet. Res.* **55(2)**, 192–198.

Pipers FS, Bonagura JD, Hamlin RL and Kittleson M (1981) Echocardiographic abnormalities of the mitral valve associated with left-side heart diseases in the dog. *J. Am. Vet. Med. Assoc.* **179**, 580–586.

Vollmar A (1991) Die Ultraschalluntersuchung des Herzens bei Hand und Katze im 2D- und M-Mode-Verfahren und ihre Konsequenzen für die Therapie der Herzerkrankungen. *Kleintierpraxis* **36**, 459–468.

10 Abdominal and Pelvic Cavity

Dirk Lüerssen and Martin Janthur

Gastrointestinal Tract

Instrumentation and Examination Technique

Gastrointestinal morphology and function are evaluated ultrasonographically by using moderate to high-frequency linear, curved-array or sector scanners. The amount and type of ingesta determine the outcome of the examination. A fluid-filled gastrointestinal tract enhances the ultrasound image.

To obtain the best results, patients should be prepared correctly for examination. Gastrointestinal air and ingesta is reduced by fasting for 12–24 hours or by administering a gas-reducing agent (Dimeticon; Lefax®, Sab Simplex Drops®). Giving water is also recommended. A stomach tube may be used to remove excess gastric air and to administer warm (20°C/68°F) water (up to 15 ml/kg). This is an excellent method for visualizing the stomach and other abdominal organs[4, 6]. Radiographic barium contrast studies should always be performed after the ultrasonographic examination. Barium causes total reflection of sound waves and degrades the image. Contrast-media containing iodine (Telebrix®) do not cause the same problems.

Normal Sonographic Findings

The gastrointestinal tract can only be visualized in separate segments. Convoluted intestines and artefacts do not permit imaging of the entire tract.

Stomach

The stomach is visualized regularly in the ultrasound image. Portions of the stomach wall seen in the near field are located caudal to the liver in the left and mid-abdomen. Wall structures in the far field are usually masked by ingesta. Animals are usually examined in dorsal recumbency, although a standing position is helpful when the stomach is partially fluid filled. Intraluminal gas is displaced dorsally by the fluid.

The normal stomach wall averages 3–5 mm in thickness and shows approximately 4–5 contractions per minute. Water intake increases peristaltic activity by an additional contraction per minute. Mucosal rugae are visible. Mural thickness of more than 6–7 mm is pathological. The rugae in an empty stomach may lead to false measurements of wall thickness[5, 6].

The normal stomach wall consists of 3–5 distinguishable layers (**357**). Ultrasonographic resolution in smaller patients may only distinguish three layers. The rugae in an empty stomach appear 'cauliflower'-like in the ultrasonographic image. This is seen more often in cats than in dogs (**358–361**). Highly echogenic gastric contents usually mask the gastric wall. Under optimal conditions, it is possible to differentiate five layers in medium-sized to large patients[5, 6].

outside ↓	1.	entering echo, hyperechoic line at the interface between surrounding tissue and serosa
	2.	hypoechoic band, muscularis propria layer
	3.	hyperechoic line, interface to the subserosa
	4.	hypoechoic band, submucosa and mucosa
inside	5.	exiting echo, hyperechoic line at the interface between the mucosal surface and the stomach lumen including ingesta.

357

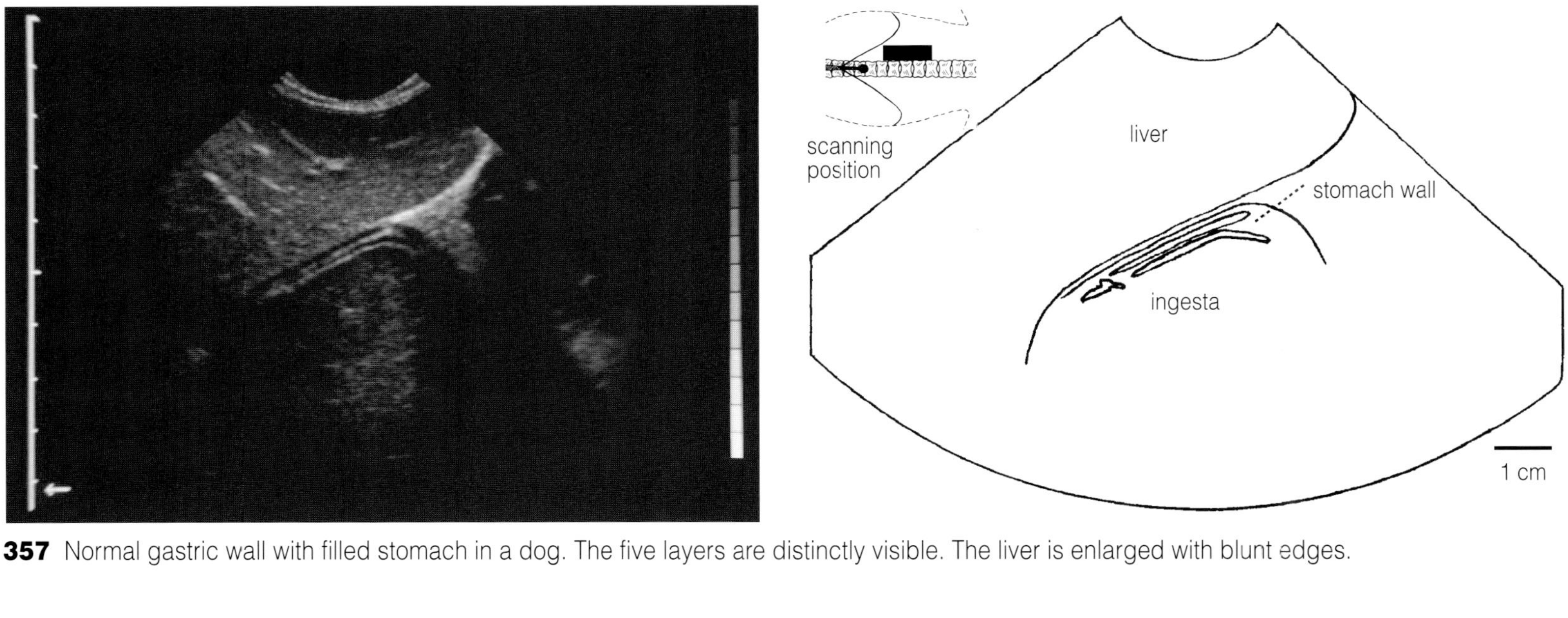

357 Normal gastric wall with filled stomach in a dog. The five layers are distinctly visible. The liver is enlarged with blunt edges.

358

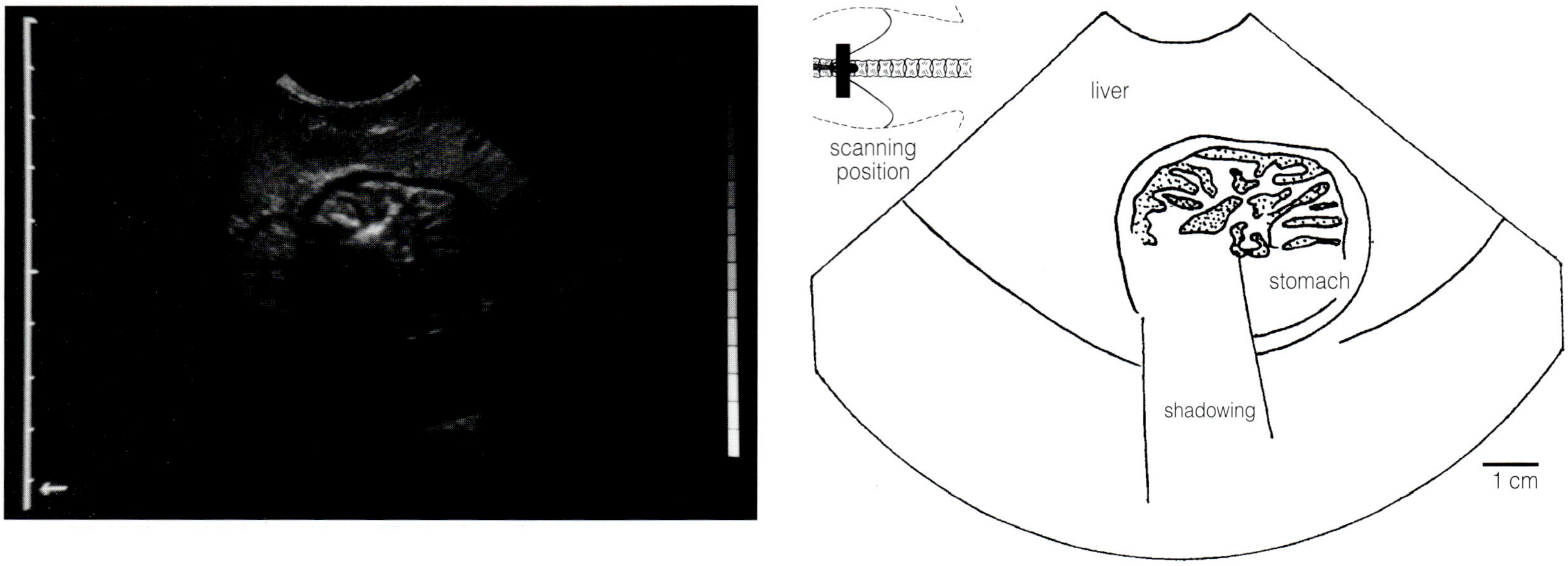

359

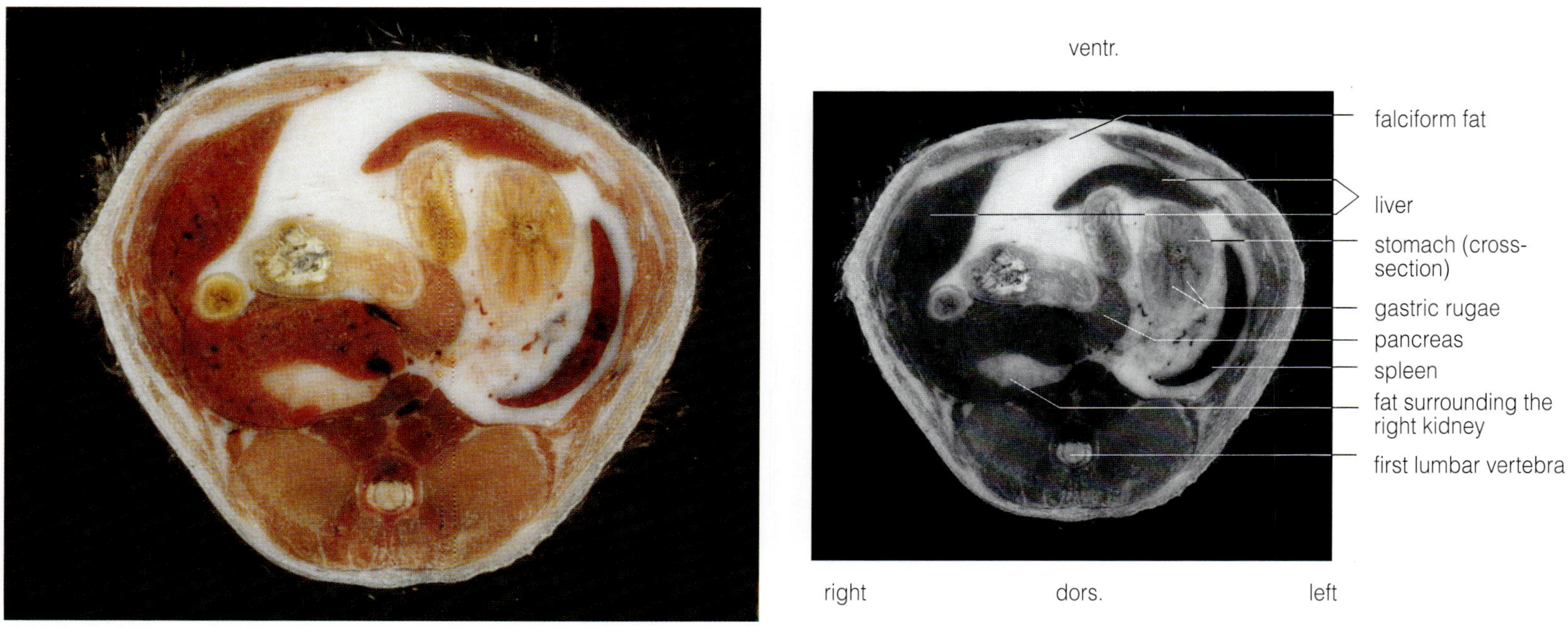

358–361 Two-dimensional sonograms (**358, 360**) and anatomical cross-sections (**359, 361**) of an empty stomach in a dog (**358, 359**) and a cat (**360, 361**). Typical mucosal rugae are seen in the transverse (**358, 359**) and longitudinal (**360, 361**) gastric body. Gas and hyperechoic ingesta cause acoustic shadowing (**358**).

Bowel

The five layers of the stomach wall are also found in the entire small bowel. Long intestinal villi make the hypoechoic fourth layer appear wider than in the stomach (362). These layers cannot be differentiated in the large bowel (366).

Duodenal contractions are the same as in the stomach. The jejunum and ileum show approximately one to three contractions per minute (363–365), while peristalsis is rarely noted in the colon. Wall thickness in the entire bowel is between 2 and 3 mm, depending on the contractions [5,6].

The descending colon is identified retrogradely. The presence of fluid, faeces and/or gas helps to distinguish the large bowel. Structures in the far field are usually masked, except when the colon is filled with fluid. The descending colon is found dorsal to the urinary bladder and can be followed cranially, left to median. While the transverse colon is identified caudal to the stomach by its diameter, the ascending colon and caecum cannot be differentiated. The cranial portion of the duodenum (located to the dorsal right of the pylorus) and the descending duodenum (covered by the rib cage) may be identified within the convoluted small intestines. The small bowel segments are imaged from the left abdominal wall with the spleen acting as an acoustic window.

360

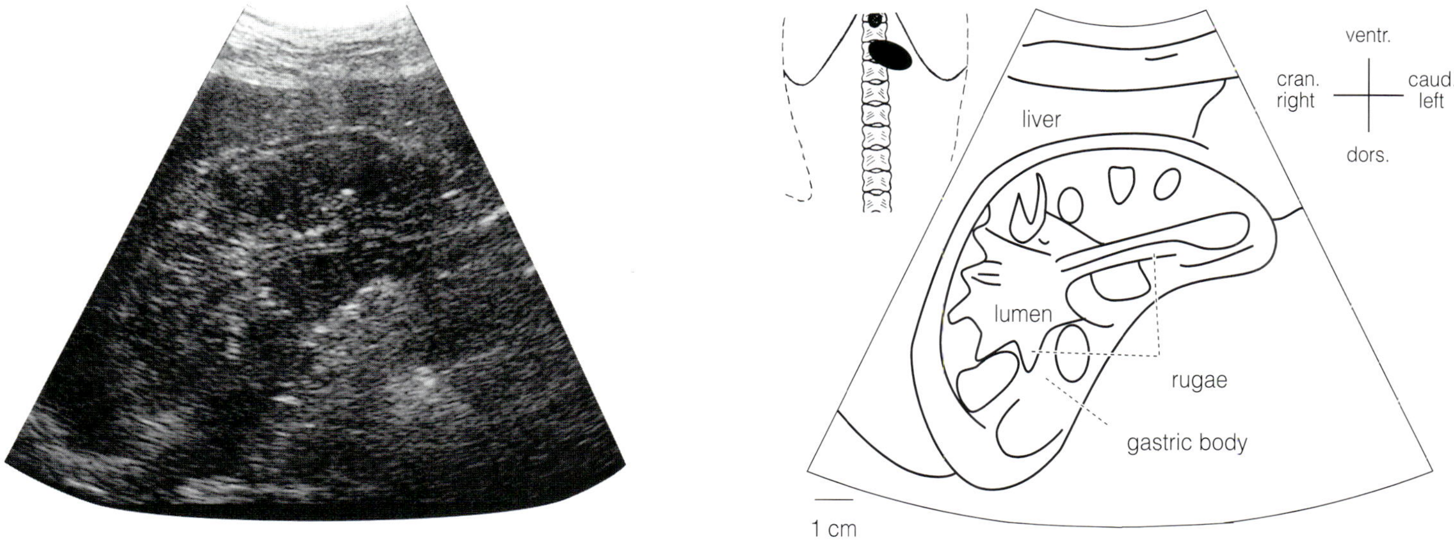

361

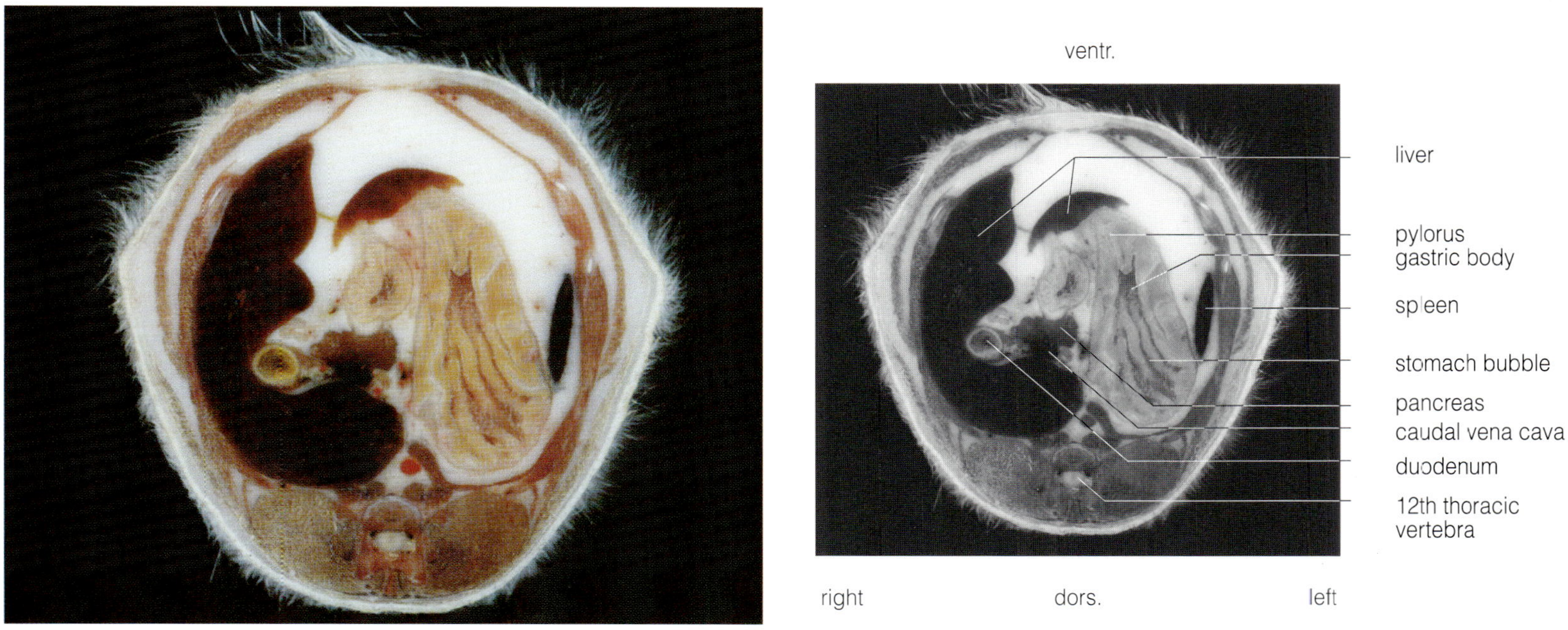

362

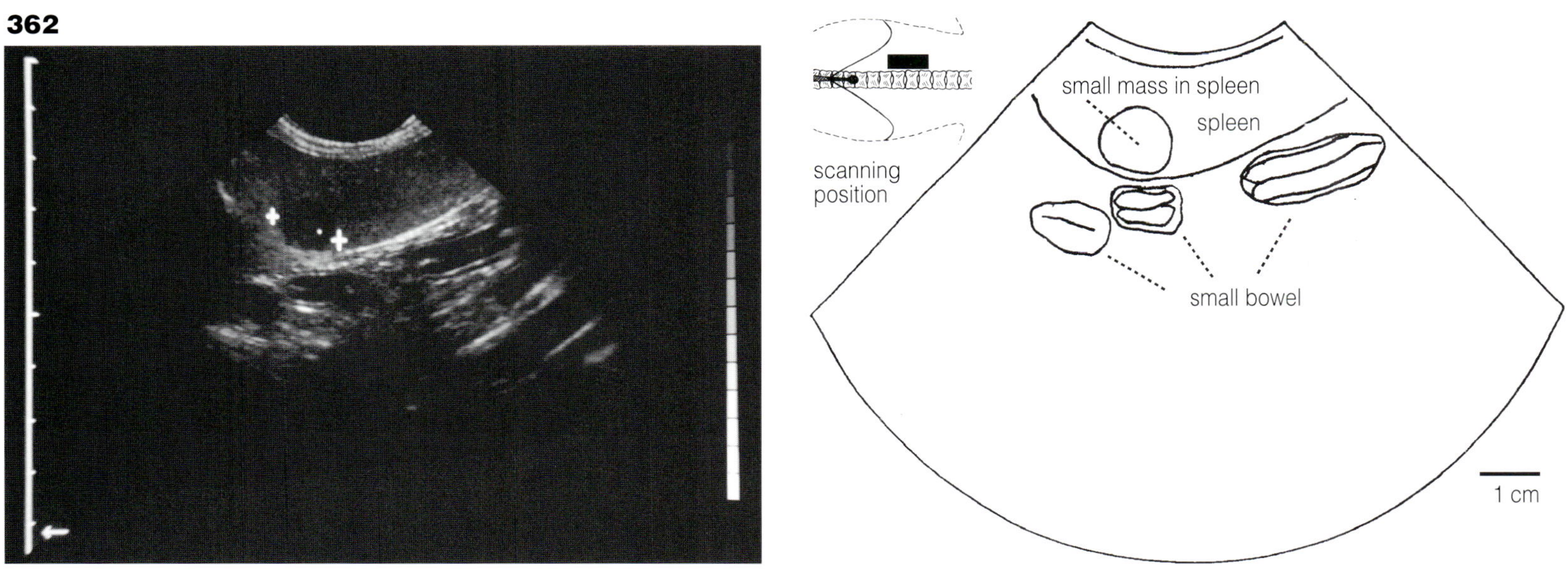

362 Normal jejunum in a dog. Using the spleen as an acoustic window, the five ultrasonographic layers of the small bowel are recognized in longitudinal and transverse planes ('coffee bean').

363

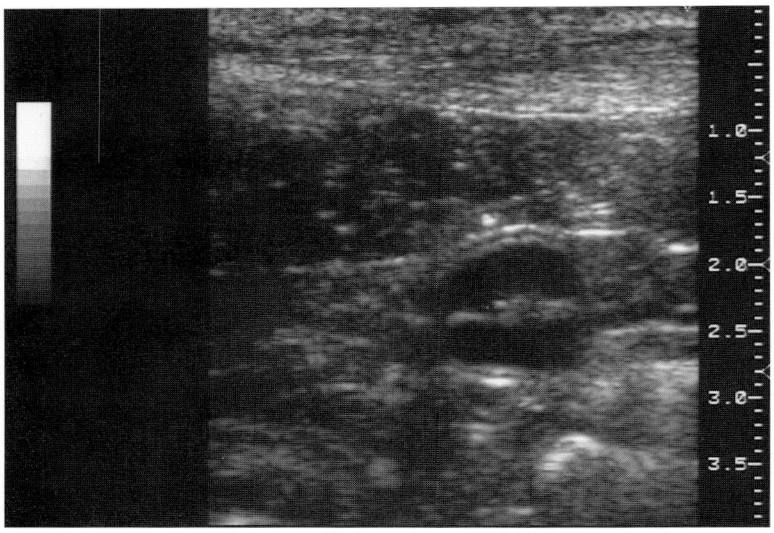

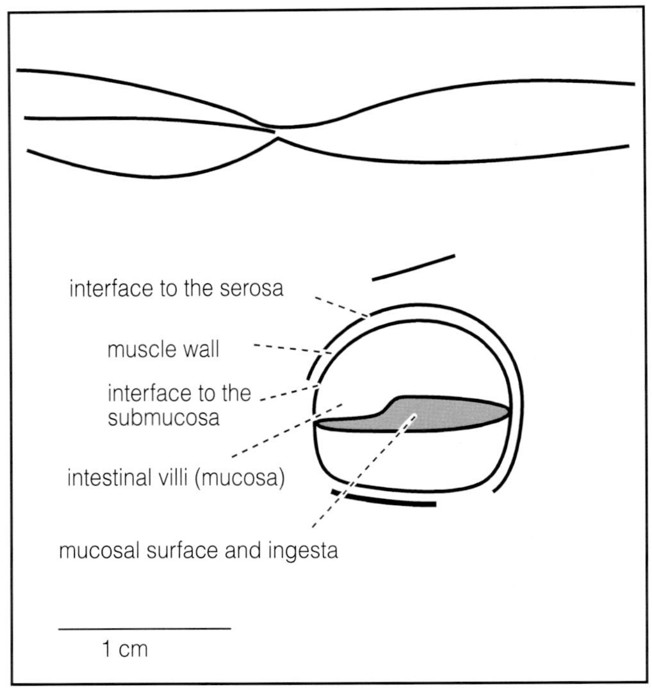

364

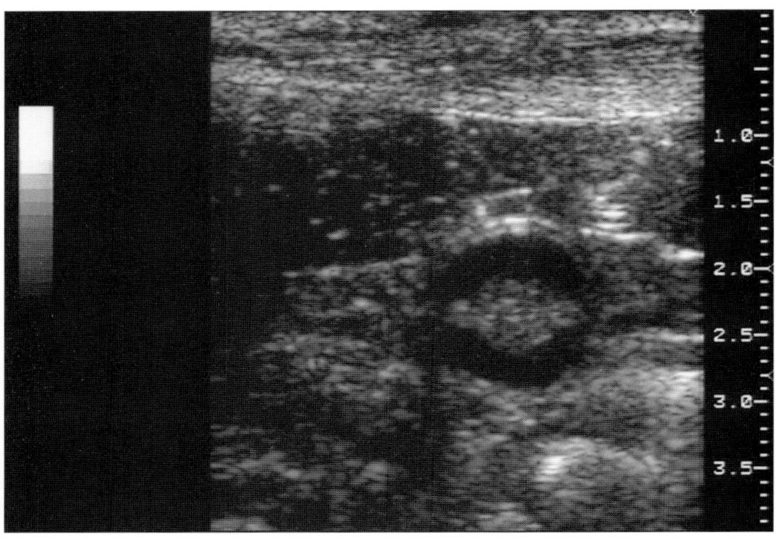

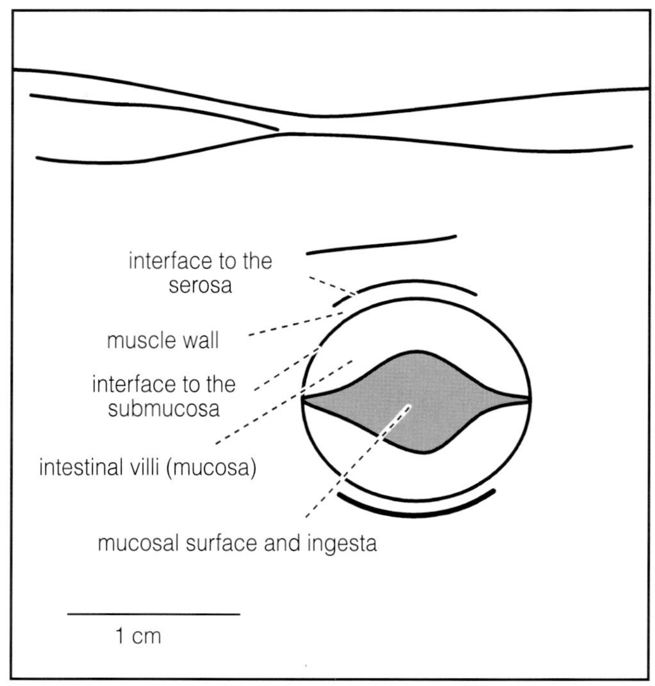

365

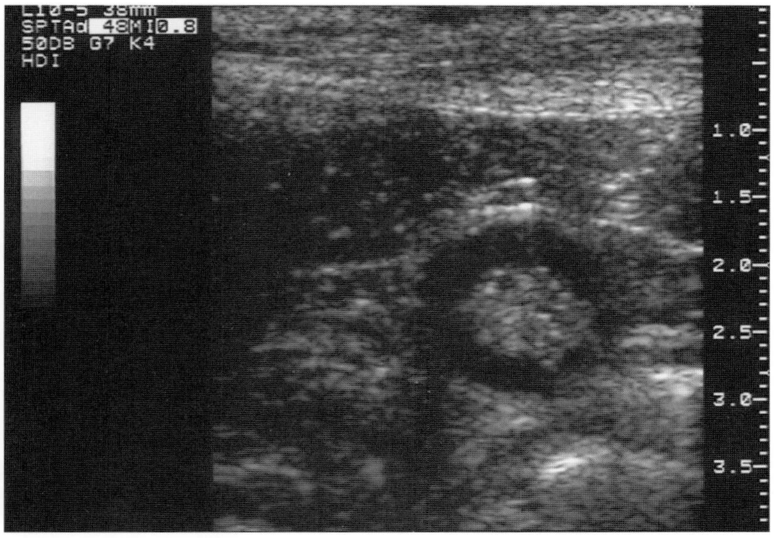

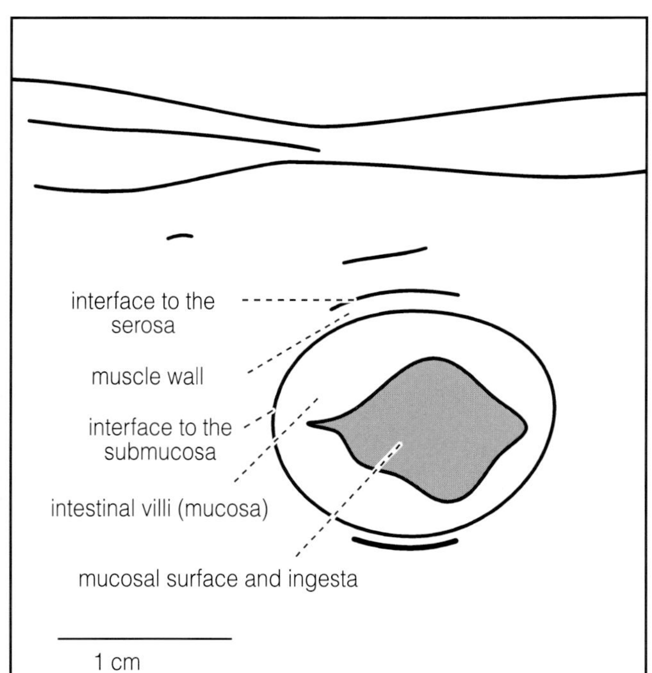

363–365 Normal jejunum during a peristaltic contraction in a dog. Cross-section of the small bowel before (**363**), at the beginning of (**364**) and during (**365**) the ingesta passage.

366

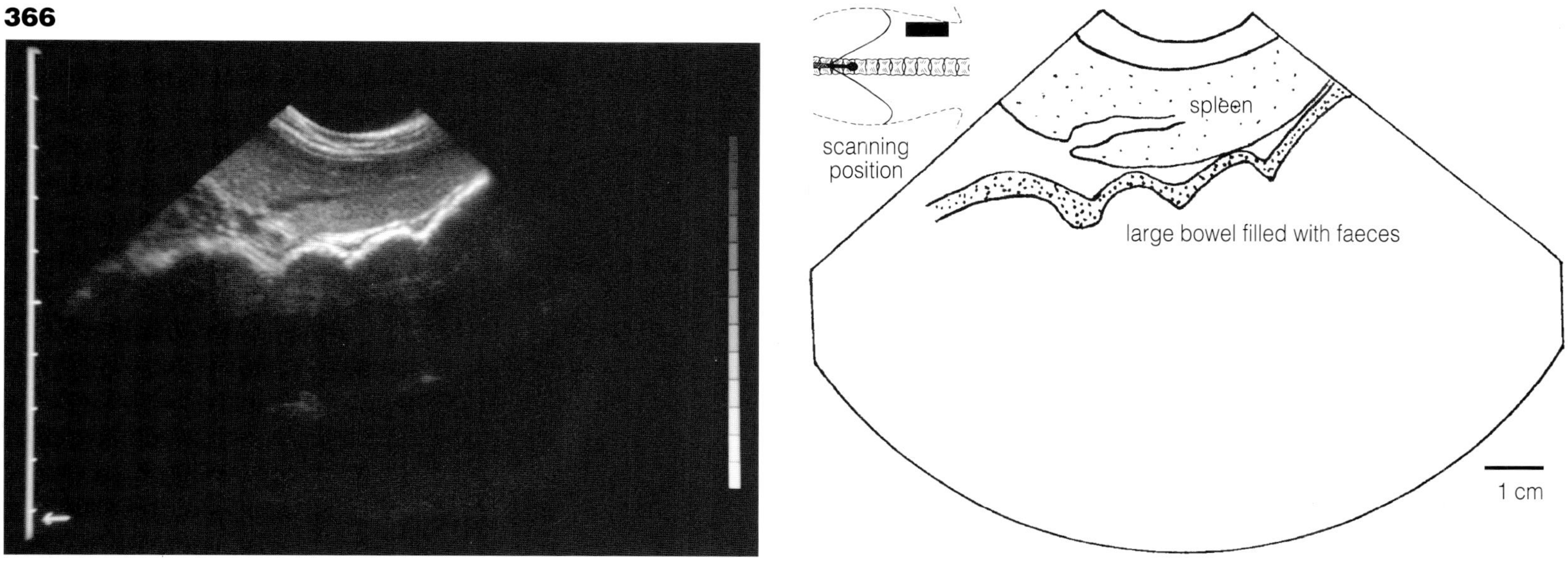

366 Descending colon of a dog. The unique appearance with distal shadowing is caused by faeces. This is not a pathological finding.

367

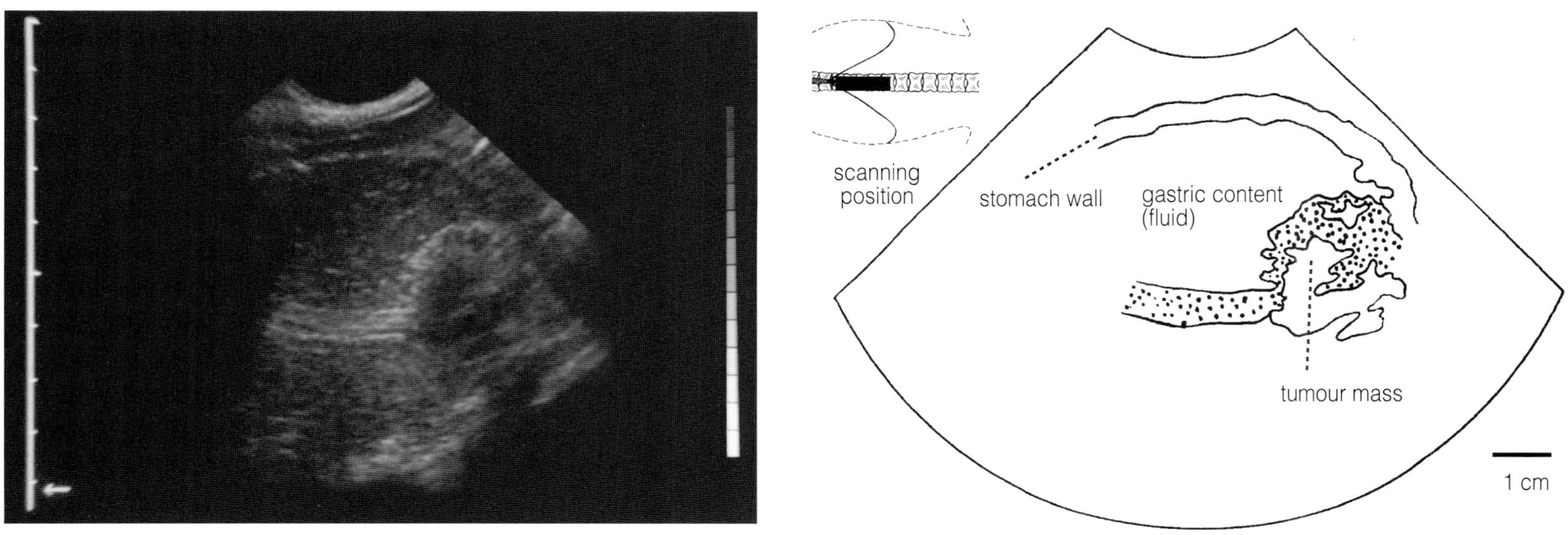

367 Stomach wall mass in a dog with vomiting. Mucosal carcinoma was found histopathologically. The stomach is filled with fluid, which favours visualization. The tumour obstructed gastric outflow and caused fluid retention.

Ultrasonography of Gastrointestinal Disorders

An ultrasonographic diagnosis of gastrointestinal disorder is only possible in conjunction with history, a clinical examination including laboratory profiles, and other imaging methods. Precise sonographic findings or pathognomonic images of the gastrointestinal tract are rarely found, apart from cases of intussusception. Wall thickening, seen with tumours and inflammation, is usually easier to interpret than circumscript thinning of the mucosal layer, e.g. with ulcerations or erosions.

Sonography of Gastric Disorders

Focal lesions (**367, 368**) of the stomach wall are recognized as wall thickening and/or an irregular wall structure. Adjacent

> *Indications for ultrasonographic examination of the gastrointestinal tract include an acute abdomen, vomiting, diarrhoea, and unclear abdominal disorders with suspected:*
>
> - Inflammatory diseases.
> - Neoplasia.
> - Foreign bodies.
> - Motility disorders.
> - Displacement, ileus and stenosis.
>
> A further indication is for monitoring treatment response.

368

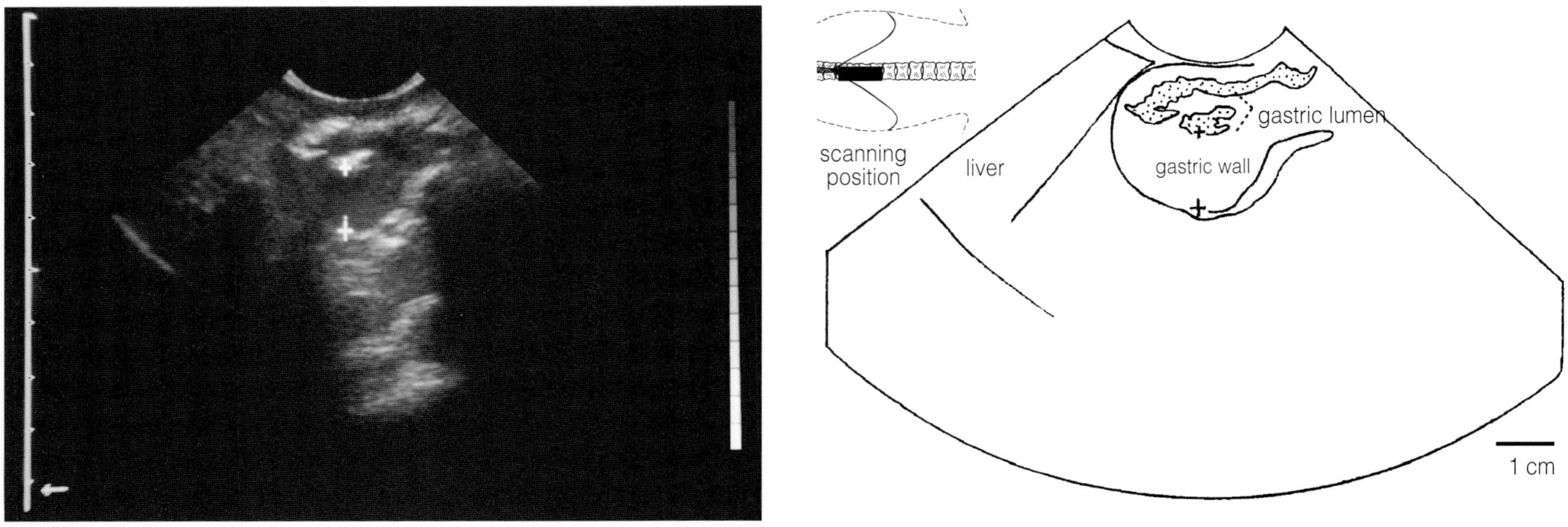

368 Decentralized gastric lumen and focal hypoechoic stomach wall lesion in a cat. Tentative diagnosis of a stomach wall tumour was confirmed histopathologically (infiltrative, solid gastric mucosal carcinoma). A similar image is found with chronic gastric ulceration.

369

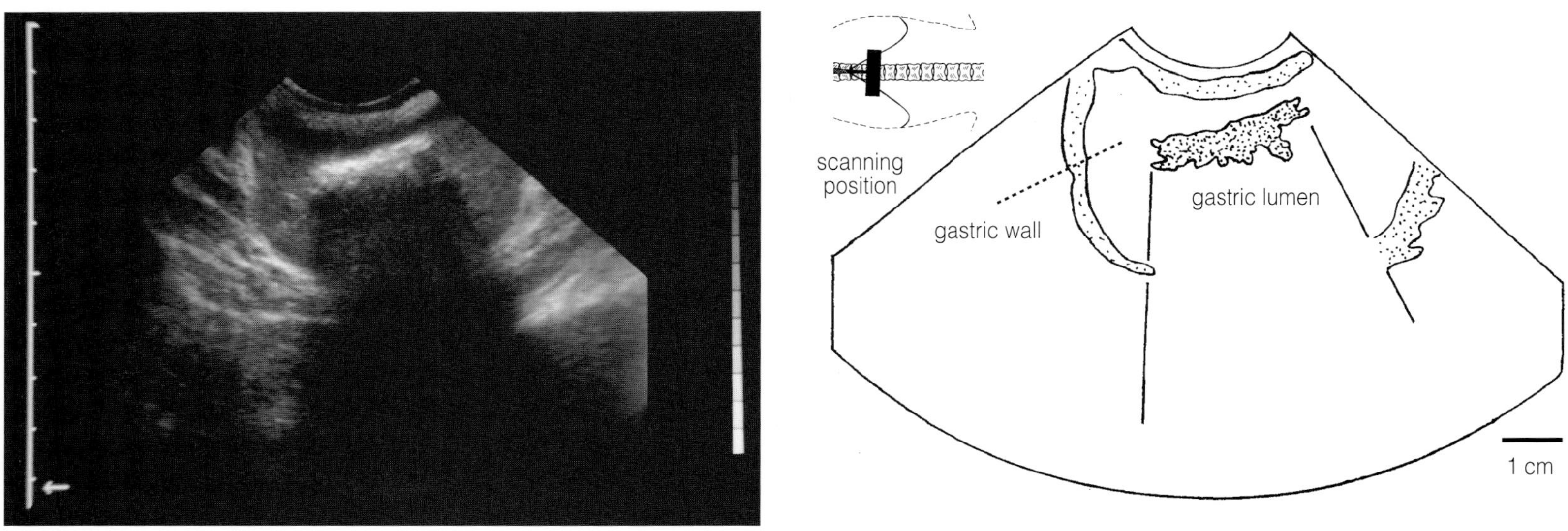

369 Generalized uniformly echogenic thickening of the stomach wall in a cat. Gastric contents produce distal shadowing. Histopathology confirmed the tumour (lymphoma). A similar image is seen with chronic gastritis.

370

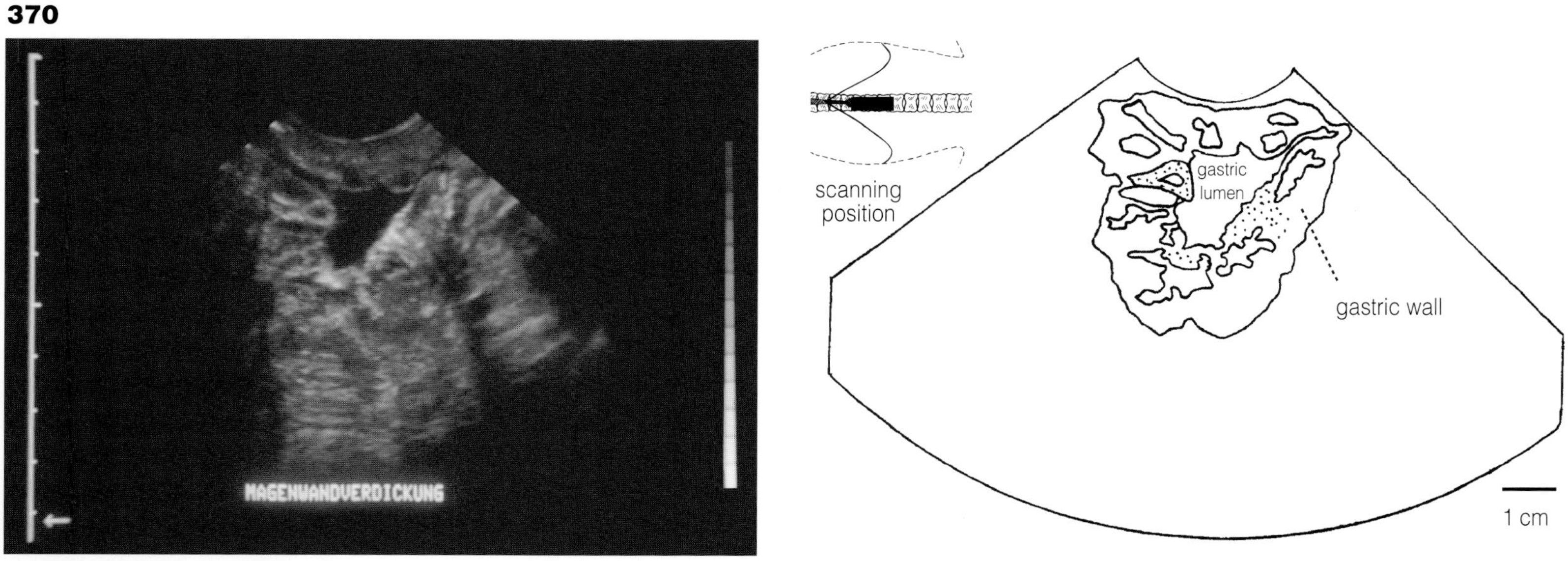

370 Fluid-filled stomach with marked generalized thickening and non-homogenous texture of the mucosa in a dog. Chronic gastritis was suggested and confirmed histopathologically (eosinophilic gastritis). Neoplasia has a similar ultrasonographic appearance.

371

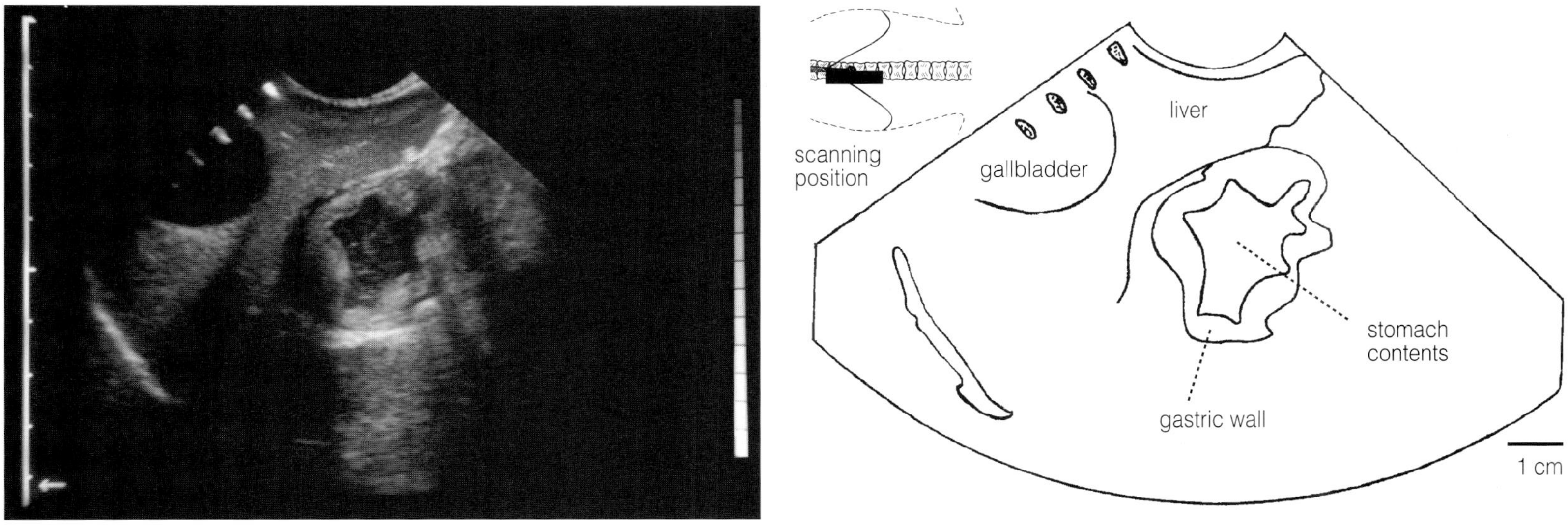

371 Fluid-filled stomach in a dog. Marked thickening and echogenicity of the wall suggests gastritis.

372

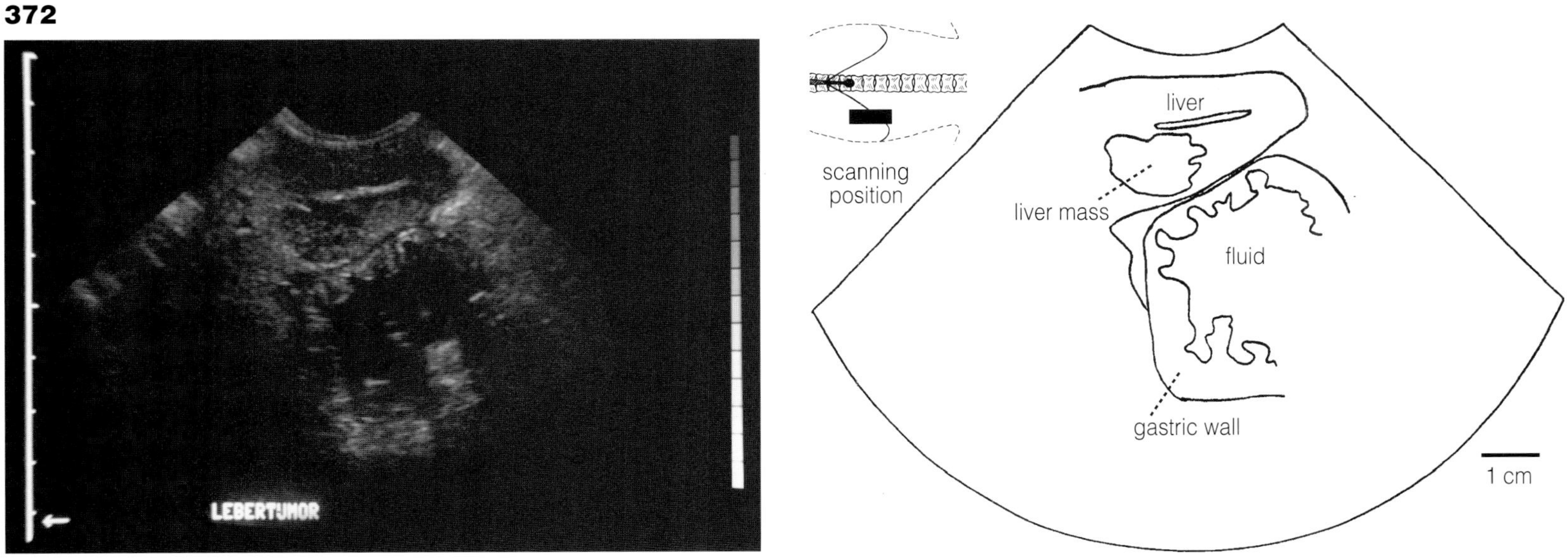

372 Fluid-filled stomach in a dog, four hours after drinking. The gastric wall is normal. The slowed passage of gastric contents is of unknown origin. A hypoechoic liver mass may be the cause of metastatic stomach lesions near the pylorus. Visualization of a stenosis is not always possible with ultrasonography.

segments show normal sonographic findings. Plaques with higher or lower echogenicity are indicative of inflammation or neoplasia.

Diffuse abnormalities affect the entire stomach wall and they are also seen with neoplasia (369) and inflammatory disease (370). Gastritis is diagnosed most commonly (371). Generalized hyperechogenicity of the mucosa is often caused by mineralization[3].

Focal or diffuse wall lesions cannot always be associated with a specific layer in the sonographic image. Further diagnostics include filling the stomach with water to test if the gastric wall is flexible and becomes thinner with fluid accumulation or remains inelastic and thickened. When a patient shows a fluid-filled stomach, the following history must be taken:

- Water intake immediately before the examination.
- Polydipsia.
- Stenosis (372).

The stenotic area is not always visible. Hypertrophic pyloric stenosis in young dogs (373, 374) and chronic hypertrophic pyloric gastropathy of the adult dog[1] can be visualized.

Gastric foreign bodies are difficult to identify ultrasonographically. Ultrasonography can give additional information to suspicious radiographic findings. Fluid stomach contents facilitate imaging, while gas and ingesta make it more difficult. Stones and needles are identified by their total reflection and distal acoustic shadowing. Balls have variable echogenicities and may be recognized by a round, capsule-like hyperechoic line[8]. A foreign body may be identified in a fluid-filled stomach and will move when the patient's position is changed.

Ingesta in the stomach may lead to a false diagnosis (375, 376). Contents in stomachs with decreased gastric motility are indicative of gastric dilation (377). Lack of gastric peristaltis is seen with chronic partial ileus (378) but also with gastritis. Hyperperistalsis is present with acute disorders. This may be caused by foreign bodies in the pyloric region, acute gastritis and ruptured stomachs.

373

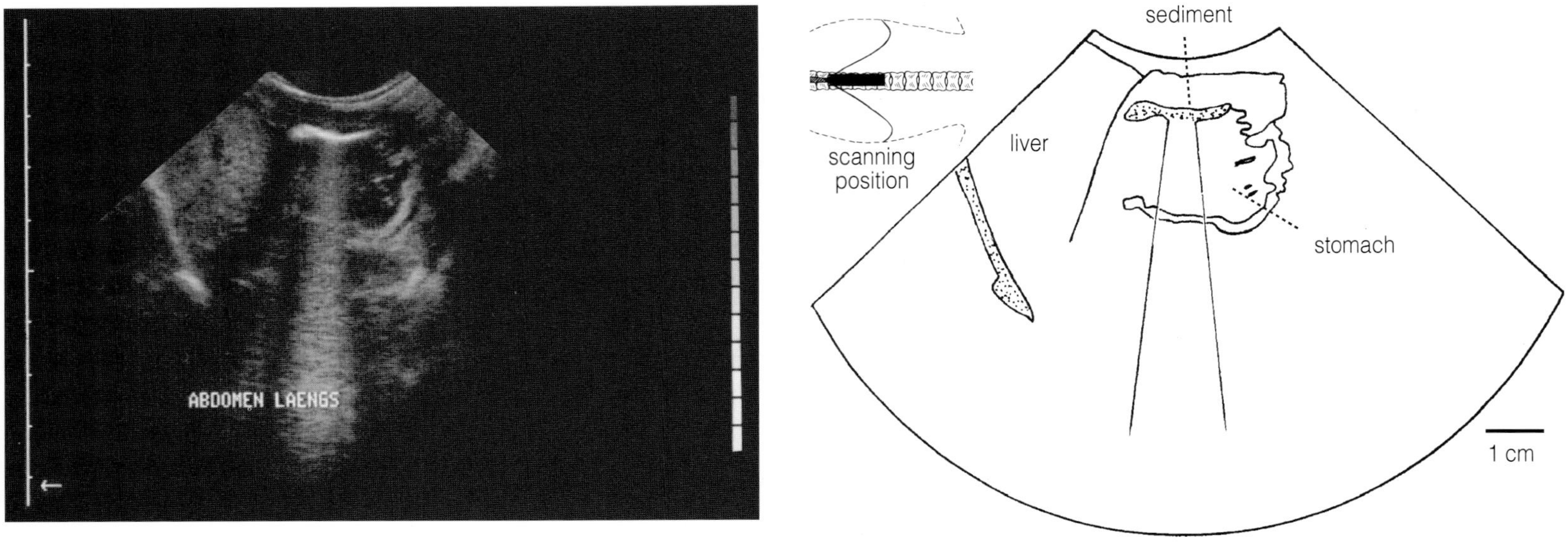

374

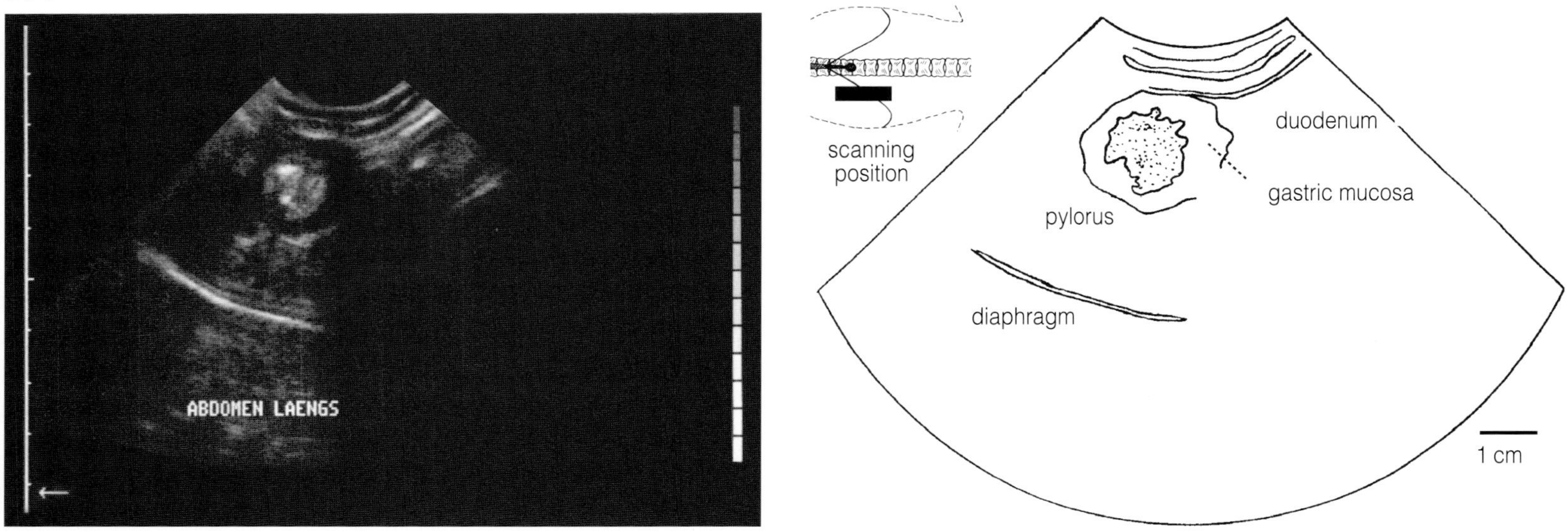

373, 374 Gastric body (**373**) and pylorus (**374**) in a standing puppy. There is fluid accumulation in the gastric body (**373**) and thickening of the pyloric mucosa (**374**). These findings indicate pyloric stenosis.

375

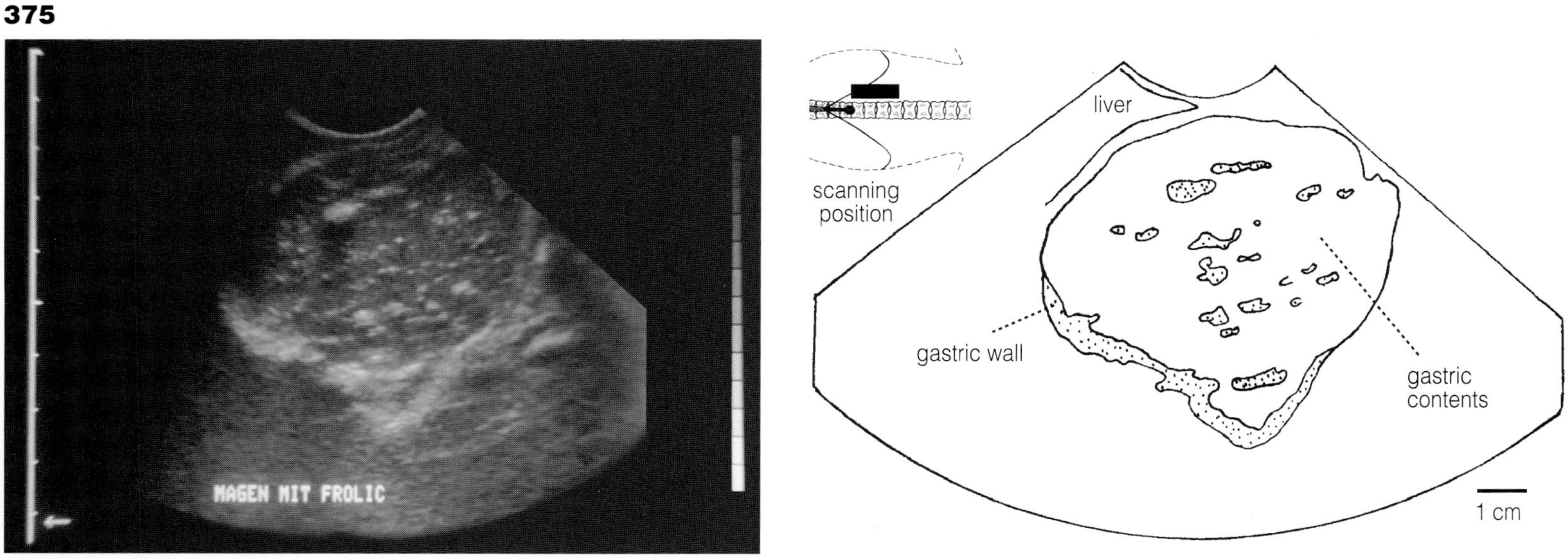

375 Stomach filled with ingesta in a dog. **NB:** These contents may simulate non-homogenous parenchyma.

376

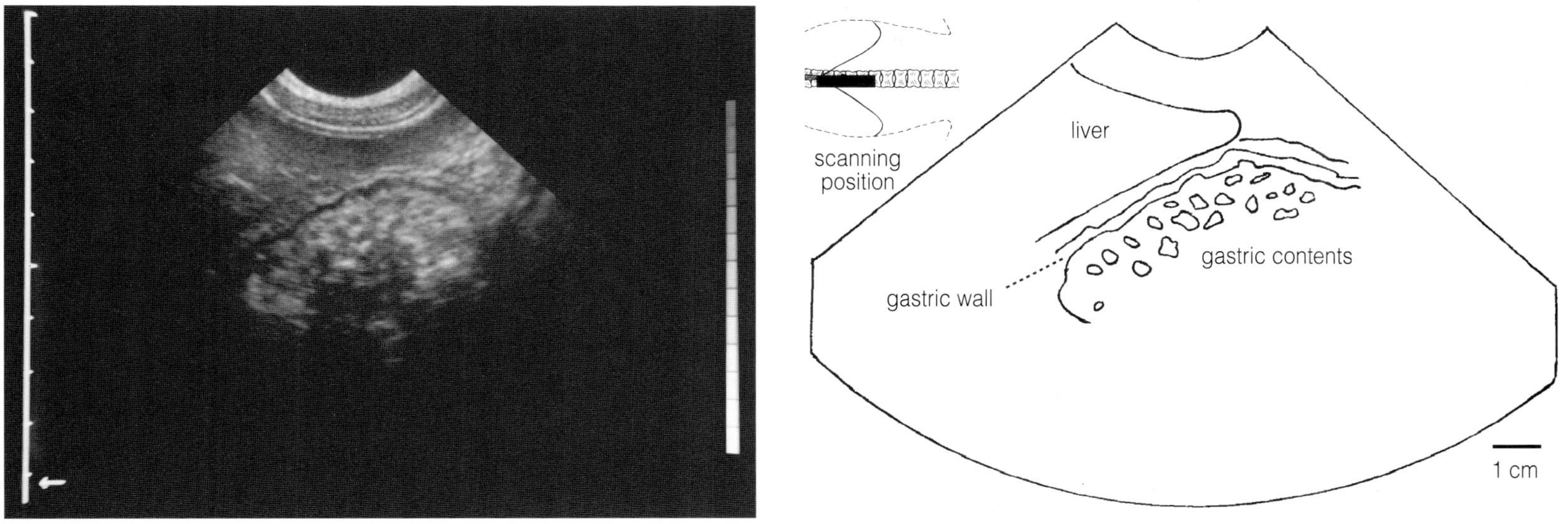

376 Stomach filled with ingesta in a dog after a rice meal. *NB:* These contents may simulate non-homogenous parenchyma.

377

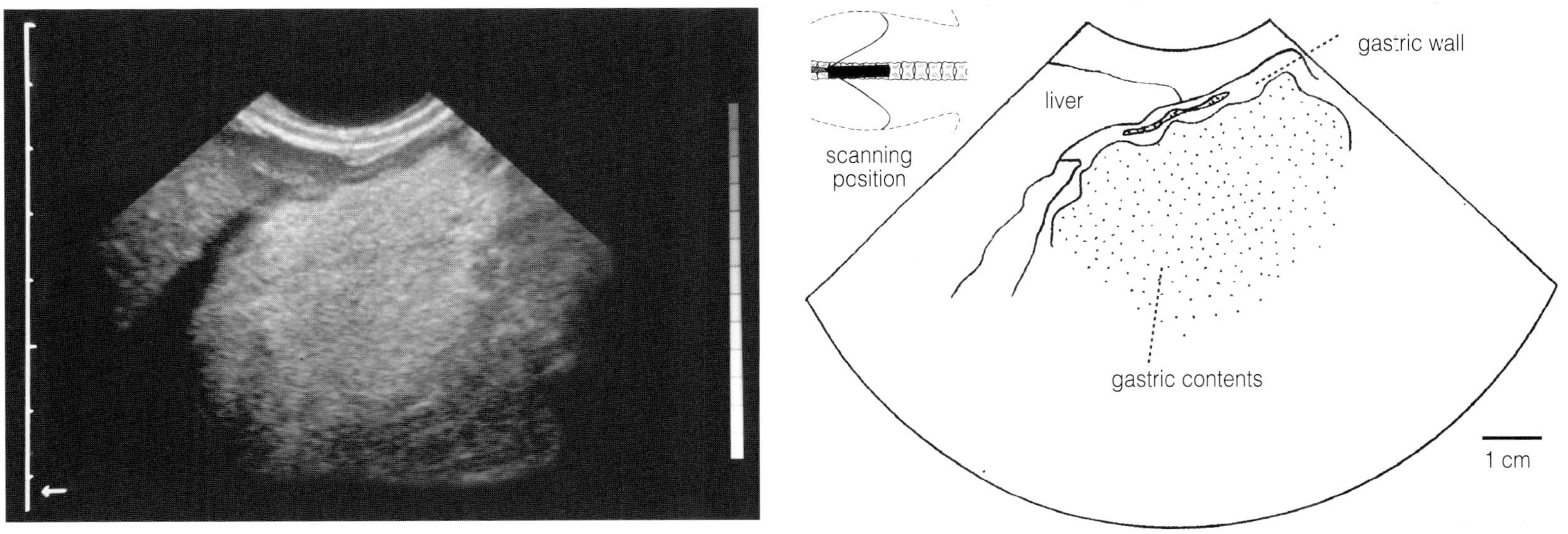

377 Severely dilated stomach filled with ingesta in a dog.

378

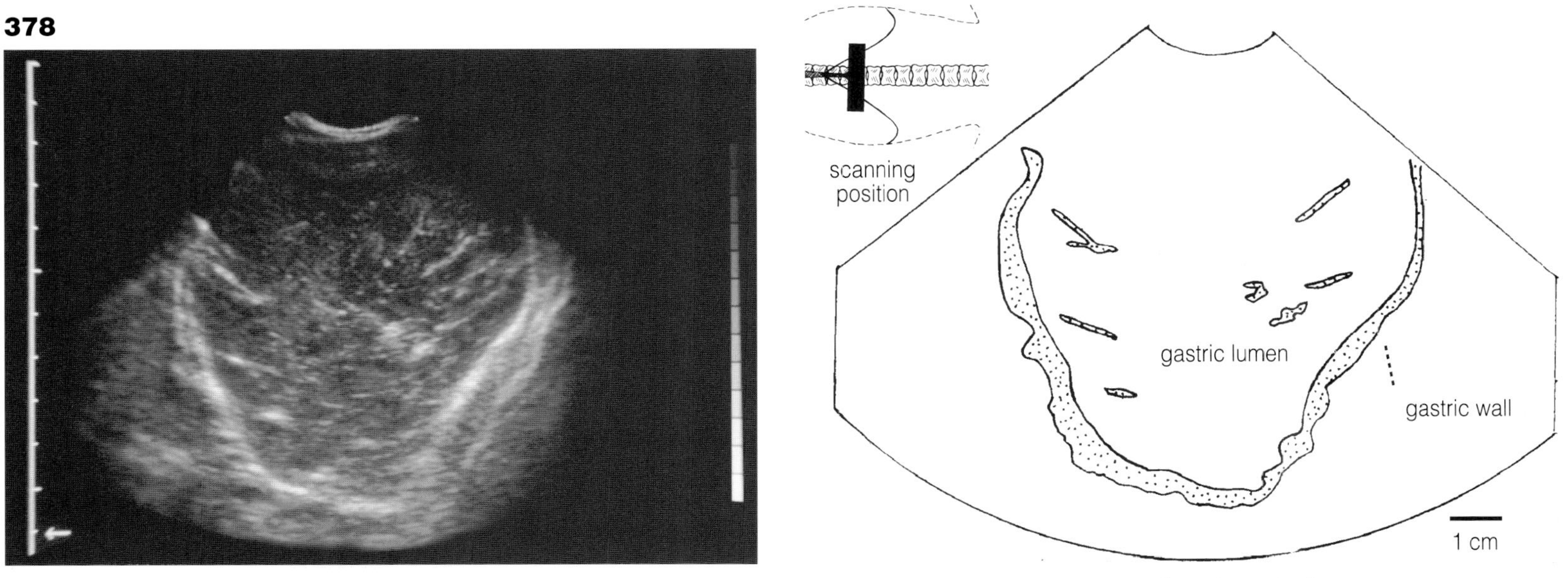

378 Severely dilated, fluid-filled stomach in a Persian cat suggesting gastric ileus. A pyloric trichobezoar was found surgically.

379

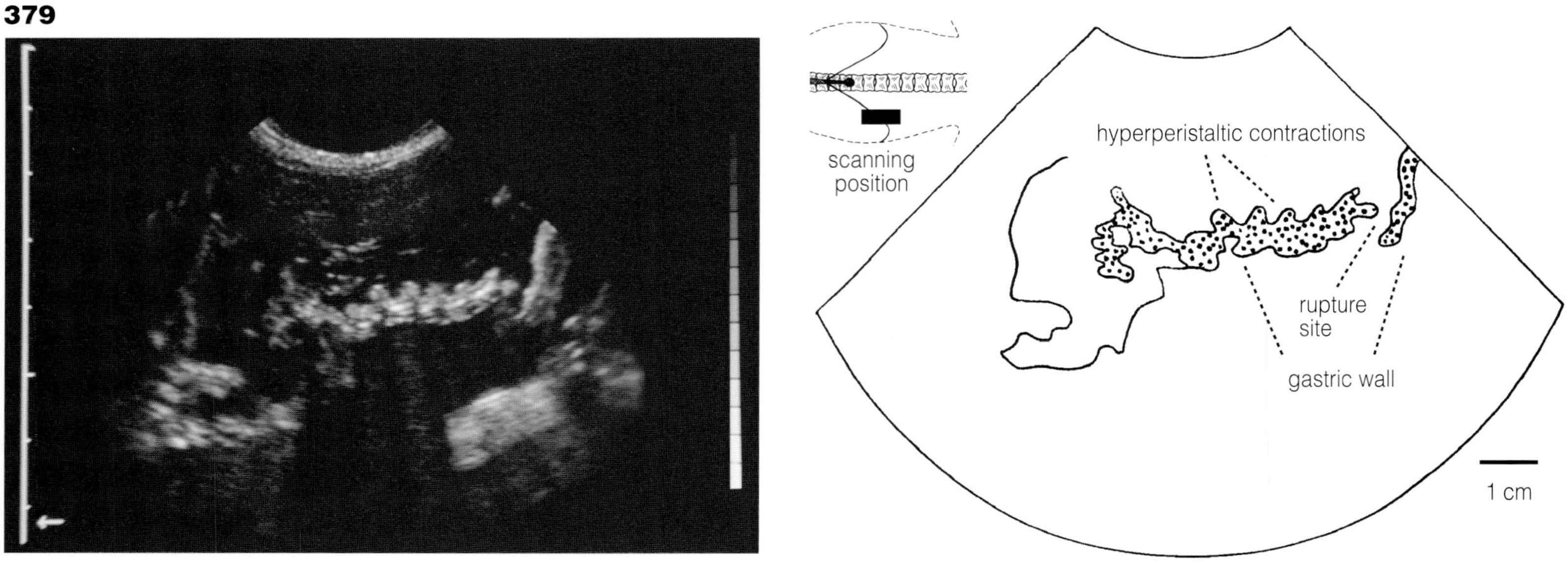

379 Ruptured stomach in a dog following a car accident. The severed stomach wall is only seen with optimal scanning conditions. Hyperperistalsis is characteristic. Free abdominal fluid and/or ingesta are seen as echogenic irregular structures, depending on the stomach contents and amount of haemorrhaging.

380

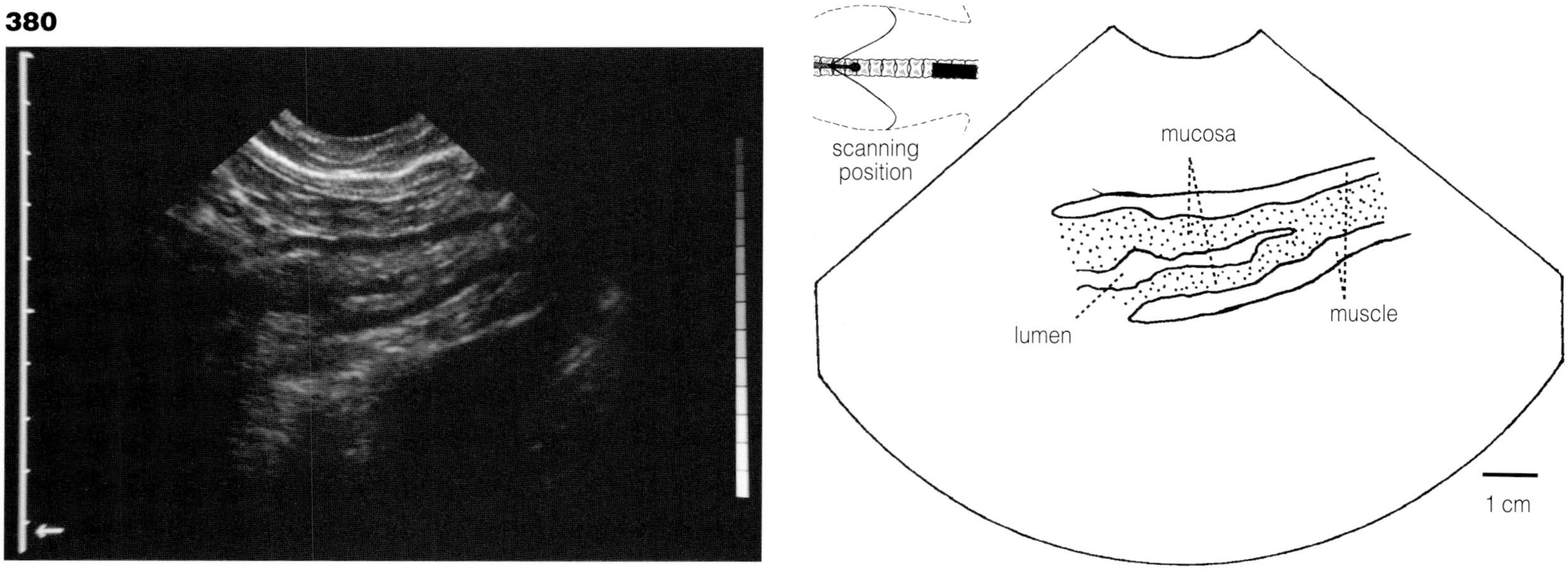

381

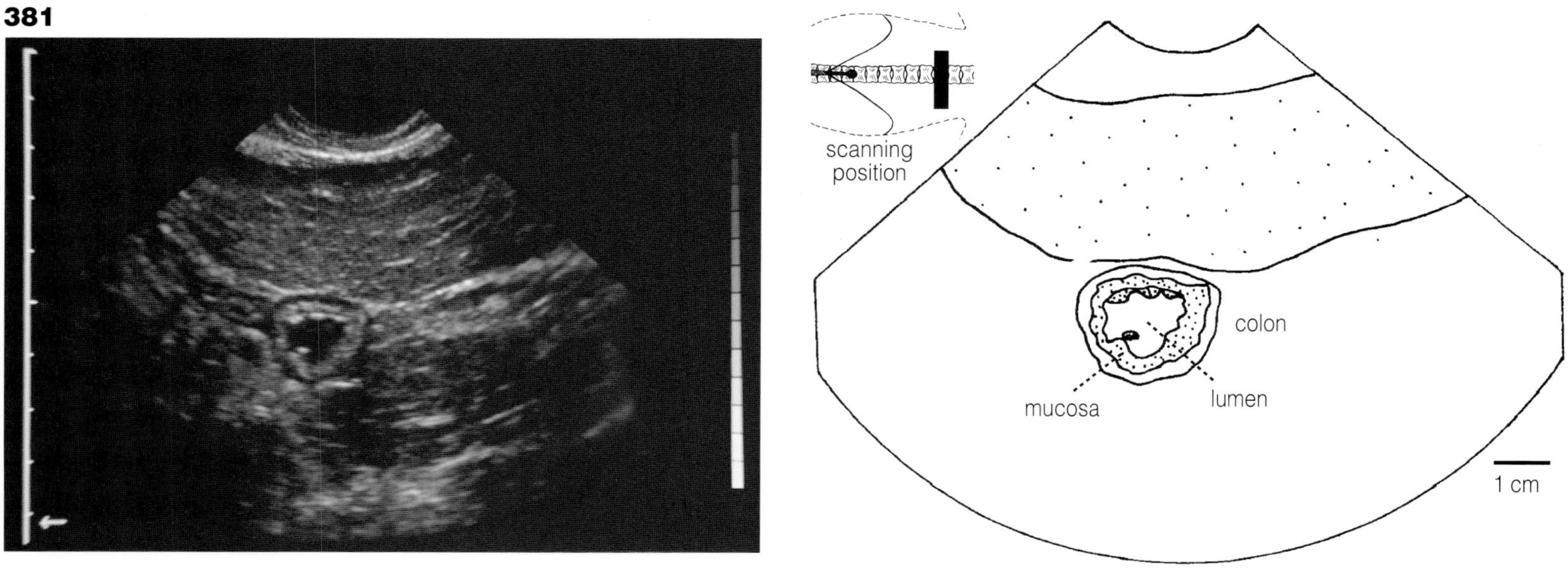

380, 381 Longitudinal (**380**) and transverse (**381**) scans of an enlarged colon in a cat. The anechoic muscle layer can easily be distinguished from the hyperechoic thickened mucosa. The lumen is filled with fluid and is anechoic. Histopathological studies of a biopsy confirmed colitis.

382

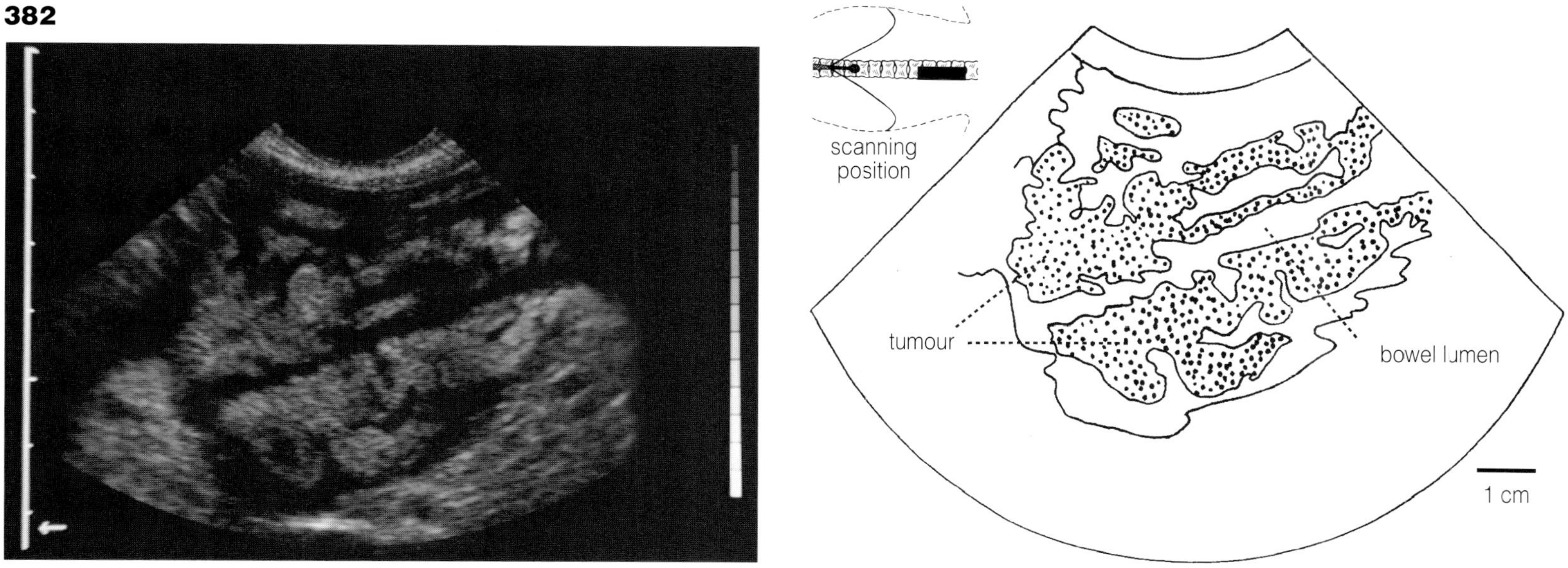

382 Mass in the rectum of a dog. The image shows the rugae-like structure of the tumour with a central anechoic lumen. Histopathology revealed mucosal carcinoma of the rectum.

383

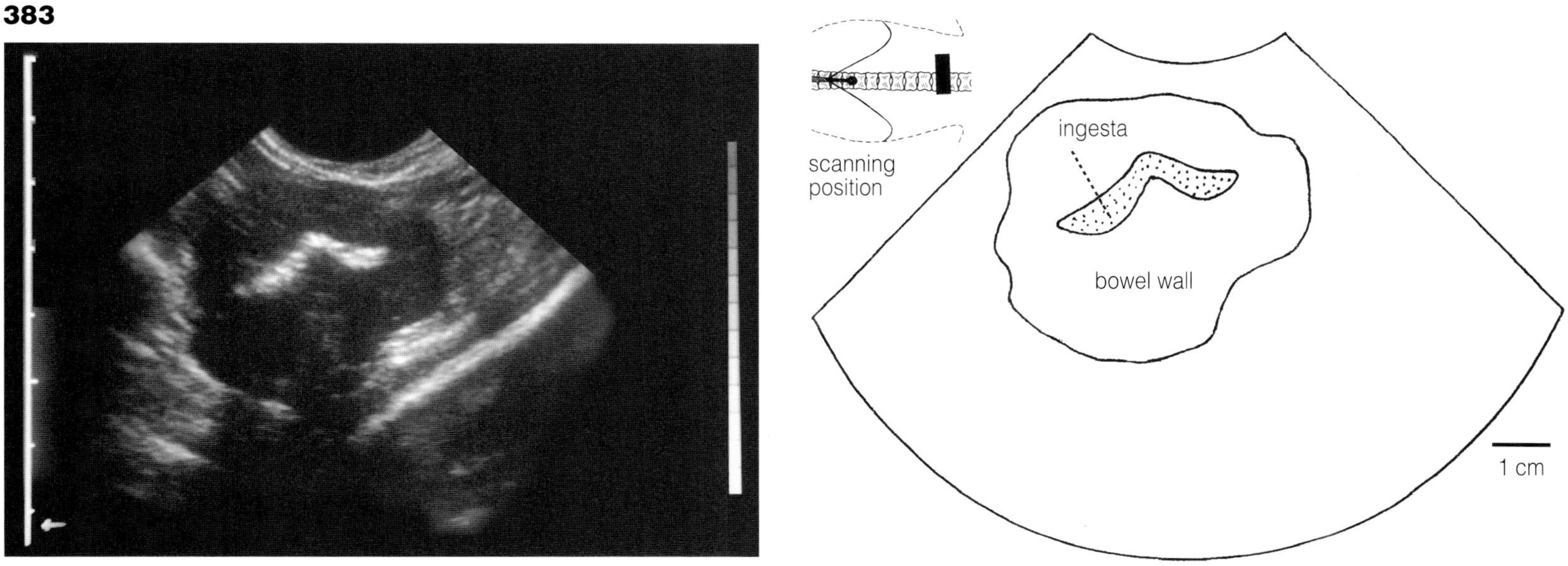

383 Severe hypoechoic thickening of the small intestinal wall with a hyperechoic central lumen in a cat with lymphosarcoma.

Ruptured stomachs cannot be imaged directly. Spontaneous hyperperistalsis of the gastric wall with irregular echoes and free peritoneal fluid in the cranial abdomen may be apparent (379).

Sonography of Intestinal Disorders

Ultrasonographic abnormalities of the bowel wall include wall thickening (380, 381) and/or changes in echogenicity.

Intestinal tumours of the large bowel may extend into the lumen (382). Small intestinal tumours are usually associated with wall thickening (383–385). Focal masses can appear as an asymmetric thickening of the wall.

Most cases of enteritis do not show impressive wall lesions (386), but have abnormal contents (387) and/or peristaltic disorders (388–390). Lymphadenopathy associated with inflammation shows the lymph nodes as anechoic to hypoechoic round structures.

The ultrasonographic pattern of intussusception is characteristic (**391, 392**). The pathognomonic image in the transverse view (391) looks like a target or onion skin layering[2, 7]. The longitudinal view (392) shows multiple wall layers. The length of the intussusception cannot always be identified. Adhesions of bowel loops may produce a similar image in longitudinal views (393).

Anechoic fluid in the bowel lumen is usually pathological. Additional gas or large amounts of ingesta restrict sonographic evaluation of the intestinal tract. Rectal fluid administration may improve visualization of the rectum and descending colon.

Foreign bodies may be identified within the bowel lumen as structures of variable shape and echogenicity[8] (**394, 395**). Diagnosis is made difficult by bowel contents. Fluid accumulation in the bowel is helpful in finding foreign bodies and evaluating an

384

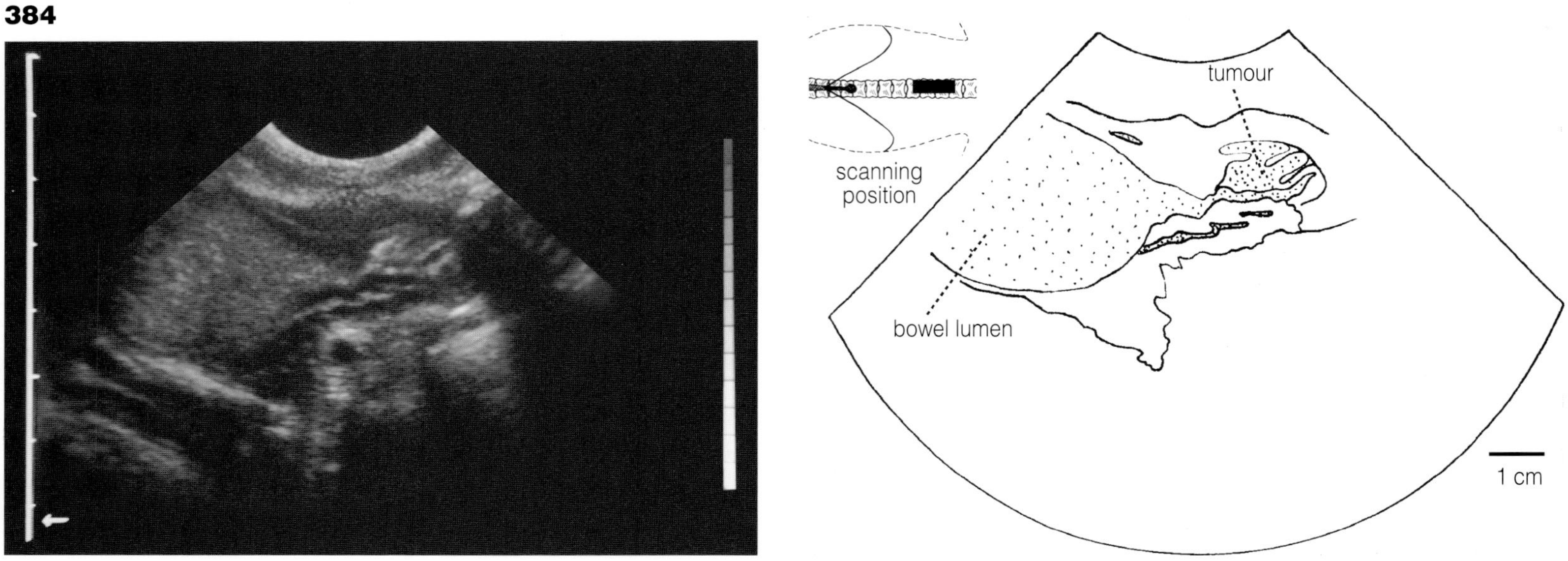

384 Dilated bowel with accumulated ingesta and partial obstruction of the lumen by a hyperechoic wall mass in a dog. The surrounding tissue shown is more echogenic. Partial ileus, caused by an intestinal tumour with peritonitis, was diagnosed. Histopathology revealed an adenocarcinoma and serositis.

385

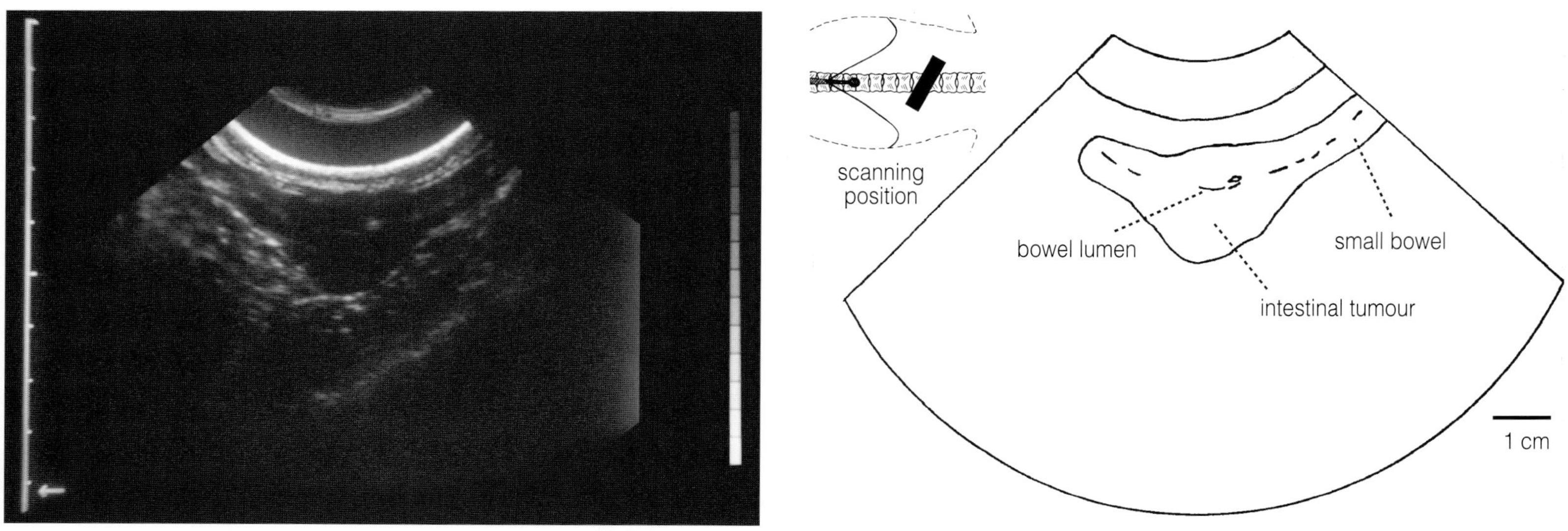

385 Longitudinal scan of a small bowel segment in a cat with myeloid leucosis. The intestinal wall shows generalized hypoechogenicity with focal distensions. The lumen is seen as a central hyperechoic line.

386

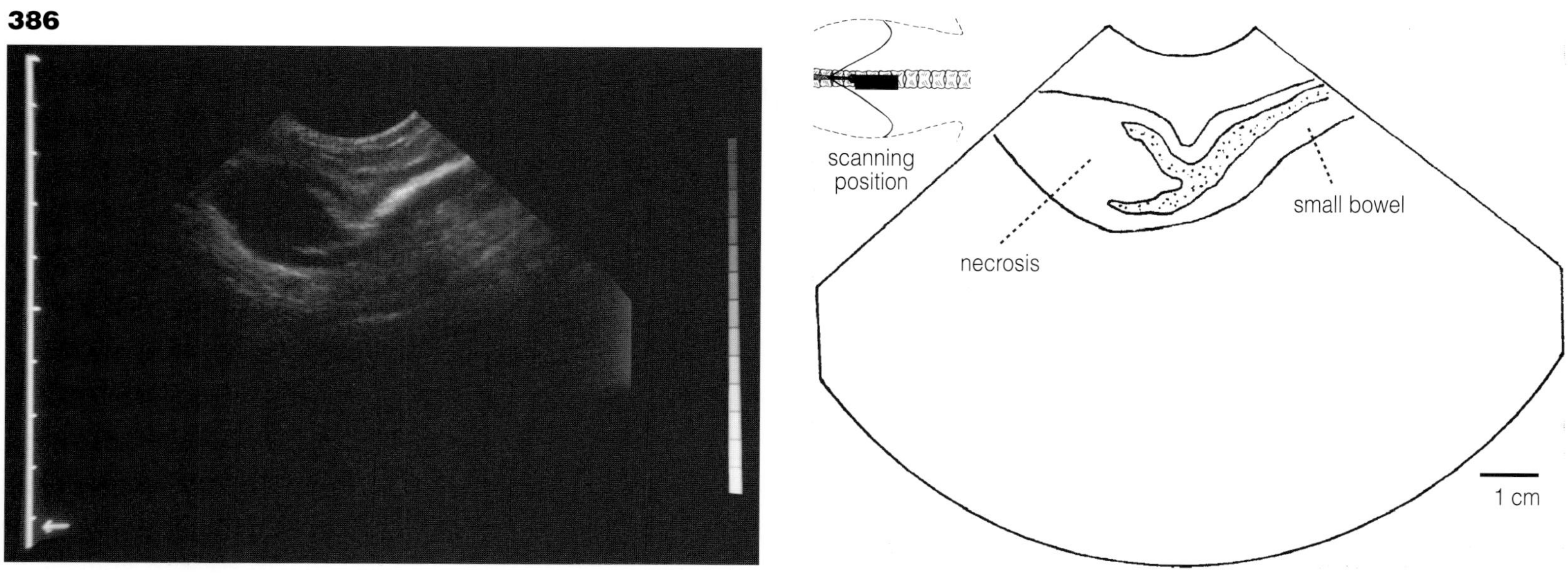

386 Distension of the small bowel with loss of wall layering in a dog. Diphteroid-necrotizing enteritis was diagnosed histopathologically. Intestinal tumours have a similar image.

387

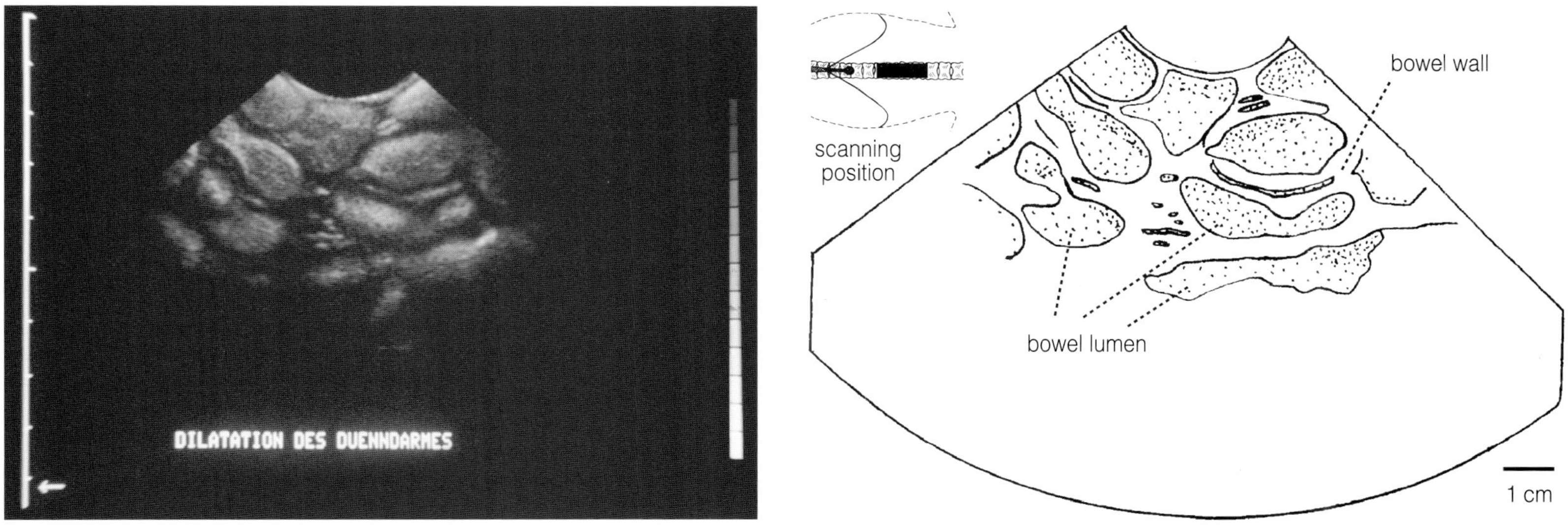

387 Hyperechoic intestinal content in dilated bowel loops of a dog. Increased intestinal motility is not appreciated in the frozen image. The dog was diagnosed with viral enteritis.

388

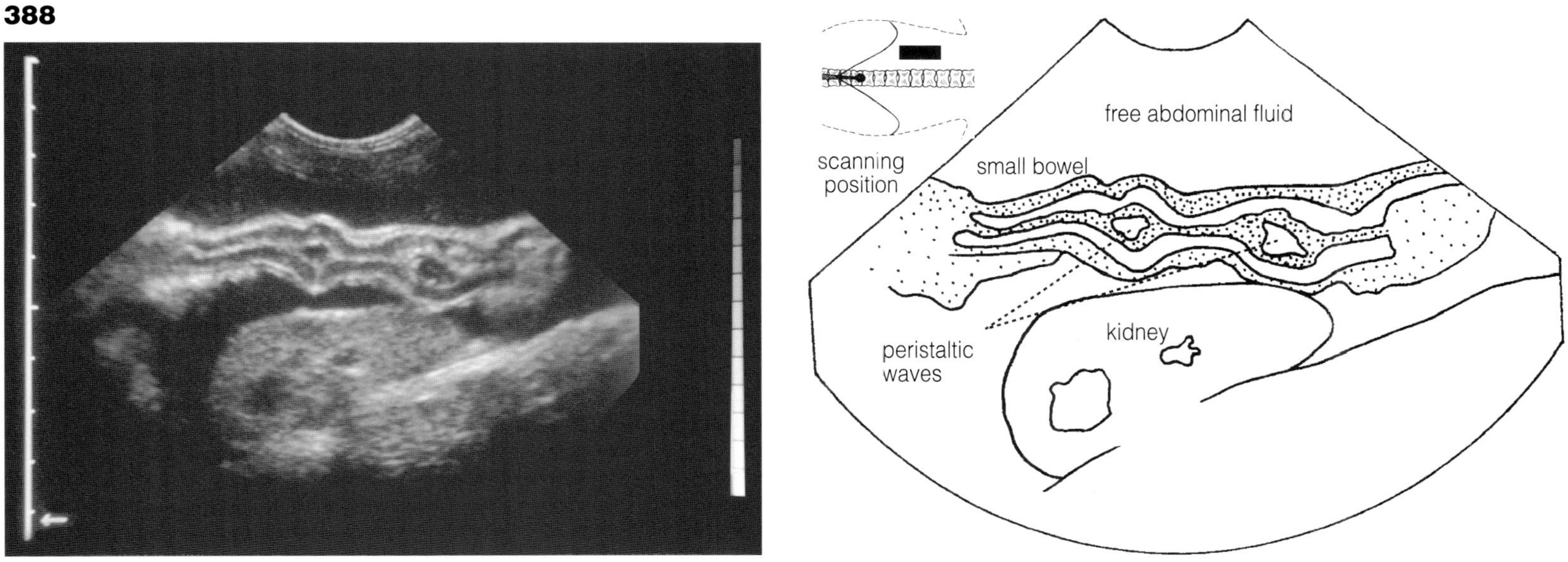

388 Ascites in a dog. Peristaltic waves are recognized in the small bowel. Intestinal contents are anechoic, similar to the free peritoneal fluid. Enteritis is suspected. The interface to the serosa is more hyperechoic than the mucosa–lumen interface. This is explained by the free abdominal fluid.

389

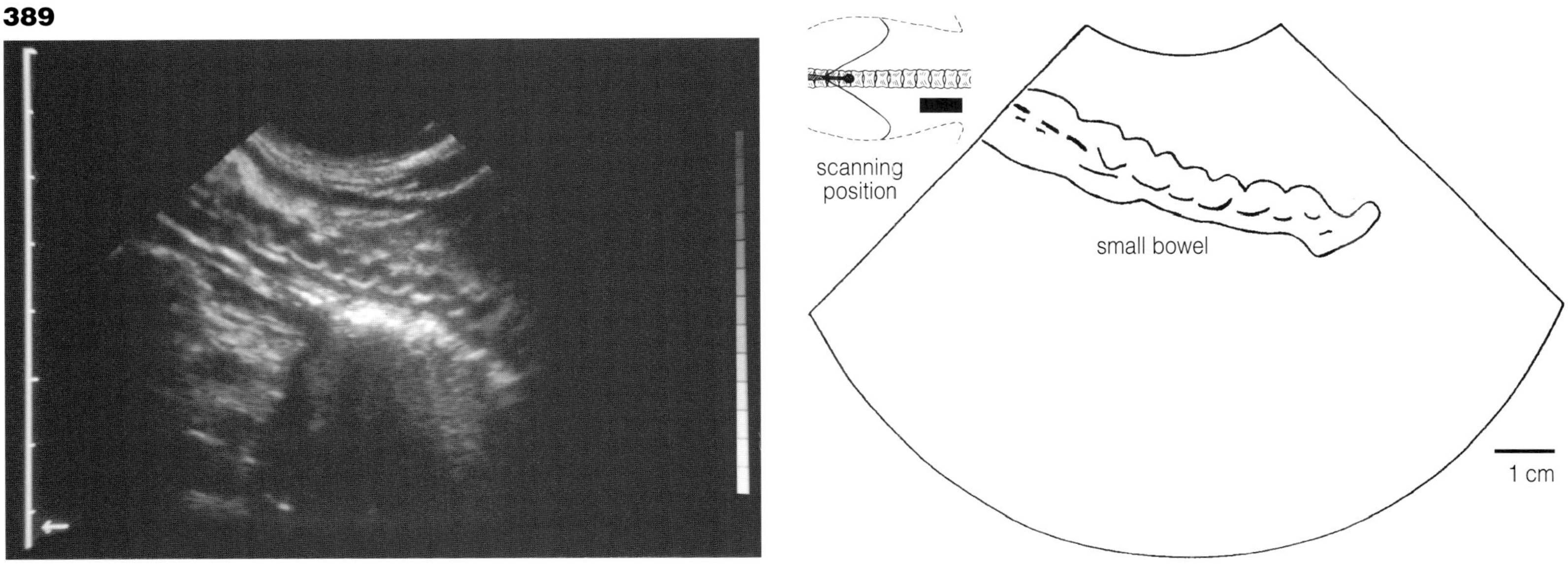

389 Marked hypermotility of the small intestine in a dog with viral enteritis. Increased peristalsis is displayed by the wavy appearance of the small bowel in the frozen image.

390

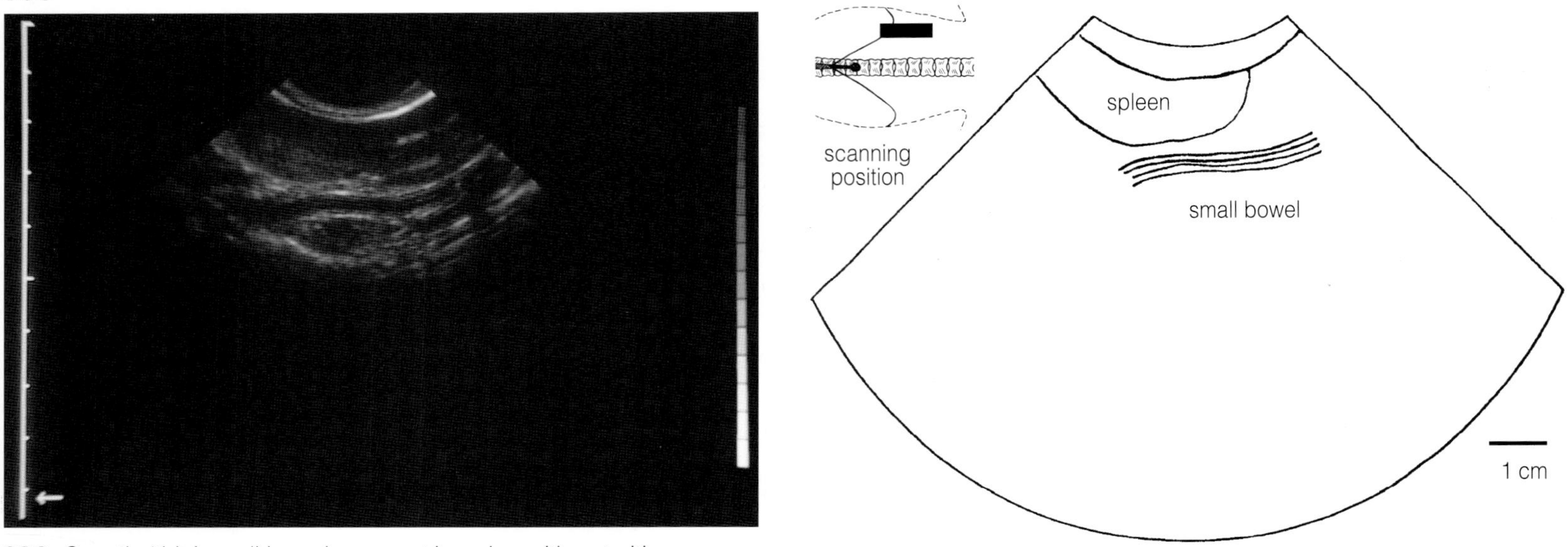

390 Spastic 'thin' small bowel segment in a dog with enteritis.

391

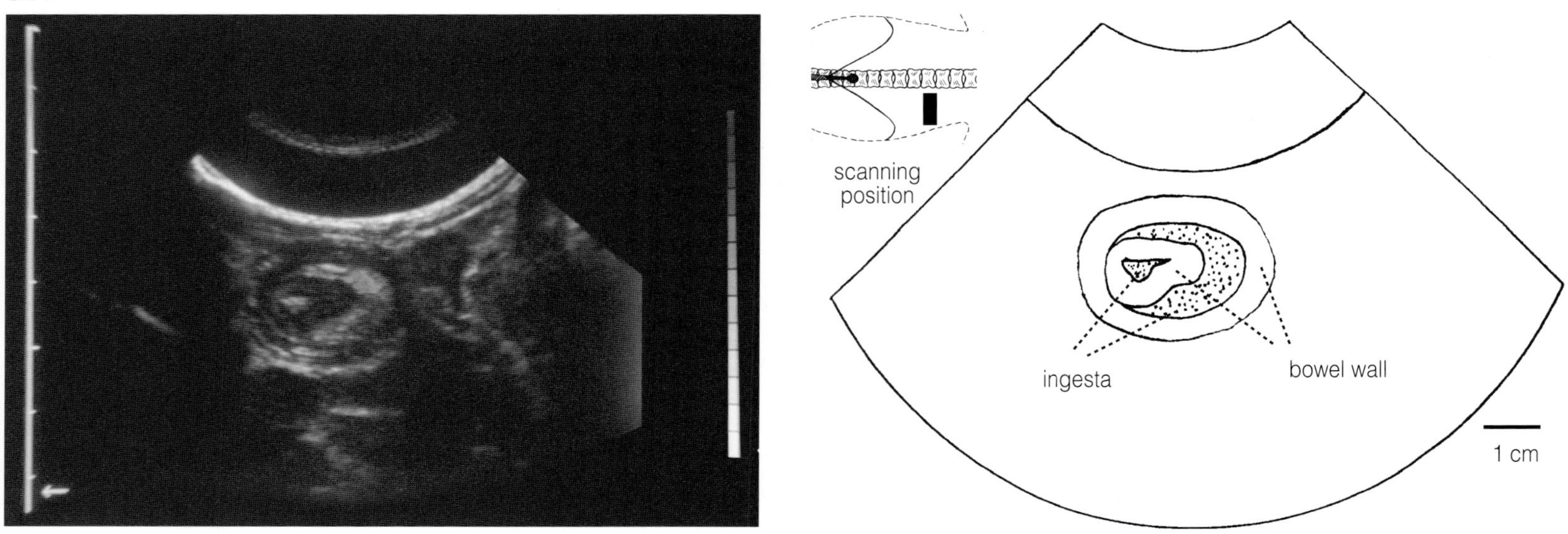

392

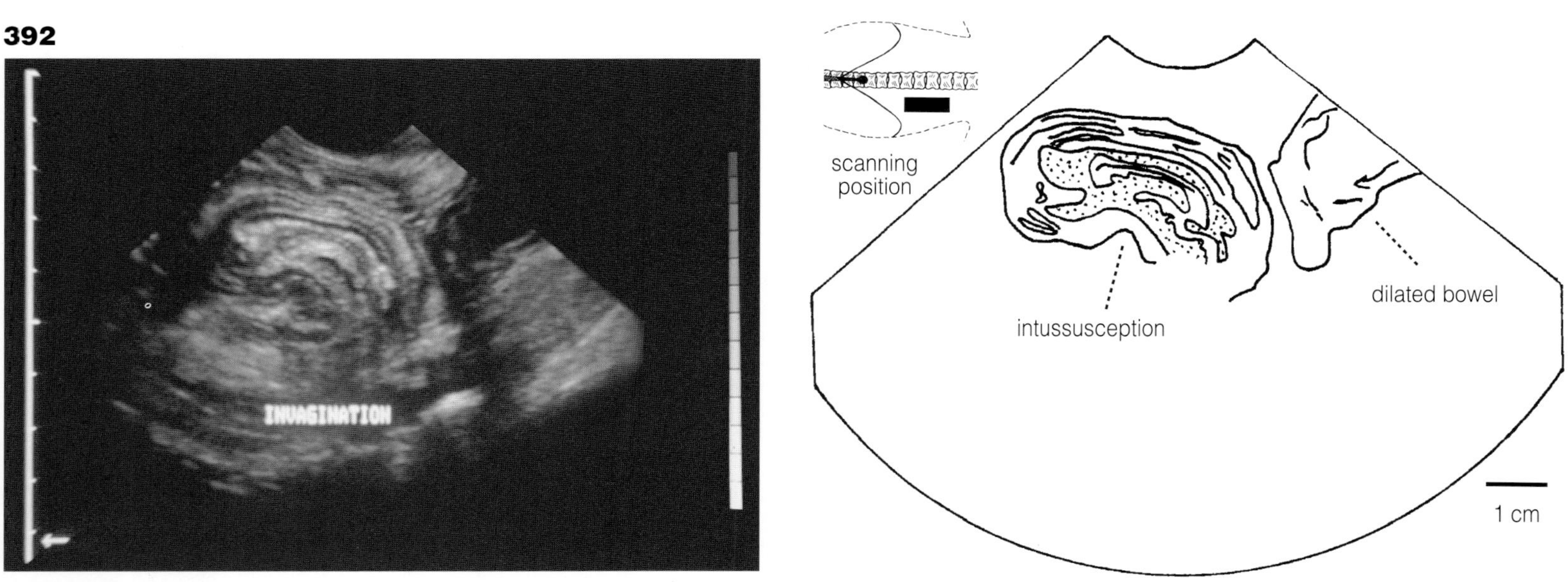

391, 392 Transverse (**391**) and longitudinal (**392**) scan of a canine intussusception. The intussusception is seen with ingesta. The transverse view (**391**) shows multilayered concentric rings of intestinal wall segments (target pattern, ring sign). Prestenotic intestinal dilation is displayed in the longitudinal view (**392**).

393

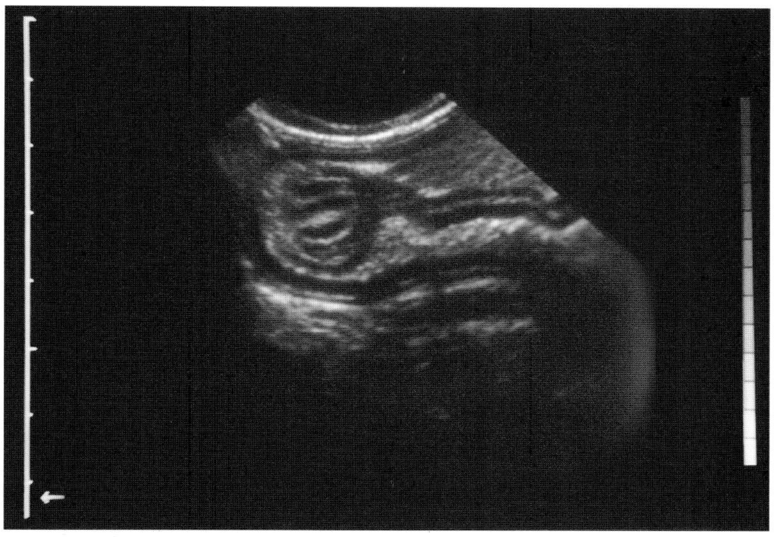

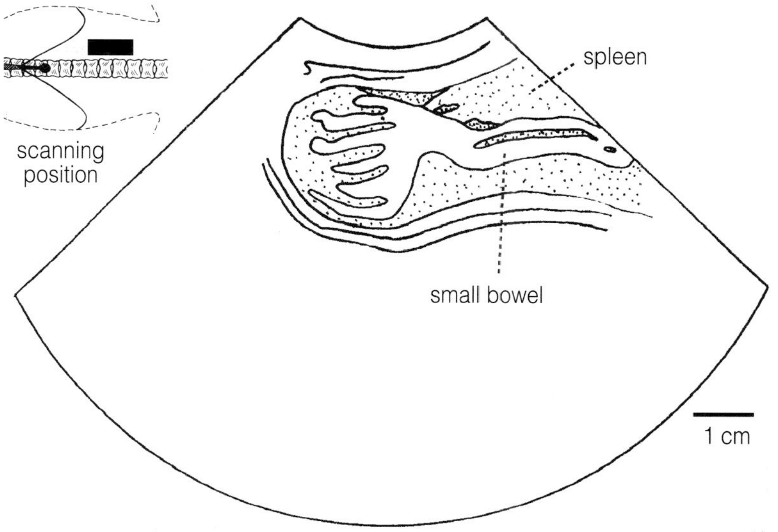

393 Irregular ring sign with bowel loop adhesions. Differential diagnosis includes intussuception.

394

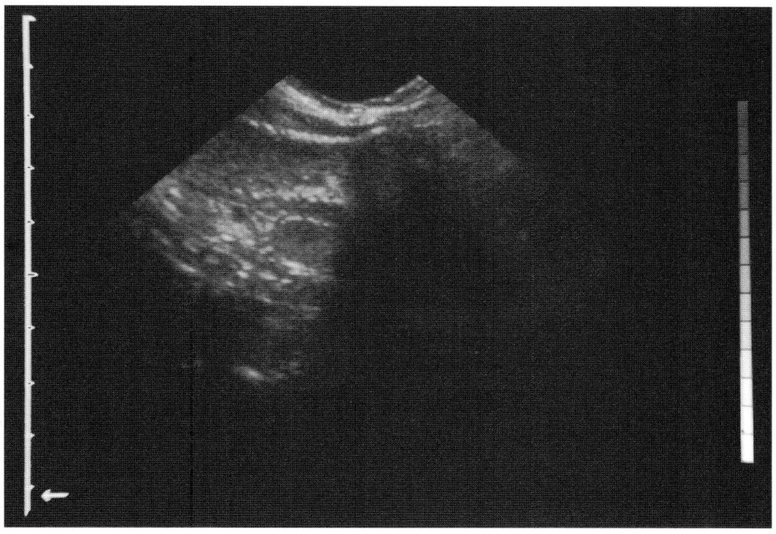

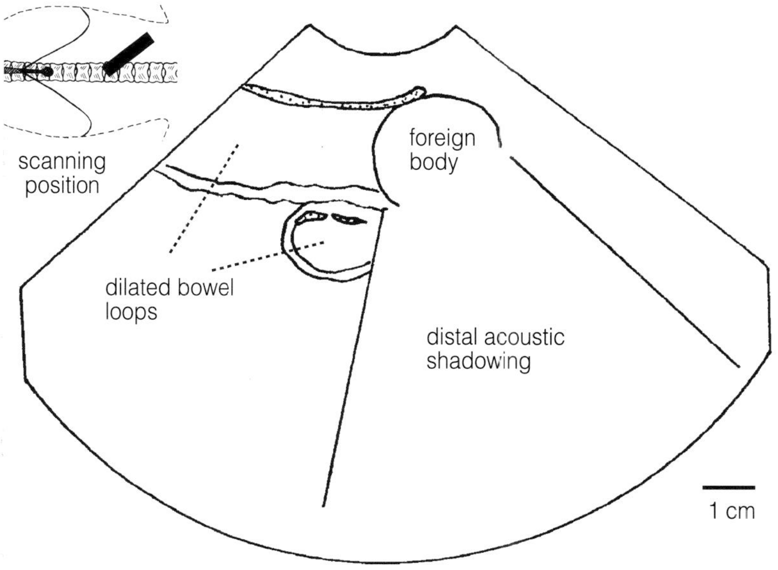

395

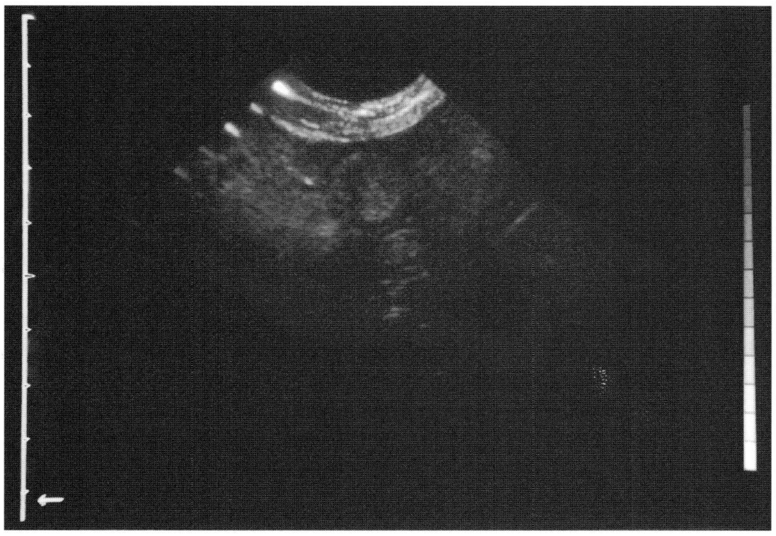

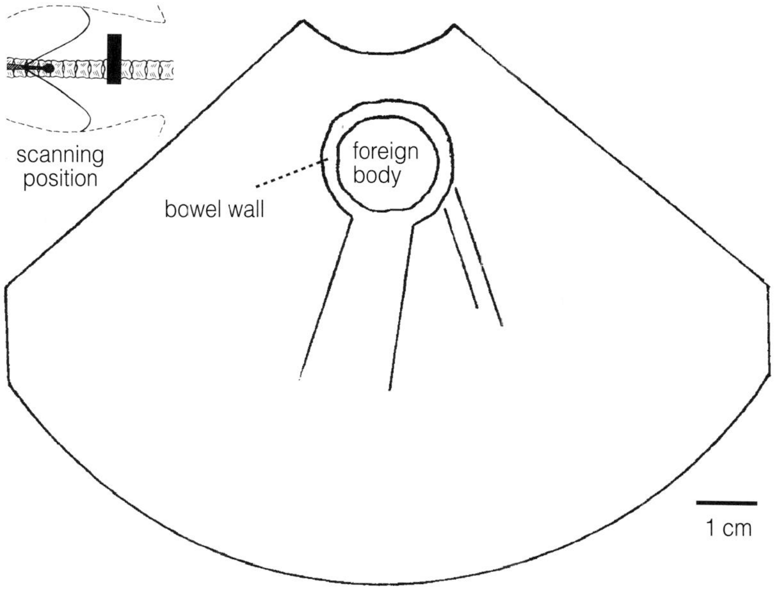

394, 395 Dilated, fluid-filled bowel loops in a dog. Dilation stops at a round, anechoic structure with distal acoustic shadowing (**394**). The structure appears more echogenic in a transverse scan (**395**). The dog was diagnosed with mechanical ileus caused by a foreign body obstruction. An acorn was found in the jejunum during surgery.

396

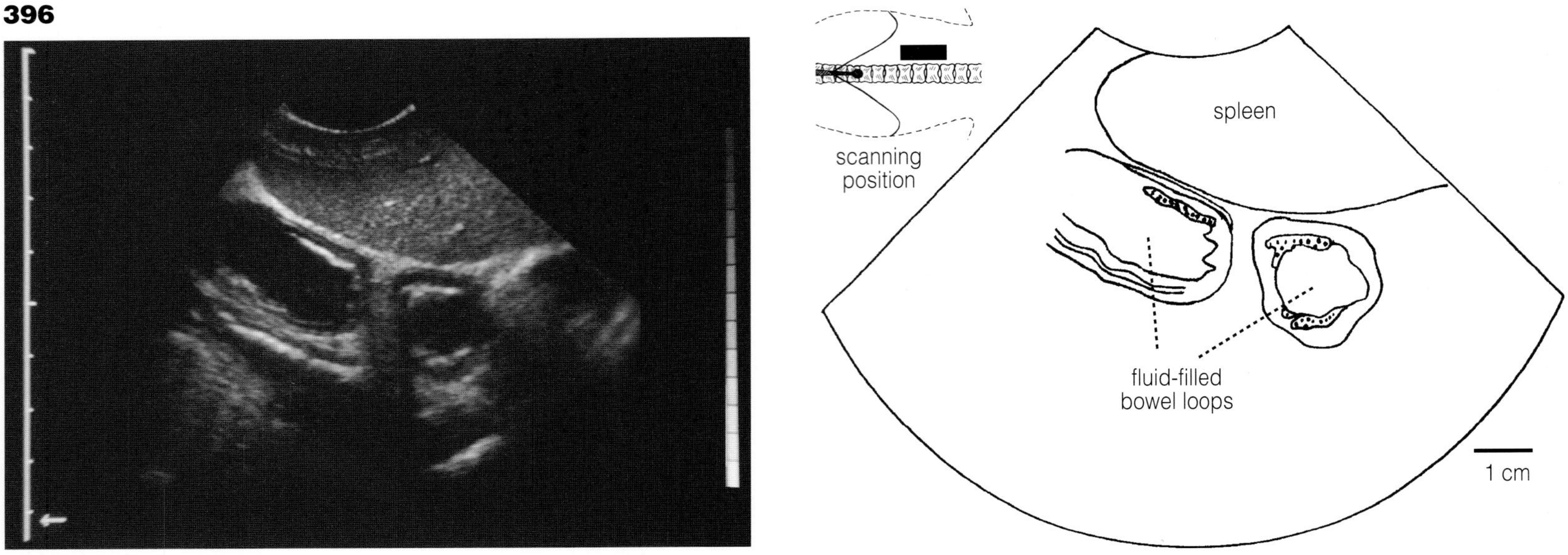

396 Fluid-filled bowel loops in a dog. Possible causes include ileus and enteritis.

397

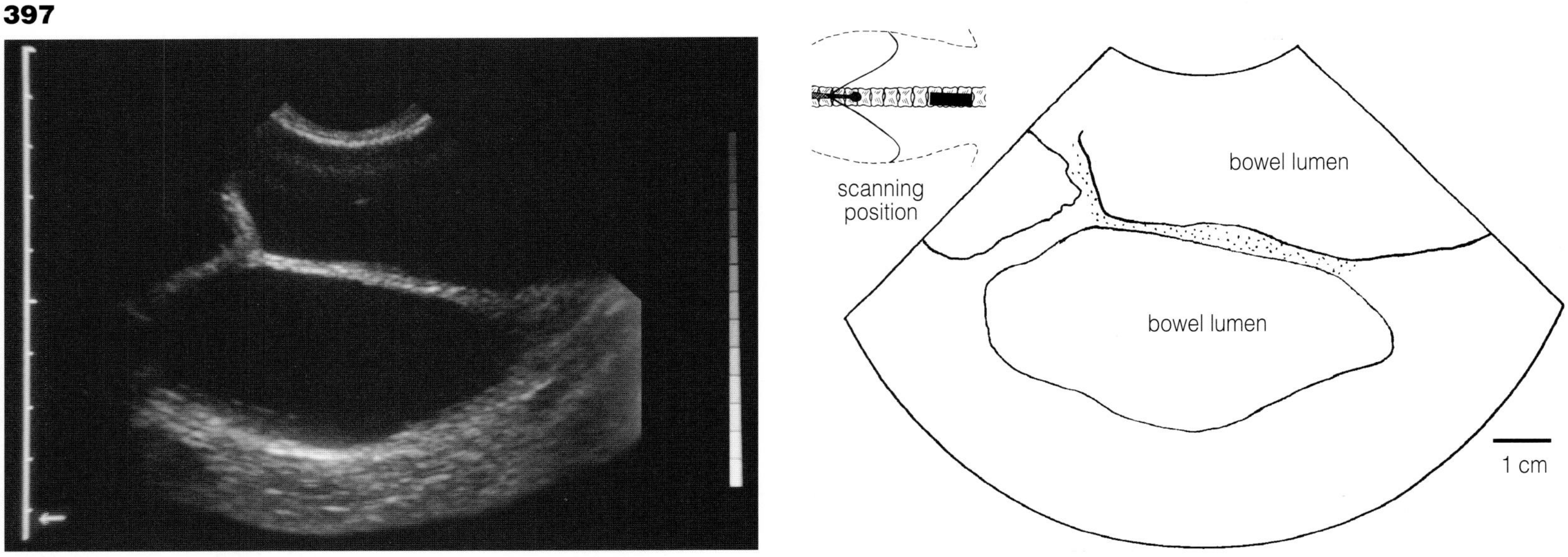

397 Dilated, atonic fluid-filled bowel loops in a dog diagnosed with ileus. Differential diagnosis includes pyometra or paraprostatic cysts.

398

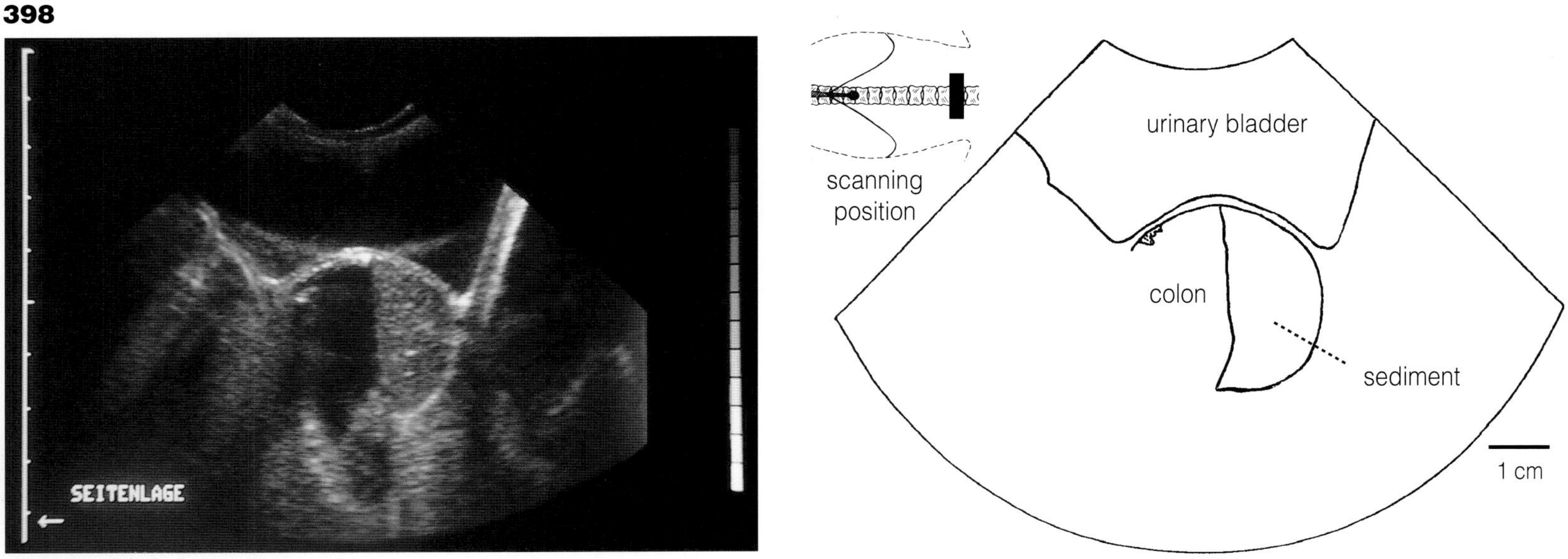

398 Transverse scan of a fluid-filled colon with deposits in a dog with enteritis, examined in lateral recumbency. Differential diagnosis includes pyometra or paraprostatic cysts.

ileus and its cause. Peristaltic activity shows contractions and flow towards the ileus with antiperistaltic waves. Dilated bowel segments (**396–398**) show loss of wall layering and fluid accumulation. This image is also found with some cases of pyometra (see Uterus and Vagina, page 260).

Hyperperistalsis is often seen with enteritis. Increased peristaltic activity is also noted with intussusception cranial to the stenosis. Lack of peristalsis is caused by various disorders and cannot be diagnosed ultrasonographically. Functional ileus is usually a reason for an exploratory laparotomy.

> **NB:** The number of peristaltic waves may be reduced physiologically in the fasted patient.

References

1. Biller DS, Partington BP, Miyabayashi T and Lveille R (1994) Ultrasonographic appearance of chronic hypertrophic pyloric gastropathy in the dog. *Vet. Radiol. Ultrasound* **35**, 30–33.
2. Flückiger M and Arnold P (1986) Die Darminvagination beim Hand – ihr sonographisches Bild. *Kleintierpraxis* **31**, 379–382.
3. Grooters AM, Miyabayashi T, Biller DS and Merryman J (1994) Sonographic appearance of uremic gastropathy in four dogs. *Vet. Radiol.Ultrasound* **35**, 35–40.
4. Kleine LJ and Lamb CR (1989) Comparative organ imaging: the gastrointestinal tract. *Vet. Radiol.* **30**, 133–141.
5. Lamb CR (1990) Abdominal ultrasonography in small animals: intestinal tract and mesentery, kidneys, adrenal glands, uterus and prostate. *J. Small Anim.Pract.* **31**, 295–304.
6. Penninck DG, Nyland TG, Fischer PE and Kerr LY (1989) Ultrasonography of the normal canine gastrointestinal tract. *Vet. Radiol.* **30**, 272–276.
7. Penninck DG, Nyland TG, Kerr LY and Fischer PE (1990) Ultrasonographic evaluation of gastrointestinal diseases in small animals. *Vet. Radiol.* **31**, 134–141.
8. Tidwell AS and Penninck DG (1992) Ultrasonography of gastrointestinal foreign bodies. *Vet. Radiol. Ultrasound* **33**, 160–169

Liver and Gallbladder

Sabine Scholz and Dirk Lüerssen

Instrumentation and Examination Technique

The liver and gallbladder should be scanned using a 5.0–7.5 MHz sector transducer. Sector scanners are able to visualize the intrathoracic cranial parts of the liver. Linear and curved-array transducers can only be used in medium-sized to large dogs. Good skin contact is difficult in smaller dogs and cats because of the narrow rib cage. The same is true for dog breeds with long and narrow chests, e.g. Whippets.

With normal feeding, dogs and cats do not have to be fasted and/or given oral gas-reducing agents before scanning the liver. A full stomach may decrease the quality of imaging in dorsally recumbent patients, which is why animals should be fasted before the examination. Normal small bowel loops are displaced dorsally or to the bottom in dorsally or laterally recumbent patients and do not interfere with the liver scan. Ultrasonographic examinations of standing cats may require fasting for one day. Longer fasting has not proven useful. These considerations depend on the type of food given to the individual animal. Commercially available canned food is less likely to cause artefacts than fresh meat, which often leads to bloating of the gastrointestinal tract.

Anatomy and Normal Sonographic Findings

Anatomy

The liver is located almost entirely within the intrathoracic portion of the abdominal cavity in dogs and cats and lies to the left and right of the median plane (**399, 400**). The cranial pole of the the convex diaphragmatic surface of the liver is situated at the level of the 8th–10th thoracic vertebrae[1]. The liver is separated from the lungs, mediastinum and pericardium by the diaphragm (**401**). The stomach, duodenum, right kidney and pancreas border the visceral surface of the liver[2] (**402**).

The porta hepatis is located to the right of the median plane at the level of the 12th thoracic vertebra. The portal vein, hepatic artery, nerves, lymphatic vessels and bile ducts enter or exit through the porta hepatis. The large portal vein (functional system) enters the liver and divides into two main branches, which continue to subdivide (**404**). The relatively thin hepatic artery (nutritive system) enters through the porta hepatis and branches into three vessels. The hepatic veins collect the functional and nutritive blood and empty into the caudal vena cava (**406**).

The gallbladder lies within a liver fossa and is located near the 8th intercostal space in dogs and cats (**406, 411**). Some cats show gallbladder duplication, septa or angulation. The cystic duct of the gallbladder collects the hepatic ducts, turns into the common bile duct and empties into the duodenum at the greater papilla.

Scanning Positions

Ultrasonographic examinations of the liver are easiest on the dorsally recumbent patient. An air-filled stomach or intestinal gas may impair visualization from a ventral position. These animals should be examined in a standing position with the scan head placed laterally.

The entire liver cannot be displayed in one ultrasound image. It is therefore important to scan the liver carefully in smaller segments. The transducer is placed directly caudal to the rib cage and sternum in sagittal or transverse planes. By angling and turning the probe, the liver contours can be imaged in their entirety.

The hepatic veins in the dog are most easily recognized in the 6th–8th intercostal space of the ventral right thoracic wall in a caudomedial scanning plane, where they empty into the caudal vena cava. Two-dimensional ultrasonography of feline hepatic veins is more difficult because of their small size.

The scanning plane for the porta hepatis with the portal vein, portal vein branches, gallbladder and large bile ducts is located caudal to the sternum, median (dog, cat) or to the right (dog) of the ventral abdominal wall. The transducer should be angled slightly to the right.

399

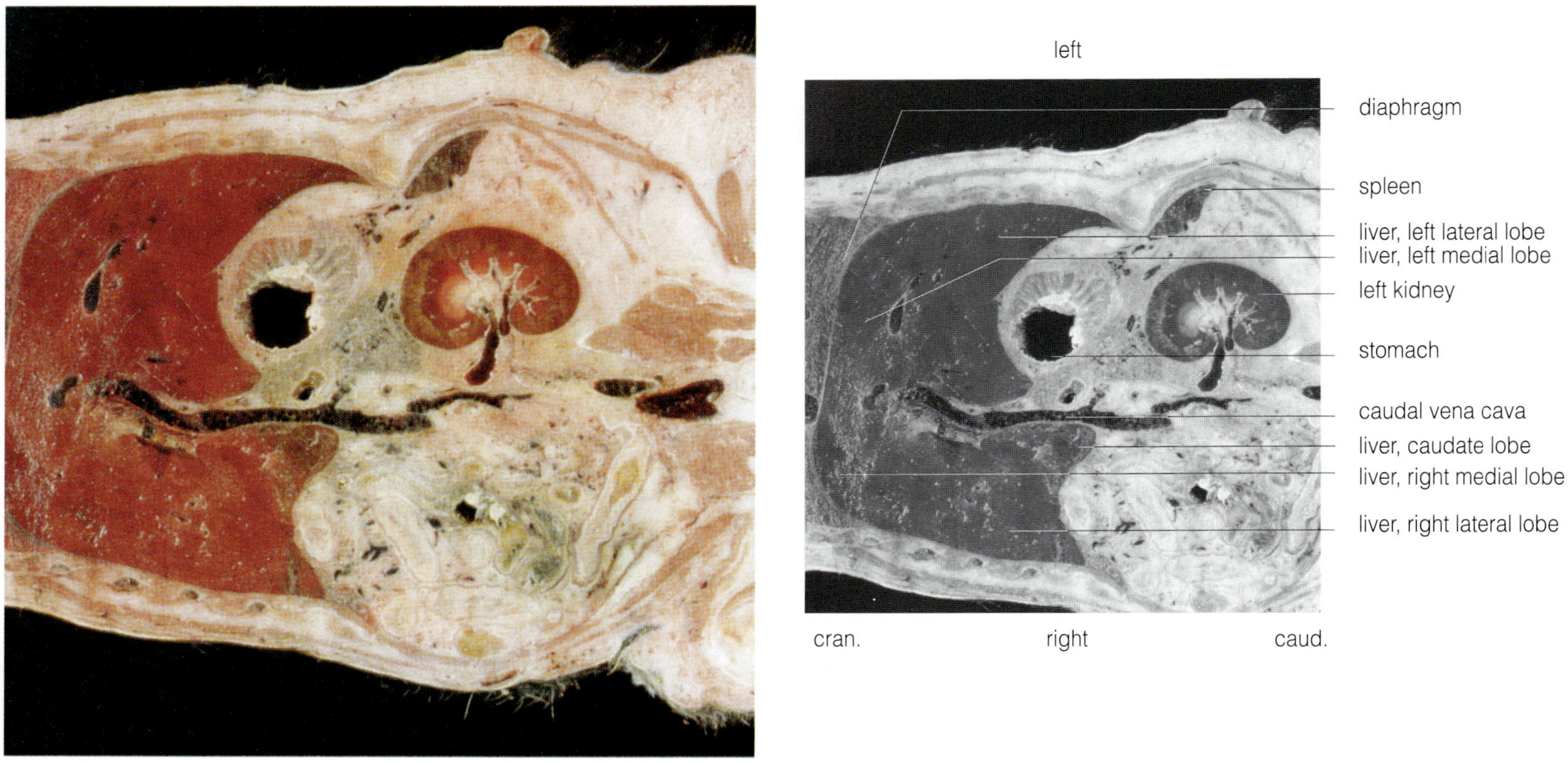

400

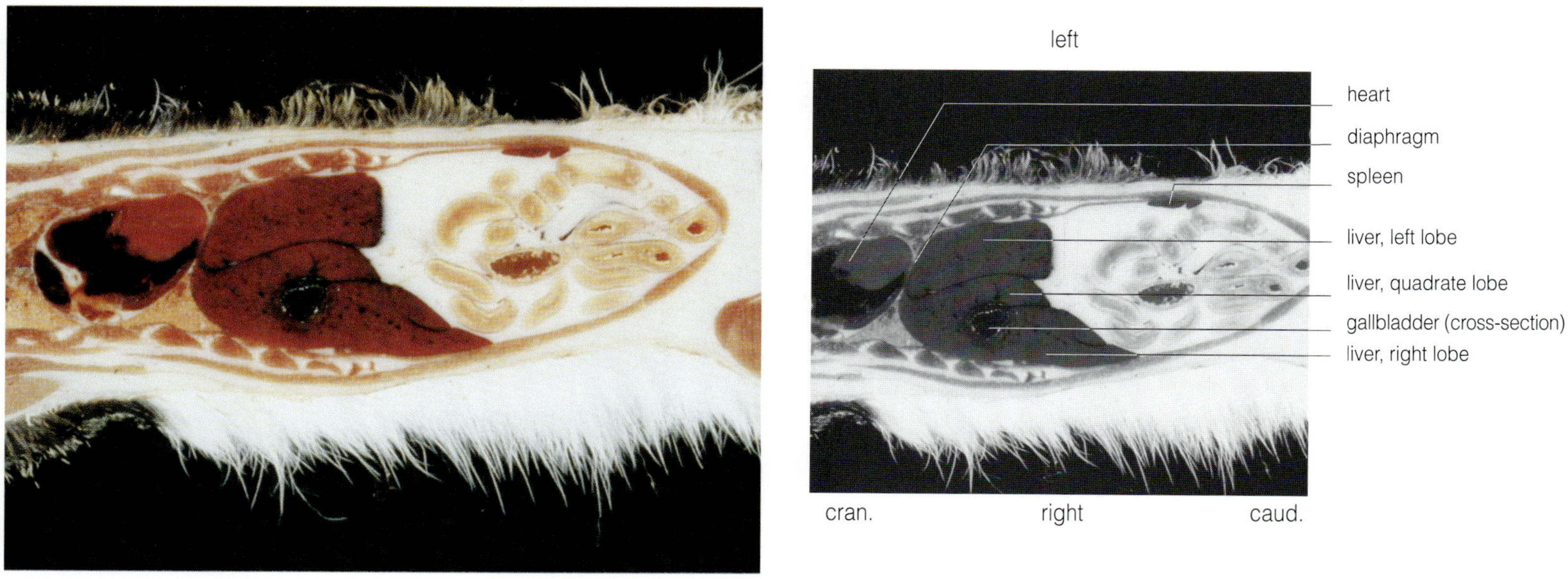

399, 400 Anatomical dorsal section of a dog (**399**) and a cat (**400**).

Normal Sonographic Findings

The normal hepatic parenchyma has a uniform echo pattern of low to medium echogenicity. To detect differences in parenchymal texture in liver ultrasonography, the gain settings should be increased. The liver lobes have clear margins and the surface is smooth. Ultrasonographic assessment of liver size is based on the ultrasonographer's experience and it is difficult to measure objectively.

The portal vein and its branches, the caudal vena cava, the hepatic veins and the gallbladder are seen as large anechoic fluid-filled structures within the hepatic parenchyma. The branches of the portal vein are anechoic with peripheral wall echoes (**403, 407**). The caudal vena cava also has echogenic walls and pulsates. The walls of the hepatic veins are usually not seen (**405, 407**) unless the sound beam is directly perpendicular. The hepatic arteries are not visualized in two-dimensional ultrasonography.

406

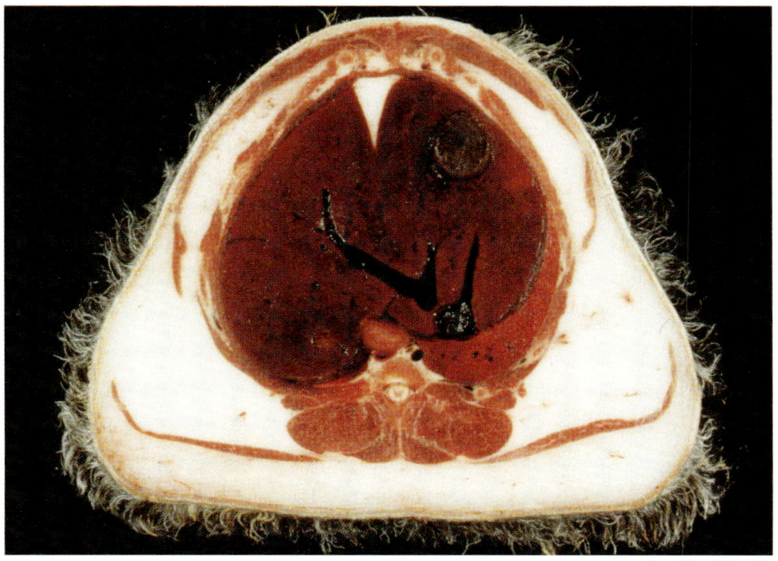

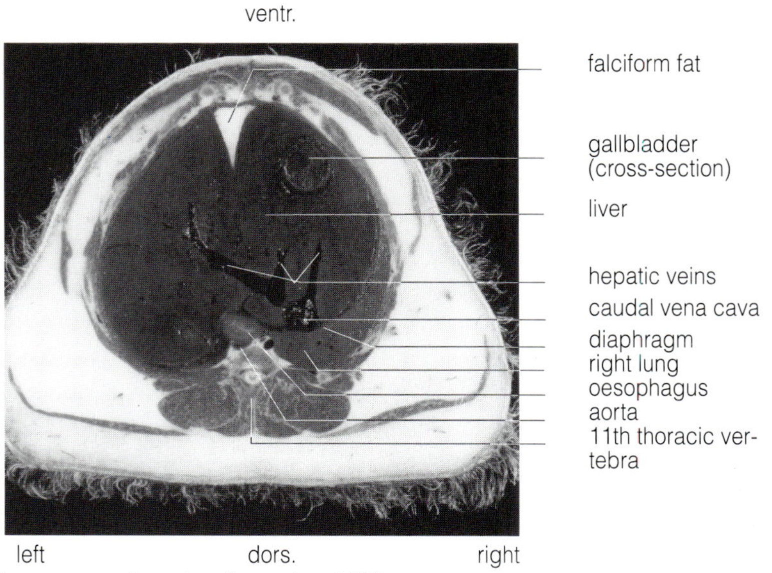

406 Anatomical cross-section of the hepatic veins emptying into the caudal vena cava in a dog (see also **405**).

407

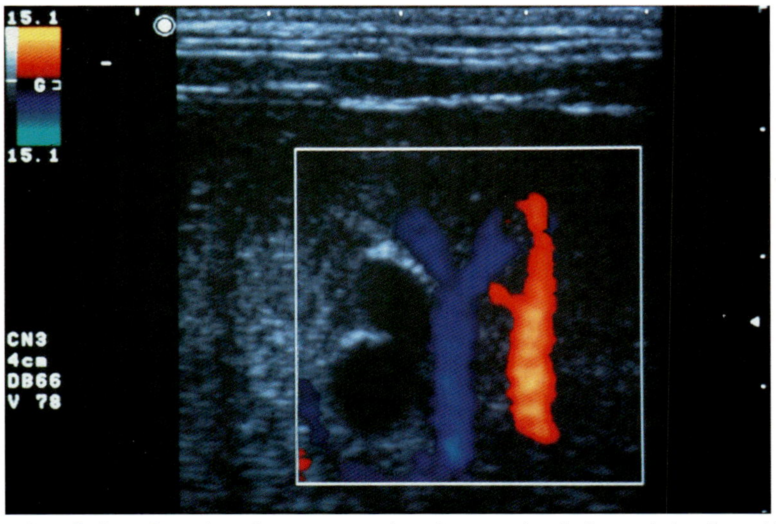

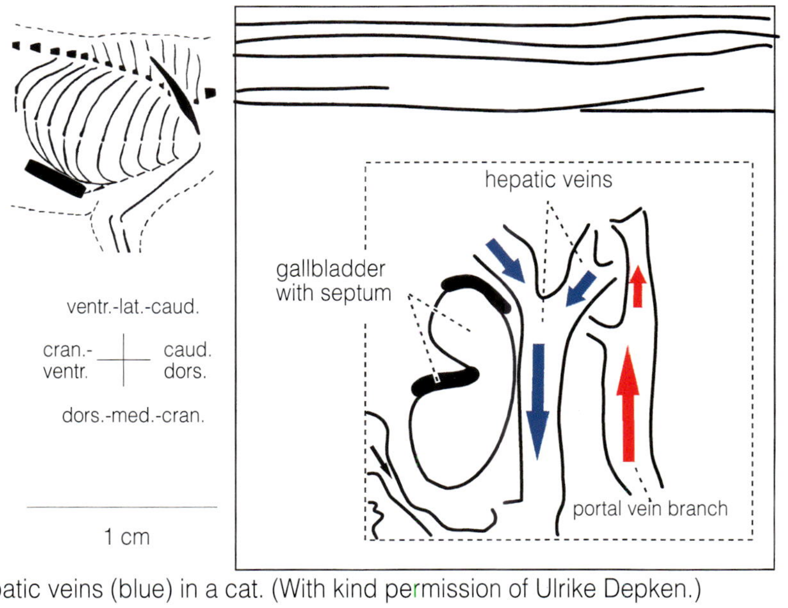

407 Colour Doppler ultrasonography of a portal vein branch (red) and hepatic veins (blue) in a cat. (With kind permission of Ulrike Depken.)

408

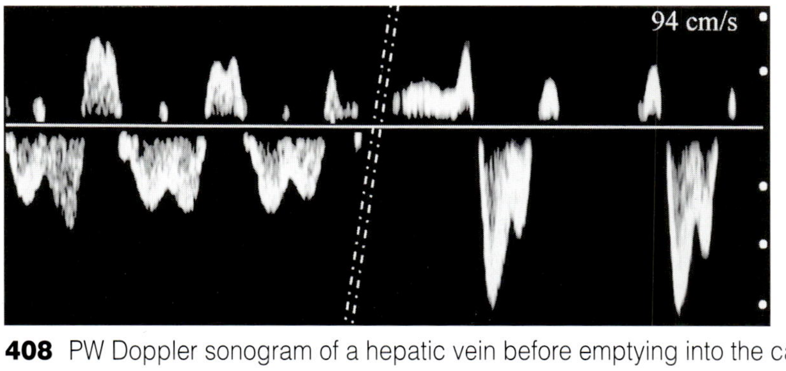

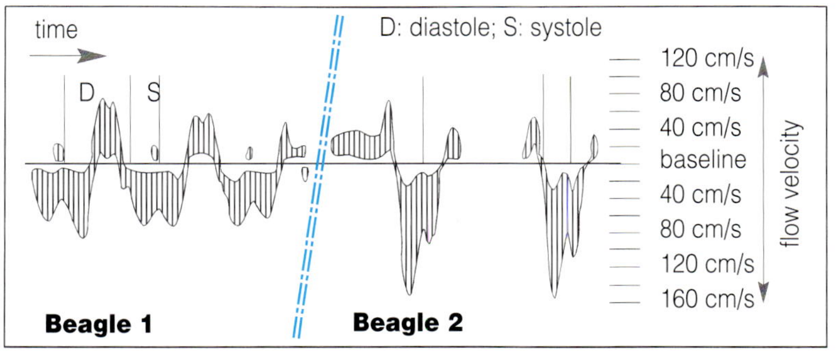

408 PW Doppler sonogram of a hepatic vein before emptying into the caudal vena cava in two dogs.

409

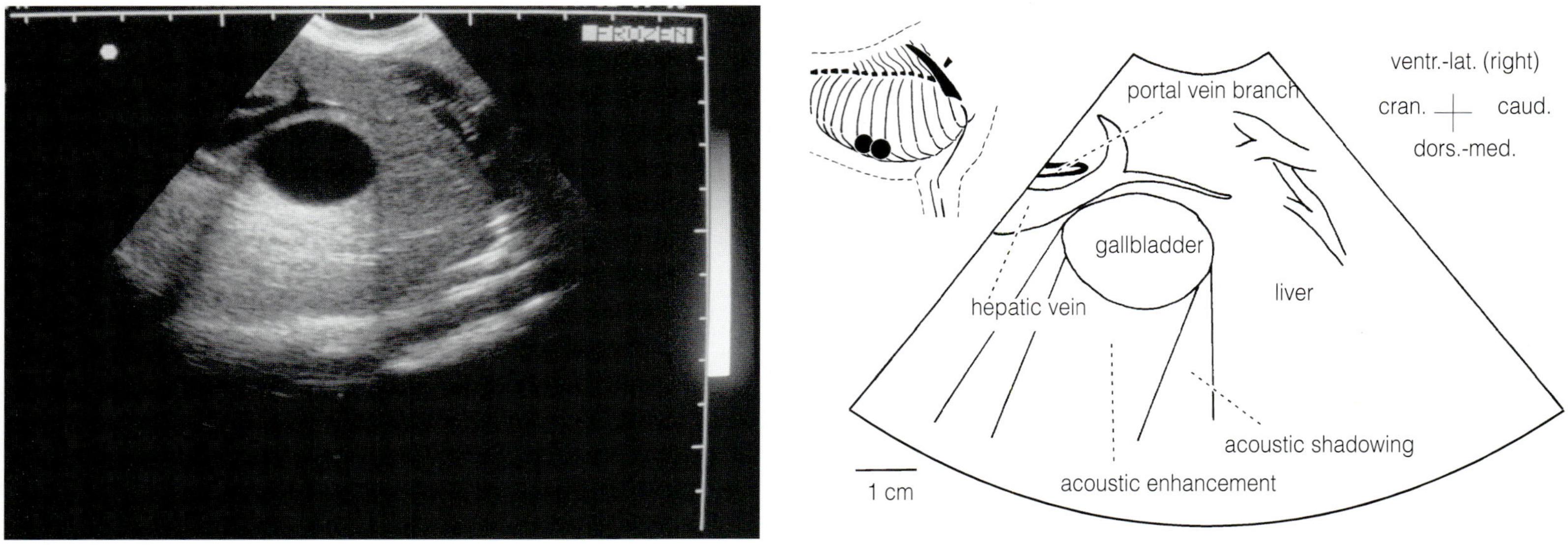

410

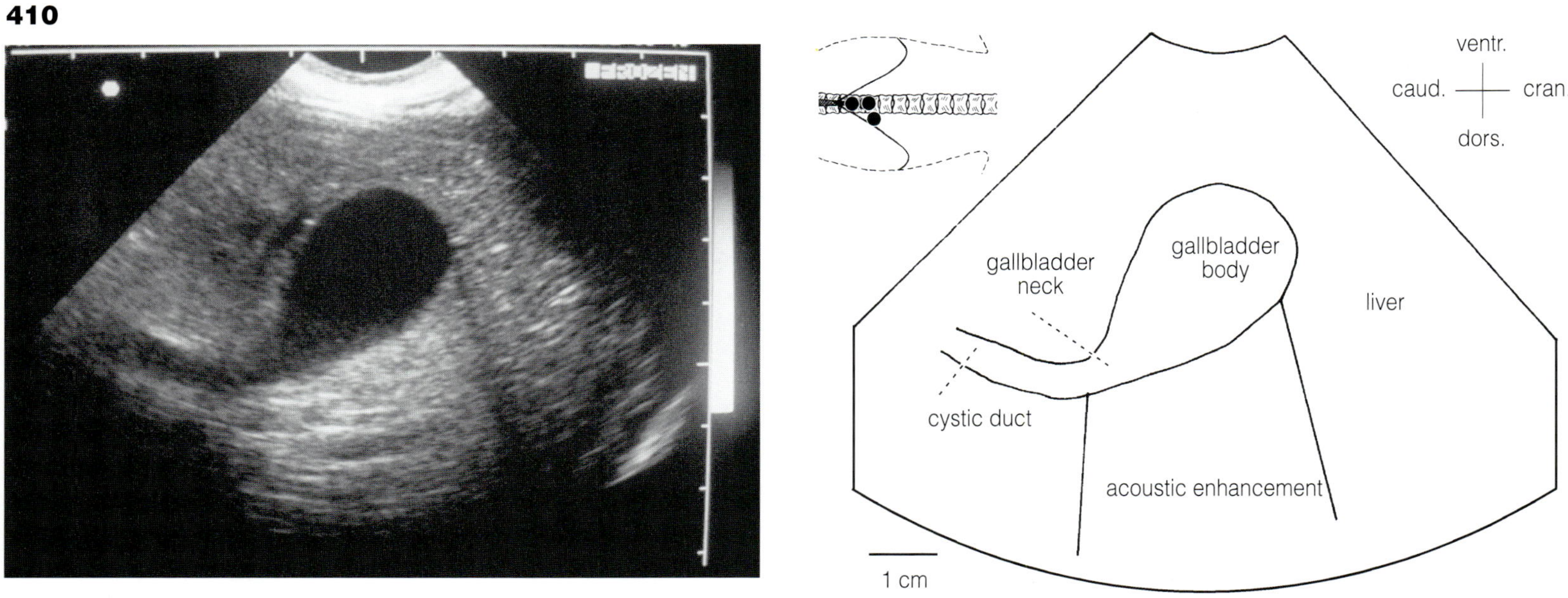

411

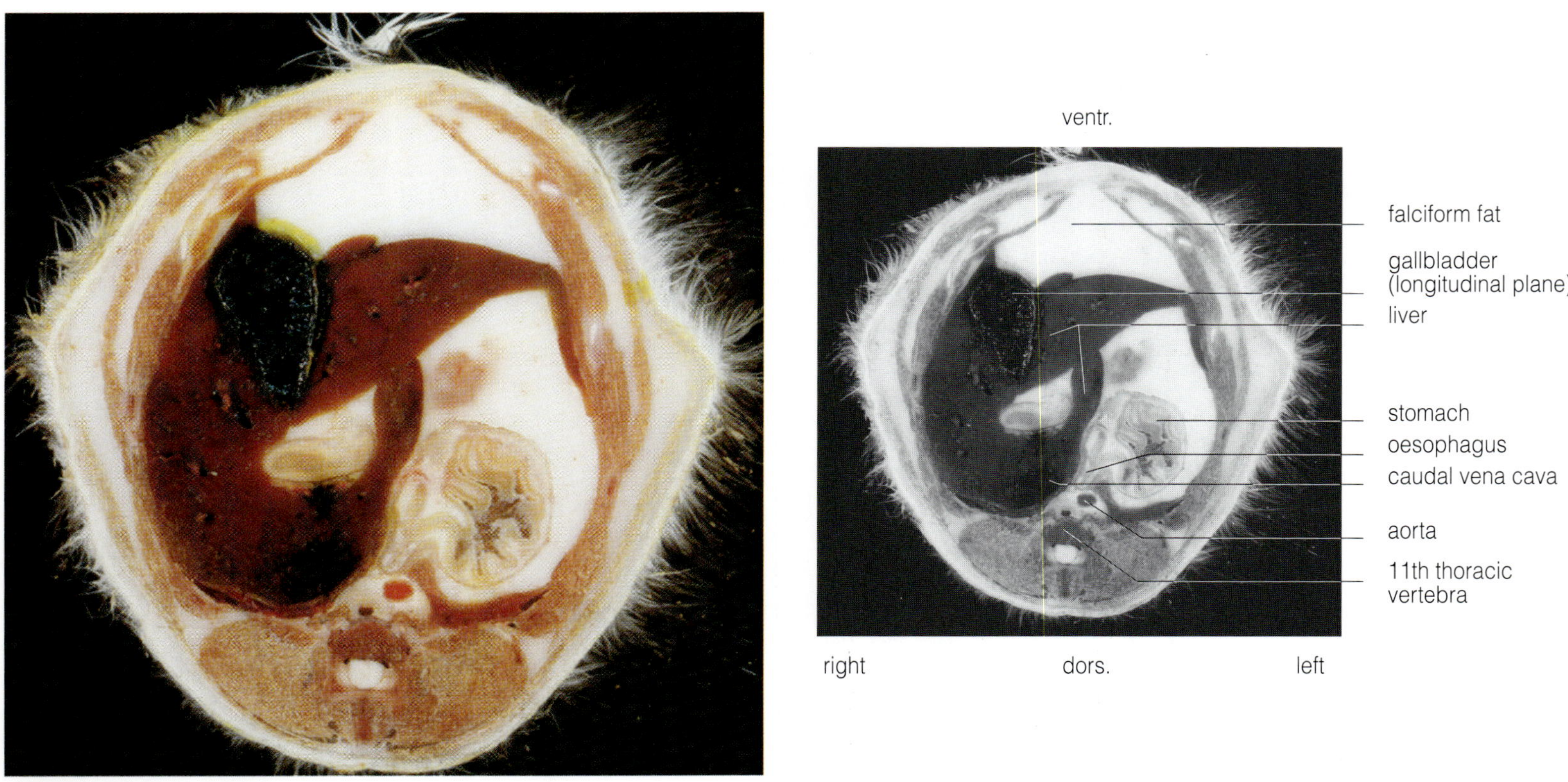

409–411 Two-dimensional sonograms (**409, 410**) and anatomical cross-section (**411**) of a filled canine gallbladder in transverse (**409**) and longitudinal (**410, 411**) views.

412

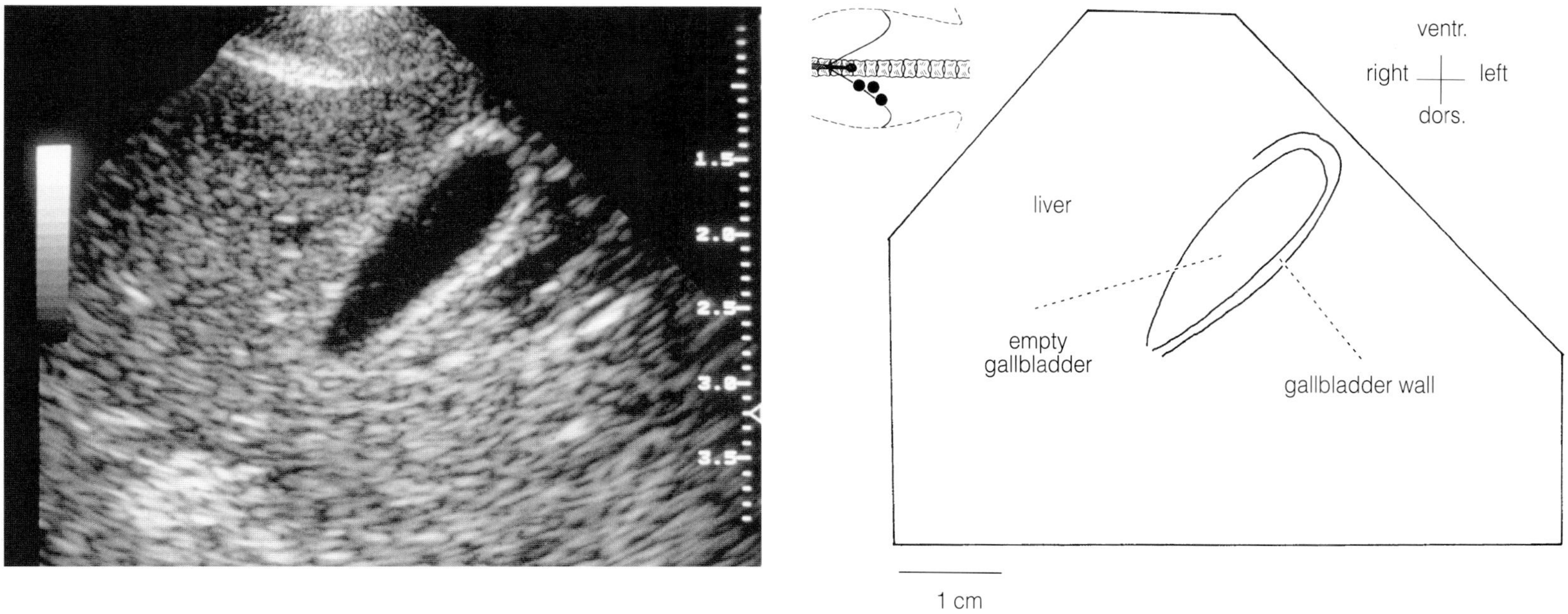

413

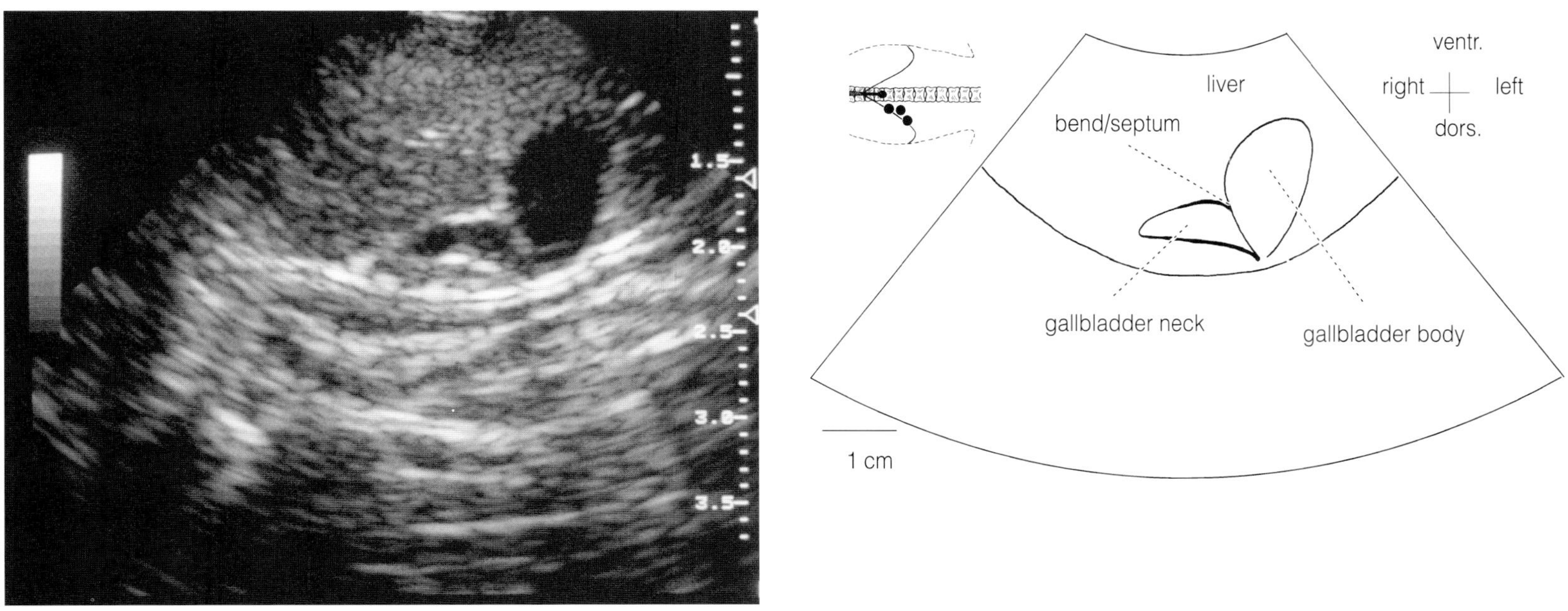

414

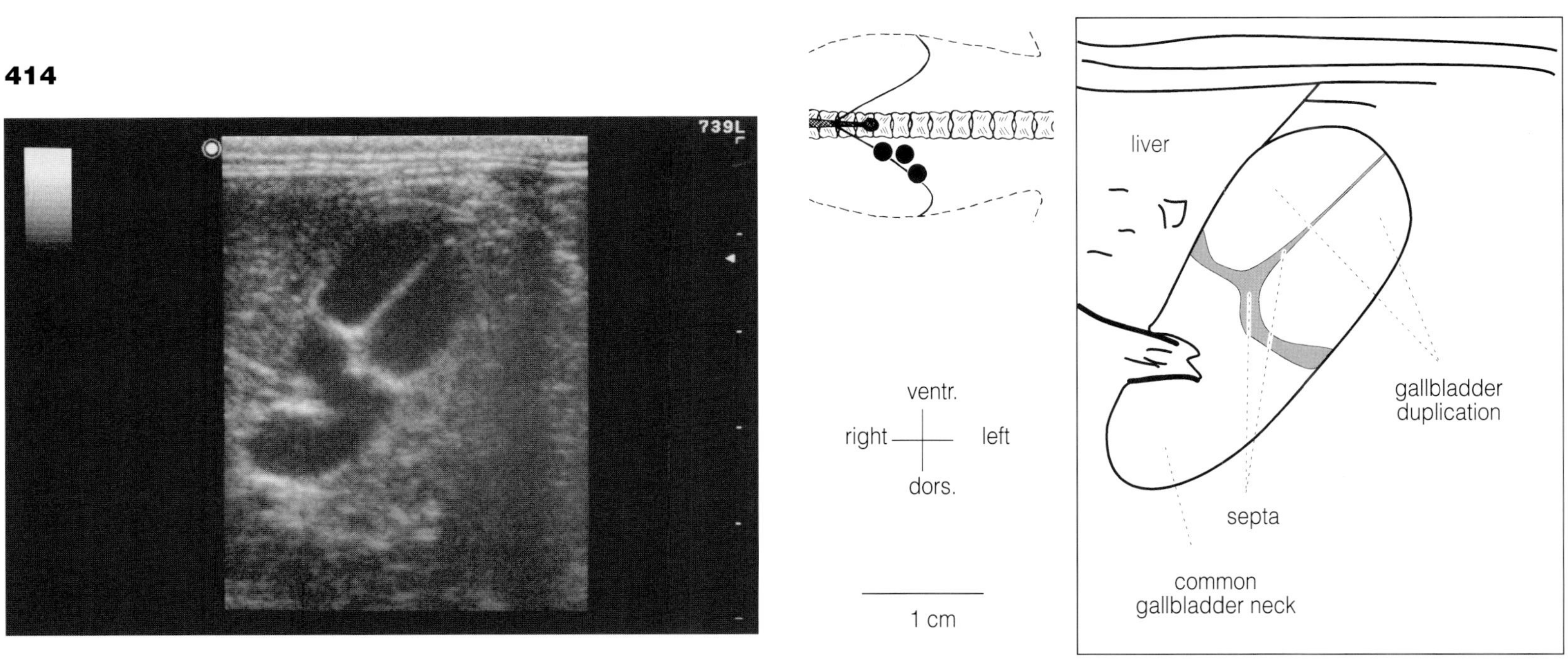

412–414 Two-dimensional sonograms of a moderately filled, oval gallbaldder (**412**), a filled, bent gallbladder (**413**), as well as an incomplete duplication (**414**) in a cat.

415

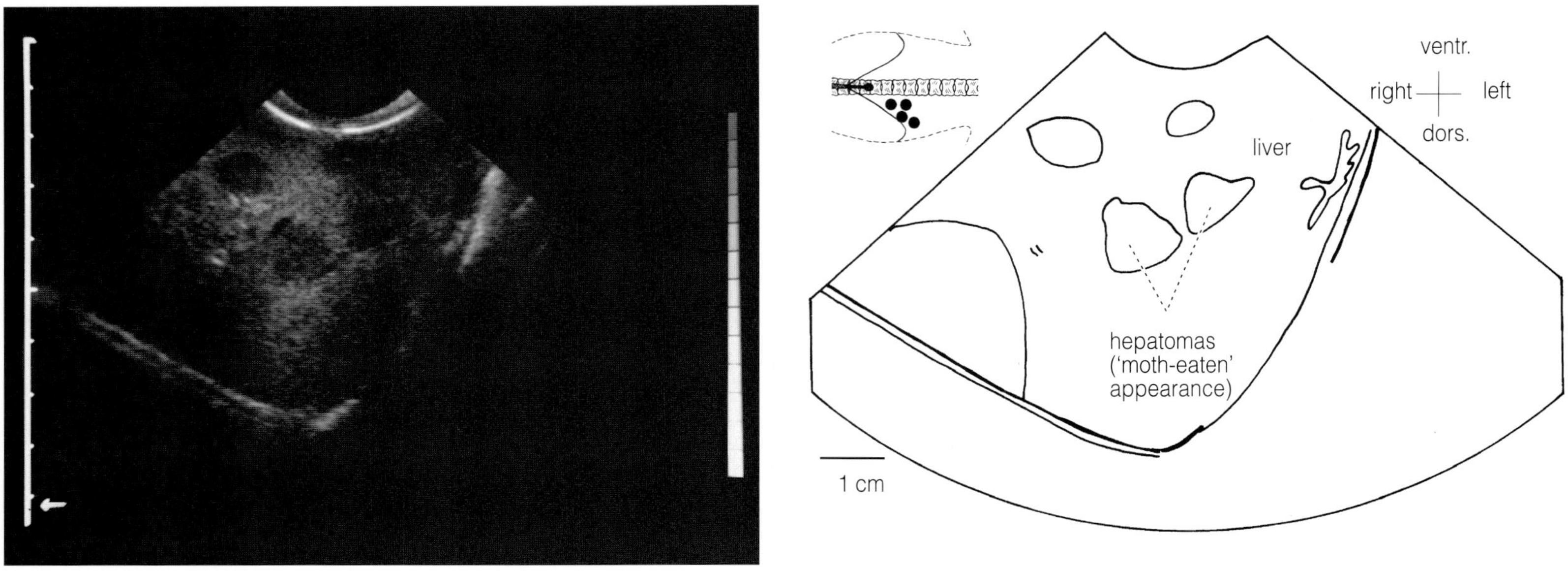

415 Hepatomegaly with focal hepatic lesions in a dog.

416

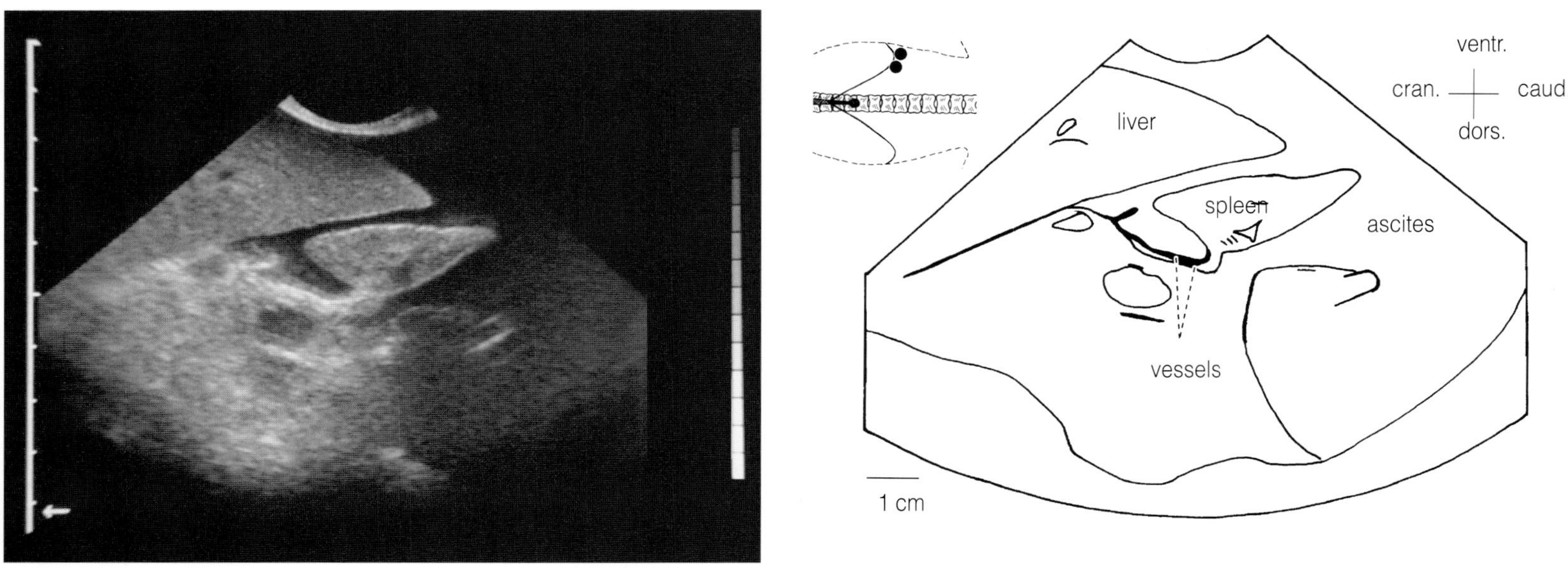

416 Hepatic lipidosis and ascites in a dog. The liver and spleen are well-demarcated by the anechoic abdominal fluid and show the same echogenicity. Diagnosis can be confirmed by a liver biopsy.

Ultrasonography of Liver and Gallbladder Disease

Hepatomegaly

Hepatomegaly is a non-specific finding that may already be seen radiographically. The liver margins are rounded and blunted in the sonogram. Hepatitis, hepatic lipidosis, cirrhosis, congestion and neoplasia may cause hepatomegaly and should be evaluated sonographically for prognosis (**415**). A liver biopsy is required with hepatomegaly for a histological diagnosis.

Diffuse Liver Disease such as Hepatic Lipidosis and Cirrhosis

Diffuse liver disease causes changes in liver echogenicity and affects the entire parenchyma. Ultrasonography cannot determine the cause or histopathological finding of diffuse liver disease. Slight variations in echogenicity do not usually show any correlation with macroscopic findings. In contrast, some macro-

Indications for liver ultrasonography include abnormal blood profiles, toxic conditions, acute abdomen, acute trauma, non-specific abdominal disease, abnormal palpation, and right heart failure with suspected:

- Hepatomegaly.
- Diffuse liver disease including hepatic lipidosis and cirrhosis.
- Focal parenchymal abnormalities such as cysts, haematomas, abscesses and hypoechoic foci.
- Hepatic neoplasia and metastases.
- Hepatic and portal vein abnormalities such as portosystemic shunts, portal hypertension and hepatic congestion.
- Gallbladder and biliary tract abnormalities such as inflammatory disease, neoplasia, sludge, calculi and polyps.

A further indication is for monitoring treatment response.

417

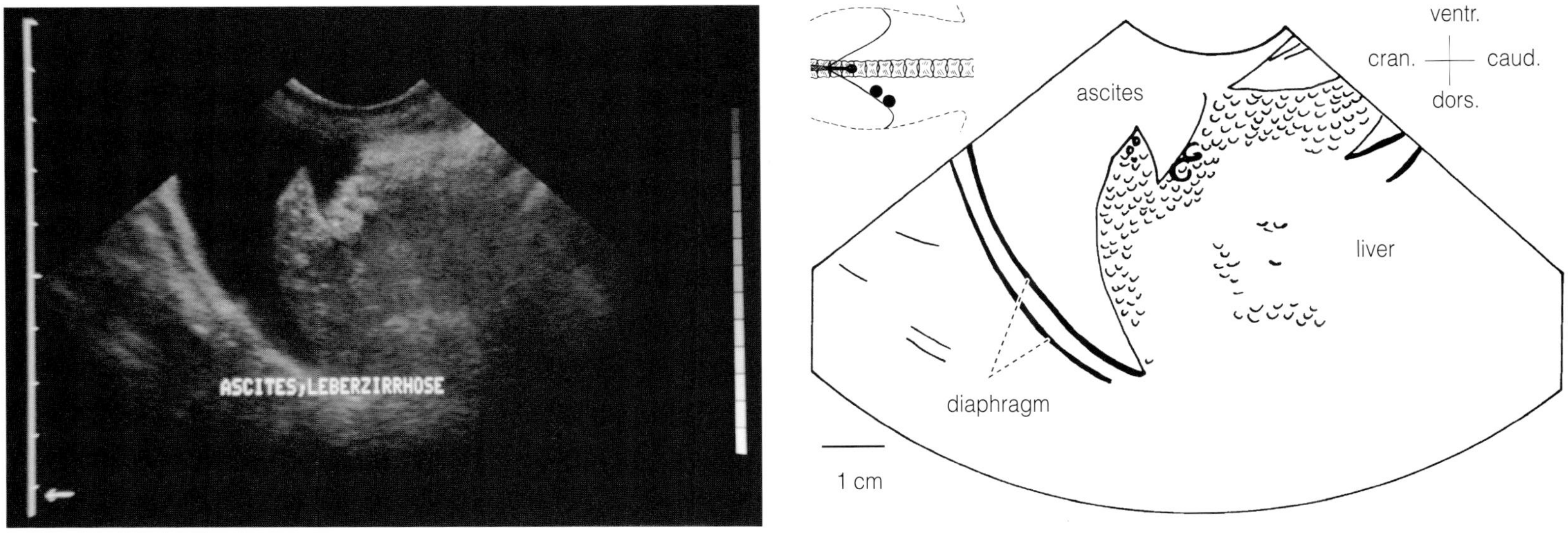

417 Hepatic cirrhosis and ascites in a dog.

418

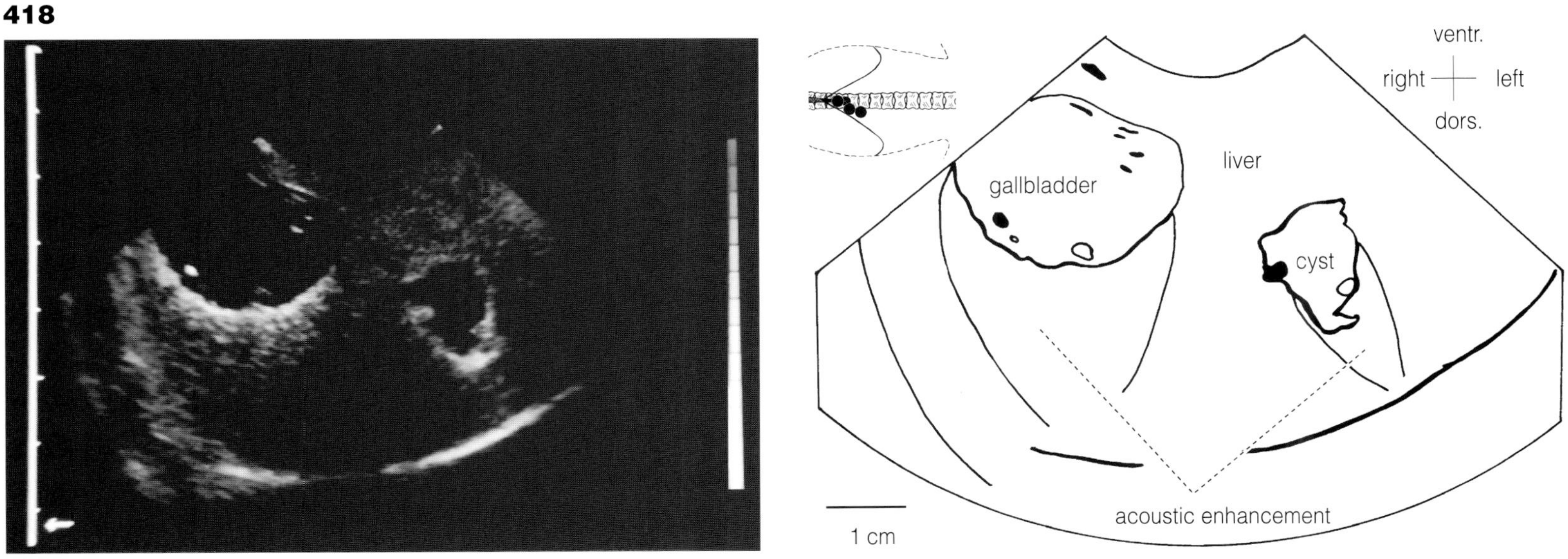

418 Hepatic cyst next to the gallbladder in a dog. The large anechoic gallbladder contains echogenic particles

scopic lesions found during a laparotomy are not seen in the sonogram. Diffuse liver disease includes hepatic lipidosis and cirrhosis.

Hepatic Lipidosis

Hepatic lipidosis is not diagnosed as often sonographically in the dog and cat as in humans. Ultrasonoghaphy shows hepatomegaly and a more or less increased echogenicity of the liver parenchyma[5]. A liver with fatty infiltration appears similar to slightly more echogenic than the normally more hyperechoic spleen (**416**).

Hepatic Cirrhosis

Ultrasonographic findings with hepatic cirrhosis vary with the current stage of the disease and other complications. Early stage cirrhosis is difficult to determine sonographically and cannot be ruled out[3]. A final diagnosis is made in conjunction with clinical examination, serum biochemistry and histological findings. End-stage cirrhosis with liver atrophy is more evident sonographically and is accompanied by a number of secondary clinical symptoms, resulting in a hepatic coma. The sonogram shows a small liver with nodular lesions and a non-uniform echo pattern[4]. The liver appears even smaller when the entire organ is involved. Hepatic cirrhosis is often accompanied by ascites (**417**).

Focal Hepatic Lesions such as Cysts, Haematomas, Abscesses and Hepatomas

Focal lesions are easily detected sonographically because the normal parenchyma provides a background with uniform echogenicity. Focal hepatic abnormalities include cysts, haematomas and abscesses, which are usually hypoechoic with some echogenic contents. Foci of at least 5 mm in size are usually easily detected. Some lesions are difficult to differentiate from others and almost impossible to differentiate from tumours. Diagnosis is made histopathologically after laparotomy. Anechoic structures such as cysts should not be mistaken for the gallbladder or a fluid-filled stomach caudal to the liver (**418**). The aetiology of a cyst (congenital, parasites, bacteria, trauma, inflammation) cannot be determined ultrasonographically.

419

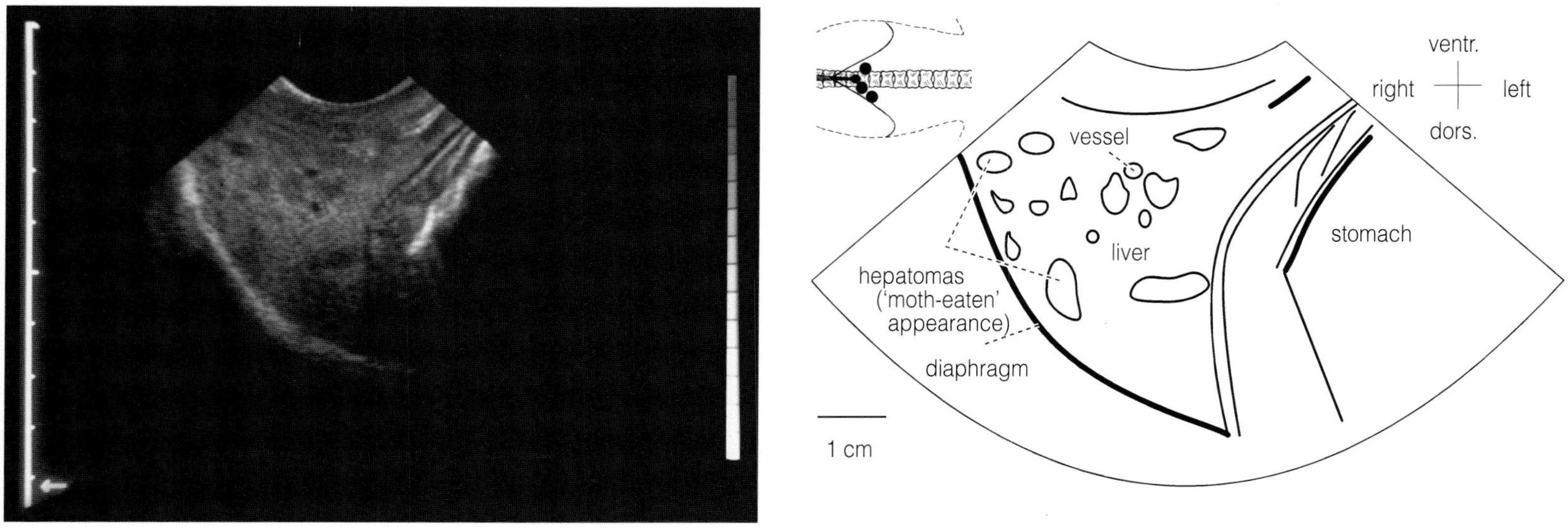

419 Liver with multiple hypoechoic focal lesions giving it a 'moth-eaten' appearance (hepatomas) in a dog.

420

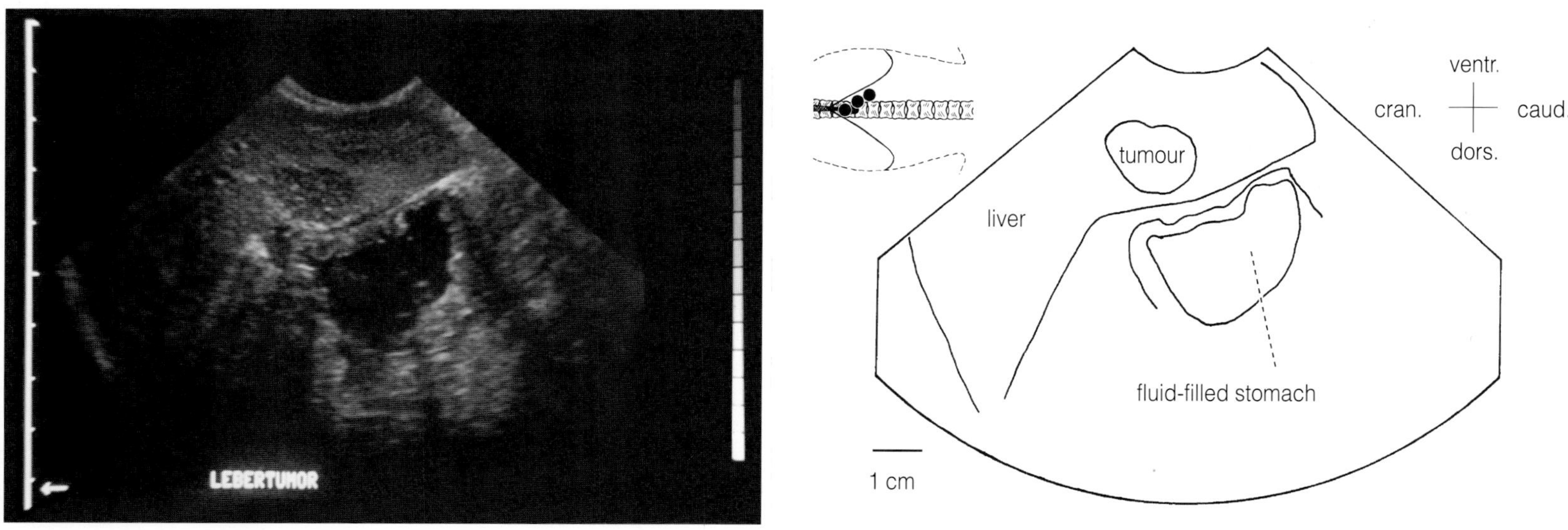

420 Liver with a well-demarcated, hypoechoic solitary tumour in a dog. The anechoic fluid-filled stomach represents a secondary finding.

Frequently, hypoechoic, well-demarcated areas with smooth to irregular contours are seen within the normal hepatic parenchyma. These multiple, benign lesions are also called hepatomas and may not be seen in follow-up examinations. Their image gives the liver a 'moth-eaten' appearance. The aetiology is unknown (**415, 419**).

Hepatic Neoplasia and Metastases

Hepatic neoplasia and metastases appear as solid to cystic focal lesions in the parenchyma. They are anechoic to hyperechoic, uniform to irregular, and more or less demarcated (**420–425**). The tumour type or malignancy cannot be differentiated ultrasonographically. Computed tomography and histology are useful in determining the diagnosis. Hepatic neoplasia is also difficult to differentiate from other focal lesions. A thorough examination is required to determine if large peripheral focal tumours involve the liver and to differentiate gastric, pancreatic and splenic tumours. A quick 'look' is not sufficient.

> **NB**: Focal lesions, e.g. tumours, may be overlooked in the cranial portion of the liver because of location and size. Diagnosis of neoplasia requires a thorough examination of the liver in various imaging planes. A definitive diagnosis is still difficult to make.

421

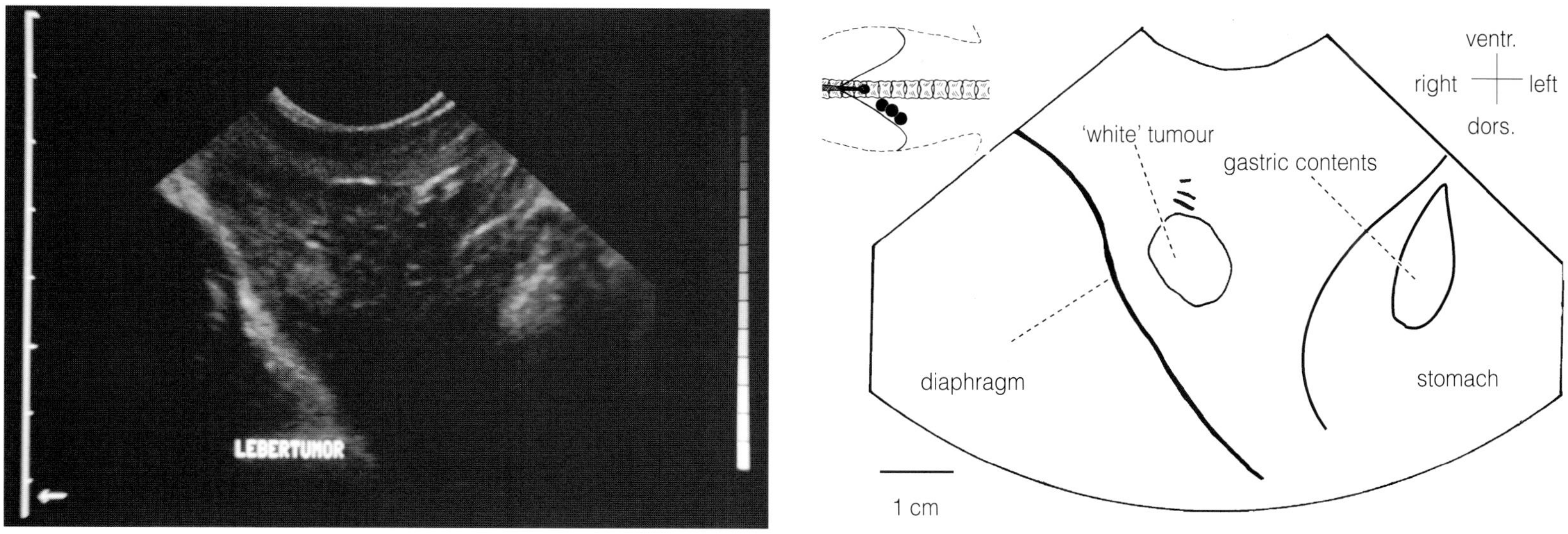

421 Canine liver with a well-demarcated, hyperechoic, so-called 'white' solitary tumour. (Hyperechoic 'white' tumours are usually diagnosed as carcinoma.)

422

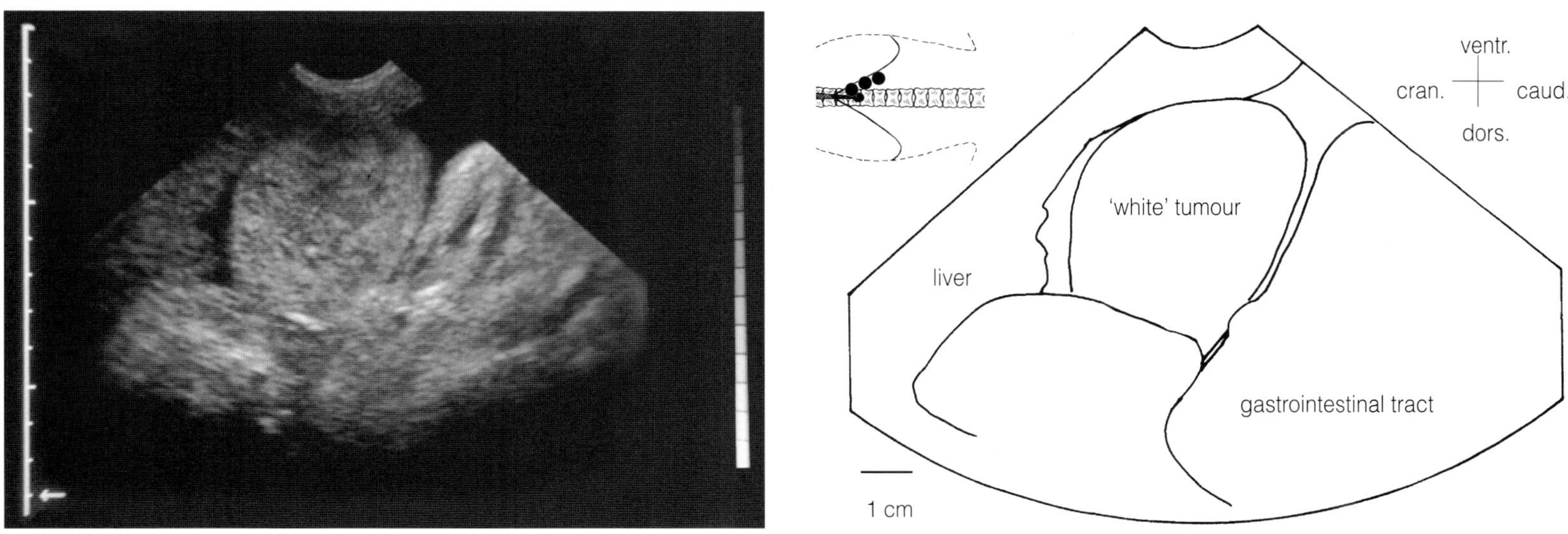

421 Canine liver with a well-demarcated, hyperechoic, so-called 'white' solitary tumour. (Hyperechoic 'white' tumours are usually diagnosed as carcinoma.)

Hepatic Vascular Abnormalities such as Portosystemic Shunts, Portal Hypertension and Liver Congestion

Ultrasonography of extrahepatic portosystemic shunts in young dogs shows a small liver with enlarged vessels near the porta hepatis[6]. Intrahepatic portal veins and hepatic veins are not seen[8]. The shunt between the portal vein branch and the caudal vena cava may be detected or visualized using colour Doppler.

The causes for portal hypertension may be prehepatic following abdominal infections, pancreatitis and peritonitis; intrahepatic with cirrhosis and severe functional liver disorders; or posthepatic with right-sided heart failure[3]. The ultrasonographic sign is a distended lumen of the portal vein and/or its branches. In some cases a portal vein thrombus may be identified. Secondary signs include splenomegaly and ascites[3]. Right-sided heart failure causes congestion of blood in the caudal vena cava and the hepatic veins and dilation of these vessels. This results in liver congestion with decreased echogenicity of the hepatic parenchyma and/or portal hypertension (**426**).

Diseases of the Gallbladder and Biliary Tract

Inflammation of the gallbladder wall results in increased echogenicity and thickening of the wall with small echogenic deposits. In acute cholecystitis the gallbladder contents are anechoic (**427**), while chronic disorders produce echogenic particles suspended in the bile fluid (**428**). Calculi in the gallbladder may also occur with cholecystitis.

423

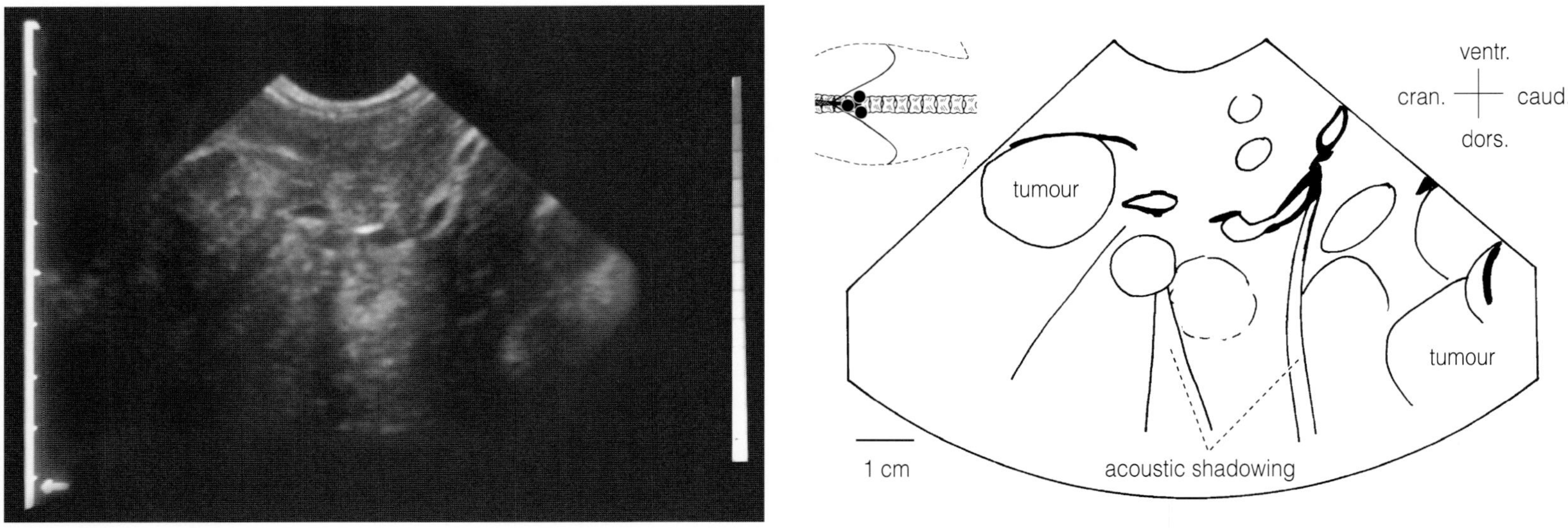

423 Canine liver with multiple, irregular 'white' tumours (tentative diagnosis: carcinoma). Hepatomegaly and distended hepatic vessels are visible.

424

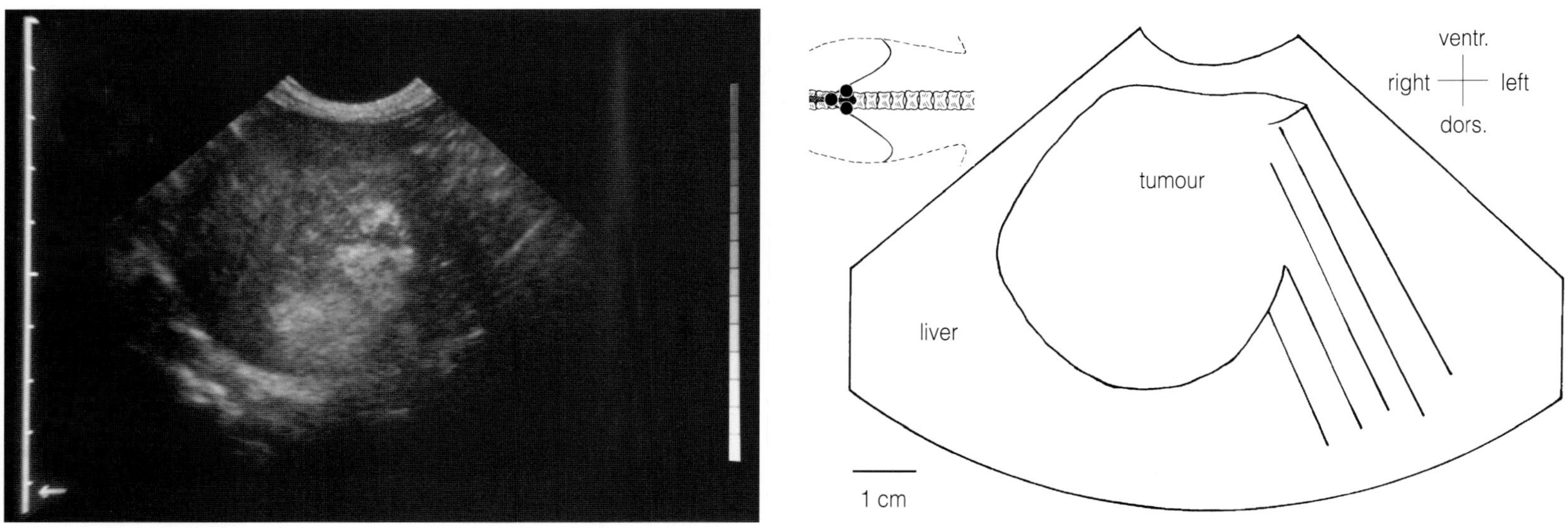

424 Canine liver with a non-uniform, irregular solitary tumour.

425

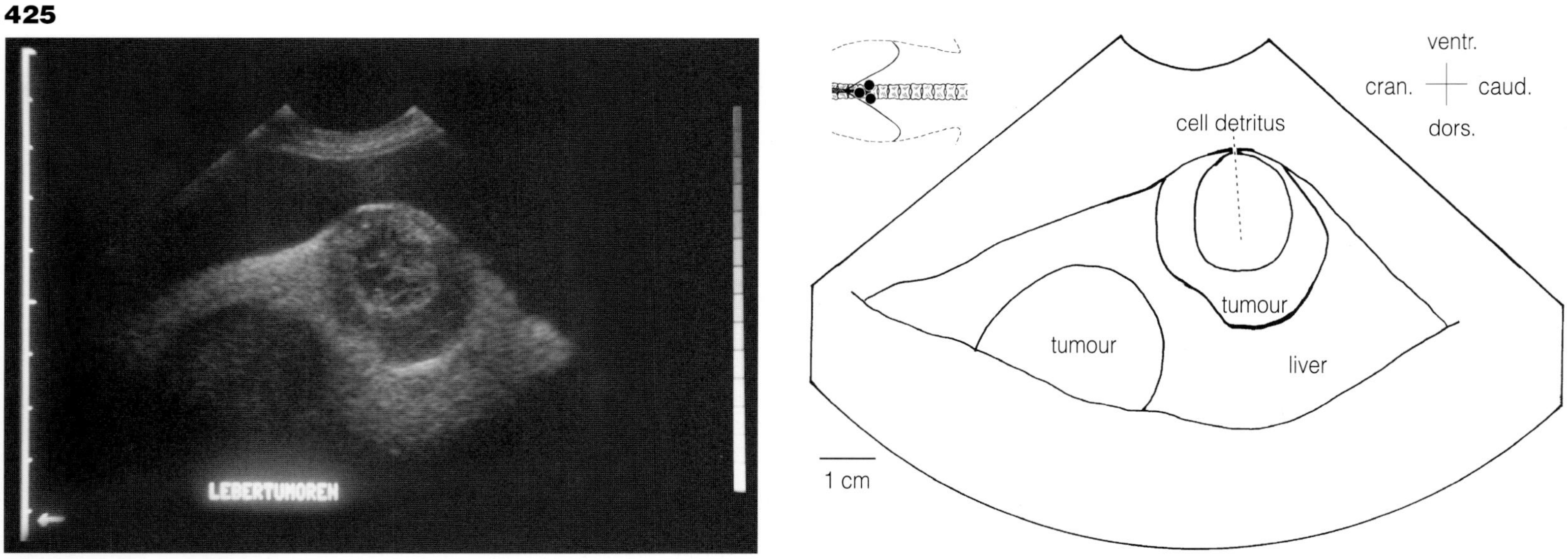

425 Canine liver with two hypoechoic irregular tumours. Anechoic, central necrosis is visible on both lesions. These findings indicate possible rupture of the tumour.

426

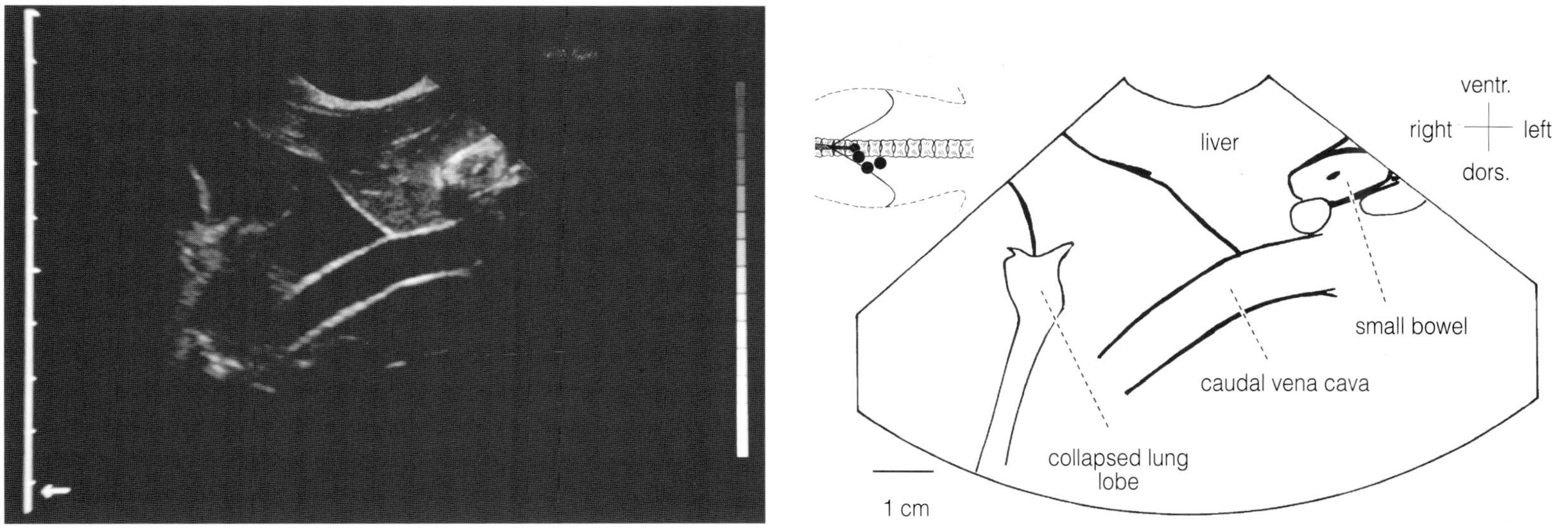

426 Canine liver with dilated caudal vena cava and free thoracic fluid.

427

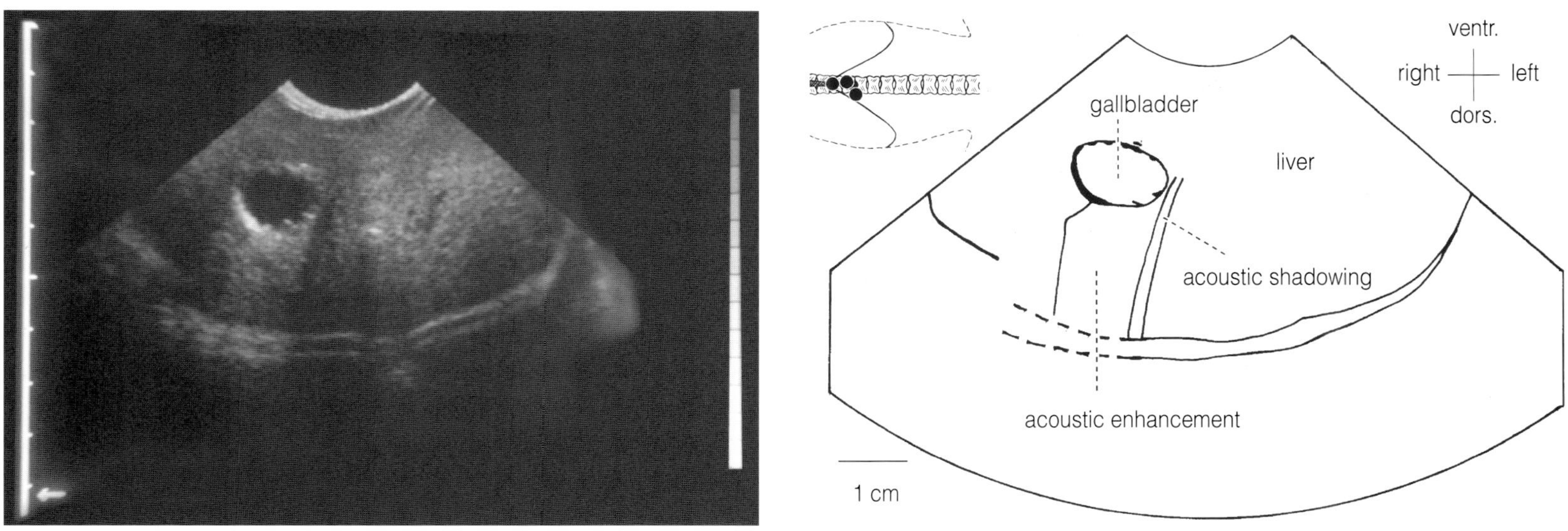

427 Acute cholecystitis with an irregular, hyperechoic gallbladder wall.

428

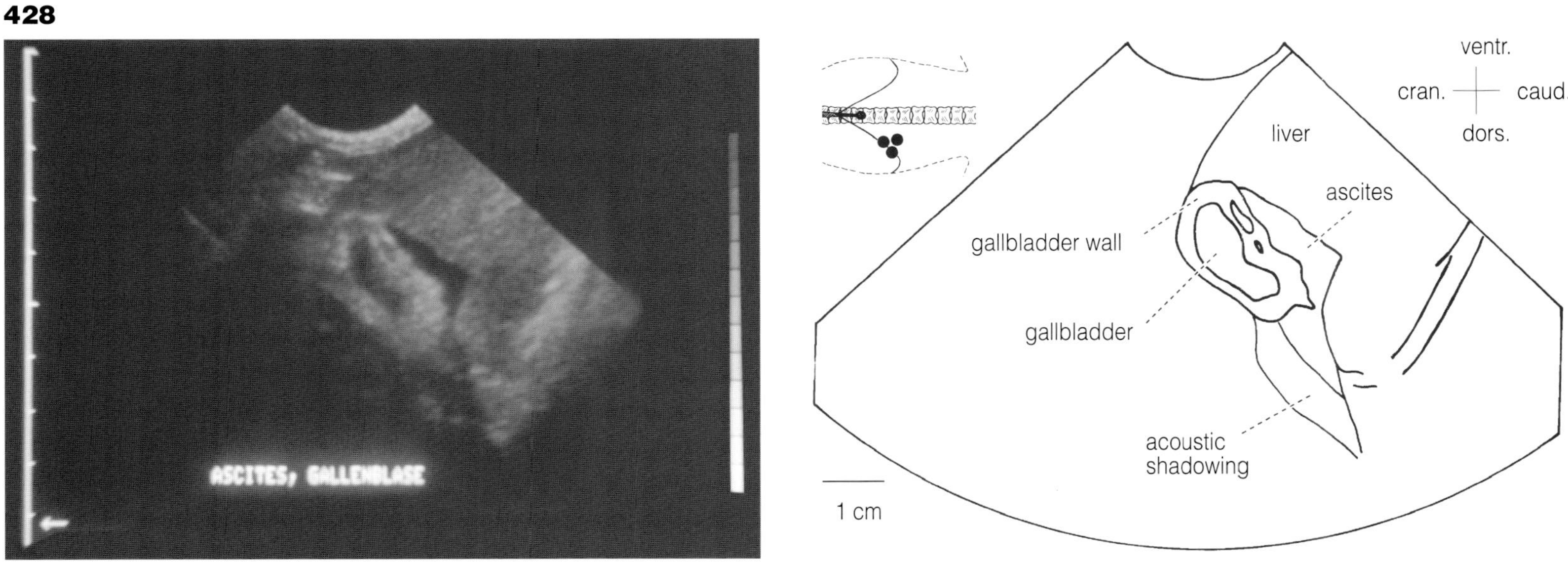

428 Chronic cholecystitis with a thickened, hyperechoic gallbladder wall and echogenic particles in a dog. Ascites is also present. Causes for the anechoic peritoneal fluid surrounding the gallbladder include a perforated or ruptured gallbladder wall or a pericholecystic abscess.

429

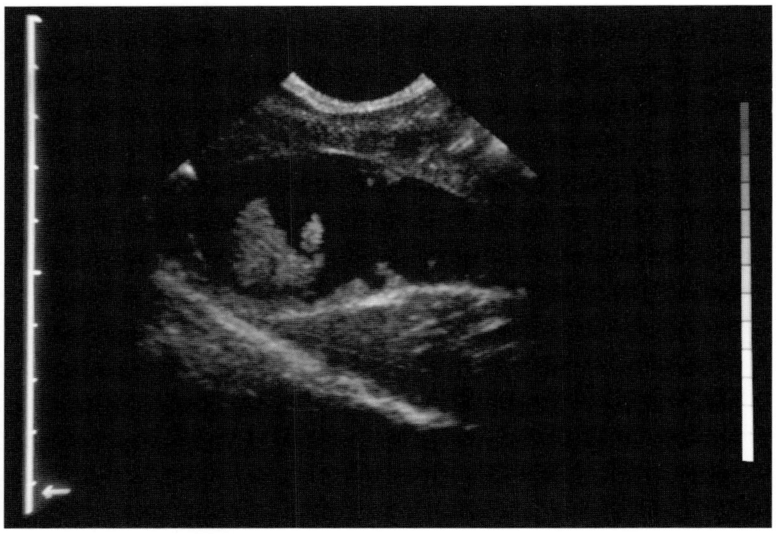

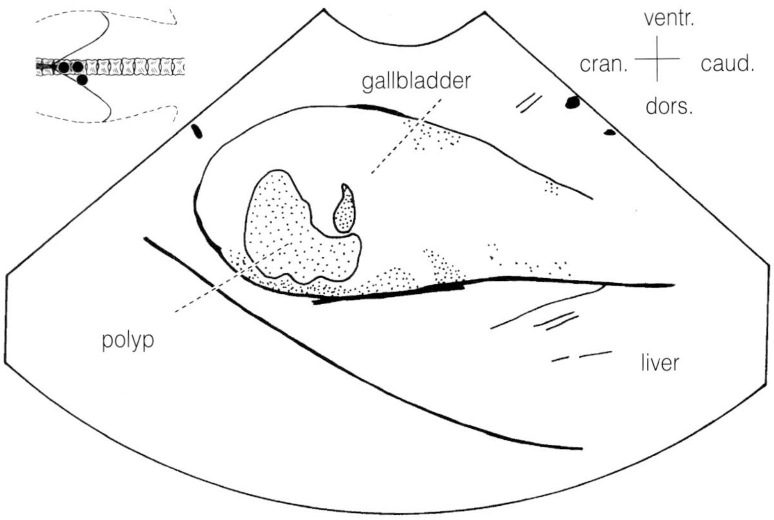

430

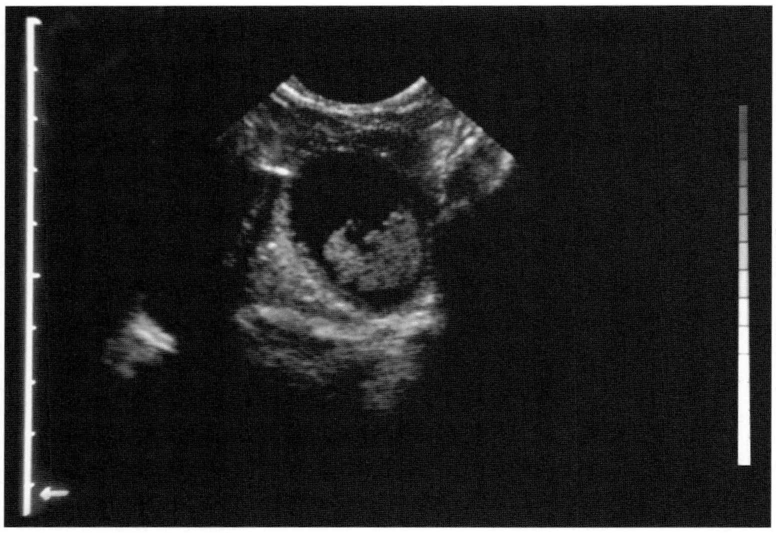

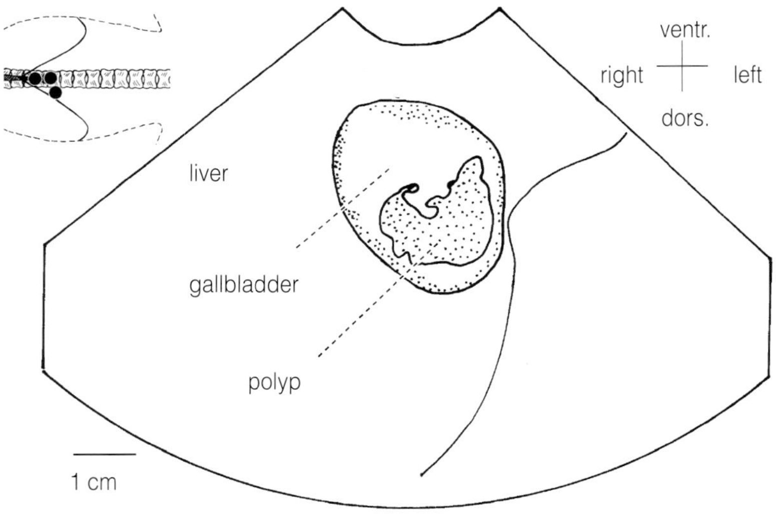

429, 430 Canine gallbladder wall with a cauliflower-like polyp extending into the lumen in a longitudinal (**429**) and transverse view (**430**). An almost identical image may be seen with sludge.

Polyps and tumours are seen as hyperechoic structures attached to the wall and extending into the gallbladder lumen (**429, 430**). Malignancy of these masses cannot be determined. Sludge is occasionally difficult to differentiate from a polyp or tumour.

The gallbladder often contains fine, homogenous sediment of medium echogenicity. The sediment settles at the bottom of the gallbladder after repositioning the animal. Gallbladder sludge is not considered pathological and is often seen in fasted dogs. Crystals and calcifications produce stronger echoes **431–433**). It is important to differentiate sludge from neoplastic lesions. This is done by repositioning the animal. When a definitive diagnosis cannot be made, follow-up examinations are indicated.

431

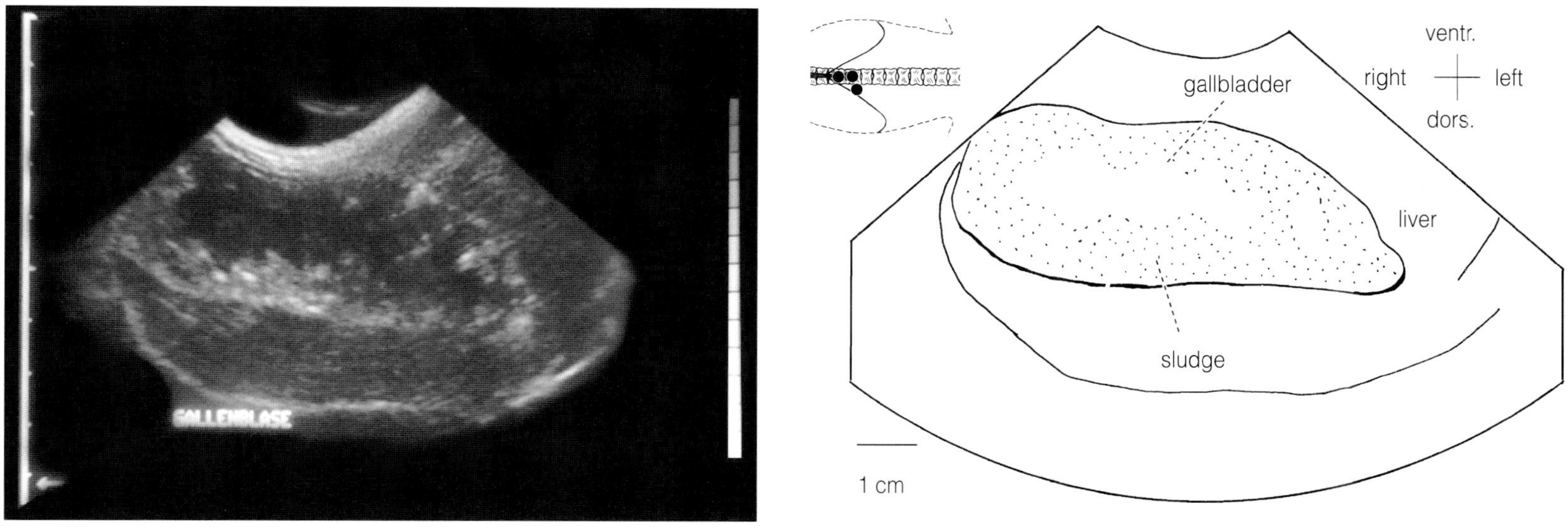

432

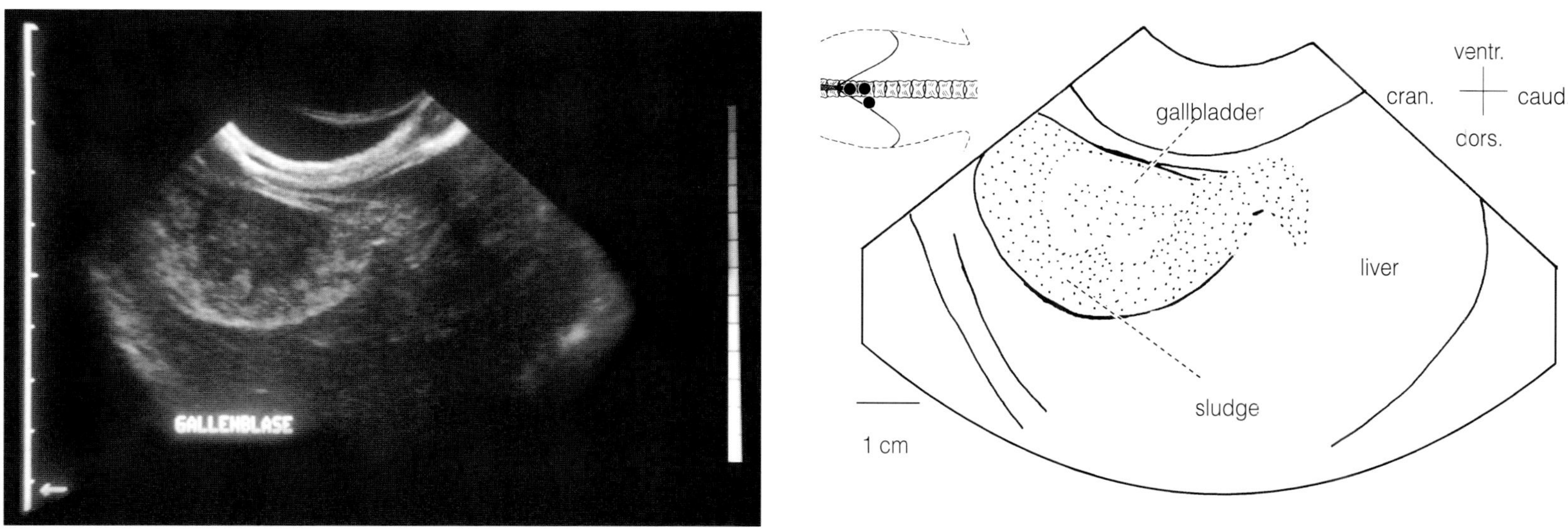

431, 432 Gallbladder sludge in a longitudinal (**431**) and transverse (**432**) view in a dog. The sludge is difficult to differentiate from the gallbladder wall. The echogenicity is indicative of crystals or calcification.

433

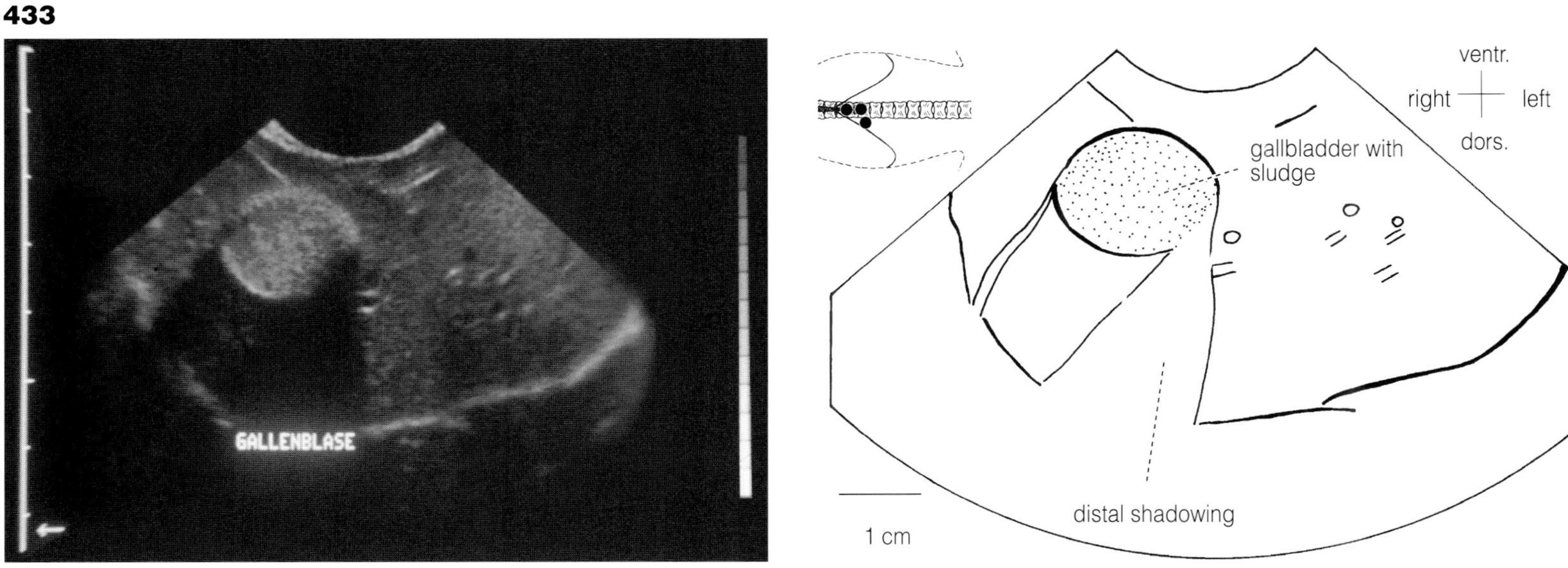

433 Echogenic gallbladder sludge with distal shadowing in a dog.

434

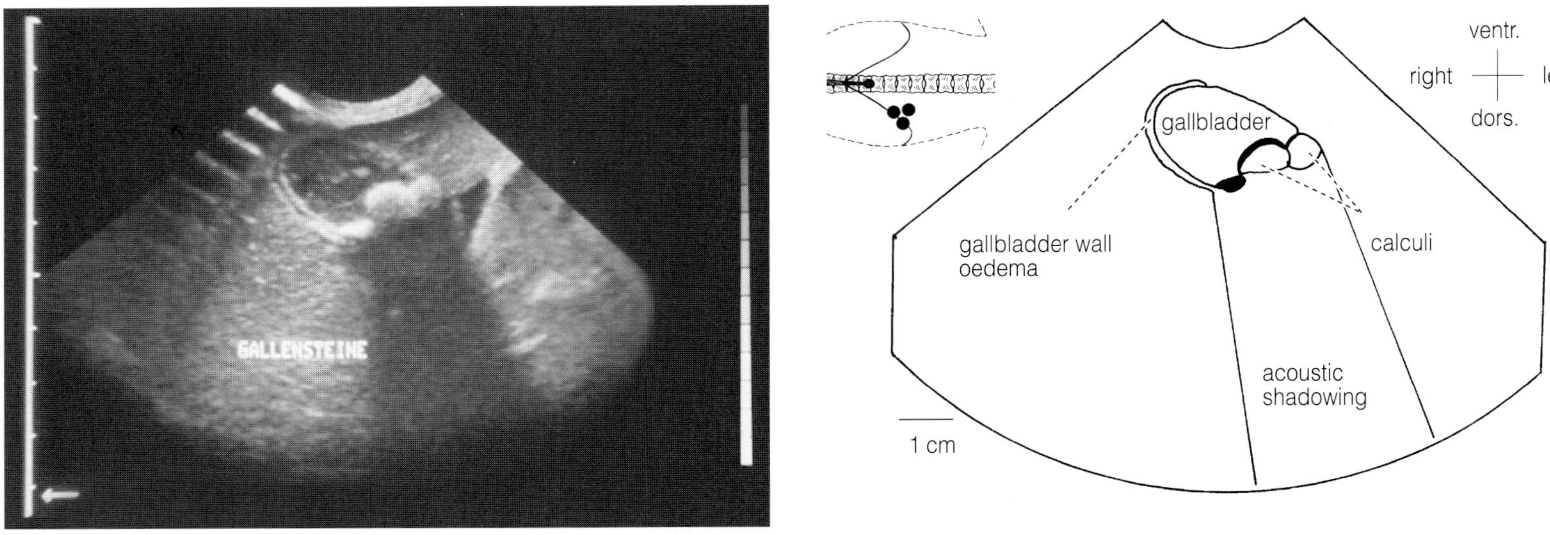

434 Cholecystolithiasis with inflammatory gallbladder wall oedema, calculi in the dorsal portion of the gallbladder and distal shadowing in a dog in dorsal recumbency.

435

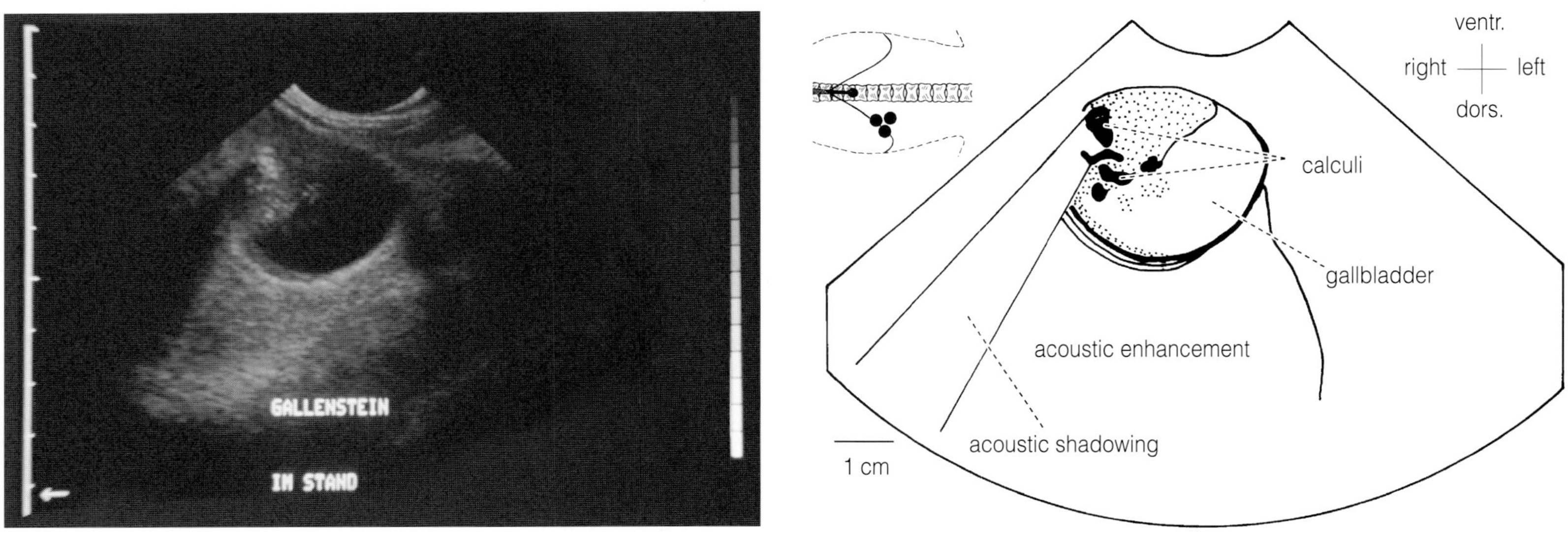

435 Cholecystolithiasis with slightly increased wall echogenicity and a calculus in the ventral portion of the gallbladder with acoustic shadowing in a standing dog.

436

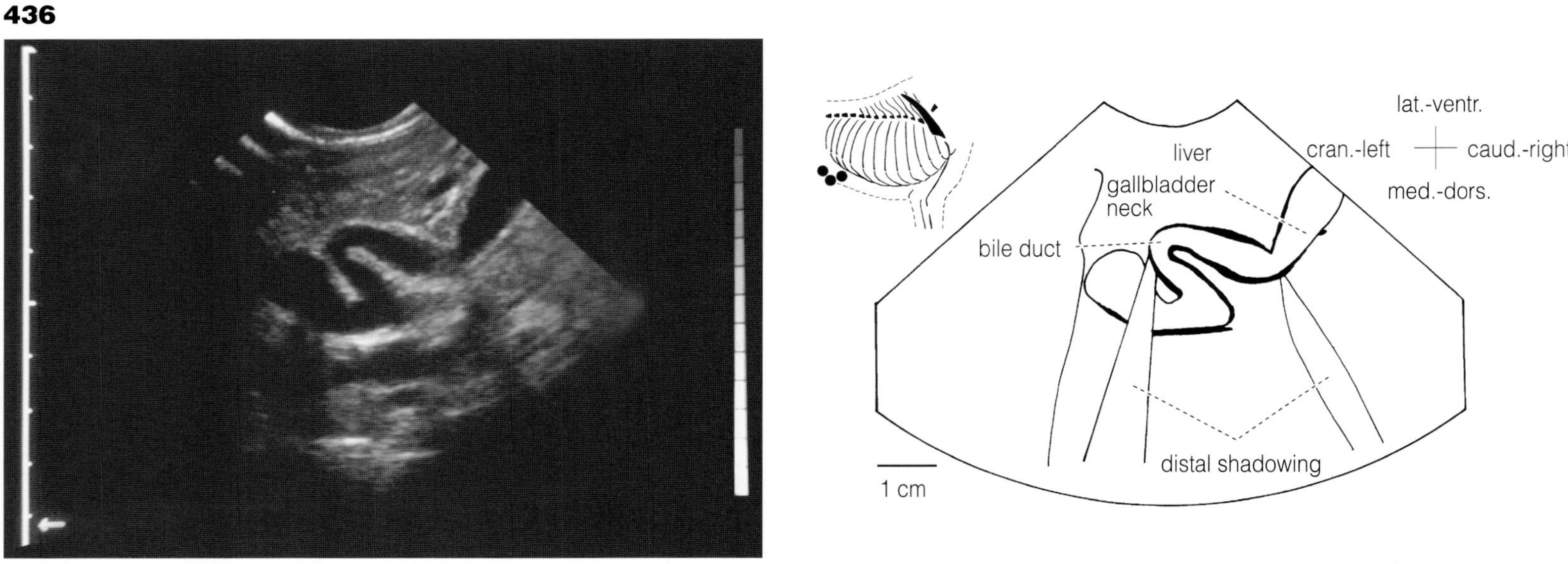

436 Severely dilated, tortuous common bile duct in a dog with duodenitis.

437

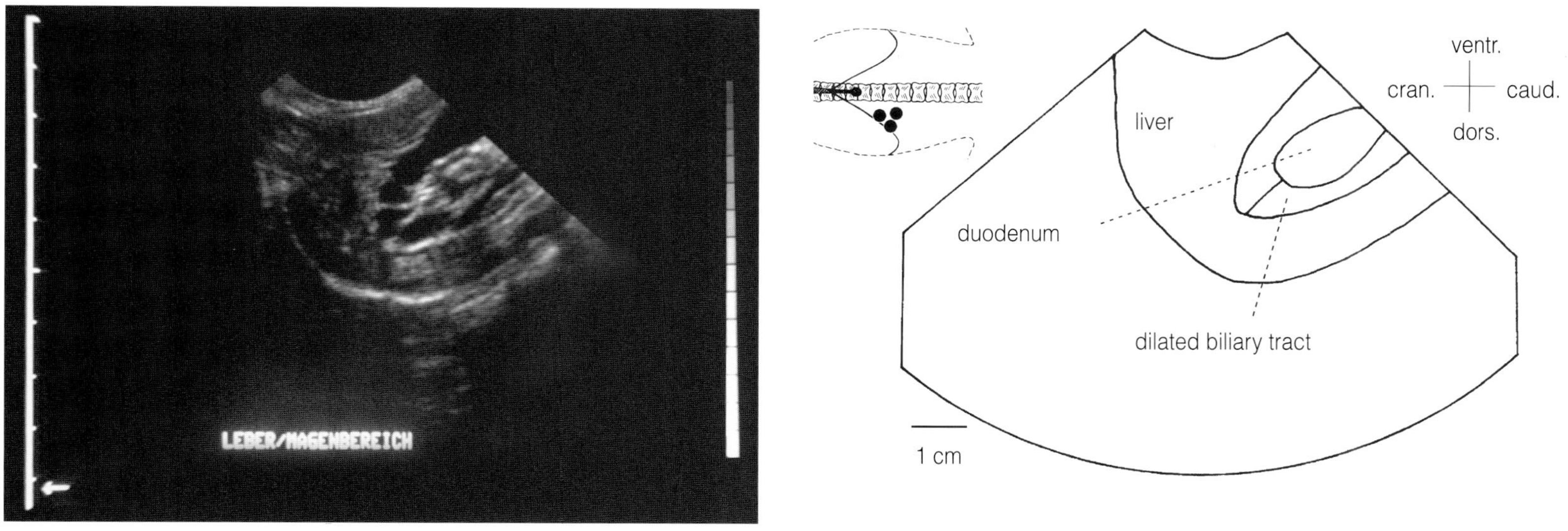

437 Gallbladder and severly distended bile ducts in a cat with a pancreatic tumour.

Calculi in the biliary tract are hyperechoic with distal acoustic shadowing. They are usually associated with an inflamed and thickened gallbladder wall (**434, 435**). Small discrete stones with poor echogenicity and without shadowing may be overlooked during routine examinations or mistaken for sludge.

Intrahepatic or extrahepatic distended bile ducts (cystic duct, common bile duct) are seen as anechoic longitudinal, sometimes tortuous, structures with distinctly echogenic walls (**436, 437**). Causes for these bile duct abnormalities or obstructions may not be determined ultrasonographically. Liver neoplasia, inflammation and tumours of the biliary tract itself, or pancreatic and duodenal lesions, may cause biliary obstruction.

References

Cited References

1 Breiling F (1994) *Vergleichende Makroskopisch-fotografische Transversale Schnittanatomie der abdominalen Organe von Hand und Katze*. Hannover, Tierärztl. Hochsch., Diss.

2 Evans HE (1993) The digestive apparatus and abdomen. In: Evans HE (Ed.) *Miller's Anatomy of the Dog*. 3rd Edn. WB Saunders, Philadelphia, London, pp. 385–462.

3 Kremer H, Dobrinski W and Schrieber MA (1992) Leber. In: Kremer H and Dobrinski W (Eds.) *Sonographische Diagnostik. Innere Medizin und Angrenzende Gebiete*. 4th Edn. Urban and Schwarzenberg, München, Wien, Baltimore.

4 Lamb CR (1990) Abdominal ultrasonography in small animals: examination of the liver, spleen and pancreas. *J. Small Anim.Pract.* **31**, 5–14.

5 Lijour L (1987) L'échotomographie hépatique chez les carnivores domestiques. 2ième partie: Images échotomographiques anormales. *Prat. Méd. Chir. Anim. Comp.* **22**, 113–127.

6 Nyland TG and Park RD (1983) Hepatic ultrasonography in the dog. *Vet. Radiol.* **24**, 74–84.

7 Poulsen Nautrup C (1995) Persönliche Mitteilung vom 09.07.1995, Hannover.

8 Wrigley RH, Konde LJ, Park RD and Lebel JL (1987) Ultrasonographic diagnosis of portacaval shunts in young dogs. *J. Am. Vet. Med. Assoc.* **191**, 421–424.

Additional Reading

Carniel P (1987) Echographie du foie du chien. *Point Vét.* **19**, 415–432.

Nyland TG and Hager DA (1985) Sonography of the liver, gallbladder and spleen. Symposium of diagnostic ultrasound. *Vet. Clin. North Am. Small Anim. Pract.* **15**, 1123–1147.

Probst A (1992) *Untersuchungen zur Sonographischen Differenzierung der Leberlappen des Handes*. Wien, Veterinärmed. Univ., Diss.

Wrighley RH (1985) Radiographic and ultrasonographic diagnosis of liver diseases in dogs and cats. *Vet. Clin. North Am. Small Anim. Pract.* **15**, 21–38.

Pancreas

Dirk Lüerssen and Martin Janthur

The pancreas is considered one of the most difficult abdominal organs to display ultrasonographically. In most cases the normal pancreas is not visualized.

Examination Technique

The examination of the patient is preceded by the usual preparations. The patient is positioned in dorsal recumbency. Repositioning the animal during the examination may improve visualization of the left or right pancreatic limb when bowel loops are displaced. The scanning field extends from the left costal arch to the 9th or 10th right rib and from the xiphoid to the umbilical area. The right pancreatic limb in the cat is usually best seen from a left paracostal scanning position[5].

Anatomy and Normal Sonographic Findings

From a ventral aspect, the pancreas resembles an upside-down L. The left pancreatic limb lies in a transverse position, extending from the spleen to the cranial duodenal flexure and adjacent to the splenic vein. The left limb lies between the greater curvature of the stomach and the transverse colon. The right limb of the pancreas is orientated longitudinally and adjacent to the descending duodenum. Dorsal to the right limb lies the right kidney and the caudate lobe of the liver. Both limbs are joined by the pancre-

438

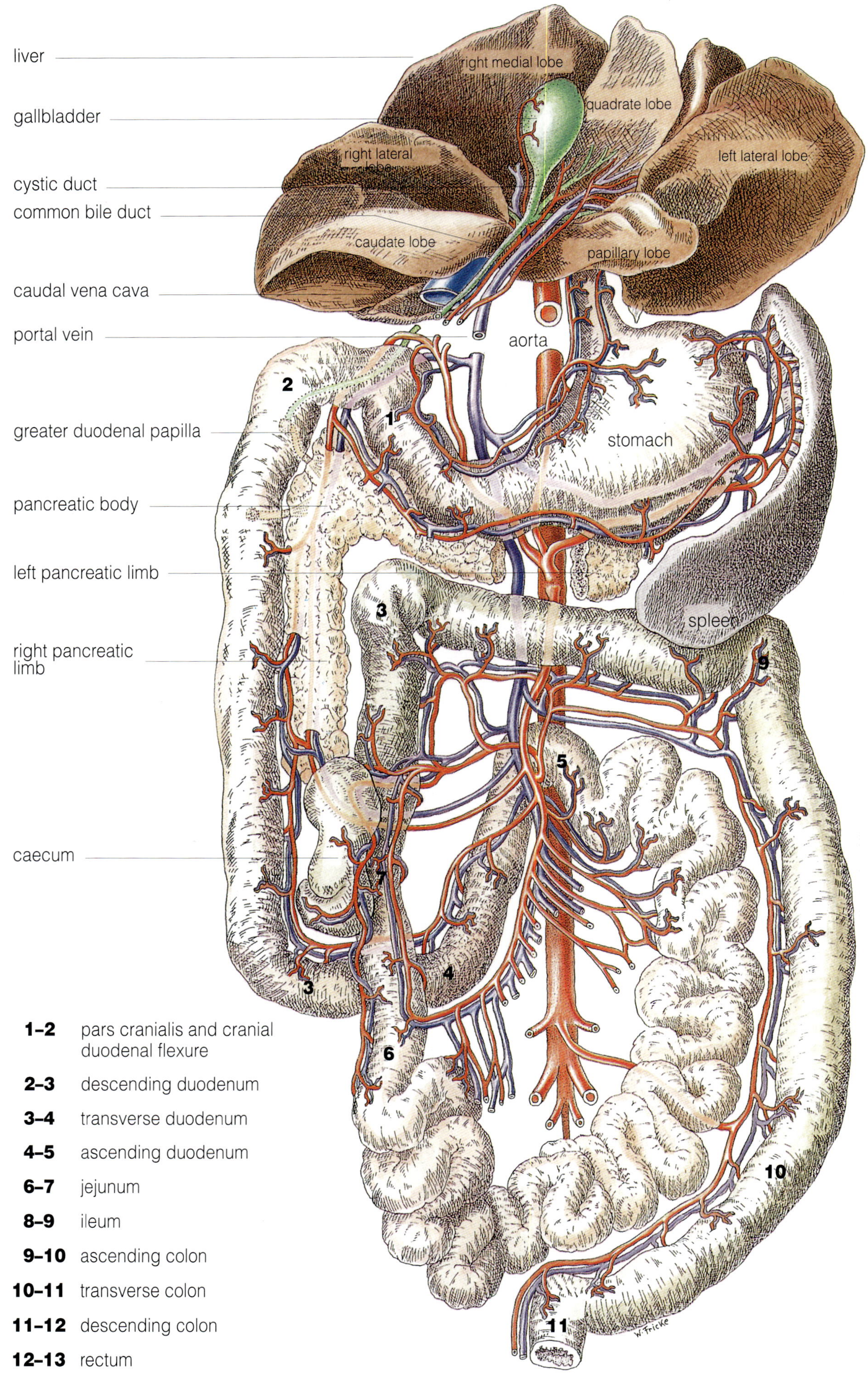

438 Schematic illustration of pancreatic topography. (Reprinted with permission from K-D Budras in: Budras K-D, Fricke W and Richter R (1996) *Atlas der Anatomie des Hundes*. 5th edn., Schluetersche Verlagsanstalt und Druckerei, Hannover.)

atic body, which lies caudal to the pylorus and ventral to the portal vein (**438**).

The pancreas is localized by using the surrounding abdominal organs as well as vessels passing through the pancreatic region. The pancreas is usually found between the stomach, the spleen and the left kidney, although a more or less full stomach will cover the pancreas from the ventral and the left side (see Stomach, page 165; **359, 360**). For this reason, patients should be fasted prior to examination. However, a fluid-filled stomach may be useful. The splenic vein passes dorsal to the left pancreatic limb and this may

439

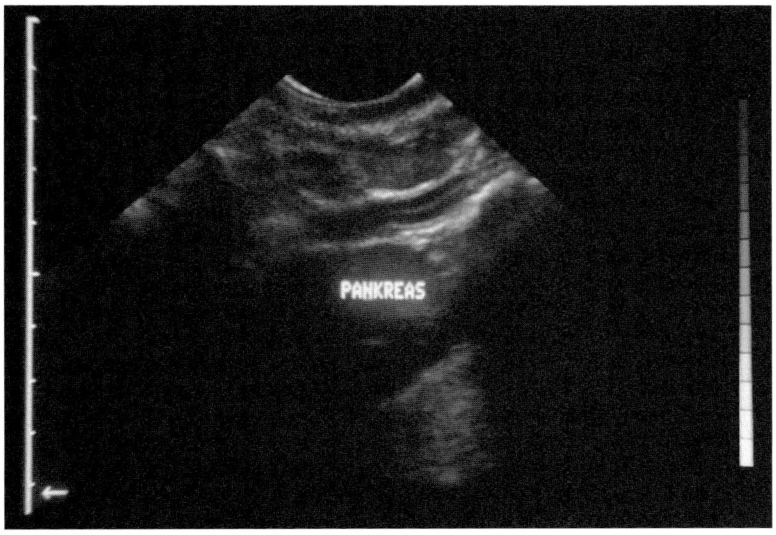

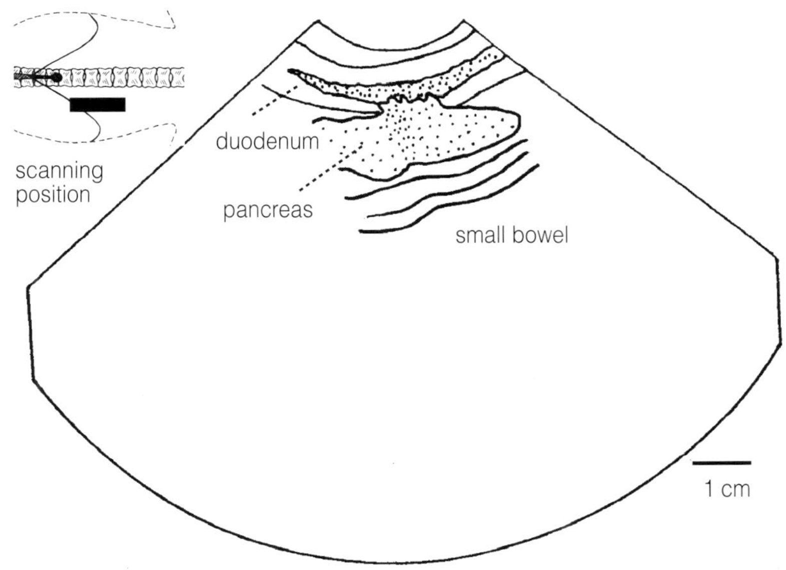

439 Long-axis scan of the right limb of the pancreas in a dog. Using a 7.5 MHz transducer, the pancreas has a finely granulated, homogenous texture.

440

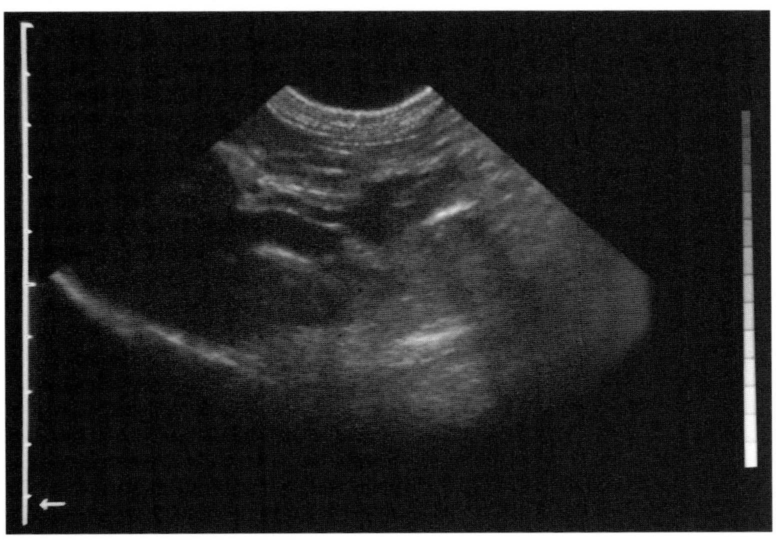

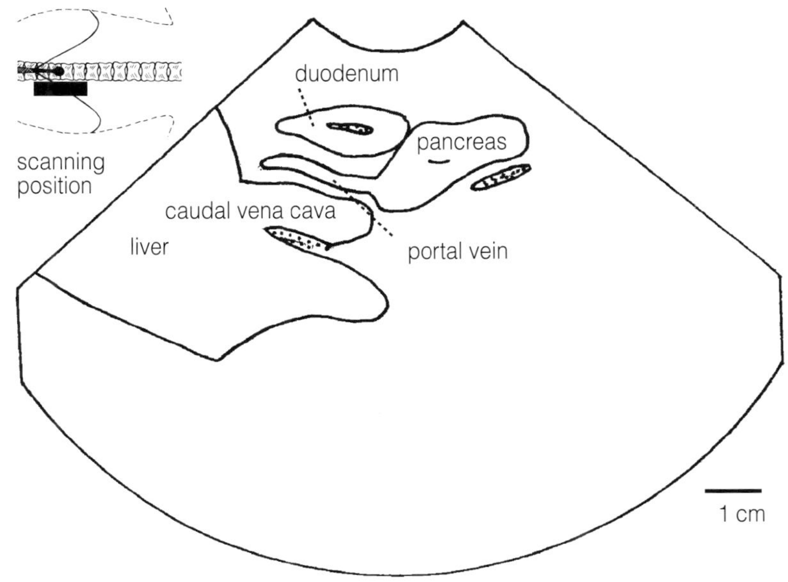

440 Right pancreatic limb in a dog. Peritonitis, caused by a ruptured pyometra, outlines the pancreas from surrounding tissue. The normal parenchyma is uniform and finely granulated.

> *Indications for pancreatic ultrasonography include digestive disorders, painful cranial abdomen, and abnormalities in pancreatic blood profiles with suspected:*
>
> - Acute pancreatitis.
> - Chronic pancreatitis.
> - Pancreatic cysts.
> - Pancreatic neoplasia.
>
> A further indication is for monitoring treatment response.

help with localization. The craniocaudal pancreaticoduodenal vein courses through the right limb of the pancreas[6]. The right limb is easier to visualize than the left limb. Pancreatic ultrasonography still remains problematic because of its close association with the gastrointestinal tract and the echogenicity of the normal pancreas, which is similar to the surrounding mesentry fat[3].

The normal pancreas appears hypoechoic, finely granulated and homogenous in the two-dimensional sonogram.

The normal pancreas is seen better ultrasonographically if there is diffuse peritonitis because of the differing echogenicities (440).

Ultrasonography of Pancreatic Disease

Acute Pancreatitis

With acute pancreatitis the pancreas has an enlarged hypoechoic structure[3]. The capsule is not visualized. Depending on the hypoechogenicity, the pancreas may be differentiated from the surrounding abdominal structures. The ultrasonographic appearance is due to oedema and shows echogenic lobulated structures within a hypoechoic, uniform net (441). Generally, lesions are visualized more efficiently in the right limb of the pancreas because of its localization. A tentative diagnosis may be made on the basis of the sonographic findings in the right cranial abdomen in association with a painful pancreatic area when applying local transducer pressure. A dilated pancreatic duct confirms the diagnosis of acute pancreatitis[2].

Chronic Pancreatitis

Chronic pancreatitis leads to a decrease in echogenicity due to necrosis (442) and abscess-formation[7], or an increase in echogenicity caused by atrophy and fibrosis[1]. Generally, a marked nonhomogenicity is expected (443).

441

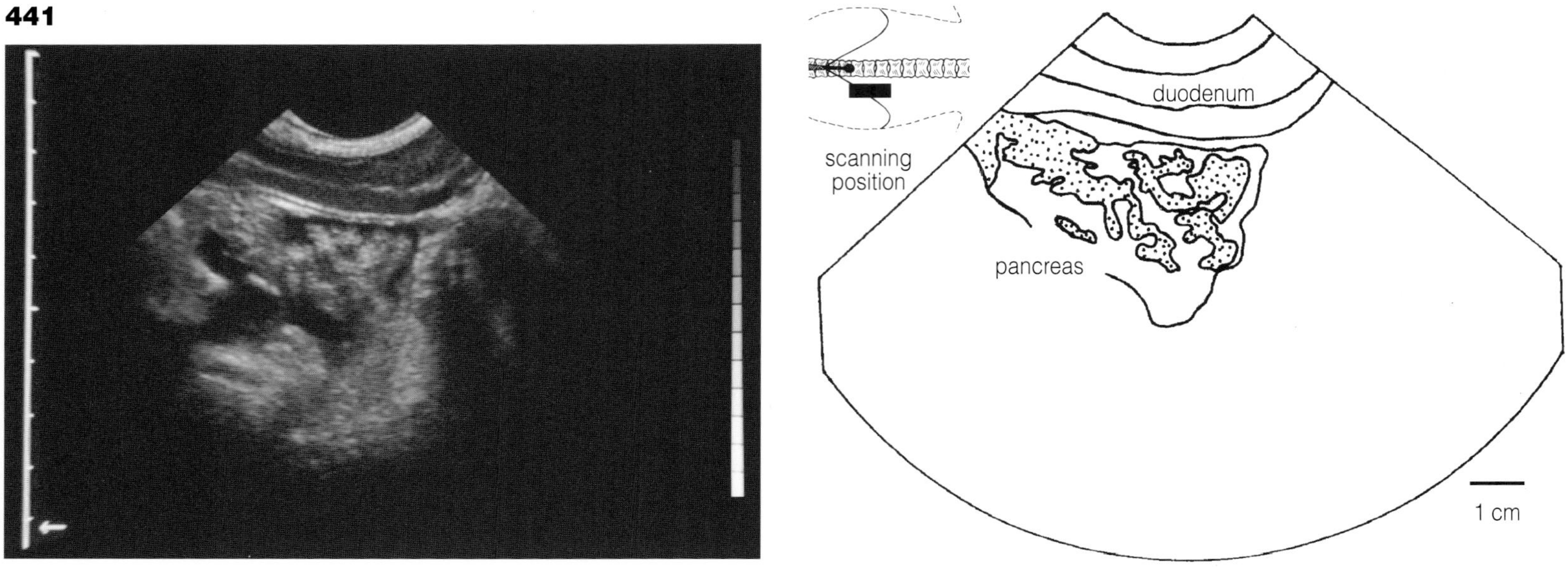

441 Oedema of the right pancreatic limb in a dog. The parenchyma is non-homogenous with a lobular, echogenic structure and a hypoechoic to anechoic margin.

442

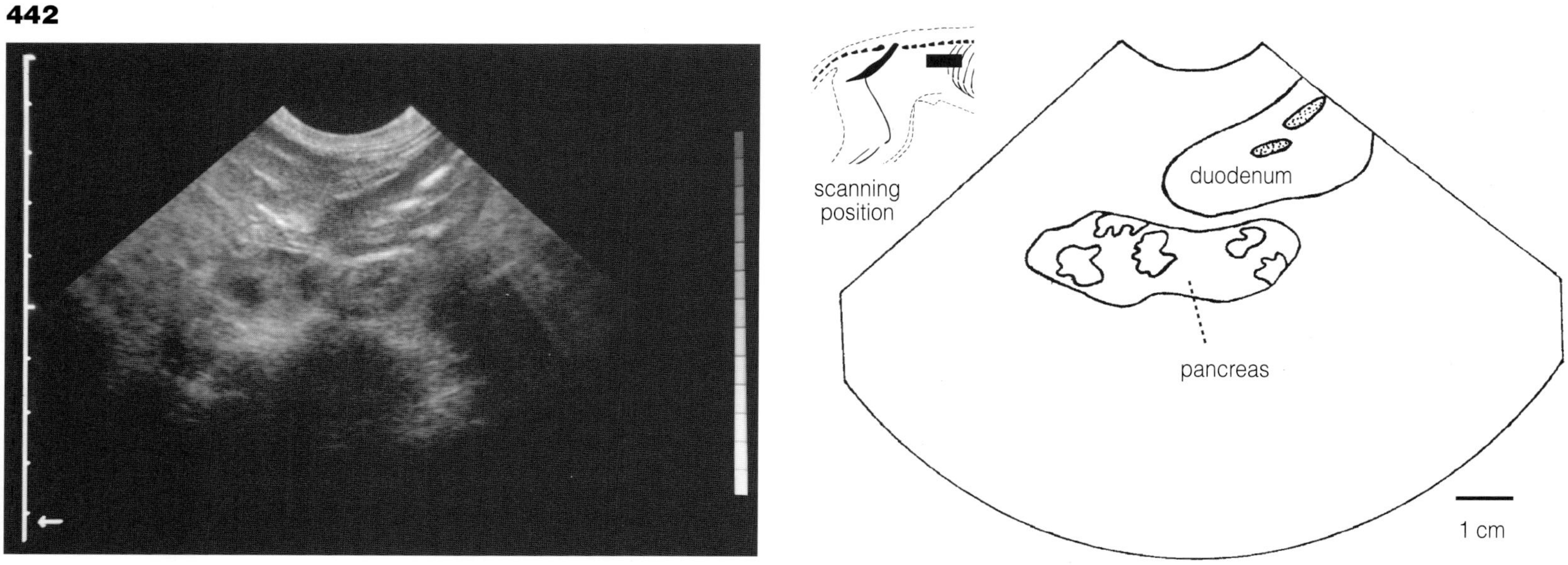

442 Chronic pancreatitis with focal necrosis in a dog. Hypoechoic, irregular areas are apparent in the right pancreatic limb. A similar ultrasonographic image is seen with mulicentric tumours.

443

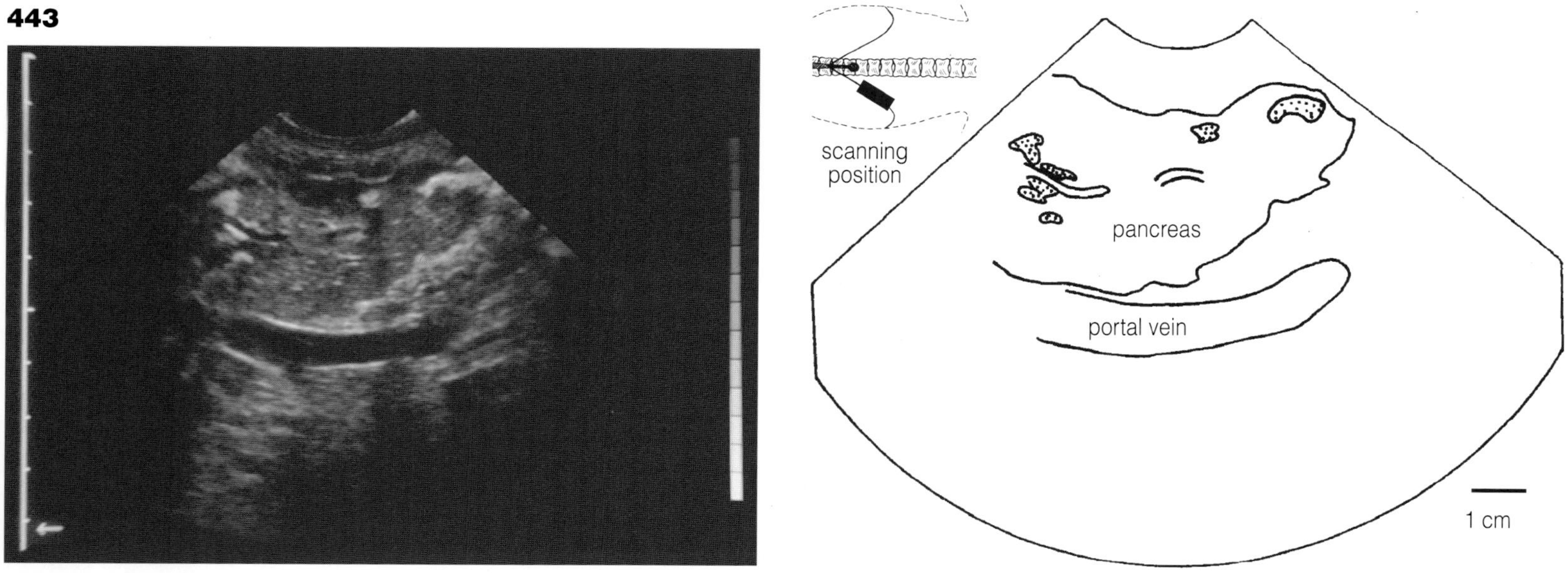

443 Chronic pancreatitis with diabetes mellitus in a dog. The parenchyma of the enlarged right pancreatic limb is finely granulated and homogenous with hyperechoic foci. The pancreas has a lobulated appearance. The pancreaticoduodenal vessels are also prominent.

444

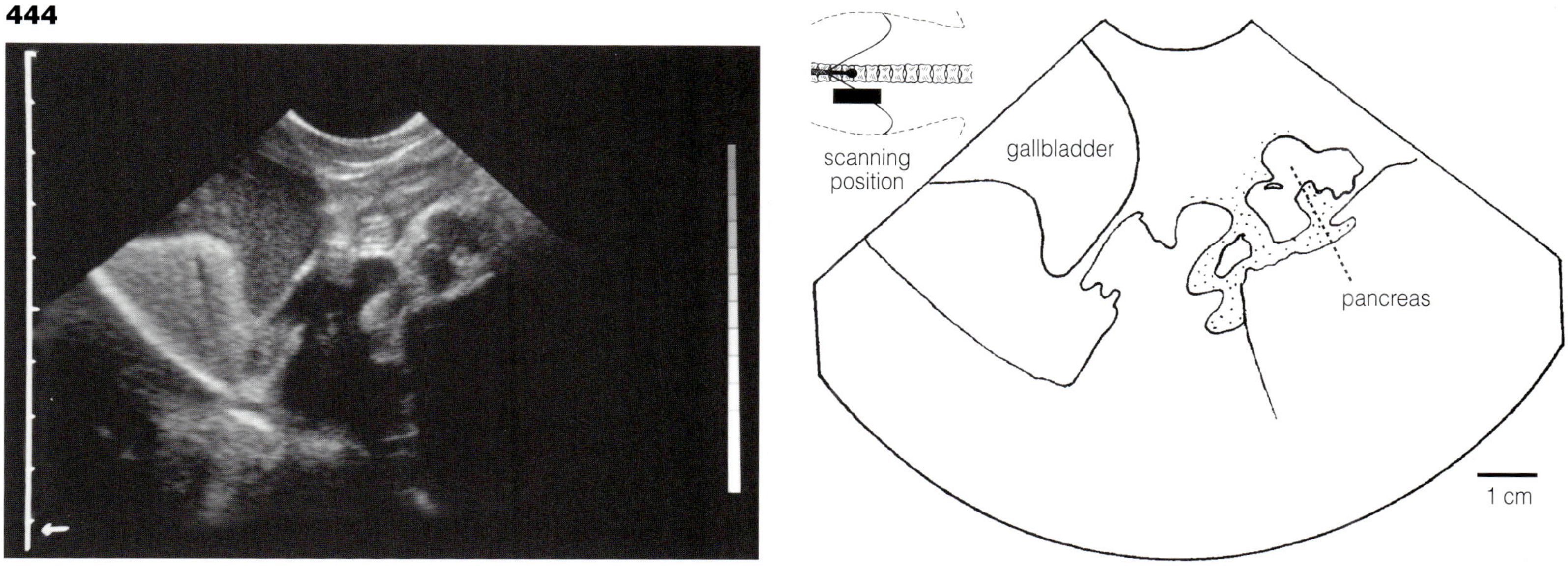

444 Pancreatitis in a cat indicated by a severely dilated gallbladder. The same secondary lesions are found with pancreatic tumours and bile duct carcinoma.

445

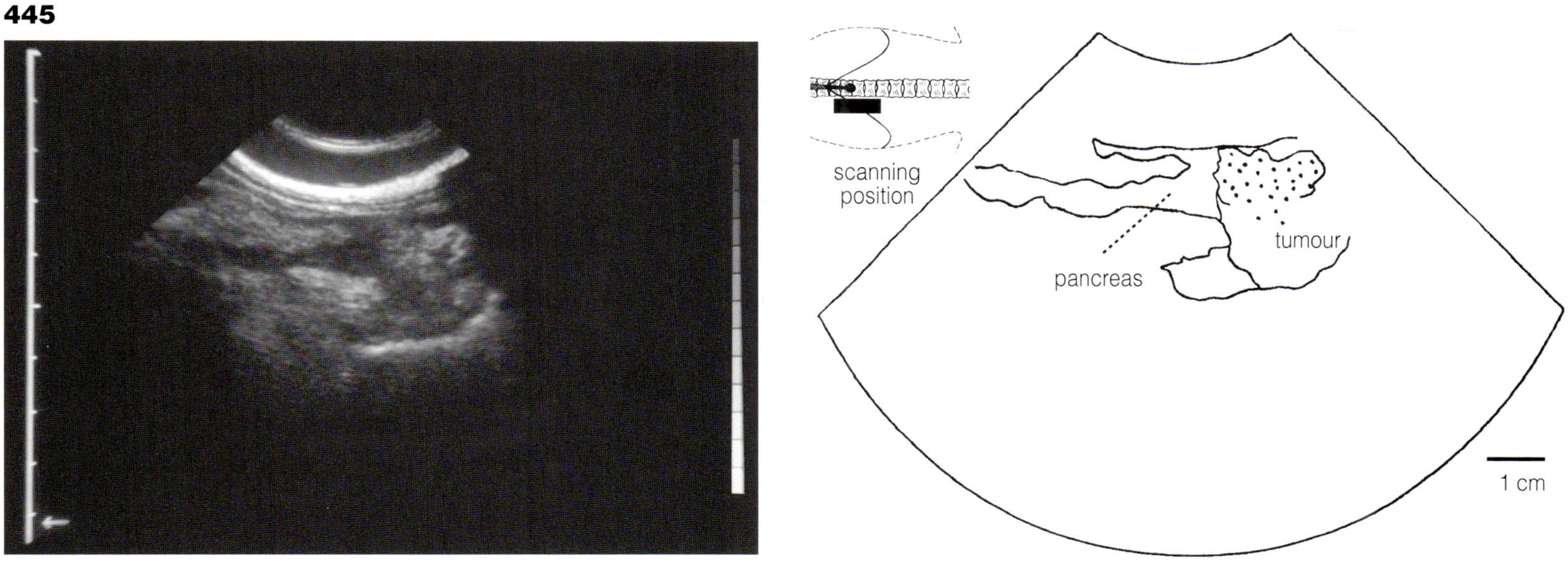

446

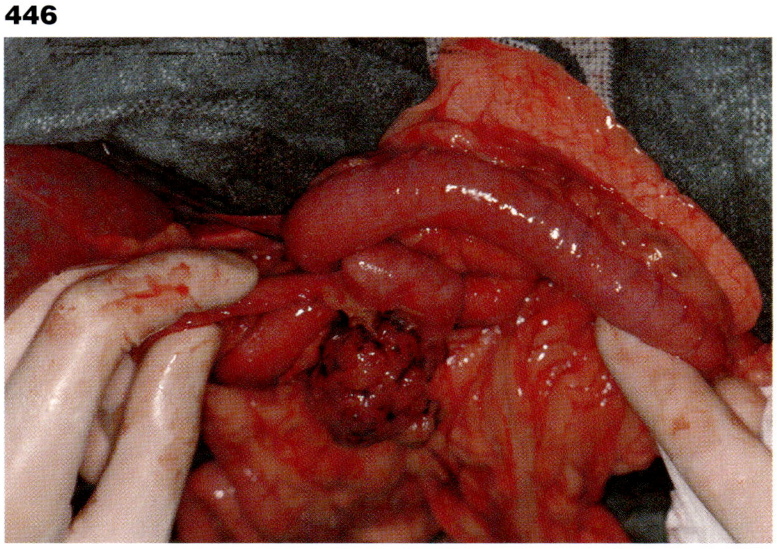

445, 446 Two-dimensional sonogram (**445**) and surgery site (**446**) of pancreatic carcinoma with peritoneal irritation in a dog. The hypoechoic right pancreatic limb shows an echogenic, non-homogenous mass in the sonogram (**445**). The surrounding structures are hyperechoic. Similar lesions are found with pancreatitis.

Tissue surrounding the pancreas may become more echogenic with spreading inflammation. The pancreas is difficult to differentiate in these cases. A diffuse increase of echogenicity in the cranial right abdomen usually indicates pancreatic disease. Secondary findings include an enlarged gallbladder with dilated biliary ducts, especially in cats (444).

Pancreatic Cysts

Cysts or pseudocysts are occasionally found with various forms of pancreatic disease. An anechoic area with distal acoustic enhancement is seen within the pancreatic parenchyma[4]. Cystic lesions of other origins must be considered.

Pancreatic Neoplasia

An enlarged gallbladder and dilated biliary ducts in the cat are also seen with pancreatic tumours not visualized ultrasonographically. Differential diagnosis includes bile duct carcinoma.

Canine and feline pancreatic tumours of a certain size are recognized as having variable echogenicities. In most cases they are too small to identify. This is also true for islet cell tumours. Large islet cell tumours are seen as well-demarcated, nodular, hypoechoic structures[5]. Carcinomas are hypoechoic and may be very large when clinical symptoms are present. Adjacent structures may also be affected. Hyperechoic carcinomas are also found (445, 446). Adenomas are usually defined and do not dissemi-

447

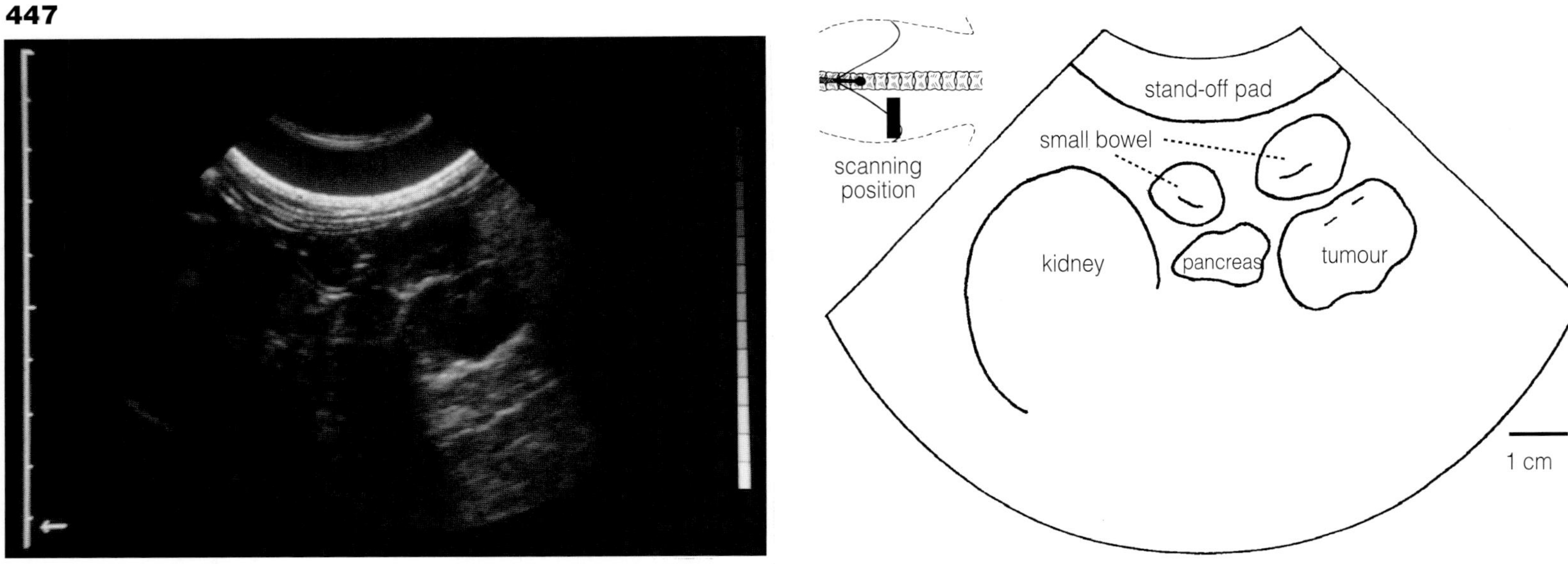

447 Carcinoma of the pancreas in a dog with normal pancreatic parenchyma and a hypoechoic mass medial to the pancreas (tentative diagnosis of enlarged metastatic lymph node). Bowel loops, mass and pancreas are separated by hyperechoic lines.

nate. The patient should be examined for metastases in adjacent lymph nodes and the liver. Lymph node metastasis may be the only finding with small, sonographically invisible pancreatic tumours (**447**). This is a clear indication for malignancy. Benign nodular hyperplasia of the pancreas produces defined areas of mixed echogenicity. These cannot be differentiated sonographically from malignant tumours.

> **NB**: Pancreatitis cannot be differentiated from pancreatic tumours solely on the basis of ultrasonographic findings.

References

1 Edwards DF, Bauer MS, Walker MA, Pardo AD, McCracken MD and Walker TL (1990) Pancreatic masses in seven dogs following acute pancreatitis. *J. Am. Anim. Hosp. Assoc.* **26**, 189–198.

2 Lamb CR (1989) Dilation of the pancreatic duct: an ultrasonographic finding in acute pancreatitis. *J. Small Anim.Pract.* **30**, 410–413

3 Lamb CR (1990) Abdominal ultrasonography in small animals: examination of the liver, spleen and pancreas. *J. Small Anim.Pract.* **31**, 6–15.

4 Rutgers C, Herring DS and Orton EC (1984) Pancreatic pseudocyst associated with acute pancreatitis in a dog: ultrasonographic diagnosis. *J. Am. Anim. Hosp. Assoc.* **21**, 411–416

5 Saunders HM (1991) Ultrasonography of the pancreas. *Prob. Vet. Med.* **3**, 583–603.

6 Saunders HM, Pugh CR and Rhodes WH (1992) Expanding applications of abdominal ultrasonography. *J. Am. Anim. Hosp. Assoc.* **28**, 369–374.

7 Simpson KW, Shiroma JT, Biller JT, Wicks J, Johnson SE, Dimski D and Chew D (1994) Antemortem diagnosis of pancreatitis in four cats. *J. Small Anim.Pract.* **35**, 93–99.

Spleen

Sabine Scholz and Dirk Lüerssen

Instrumentation and Examination Technique

Ultrasonography of the superficially located spleen does not require any special preparation. A small, medium to high-frequency (7.5 MHz), curved-array or linear transducer is recommended for the examination. A stand-off pad is helpful when using a 5 MHz sector scanner in small dogs and cats,

The patient should be placed in dorsal or right lateral recumbency for the examination. Splenic ultrasonography in cats can be performed on the standing patient. Cats should always be placed in the most comfortable position for the examination.

Anatomy and Normal Sonographic Findings

The spleen in dogs and cats is located to the left and cranial in the abdominal cavity. It lies immediatedly beneath the abdominal wall, extending from dorsal to ventral. Because of its loose attachment, the exact location of the spleen depends on the amount of gastric contents[3]. The longitudinal plane of the spleen is caudoventral (**448, 449**). The craniodorsal portion lies intercostally with normal gastric filling. The caudoventral part is intrathoracic with normal gastric filling in the dog and extrathoracic with gastric distension. In the cat the caudoventral spleen is always extrathoracic[2].

The canine spleen crosses the ventral midline to the right side. The spleen is in contact with the diaphragm, stomach, liver,

448

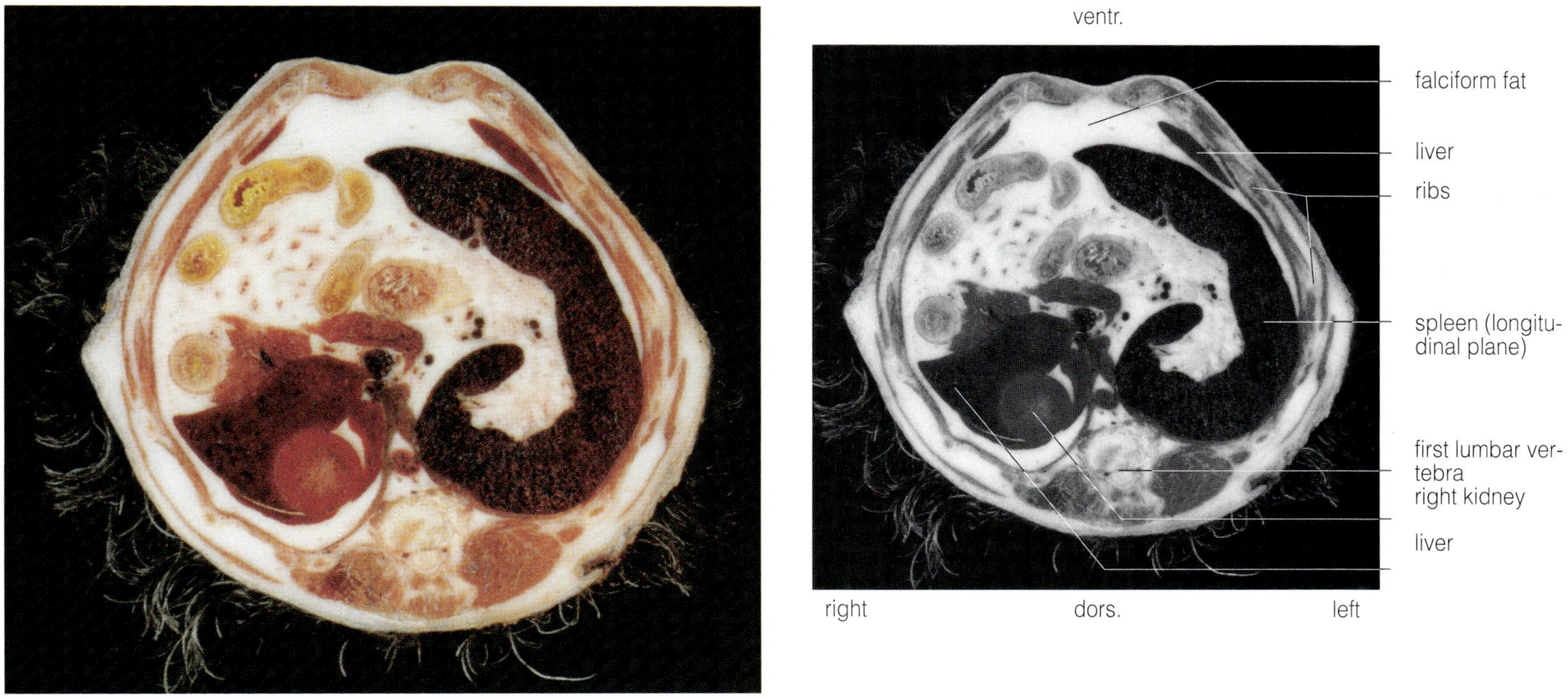

449

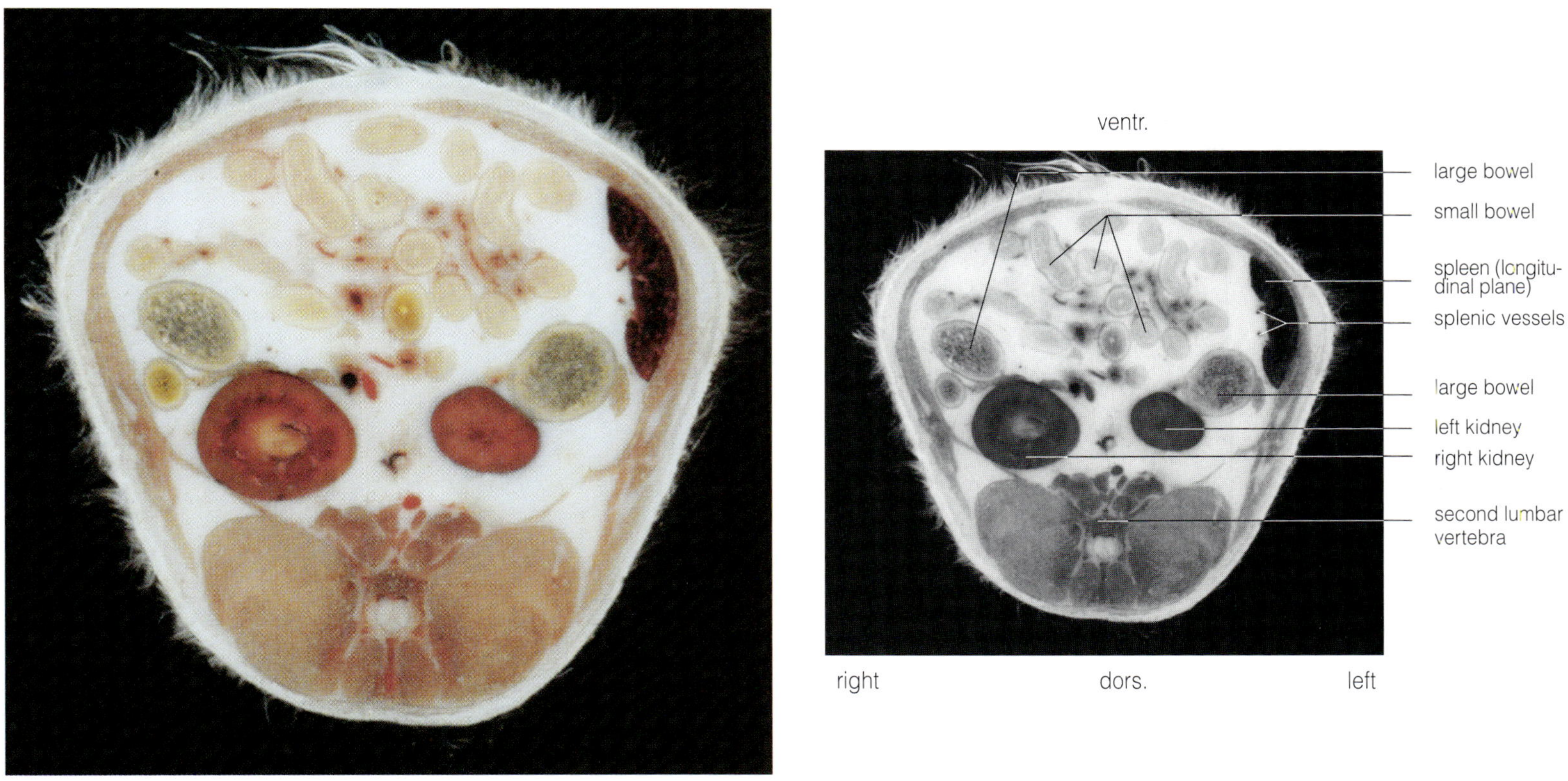

448, 449 Transverse anatomical cross-sections of the longitudinal spleen in the dog (**448**) and cat (**449**).

pancreas, left kidney and small and large bowel. The absolute and relative size of the spleen is variable and depends on the breed. Some adult, middle-aged German Shepherd Dogs have large spleens[4, 5]. Numerous splenic arteries and veins enter the spleen through the hilus (450).

Because of the spleen's variable size and location, it is not possible to give an exact scanning position.

In the dog the transducer is placed directly behind the costal arch. The spleen is scanned in sagittal and transverse planes from the left lateral or ventral abdominal wall. An empty or slightly full stomach requires moving the probe into the last intercostal spaces with the sound beam directed medially. Respiratory movement, especially panting, may lead to displacement of the spleen[5]. Full-term pregnancy pushes the spleen cranially, which also requires an intercostal approach.

In cats and small dogs the transducer is placed on the left lateral abdominal wall, directly caudal to the costal arch and ventral to the long dorsal muscles in the standing patient. The probe is then moved ventrally according to the position of the spleen. The transducer should be angled cranially for subcostal scanning. Because of the superficial location of the spleen, it can be used as an acoustic window for the stomach (449), intestinal tract and left kidney (450).

In a transverse view the normal canine spleen has a triangular shape with smooth margins (450). In the cat the spleen appears more oval. The longitudinal plane of the spleen appears more rounded or rectangular, with thin margins and a wider hilus. The spleen may have a crescent shape in some longitudinal planes

450

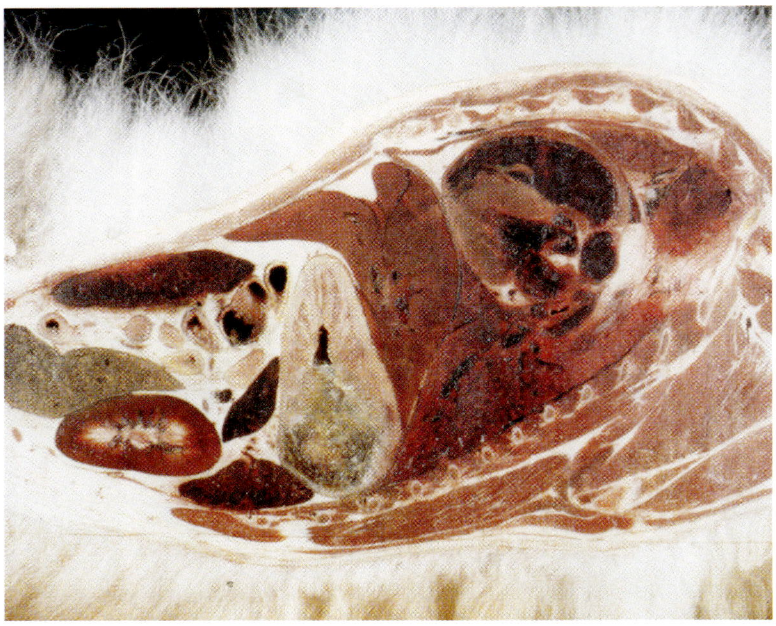

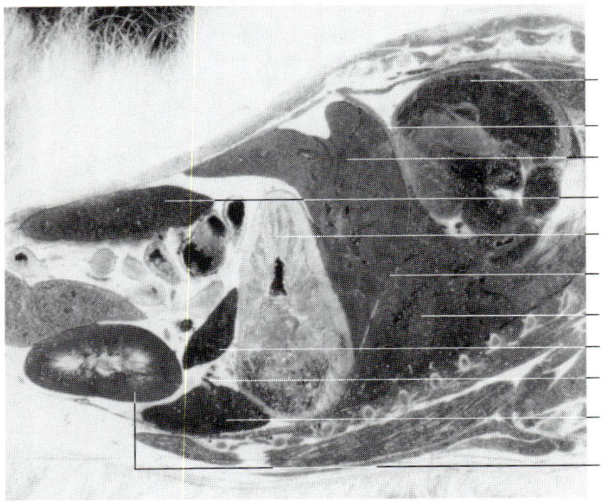

450 Left paramedian anatomical section of the splenic hilar region with a vessel in a dog.

451

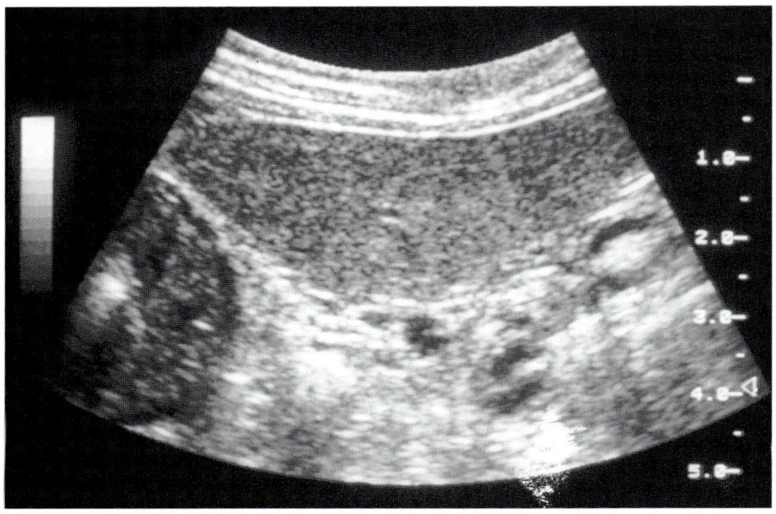

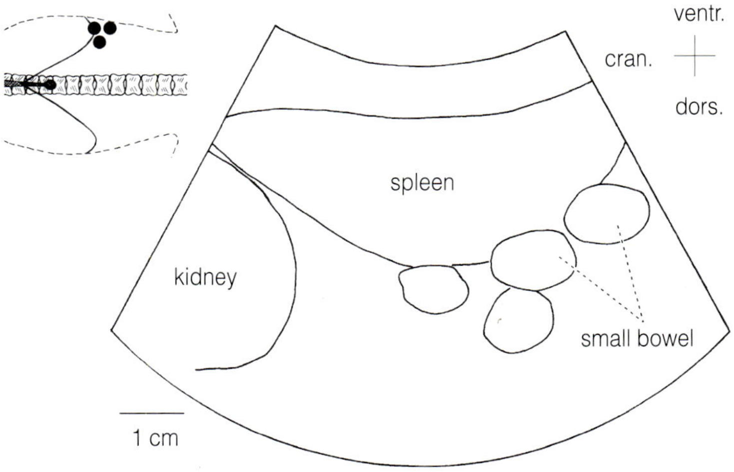

452

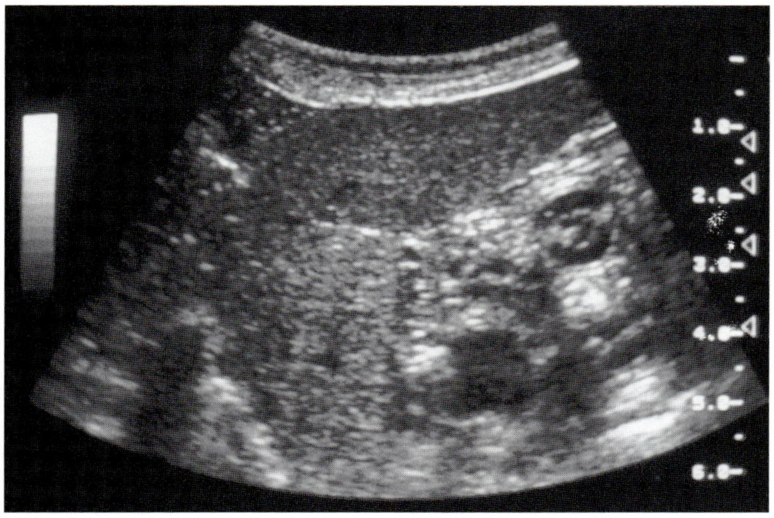

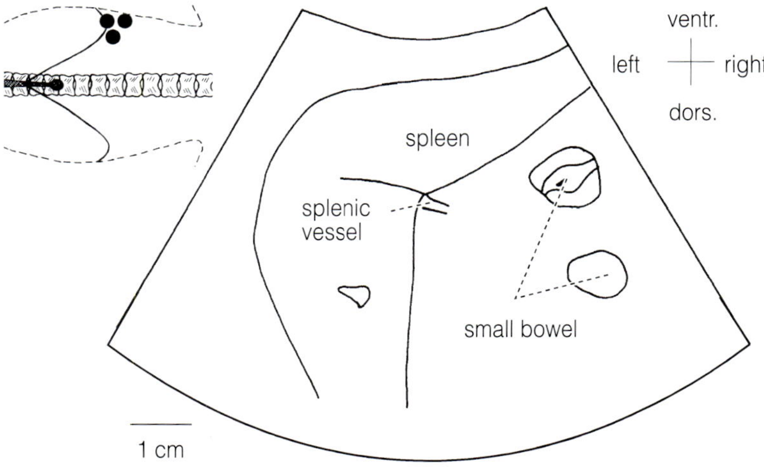

451, 452 Two-dimensional sonograms of a dog. Normal spleen in a sagittal (**451**) and a transverse (**452**) view.

(451). With a directly perpendicular sound beam, a thin splenic capsule with smooth contours is visualized (451–454). The splenic parenchyma is more echogenic, uniform and more finely textured than the liver. The spleen is more echogenic than the cortex of the left kidney in dogs and in most cats[6, 10]. In the blue European domestic cat the renal cortex may appear more echogenic than the splenic parenchyma. The splenic vessels are identified at the splenic hilar region (452–454). The vessels usually do not have a wall echo. Colour Doppler may be used to differentiate arteries from veins (453–455). Arteries have a typical orthograde blood flow with early-systolic maximal velocities and continuously slower diastolic flow. Systolic and diastolic blood flow velocities in the trabecular arteries rise and fall in cycles which creates an undulating flow (455).

453

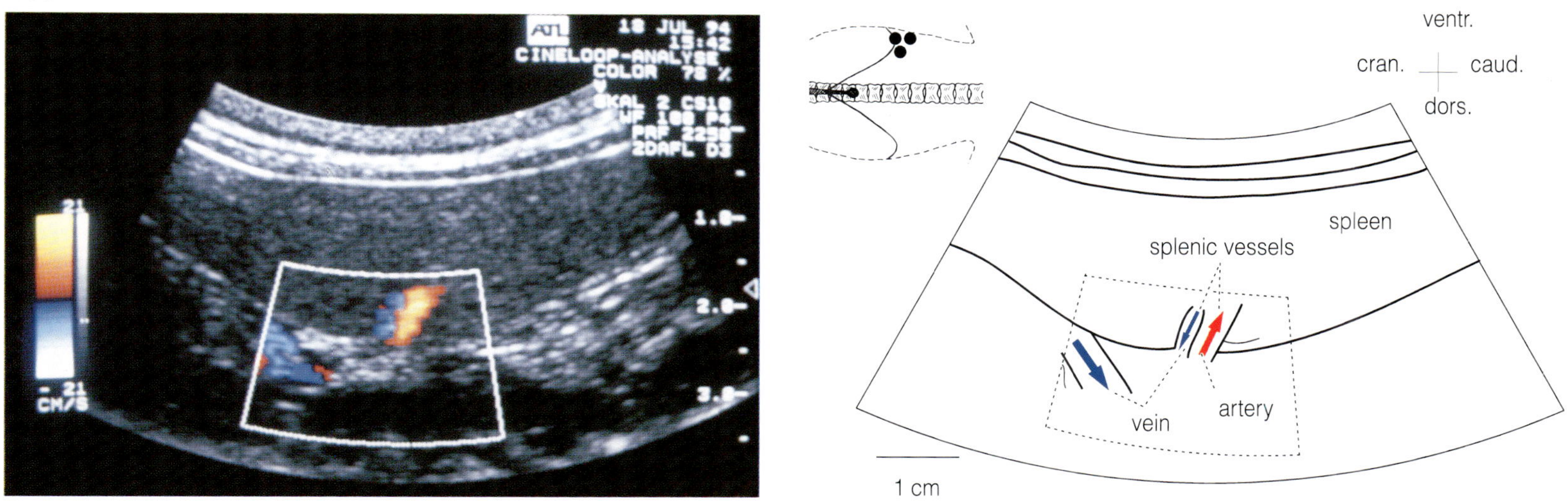

454

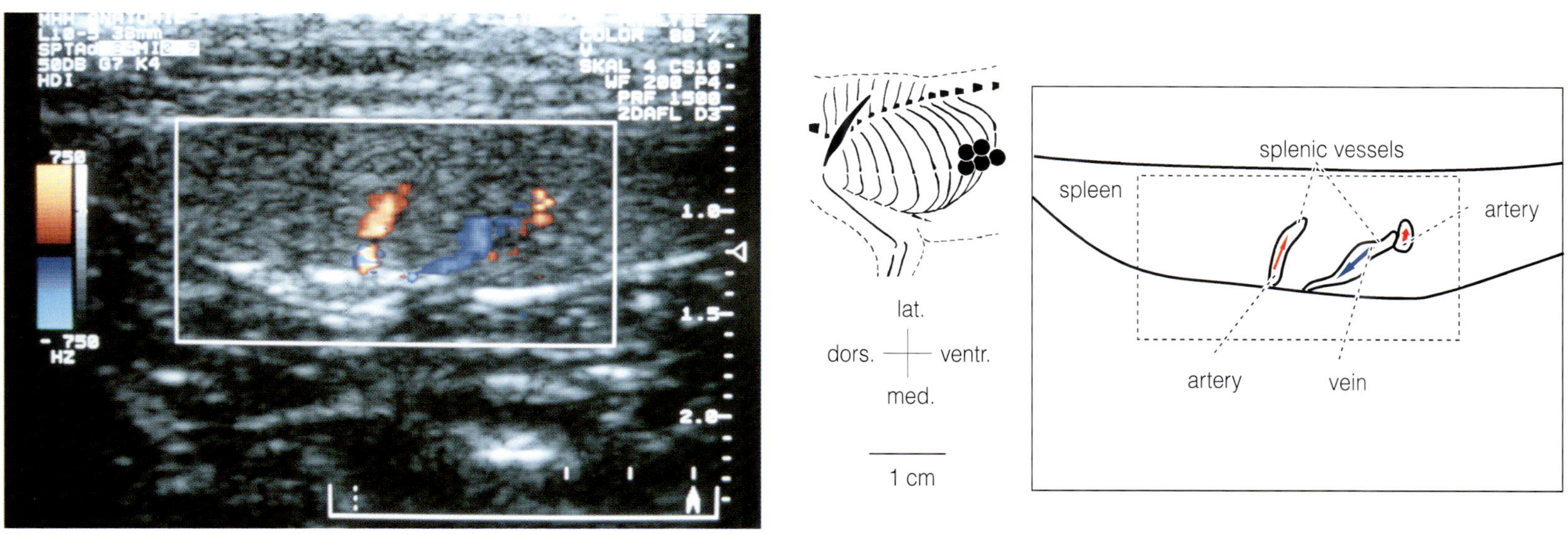

453, 454 Two-dimensional sonograms with colour Doppler display in a dog (**453**) and a cat (**454**). Normal spleen with vessels in a transverse (**453**) and a longitudinal (**454**) view.

455

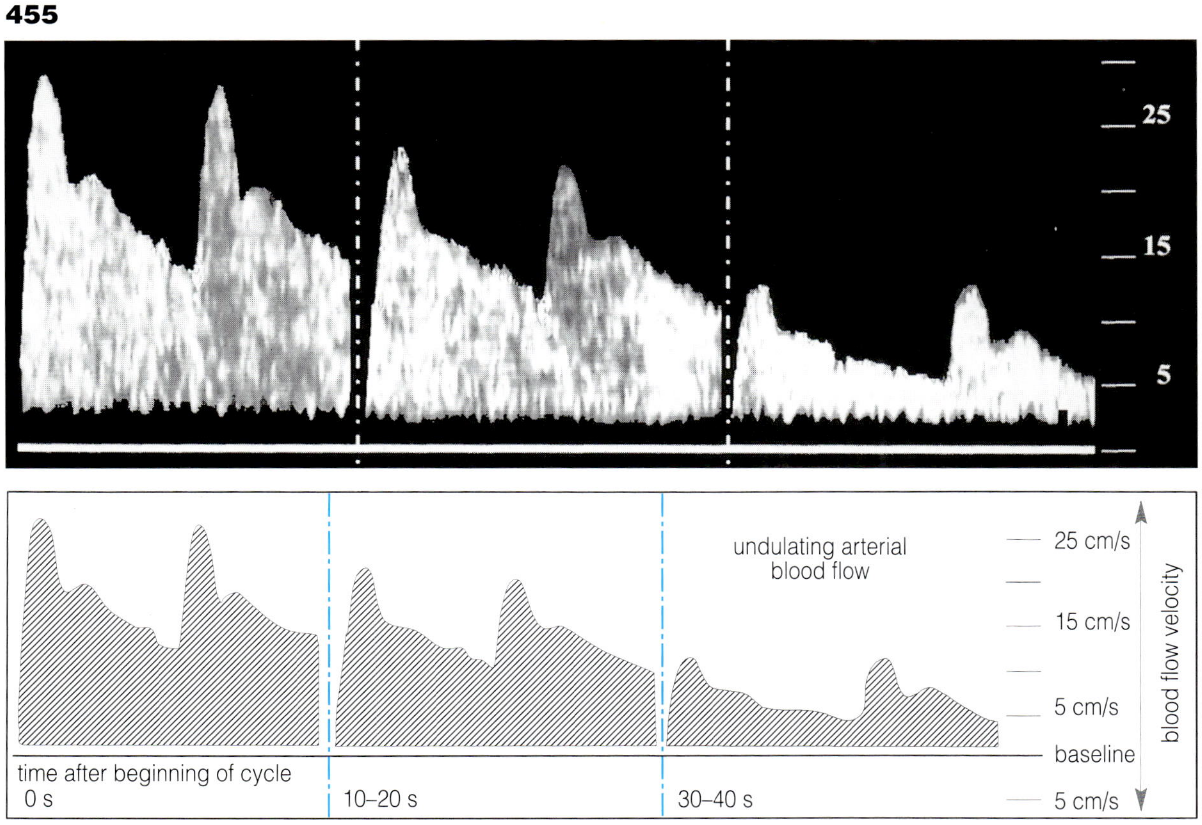

455 PW Doppler ultrasonography of a trabecular artery in a dog with normal, systolic and diastolic, orthograde blood flow as well as characteristic undulating velocities. (With permission from Isabelle von Goetz.)

456

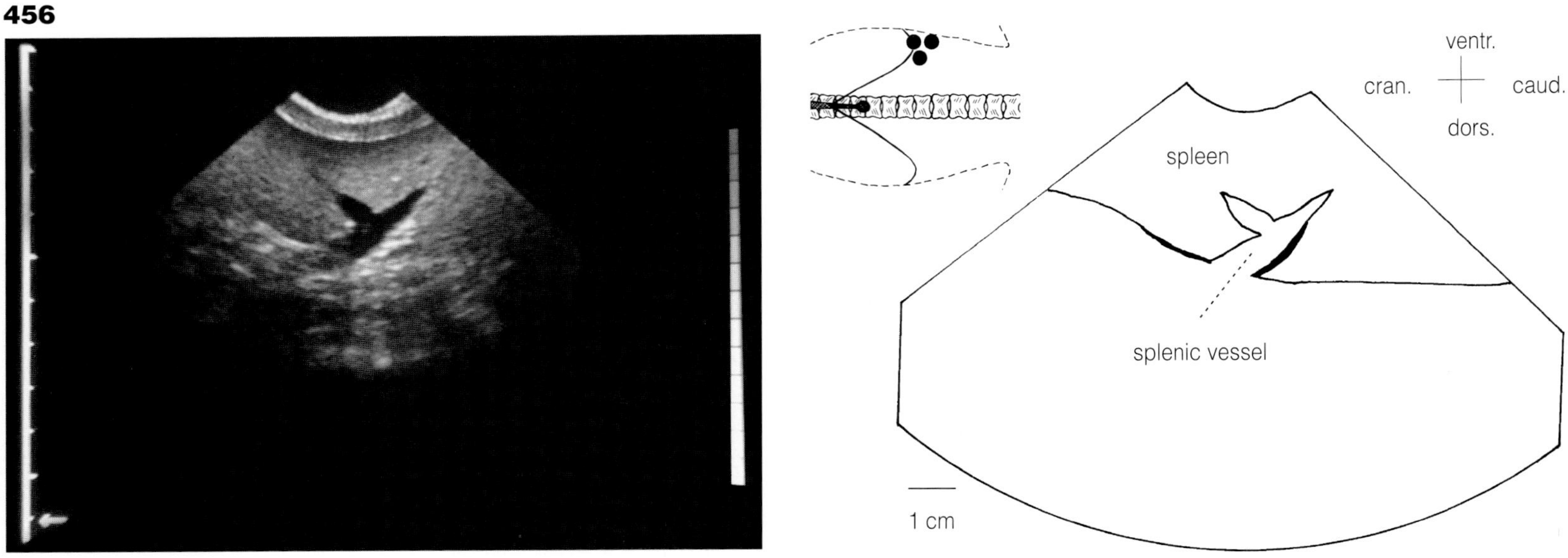

456 Splenomegaly with dilated splenic vessels in a dog. The vessel diameter is over 1 cm, which indicates congestion.

457

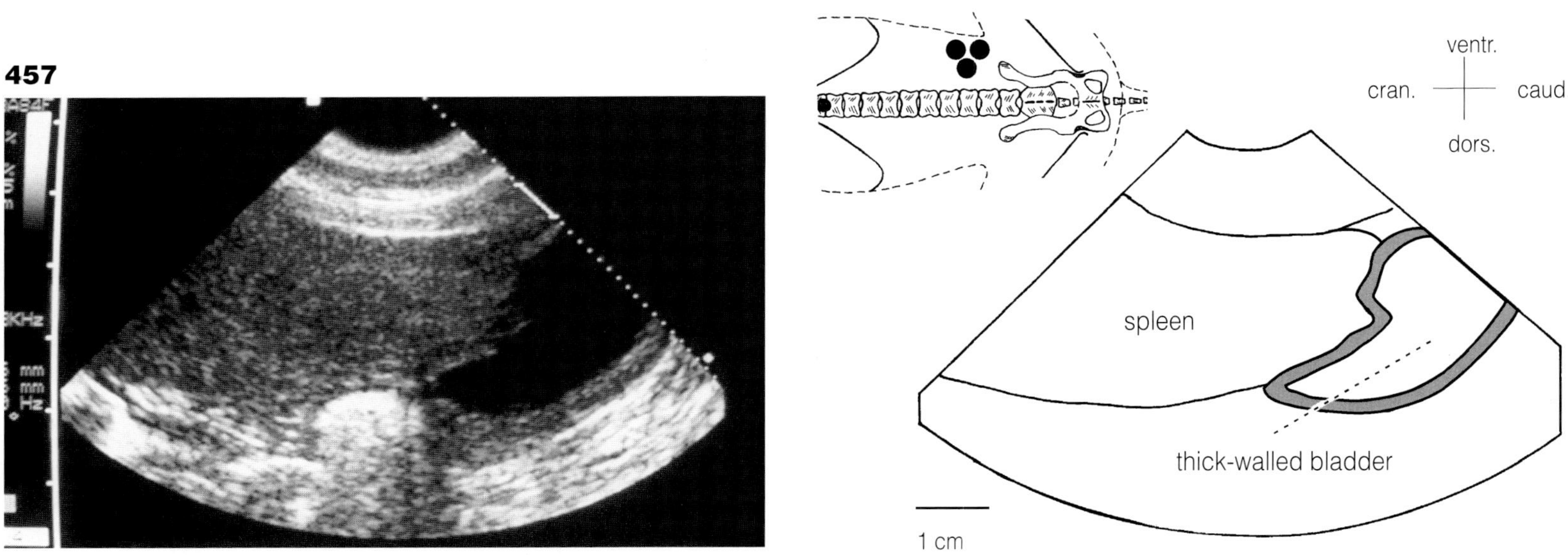

457 Splenomegaly in a six-year-old, healthy German Shepherd Dog. The enlarged, poorly echogenic, uniform spleen is adjacent to the urinary bladder.

Indications for ultrasonography of the spleen include blood profile abnormalities such as anaemia or leucocytosis, an acute abdomen, acute trauma, abdominal disorders of unknown origin, and palpable masses with suspected:

- Splenomegaly.
- Splenic torsion and ruptured spleen.
- Focal and diffuse splenic lesions such as cysts, haematomas, abscesses, infarcts, necrosis and calcifications.
- Splenic neoplasia.

A further indication is for monitoring treatment response.

Ultrasonography of Splenic Disease

Splenomegaly

Splenomegaly is usually associated with rounded contours and enlargement of the spleen with normal homogenous splenic parenchyma (**456**)[7]. When the spleen is enlarged, it may extend caudally to the normal or empty urinary bladder (**457**). In addition, dilated blood vessels are often found. The adult, middle-aged German Shepherd Dog often shows physiological splenomegaly with moderately dilated blood vessels[4, 5].

Splenic Torsion and Rupture

Splenic torsion gives the spleen a three-dimensional appearance in the ultrasound image. The spleen is enlarged with retraction of the hilus caused by parenchymal swelling. The splenic parenchyma is hypoechoic with a non-uniform echo pattern. The surface is irregular with hyperechoic borders (**458**).

Splenic rupture shows non-homogenous parenchyma at the site of the rupture, which is often not distinguished with ultrasound. A hypoechoic subcapsular haematoma is seen with intraperitoneal haemorrhaging, i.e. anechoic free abdominal fluid (**459**)[8].

Focal and Diffuse Splenic Lesions

Focal and diffuse splenic abnormalities are easily detected within the normal parenchyma and include cysts, haematomas, abscess-

458

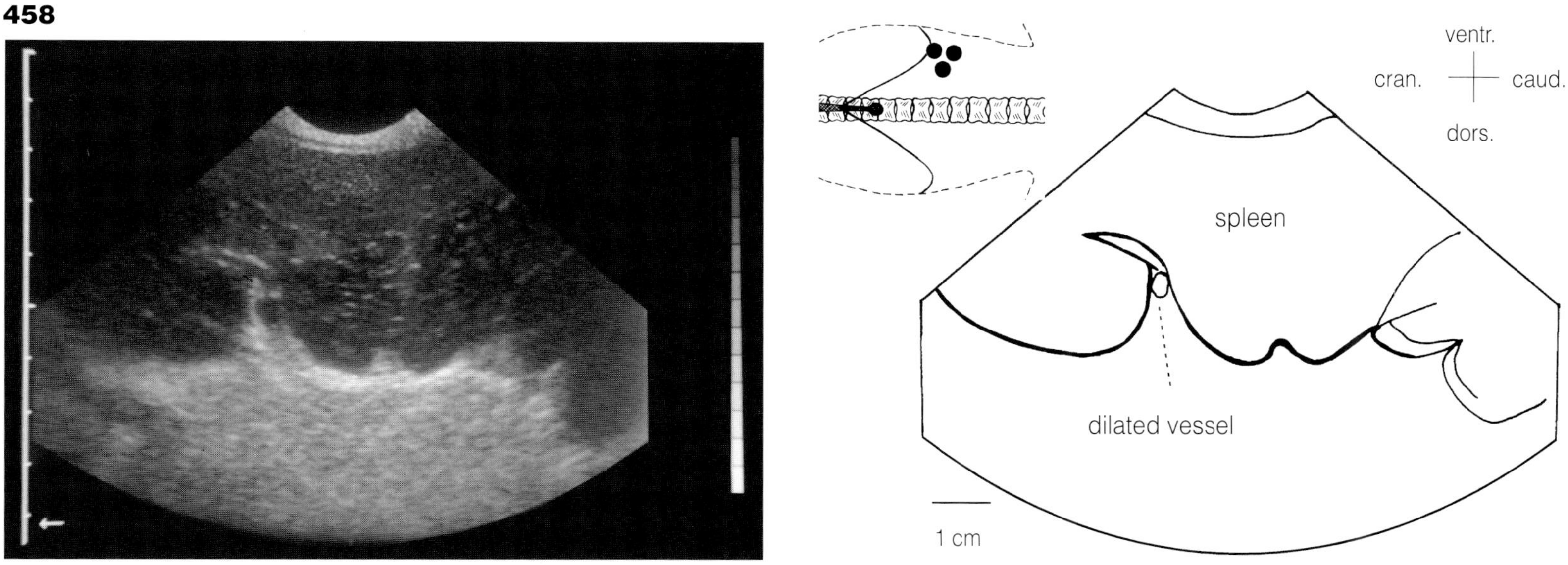

458 Splenic torsion in a dog.

459

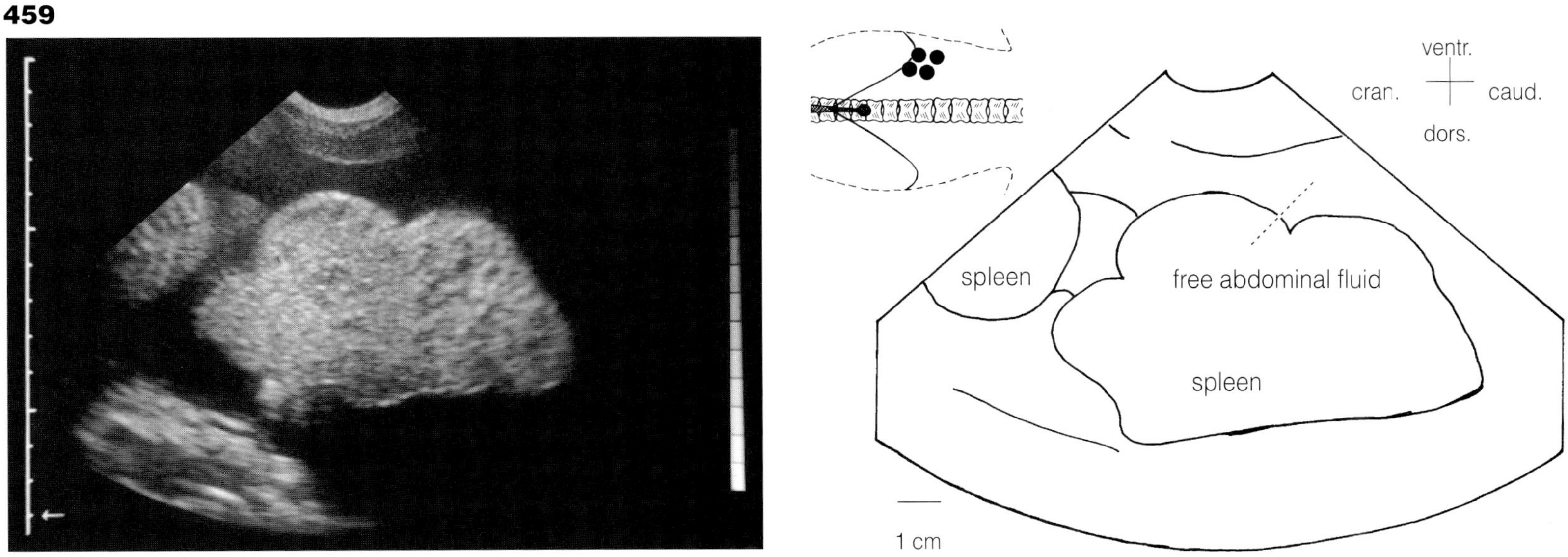

459 Ruptured spleen in a dog. The splenic parenchyma appears non-homogenous with an irregular surface. Free fluid is seen in the abdominal cavity. Differential diagnosis includes splenic neoplasia, since a subcapsular haematoma is not visible on this frozen image.

es, infarcts, necrosis and calcifications. Cysts are typically hypoechoic with distal acoustic enhancement. Acute haematomas are also hypoechoic. The echogenicity increases with progressive resorption and organization. Echogenic septa produce cavitation. Splenic abscesses are hypo- to hyperechoic with echogenic contents (cell detritus). Infarcts of the spleen are usually caused by embolism following valvular endocarditis and neoplasia. They are round or wedge-shaped, hypoechoic structures close to the splenic margins. Scar formation and calcification of splenic infarcts produce more echogenic lesions[8]. Splenic necrosis may be seen secondary to septicaemia with or without infarction and splenic torsion. Ultrasonography shows anechoic and occasionally echogenic, poorly marginated structures around the splenic vessels. It is not possible to distinguish abscesses, cysts, haematomas, necrosis and tumours from other focal lesions based on ultrasonographic appearance. A definitive diagnosis can be made histologically following laparotomy[7, 9]. Focal or diffuse splenic calcifications are caused by calcified haematomas, abscesses, infarcts and necrosis[1] and they produce a strong echo with distal acoustic shadowing (**460**).

Splenic Neoplasia

The ultrasonographic appearance of splenic tumours varies greatly. Most benign and malignant neoplastic lesions are detected easily as hypo- to hyperechoic, homogenous to non-homogenous parenchymal abnormalities. These tumours are usually incidental findings with routine abdominal scans; there are no clinical symptoms and laboratory and radiographic findings are normal. Follow-up examinations every four weeks may determine tumour malignancy.

Benign tumours (haemangiomas) produce thick echogenic (white) vascular sheaths. Depending on the scanning plane, they often

460

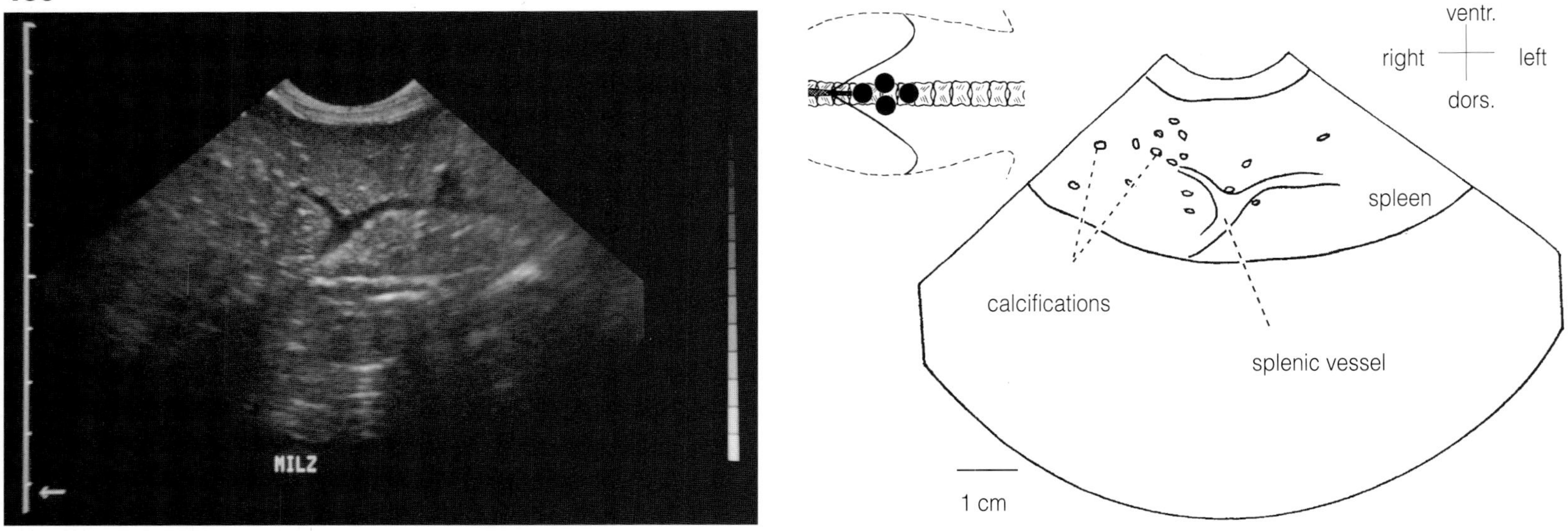

460 Multifocal calcifications in the spleen of a dog.

461

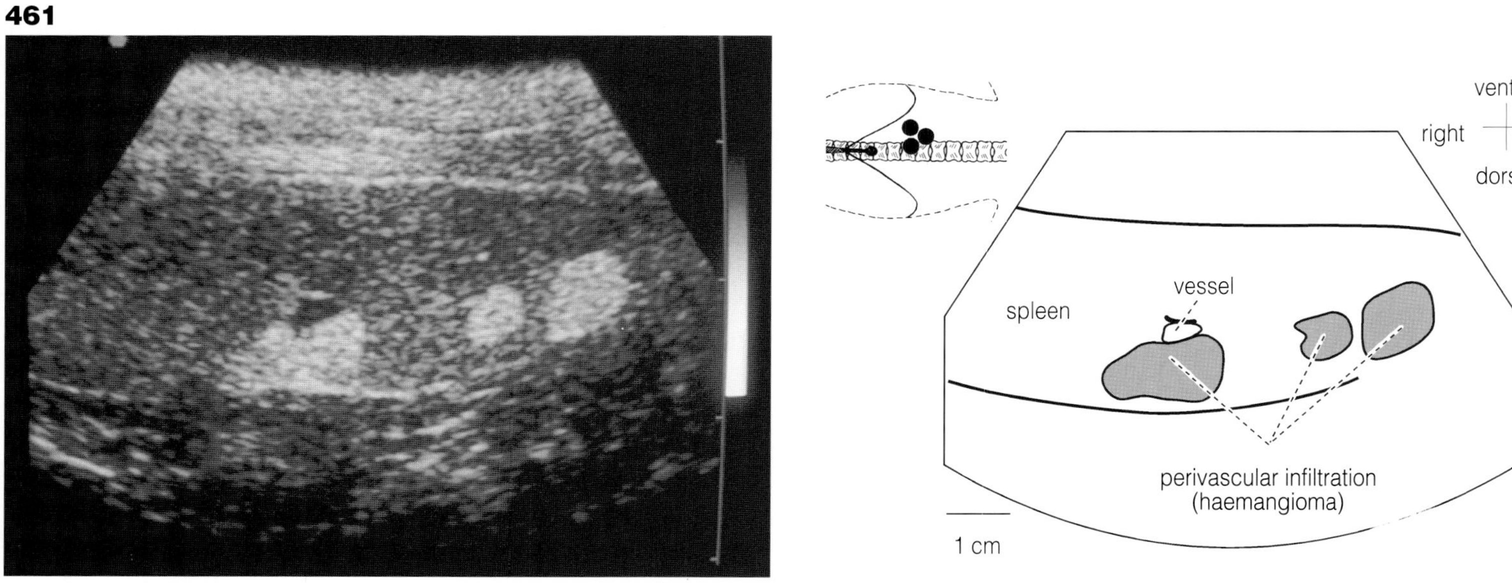

462

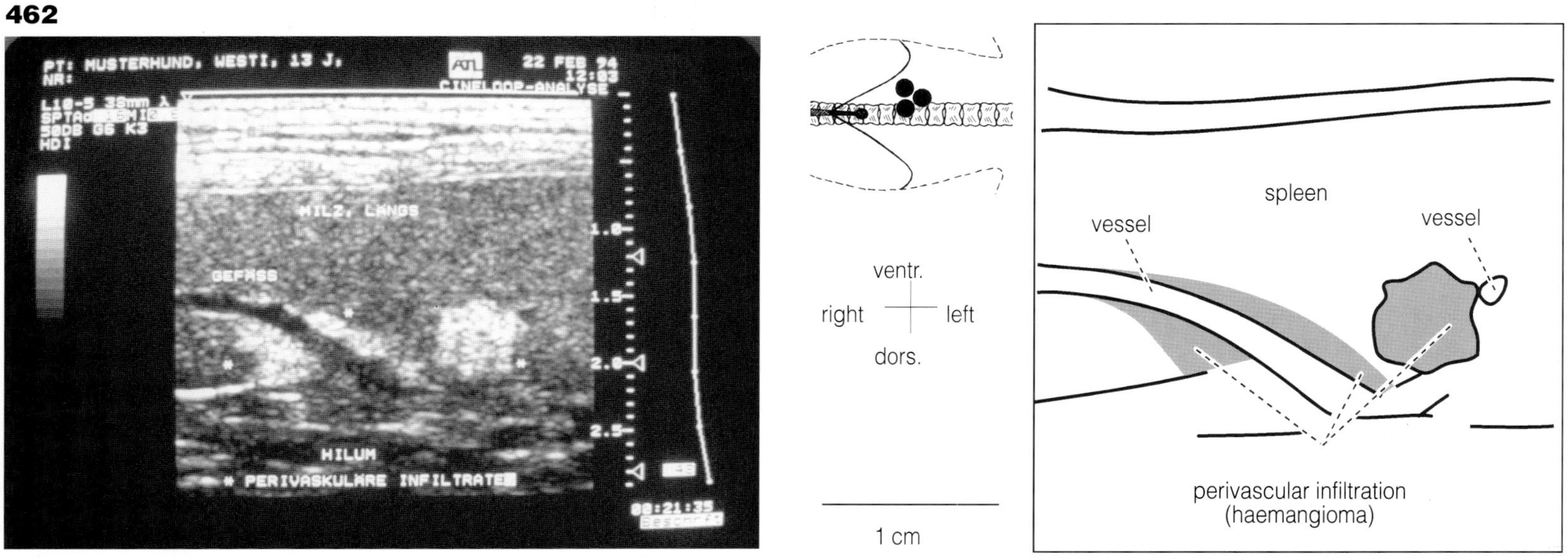

461, 462 Haemangioma in an old dog, seen as a solid echogenic structure in the transverse view (**461**) and as a 'vessel sheath' in the longitudinal plane (**462**).

appear as round to irregularly shaped, solid areas in the hilar region of the spleen in middle-aged to older dogs. By angling and turning the transducer, the central vessel can be distinguished (461, 462). Ultrasonographic follow-ups every six months are recommended.

Malignant splenic tumours are commonly hypoechoic haemangiosarcomas of variable size and margination (463, 464). Metastasis, fibrosarcoma, lymphosarcoma and malignant haemangioendothelioma have also been found. Splenic lymphosarcoma produces a non-homogenous parenchyma with multifocal, round, hypoechoic lesions (465).

463

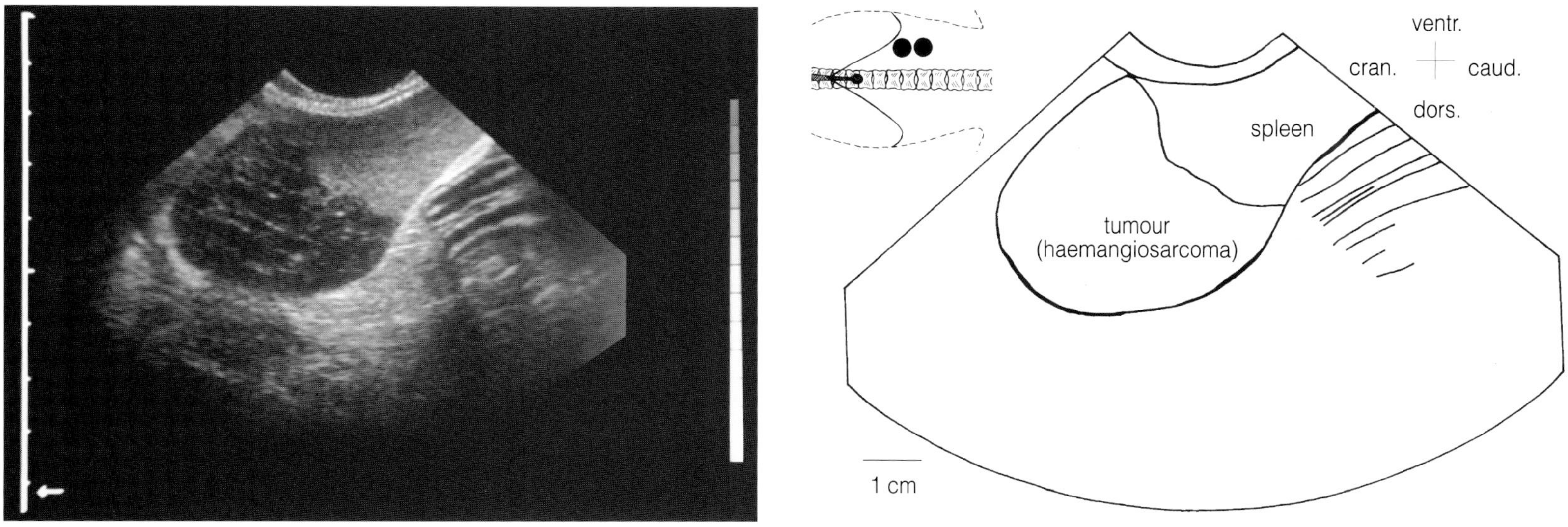

463 Haemangiosarcoma in a dog. A hypoechoic mass is seen extending from normal splenic parenchyma. Differential diagnosis includes a haematoma or an abscess.

464

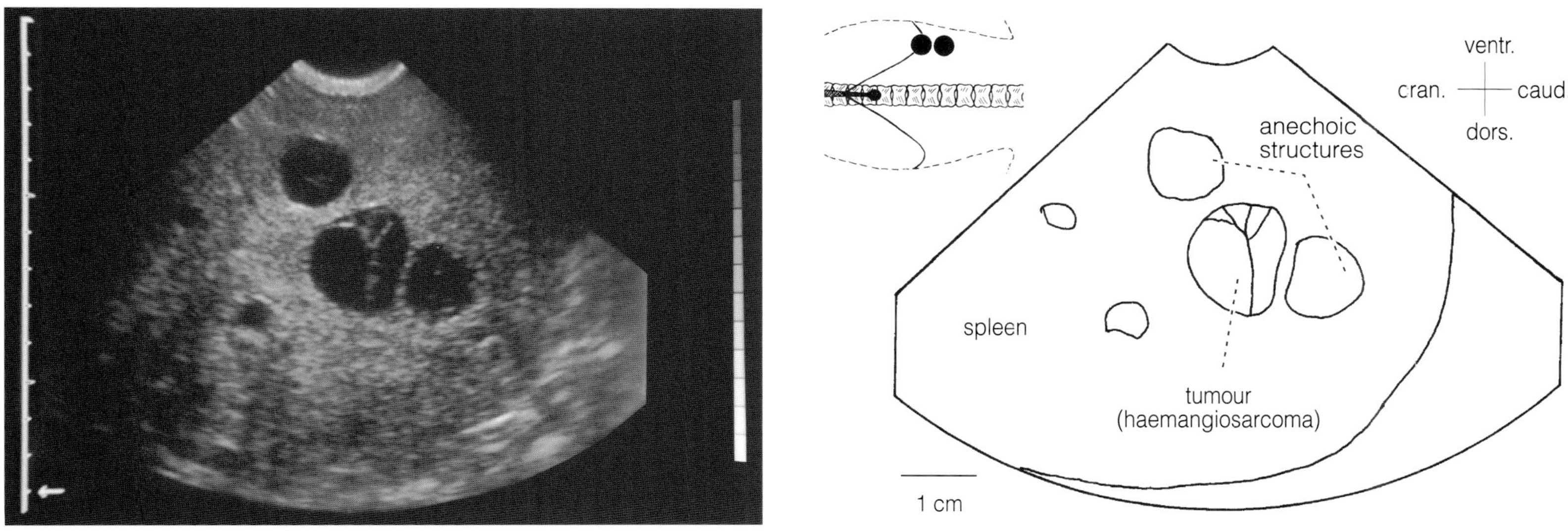

464 Haemangiosarcoma in a dog. Hypoechoic to anechoic cavitations. Differential diagnosis includes cysts, haematomas, abscesses and neoplasia. Ultrasonographic follow-up examinations are indicated every 2–4 weeks.

465

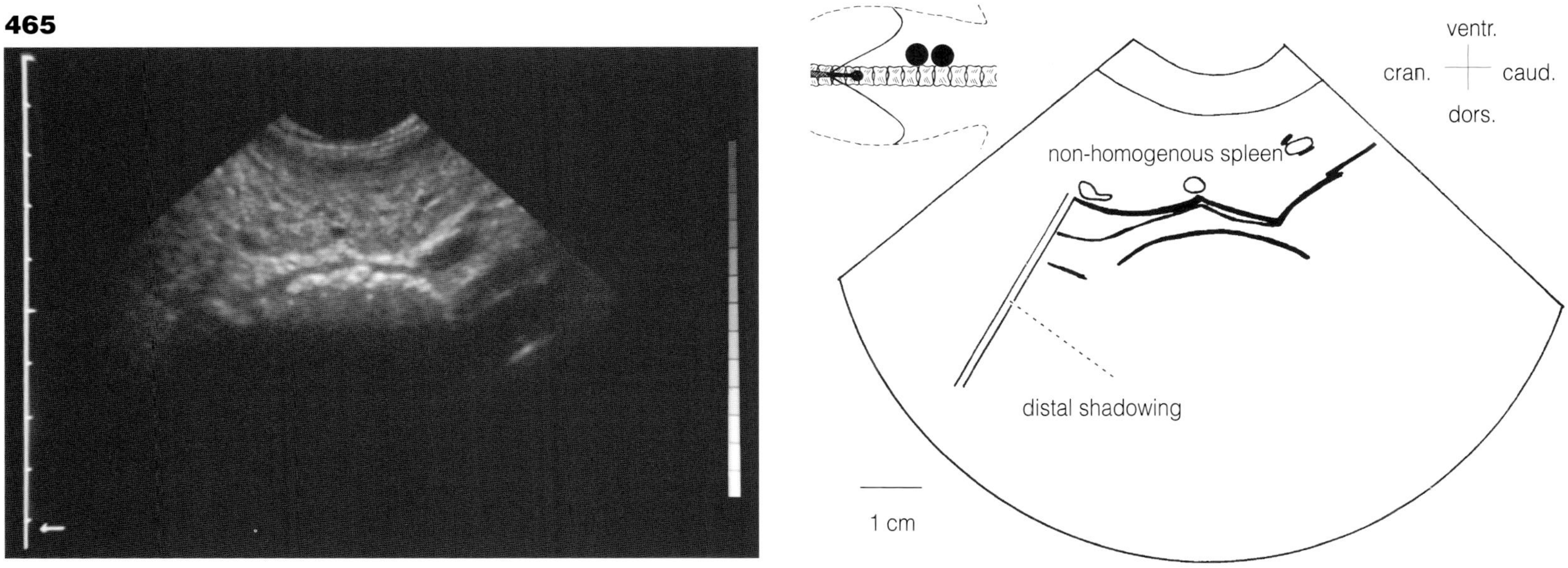

465 Splenic lymphosarcoma in a cat. The parenchyma is non-homogenous with anechoic lesions and a retracted hilar region.

References

1 Banholzer P (1993) Milz. In: Kremer H and Dobrinski W (Eds.) *Sonographische Diagnostik. Innere Medizin und Angrenzende Gebiete*. 4th Edn. Urban and Schwarzenberg, München, Wien, Baltimore, pp. 145–155.

2 Breiling F (1994) *Vergleichende Makroskopisch-fotografische Transversale Schnittanatomie der Abdominalen Organe von Hand und Katze*. Hannover, Tierärztl. Hochsch., Diss.

3 Dyce KM, Sack WO and Wensing CJG (1991) *Anatomie der Haustiere*. Enke Verlag, Stuttgart.

4 Fritsch R and Gerwing M (1991) *Sonographie bei Hand und Katze*. Enke Verlag, Stuttgart.

5 Gerwing MF (1989) *Sonographische Darstellung von Milz und Prostata des Handes unter Besonderer Berücksichtigung der Messung ihrer Länge und Größe Sowie des Sonographischen Bildes der Pathologischen Veränderungen. Das Hydroperitoneum zur Besseren Differenzierung Abdominaler Organe*. Gießen, Justus-Liebig-Univ., Veterinärmed. Fak., Diss.

6 Heitz FB, Carlier P, Guinet P, Legrand JJ and Viard PF (1980) Exploration échotomographique du rein normale et pathologique du chien et du chat. *Recl. Méd. Vét.* **156**, 363–369.

7 Konde LJ, Wrigley RH, Lebel JL, Park RD, Pugh C and Finn S (1989) Sonographic and radiographic changes associated with splenic torsion in the dog. *Vet. Radiol.* **30**, 41–45.

8 Nyland TG and Hager DA (1985) Sonography of the liver, gallbladder, and spleen. Symposium on diagnostic ultrasound. *Vet. Clin. North Am. Small Anim. Pract.* **15**, 1123–1147.

9 Schelling CG, Wordman JA and Saunders HM (1988) Ultrasonic detection of splenic necrosis in the dog. *Vet. Radiol.* **29**, 227–233.

10 Walter PA, Johnston GR, Feeney DA and O'Brien TD (1987) Renal ultrasonography in healthy cats. *Am. J. Vet. Res.* **48**, 600–607.

Kidneys and Ureters

Martin Janthur and Dirk Lüerssen

Instrumentation and Examination Technique

A 7.5 MHz transducer is optimal for ultrasonography of the kidneys in cats and small to medium-sized dogs, while large breed dogs may require a 5 MHz probe. The kidneys are examined with the animal in dorsal recumbency. Uncooperative patients can also be scanned from the lateral abdomen or in a standing position.

The left canine kidney is scanned left of midline, caudal to the rib cage, with the spleen providing an acoustic window. The right canine kidney is more difficult to visualize because of its position within the rib cage. The cranial pole is often hidden under the stomach or bowel. Scanning from the 11th or 12th intercostal space from the lateral abdomen makes the right kidney more accessible. Feline kidneys are easier to examine because of their more caudal location. The left kidney in the cat is more mobile than in the dog. Too much transducer pressure on the abdomen results in displacement of feline kidneys. In these cases the pressure should be reduced or the transducer placed ventral to the dorsal muscles on the lateral abdomen. The sonographer can also use a free hand to push the feline kidneys into view. Canine kidneys are not as mobile, except in anorexic dogs.

A complete scan of both kidneys should always be performed in transverse and longitudinal planes before making a diagnosis. Focal lesions may otherwise be overlooked.

Anatomy and Normal Sonographic Findings

In a sagittal plane (**466–472**) the canine kidney has an oval shape, while it appears more bean-shaped in a dorsal view (**473–477**). Feline kidneys are rounder in sagittal and dorsal planes than those of the dog (**483–484**). In a transverse plane (**478–482**) the kidneys are oval at the renal hilus and round near the poles[15]. (*Tables 34* and *35*, page 219, give ultrasonographic measurements of normal kidney size in the dog and in the cat.)

The normal renal cortex is finely granulated, homogenous and more hypoechoic than the parenchyma of the adjacent liver and spleen[5, 9]. In some blue-coloured European domestic cats the normal renal cortex is similar or more echogenic compared to the splenic or hepatic parenchyma[16]. The relationship of kidney echogenicity to that of the liver and spleen is important for ultrasonographic evaluation. The renal cortex is the least echogenic, while the spleen has the highest echogenicity.

The renal medulla is hypoechoic. In a sagittal view the hypoechoic to anechoic medullary pyramids are separated by renal columns. In the dorsal plane the anechoic renal medulla is separated by the renal columns and echogenic pelvic diverticula and shows a typical butterfly shape. This shape is most apparent in the cat with a relatively large renal medulla.

The pelvic recesses or diverticula appear hyperechoic because of the surrounding fat and fibrous tissue. In a sagittal and dorsal longitudinal plane they are crescent-shaped. In older animals the diverticula are more echogenic and more apparent. This is an incidental finding without clinical relevance (**491**).

The renal sinus is hyperechoic due to peripelvic fat and this creates a so-called central sinus reflex[15]. The renal pelvis within the renal sinus is normally not visualized. In some dogs with good sonographic images, such as Whippets, the renal pelvis may be identified in a dorsal view as an anechoic Y-shaped structure (**474–477**).

466

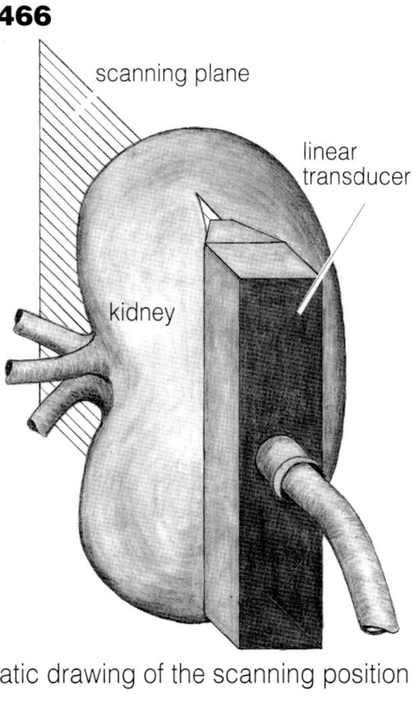

466 Schematic drawing of the scanning position for a sagittal view.

467

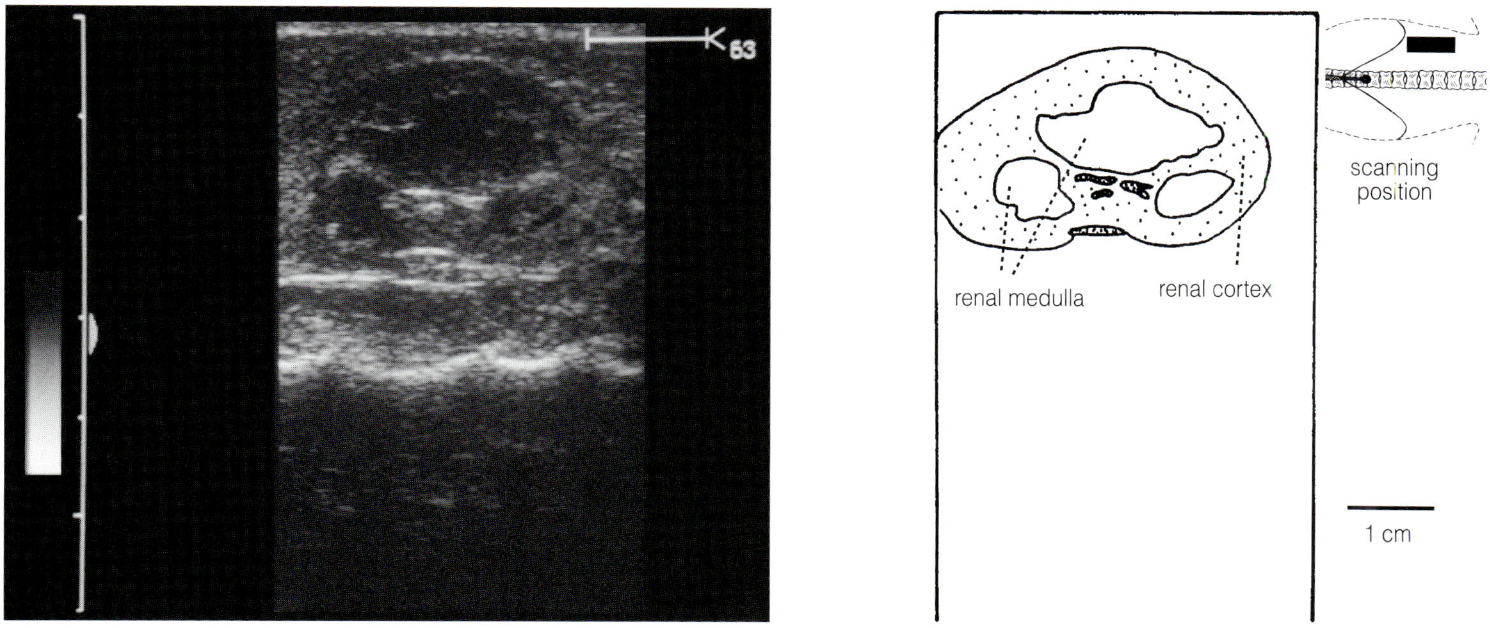

468

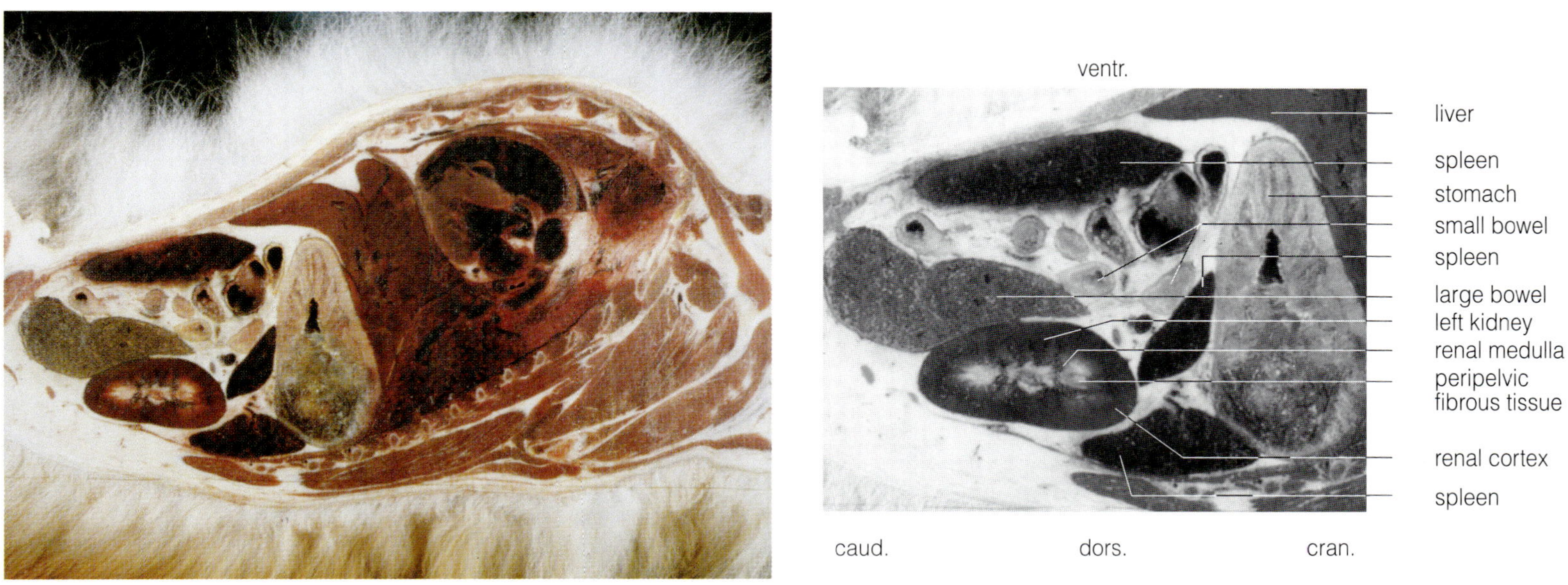

469

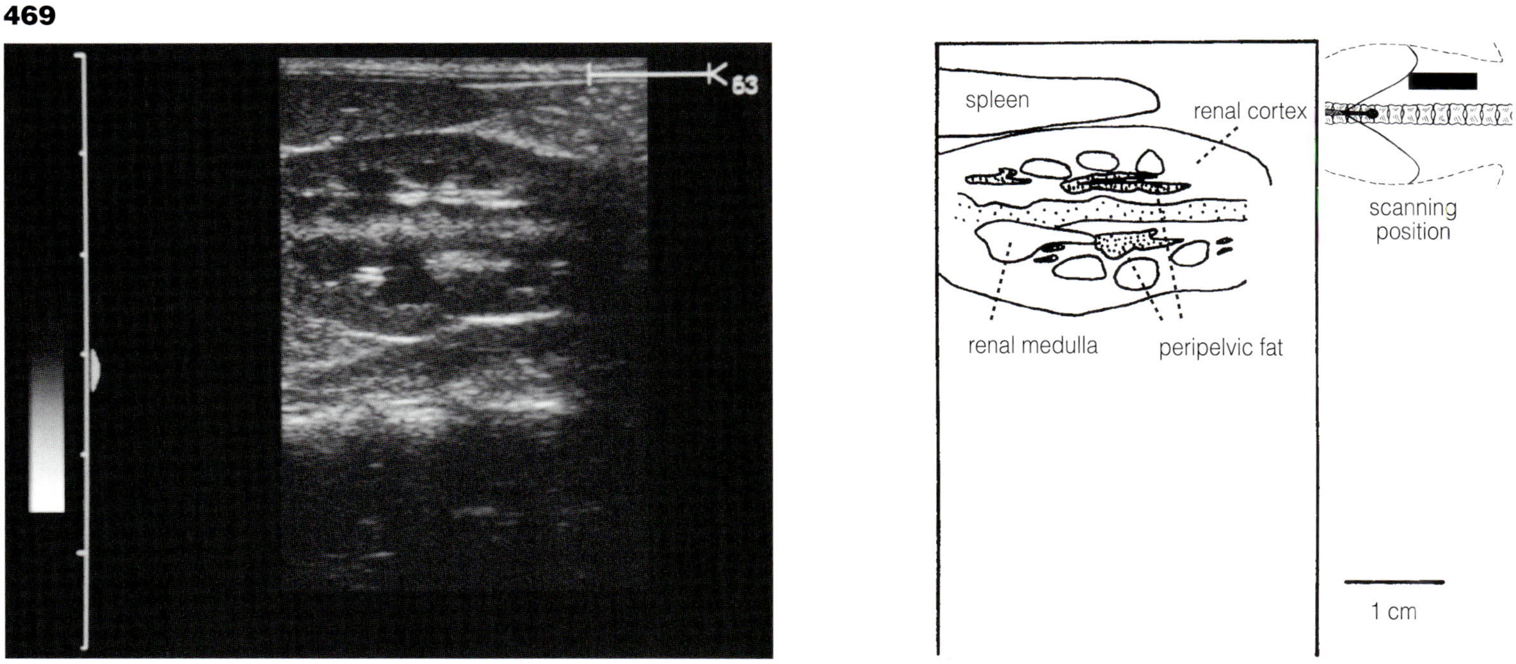

467–472 Sagittal sonograms (**467, 469, 471**) and corresponding anatomical sagittal sections (**468, 470, 472**) of left canine kidneys. The slices are exactly in the centre (**467, 468**), slightly lateral (**469, 470**) and at the level of the pelvic diverticula (**471, 472**).

470

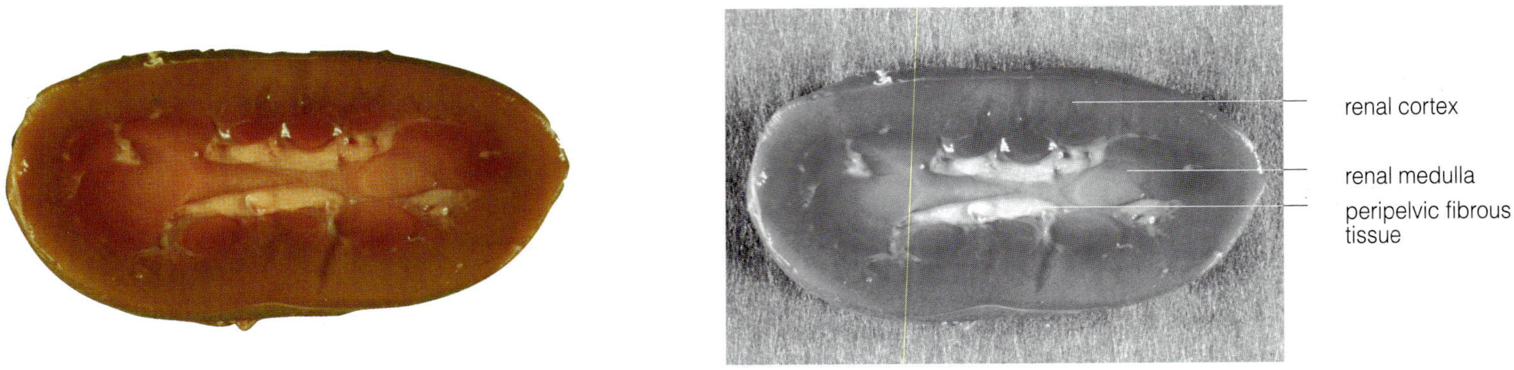

471

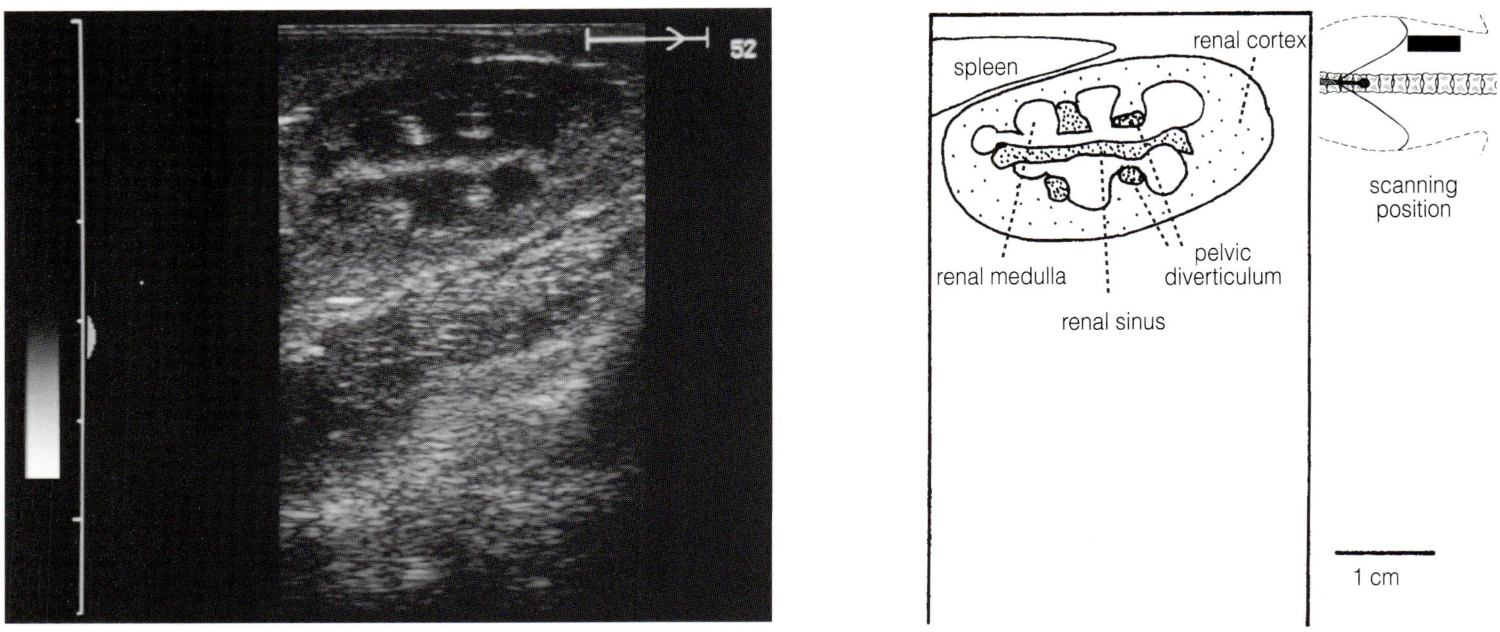

472

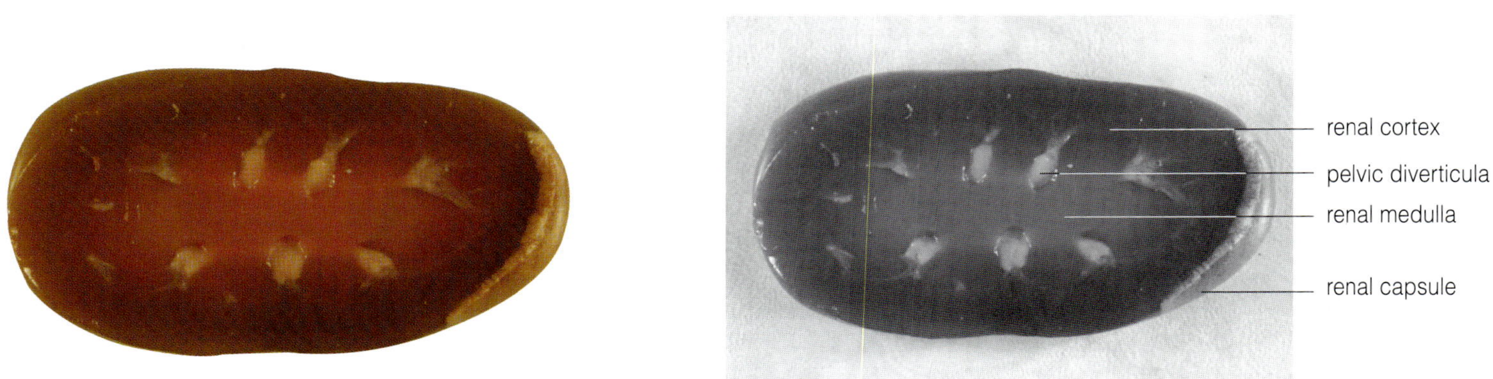

470–472 Sagittal sonogram (**471**) and corresponding anatomical sagittal sections (**470, 472**) of left canine kidneys (see also **467–469**).

473

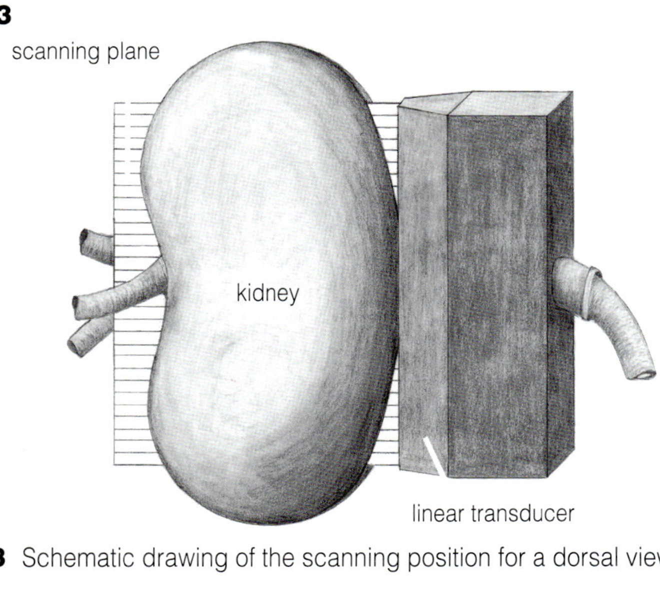

473 Schematic drawing of the scanning position for a dorsal view.

474

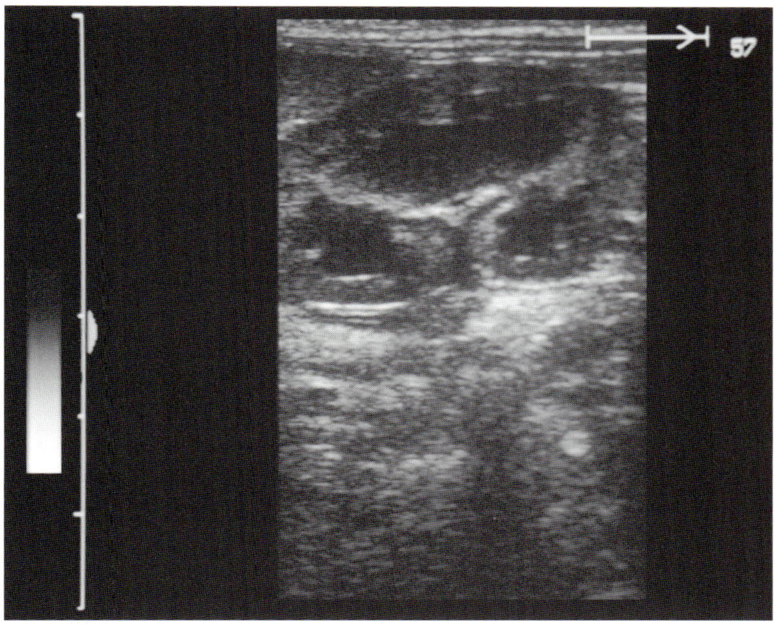

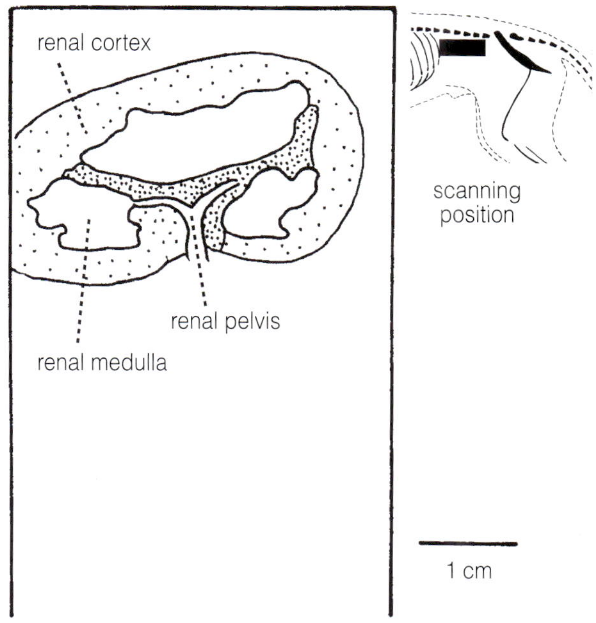

475

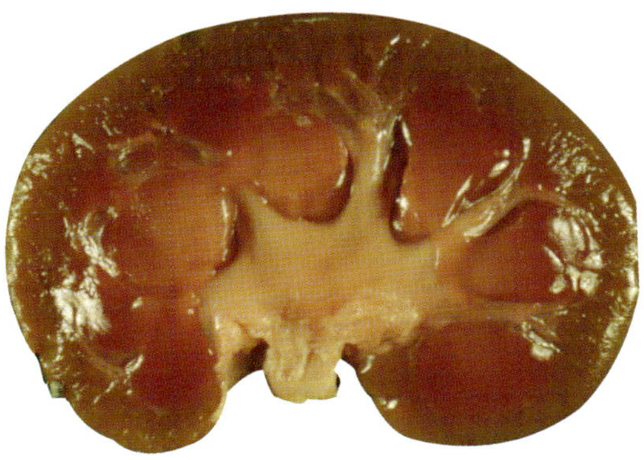

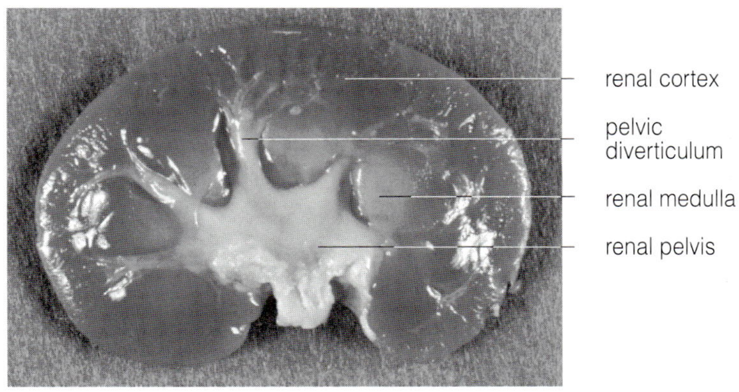

476

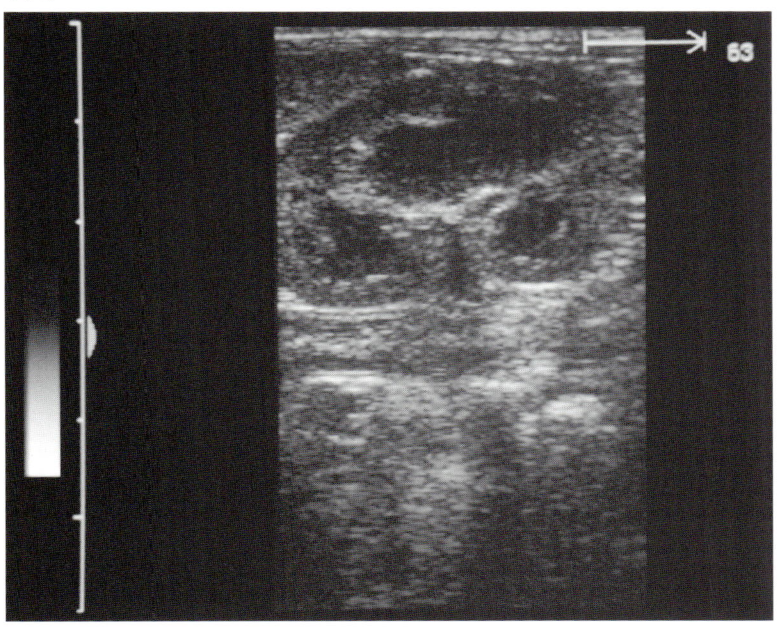

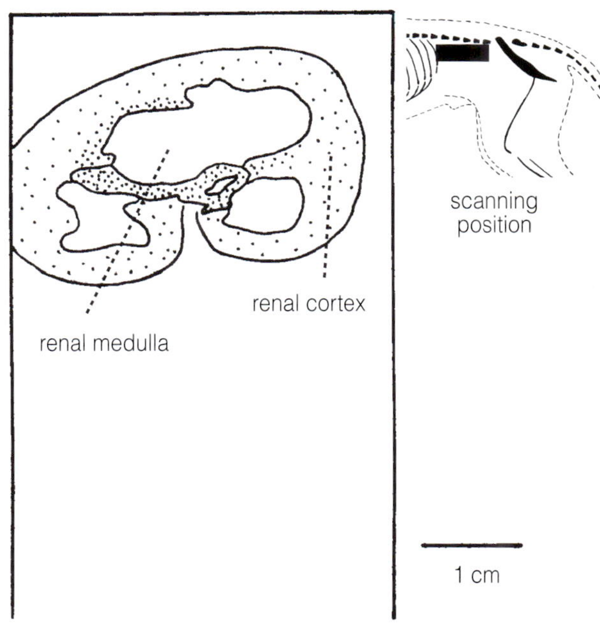

474–477 Dorsal sonograms (**474, 476**) and corresponding anatomical dorsal sections (**475, 477**, overleaf) of left canine kidneys. The slices are exactly in the renal sinus (**474, 475**) and slightly peripheral near the renal vessels (**476, 477**).

477

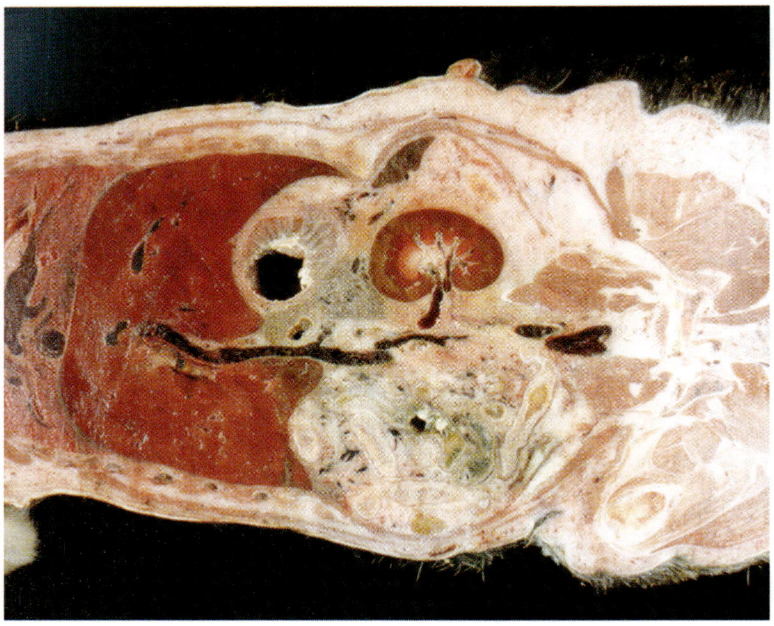

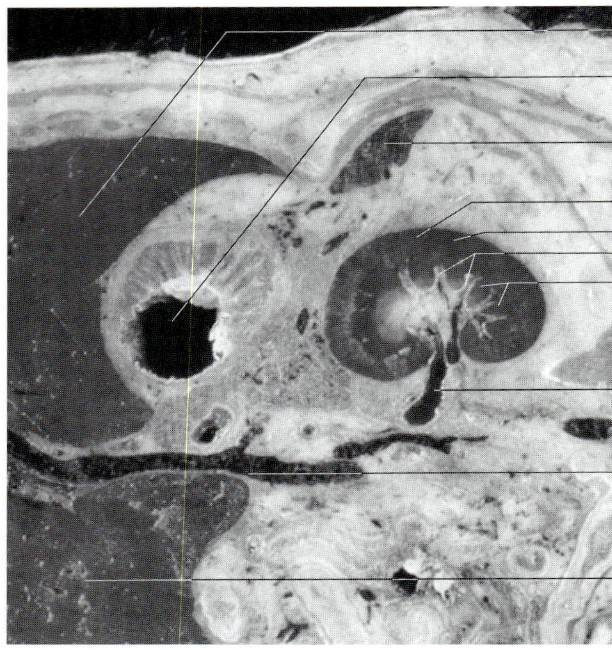

477 Anatomical dorsal section of left canine kidney (see **474–476**).

478

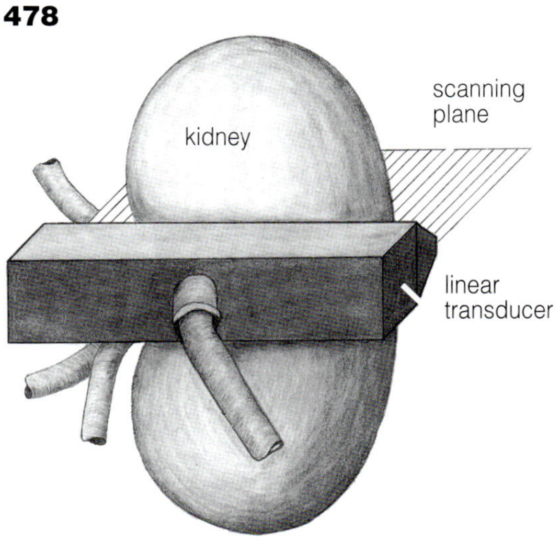

478 Schematic drawing of the scanning position for a transverse view.

479

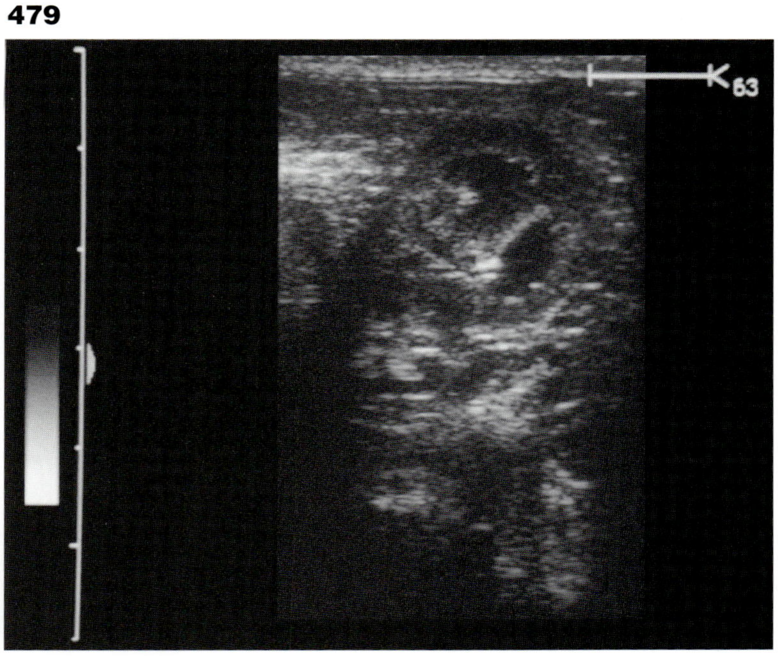

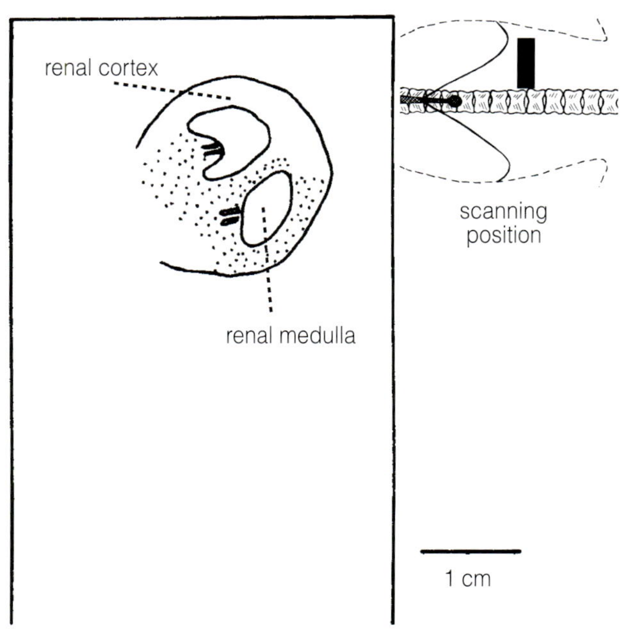

480

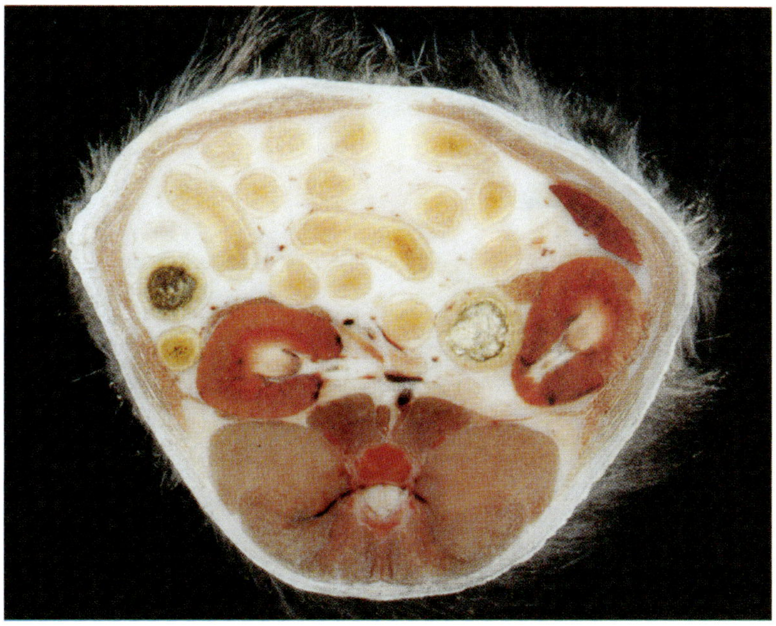

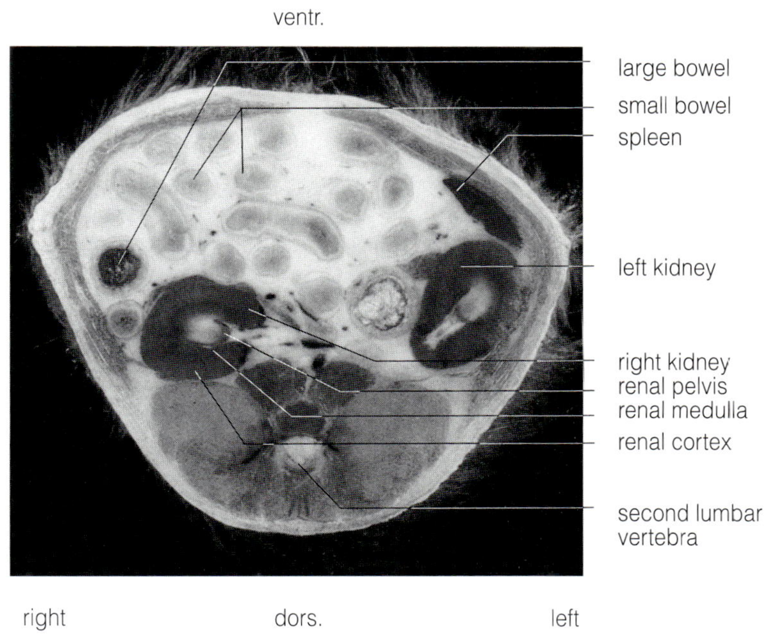

481

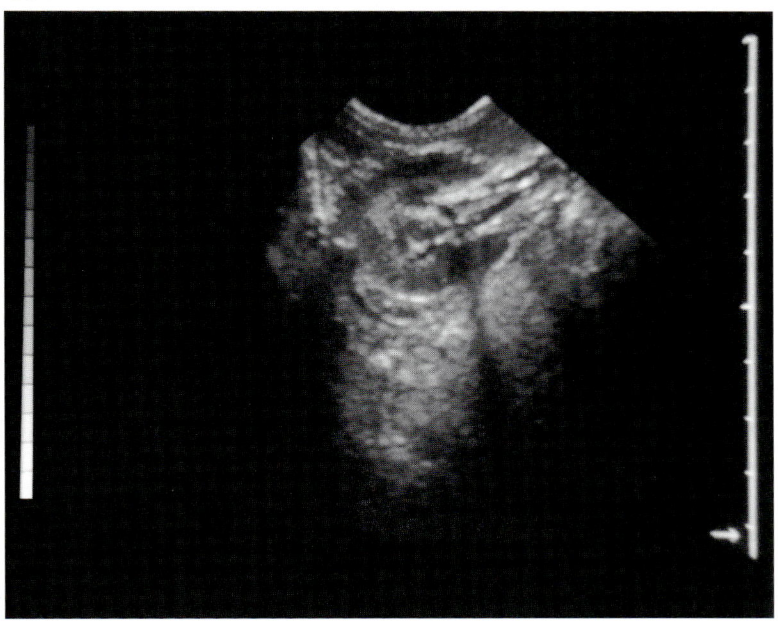

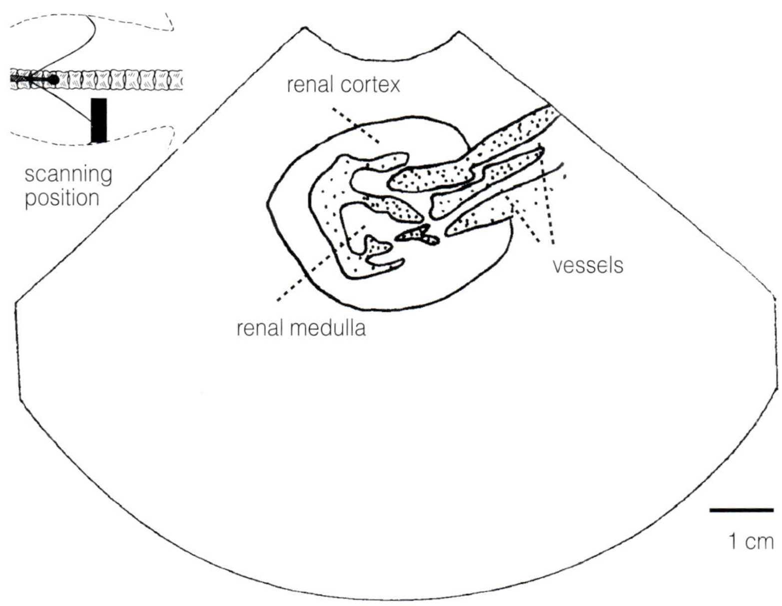

482

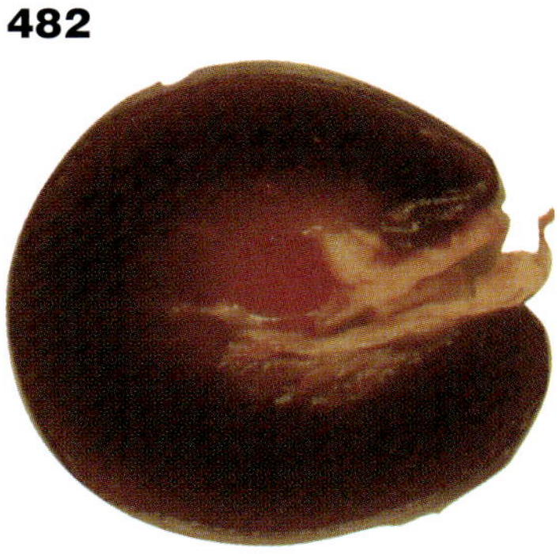

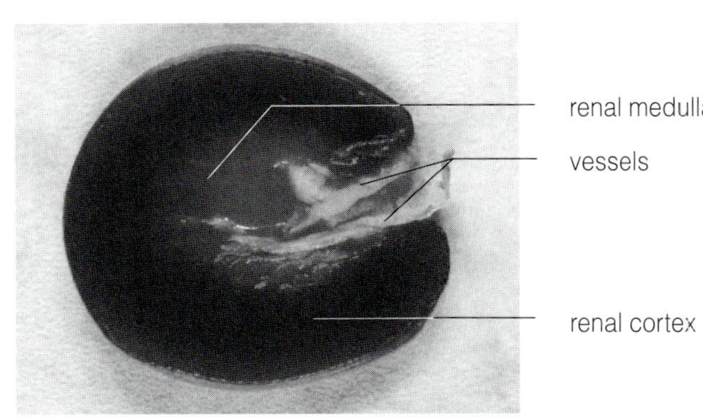

479–482 Transverse sonograms (**479, 481**) and corresponding anatomical transverse sections (**480, 482**) of a canine kidney. The slices are exactly in the renal sinus (**479, 480**) and slightly caudal near the renal vessels (**481, 482**).

483

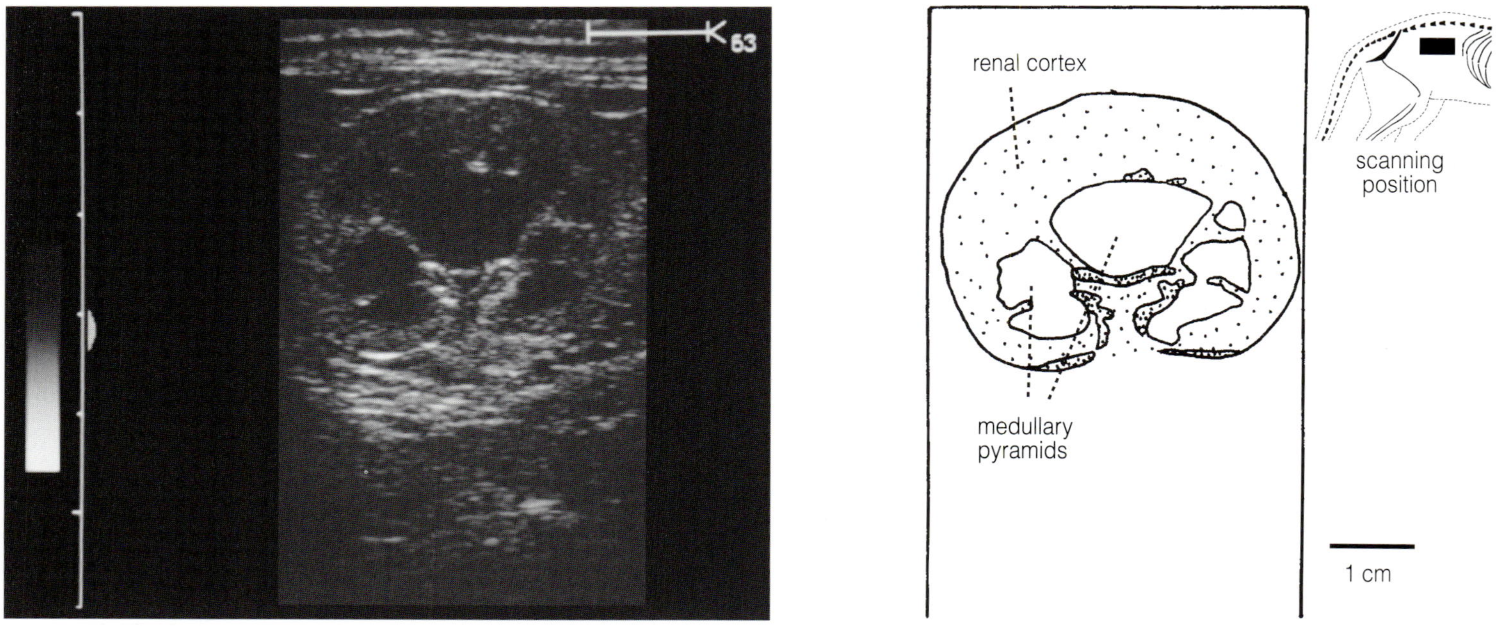

484

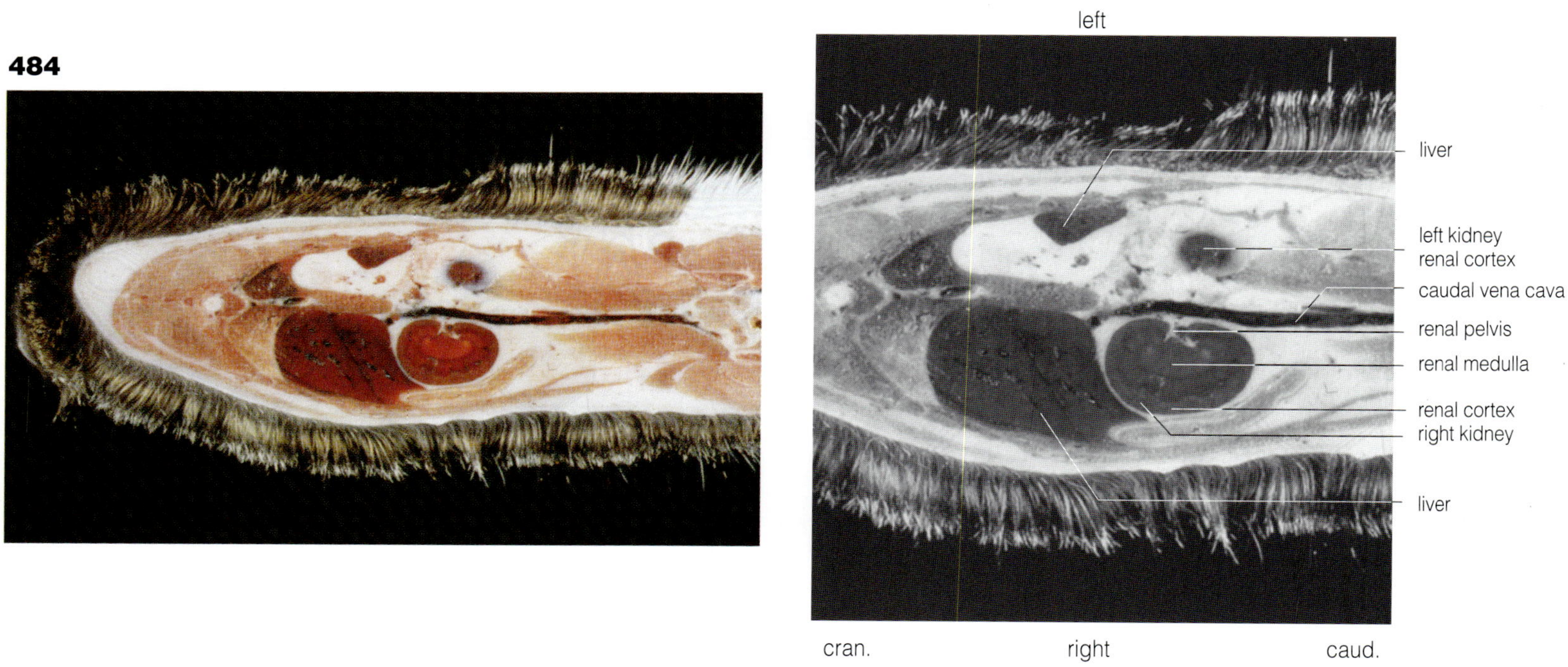

483, 484 Sonogram (**483**) and anatomical dorsal section (**484**) of a feline kidney.

485

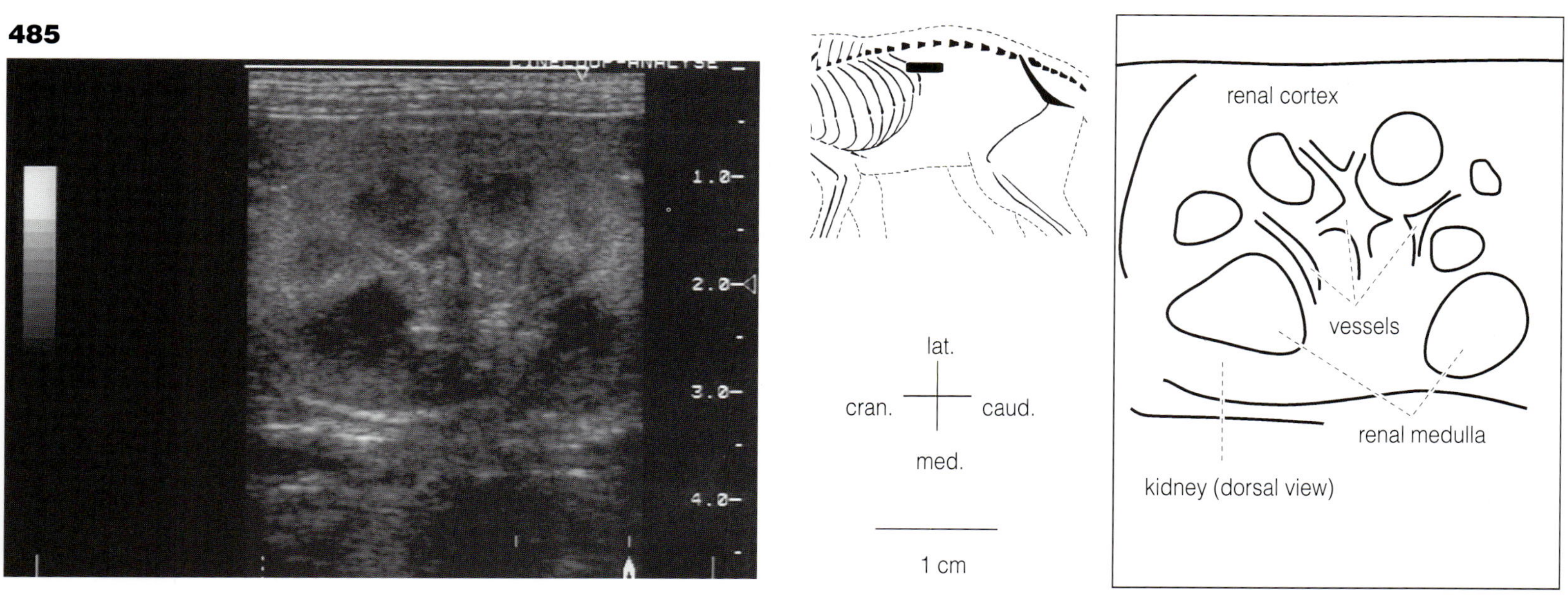

486

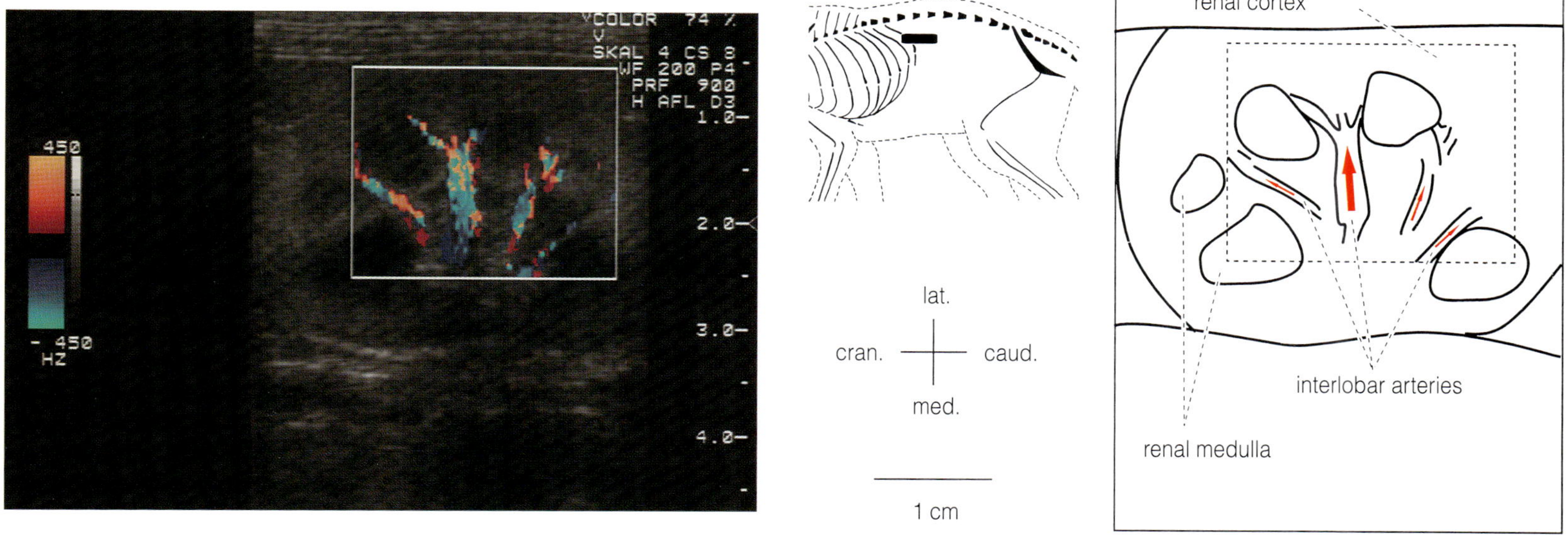

487

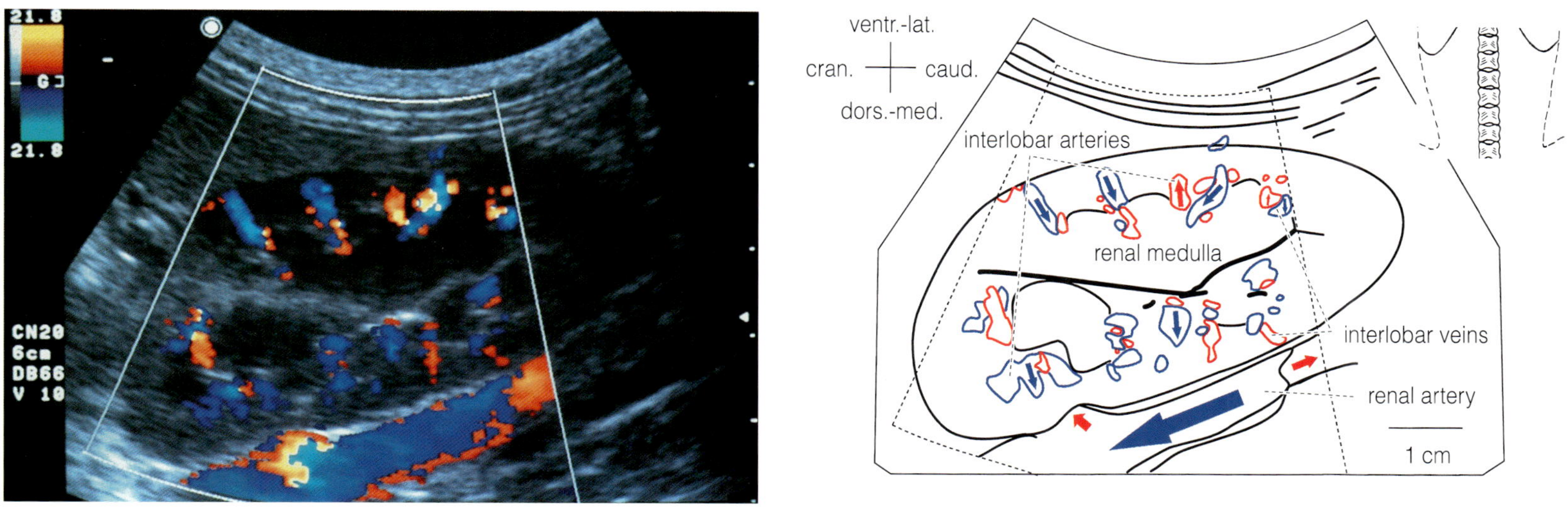

488

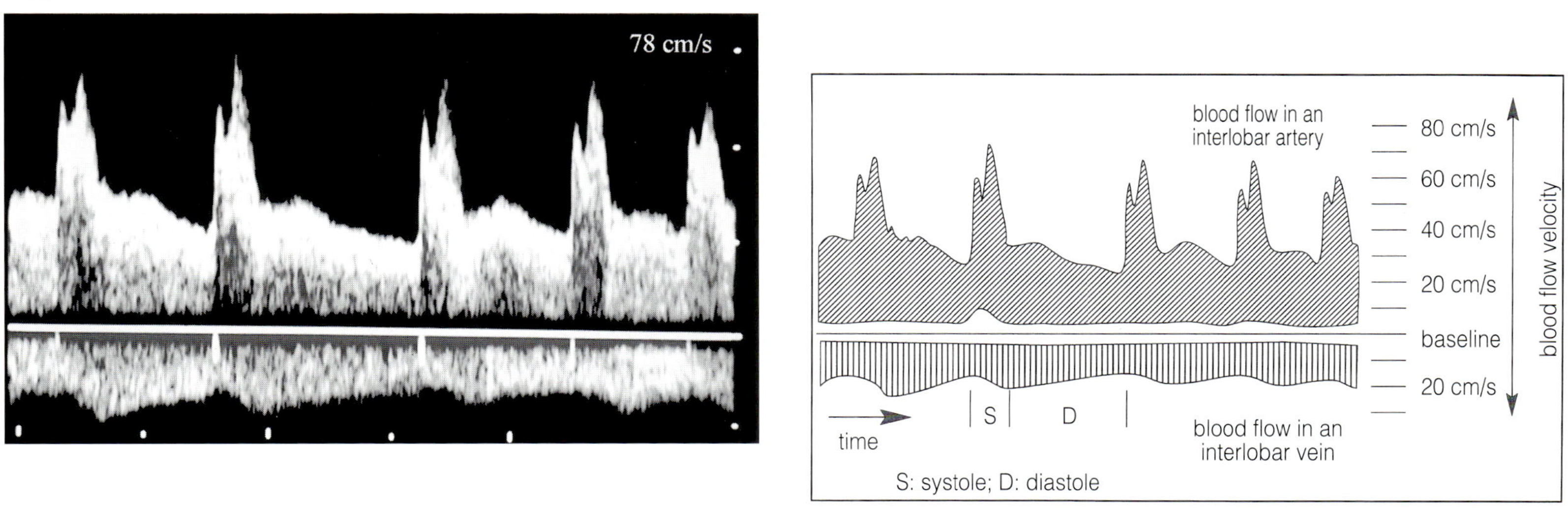

485–488 Two-dimensional sonogram (**485**) and colour Doppler echogram (**486, 487**) of normal renal vessels and their blood flow in a dorsal view in a cat (**485, 486**) as well as a sagittal view in a dog (**487**). PW Doppler display of blood flow in a branch of the renal artery and vein in a dog (**488**). (With permission from Isabelle von Goetz.)

The normal ureters cannot be visualized ultrasonographically. Two-dimensional sonography of renal vessels is usually possible in one of the three planes. They are identified by an anechoic lumen with an echogenic wall and are located directly lateral to the central renal pelvic area. Intrarenal vessels are usually the same size and run symmetrically. Renal arteries and veins can be differentiated using colour Doppler sonography (485–488).

489

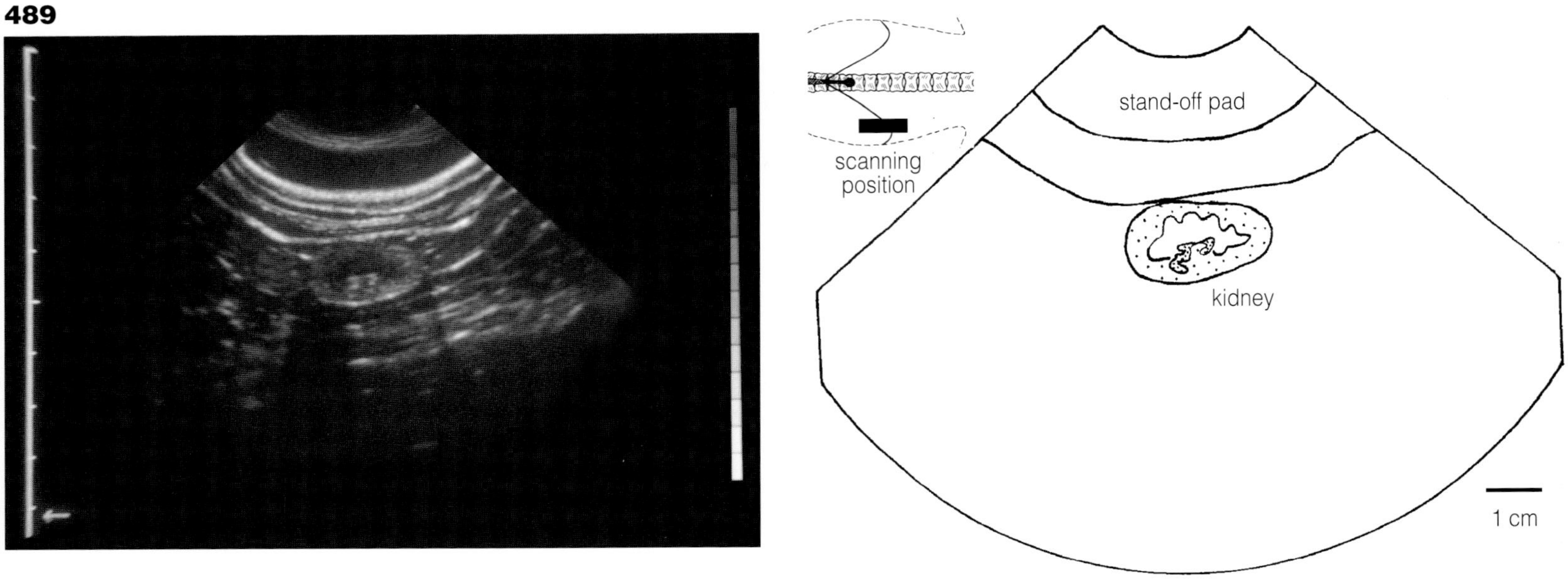

490

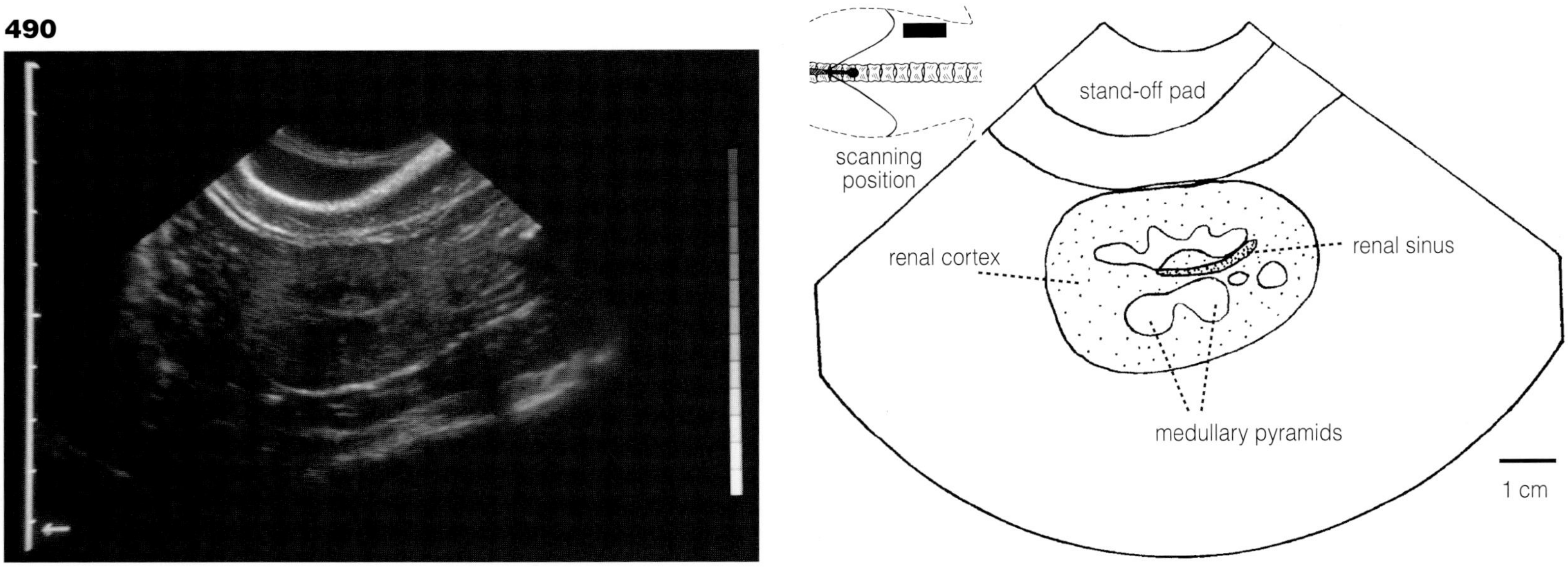

489, 490 Hypoplastic right kidney in a cat (**489**) compared to the normal opposite kidney (**490**) in sagittal views. Kidney shape and structure is identical and normal in both sonograms.

491

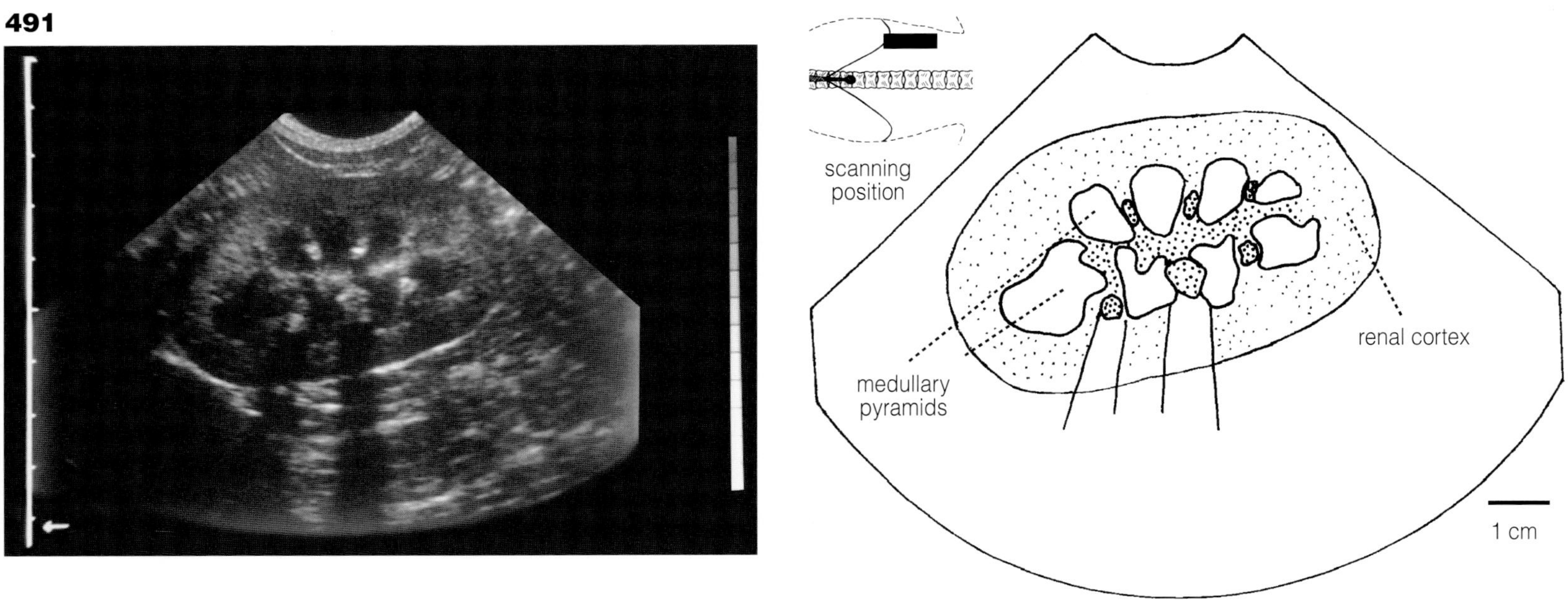

491 Left kidney with hyperechoic pelvic diverticula and distal acoustic shadowing. These findings signify fibrous tissue lesions. The dog was diagnosed with chronic interstitial nephritis.

492

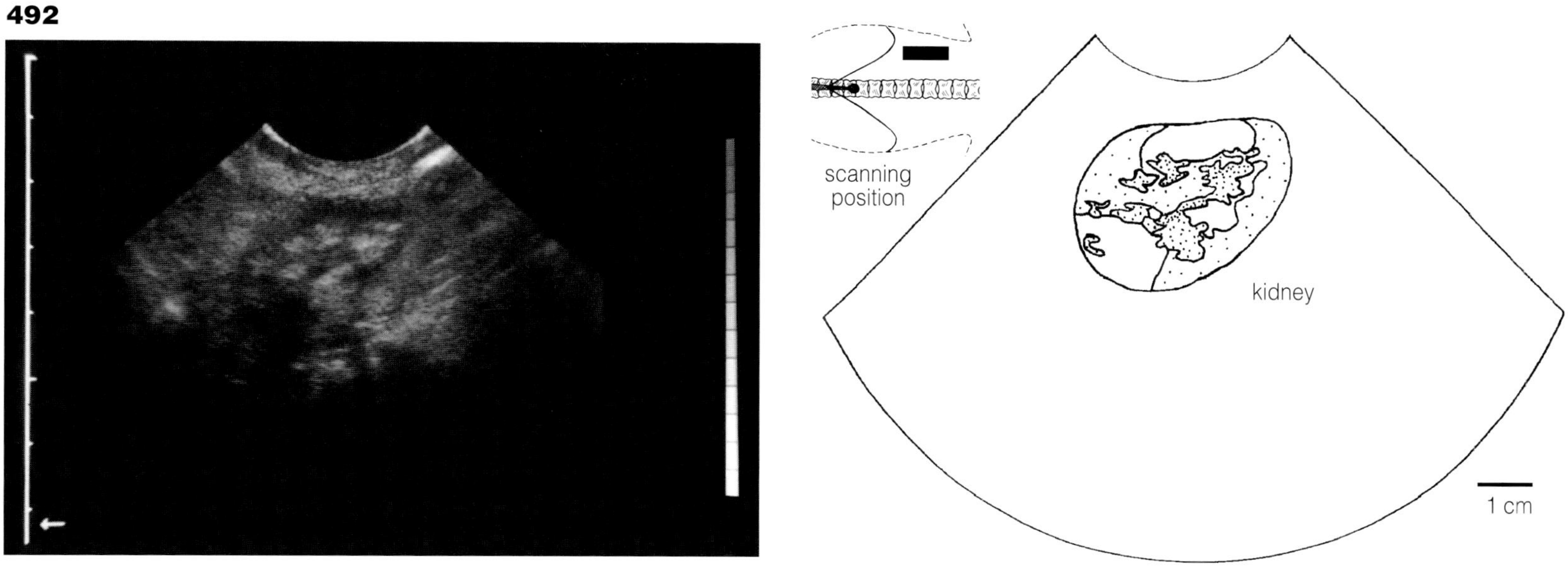

492 Sagittal view of an end-stage kidney in a dog. Compared to the opposite organ, this kidney is small with a non-homogenous structure and loss of corticomedullary definition.

Table 34 Ultrasonographic measurements of normal kidney size in the dog (from Barr, 1990[4]).

Weight (kg)	Kidney length (cm) Minimum value	Maximum value	Average value
0–4	3.2	3.3	3.2
5–9	3.2	5.2	4.4
10–14	4.8	6.4	5.6
15–19	5.0	6.7	6.0
20–24	5.2	8.0	6.5
25–29	5.3	7.8	6.9
30–34	6.1	8.7	7.2
35–39	6.6	9.3	7.6
40–44	6.3	8.4	7.6
45–49	7.6	9.1	8.5
50–59	7.5	10.6	9.1
60–69	8.3	9.8	9.0
90–99	8.6	10.1	9.4

Table 35 Ultrasonographic measurements of normal kidney size in the cat (modified from Scholz, 1992[16]).

	Minimum value	Maximum value	Average value
Length (cm)	2.7	4.7	3.5
Width (cm)	1.7	2.8	2.1

Indications for ultrasonography of the kidneys and ureters include polydipsia, polyuria, vomiting of unknown cause, acute abdomen, palpable organ abnormalities, as well as blood and urine profile disorders with suspected:

- Hypoplastic kidney and renal aplasia.
- Nephritis.
- End-stage kidney.
- Renal abnormalities with ethylene glycol toxicity.
- Renal infarcts.
- Renal calcifications.
- Trauma to the kidney.
- Renal abscess.
- Renal neoplasia.
- Renal cysts.
- Polycystic renal disease.
- Renal pelvic dilation and hydronephrosis.
- Renal calculi.
- Ureteral dilation.

A further indication is for monitoring treatment response.

Ultrasonography of Renal and Ureteral Disease

Renal Hypoplasia and Renal Aplasia

In one-sided renal hypoplasia a smaller, normally structured kidney is visualized (**489, 490**). The number of medullary pyramids may be reduced.

Displacement or aplasia of a kidney is diagnosed when one kidney is not found.

Nephritis

Chronic nephritis (**491**) shows an increased echogenicity of the renal cortex, rarely of the renal medulla[14, 17, 18]. Loss of corticomedullary definition with increased overall echogenicity and non-homogenous renal architecture are also recognized with chronic nephritis. Depending on the disease stage, the kidneys may be of normal size, or larger or smaller. Diffuse parenchymal renal diseases are difficult to diagnose or are not recognizable ultrasonographically[5, 10, 14, 17]. Diffuse inflammatory abnormalities of the kidneys may look normal in the ultrasound image. Histological examinations are needed to differentiate the various forms of nephritis.

End-stage Kidneys

End-stage kidneys are usually caused by chronic interstitial nephritis. They are typically small in size with loss of corticomedullary detail. Renal parenchyma cannot be differentiated from surrounding tissue. The diagnosis is made by the localization of the abnormality or the absence of an intact kidney[11] (**492**).

493

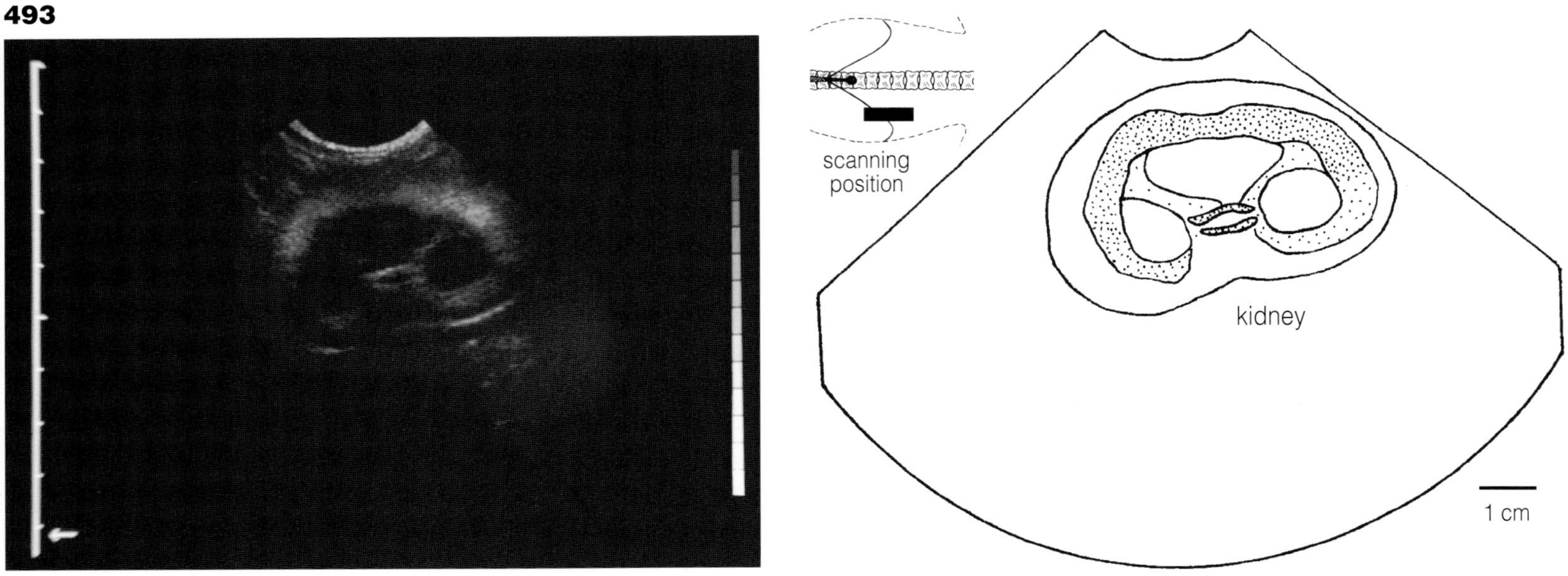

493 Nephropathy with ethylene glycol toxicosis in a dog. Right kidney in a dorsal longitudinal view. Renal shape and size are normal as well as cortical and medullary architecture. The renal cortex is divided into a thin hypoechoic outer layer and an inner hyperechoic layer.

494

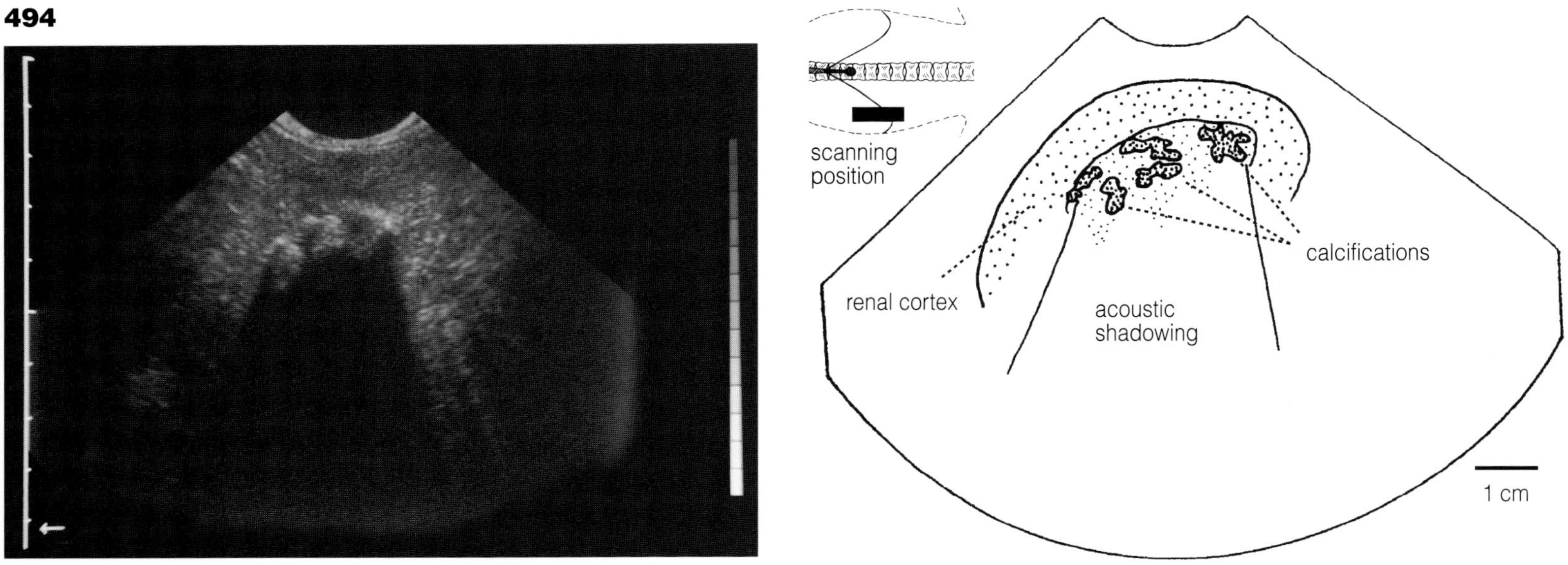

494 Diffuse renal calcifications associated with an osteorenal syndrome in a dog. The right kidney is seen in a sagittal long-axis view. Hyperechoic structures with distal shadowing are recognized at the corticomedullary junction.

Nephropathy with Ethylene Glycol Toxicosis

Increased cortical echogenicity is found with ethylene glycol poisoning. Corticomedullary definition is decreased (**493**) [1, 2, 13]. Differential diagnosis includes other inflammatory diseases.

Renal Infarcts

Renal infarcts may be caused by embolism. Renal artery occlusion produces kidney infarcts that have a wedge-shaped appearance with a peripheral broader base, narrowing towards the corticomedullary junction[7]. Acute infarcts are usually hypoechoic with a slightly protruding renal capsule, while older infarcts and scarring are hyperechoic with retraction of the renal surface[5].

Nephropathy

Renal calcifications are seen as focal or diffuse hyperechoic areas with or without distal acoustic shadowing. These calcifications may be recognized ultrasonographically before they are visualized on radiographs (**494**)[14].

A finely hyperechoic band may be observed at the corticomedullary junction and this is caused my mineral deposits. This medullary rim sign is visualized with a number of nephropathies (**495**)[3, 8].

Renal Trauma

Ultrasonography is useful in detecting renal trauma and evaluating any lesions (**496, 497**). Anechoic subcapsular or perirenal fluid accumulation is easily recognized with haemorrhaging[5, 12].

Immediately after trauma to the kidney, differentiation between haemorrhaging and urine from a ruptured ureter or renal pelvis is difficult. Follow-up examinations will show resorption and organization of the haemorrhage, while the amount of free urine will increase. Ultrasound-guided aspiration is useful for determining the type of fluid.

495

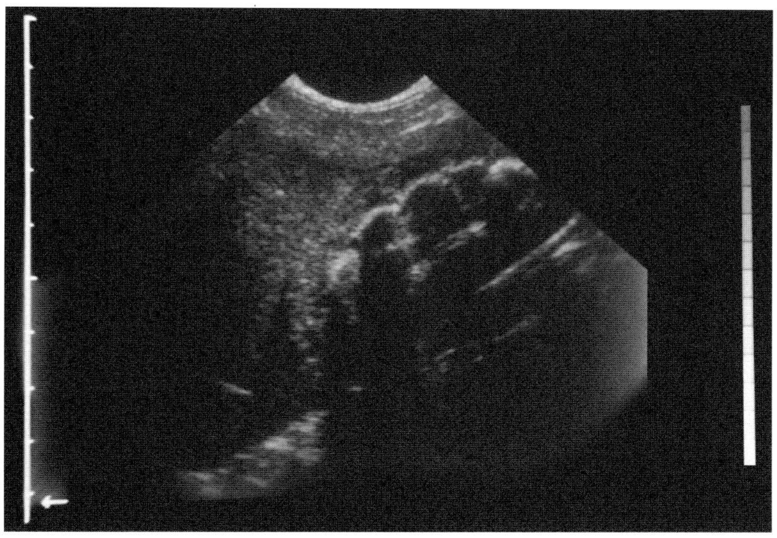

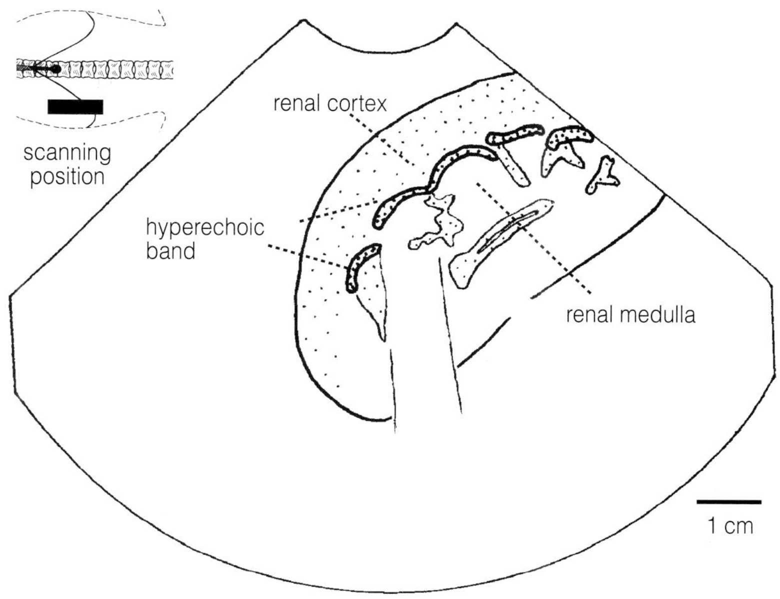

495 Medullary rim sign in a right canine kidney. Tubular calcification and glomerulonephritis caused these lesions.

496

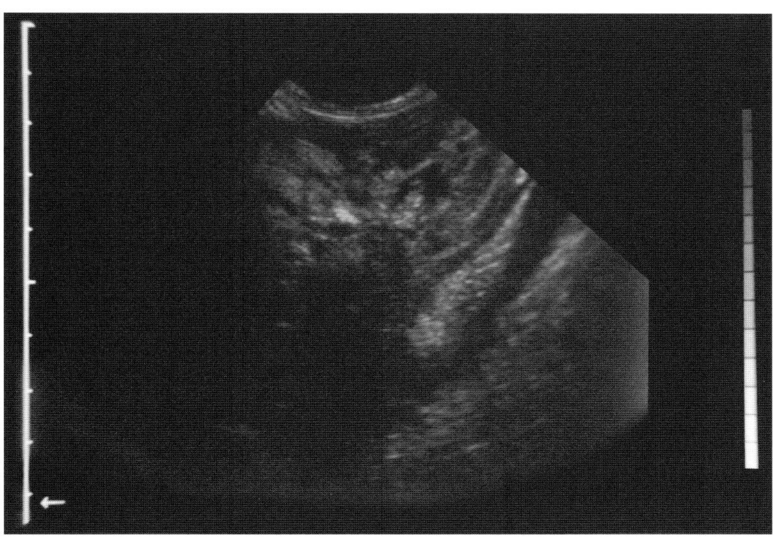

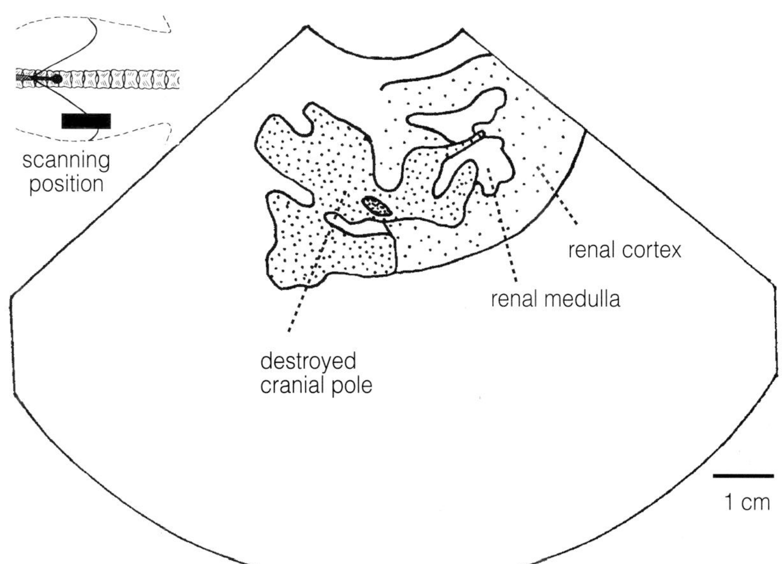

497

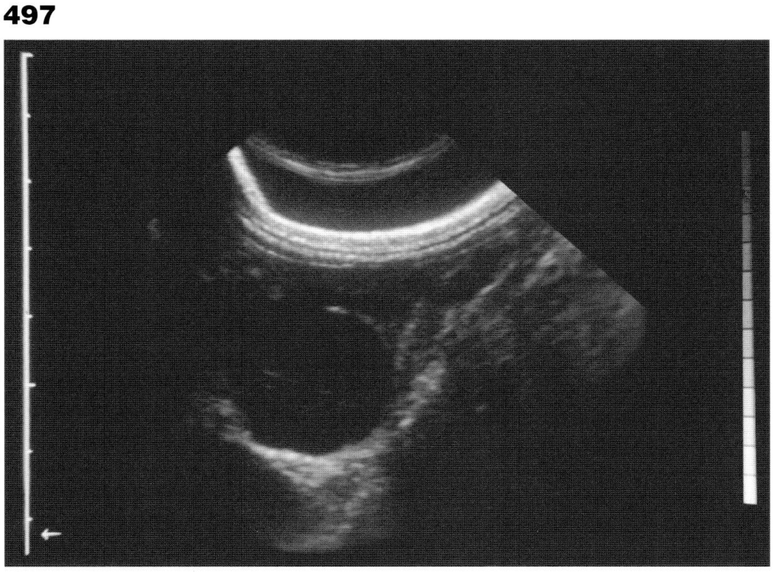

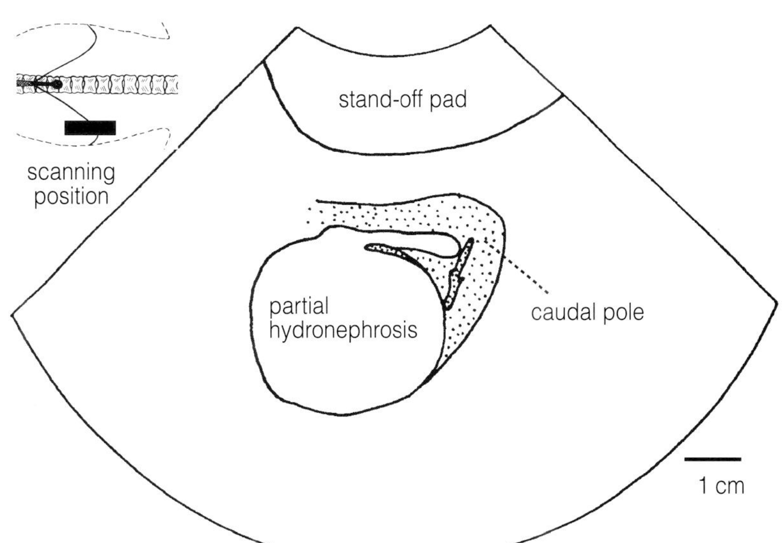

496, 497 Partial trauma to the kidney of a dog following a bite wound. In a sagittal long-axis view of the right kidney the caudal pole is normal, while the cranial pole is completely destroyed. A hypoechoic rim surrounds the hyperechoic, irregular centre (**496**). Four weeks later the renal tissue is altered (**497**). The cranial pole is replaced by a round, almost anechoic structure with distal enhancement.

498

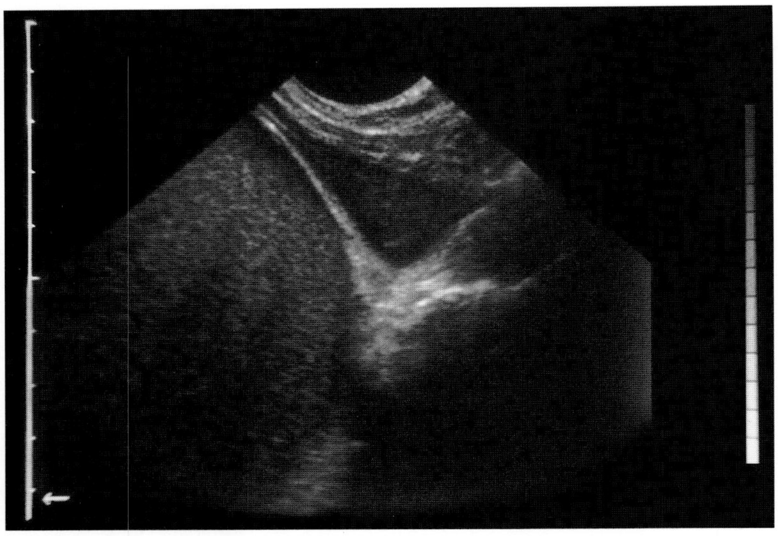
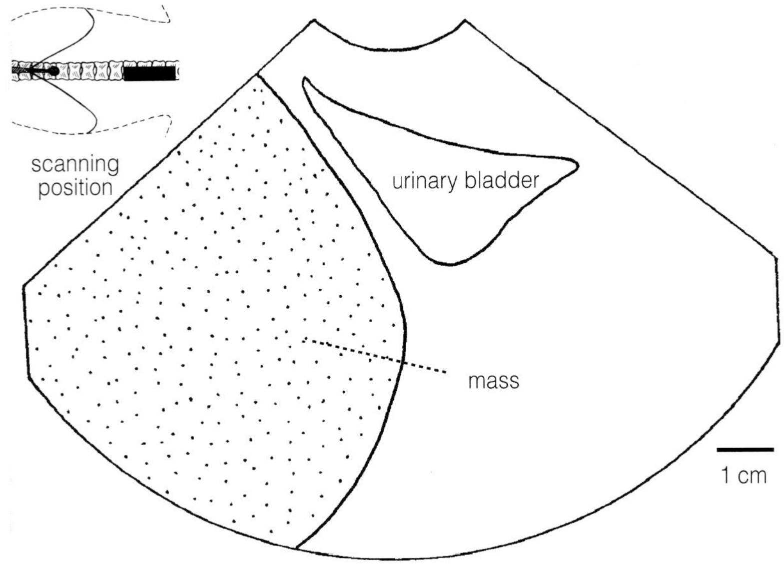

498 Pyonephrosis in a dog following ovariohysterectomy. An 18 cm oval mass is seen cranial to the urinary bladder with granulated, echogenic, floating contents. The right kidney was not found after extensive abdominal ultrasonography.

499

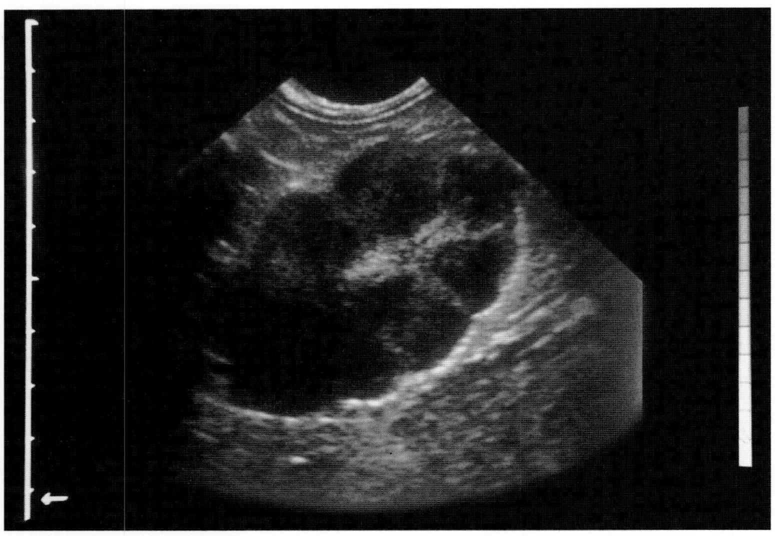
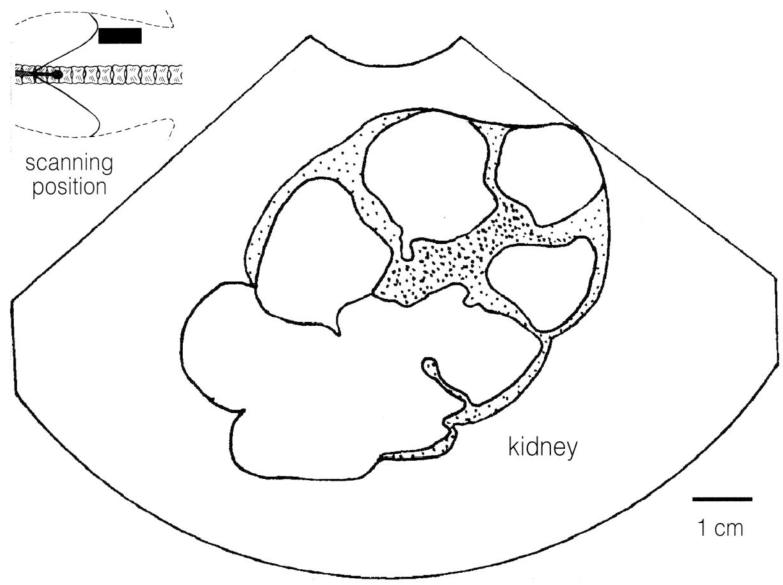

499 Renal tumour with lymphosarcoma in a dog. The left kidney is seen in a sagittal long-axis view. The kidney shape is recognizable; the renal parenchyma is altered. Hypoechoic round lesions are seen within the kidney.

Post-traumatic abscess formation or hydronephrosis may occur in the kidney (**497**). These lesions may affect parts of the kidney or the entire organ.

Renal Abscesses

Renal abscesses are rare but they may be found after pyelonephritis or after renal trauma such as perforating bite wounds. Abscesses are usually focal, well-demarcated, hypoechoic lesions with echogenic contents. In cases of pyonephrosis the entire kidney is affected. Differential diagnosis includes a haematoma or tumour. Compared to renal cysts, an abscess contains echogenic particles and a thicker, hyperechoic capsule. Distal enhancement may not be present or may be less obvious[5, 14].

Pyonephrosis causes a marked increase in renal size and complete loss of renal architecture (**498**). A tentative diagnosis is made by not finding a second kidney. This abnormality is difficult to differentiate from hydronephrosis.

Renal Neoplasia

Tumours of the kidney are seen with variable images in the dog and cat. Primary renal tumours usually originate from carcinomas and they are seen in the renal cortex and closer to the poles of the kidney. The sonogram usually shows a hypoechoic, solitary, round mass. At an early stage they may appear similar in echogenicity to the renal cortex and they are recognized only by a slight protrusion of the renal capsule. With increasing size, cell necrosis and

500

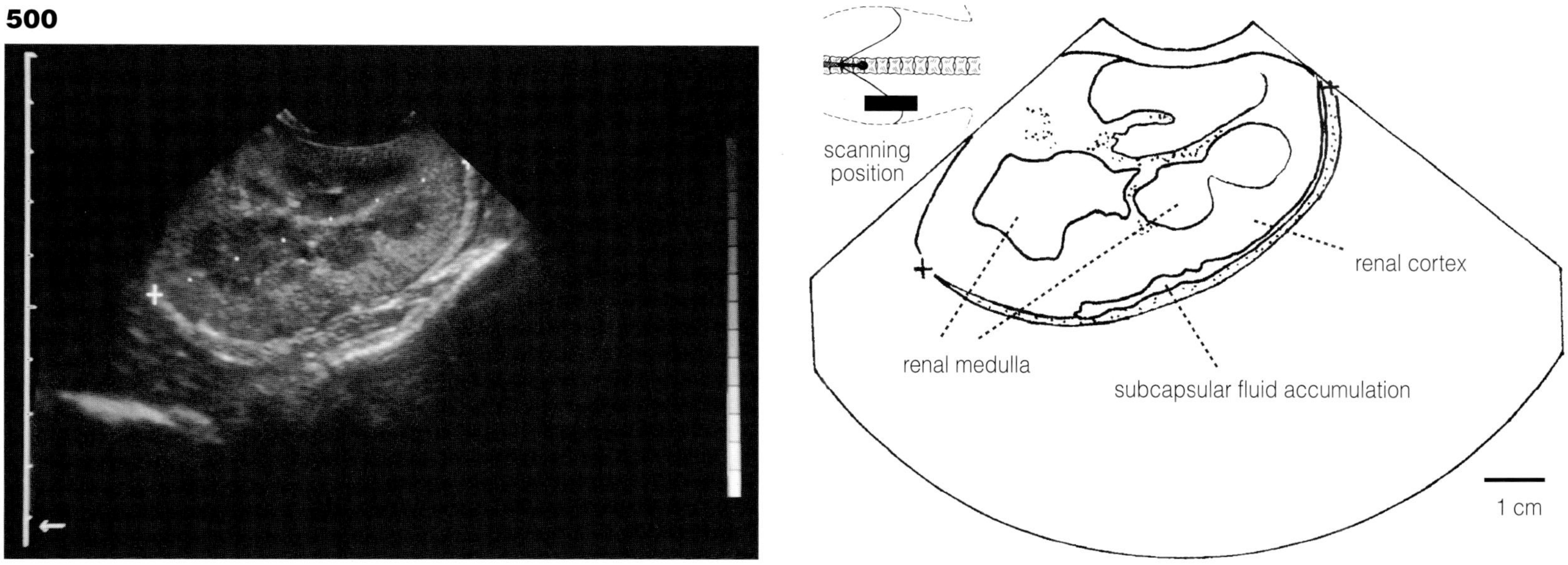

500 Lymphosarcoma of the right kidney in a cat. The enlarged kidney is echogenic with a coarsely granulated cortex. The kidney is surrounded by a thin anechoic rim.

501

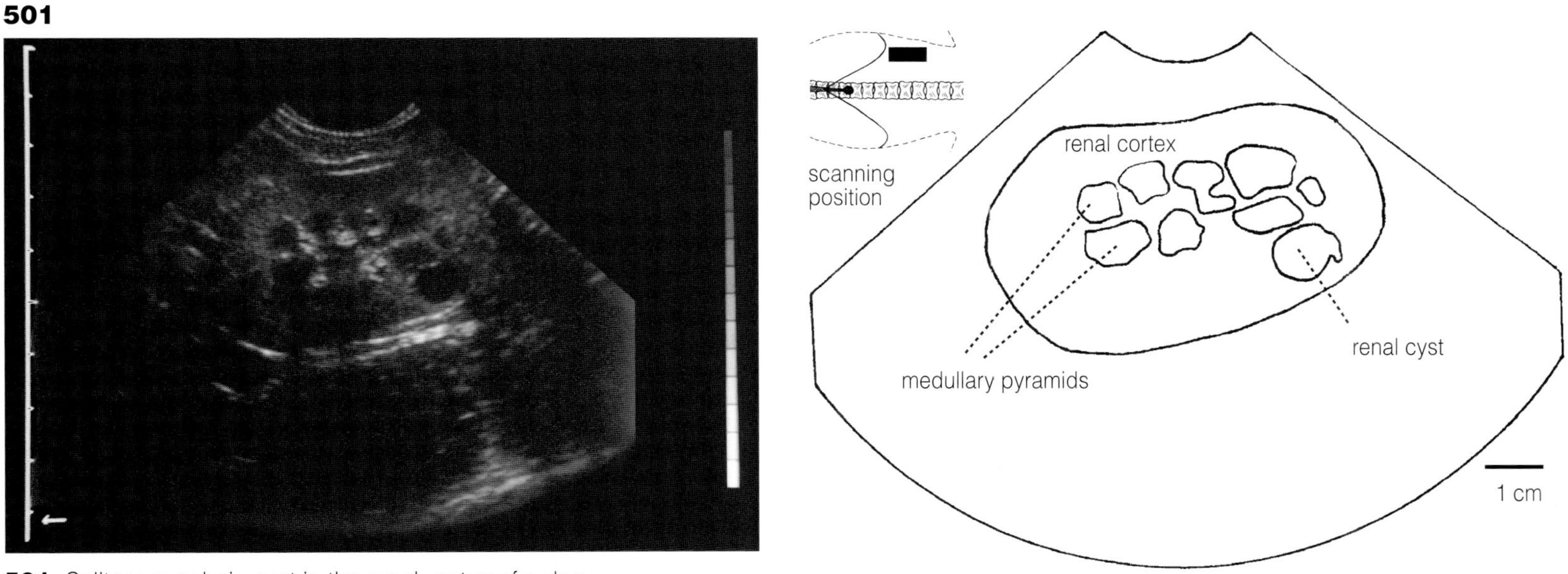

501 Solitary anechoic cyst in the renal cortex of a dog.

non-homogenicities occur. Secondary renal tumours are caused by lymphosarcoma or lymphoma. While the dog usually shows hypoechoic masses within the renal cortex (**499**) or diffuse enlargement with loss of renal architecture, cats with lymphosarcoma have enlarged kidneys with more or less normal structural detail. Echogenicity and homogenicity are occasionally normal (**500**). The types of tumours cannot be differentiated ultrasonographically.

Renal Cysts

Renal cysts are congenital abnormalities of the kidney. The sonogram visualizes cysts in the renal cortex as round anechoic structures with distal acoustic enhancement[14, 18] (**501**). They may be solitary or multiple. In most cases, cysts are incidental findings without clinical symptoms.

Polycystic Kidney Disease

Polycystic renal disease involves the entire or a greater part of the kidney. In an advanced stage the cortex and medulla are not distinguishable and anechoic cystic lesions are found within the entire kidney. The kidney outline is irregularly deformed. Uraemia is clinically apparent in patients with these cystic lesions. Cysts may have cellular contents and appear more echogenic. Polycystic renal disease is an inherited disease in Persian cats (**502**)[6]. The cystic lesions are visualized in both kidneys. In some cases, concurrent hepatic cysts are observed.

502

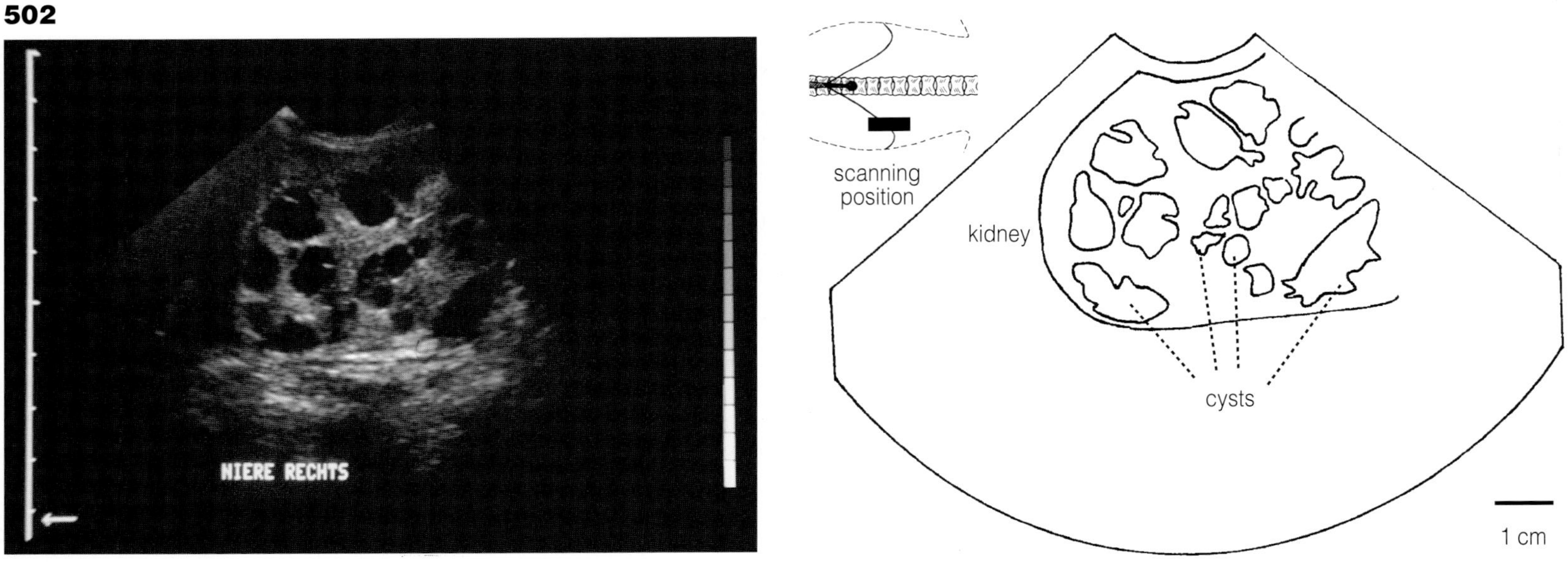

502 Polycystic renal disease in a Persian cat.

503

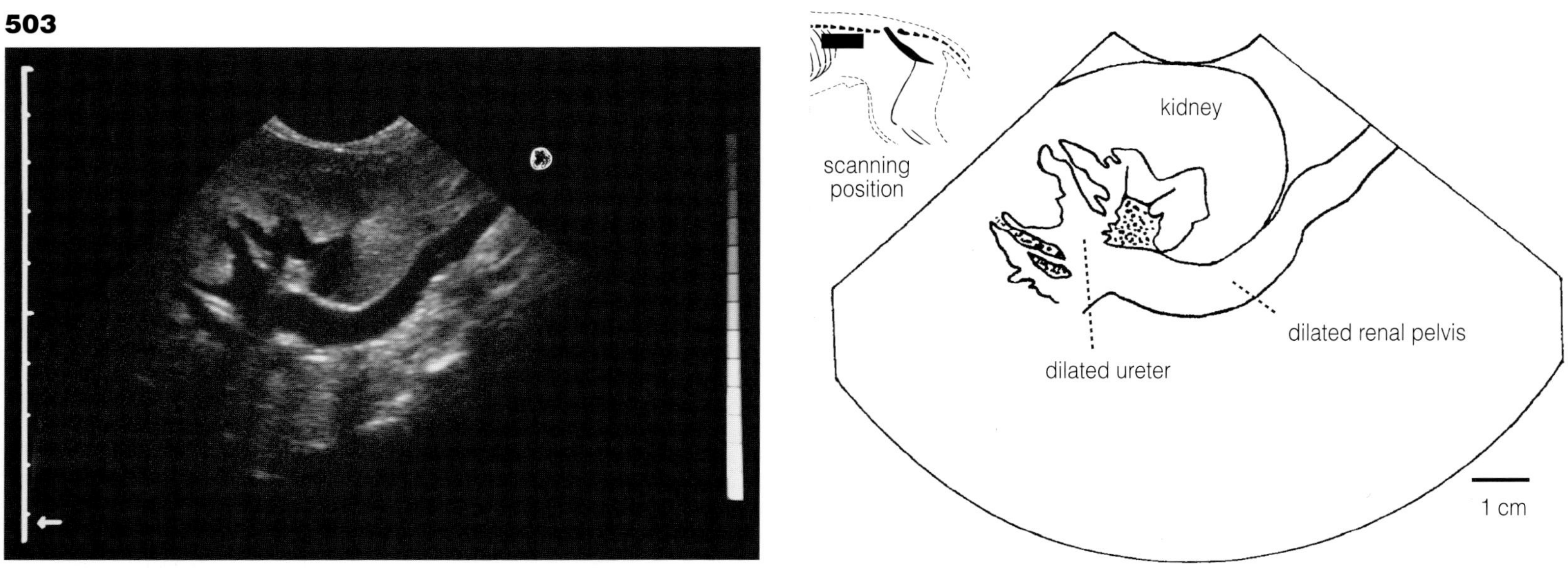

503 Mild hydronephrosis and ureteral dilation in a dog with ureteral obstruction caused by metastasis from a prostatic carcinoma.

Renal Pelvic Dilation and Hydronephrosis

Renal Pelvic Dilation

Dilation of the renal pelvis is caused by ureteral obstruction and urine accumulation (**503**). The central renal sinus is separated by an anechoic space. In a transverse view the V-shaped, hyperechoic renal pelvis shows a central anechoic area that can be traced to the proximal ureter[14]. Congenital pelvic dilation is caused by an ectopic ureter. Aquired dilation of the renal pelvis may be found with obstruction of the ureter by calculi or a bladder tumour. Dilation of the renal pelvis may also be caused by surgical complications (**504**).

Hydronephrosis

Longstanding ureteral obstruction leads to marked renal pelvic dilation and atrophy of renal parenchyma (**505**). The renal medulla is affected first, followed by the renal cortex. Severe hydronephrosis is characterized by a renal capsule with fibrous spokes extending into the lumen (**506**). These spokes are from the remaining pelvic diverticula. Causes for hydronephrosis are usually not determined ultrasonographically; they include tumours, congenital abnormalities, surgeries and ureteral calculi.

Renal Calculi

Renal calculi are rare and are usually located in the renal pelvis with total reflection and strong distal acoustic shadowing. A small amount of fluid is sometimes seen above the calculus nearer to the transducer. Very large calculi are difficult to image because the compressed medulla cannot be visualized, and the remaining renal cortex is masked by the strong echoes (**507**). Smaller calculi with normal renal architecture are easier to distinguish (**508**).

Ureteral Dilation

Obstruction of the ureter produces prestenotic dilation which is seen best near the renal hilus. A dilated ureter cannot be traced all the way to the bladder because of overlying bowel loops and

504

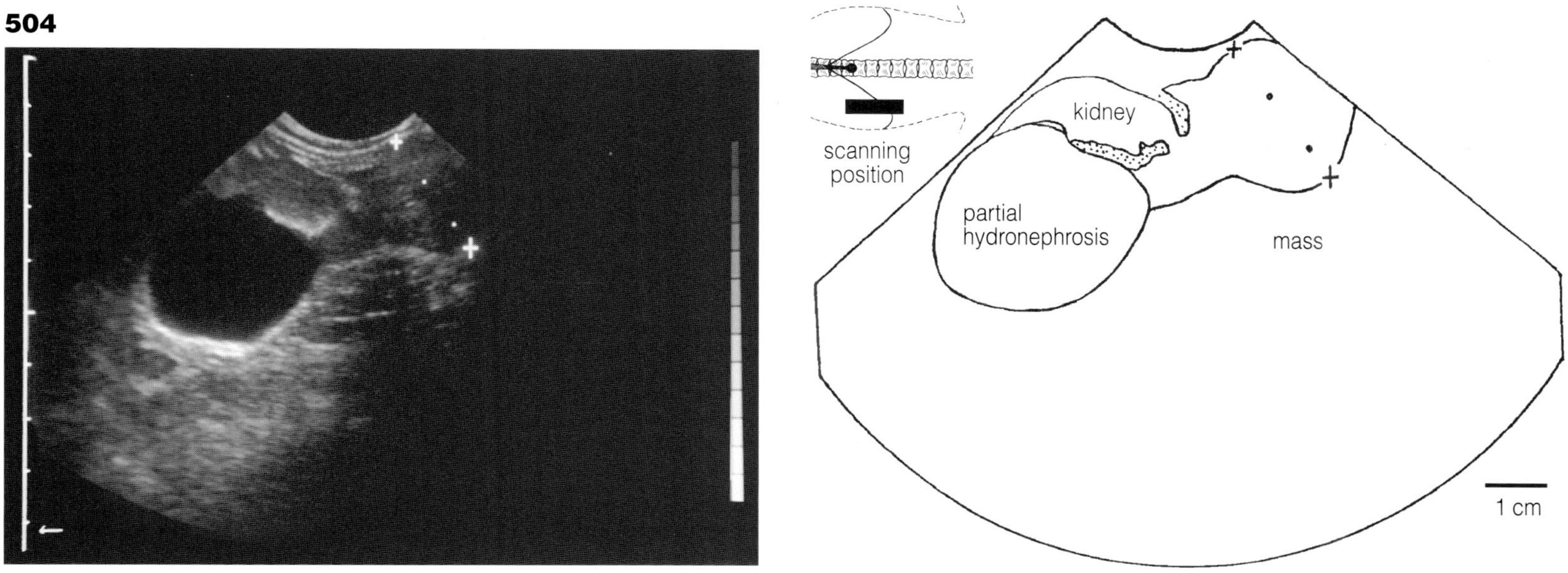

504 Atypical, early hydronephrosis following ovariohysterectomy in a bitch. The cranial pole shows a large anechoic lesion with distal acoustic enhancement, while the caudal pole has normal architecture. A round hypoechoic mass is seen caudal to the kidney. A granuloma from suture material caused obstruction of the ureter.

505

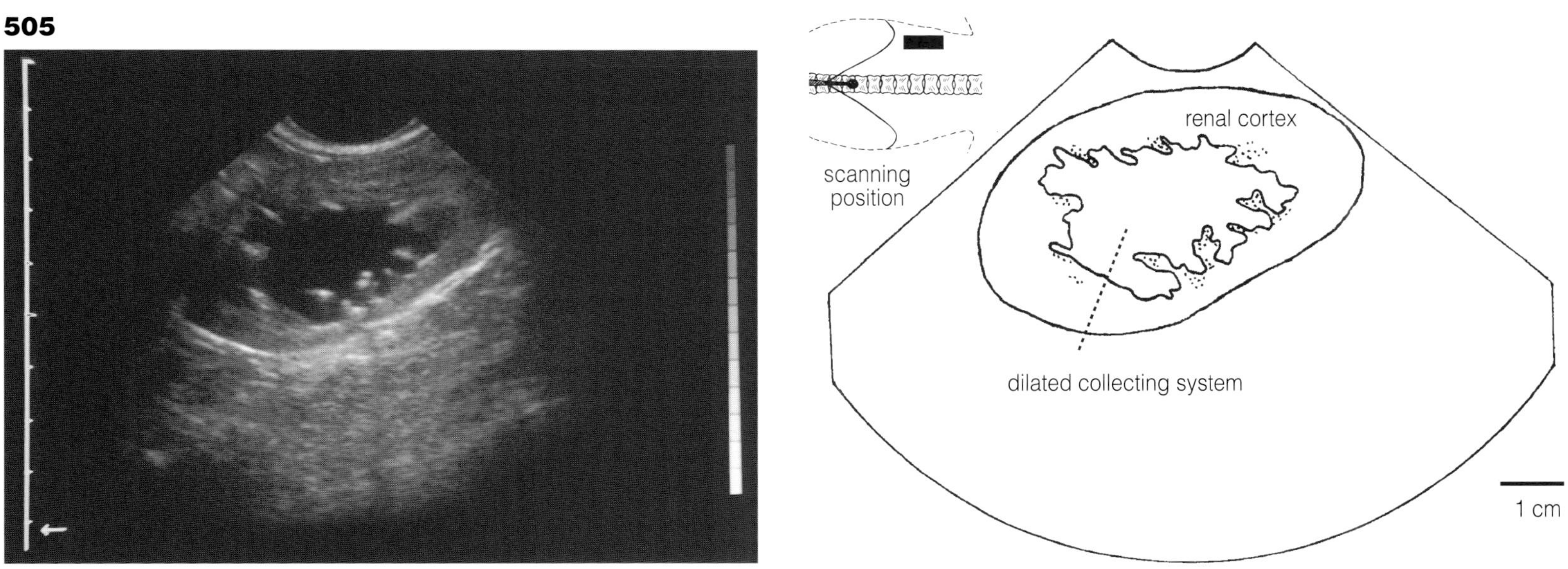

505 Hydronephrosis in a dog. The renal cortex is visible.

506

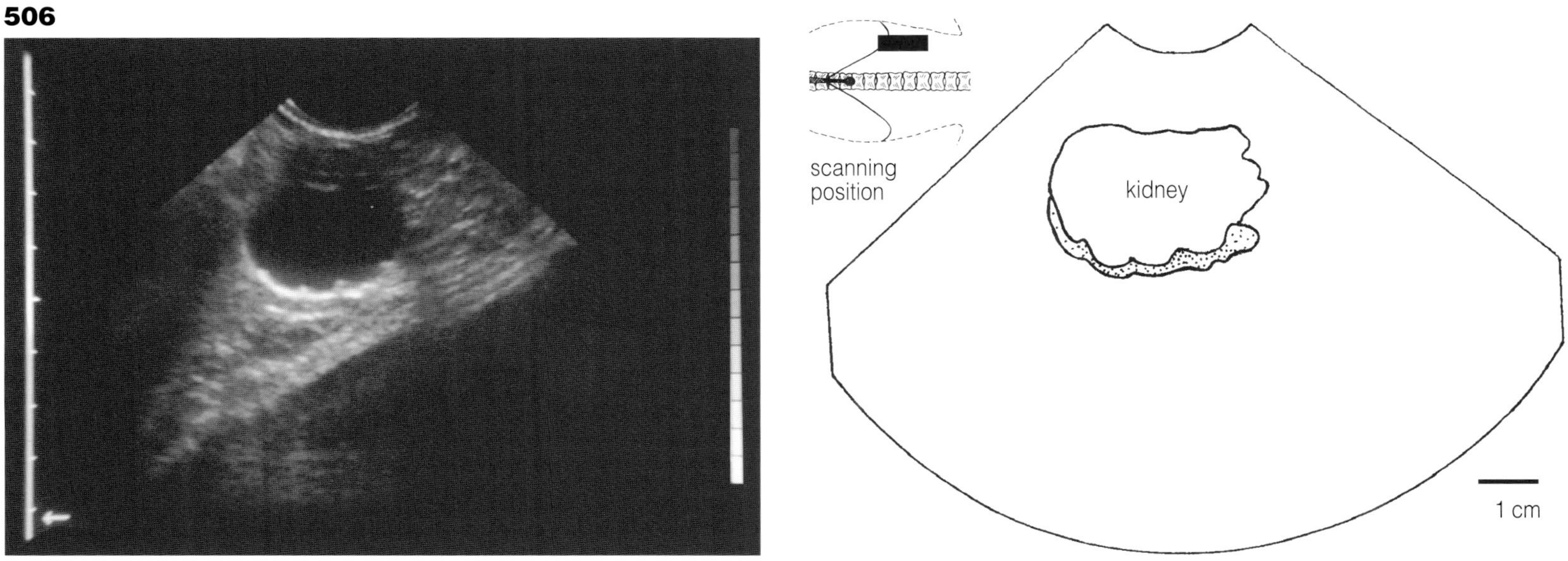

506 Hydronephrosis of a left feline kidney. Kidney shape and spoke-like fibrous septa are seen in a sagittal long-axis plane. An anechoic space with distal acoustic enhancement has replaced medullary and cortical parenchyma.

507

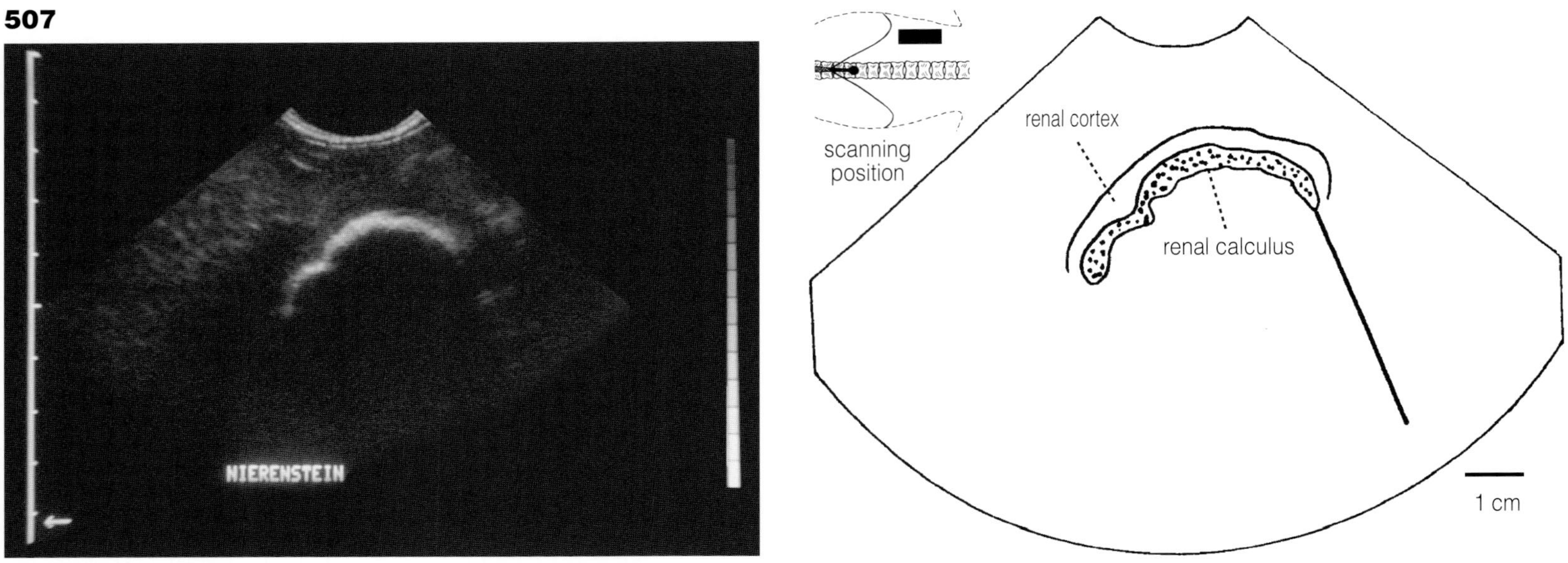

507 Renal pelvic calculus with compression of the renal parenchyma in a dog. Sagittal long-axis view of the left kidney with suggested oval shape and loss of architectural definition. The renal cortex remains as a thin rim.

508

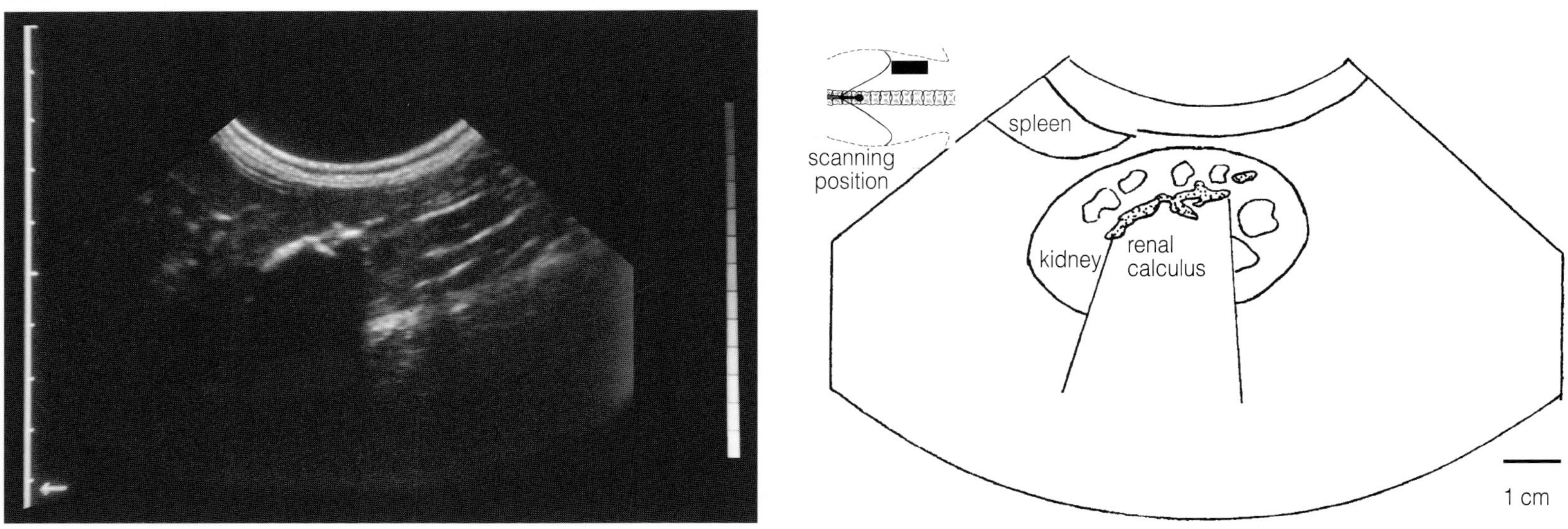

508 Renal calculus in a dog. Sagittal long-axis view of the left kidney. Renal shape and architecture are normal. An echogenic line with distal acoustic shadowing is seen in the central renal sinus.

509

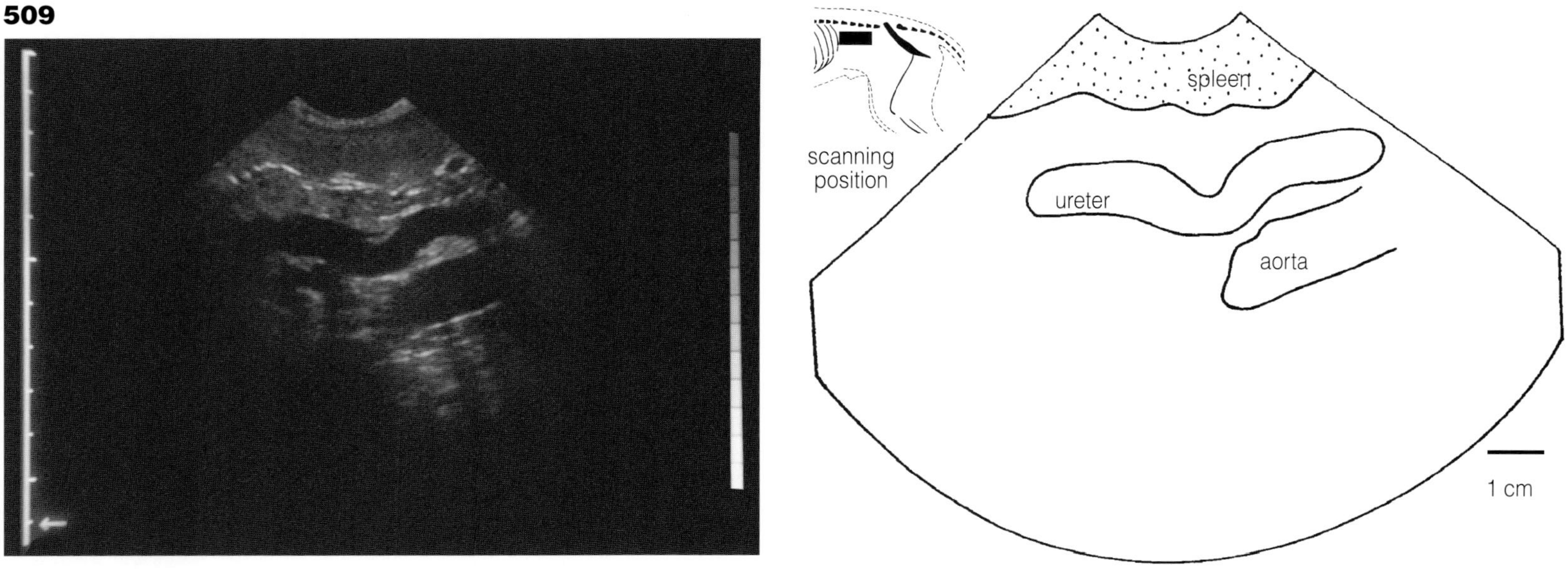

509 Ureteral dilation with typical tortuous course and partial visualization.

510

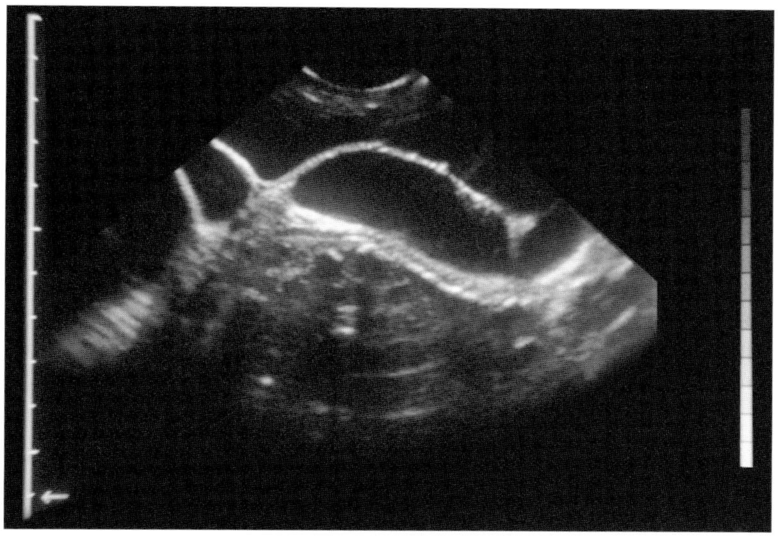

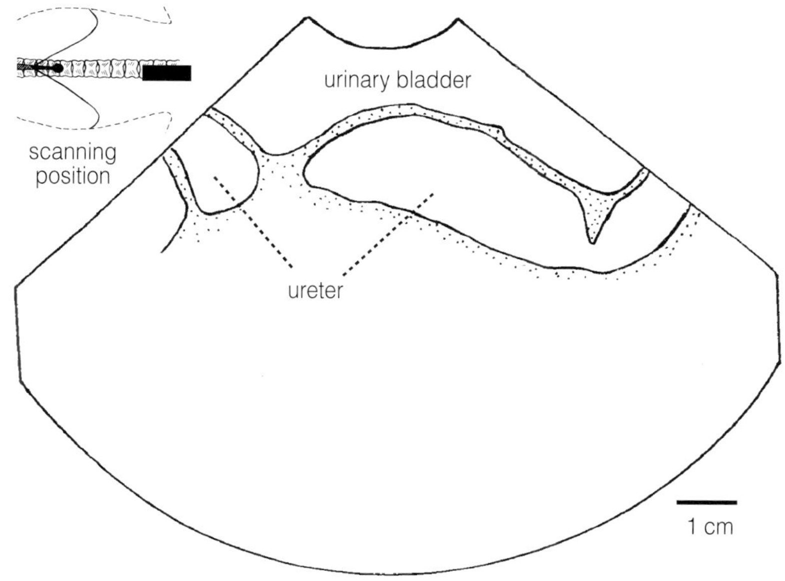

511

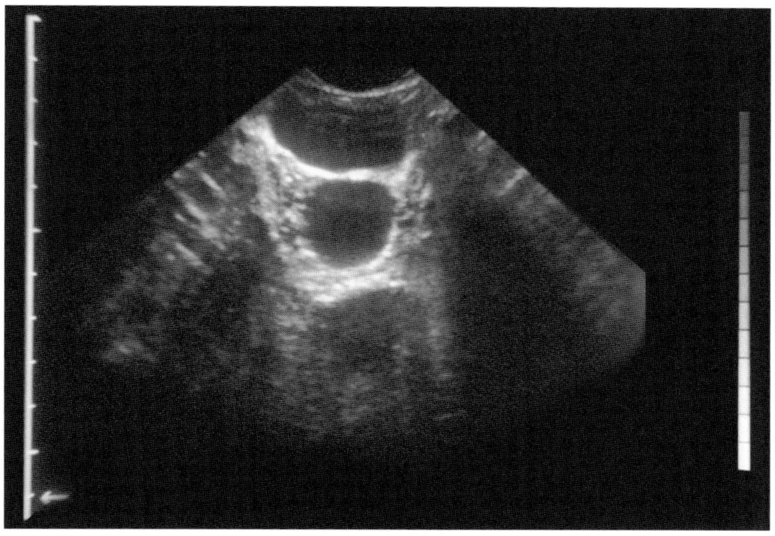

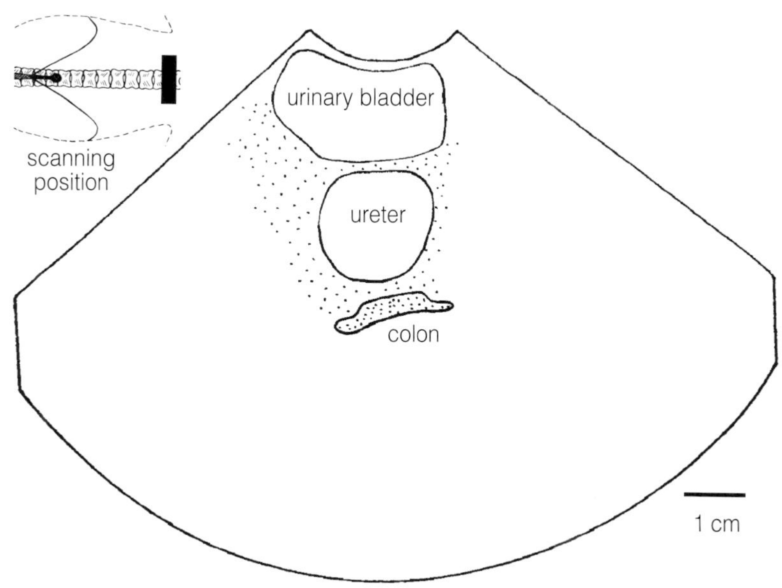

510, 511 Dilation of the ureter with an ectopic ureter in a dog in a longitudinal (**510**) and a transverse (**511**) view. The tortuous course allows partial visualization of the ureter. The wall of the ureter is thin. The urinary bladder is normal and small with a thin wall. The ureteral junctions are not visible.

acoustic shadowing. Portions of the distended ureter may be identified in mid-abdomen by its tortuous course (**509**). The ureteral junction at the bladder is occasionally visualized. Obstruction with ectopic ureters produces the same findings (**510, 511**).

References

1 Adams WH, Toal RL, Walker MA and Breider MA (1989) Early renal ultrasonographic findings in dogs with experimentally induced ethylene glycol nephrosis. *Am. J. Vet. Res.* **50**, 1370–1376.

2 Adams WH, Toal RL and Breider MA (1991) Ultrasonographic findings in dogs and cats with oxalate nephrosis attributed to ethylene glycol intoxication: 15 cases (1984–1988). *J. Am. Vet. Med. Assoc.* **199**, 492–496.

3 Barr FJ, Patteson MW, Lucke VM and Gibbs C (1989) Hypercalcemic nephropathy in three dogs: sonographic appearance. *Vet. Radiol.* **30**, 169–173.

4 Barr FJ, Holt PE and Gibbs C (1990) Ultrasonographic measurement of normal renal parameters. *J. Small Anim.Pract.* **31**, 180–184.

5 Barr FJ (1992) Harnapparat: Nieren. In: Barr FJ. *Ultraschalldiagnostik bei Hand und Katze*. Gustav Fischer Verlag, Stuttgart, Jena, New York.

6 Biller DS, Chew DJ and Dibartola SP (1990) Polycystic kidney disease in a family of Persian cats. *J. Am. Vet. Med. Assoc.* **196**, 1288–1290.

7 Biller DS, Schenkman DI and Bortnowsski H (1991) Ultrasonographic appearance of renal infarcts in a dog. *J. Am. Anim. Hosp. Assoc.* **27**, 370–372.

8 Biller DS, Bradley GA and Partington BP (1992) Renal medullary rim sign: ultrasonographic evidence of renal disease. *Vet. Radiol.Ultrasound* **33**, 286–290.

9 Feeney DA, Johnston GR and Walter PA (1991) Ultrasonography of the kidney and prostate gland. *Prob. Vet. Med.* **3**, 619–646.

10 Flückiger M (1991) Ultraschalldiagnostik bei Hand und Katze. 2. Klinische Anwendung – Eine. *Übersicht. Schw. Arch. Tierheilk.* **133**, 101–111.

11 Gerwing M (1993) Niere. In: Fritsch R and Gerwing M (Eds.) *Sonographie bei Hand und Katze*. Ferdinand Enke Verlag, Stuttgart.

12 Heitz F, Carlier B, Guinet P, Legrand JJ and Viard PF (1980) Exploration échotomographique du rein normal et pathologique du chien et du chat. *Rec. Méd. Vét.* **156**, 363–369.

13 Kantrowitz BM, Dimski D, Swalec K and Biller DS (1988) Ultrasonographic detection of jejunal intussusception and acute renal failure due to ethylene glycol toxicity. *J. Am. Anim. Hosp. Ass.* **24**, 697–700.

14 Konde LJ (1989) Renal sonography. *Semin. Vet. Med. Surg.* **4**, 32–43.

15 Probst A and Künzel W (1993) Sonographisch-anatomische Untersuchungen an den Nieren des Handes. *Wien Tierärztl. Mschr.* **80**, 338–344.

16 Scholz S (1992) *Sonographisch-anatomische Darstellung der Bauchhöhlenorgane Leber, Gallenblase, Milz und Nieren bei der Katze (Felis domestica)*. Hannover, Tierärztl. Hochsch., Diss.

17 Walter PA, Feeney DA, Johnston GR and O'Leary TP (1987) Ultrasonographic evaluation of renal parenchymal diseases in dogs: 32 cases (1981–1986). *J. Am. Vet. Med. Assoc.* **191**, 999–1007.

18 Vörös K, Vrabély T, Papp L, Horvath L and Karsai F (1991) Beitrag zur Ultraschalldiagnostik des Harnapparates bei Hand und Katze. *Wien Tierärztl. Mschr.* **79**, 20–29

Urinary Bladder and Urethra

Urinary Bladder

Dirk Lüerssen, Adelheid Prüfer and Martin Janthur

Instrumentation and Examination Technique

Ultrasonographic evaluation of the urinary bladder is performed on patients in dorsal recumbency. This position allows optimal visualization of the urinary bladder. In some cases the patient can also be examined in lateral recumbency or in a standing position[5]. A 5 MHz transducer can be used for the examination, although a 7.5 MHz probe is usually more suitable. The urinary bladder is scanned in two planes from the navel to the pubic bone. The bladder should be moderately distended with urine[1]. Empty bladders cannot be evaluated. An intact bladder can be filled within a short time by giving a diuretic (furosemide 1–2 mg/kg body weight) (**512, 513**). Bladder catheterization with retrograde fluid application is contraindicated because air bubble injection causes numerous artefacts. A stand-off pad may assist in evaluating the ventral bladder wall when using sector transducers. The urinary bladder itself can be used as an acoustic window to visualize dorsal structures such as the uterus and colon.

Normal Sonographic Findings

The normal sonogram of the urinary bladder is pear-shaped in the longitudinal plane and round in the transverse view (**514–516**). A full colon or masses near the bladder can change this shape[2]. The bladder wall should only be evaluated with a directly perpendicular sound beam and with fluid in the lumen. The bladder wall

512

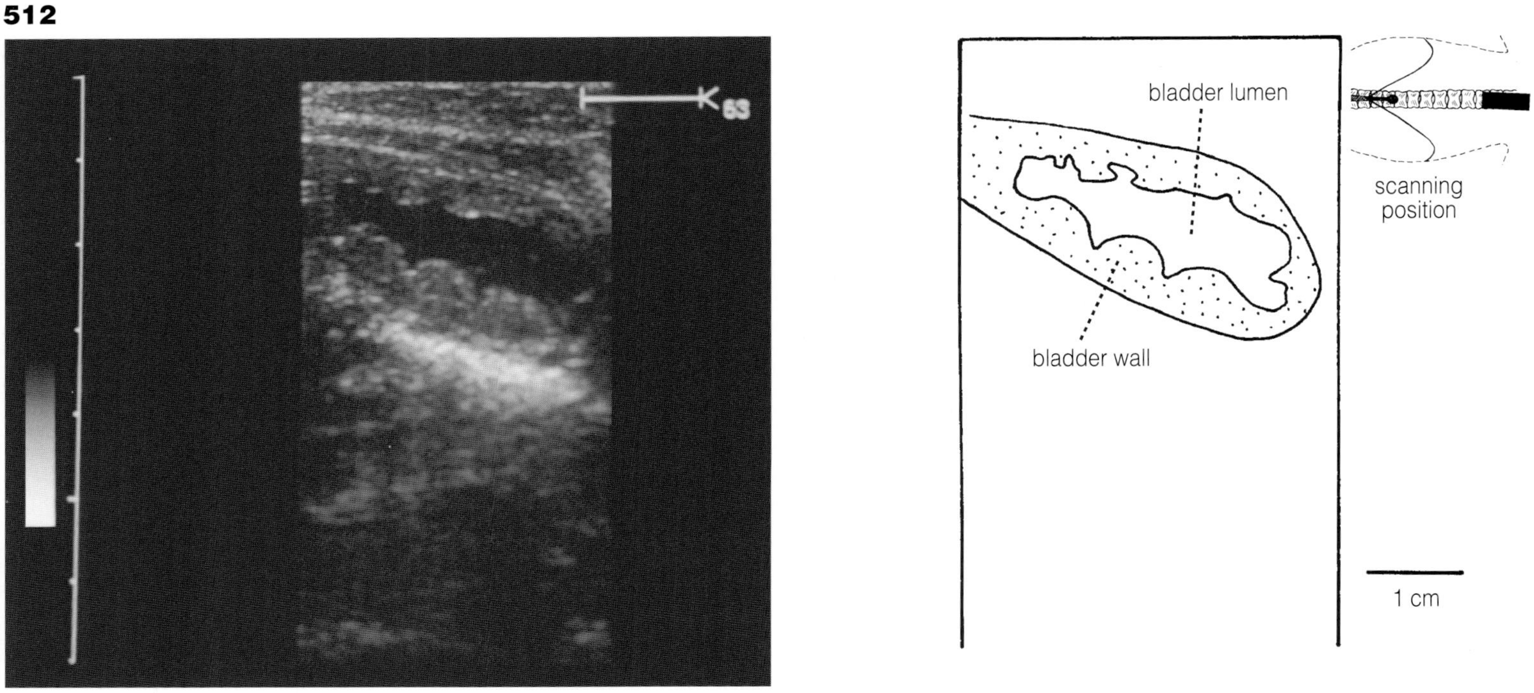

513

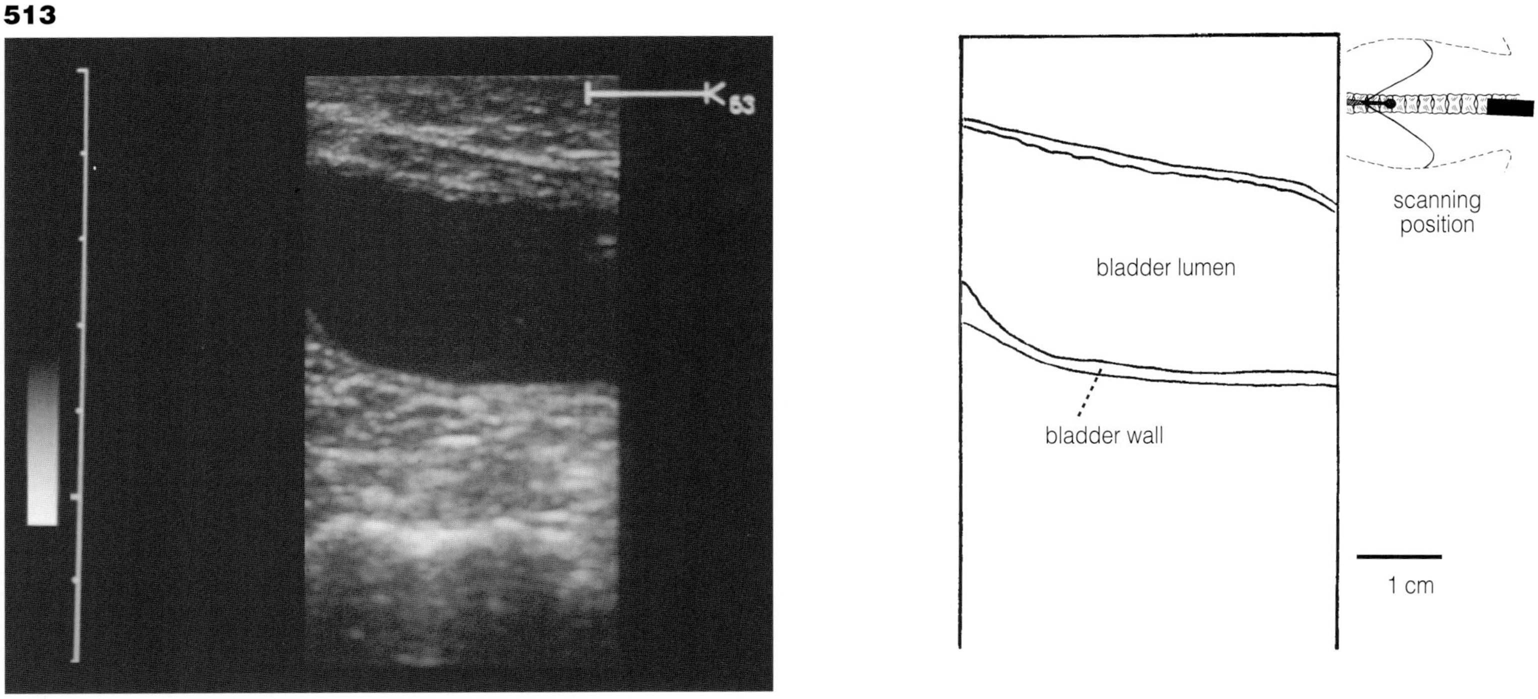

512, 513 Empty urinary bladder with an irregularly thickened wall (**512**) in a healthy dog. The same bladder 20 minutes after intravenous injection of a diuretic (**513**).

514

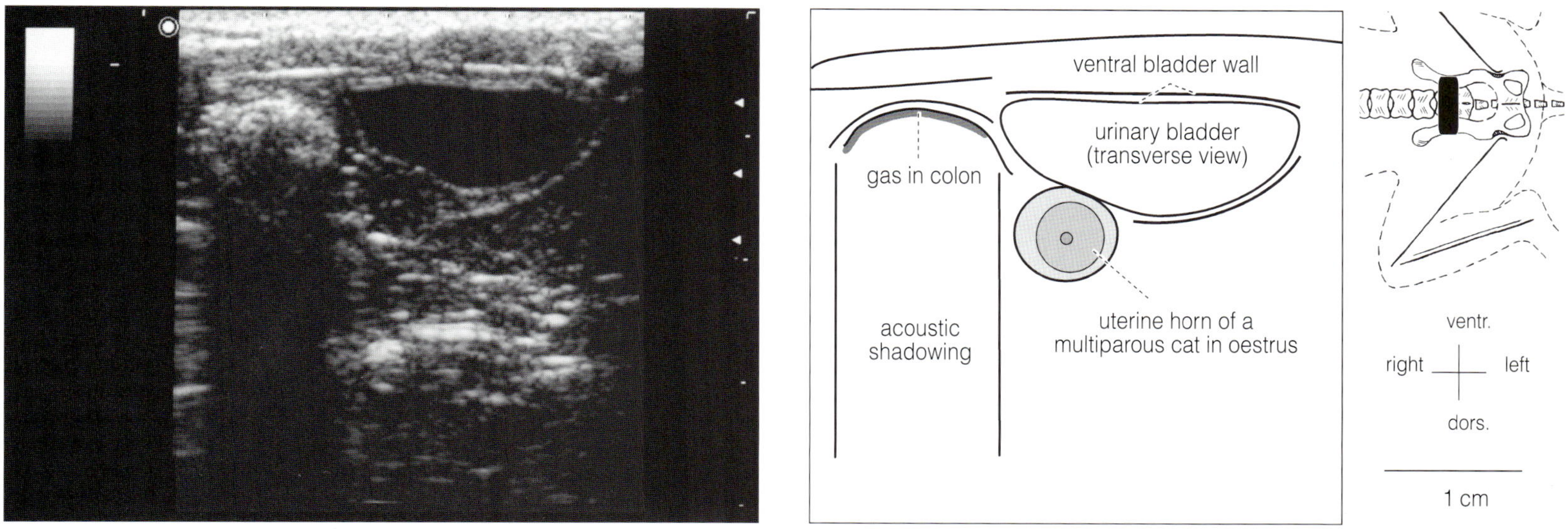

515

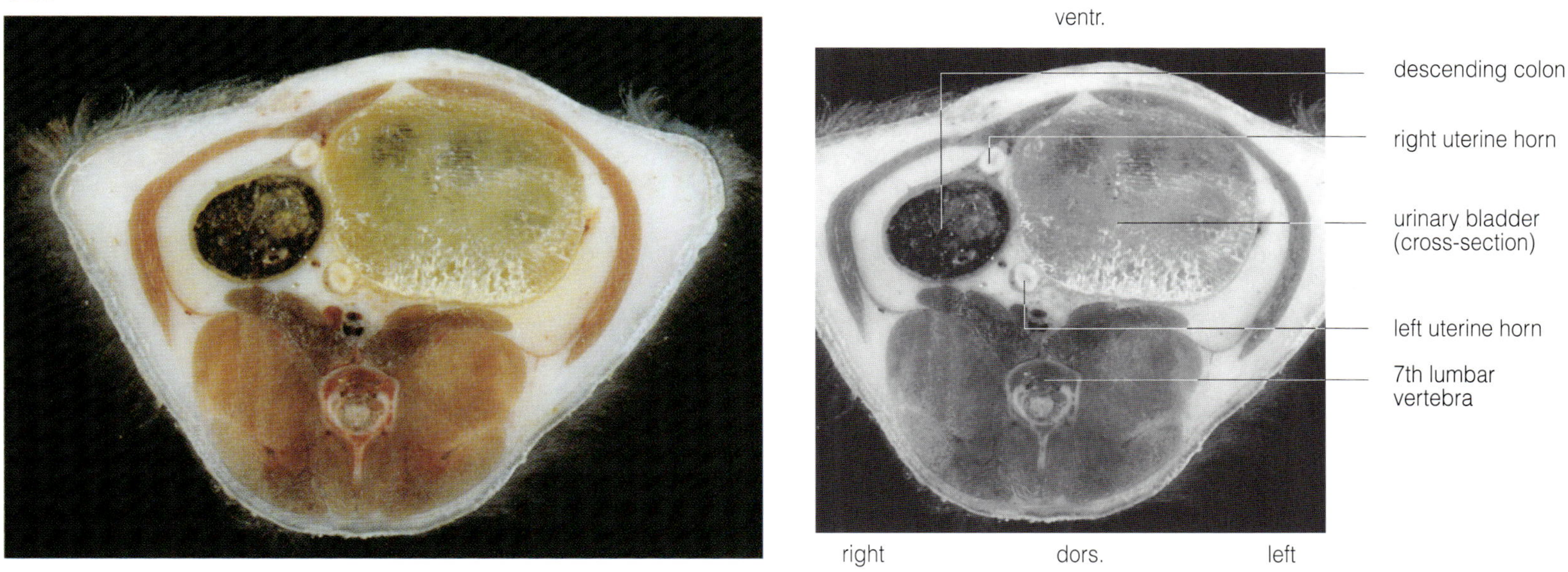

516

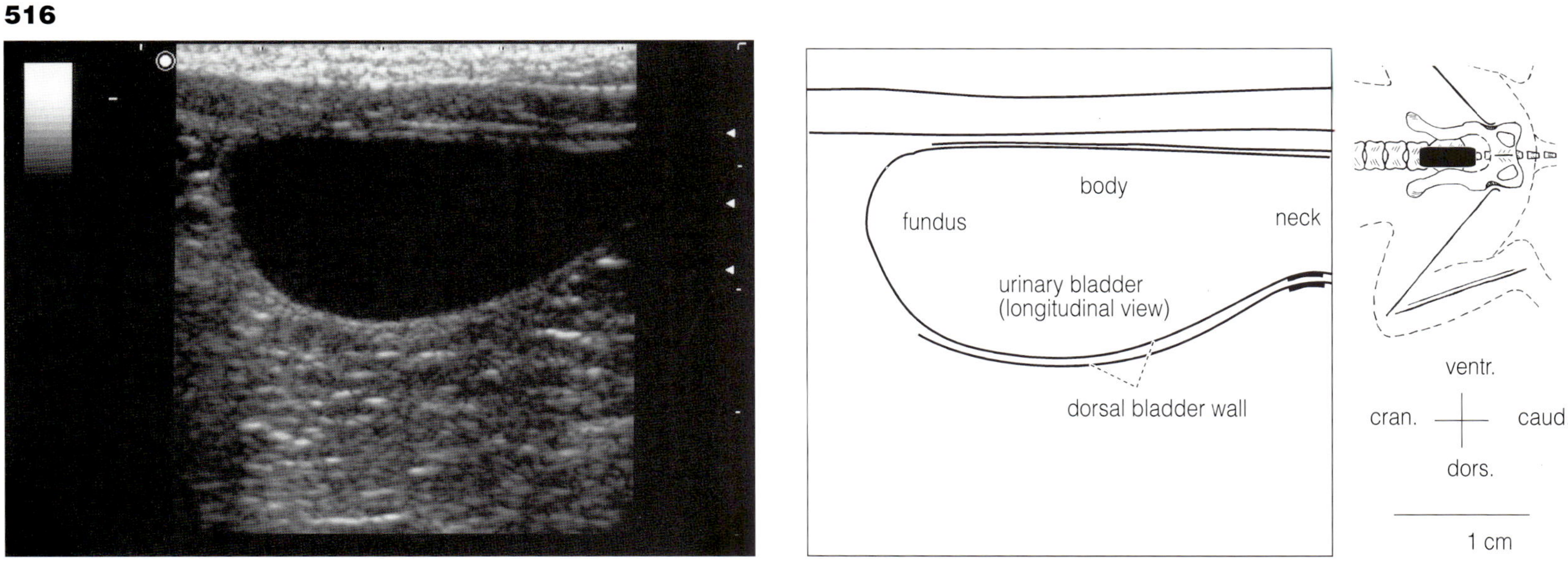

514–516 Sonograms (**514, 516**) and anatomical cross-section (**515**) of a filled urinary bladder of a cat in a transverse (**514, 515**) and longitudinal (**516**) view. The urinary bladder functions as a stand-off to visualize the uterus during oestrus.

517

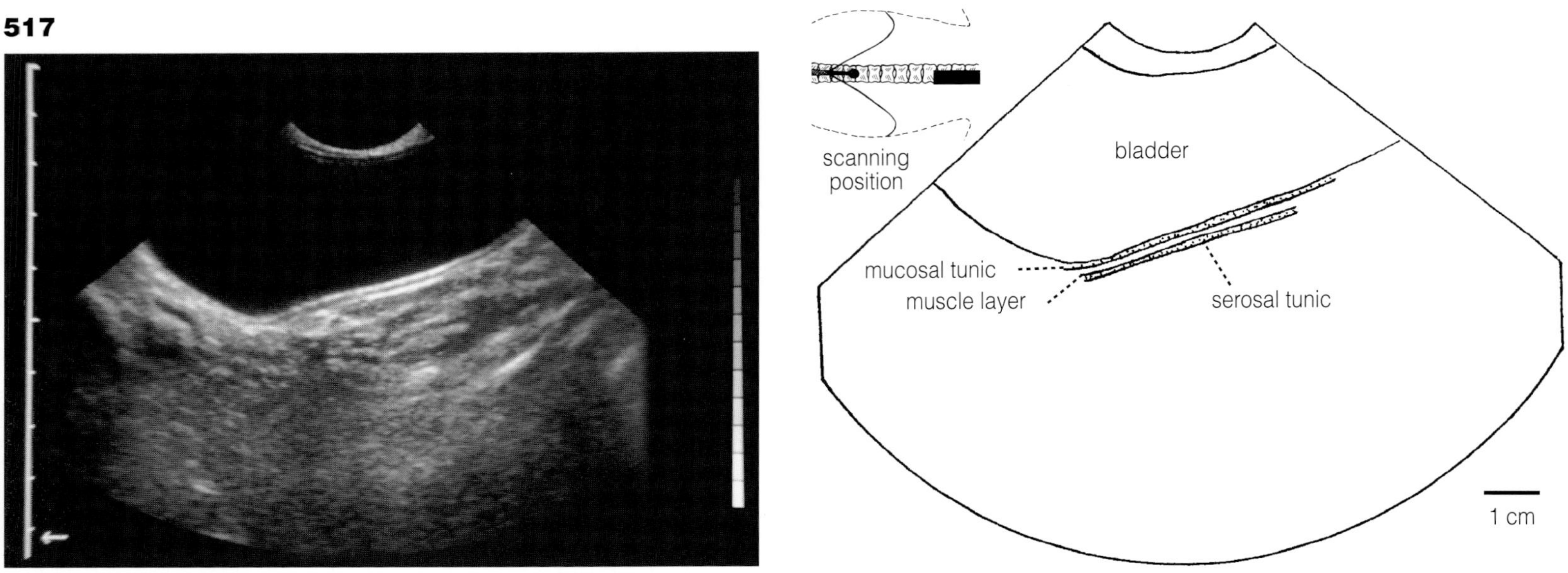

517 Moderately filled canine bladder in a longitudinal view. The bladder wall is characteristically three-layered in the focal zone when the sound beam is perpendicular. A stand-off pad was used to visualize the ventral wall. The transducer is repositioned to evaluate other portions of the bladder.

518

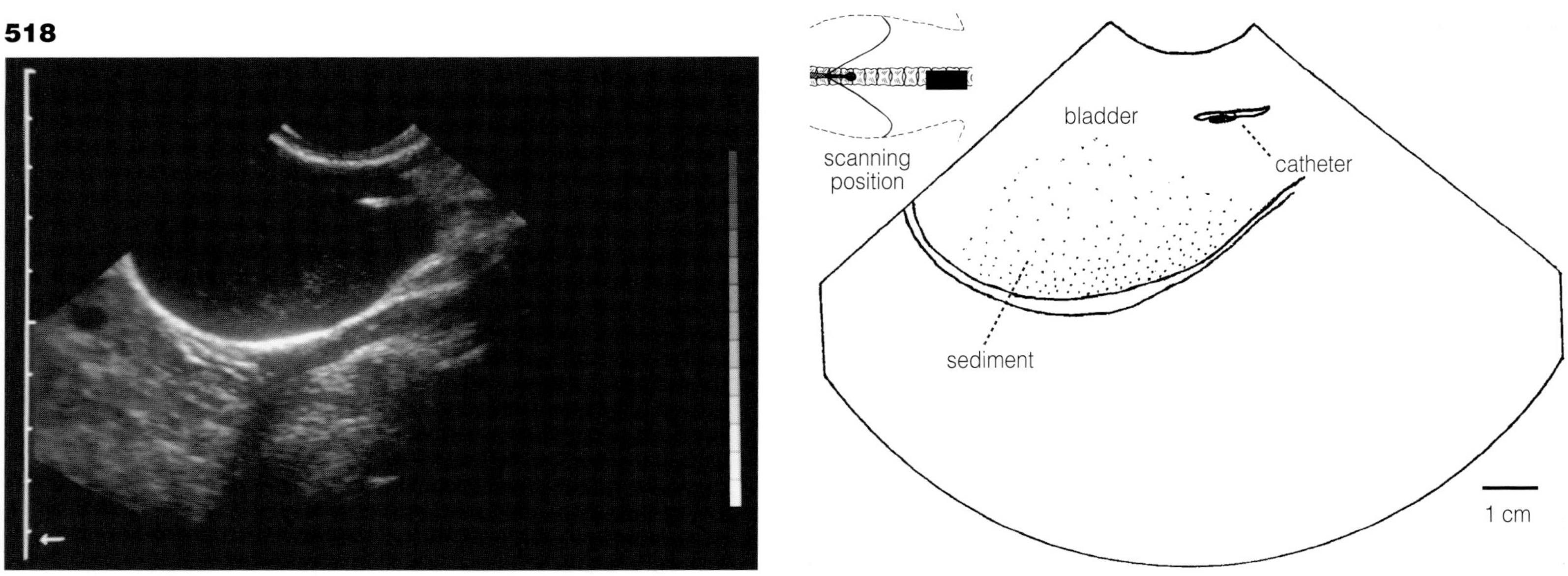

518 Acute cystitis in a cat with dysuria. Echogenic particles are visible in the distal portion of the bladder. The bladder wall is not thickened and only slightly irregular. A catheter is visible as two echogenic lines in the bladder neck region.

appears as an echogenic double line (**517**). The inner line is caused by the sound beam meeting the mucosal surface, and it is normally thin and regular in a distended bladder. The outer line represents the acoustic interface between the bladder wall and its surroundings. A thin hypoechoic muscle layer is seen between these echogenic lines. The width of the muscle layer depends on the distension of the urinary bladder. Bladder contents should be anechoic.

Indications for urinary bladder ultrasonography include every form of dysuria with suspected:

- Acute or chronic cystitis.
- Bladder sediment.
- Bladder calculi.
- Bladder neoplasia.
- Bladder displacement.
- Bladder diverticulum.
- Bladder rupture.

A further indication is for monitoring treatment response.

Ultrasonography of Bladder Disease

Acute Cystitis

With early-stage acute cystitis the bladder contains more or less numerous, small echogenic particles. These are caused by bacterial or blood cell accumulations, epithelial cells and/or crystals (**518**). The echogenicities may settle to the dependent portion of the bladder during the examination. This intensifies the echogenicity of the bladder wall (**519, 520**). The particles can be resuspended by changing transducer pressure to the abdominal wall (**521, 522**). In early acute cystitis the bladder wall is thin with a regular mucosa. The mucosa becomes irregular with progressive cystitis, and the bladder wall becomes thickened. The transition stays unnoticed.

519

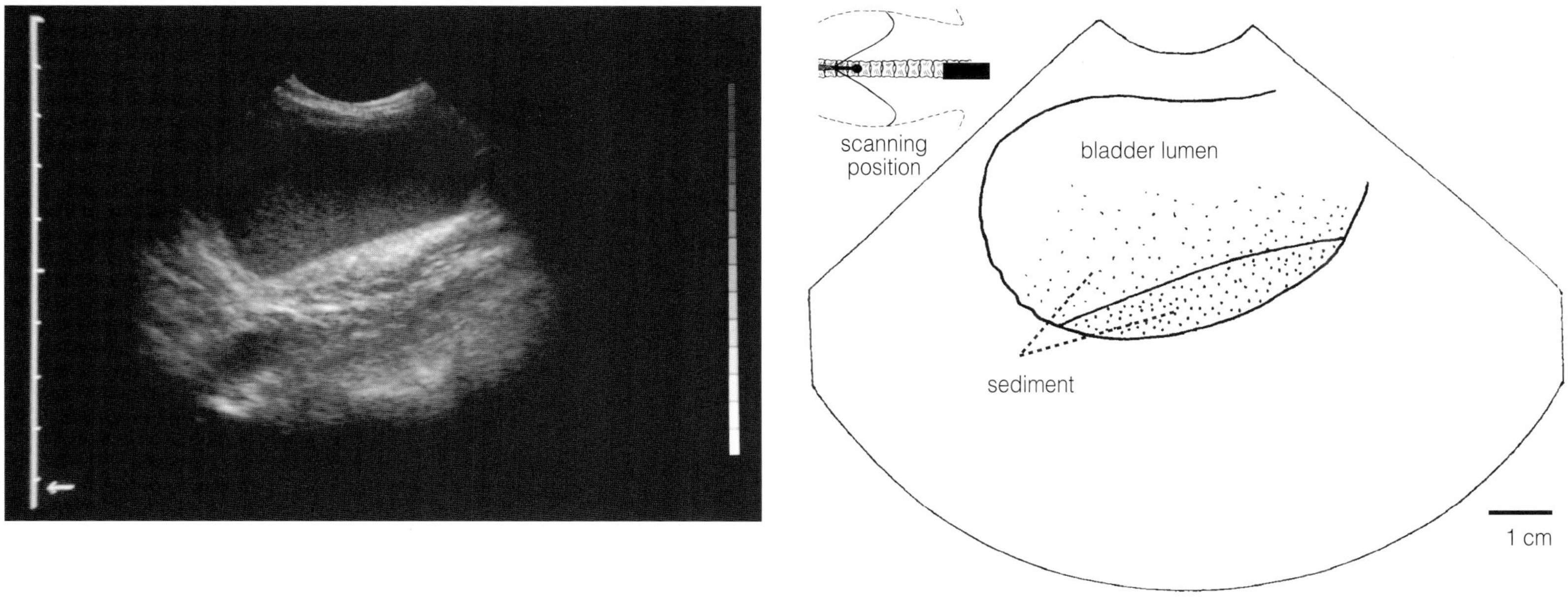

520

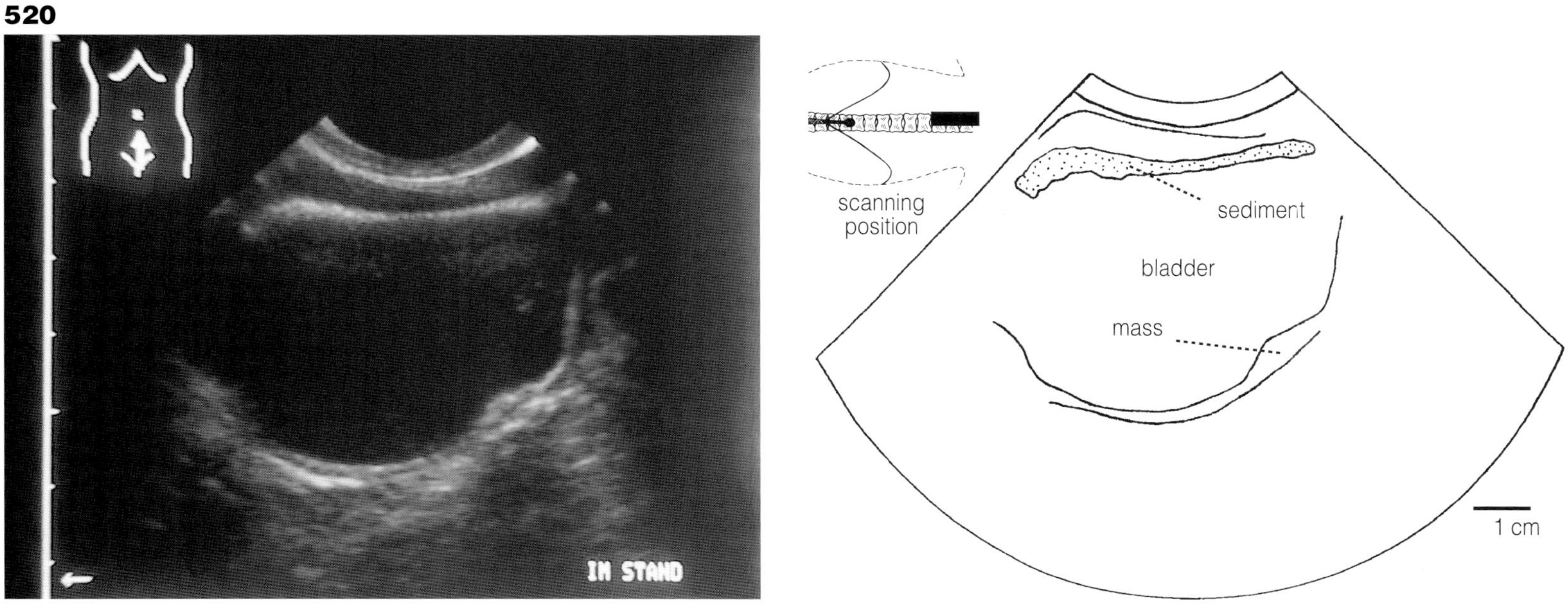

519, 520 Cystitis in a dog. The fine echogenic particles in the bladder lumen settle to the dependent portion of the bladder in the dorsally recumbent patient (**519**), while they are seen adjacent to the ventral wall in the standing patient (**520**). In the latter case a small dorsal mural mass is visible.

521 Cystitis in a cat. The echogenic particles are resuspended with transducer agitation and settle to the dependent portion of the bladder (see **522**).

521

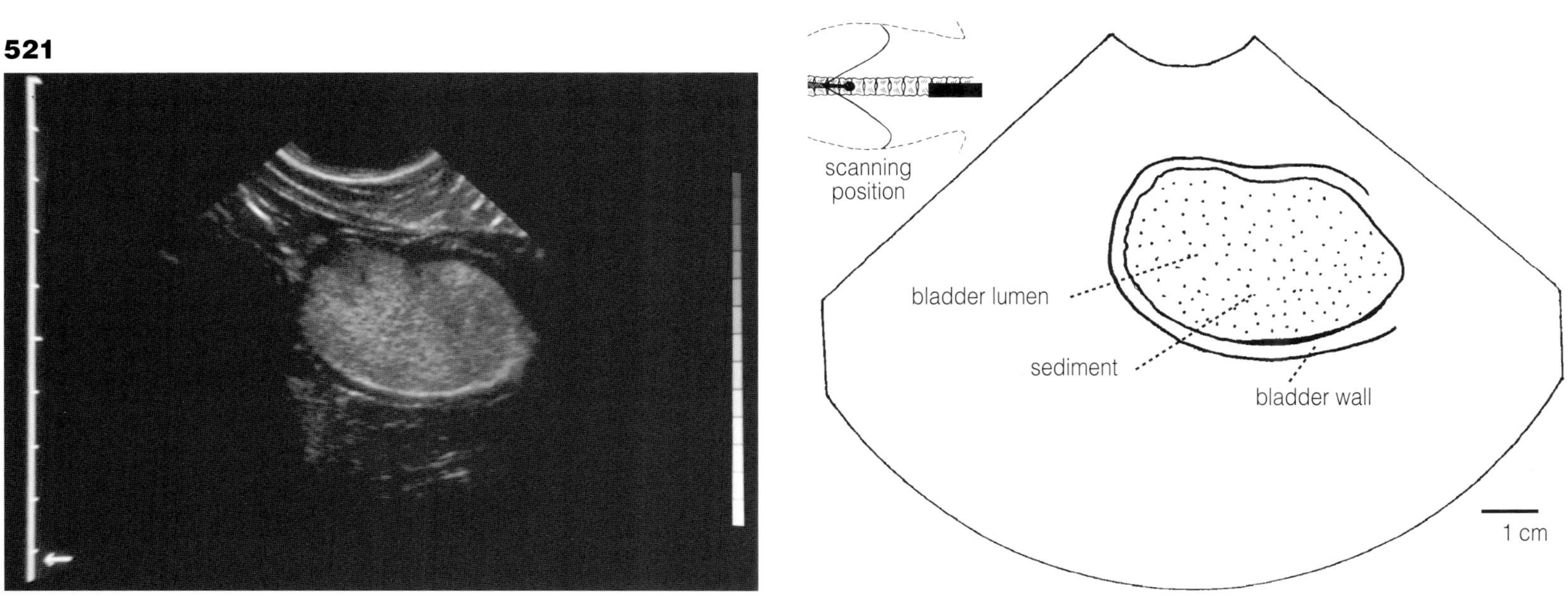

522

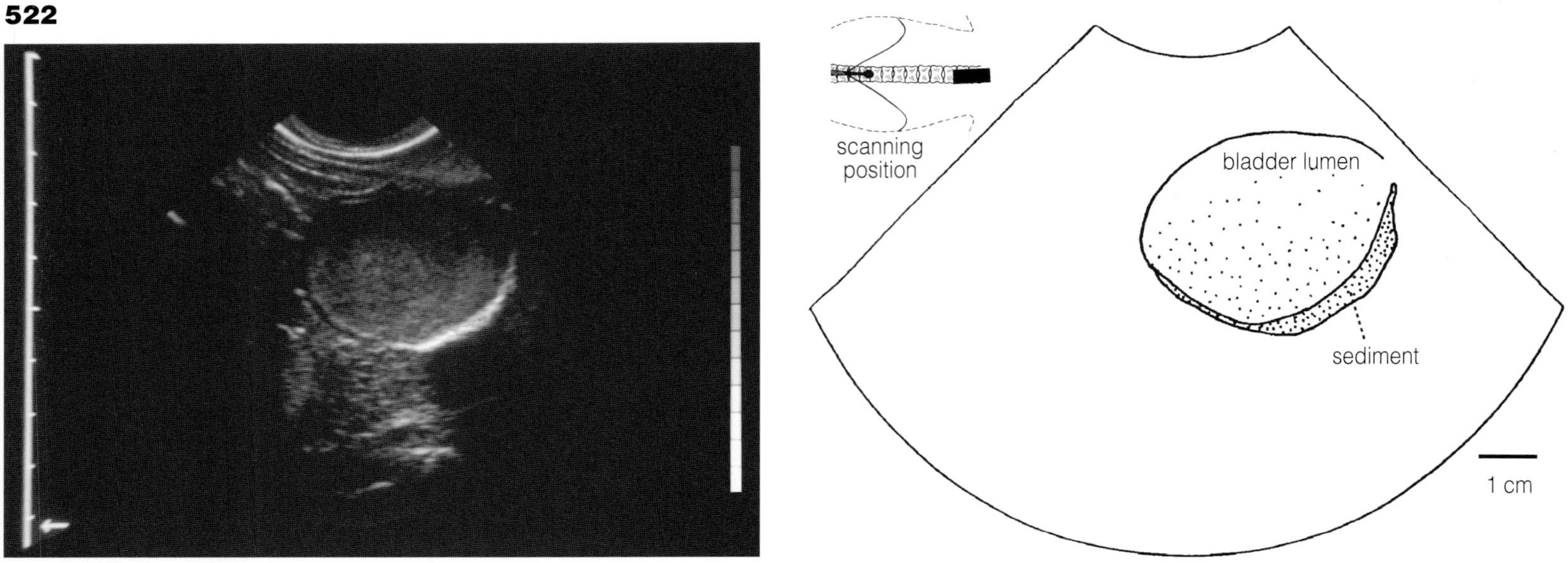

522 Cystitis in a cat. The echogenic particles settle to the dependent portion of the bladder (see also **521**).

523

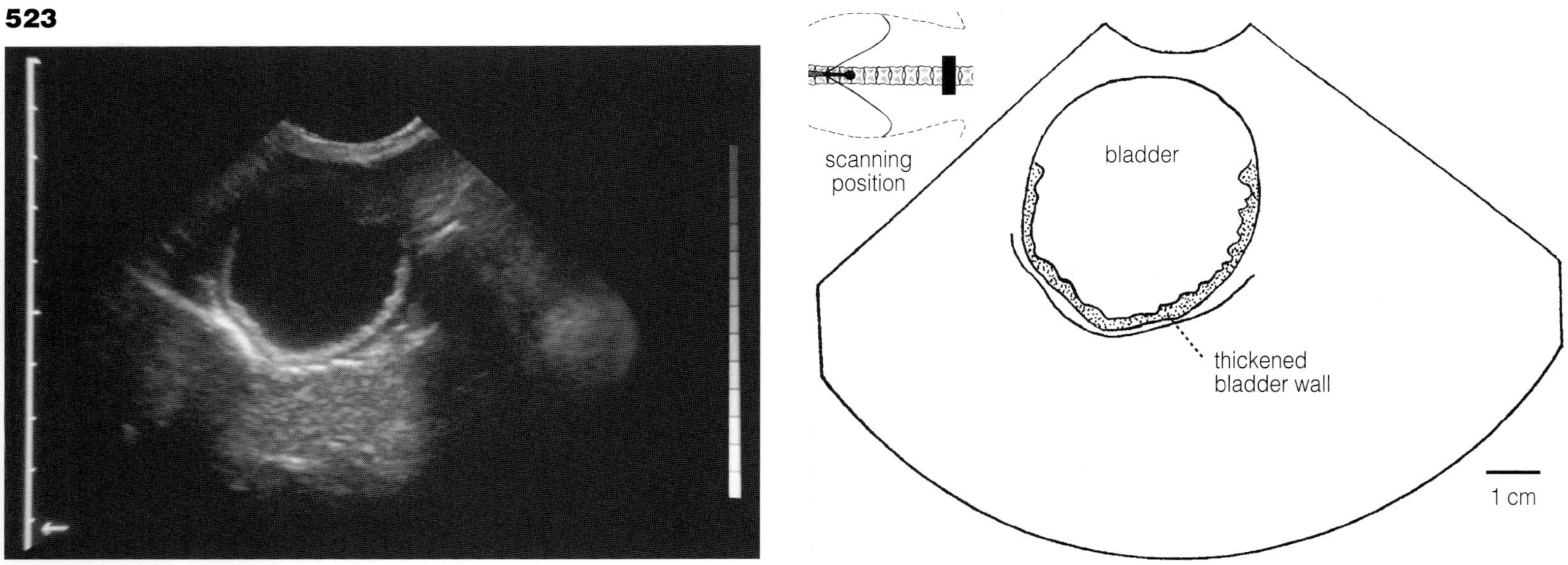

523 Chronic cystitis during healing in a dog with a thick, hyperechoic, irregular mucosa and anechoic bladder contents.

524

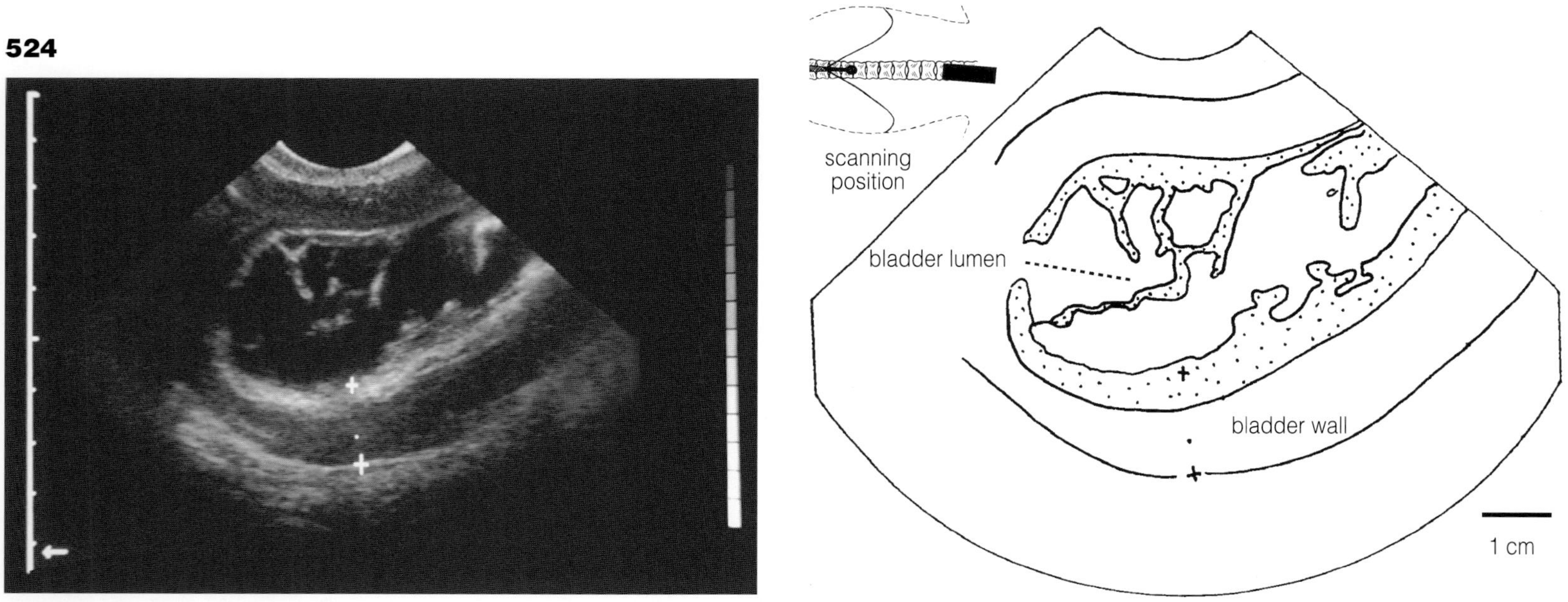

524 Chronic cystitis in a dog with generalized thickening of the bladder wall (trabeculated bladder) and echogenic structures in the lumen.

525

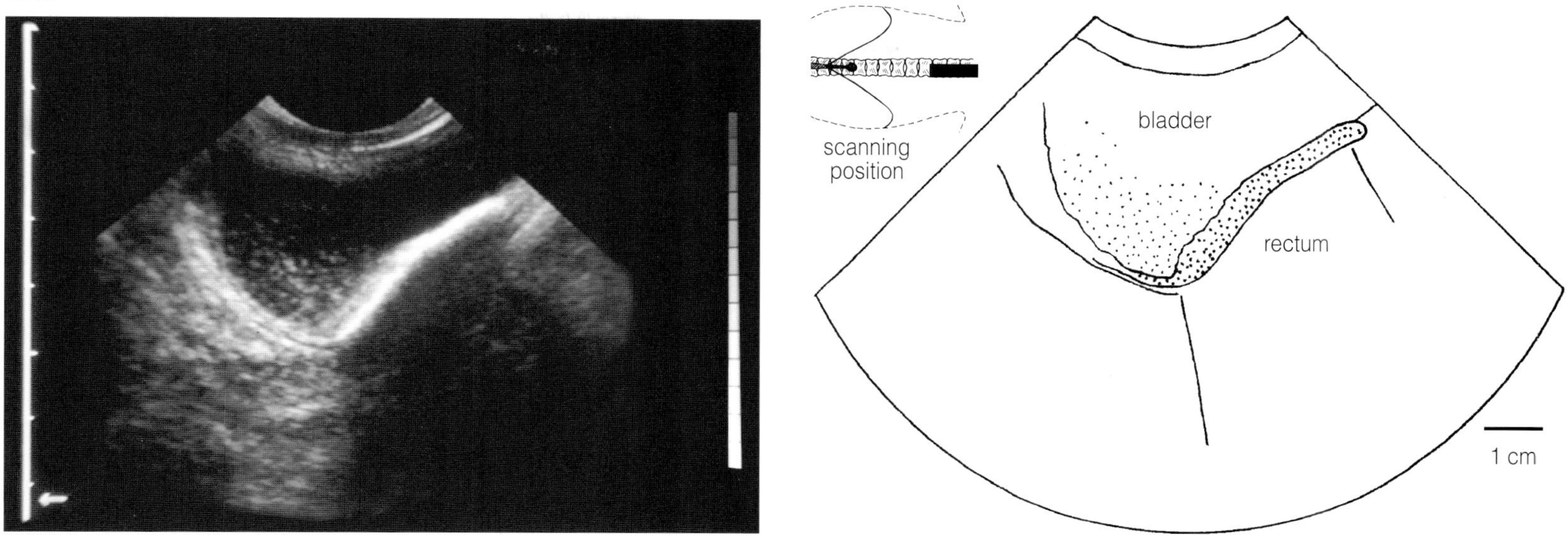

525 Chronic cystitis in a dog with moderate, generalized thickening of the bladder wall. The bladder lumen contains echogenic particles. An echogenic structure with distal shadowing is visible in the dependent portion of the bladder. This is not a calculus, but rather a filled rectum. The contours of separate calculi are not apparent and sedimentation is not present in the standing patient.

526

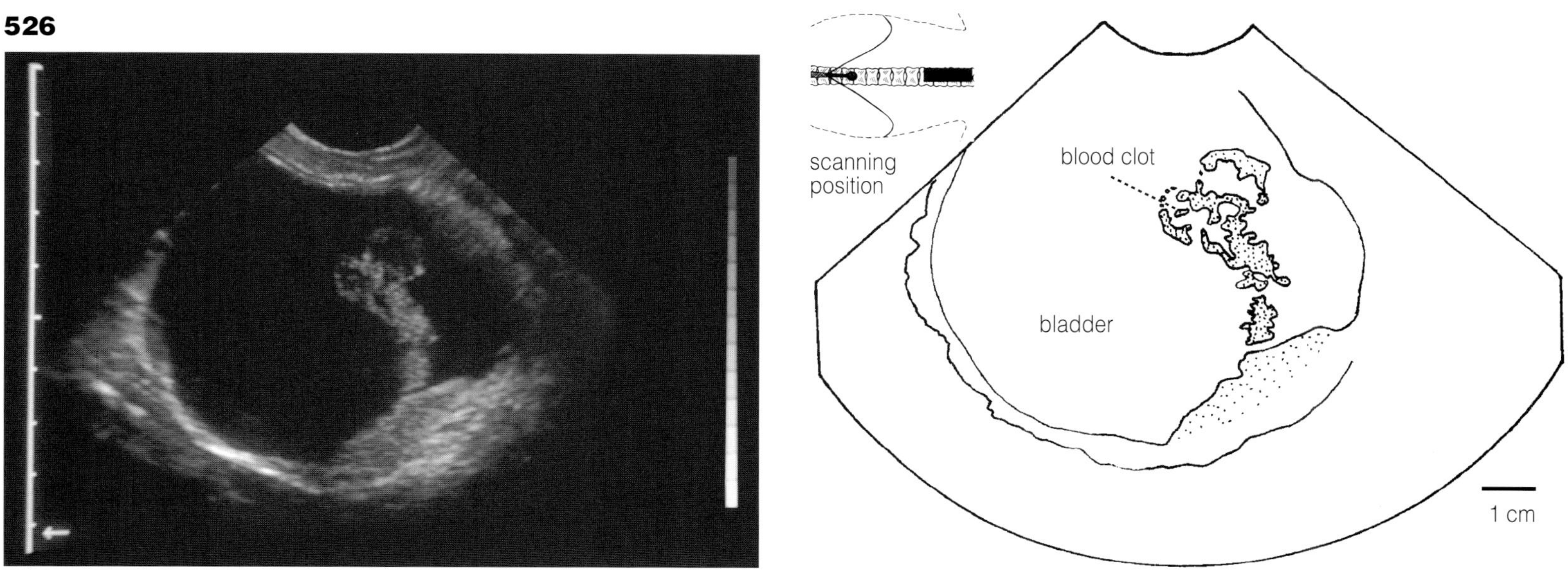

526 Wall-based, floating structure with medium echogenicity in the anechoic bladder of a dog. A blood clot was diagnosed. Similar images are seen with polyps or tumours with attached blood clots.

Chronic Cystitis

Chronic cystitis causes marked thickening of the bladder wall. Wall thickness may become pronounced depending on the severity of the disease (**523, 524**). The mucosa is seen as an echogenic, irregular line (**525**). The bladder contains multiple, hyperechoic particles as seen with acute cystitis. Haemorrhagic cystitis causes blood clot formation within the bladder. These blood clots are hypo- to hyperechoic and may adhere to the mucosal surface, extending into the bladder lumen. Their size varies and can become quite large. Depending on blood clot organization, the echogenicity may become irregular and non-homogenous. Blood clots are difficult to differentiate from a mural mass (**526, 527**). Following examinations after surgery are recommended.

A trabeculated bladder causes thickening and atonia of the bladder wall (**524**). The mucosal surface becomes irregular with concurrent cystitis. Residual urine is found after bladder emptying, and the bladder shape remains unchanged in subsequent examinations.

Bladder Sediment

The sonographic appearance of bladder sediment is that of hyperechoic particles within the bladder. The echoes settle to the dependent portion of the bladder (**521, 522**). An echogenic layer with distal shadowing is seen. The sediment can be resuspended by varying transducer pressure on the abdominal wall. Smaller flashing particles may also be seen. Wall lesions are the same as with acute or chronic cystitis.

Cystic Calculi

Calculi are easily diagnosed sonographically, regardless of their composition. Even cystine calculi, not detected on radiographs, are identified with ultrasound. Cystic calculi fall to the dependent portion of the bladder and produce strong echoes with distal acoustic shadowing. A solitary round calculus is seen as a semicircular, hyperechoic line with distal diverging shadowing (**528**). Multiple calculi produce linear distal shadows (**529, 530**). To evaluate the size and number of cystic calculi, it is necessary to mobilize the stones. This is done by repositioning the patient from a recumbent to a standing position; this also helps to distinguish calculi from mural calcifications and a full rectum.

527

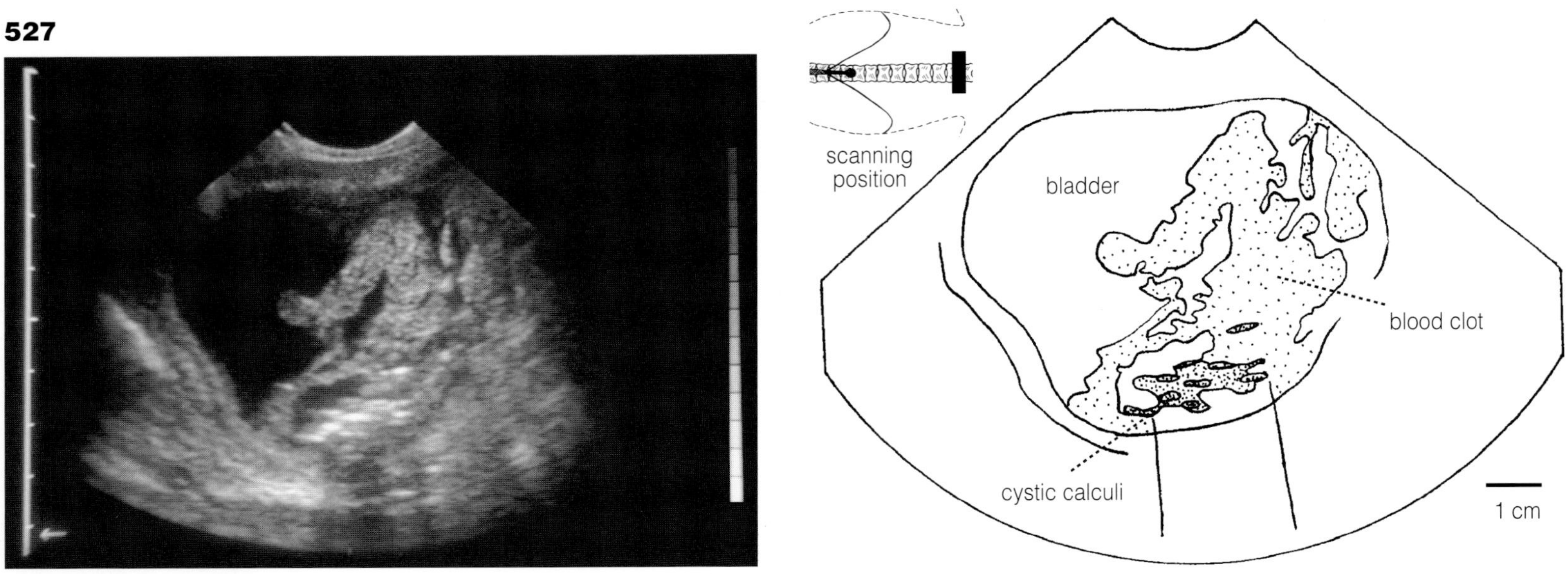

527 Large, wall-based, moderately echogenic structure and small hyperechoic calcifications with distal shadowing in the dependent portion of the bladder. The tentative diagnosis was a blood clot in association with cystitis and calculi.

528

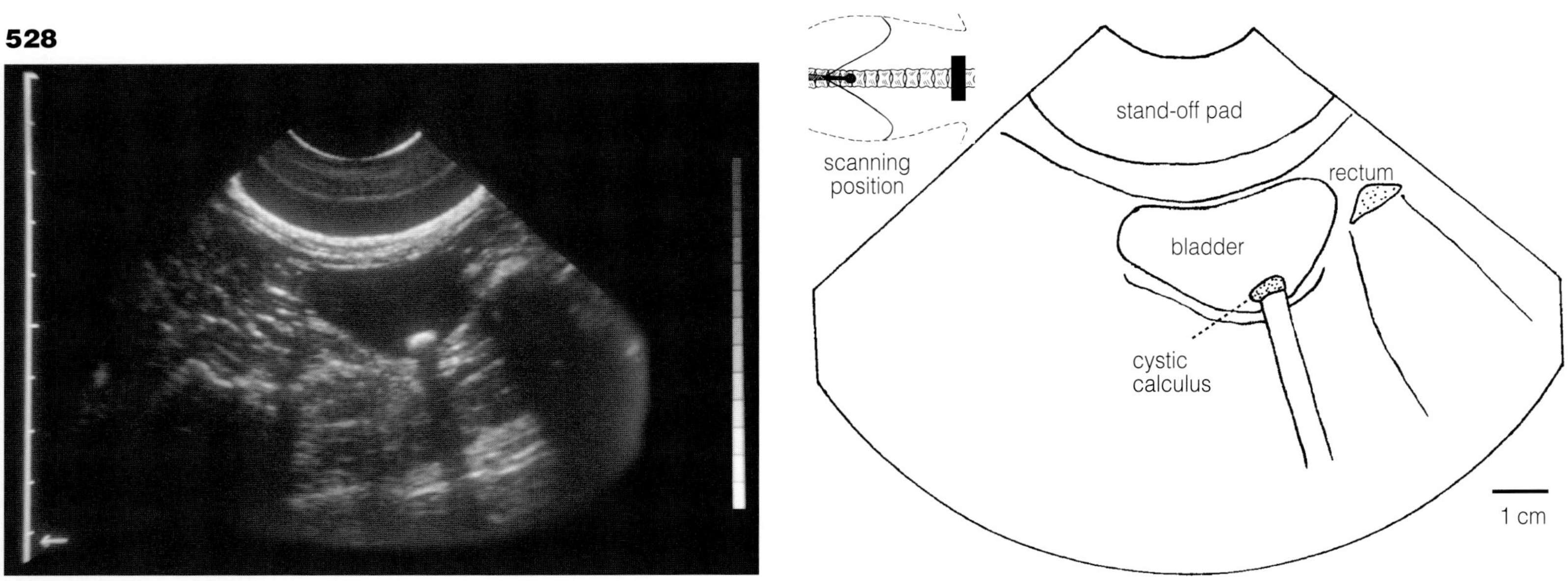

528 Hyperechoic calculus with diverging distal shadowing in a recumbent cat.

529

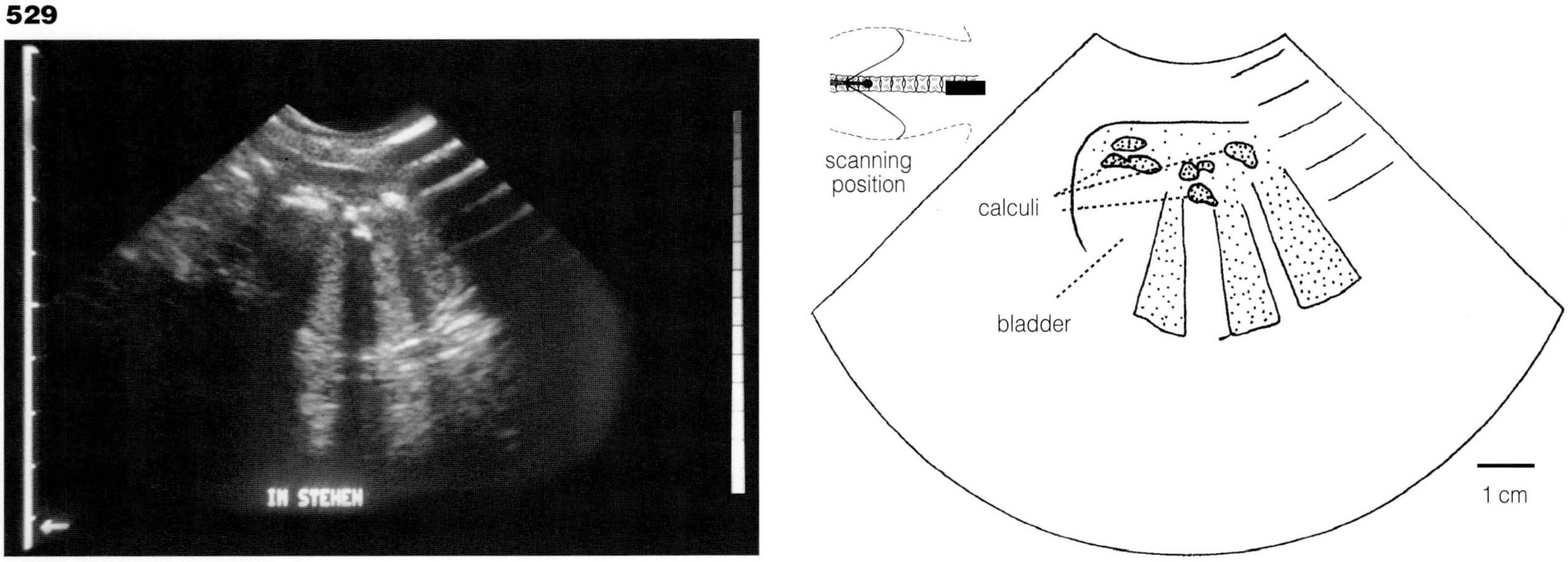

529 Cystic calculi near the transducer with linear shadowing in a standing dog.

530

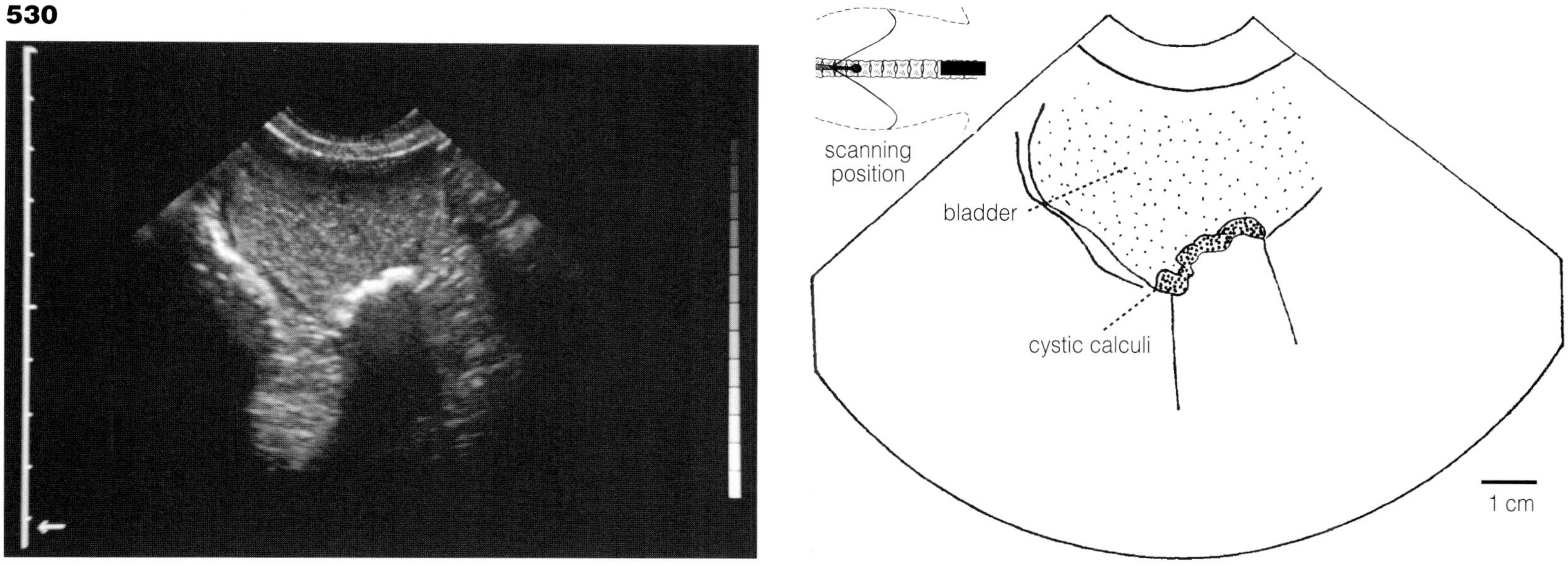

530 Cystic calculi in the dependent portion of the bladder with distal acoustic shadowing in a recumbent dog. The bladder contents are echogenic.

531

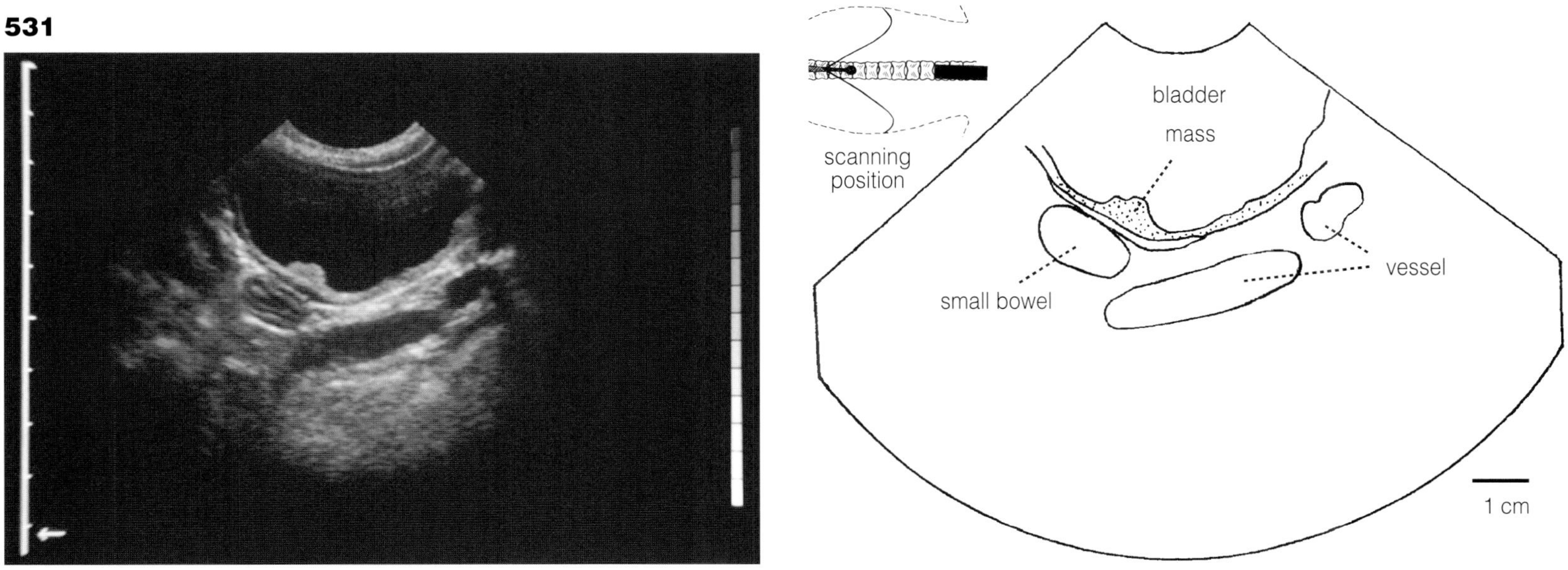

531 Small mucosal mass projecting into the bladder lumen of a dog. A polyp was diagnosed.

532

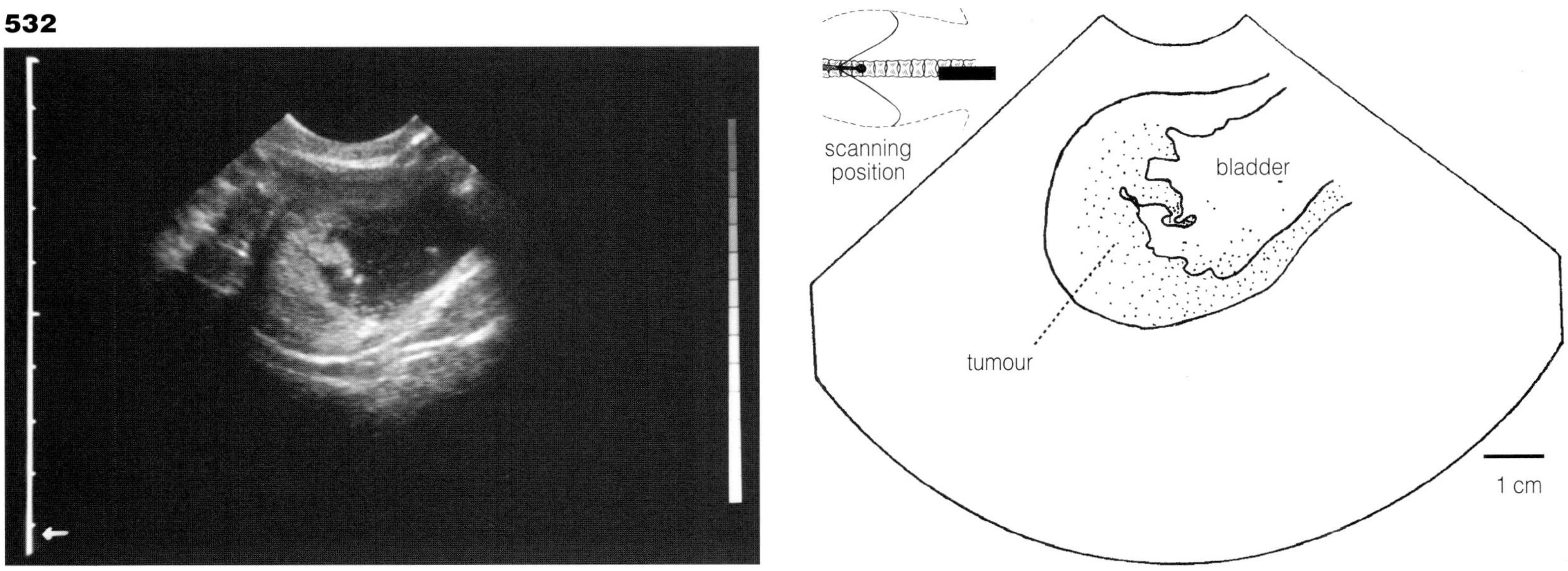

532 Cranial portion of the bladder with marked, irregular thickening of the wall. Histopathology confirmed a tumorous mass (mucosal carcinoma). Blood clots show similar sonograms.

533

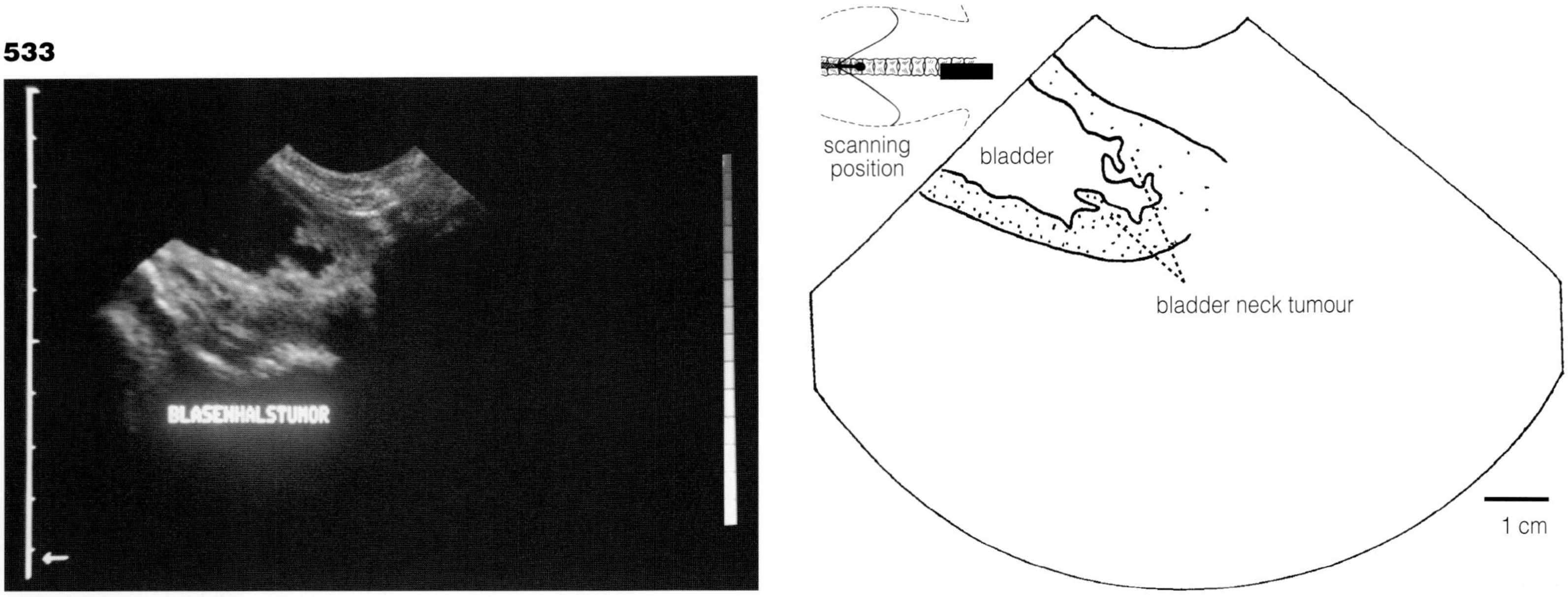

533 Hyperechoic irregular tumour in the bladder neck region of a dog. The remaining bladder wall and lumen are normal.

534

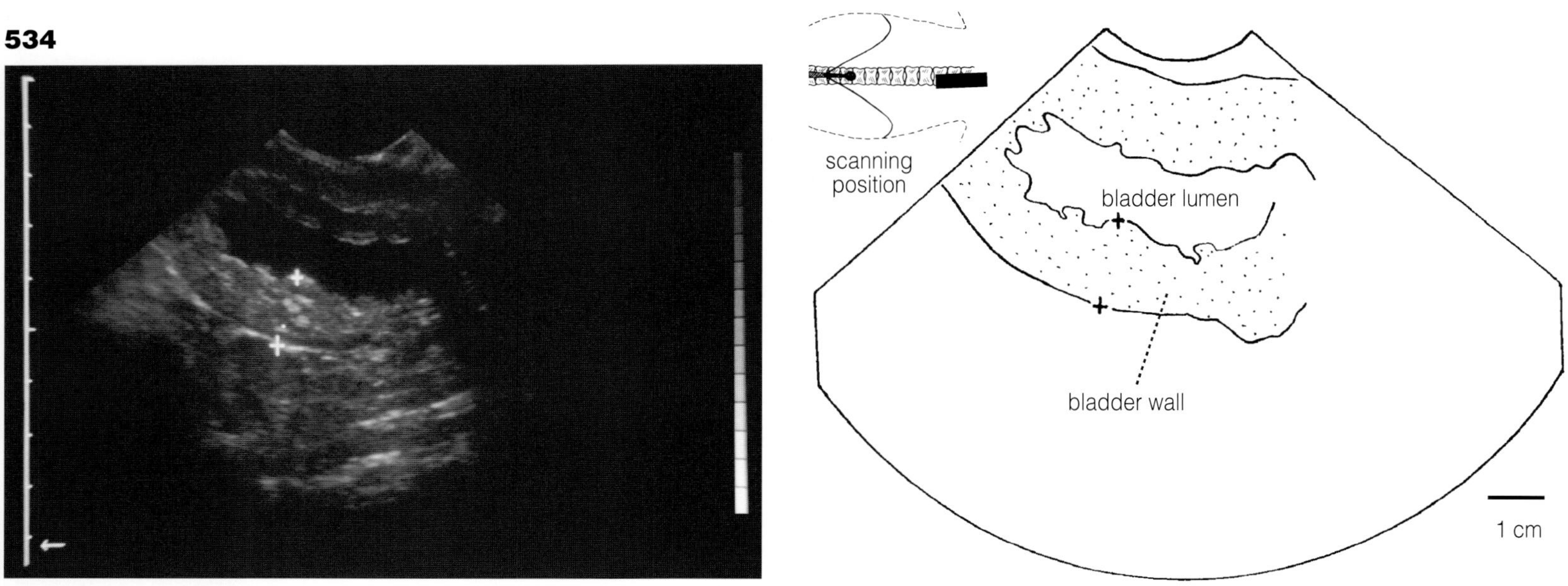

534 Irregularly thickened and non-uniform bladder wall in a cat with lymphosarcoma. The bladder contents are normal. A similar image is seen with chronic cystitis.

535

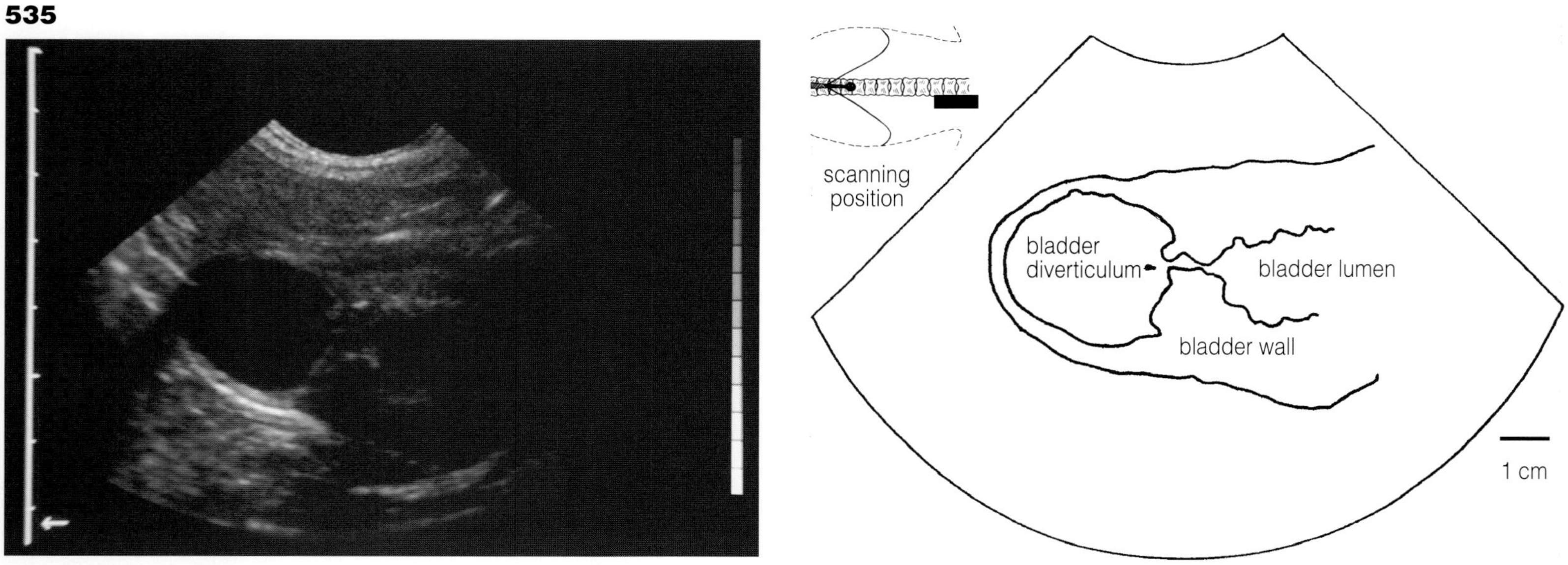

535 Moderately distended bladder in a longitudinal view in a dog with an irregularly thickened wall. A smooth, thin-walled, anechoic structure is connected to the bladder lumen. Diagnosis was chronic cystitis in association with a bladder diverticulum.

Bladder Neoplasia

Ultrasonography is the non-invasive method of choice for diagnosing bladder neoplasia. High frequency transducers of at least 7.5 MHz can detect small masses measuring only a few millimetres. Very small tumours may already be causing haematuria. Bladder tumours are identified by discontinuity of the inner hyperechoic mucosal interface (**520, 531**). The tumour projects into the bladder lumen. Instrument settings should be adjusted for this sonographic plane.

The sonographic appeareance of bladder neoplasia is variable. Some tumours have a wide base of attachment (**532**), while others are more pedunculated. Malignancies cannot be determined by homogenous or non-homogenous echogenicities. Neoplasia near the bladder neck can also be distinguished sonographically. These tumours are usually extensive and involve the entire bladder neck region (**533**). Generalized bladder wall neoplasia causes thickening of the wall similar to chronic cystitis and it is seen with feline lymphosarcoma (**534**).

Bladder Diverticulum

Bladder diverticuli are seen as fluid-filled, anechoic structures extending from the bladder lumen and producing a discontinuity of the bladder wall (**535**). These diverticuli may be congenital or be caused by continuous dysuria.

Bladder Rupture

Traumatic rupture of the bladder is difficult to diagnose ultrasonographically because the defect is often masked and residual urine remains within the bladder. Free abdominal fluid may indirectly indicate a ruptured bladder. Air insufflation produces echogenic microbubbles that escape through the rupture site.

Urethra

Cordula Poulsen Nautrup and Dirk Lüerssen

Instrumentation and Examination Technique

The urethra is scanned directly caudal to the bladder using a 5 MHz or 7.5 MHz transducer. The probe is moved caudally after evaluating the bladder. In the male the urethral portion caudal to the prostate may be visualized.

The penile urethra in the male is visualized using a 7.5 MHz or higher frequency transducer in addition to a stand-off pad. The dog should be positioned in dorsal recumbency for the examination. The transducer is placed exactly on the ventral aspect of the penis and the urethra scanned from its opening to the caudal portion in longitudinal and transverse views. The penile bone is located dorsal to the urethra or may surround it, which makes visualization difficult.

Transcutaneous ultrasonography of the caudal portion of the urethra in the pelvic cavity is not possible in the male or female because the surrounding bones cause total reflection of the sound waves. Transrectal ultrasonography (see Transrectal and Transvaginal Ultrasongraphy, page 392) makes visualization possible.

Normal Sonographic Findings

The normal urethra is round and double-layered, with a narrow anechoic centre in the transverse view. The inner echogenic margin represents the interface to the mucosa and it has a rosette-like appearance (**536, 537**). The surrounding hypoechoic layer is smooth. In a longitudinal view the layers are not clearly seen. The urethra appears as a hypoechoic band (**538, 539**). The urethra is made visible by inserting a catheter (**540**).

Urethral patency can be evaluated with the help of colour Doppler using slow manual injection or infusion of agitated saline solution. The microbubbles are detected and displayed in colour (**541**).

536 Two-dimensional sonogram of the normal urethra at the level of an enlarged prostate with cysts in a dog. Transverse view. (See also **537**.)

536

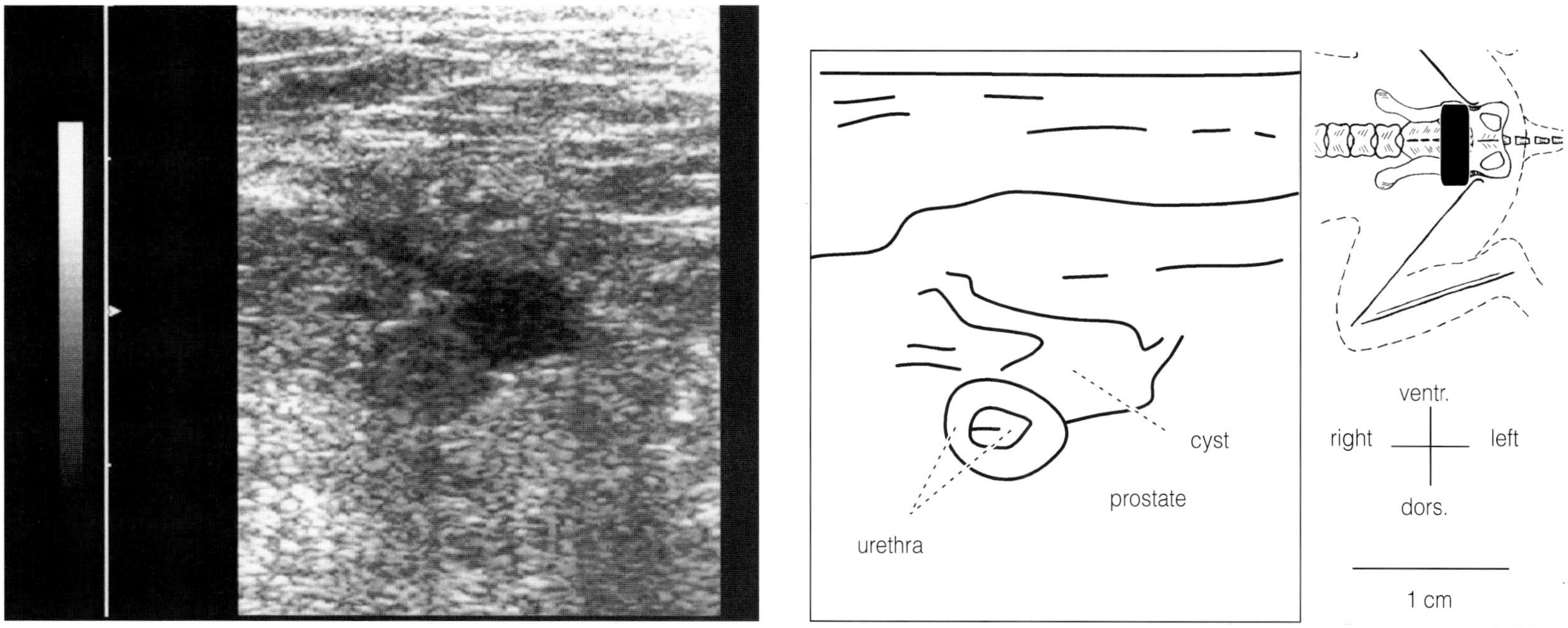

537

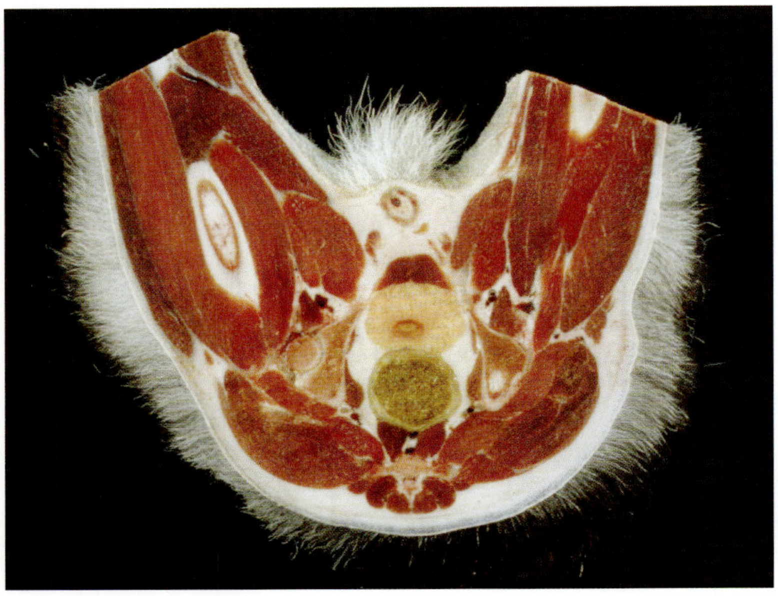

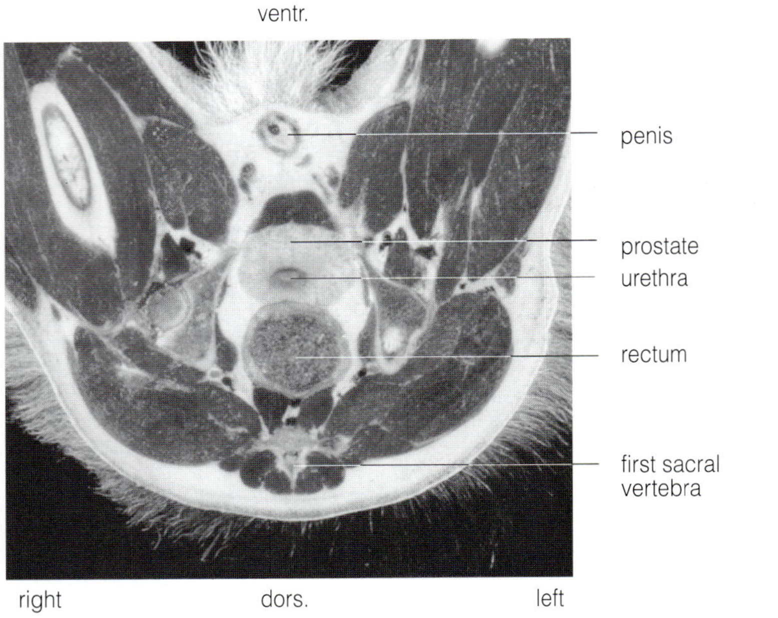

537 Anatomical cross-section of the normal urethra at the level of an enlarged prostate with cysts in a dog. Transverse view. (See also **536**.)

538

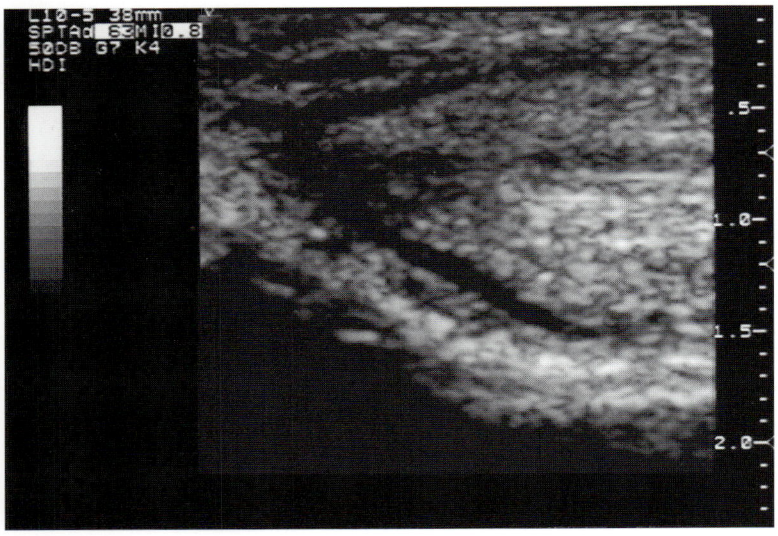

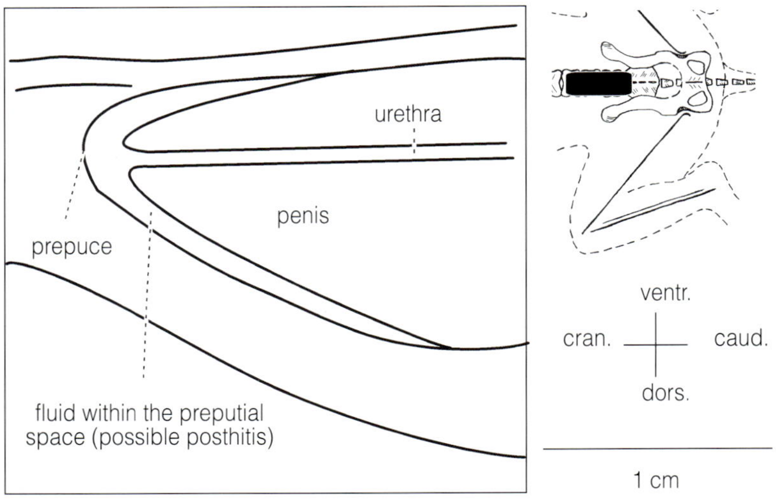

539

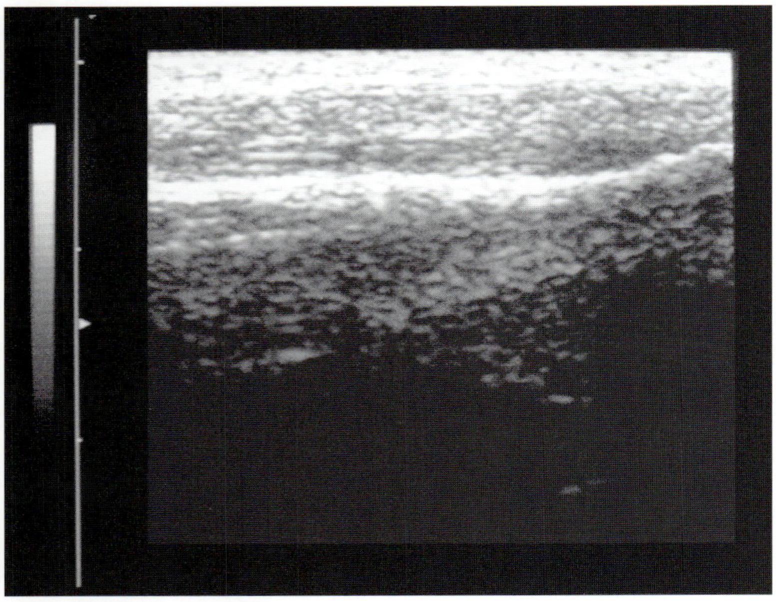

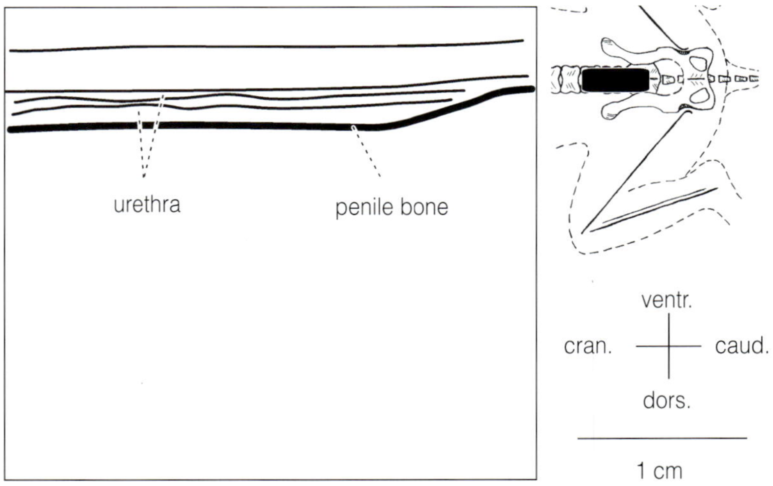

538, 539 Normal canine urethra near the tip of the penis (**538**) and with the penile bone (**539**) in a longitudinal view.

540

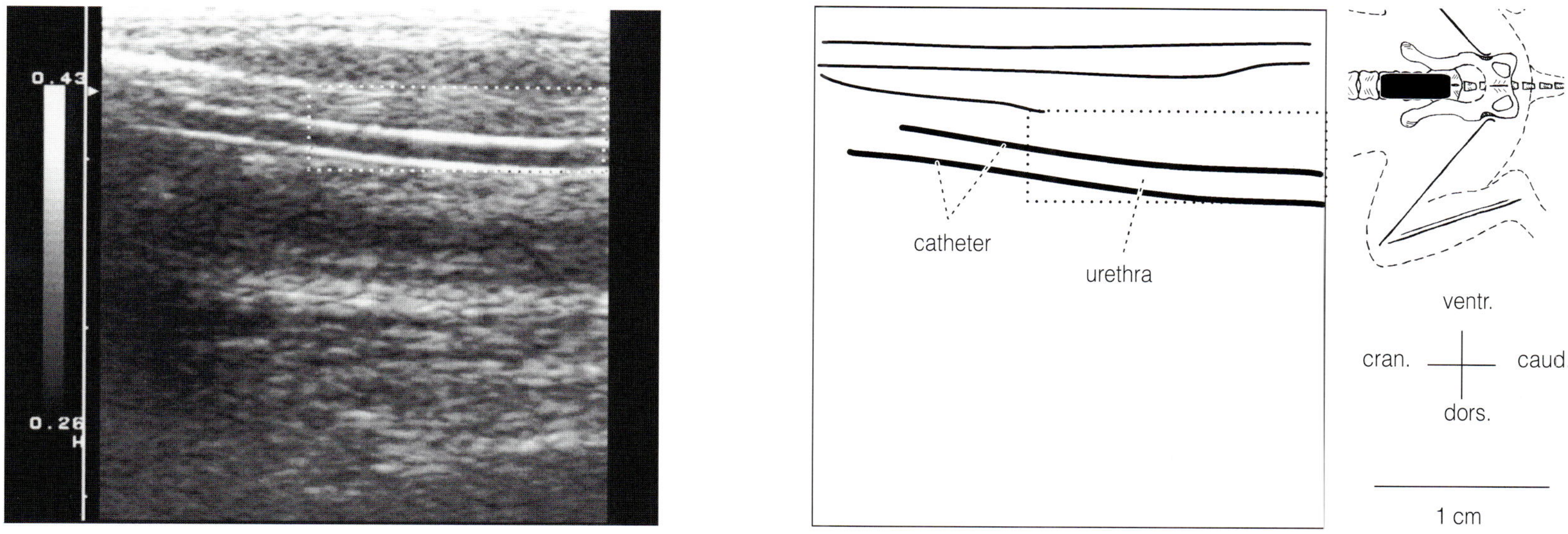

540 Normal canine urethra at the level of the penile bone with a catheter in a longitudinal view.

541

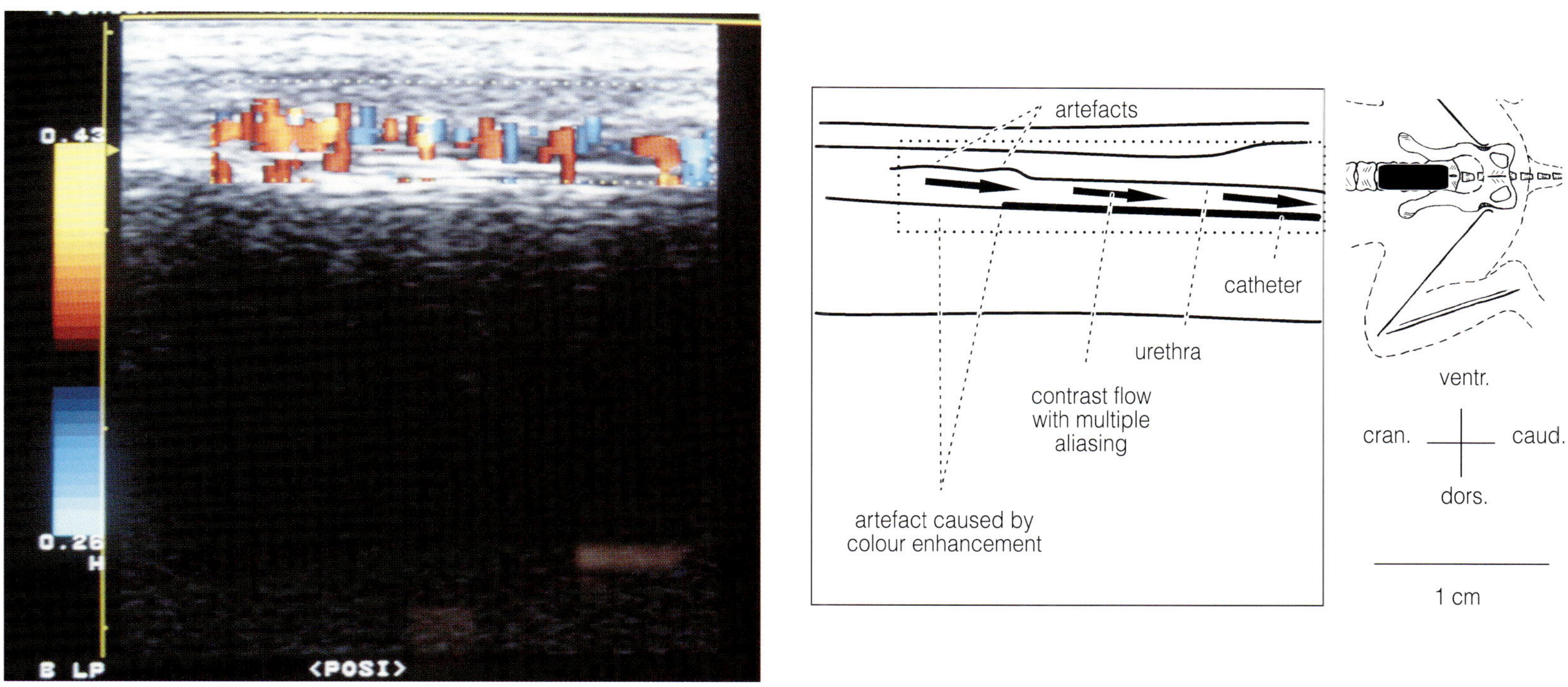

541 Colour Doppler of the normal canine urethra and penile bone during manual injection of agitated saline solution.

542

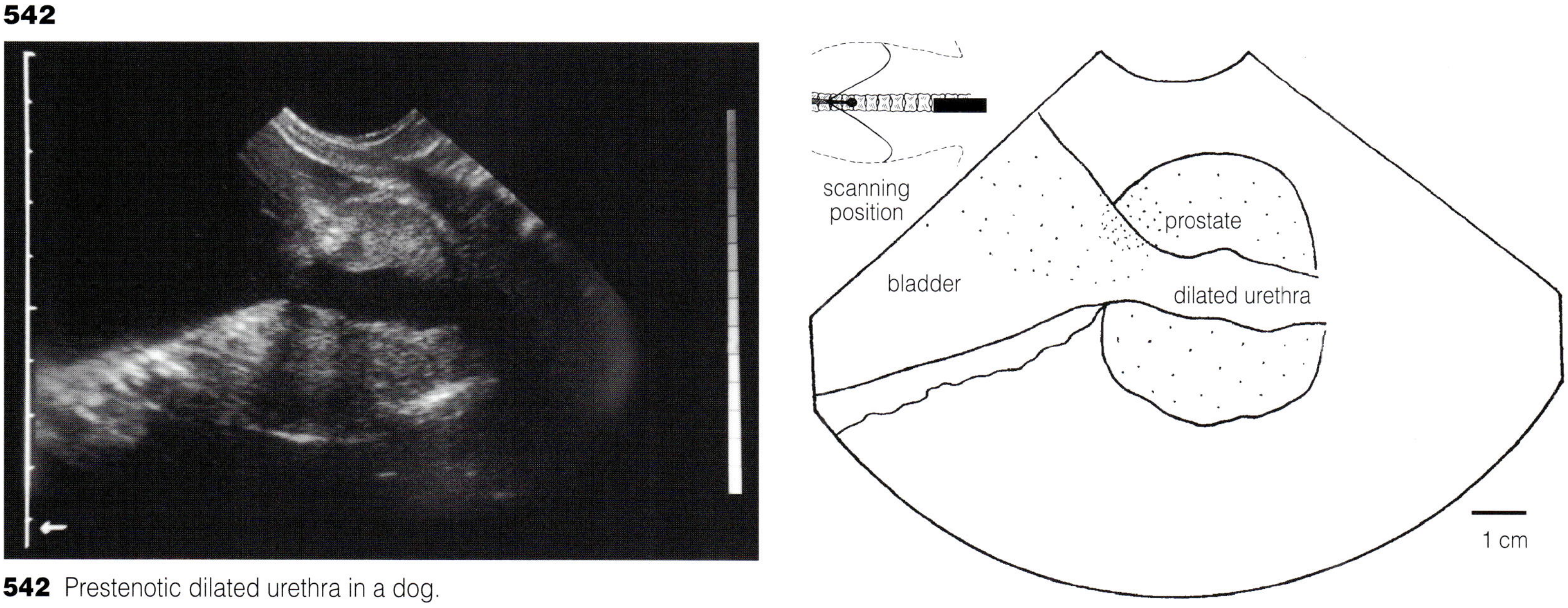

542 Prestenotic dilated urethra in a dog.

543

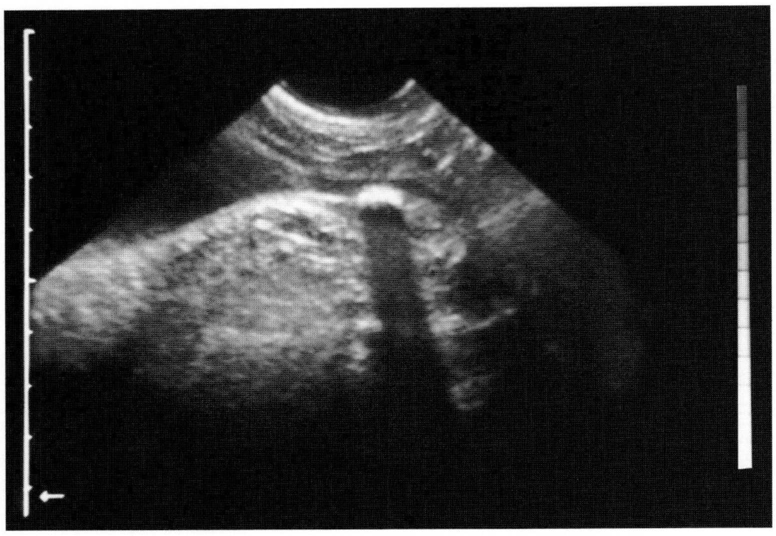

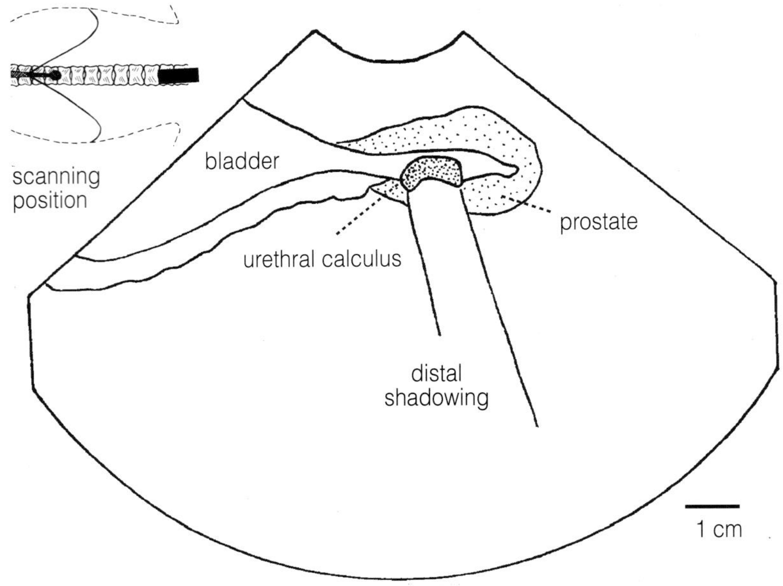

543 Urethral calculus with distal shadowing in the prostate of a dog.

Urethral Pathology

> *Indications for urethral ultrasonography include every form of dysuria with suspected:*
>
> - Urethral obstruction and dilation.
>
> A further indication is for monitoring treatment response.

Urethral Obstruction and Dilation

Urethral obstruction causes urine stasis in the dilated prestenotic portion of the urethra, which has a wide anechoic centre (**542**). The obstruction site may be identified by using a catheter and/or injection of a contrast medium (air). The obstruction may be caused by inflammation, tumours, sediment or calculi (**543**). The exact location of the obstruction cannot always be detected, especially when the intrapelvic or penile portion is affected.

Urethral tumours usually surround the urethra symmetrically and extend into the bladder neck region. In this way they are generally detected during bladder ultrasonography (**533**). These lesions are found in older female dogs[4].

Anechoic areas near the urethra should be examined for a communication. These anechoic structures are often found within the prostate (cyst, abscess), directly adjacent to the urethra (**536**).

Transcutaneous urethral ultrasonography is of limited value in the dog and cat[3].

References

1 Biller DS, Kantrowitz B, Partington BP and Miyabayashi T (1990) Diagnostic ultrasound of the urinary bladder. *J. Am. Anim. Hosp. Assoc.* **26**, 397–402.

2 Fritsch R and Gerwing M (1991) *Sonographie bei Hand und Katze*. Enke Verlag, Stuttgart.

3 Nyland TG, Mattoon JS and Wisner ER (1995) Ultrasonography of the urinary tract and adrenal glands. In: Nyland TG and Mattoon JS (Eds.) *Veterinary Diagnostic Ultrasound*. WB Saunders, Philadelphia, London, Toronto, pp. 95–124.

4 Tarvin G, Patnaik A and Greene R (1978) Primary urethral tumors in dogs. *J. Am. Vet. Med. Assoc.* **172**, 931–933.

5 Vörös K, Wladàr S, Vrabély T and Fenyves B (1993) Ultrasonographic diagnosis of urinary bladder calculi in dogs. *Canine Pract.* **18**, 29–33.

Adrenal Glands

Dirk Lüerssen and Martin Janthur

Instrumentation and Examination Technique

Ultrasonography of adrenal glands requires high frequency transducers of 7.5 MHz. These high frequencies are needed because the normal canine adrenal gland measures 2.2 to 2.3 cm in length and approximately 1 cm in width[5]. Visualization of normal left and right adrenal glands has been reported in 90% and 70% of canine glands, respectively[1].

The left adrenal is best seen from the left lateral or median ventral abdomen with the transducer angled slightly to the left. While the ribs may interfere with the examination from the lateral abdomen, overlying bowel loops make visualization difficult from the ventral abdomen. Bowel loops can be displaced laterally with transducer pressure on the abdomen, especially when using a sector scanner. The pyloric region and the transverse colon may interfere with visualization of the right adrenal from the ventral abdomen using a right lateral angulation. Evaluation of the right adrenal through the 9th to 11th intercostal space is sometimes possible. The right adrenal is often outside the focal zone of a 7.5 MHz probe or masked by acoustic shadowing. Increasing the transducer pressure is usually not effective.

Anatomy and Normal Sonographic Findings

The left adrenal gland is located more caudal than the right without the rib cage interfering with the examination. The aorta runs medial or ventromedial. The cranial mesenteric artery is located cranial to the left adrenal and the left kidney is caudolateral. The right adrenal gland is usually more difficult to distinguish than the left[4, 6]; it can be identified cranial to the origin of the mesenteric artery, lateral or dorsolateral to the caudal vena cava, and craniomedial to the right kidney[7].

The left adrenal has a dumb-bell or flat oval shape (**544, 545**), while the right adrenal is comma- or wedge-shaped (**546**)[6]. The left phrenicoabdominal vein passes over the constricted area of the left adrenal.

The normal adrenals are more hypoechoic than surrounding

544

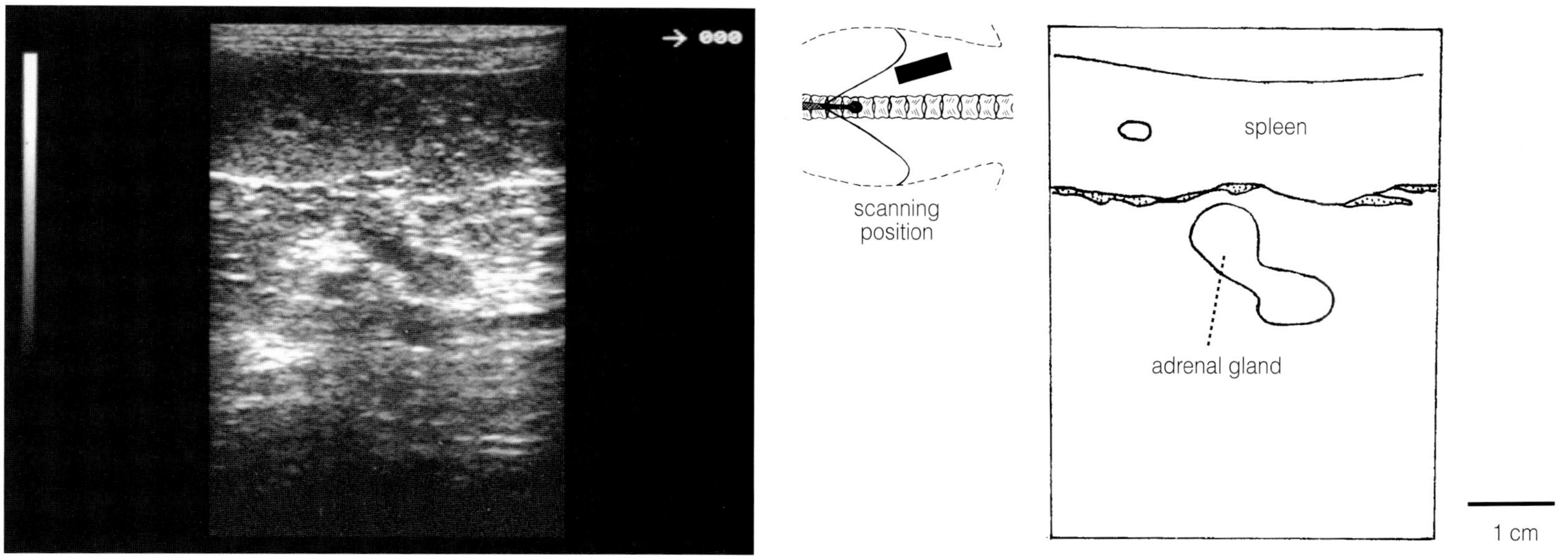

544 Normal left canine adrenal gland in a longitudinal view with a characteristic dumb-bell shape. The spleen is used as an acoustic window.

545

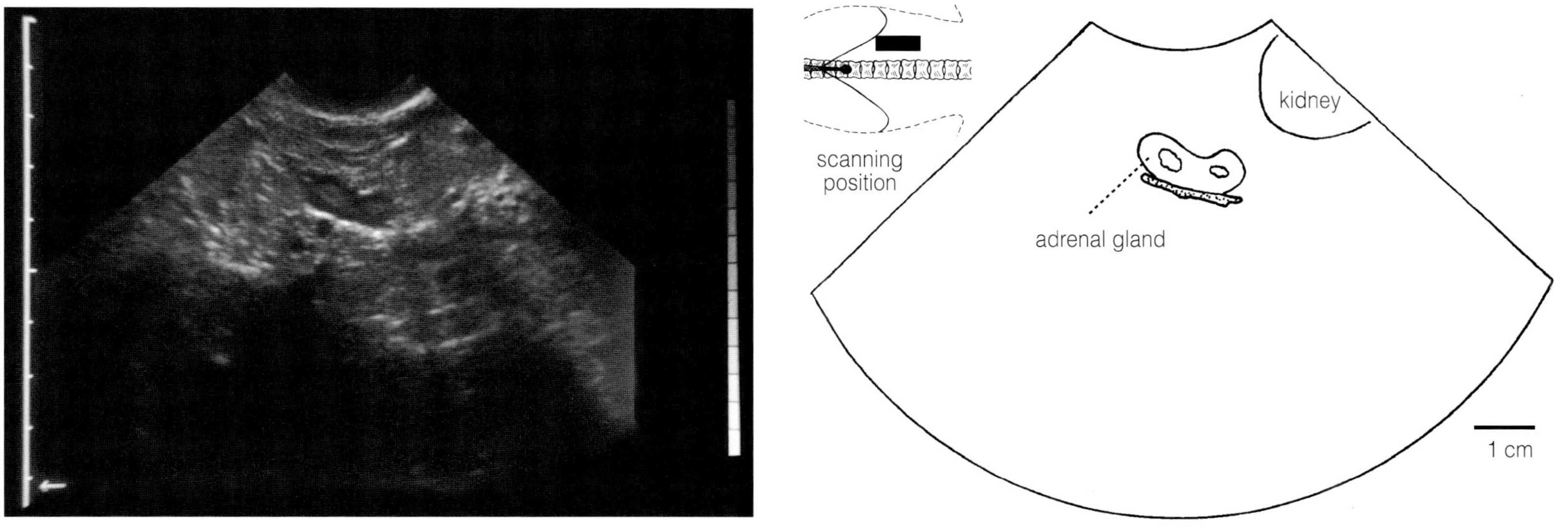

545 Normal left canine adrenal gland in a longitudinal view. Dumb-bell shape with a hypoechoic cortex and a more echogenic medulla.

structures. A hypoechoic outer ring with a more echogenic centre can be distinguished. A hyperechoic ring surrounds the periphery of the adrenal (**544**). This is thought to be due to supra-adrenal fat.

The normal left and right adrenal sizes in various dog breeds are listed in *Table 36*. The adrenal length and width in dogs with non-endocrine diseases are not significantly different from measurements in healthy dogs[2].

Table 36 Adrenal size in healthy dogs, weighing 2.5–32 kg and 1–11 years old (from Hörauf and Reusch, 1995[2]).

	Length (mm) minimum/maximum	Length (mm) mean value	Width (mm) minimum/maximum	Width (mm) mean value
Left adrenal gland	13.2 / 26.3	17.4	3.0 / 5.2	4.1
Right adrenal gland	12.4 / 22.6	16.7	3.1 / 6.0	4.3

Ultrasonography of Adrenal Disease

Indications for adrenal ultrasonography include clinical and laboratory work-ups referring to hyperadrenocorticism with:

- Hyperplasia.
- Neoplasia.
- Inflammation.
- Calcification.

A further indication is for monitoring treatment response.

Apart from hyperadrenocorticism, most adrenal lesions are incidental findings during abdominal ultrasonography.

Adrenal enlargement may be unilateral or bilateral. Both adrenal glands must always be examined ultrasonographically to complete the findings. Adrenal lesions can be differentiated

546

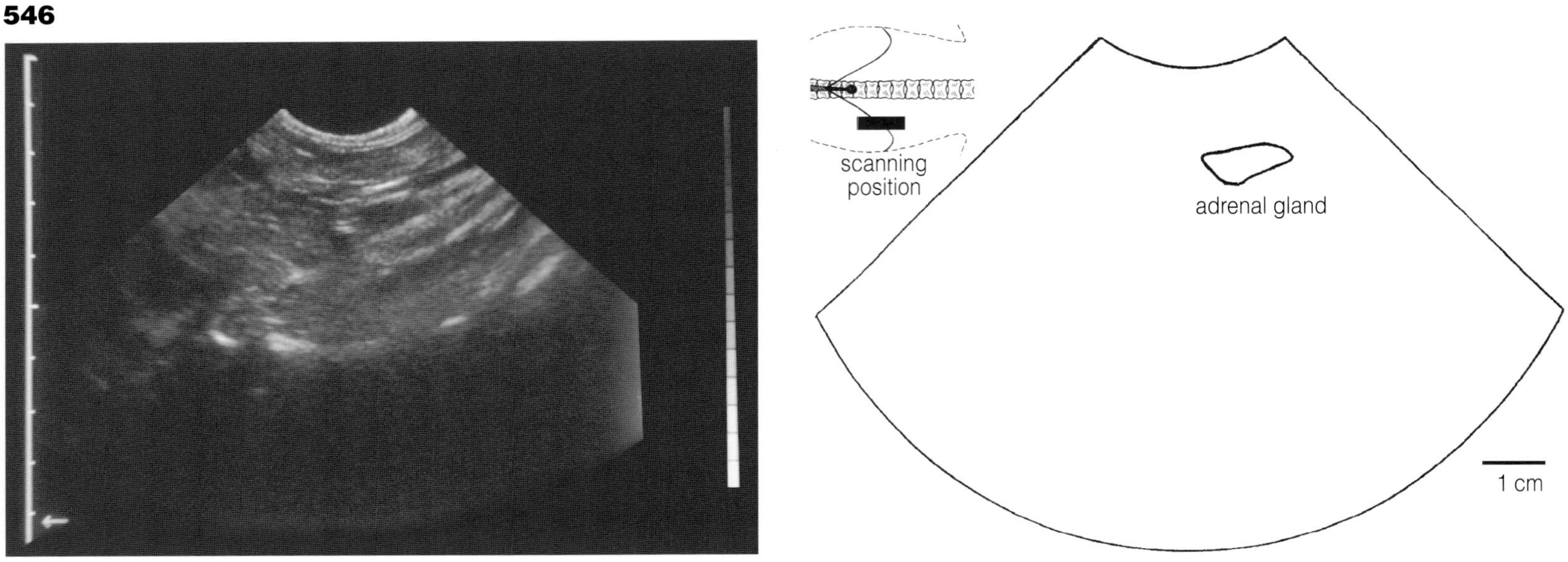

546 Normal right canine adrenal gland in a longitudinal view. The adrenal is hypoechoic with a triangular shape.

547

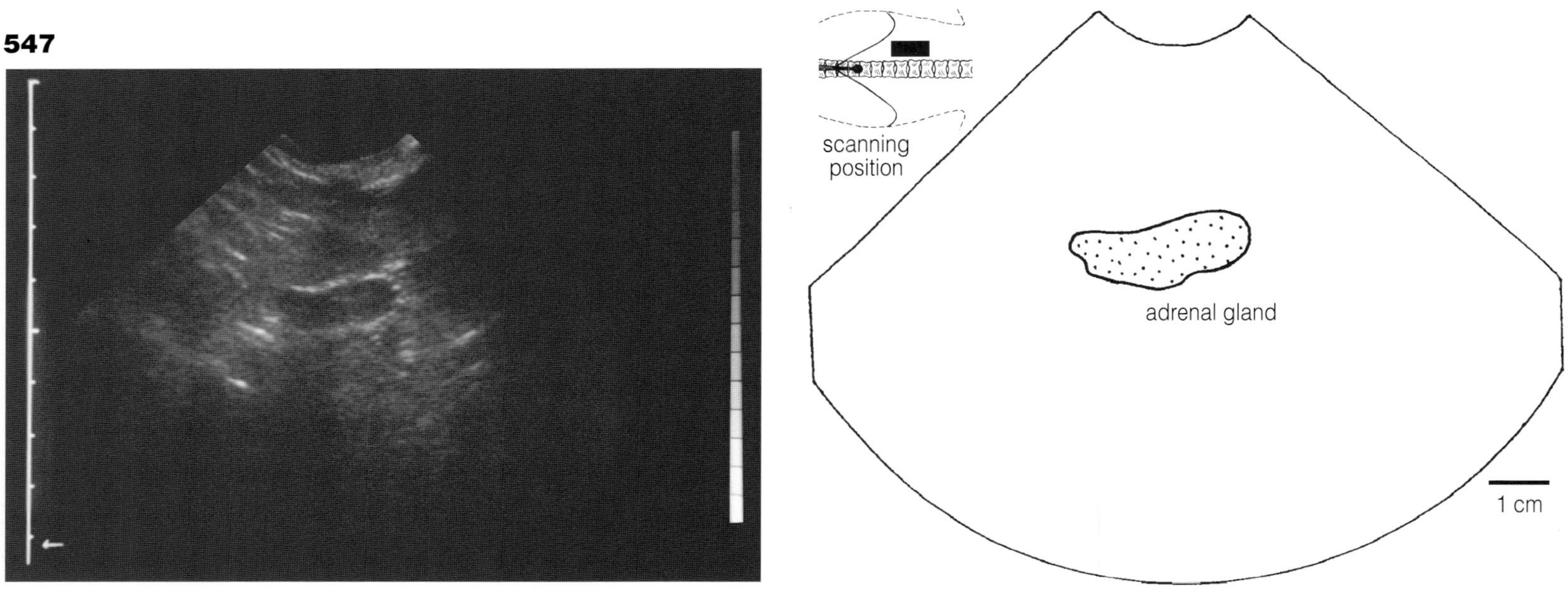

547 Adrenal hyperplasia in a dog. The enlarged adrenal gland has a normal shape and shows decreased echogenicity. The other adrenal gland showed the same findings.

from other lesions because of their typical anatomical location. Round masses cranial to the kidneys are usually caused by adrenal disease. Differential diagnosis may include lymph node disease.

Adrenal Hyperplasia

Hyperplasia is diagnosed when both adrenals are enlarged. The adrenal glands may be enlarged uniformly or become longer or wider. The echogenicity is generally reduced. Layering within the adrenal gland is not apparent (**547**).

Adrenal Neoplasia

Adrenal tumours are generally unilateral, but they may be present in both glands. The tumours include carcinomas, pheochromocytomas (**548**) and adenomas. While the echogenicity is usually increased with adenomas (**549, 550**), it decreases with carcinomas. Ultrasonography of adrenal tumours that invade the caudal vena cava is usually indicative of a malignancy. The malignancy of a tumour must be confirmed histopathologically. The texture of all tumours is generally finely granulated and more or less uniform. Large tumours appear more non-homogenous[3]. Hormonally active tumours often cause contralateral adrenal atrophy.

548

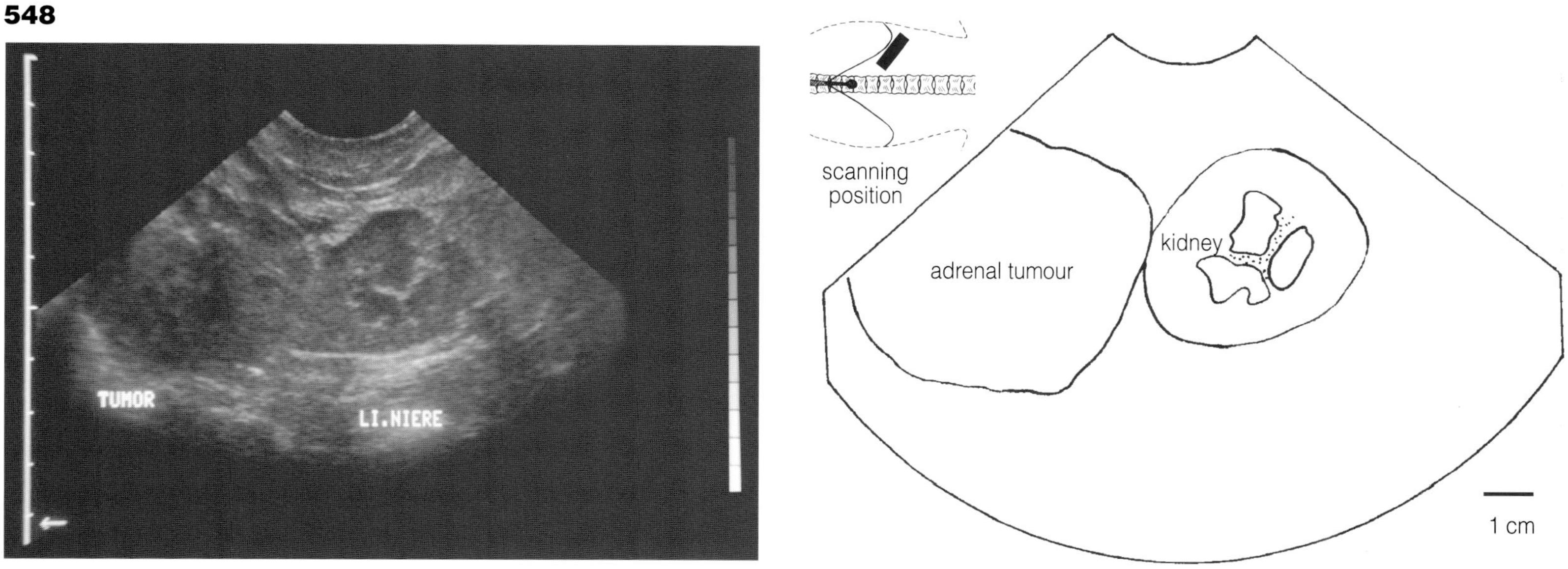

548 Pheochromocytoma in a dog. The non-homogenous mass is located craniomedial to the left kidney. The only differential diagnosis is lymph node neoplasia.

549

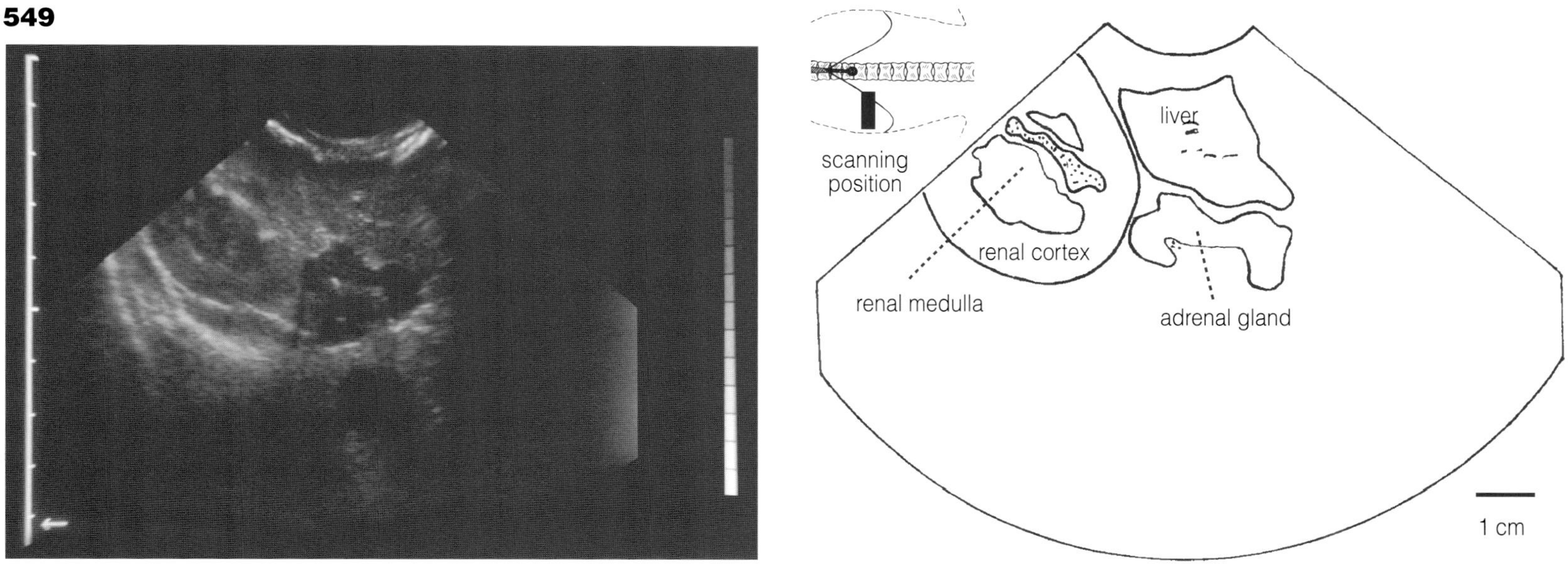

549 Adrenal adenoma in a dog.

550

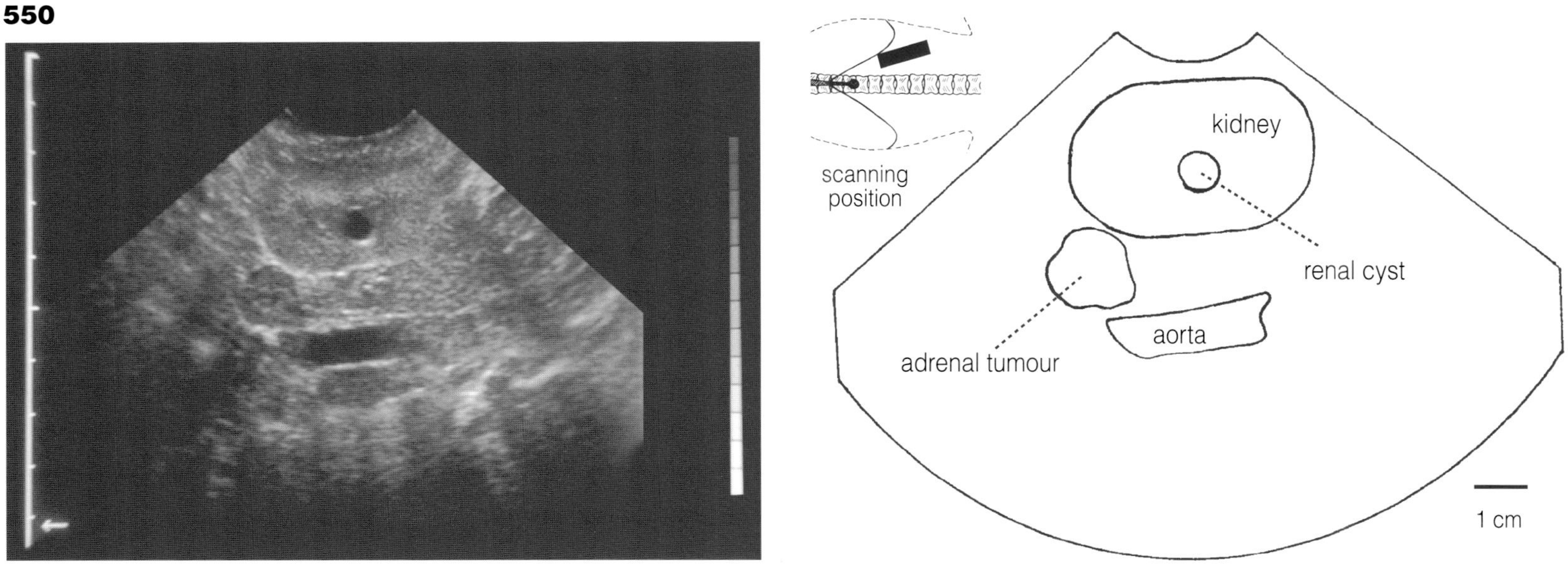

550 Adenoma of the left adrenal in a dog. The adrenal appears almost round in a longitudinal view. The centre of the adrenal is more echogenic than its borders. A renal cyst is seen as an additional finding.

551

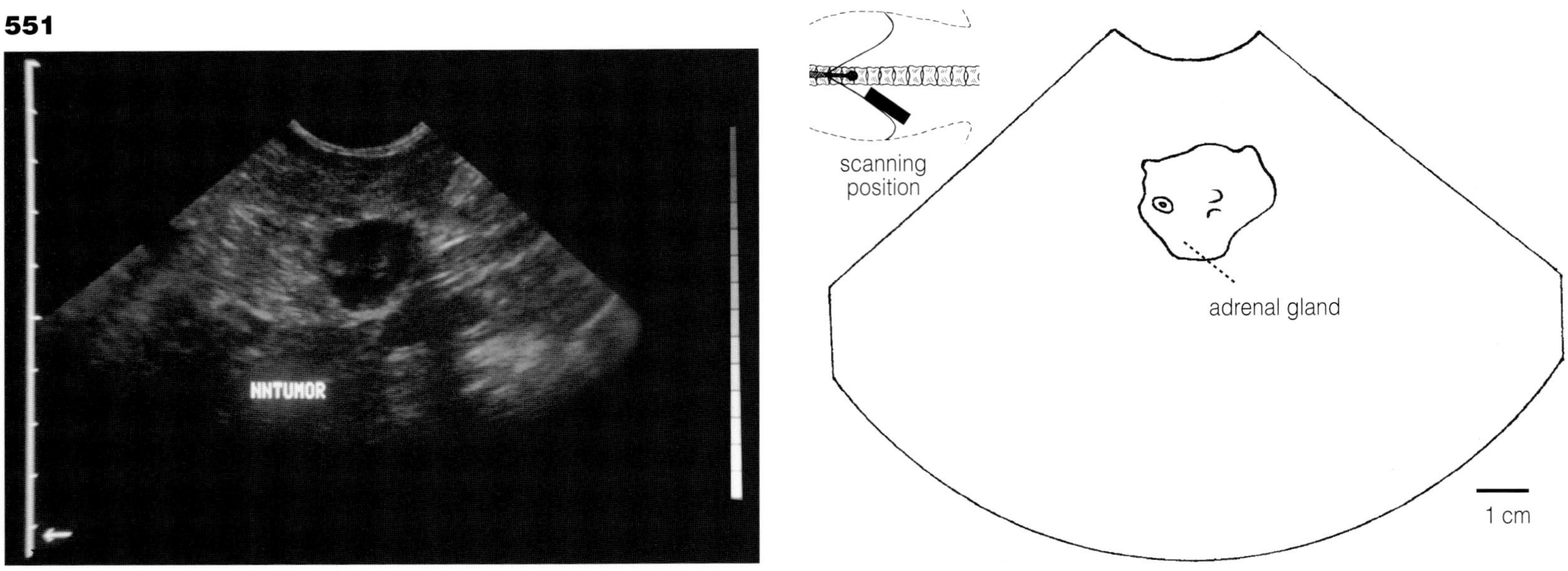

551 Adrenalitis with necrosis in a dog. Small hypo- to anechoic mass craniomedial to the right kidney. Differentials include an adrenal tumour or a tumour of other origin.

Adrenalitis

This rare adrenal disorder is seen in conjunction with a decrease in echogenicity and a change in shape (**551**). Distal acoustic enhancement may be present. A definitive differentiation from neoplasia is not possible.

References

1 Grooters AM, Biller DS, Miyabayashi T and Leveille R (1994) Evaluation of routine abdominal ultrasonography as a technique for imaging the canine adrenal glands. *J. Am. Anim. Hosp. Assoc.* **30**, 457–462.

2 Hörauf A and Reusch C (1995) Darstellung der Nebennieren mittels Ultraschall: Untersuchungen bei gesanden Handen, Handen mit nicht-endokrinen Erkrankungen sowie mit Cushing-Syndrom. *Kleintierpraxis* **40**, 351–360.

3 Kantrowitz BM, Nyland TG and Feldman EC (1986) Adrenal ultrasonography in the dog – detection of tumors and hyperplasia in hyperadrenocorticism. *Vet. Radiol.* **27**, 91–96.

4 Lamb CR (1990) Abdominal ultrasonography in small animals: intestinal tract and mesentery, kidneys, adrenal glands, uterus and prostate. *J. Small Anim.Pract.* **31**, 295–304.

5 Nickel R, Schummer A and Seiferle E (1991) (Eds.) *Lehrbuch der Anatomie der Haustiere, Vol.IV*. Verlag Paul Parey, Berlin and Hamburg.

6 Schelling CG (1991) Ultrasonography of the adrenal gland. *Prob. Vet. Med.* **3**, 604–617.

7 Voorhout TG (1990) X-ray-computed tomography, nephrotomography, and ultrasonography of the adrenal glands of healthy dogs. *Am. J. Vet. Res.* **51**, 624–631.

Lymph Nodes

Dirk Lüerssen and Martin Janthur

Instrumentation, Examination Technique and Normal Sonographic Findings

Ultrasonographic evaluation of lymph nodes requires high-resolution transducers with a frequency of at least 7.5 MHz. Normal abdominal lymph nodes are still difficult to visualize because their echogenicity is similar to that of surrounding tissues such as muscles, fat or mesentery[2, 3]. Lymph nodes can be identified and recognized by their proximity to blood vessels. Although visualization of these structures is generally difficult, deep lymph nodes are as 'easy' to identify as more superficial ones. Transducer pressure, especially with sector scanners, may help to displace 'interfering' organs such as gas-filled bowel loops. This ensures better visualization of lymph nodes. Superficial, palpable lymph nodes such as the mammary or scrotal lymph nodes can always be evaluated using a stand-off pad.

Normal lymph nodes are round (solitary lymph nodes) to elongated (jejunal lymph nodes) and uniformly hypoechoic to moderately echogenic. A hypoechoic margin with a more echogenic centre may be differentiated in mesenteric lymph nodes (**552**). Jejunal lymph nodes have a fusiform appearance that reaches up to 20 cm[1] and may be mistaken for pancreatic abnormalities.

Ultrasonography of Lymph Node Disease

Indications for lymph node ultrasonography include associated blood profile abnormalities, disorders of the lymphatic system, and lesions of palpable lymph nodes with suspected:

- Lymphadenitis and lymph node abscesses.
- Lymph node neoplasia and metastasis.
- Lymphoma.

A further indication is for monitoring treatment response.

Lymphadenitis and Lymph Node Abscess

Lymphadenitis is characterized by enlarged lymph nodes with a homogenous parenchymal texture (**553**). The hypoechoic to almost anechoic lymph nodes are round and well-demarcated and are usually close to the large abdominal vessels or in the mesentery. They can be anatomically differentiated by their location[2].

Abscessed lymph nodes show a more non-homogenous echogenicity. They contain irregular anechoic areas of a few centimetres in diameter. Differential diagnosis includes cross-sections of vessels, haematomas, abscesses of other origin, necrosis, non-lymphatic tumours and iatrogenic induced lesions (**554–557**).

552

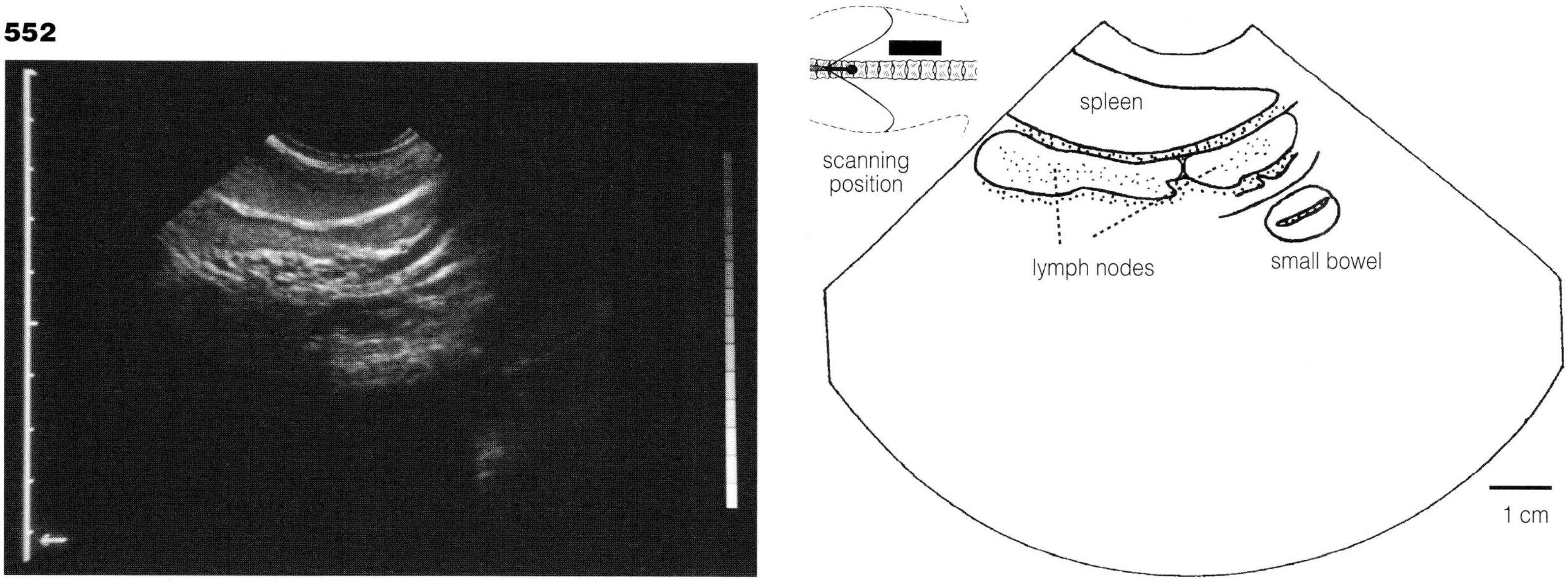

552 Normal jejunal lymph node in a dog. The elongated structure is located below the spleen. An echogenic centre is surrounded by a hypoechoic outer rim. Adjacent vessels help to identify the lymph nodes.

553

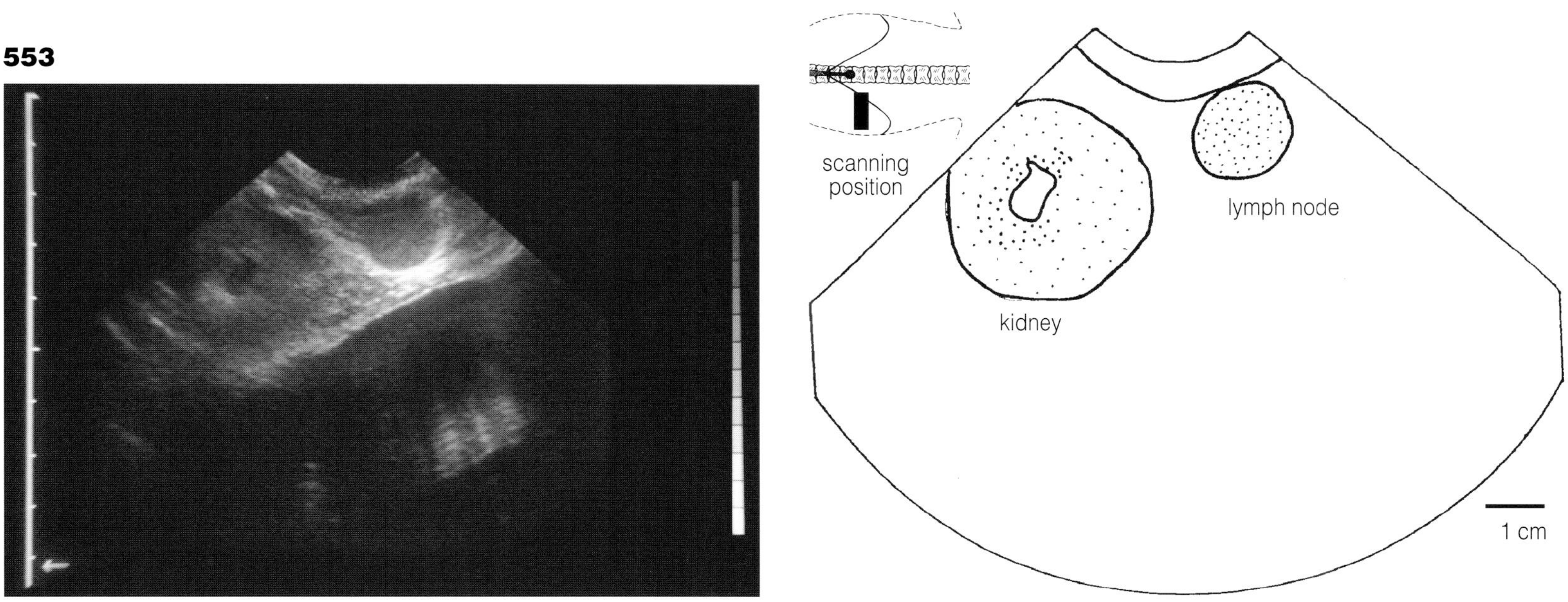

553 Lymphadenitis (histopathology: pyogranulomatous lymphadenitis) with local peritonitis in a male cat. The round, homogenously enlarged lymph node is located medial to the right kidney. The surrounding tissue is more echogenic.

554

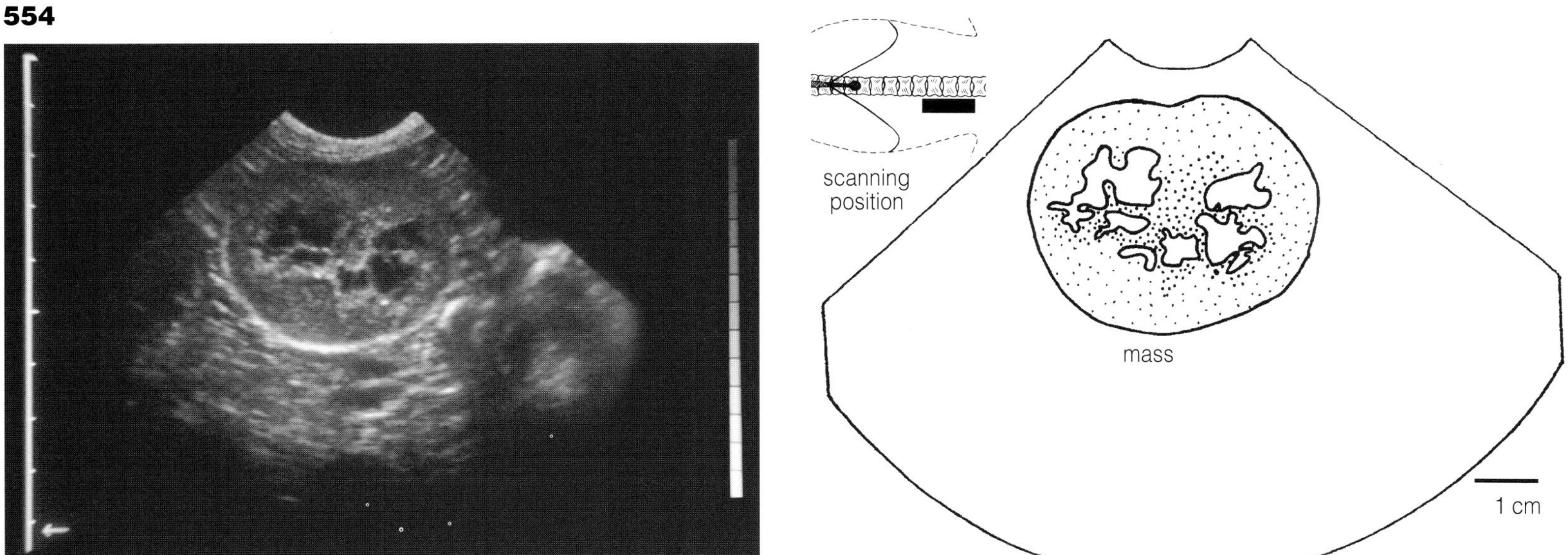

554 Round mass with an anechoic, complex centre and clear demarcation to the adjacent vessels (cranial mesenteric artery and vein). This lesion is characteristic of a lymph node abscess. The mass was actually an organized haematoma in the mesentery.

555

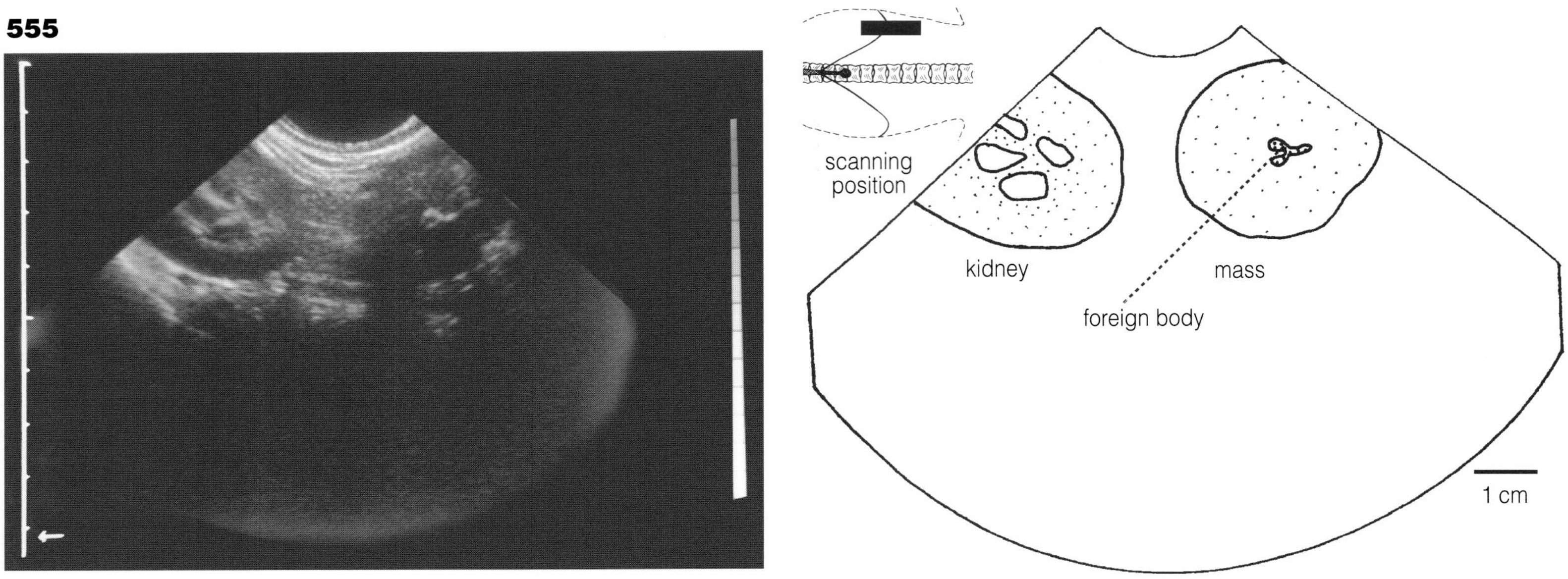

555 Round, moderately echogenic mass with a hypoechoic centre caudal to the left kidney. While the lesion appears typical for a lymph node abnormality, the scanning position is not. This mass is actually a foreign body granuloma, caused by non-resorbed suture material.

556

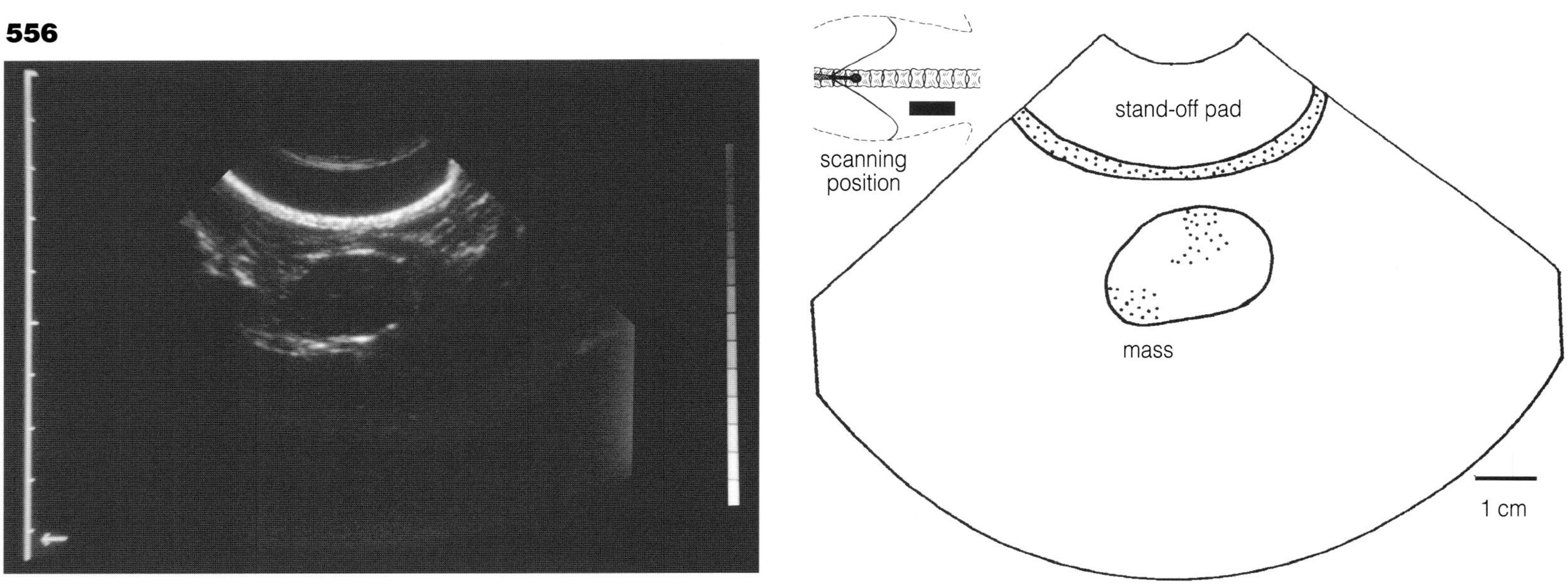

556 Round, almost anechoic mass without distal enhancement caudal to the right kidney. While the lesion appears typical for a lymph node abnormality, the scanning position is not. This mass is actually necrosis of fatty tissue, cause by ligation in a spayed bitch.

557

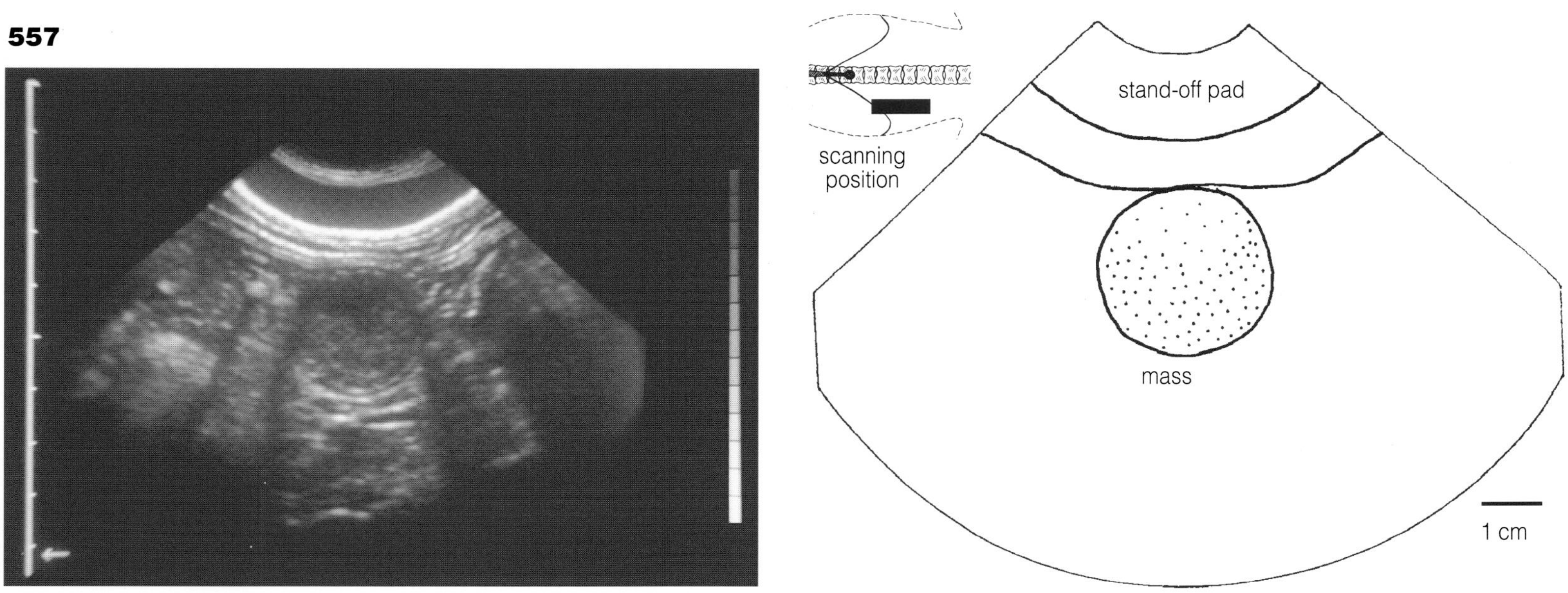

557 Round, complex mass of medium echogenicity with a capsule near the intestinal vessels. While the echogenicity, appearance and location of the lesion appear typical for a lymph node abnormality, the capsule is not. This mass is actually a mesenteric abscess of unknown origin in a spayed cat.

561

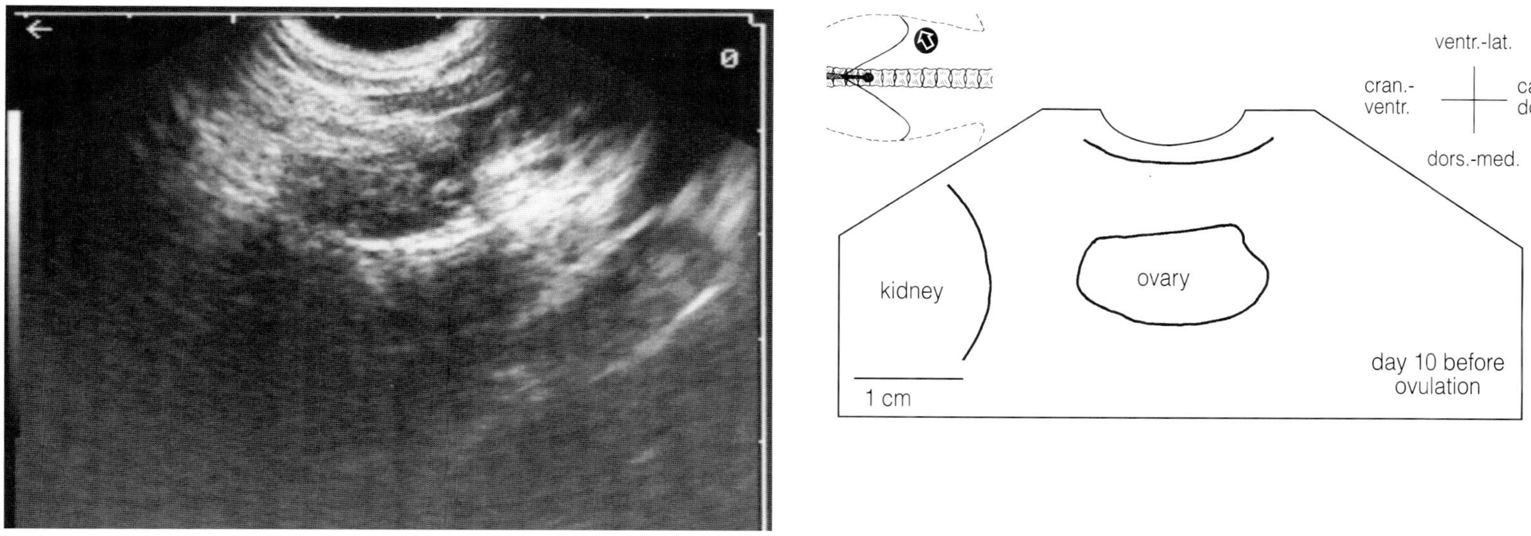

561 Left ovary of a Beagle in early follicular maturation (length 16 mm, width 10 mm) with non-uniform parenchyma due to small hypoechoic structures: 6.5 MHz.

562

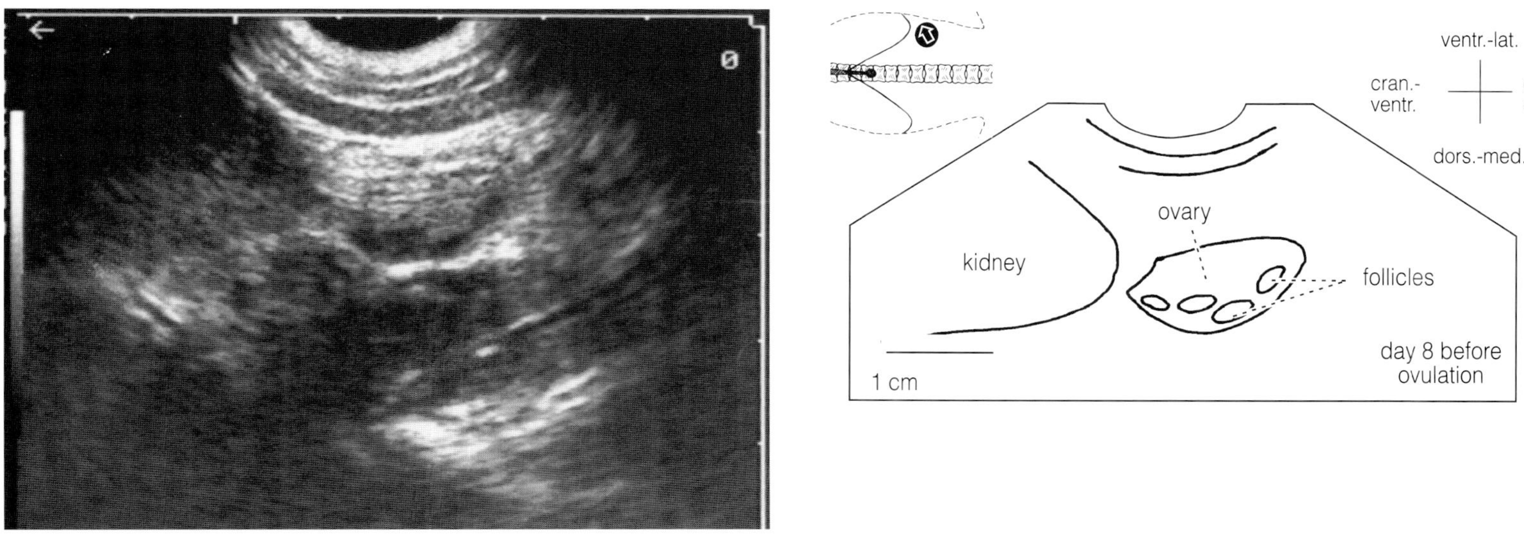

563

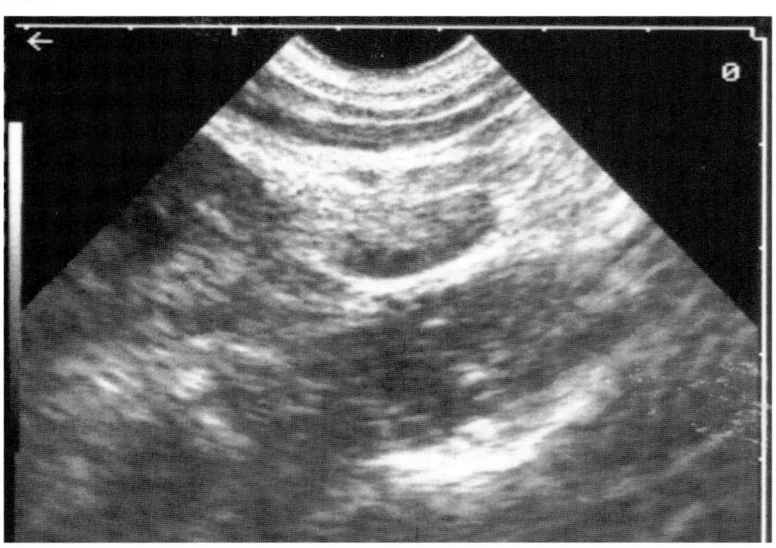

562, 563 Left ovary of a Beagle eight days before ovulation (length 17 mm, width 10 mm) with four follicles; transducer frequency: 6.5 MHz (**562**) and 5.0 MHz (**563**).

564

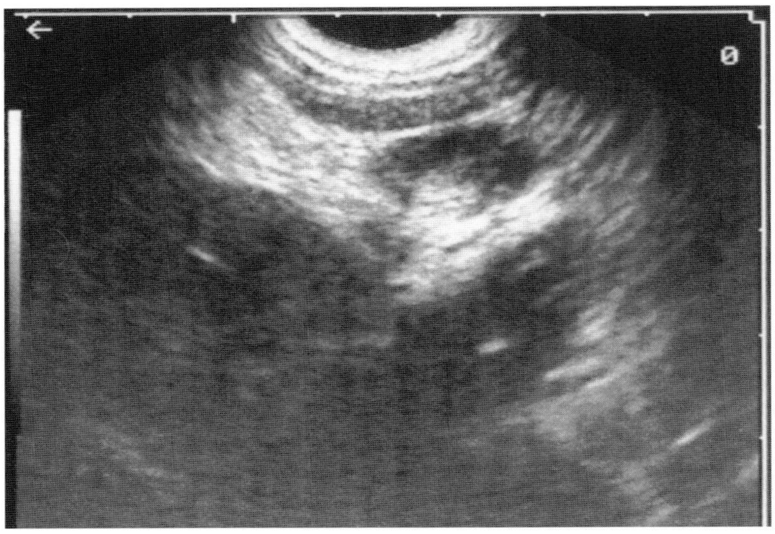

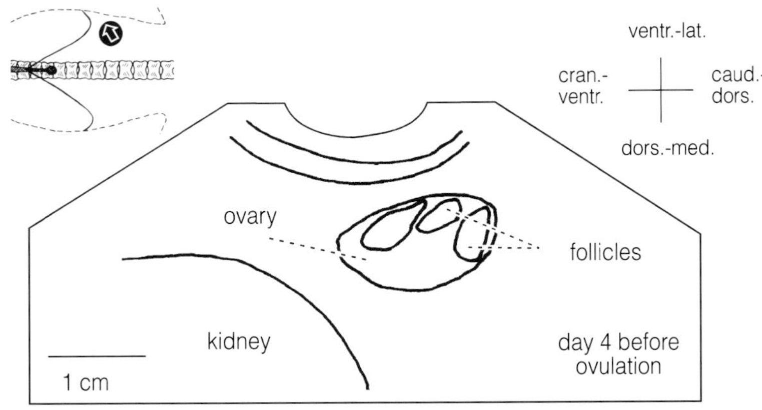

565

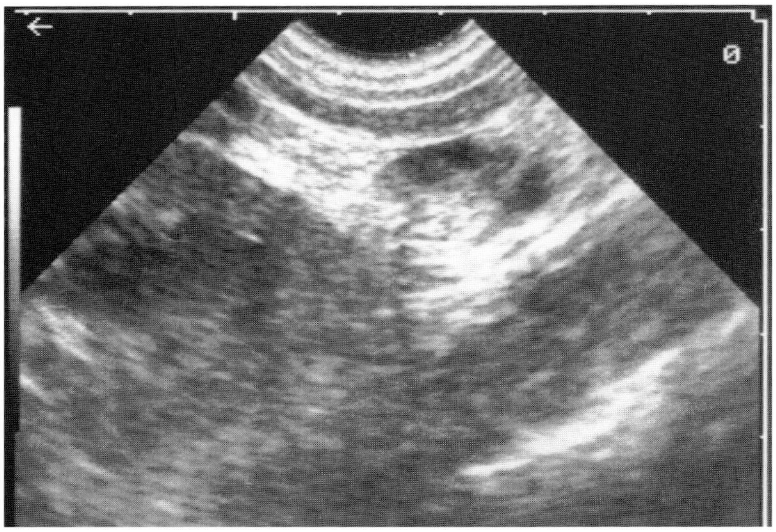

564, 565 Left ovary of a Beagle four days before ovulation (length 18 mm, width 10 mm) with three follicles measuring up to 6 mm in diameter; transducer frequency: 6.5 MHz (**564**) and 5.0 MHz (**565**).

566

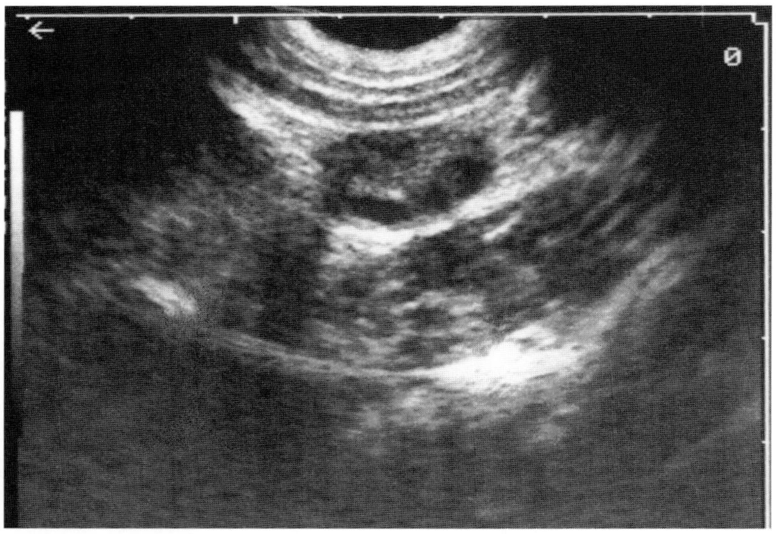

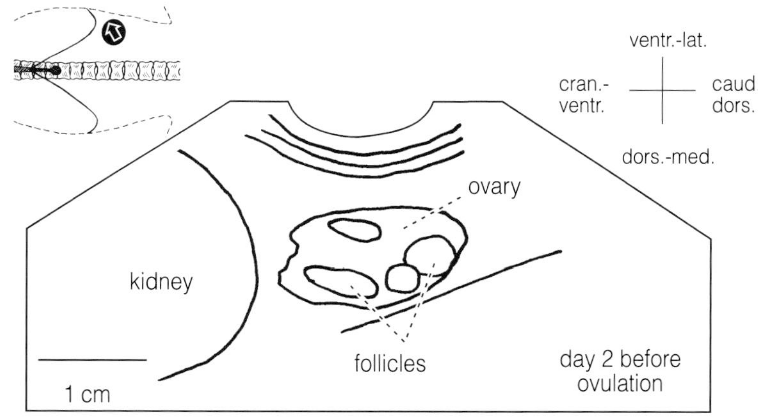

566 Left ovary of a Beagle two days before ovulation (LH-peak) (length 21 mm, width 11 mm) with four follicles measuring up to 7 mm in diameter; transducer frequency: 6.5 MHz (see also **567**).

567

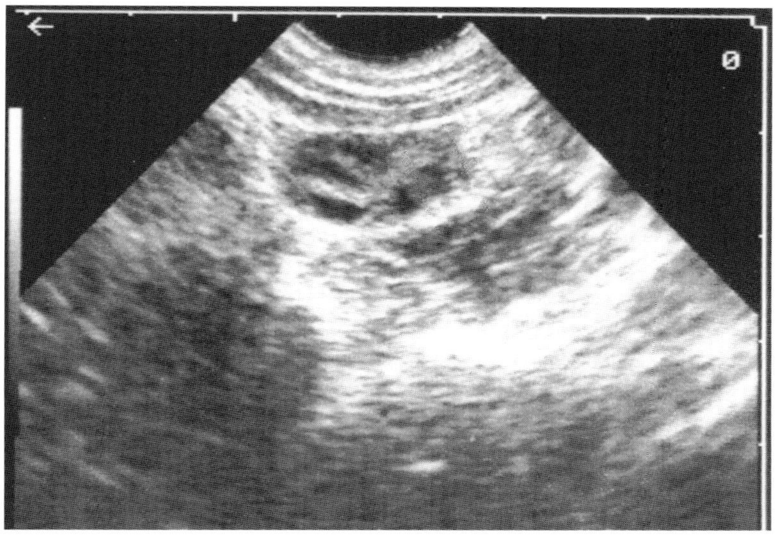

567 Left ovary of a Beagle two days before ovulation (LH-peak) (length 21 mm, width 11 mm) with four follicles measuring up to 7 mm in diameter; transducer frequency: 5.0 MHz (see also **566**).

568

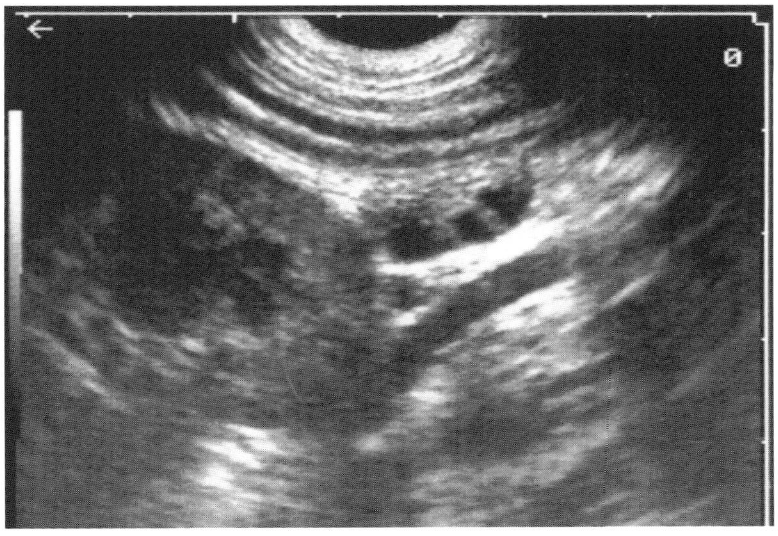

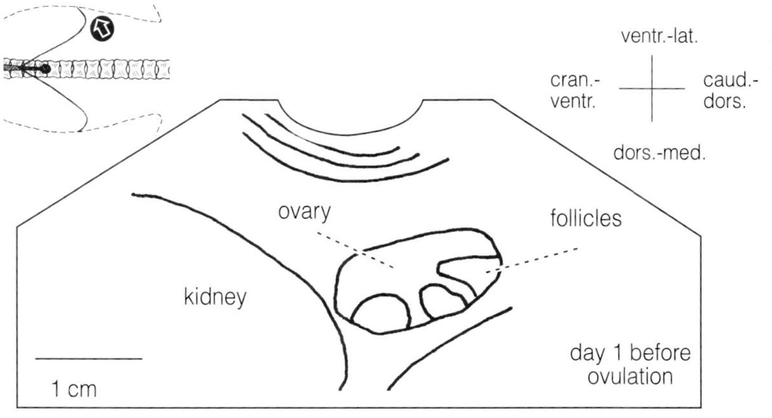

569

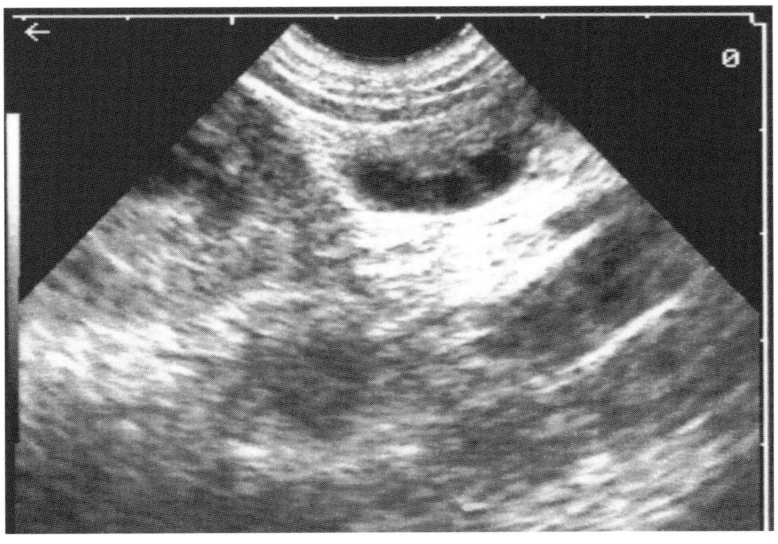

568, 569 Left ovary of a Beagle one day before ovulation (length 22 mm, width 12 mm) with three follicles measuring up to 7 mm in diameter; transducer frequency: 6.5 MHz (**568**) and 5.0 MHz (**569**).

570

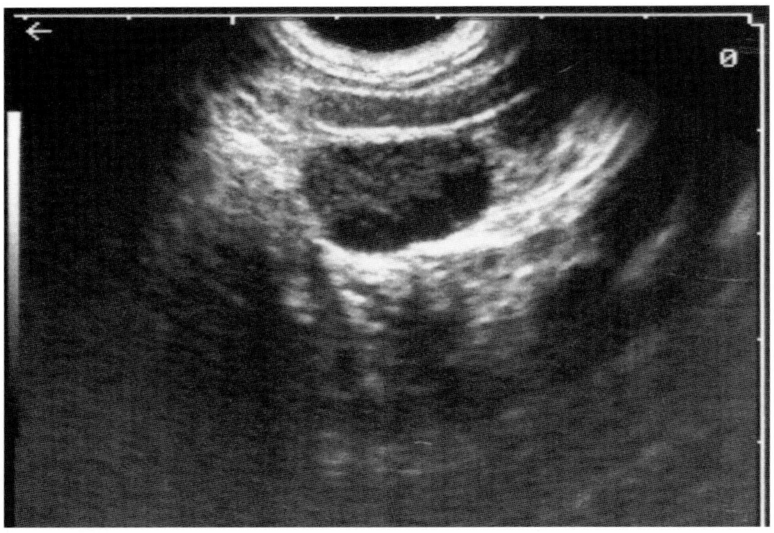

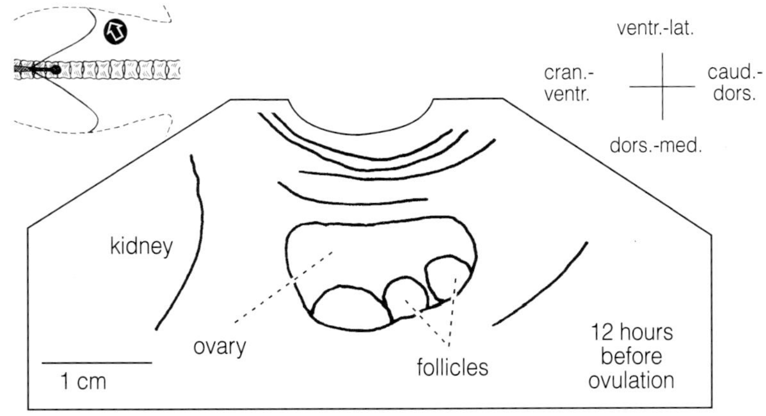

571

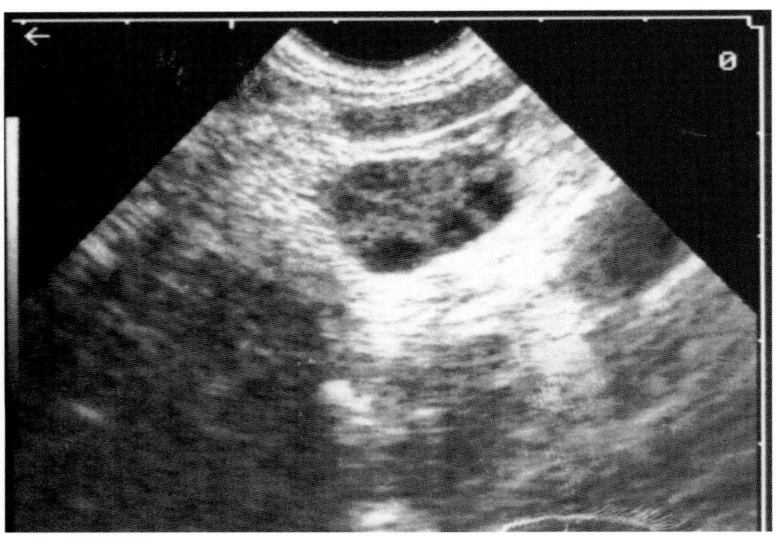

570, 571 Left ovary of a Beagle 12 hours before ovulation (length 22 mm, width 12 mm) with three follicles measuring up to 8 mm in diameter; transducer frequency: 6.5 MHz (**570**) and 5.0 MHz (**571**).

572

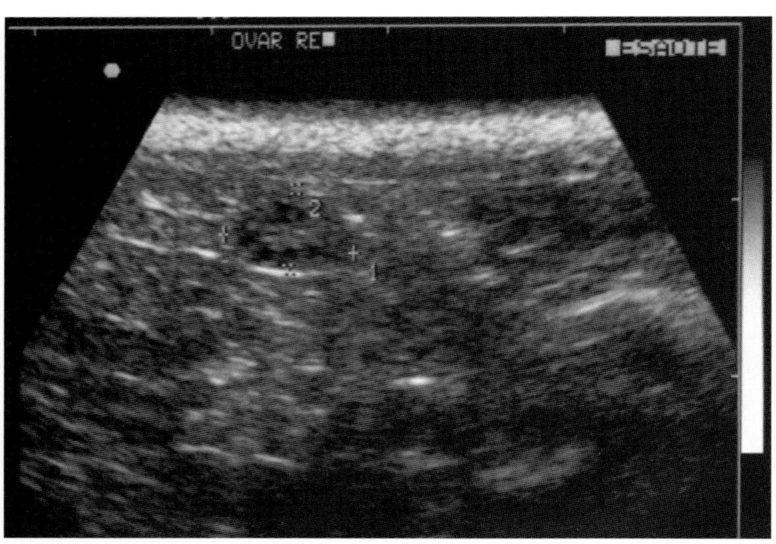

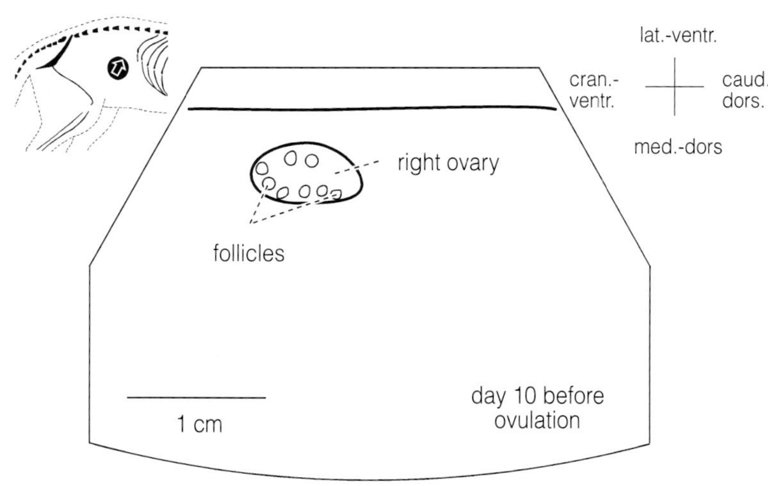

572 Right ovary of a cat in early follicular maturation (length 7.4 mm, width 4.5 mm) with small, round, hypoechoic structures; transducer frequency: 13 MHz. (Reprinted with permission from Ryoko Kawauchi, Hannover.)

573

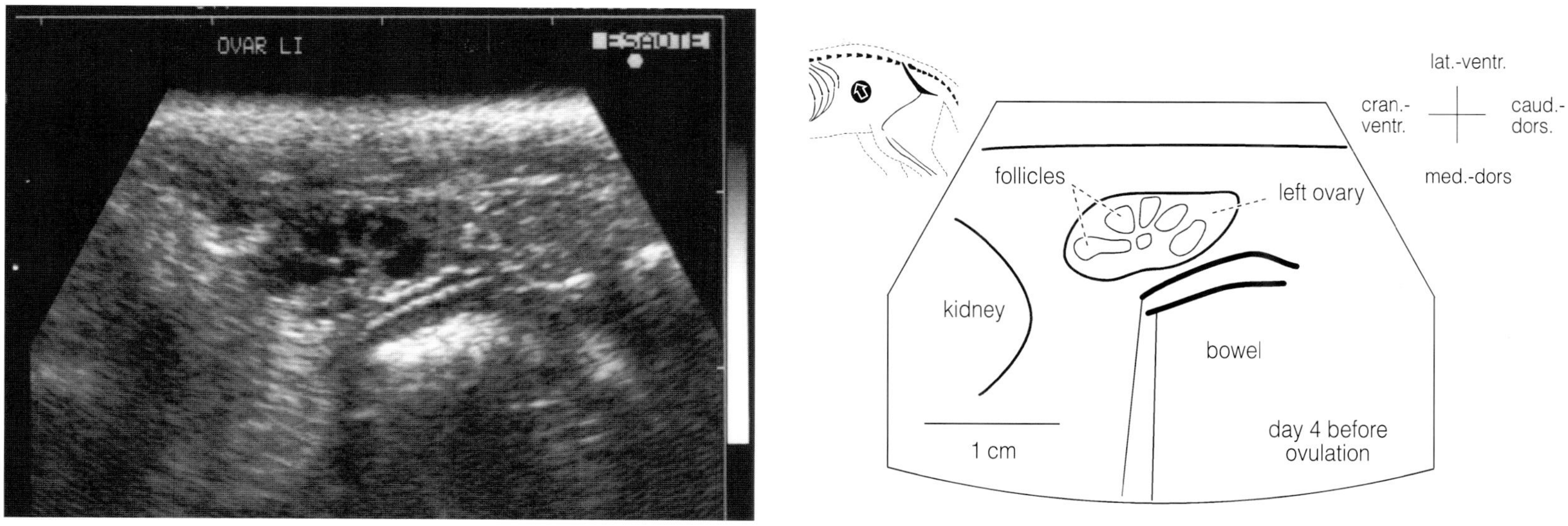

573 Left ovary of a cat four days before ovulation (length 9.8 mm, width 6.0 mm) with five follicles measuring up to 2.4 mm in diameter; transducer frequency: 13 MHz. (Reprinted with permission from Ryoko Kawauchi, Hannover.)

574

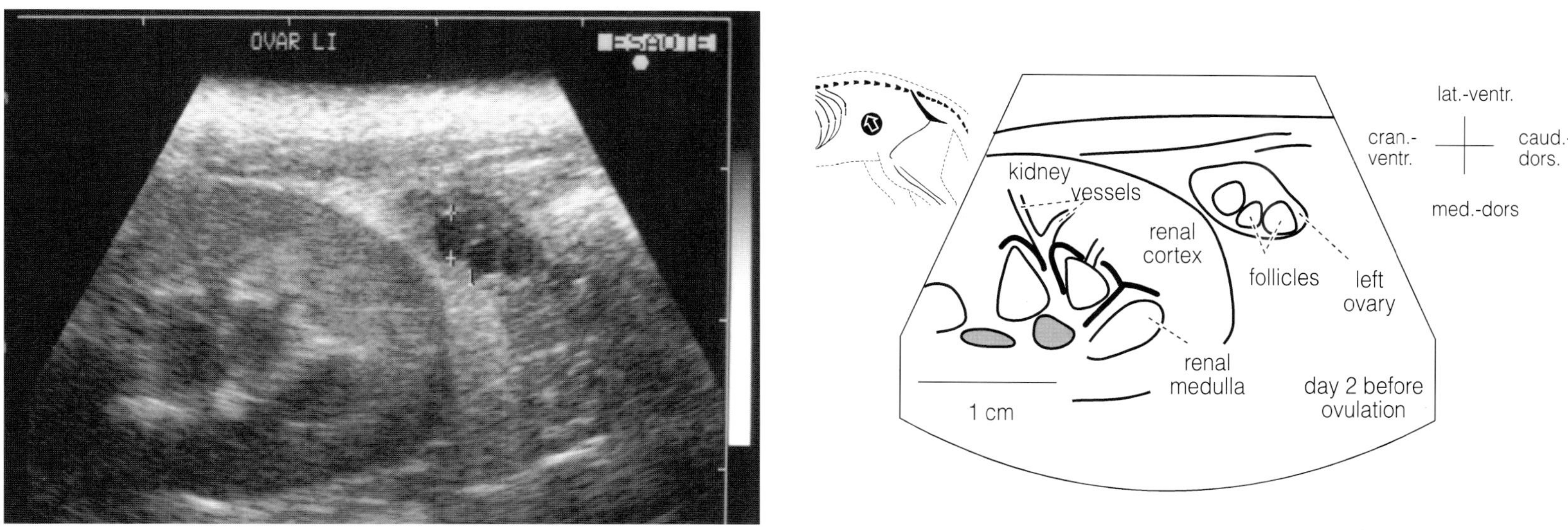

574 Left ovary of a cat two days before ovulation (length 11.3 mm, width 5.6 mm) with three follicles measuring up to 3 mm in diameter; transducer frequency: 13 MHz. (Reprinted with permission from Ryoko Kawauchi, Hannover.)

575

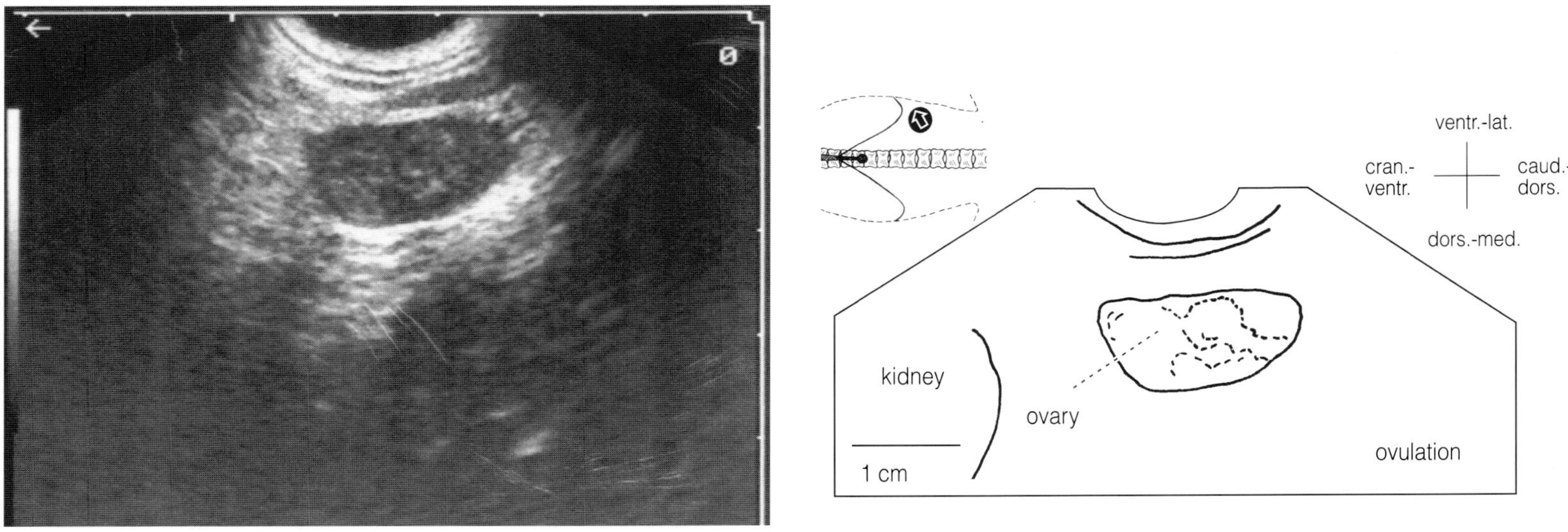

576

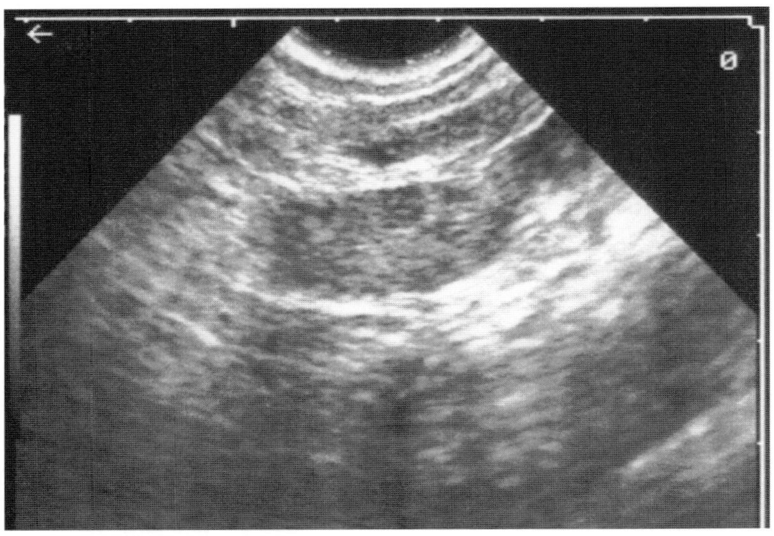

575, 576 Left ovary in a Beagle during ovulation (length 23 mm, width 12 mm), seen as a compact, echogenic structure; transducer frequency: 6.5 MHz (**575**) and 5.0 MHz (**576**).

577

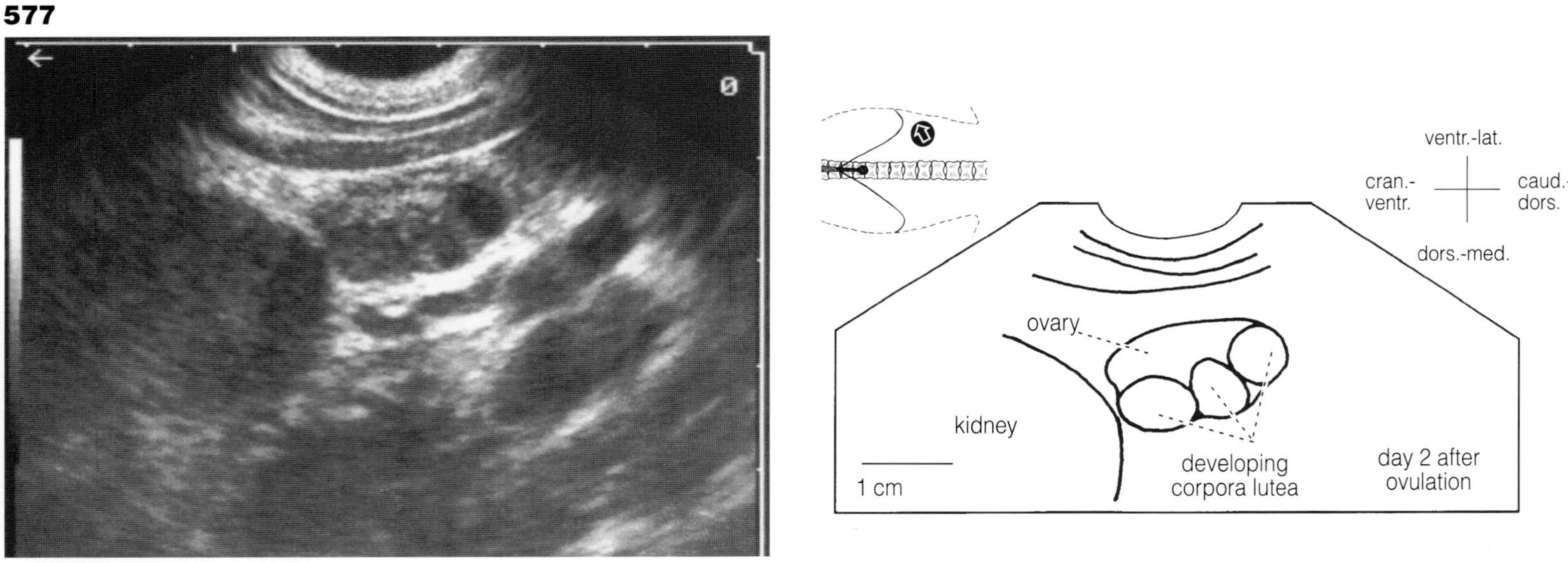

577 Left ovary in a Beagle two days after ovulation (length 28 mm, width 14 mm), showing three developing corpora lutea with partially anechoic cavities; transducer frequency: 6.5 MHz (see also **578**).

578

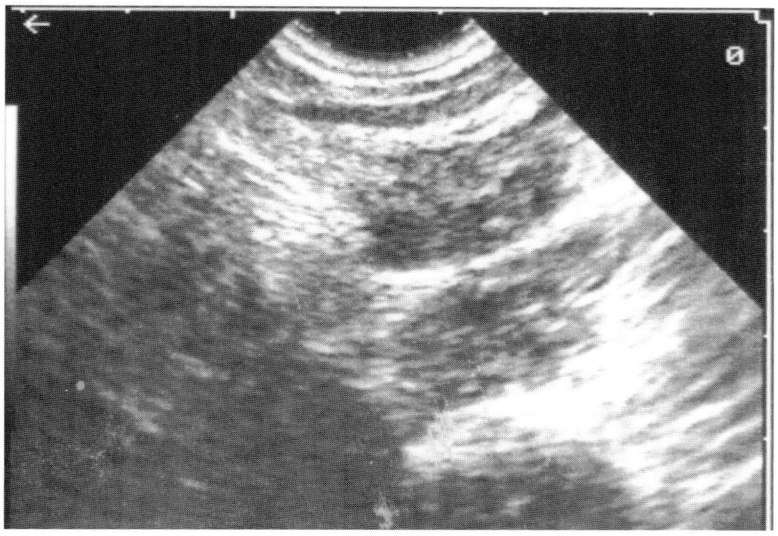

578 Left ovary in a Beagle two days after ovulation (length 28 mm, width 14 mm), showing three developing corpora lutea with partially anechoic cavities; transducer frequency: 5.0 MHz (see also **577**).

579

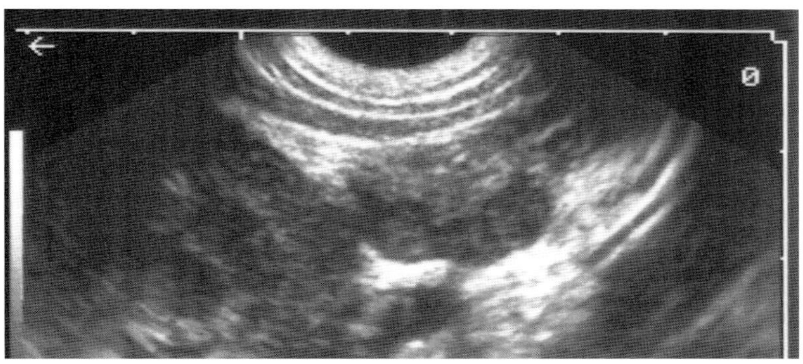

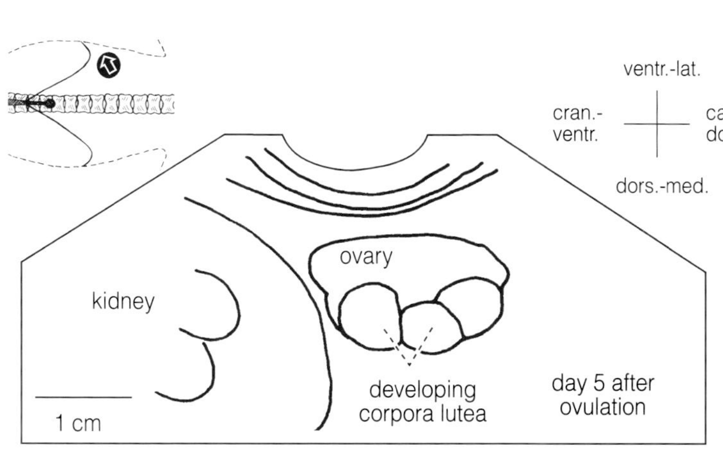

579, 580 Left ovary in a Beagle five days after ovulation (length 28 mm, width 15 mm) with three solid corpora lutea, protruding over the surface, and measuring 4 to 7 mm; transducer frequency: 6.5 MHz (**579**) and 5.0 MHz (**580**).

580

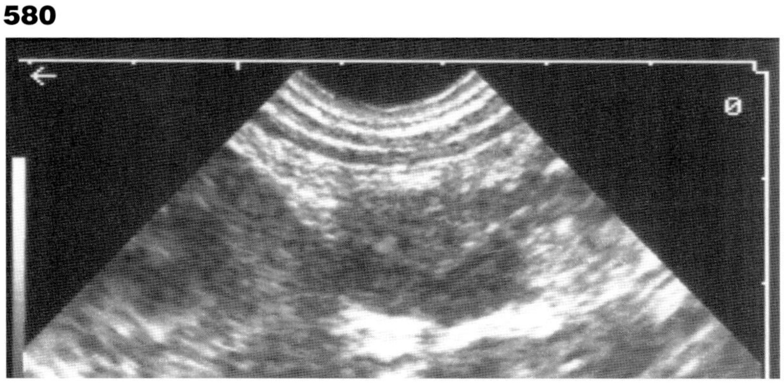

Ovulation

The oestrogen-secreting follicles in the bitch are slowly transformed into progesterone-producing corpora lutea[1, 4, 17, 18]. The mature canine follicles contain little fluid, keeping them from collapsing during ovulation. The emptying follicular cavities refill immediately, which causes an additional increase in ovary size (**575, 576**)[3, 5, 6, 8, 10]. Ovulation does not cause a marked change in the ultrasonographic image. When pre-ovulatory luteinization takes place, the follicular wall becomes more echogenic. During ovulation the ovaries are recognized as relatively echogenic, uniform structures (**575, 576**). This characteristic image is seen only for 12 hours.

Ovulation can only be safely detected with serial examinations towards the end of follicular maturation. Beginning with the initial pre-ovulatory progesterone increase, the ovaries should be scanned twice a day in 12 hour intervals.

Because of these time-consuming and costly examinations, the indications for direct ultrasonographic evaluation of ovulation are limited in veterinary practice. In cases of artificial insemination with frozen sperm, the ideal date for conception can be determined. Frozen sperm is less fertile than fresh sperm. The ideal date for fertilization is 2–4 days post ovulation.

Corpus Luteum Formation

The corpora lutea develop immediately after ovulation, which causes an increase in ovary size (**577–582**). Round, hypoechoic structures resembling follicles are scanned 24–48 hours post ovulation[5, 6, 10, 21]. The difference is their characteristically thicker hyperechoic wall and the fact that the corpora lutea protrude over the margins of the ovary. The ovary shows an irregular surface. An exact differentiation between corpora lutea and pre-ovulatoy follicles can only be made with frequent examinations and additional methods such as vaginoscopy and vaginal cytology. Even towards the end of oestrus, i.e. 6–8 days post ovulation, most of

581

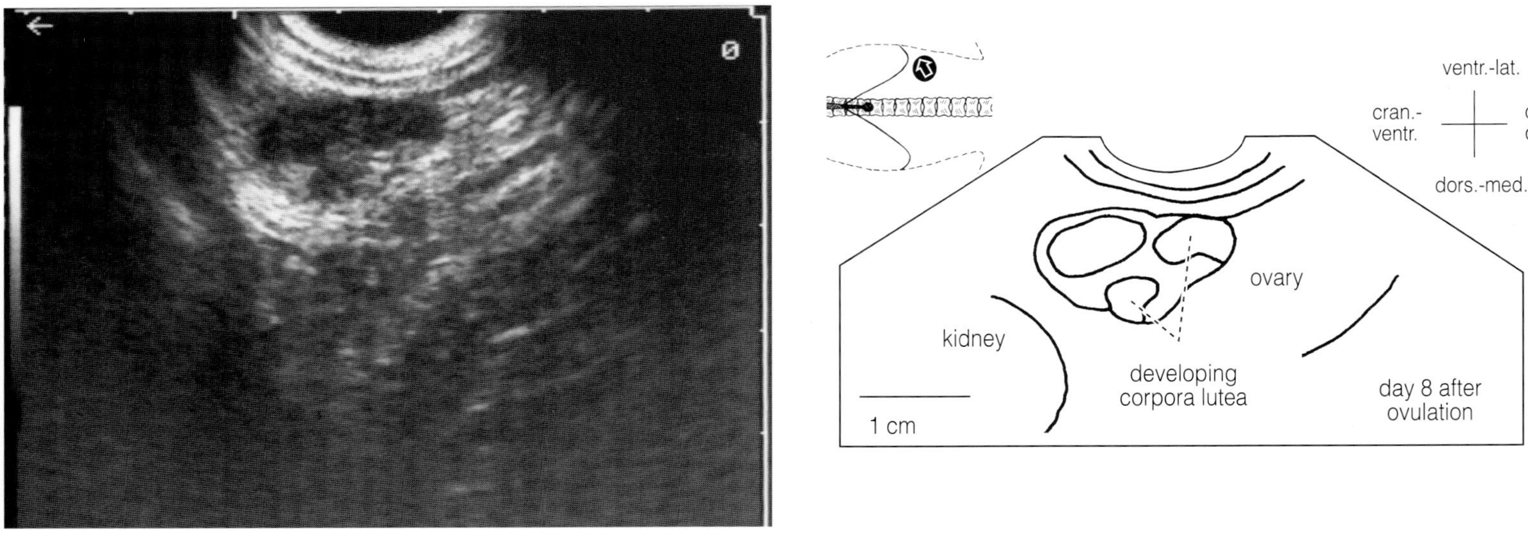

582

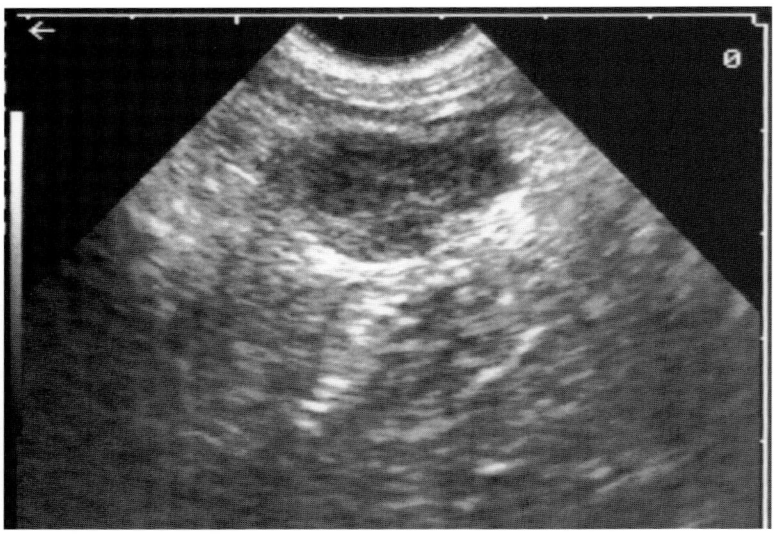

581, 582 Left ovary in a Beagle eight days after ovulation and the end of oestrus (length 28 mm, width 15 mm) with three hypoechoic corpora lutea, measuring 4 to 7 mm; transducer frequency: 6.5 MHz (**581**) and 5.0 MHz (**582**).

583

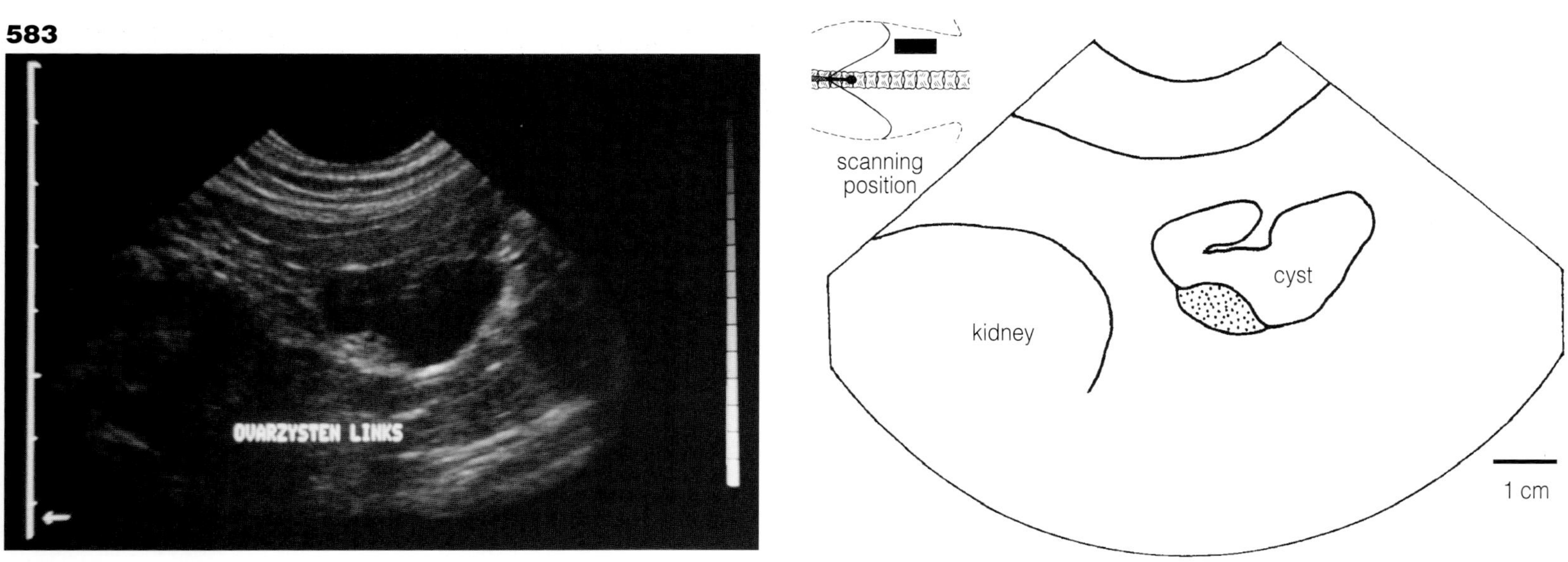

583 Ovarian cysts with distal acoustic enhancement, characteristically near the abdominal wall, caudal to the kidney in a bitch. Cyst walls are not visible and the cysts seem to be confluent, which produces an irregular organ shape.

584

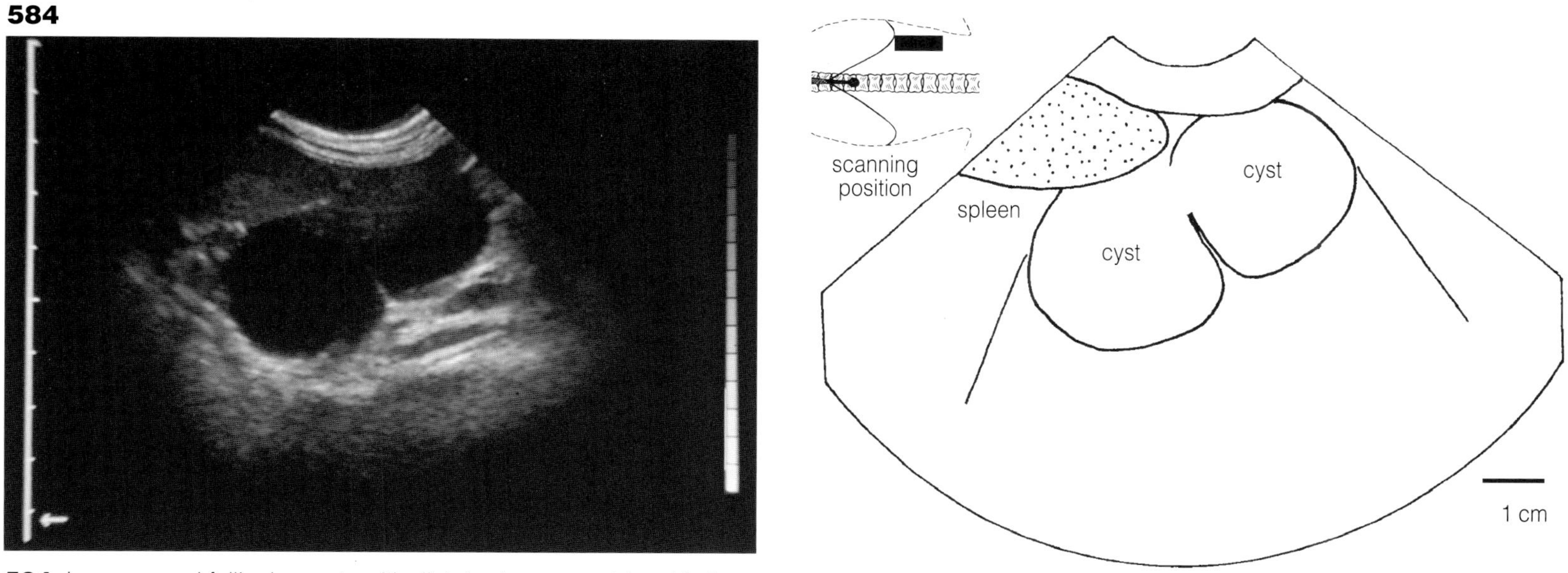

584 Large, round follicular cysts with distal enhancement in a bitch.

585

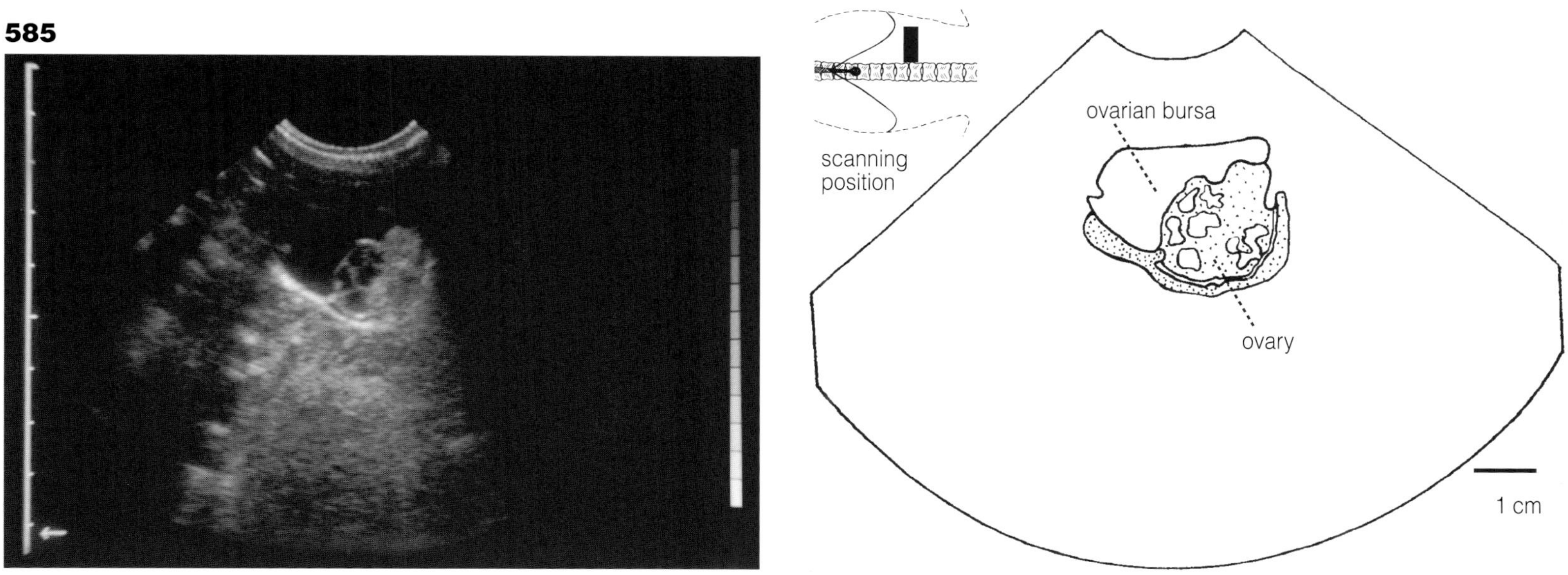

585 Fluid-filled ovarian bursa and small ovarian cysts in a bitch. This rare finding is from a freshly ruptured cyst. A similar sonogram is seen with retrograde fluid loss from a diseased uterus.

the corpora lutea still have an anechoic cavity (**581, 582**). The ovaries finally decrease in size with corpus luteum maturation.

The sonographic images of follicles, corpora lutea and pathological ovarian cysts are very similar. Differentiation is only possible by considering the oestrus cycle and using additional examination methods such as vaginoscopy, vaginal cytology and endocrinological findings.

Ultrasonography of Ovarian Disease

Dirk Lüerssen and Martin Janthur

Ovarian Cysts

Ovarian cysts appear as anechoic, well-demarcated, round to irregular structures with distal acoustic enhancement, uni- or bilaterally caudal to the kidneys[2, 16] (**583**). The wall of the cyst is very thin and it is seen occasionally. Multiple cysts may seem to flow together and produce irregular ovarian margins (**584**). Ovarian cysts are not associated with the oestrus cycle and may measure up to 20 cm in diameter or larger. Follicular cysts are rare in the dog and have the same shape as tertiary follicles, although they are larger in size. Follicular cysts are round (**584**). The ovarian bursa may be visualized when free fluid is present from ruptured cysts (**585**). In these cases, additional cysts are usually recognized. A similar sonographic image is found with retrograde fluid loss from a diseased uterus.

> *Indications for ultrasonography of the ovaries include monitoring the oestrus cycle (see Follicular Maturation, Ovulation and Corpus Luteum Formation with Oestrus and Fertility Monitoring, page 248) as well as all reproductive disorders in the bitch with suspected:*
>
> - Ovarian cysts.
> - Ovarian tumours.
>
> A further indication is for monitoring treatment response.

586

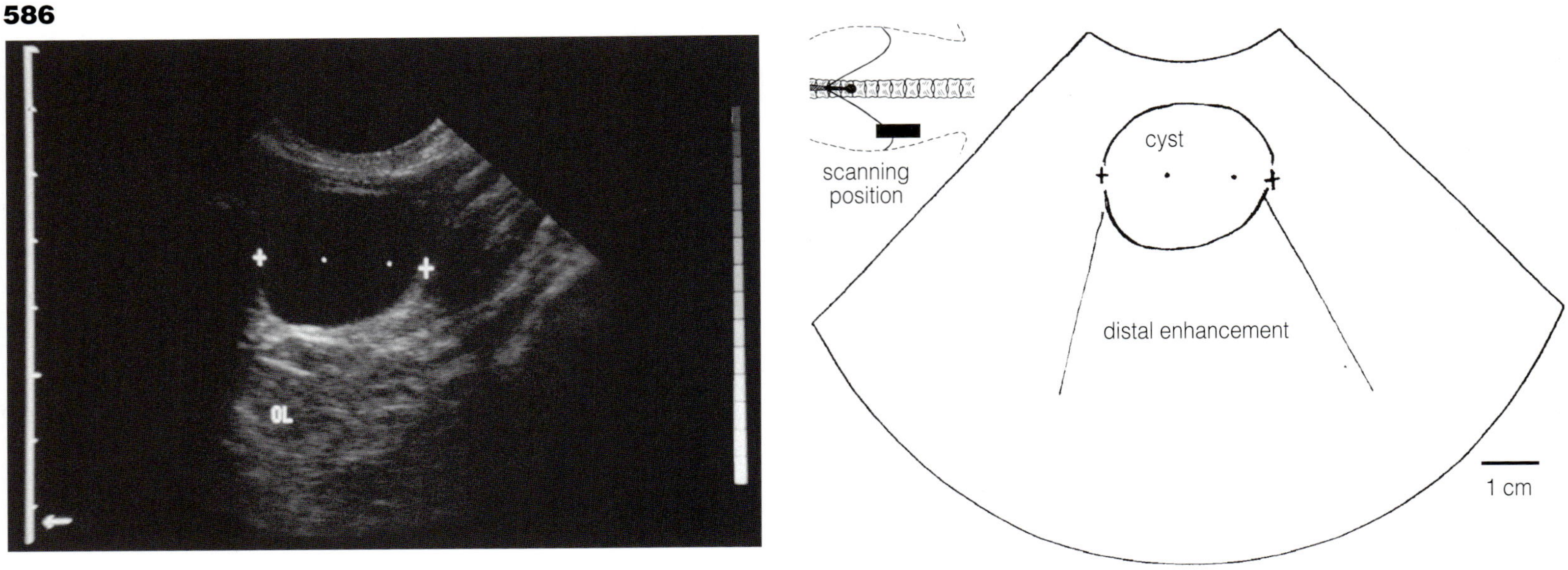

587

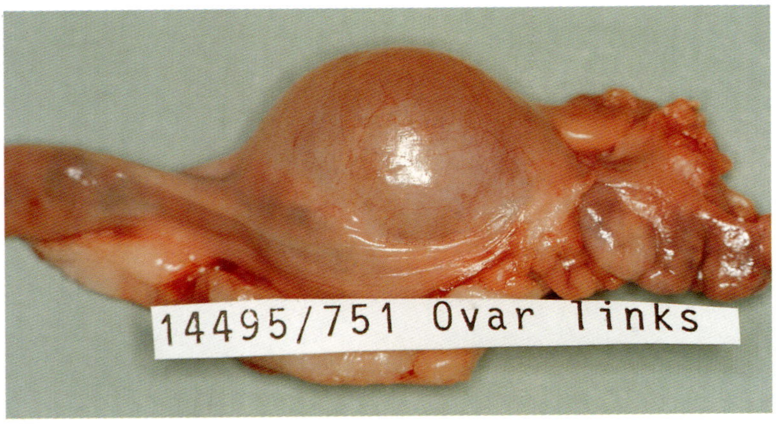

586, 587 Two-dimensional sonogram (**586**) and pathological specimen (**587**) of a canine ovary and uterus. Anechoic round mass with distal enhancement caudal to the right kidney (**586**). Because of the shape and location, an ovarian cyst was diagnosed. Final diagnosis was a pseudocyst in the uterine horn (**587**).

588

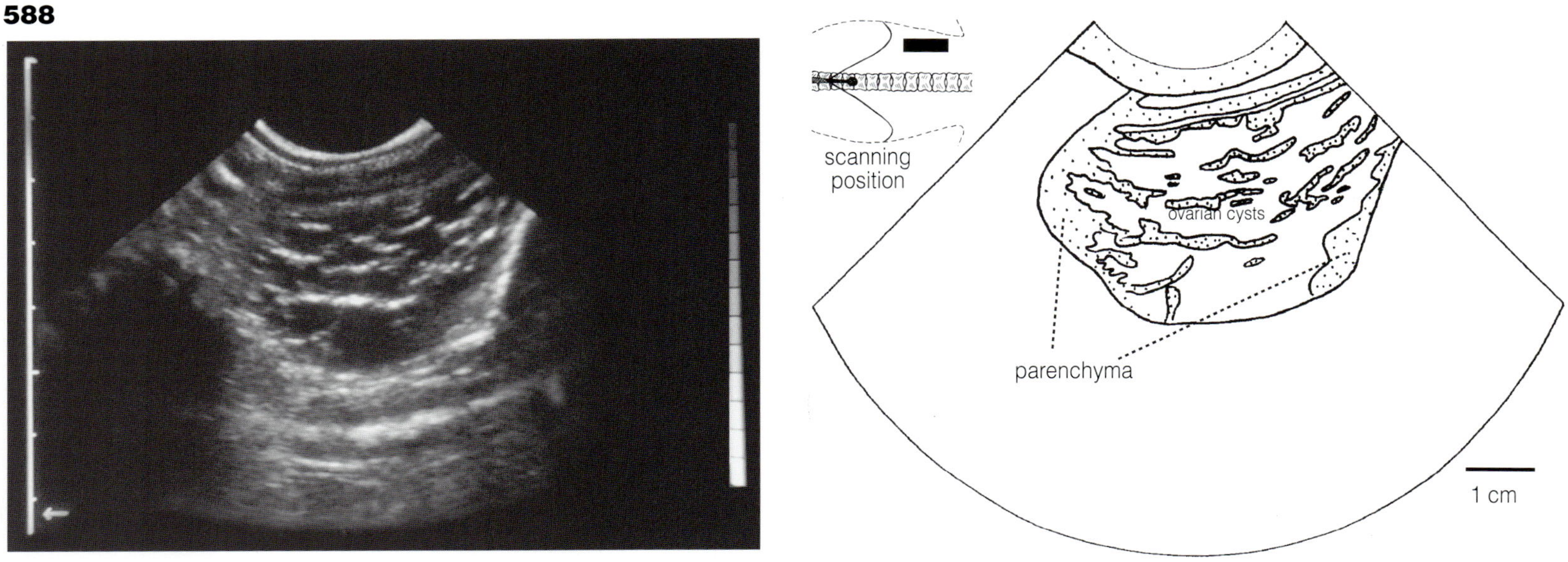

588 Cystic ovary in a bitch. The small, demarcated and septated mass lesions with surrounding tissue indicate an ovarian tumour. Differential diagnosis includes cystic tumours of another origin.

Differential diagnosis of ovarian cysts should include all fluid-filled structures, since cystic structures are often difficult to associate with a particular organ (**586, 587**). A fluid-filled uterus or bowel loop must be ruled out by history, ultrasonography in various planes and visualization of a wall. The differential diagnosis of a multicystic ovary with a large amount of tissue must always include a tumour (**588**)[15].

Ovarian Tumours

Ovarian tumours are well-demarcated from the surrounding tissue. Echogenicity may vary. The internal architecture may be complex and contain hypoechoic as well as hyperechoic areas (**589, 590**). Hyperechoic, solid masses are also seen. The tumours may be unilateral or bilateral. Large ovarian tumours may shift to another location because of their weight. Other mass lesions must be ruled out.

589

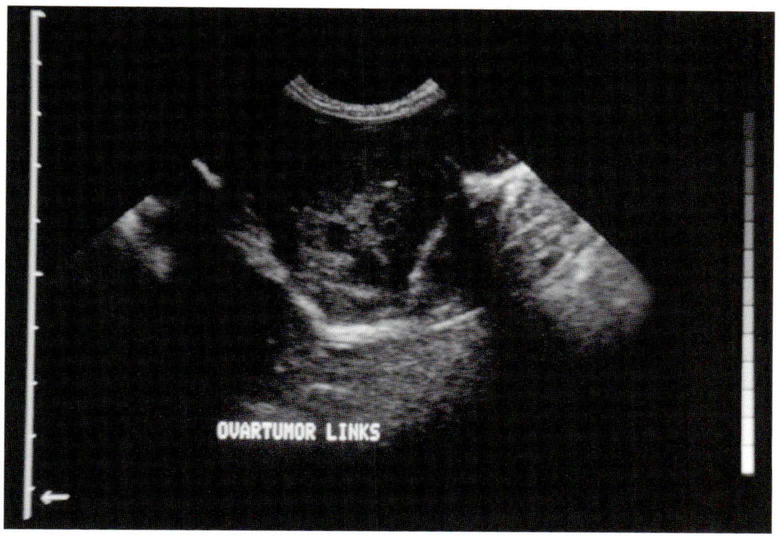

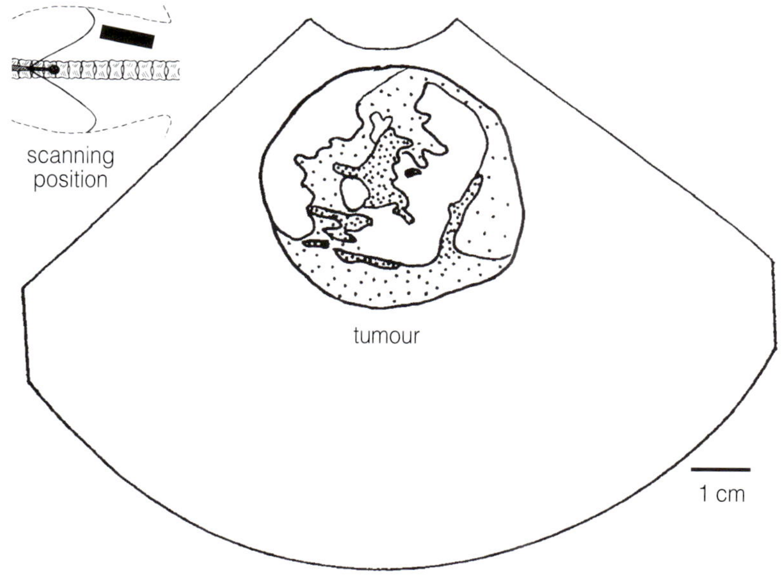

590

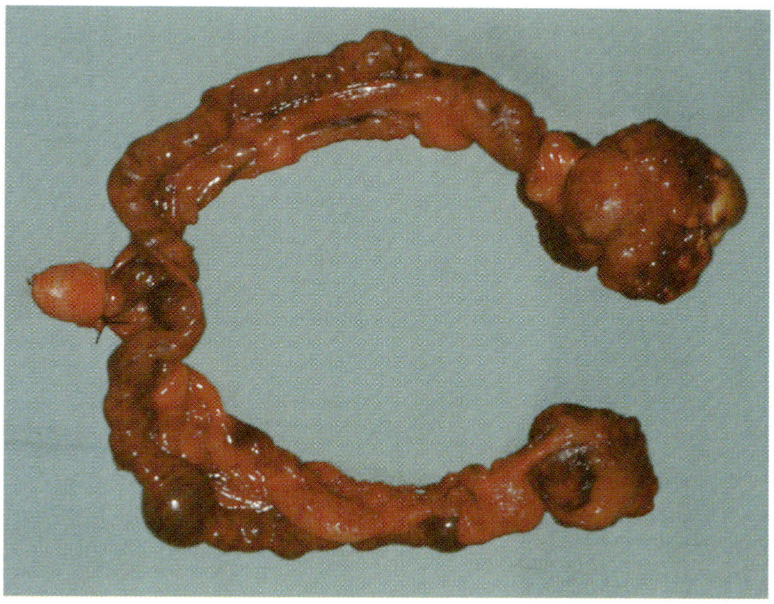

589, 590 Two-dimensional sonogram (**589**) and pathological specimen (**590**) of a canine ovary and uterus. Ovarian tumour in the shape of a small, irregular, well-demarcated mass caudal to the left kidney.

References

1 Andersen AC and Simpson ME (1973) *The Ovary and Reproductive Cycle of the Dog (Beagle)*. Geron-X Inc., Los Altos, California.

2 Barr FJ (1992) Das Ovar. In: Barr FJ: *Ultraschalldiagnostik bei Hand und Katze*. Gustav Fischer Verlag, Stuttgart, Jena, New York.

3 Boyd JS, Reton RP, Harvey MJ, Nixon D, Eckersall PD and Ferguson JM (1993) Problems associated with ultrasonography of the canine ovary aroand the time of ovulation. *J. Reprod. Fert.* **Suppl. 47**, 101–105.

4 Concannon PW, Hasel W and McEntee K (1977) Changes in LH, progesterone and sexual behaviour with preovulatory luteinization in the bitch. *Biol. Reprod.* **17**, 604–613.

5 Dieterich J (1994) *Anwendung der Sonographie zum Direkten Ovulationsnachweis and zur Erhebung Zyklischer Ovarbefande bei der Hündin*. Hannover, Tierärztl. Hochsch., Diss.

6 Dieterich J, Günzel-Apel A-R and Hoppen H-O (1994) Ultrasonographische Ovulationsdiagnostik bei der Hündin. *Reprod. Dom. Anim.* **Suppl. 3**, 261.

7 England GCW and Allen WE (1989) Real-time ultrasonic imaging of the ovary and uterus of the dog. *J. Reprod. Fert.* **Suppl. 39**, 91–100.

8 England GCW and Yeager AE (1993) Ultrasonographic appearance of the ovary and uterus of the bitch during oestrus, ovulation and early pregnancy. *J. Reprod. Fert.* **Suppl. 47**, 107–117.

9 Hayer P (1991) *Untersuchungen zur Sonographischen Darstellbarkeit der Follikelreifung, Ovulation und Gelbkörperanbildung beim Hand*. Hannover, Tierärztl. Hochsch., Diss.

10 Hayer P, Günzel-Apel A-R, Lüerssen D and Hoppen H-O (1993) Ultrasonographic monitoring of follicular development, ovulation and early luteal phase in the bitch. *J. Reprod. Fert.* **Suppl. 47**, 93–100.

11 Holst P and Phemister RD (1975) Temporal sequence of events in the estrous cycle of the bitch. *Am.J. Vet.Res.* **36**, 705–706.

12 Linde-Forsberg C and Forsberg M (1989) Fertility in dogs in relation to semen quality and the time and site of insemination with fresh and frozen semen. *J. Reprod. Fert.* **Suppl. 39**, 299–310.

13 Lüerssen D (1992) Untersuchung zur sonographischen Darstellbarkeit des Handeovars. *Kleintierpraxis* **37**, 809–816.

14 Lüerssen D (1994) Ultraschalldiagnostik des weiblichen Genitals des Handes. *Kleintierpraxis* **39**, 539–552.

15 Peter AT and Jakovljevic S (1992) Real-time ultrasonography of the small animal reproductive organs. *Compend. Contin. Educ. Pract. Vet.* **14**, 739–747.

16 Poffenbarger EM and Feeney DA (1986) Use of gray-scale ultrasonography in the diagnosis of reproductive disease in the bitch: 18 cases (1981–1984). *J. Am. Vet. Med. Assoc.* **189**, 90–95.

17 Renton JP, Boyd JS, Harvey MJ, Ferguson JM, Nickson DA and Eckersall PD (1992) Comparison of endocrine changes and ultrasound as means of identifying ovulation in the bitch. *Res. Vet. Sci.* **53**, 74–79.

18 Shille VM and Stabenfeldt GH (1980) Current concepts in reproduction of the dog and cat. *Adv. Vet. Sci. Comp. Med.* **24**, 211–243.

19 Tsutsui T (1989) Gamete physiology and timing of ovulation and fertilization in dogs. *J. Reprod. Fert.* **Suppl. 39**, 169–175.

20 Tsutsui T and Shimizu T (1975) Studies on the reproduction in the dog. IV: On the fertile period of the ovum after ovulation. *Jap. J. Anim. Reprod.* **21**, 65–69.

21 Wallace SS, Mahaffey MB, Miller DM, Thompson FN and Chakraborty PK (1992) Ultrasonographic appearance of the ovaries of dogs during the follicular and luteal phases of the estrus cycle. *Am. J. Vet. Res.* **53**, 209–215.

Uterus and Vagina

Dirk Lüerssen and Martin Janthur

Instrumentation and Examination Technique

Ultrasound is used to evaluate the normal, gravid and diseased uterus. The following sections deal with ultrasonography of the non-gravid uterus. Pregnancy diagnosis, birth and the postpartum uterus are discussed in Normal Pregnancy, page 290; Early Pregnancy, page 293; Parturition, page 312; Postpartum Uterus, page 313.

Because of the elongated shape of the bicornuate uterus, the patient's hair coat should be clipped extensively before the examination. The patient is positioned in dorsal or lateral recumbency. The standing patient is examined caudoventral to the last rib.

The normal vagina cannot be examined via a transabdominal approach because of the interfering pelvic bone. The proximal part of the vagina may be identified, if it is not shadowed by bone. Transrectal or transvaginal transducers may be employed, although simpler methods such as direct visualization or vaginal cytology are usually used.

The normal genital tract in the female cat requires the use of high-frequency 7.5–13 MHz transducers for a detailed image (see **515**).

The following descriptions of normal organs are limited to the dog.

Anatomy and Normal Sonographic Findings

The normal uterus is often identified by its body after one or more oestrous cycles. The cervix is seen with good visualization of the uterine body. The juvenile uterus is not seen when transducers lower than 7.5 MHz are used[1]. The uterine size increases as the animal gets older, after previous pregnancies and during the oestrous cycle (**591**).

A full urinary bladder facilitates the examination[6, 7]. The uterine body is identified through this acoustic window, ventral to the rectum. In some cases the uterine body may be displaced lateral to the bladder. With high-resolution transducers, the uterine horns are seen lateral and dorsal to the distended bladder. The uterine horns can occasionally be followed along the left or right abdominal wall, ending caudal to the respective kidney (**592**).The spleen may be used as an acoustic window to visualize the left uterine horn (**593**). Visualization of the bifurcation helps to identify the uterus (**594**). For this purpose the uterine body is followed cranially, until the uterine horns divide.

The uterine wall layers cannot usually be differentiated. The echo pattern is finely textured and moderately echogenic to hypoechoic. During oestrus, the uterine body and horns show oedematous swelling and decreased echogenicity and are easier to recognize (**594**).

The transition from a normal to a diseased uterus is usually not apparent.

Ultrasonography of Uterine Disease

Indications for ultrasonography of the uterus include oestrous cycle disorders, vaginal discharge, polydipsia, leucocytosis, as well as non-specific symptoms associated with the abdomen with suspected:

- Endometritis–pyometra complex.
- Postsurgical complications.
- Uterine cysts.
- Uterine tumours.

A further indication is for monitoring treatment response.

Endometritis–Pyometra Complex

Endometritis

Ultrasonographic diagnosis of endometritis with only a slightly enlarged uterus is difficult. Decreased echogenicity of the uterus is usually noticed. The parenchyma is finely textured and homogenous. As the disease progresses, an increased non-homogenicity of

591

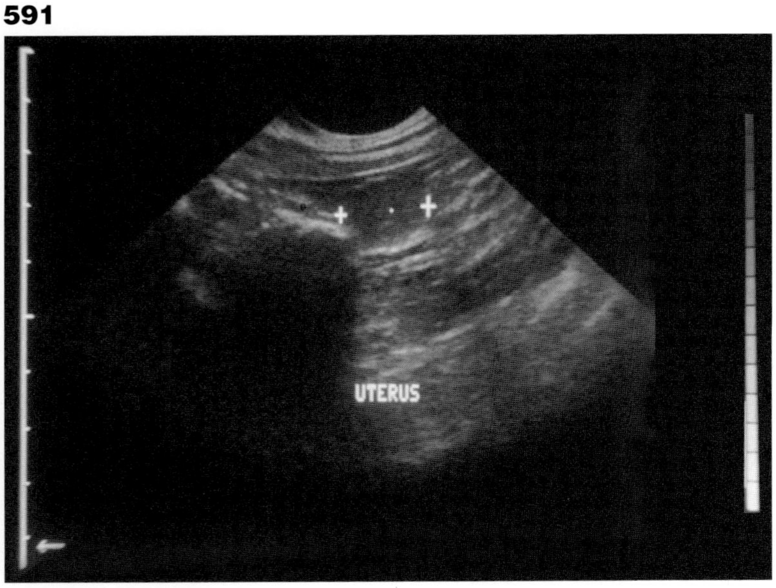

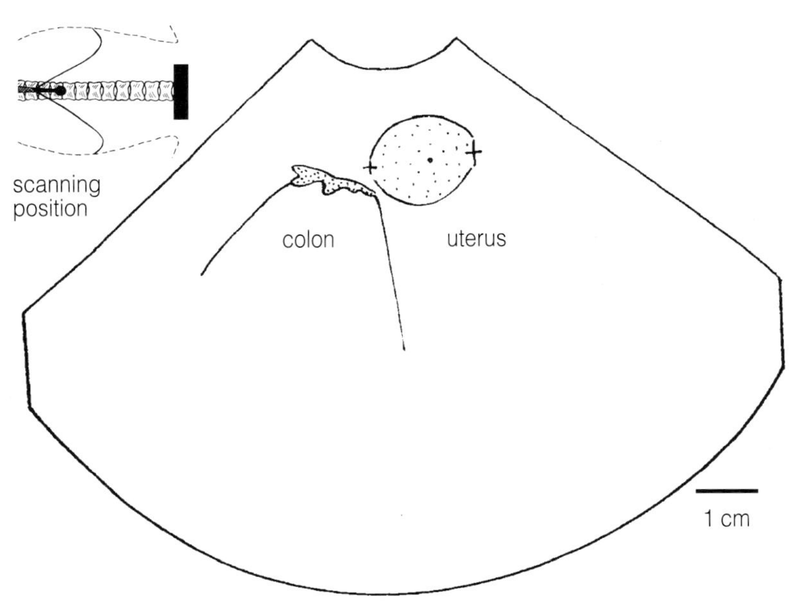

591 Canine uterine body in anoestrus. The transverse uterine body is 1.7 cm in diameter. This is a normal finding in large-breed dogs after the first oestrous cycle. A uterine lumen is not visible.

592

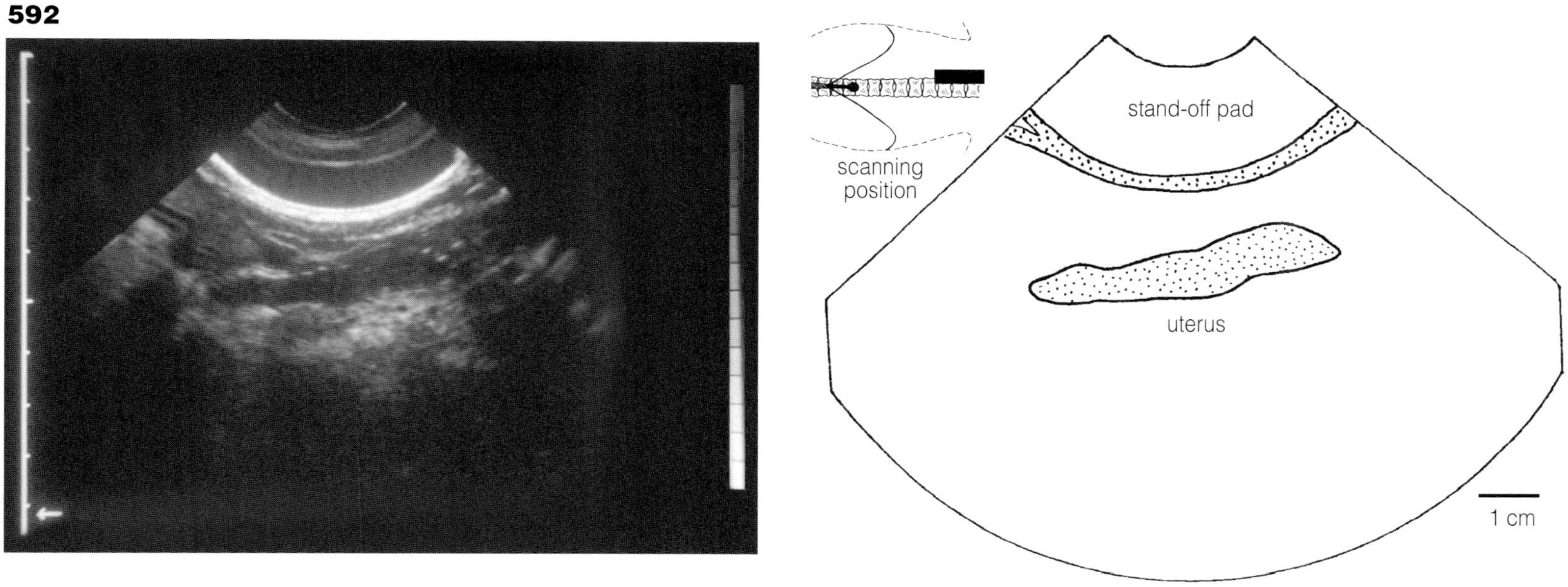

593

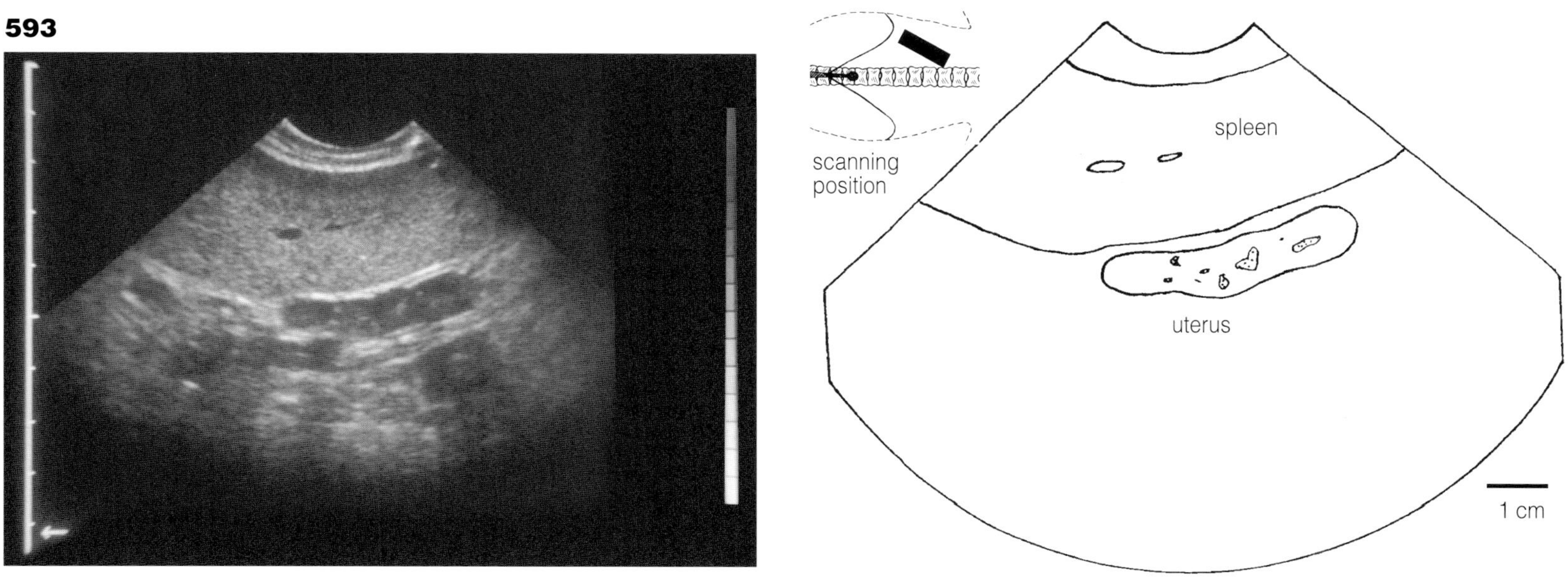

592, 593 Normal uterine horns in a longitudinal view in two bitches. While the uterine horn is homogenous and slightly echogenic in the first bitch (**592**), the second bitch shows a hypoechoic rim and a more echogenic inner architecture (**593**). Similar images are seen during the oestrous cycle, with a postpartum uterus, or with early endometritis.

594

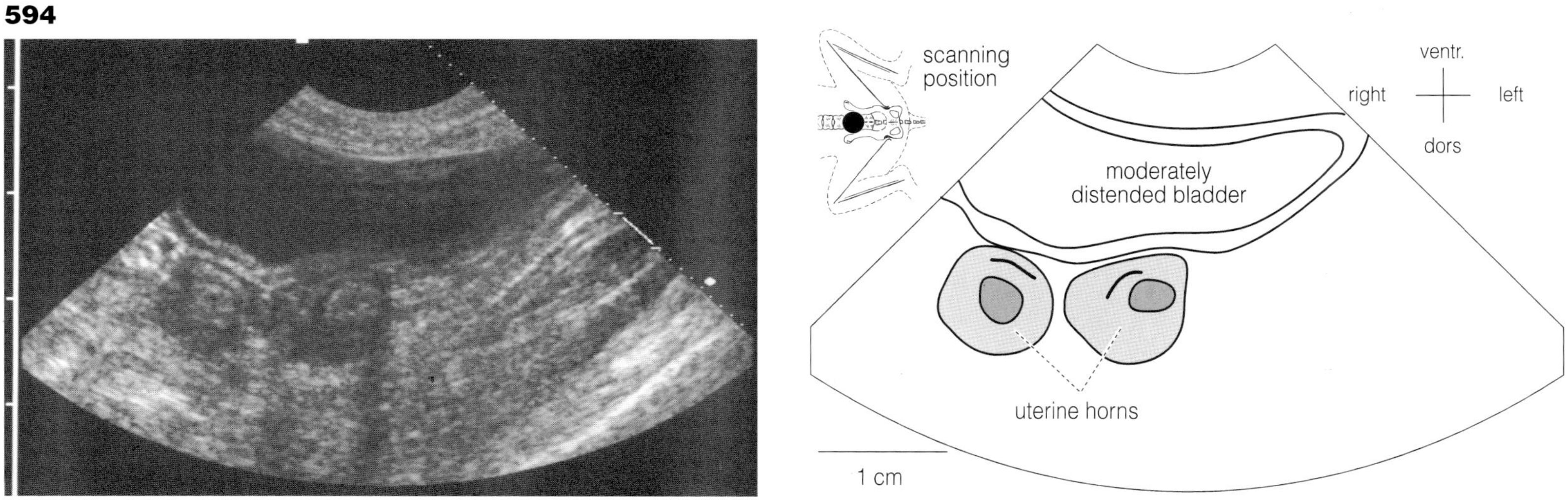

594 Normal uterine horns of a bitch in heat directly cranial to the bifurcation in a transverse view.

595

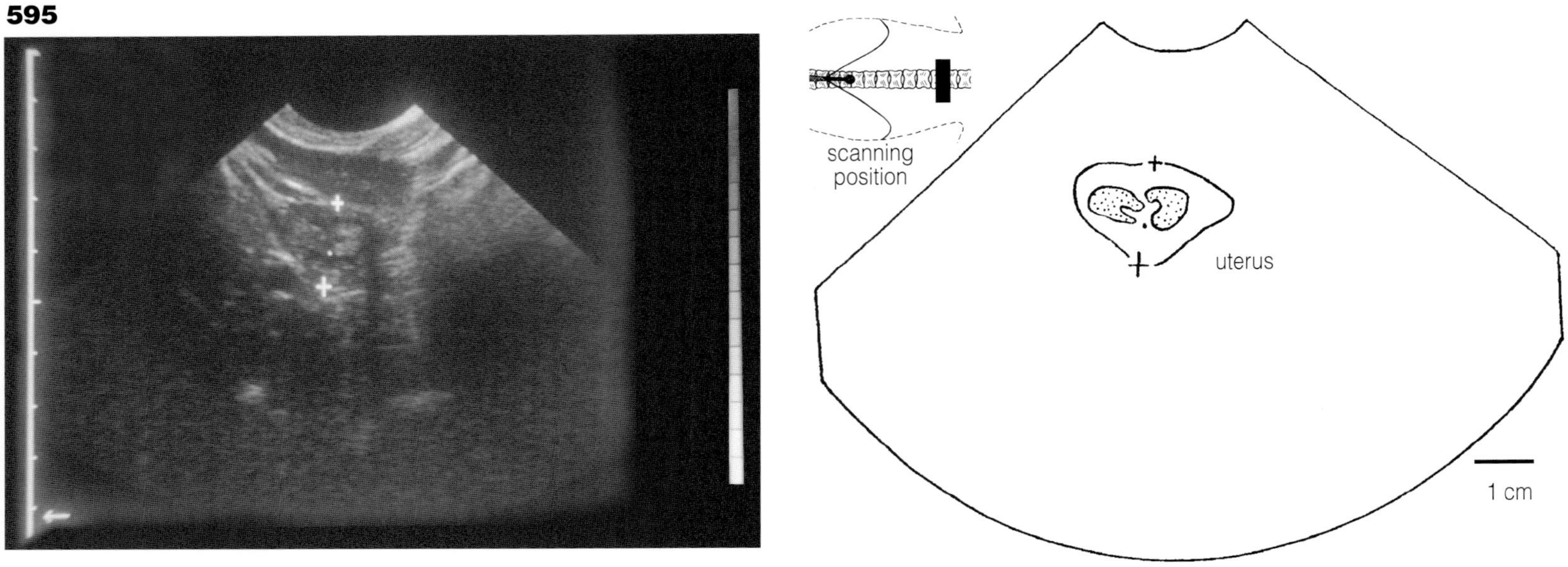

596

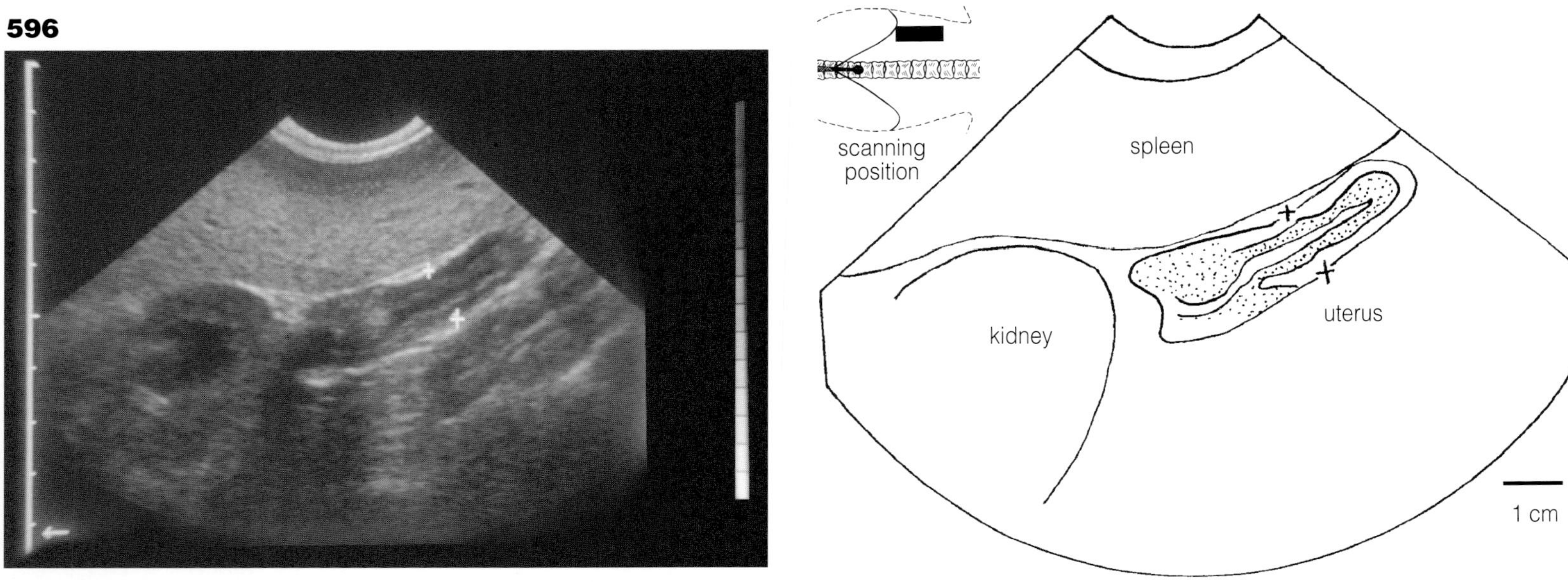

595, 596 Endometritis in a small dog in a transverse (**595**) and longitudinal (**596**) view. The transverse uterine body (**595**) has a heterogenous echo pattern and is relatively large for a small dog with a diameter of 1.7 cm. The anechoic lumen is barely visible. The left uterine horn in a longitudinal view (**596**) shows an anechoic lumen in contrast to the hyperechoic endometrium.

597

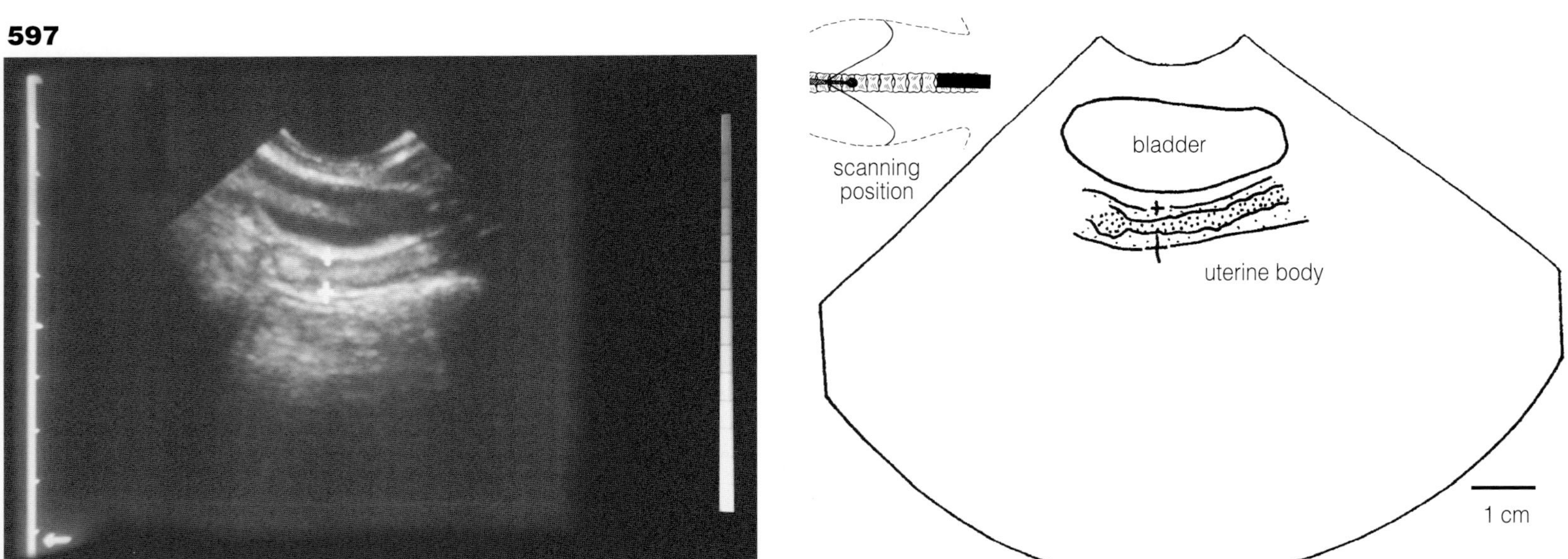

597 Early endometritis in a dog. The uterine body in a longitudinal view is clearly visible through the acoustic bladder window. A hypoechoic rim surrounds a hyperechoic centre. The lumen is more echogenic than in **594**. This indicates a pathological finding. Early endometritis can only be differentiated from a normal uterus during oestrus or from an early postpartum uterus in conjunction with history and a clinical examination.

598

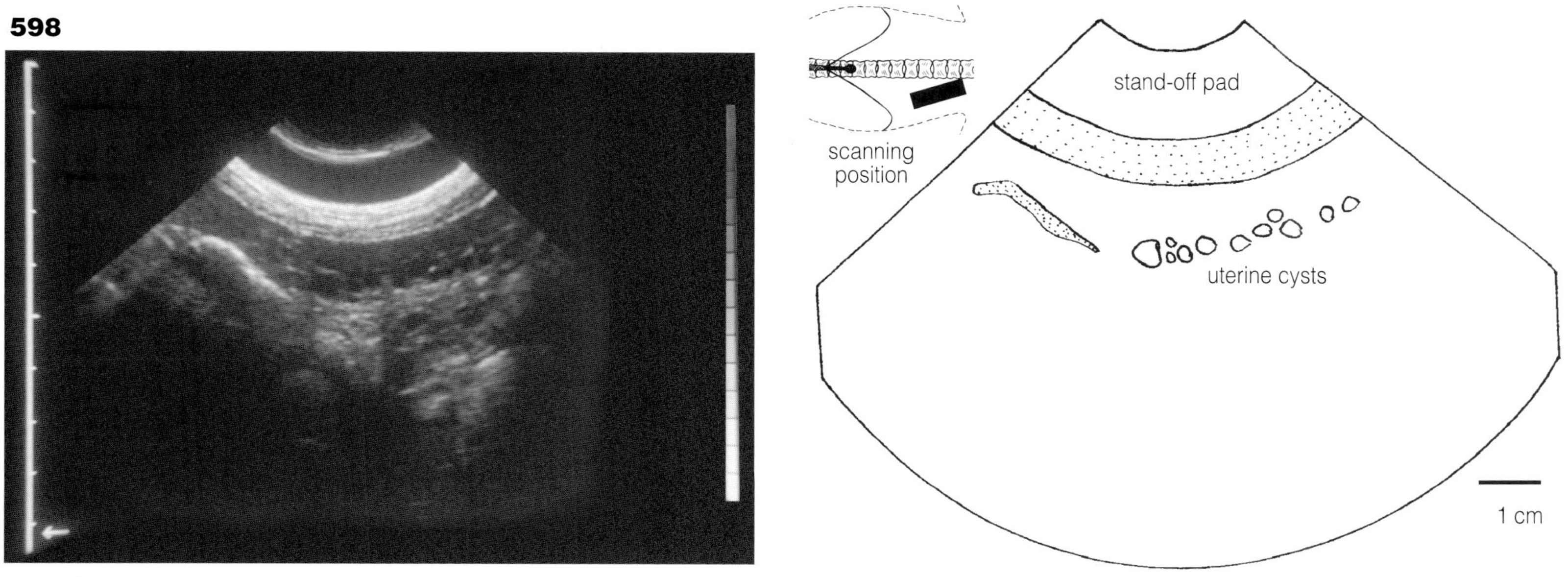

598 Glandular cystic endometritis in a dog. The right uterine horn adjacent to the abdominal wall shows a row of small, anechoic, round foci. (Sector transducers require a stand-off pad to visualize these superficial organ lesions).

599

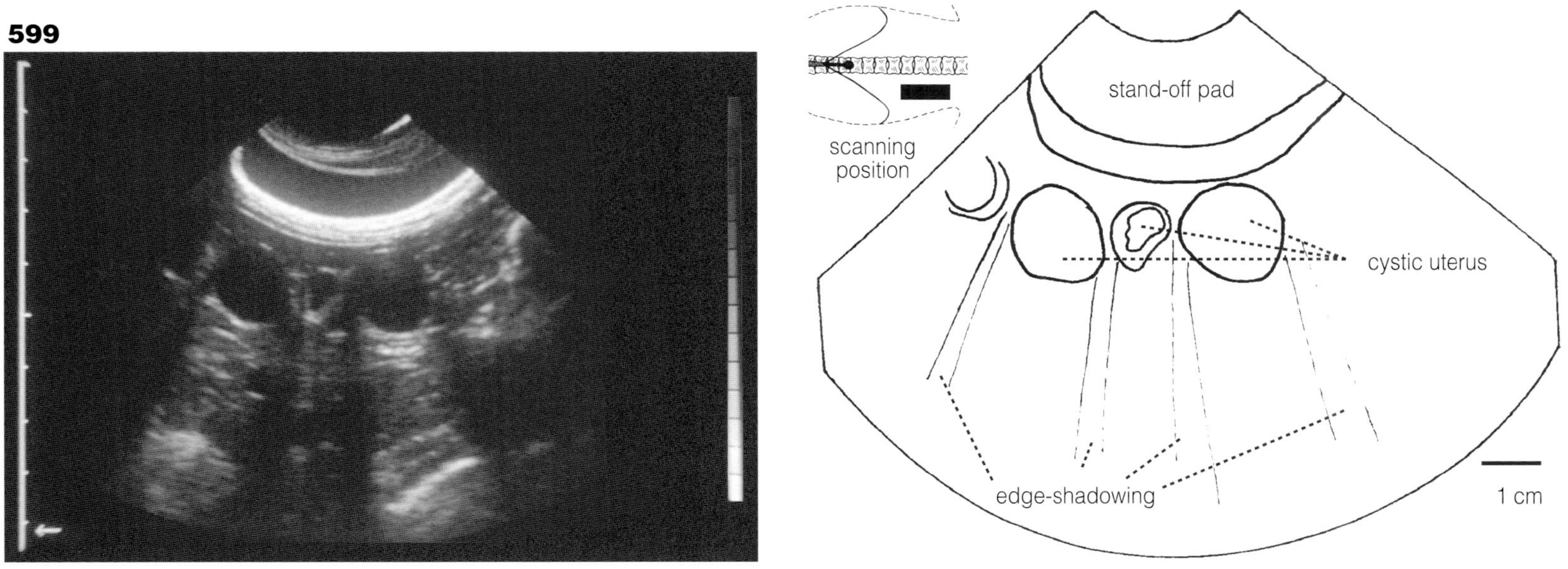

599 Glandular cystic endometritis in a dog. The right uterine horn adjacent to the abdominal wall shows a row of large anechoic, round foci. (Sector transducers require a stand-off pad to visualize these superficial organ lesions).

the echo pattern is not unusual (**595, 596**). Early-stage endometritis cannot be differentiated from a normal uterus or a uterus during oestrus (**597**).

As the uterus becomes larger, endometritis is easier to diagnose. The sonographic image may vary. Cystic, anechoic structures or more hyperechoic areas are seen in the uterine parenchyma. An anechoic or hypoechoic lumen may be distinguished as an fine line.

Glandular-cystic hyperplasia is seen as anechoic, round islets in the endometrium (**598–600**). In some rare cases the uterine parenchyma cannot be distinguished between the cysts (**598**). Conservative treatment should not be used with glandular-cystic hyperplasia.

Pyometra, Hydrometra, Haemometra and Mucometra

Pyometra, hydrometra, haemometra and mucometra are easier to diagnose than endometritis as the lumen contains more fluid. Ultrasonographic differentiation of the contents and each individual disease is only partially possible.

The echogenicity of the uterine contents with **pyometra** ranges from anechoic to 'textured' or hyperechoic (**601–607**). The number of cells or viscosity of the luminal contents do not always correlate with a certain echogenicity. The uterine contents may show areas of varying echogenicity (**605**). The fluid can mimic parenchymal texture[4]. This form of pyometra cannot be differentiated from endometrial hyperplasia.

600

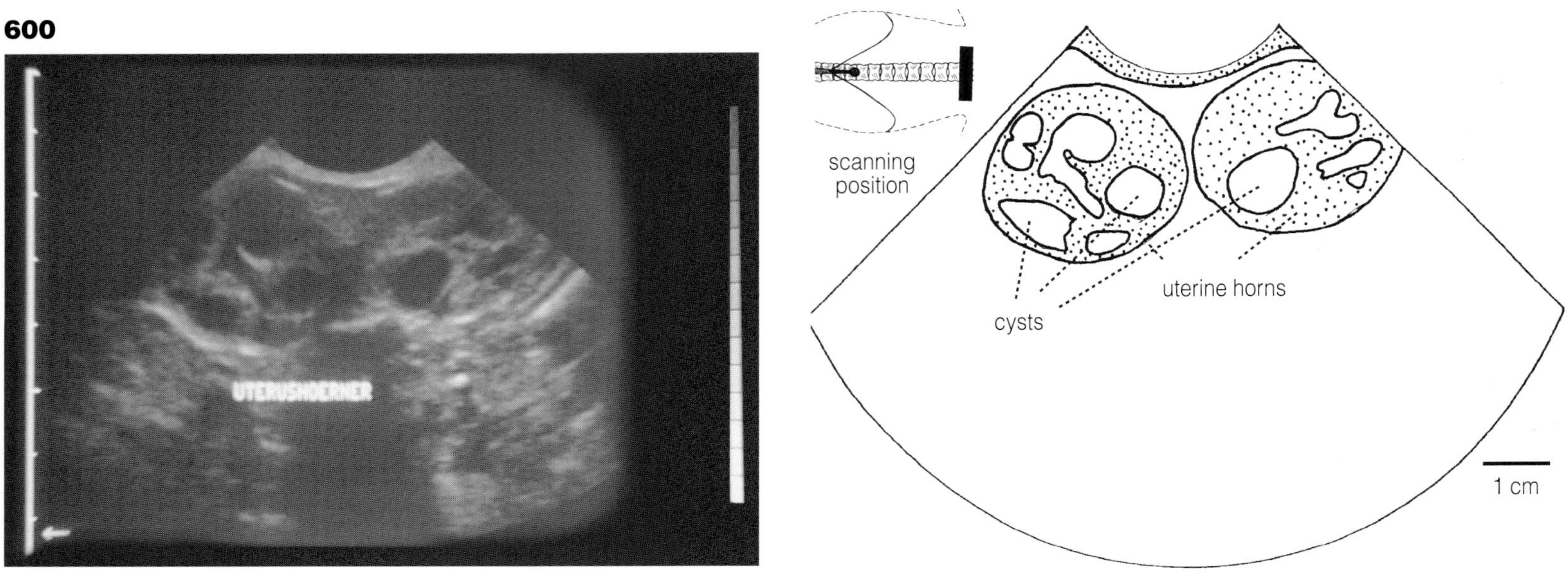

600 Glandular cystic endometritis in a dog. Both transverse uterine horns are non-homogenous and show multiple anechoic foci within the parenchyma.

601

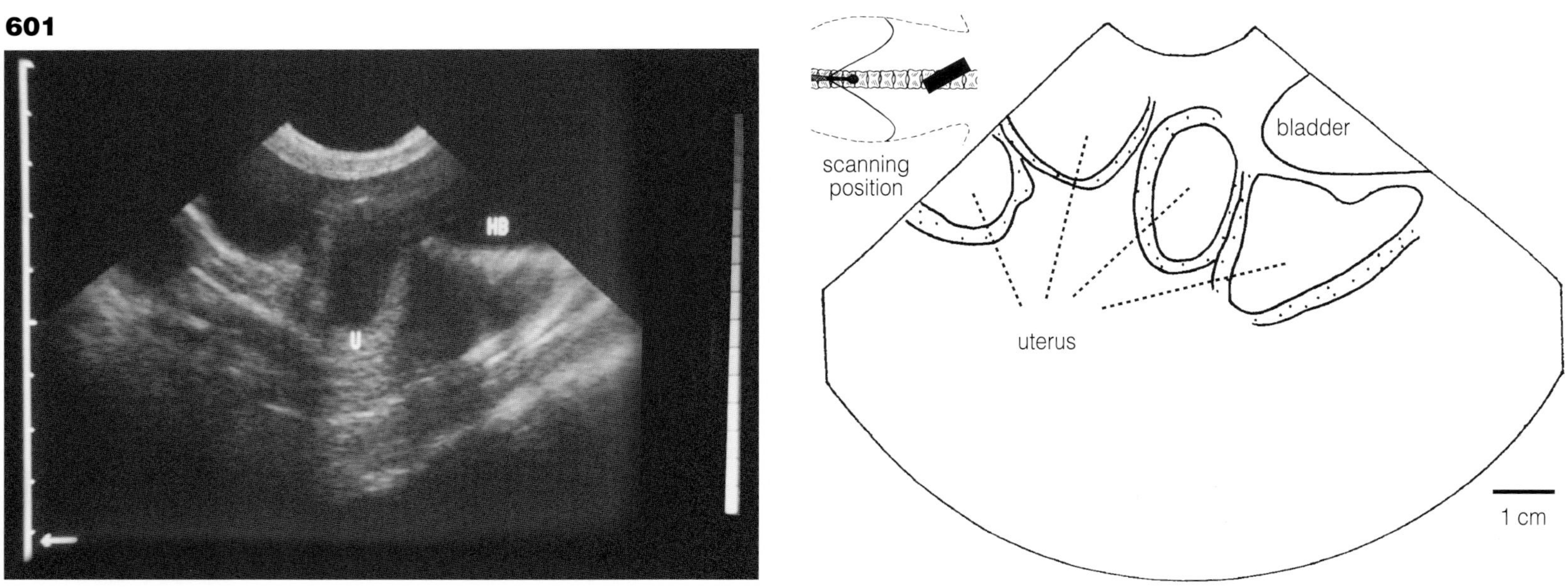

601 Pyometra in a dog. The pus-filled uterus is often seen as anechoic round structures dorsal, lateral and cranial to the bladder. Differential diagnosis includes intestinal atony.

602

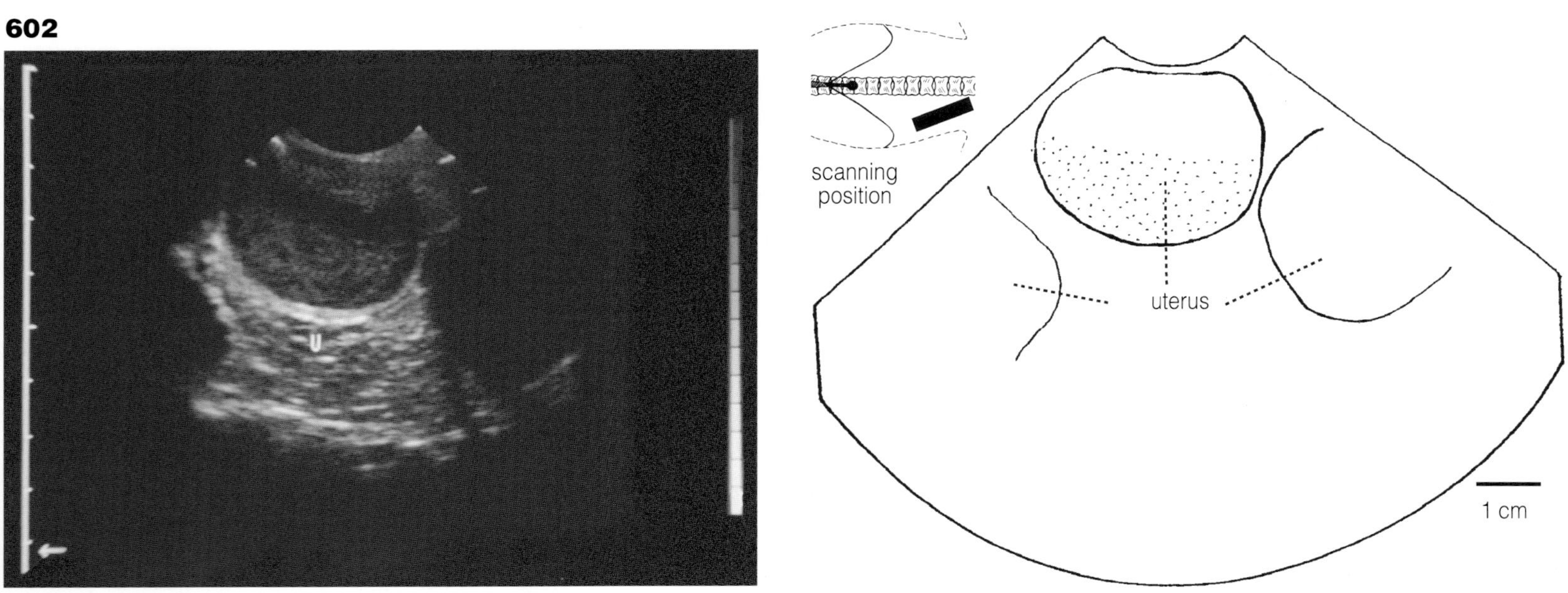

602 Pyometra in a dog. The three segments of the pus-filled uterus can be connected in real-time ultrasonography. The contents vary from anechoic to finely granulated and hypoechoic.

603

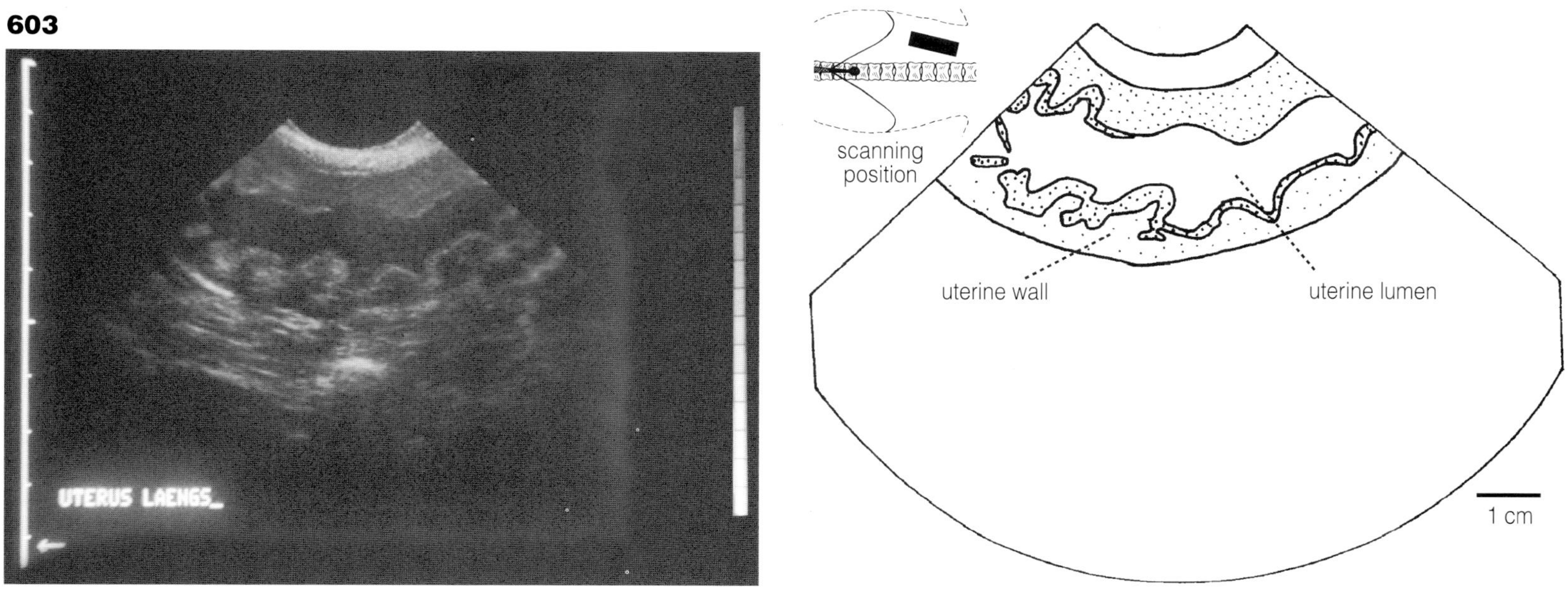

603 Pyometra in a dog. The thickened wall and anechoic lumen are seen in a longitudinal view. The wall appears non-homogenous with an irregular inner surface.

604

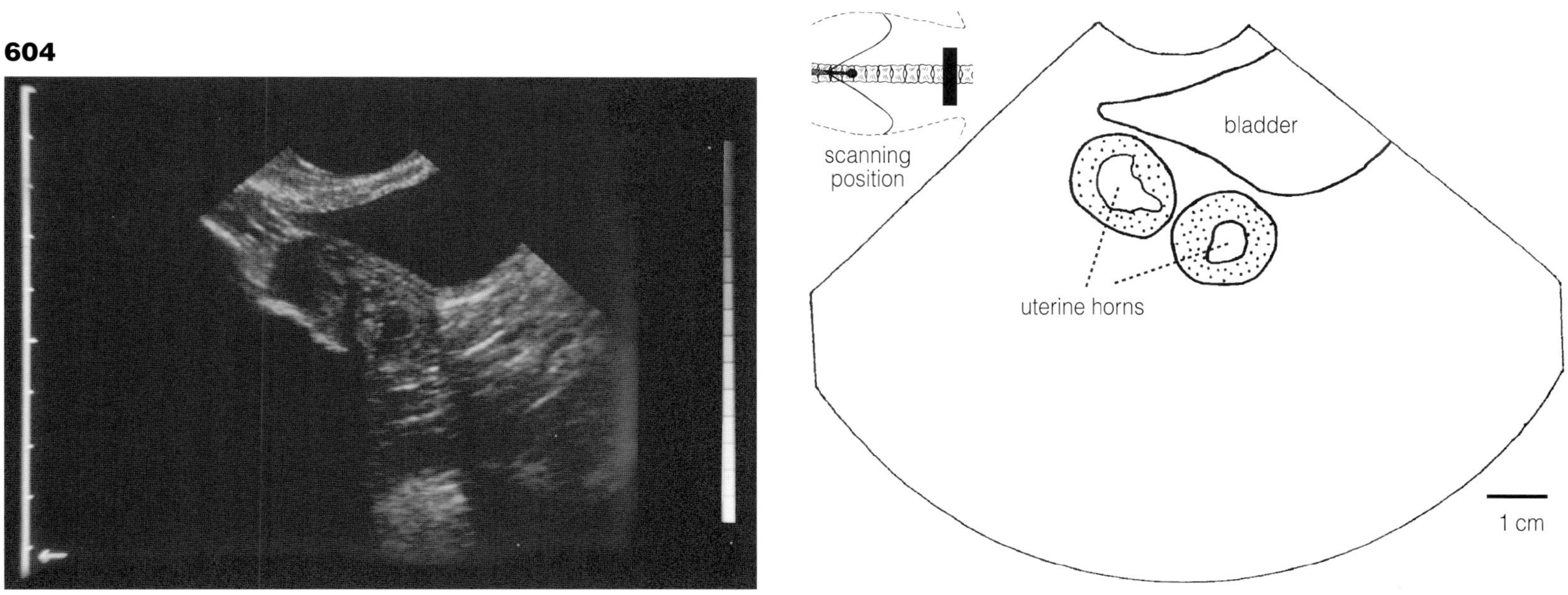

604 Pyometra in a dog. Transverse view of the uterine horns with a thickened wall and anechoic lumen dorsal to the bladder.

605

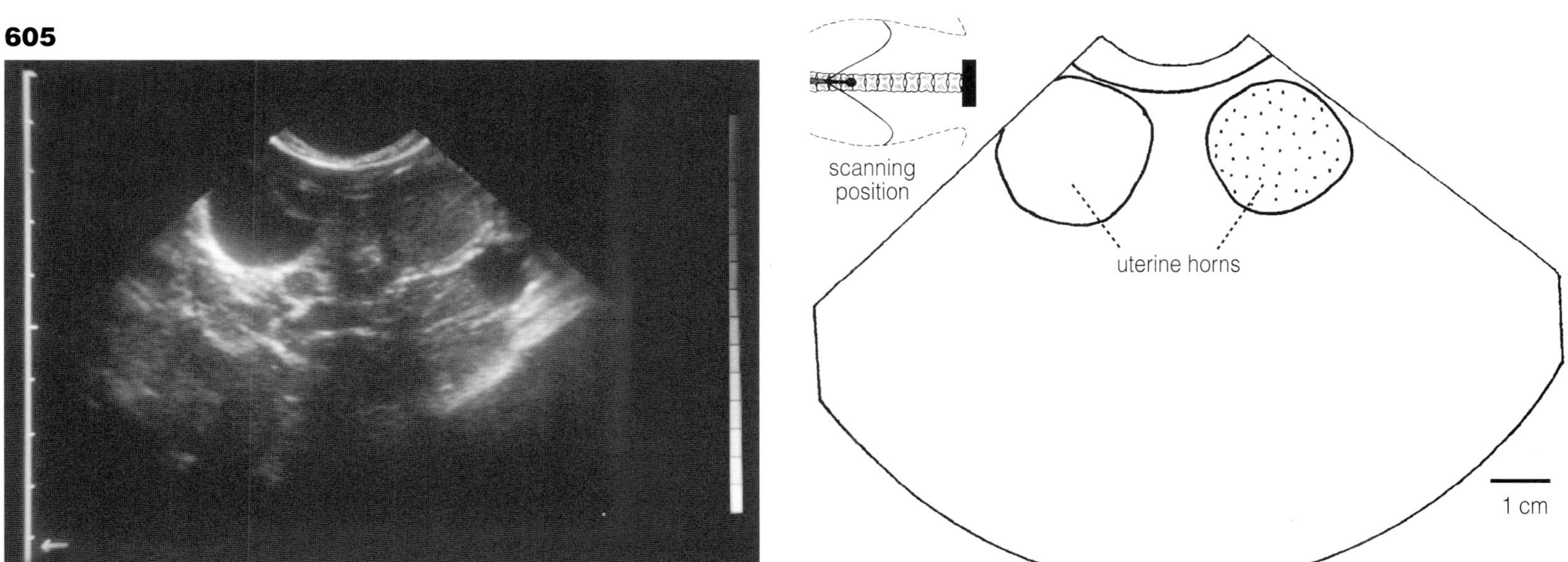

605 Pyometra in a dog. Transverse view of the uterine horns with a thin wall and a mixed echogenic lumen.

606

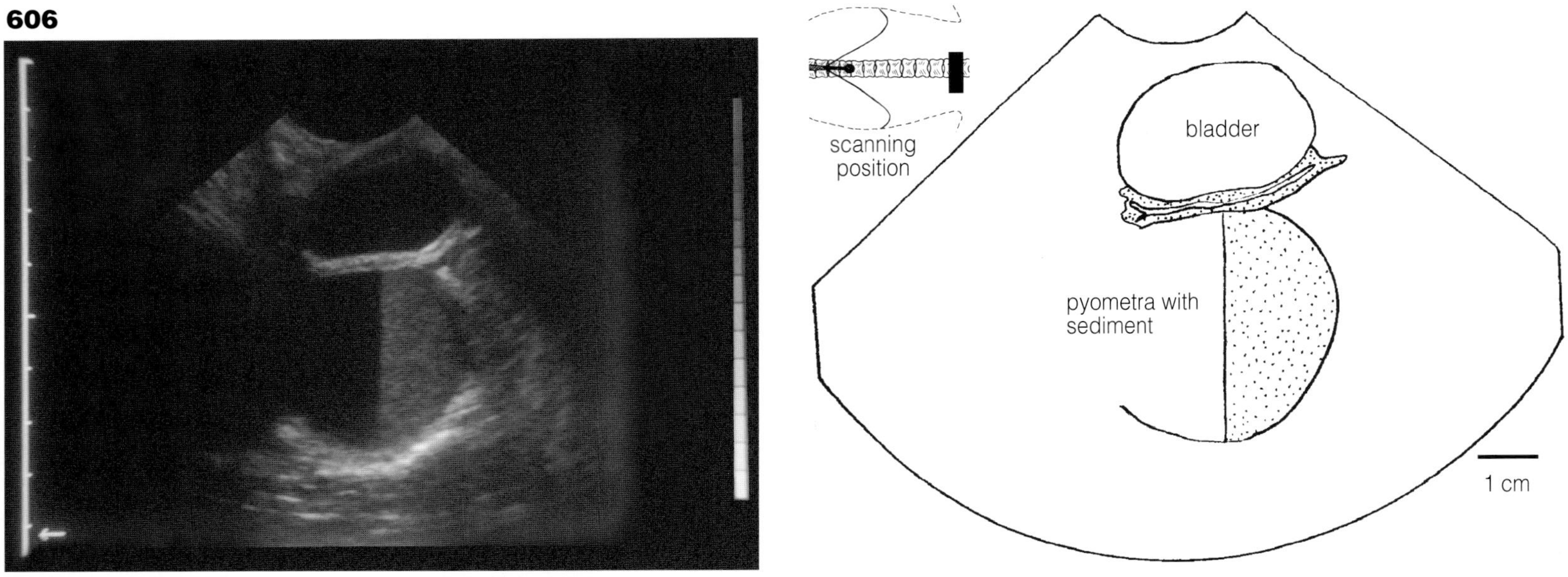

606 Pyometra with abnormal sediment in a dog. The animal was in lateral recumbency with the transducer applied to the ventral abdominal wall. A large round structure with sediment is seen distal to the anechoic bladder. Differential diagnosis includes a fluid-filled bowel with sediment.

607

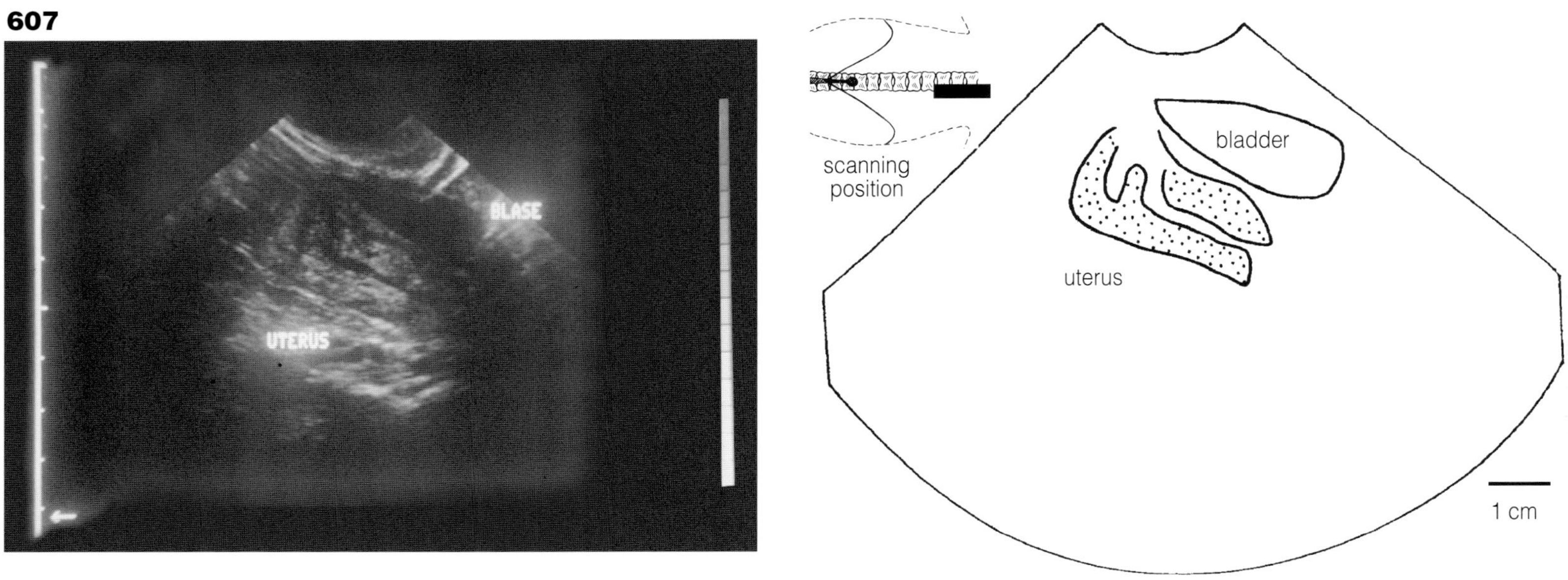

607 Pyometra in a cat. The longitudinal uterus shows wall thickening and a narrow fluid-filled lumen.

The entire uterus must be scanned to detect local lesions. The lumen of the uterus may be enlarged in its entirety or focally[2]. The tortuous uterine horns often do not have a fluid-filled tubular appearance in a longitudinal plane. Round, fluid-filled cavities are seen and these are produced by multiple views through the uterine horn (**607**). The uterine wall should be evaluated in its entirety as it may vary segmentally.

Ultrasonographic monitoring of conservative therapy should include measuring the uterine lumen as well as evaluating wall thickness. Measurements should only be made with the sound beam perpendicular to the uterine wall.

Differential diagnoses include other diseases of the endometritis–pyometra complex (**608**), blood vessels and fluid-filled bowel loops. Arterial vessels are recognized by their pulsations, while veins are identified by small echoes caused by blood flow. Blood vessels characteristically have a uniform lumen and/or branching and bifurcation[3]. Fluid-filled bowel loops may be difficult to differentiate, especially in the large bowel area (**609**).

A gas-filled uterus shows shadowing of the sound waves distal to the near uterine wall. In conjunction with a thin wall, the uterus may be mistaken for small or large intestines. In these cases, survey radiographs are more accurate.

Hydrometra is recognized by an anechoic lumen and a thin uterine wall (**610–612**). This rare disease is seen more frequently than pyometra in the cat.

Compared to hydrometra, **haemometra** has identical anechoic contents with a distinctly thicker wall. As the disease progresses, the luminal contents become more non-homogenous and echogenic. Ultrasonographic differentiation from pyometra is not possible.

Mucometra cannot be differentiated from other diseases of the endometritis–pyometra complex.

608

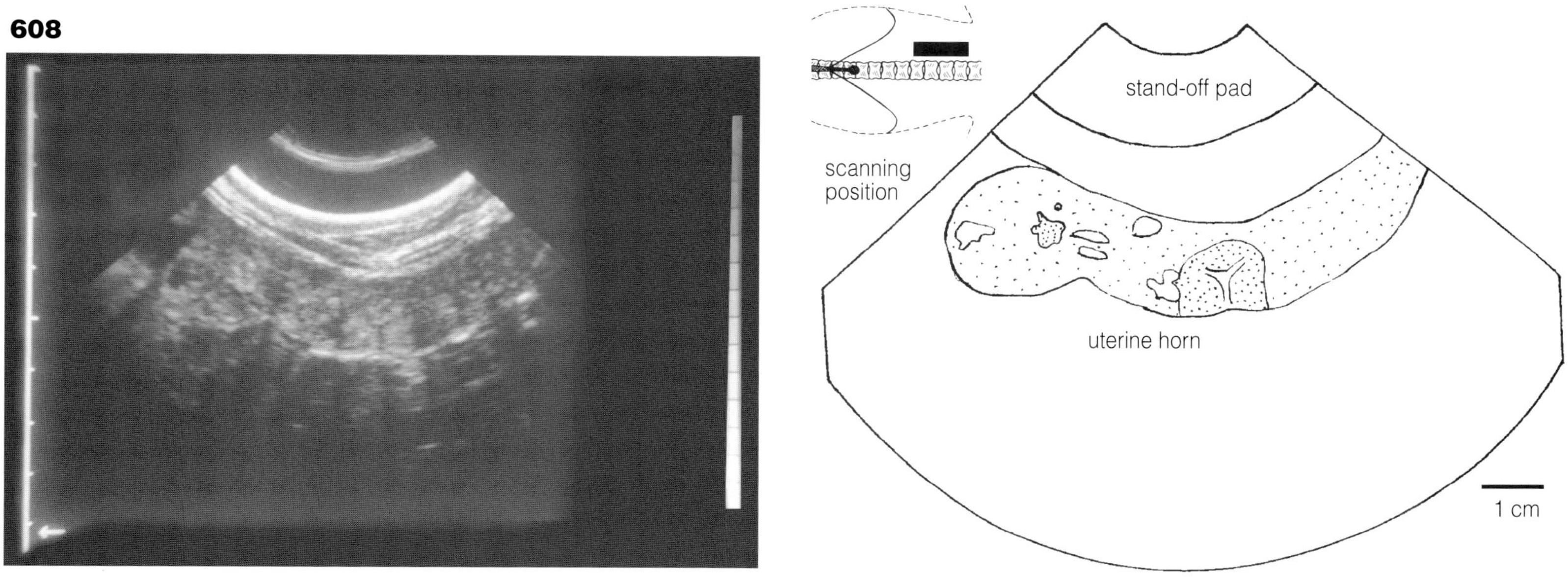

608 Endometritis–pyometra complex in a dog. A tubular, non-homogenous mass is seen to the left and right in the abdomen. Histopathology revealed an autolytic–necrotising placenta with complete atrophy of the endometrium.

609

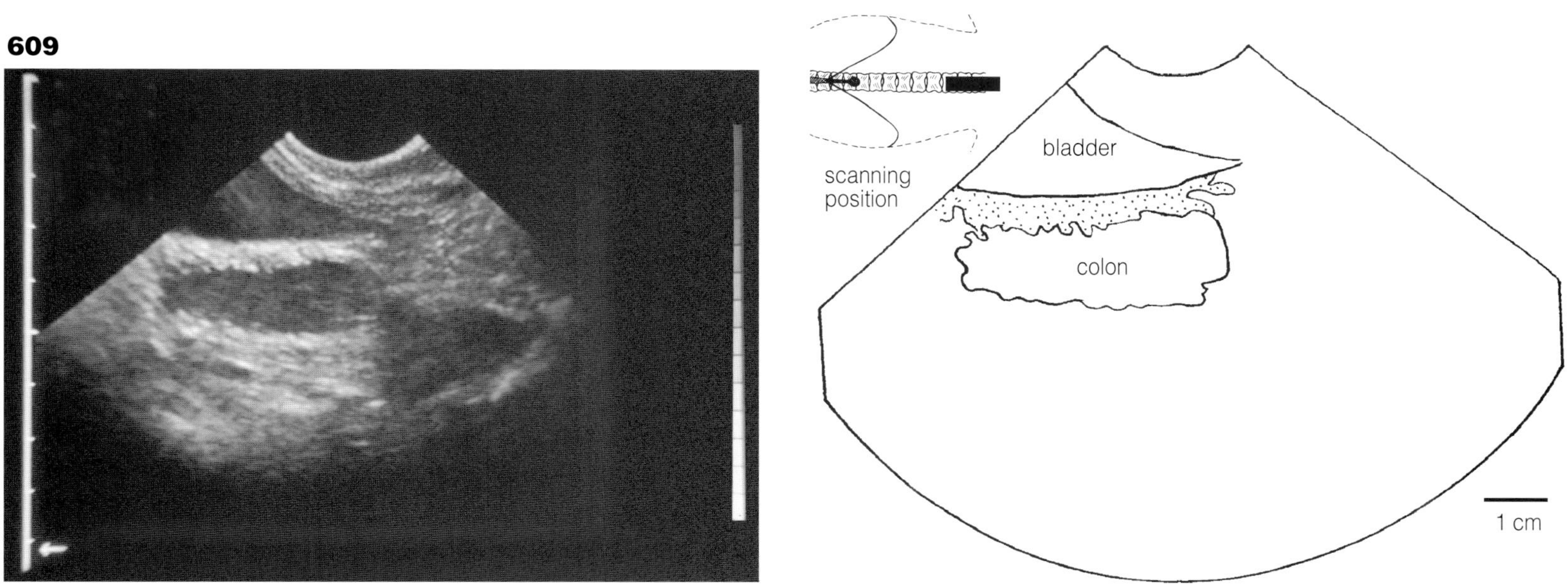

609 Longitudinal view of a fluid-filled colon with hypoechoic contents in a dog. This sonogram is similar to a pyometra or stump pyometra.

610

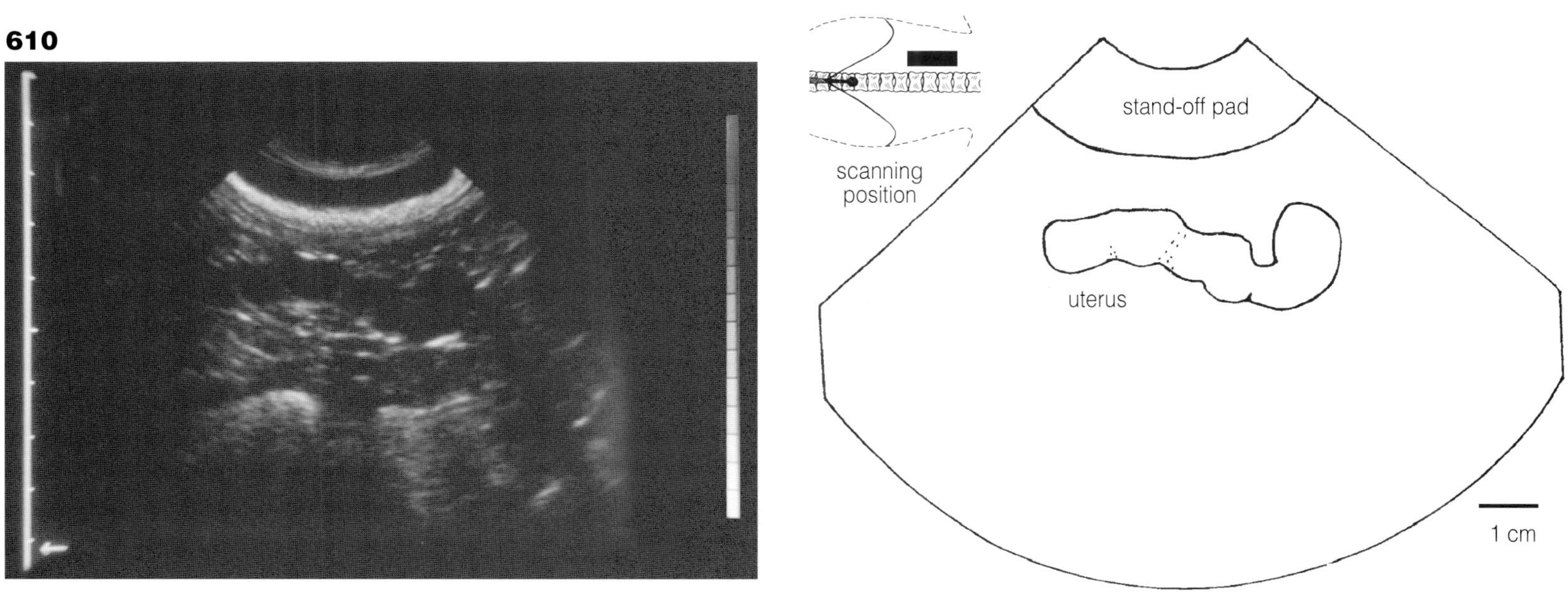

610 Longitudinal view of hydrometra in a dog. The uterus shows a characteristic thin wall, anechoic lumen and an almost straight course. Differential diagnoses include other diseases associated with the endometritis–pyometra complex, as well as fluid-filled organs such as vessels or intestines.

611

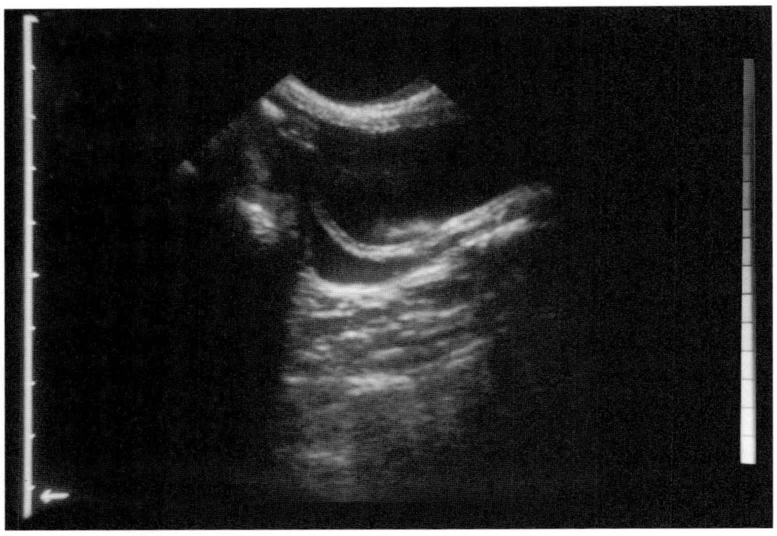

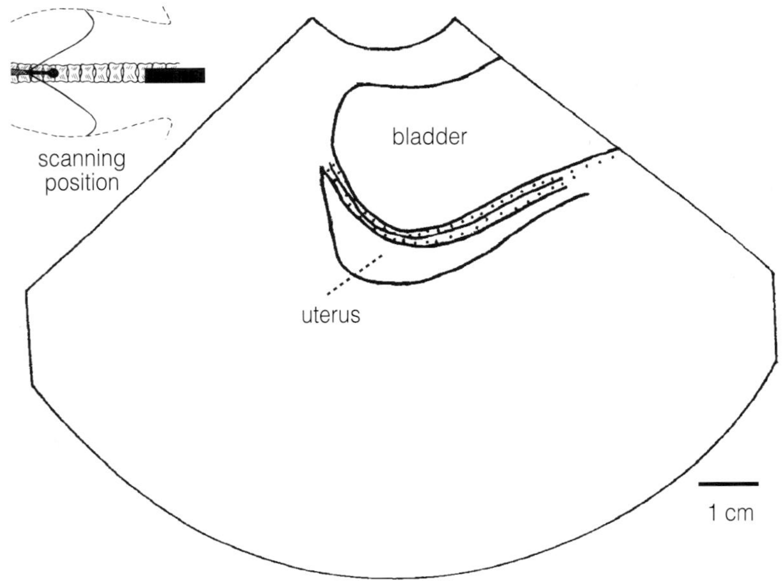

612

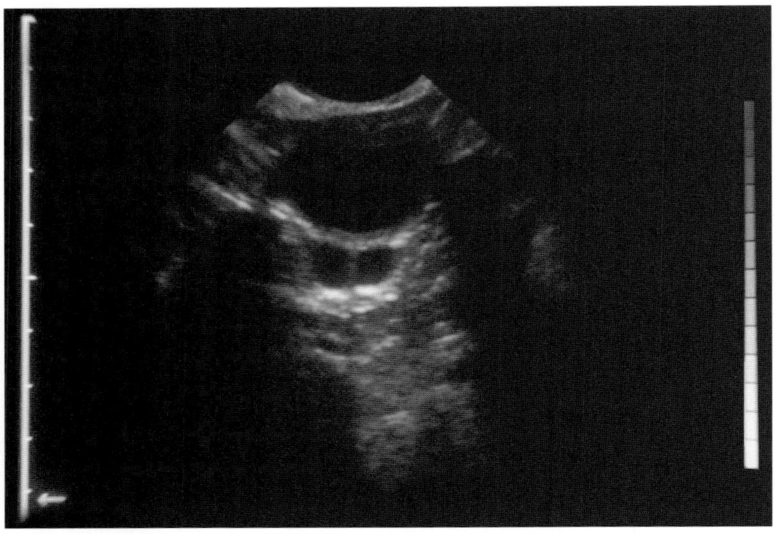

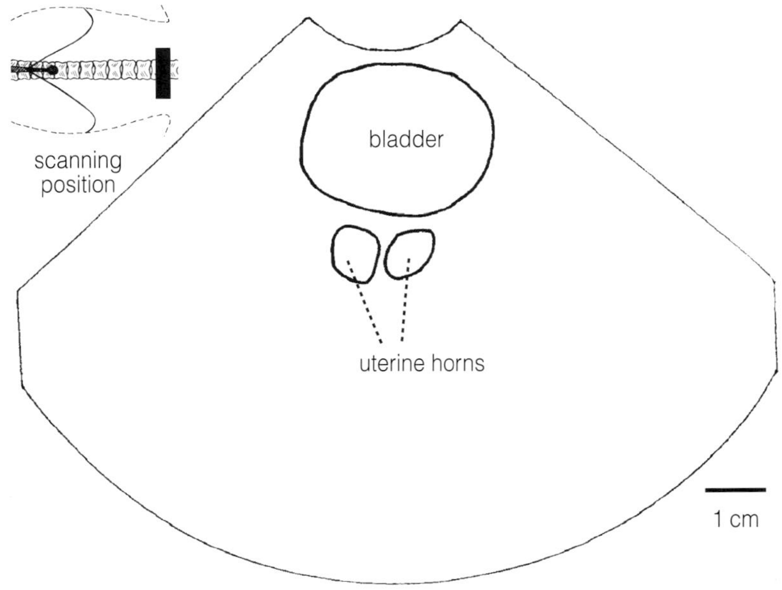

611, 612 Hydrometra in a dog in a longitudinal (**611**) and a transverse (**612**) view with a thin uterine wall, anechoic lumen and distal acoustic enhancement. The uterus was identified by locating the bifurcation.

Complications with the Endometritis–Pyometra Complex

Complications associated with the endometritis–pyometra complex include displacement of the enlarged uterus and perforation. Displacement of the enlarged uterine horn occurs with inguinal hernias (**613**). A perforated wall causes fluid accumulation and/or hyperechoic tissue around the uterus, which is indicative of local peritonitis (**614**). Ascites is characteristic of generalized peritonitis (**615**).

Postoperative Complications following Hysterectomy

Postoperative complications following hysterectomy include stump granuloma and stump pyometra. The granuloma is located dorsal to the bladder neck. This complex mass has a round shape and is well-demarcated (**616**)[5]. Stump pyometra is located in the same position, but shows a hypoechoic to anechoic lumen with a distinct wall (**617**). For additional lesions associated with ovariohysterectomy see Lymphadenitis and Lymph Node Abscess, page 244; **555, 556**.

Uterine Cysts

Subserosal uterine cysts often appear as an incidental finding in the normal uterus (see Ovarian Cysts, page 257; **586, 587**). These cysts are usually located in the tips of the uterine horns and are difficult to differentiate from ovarian cysts. Solitary cysts within the uterine wall are rarely seen (**618**).

Uterine Tumours

Uterine tumours of considerable size are visualized as incidental findings in the middle to caudal abdomen. The ultrasonographic appearance varies. Large tumours appear as complex masses (**619**), while smaller tumours have a more uniform structure. The surface is usually smooth. Cystic structures may be seen as hypoechoic to anechoic cavities within the tumour. Large tumours are often difficult to connect with the uterus, although tumours of this size, without any clinical symptoms, are generally not associated with vital organs. Smaller tumours are easier to differentiate ultrasonographically.

613

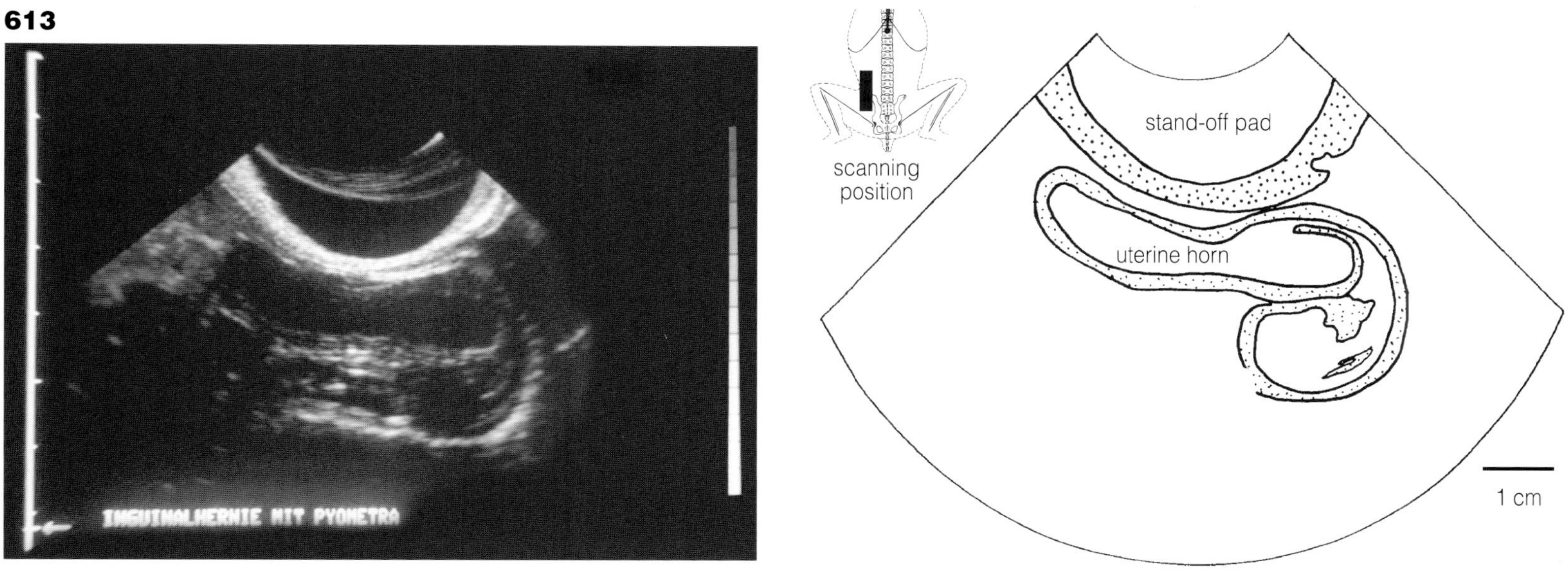

613 Inguinal hernia and pyometra in a dog. The anechoic, tubular body within the mass is apparent. Diagnosis was made by locating the other fluid-filled uterine horn, which ruled out an inguinal hernia with fluid-filled intestines.

614

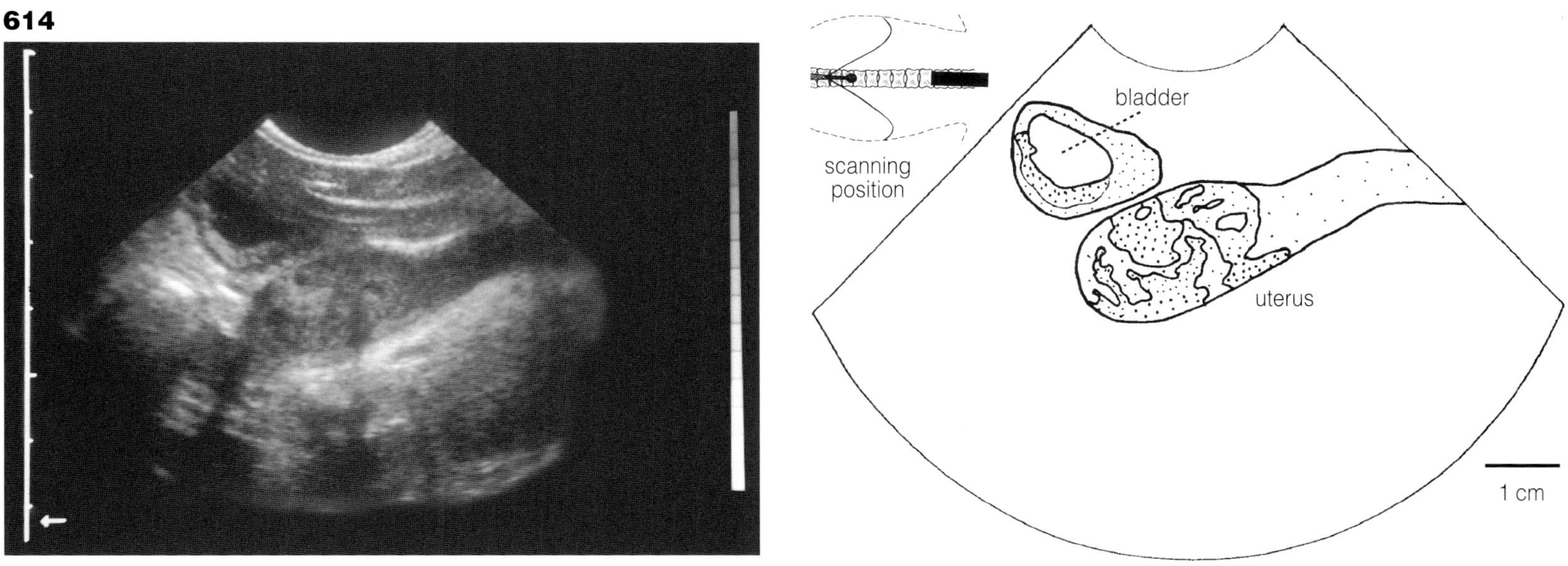

614 Pathological uterus and local peritonitis in a dog. The echogenic tissue surrounding the hypoechoic, non-homogenous uterus is characteristic of this finding. A similar image is seen with anorexic animals.

615

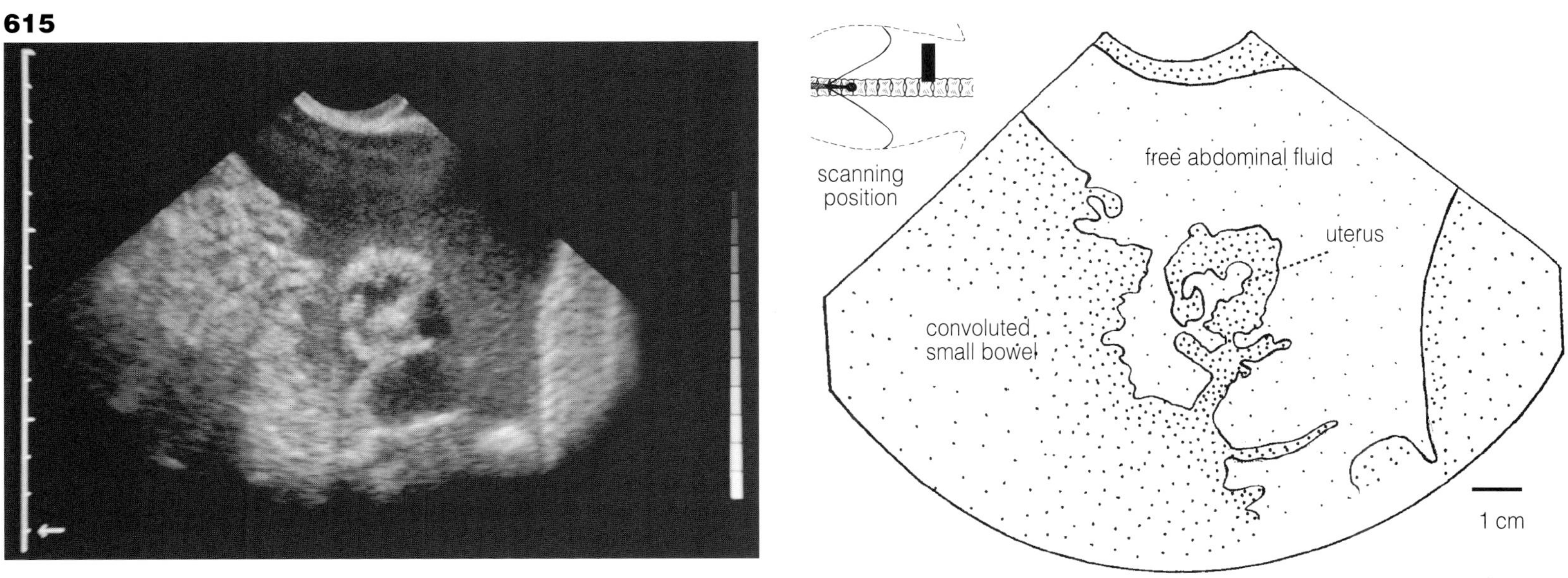

615 Generalized peritonitis caused by a perforated pyometra in a dog. The convoluted bowel loops around the mesentery are indicative of chronic peritonitis. The free abdominal fluid is not completely anechoic and it contains echogenic particles. The round mass with an anechoic lumen in the middle of the image is the uterus. Differential diagnosis includes ascites of another inflammatory origin.

616

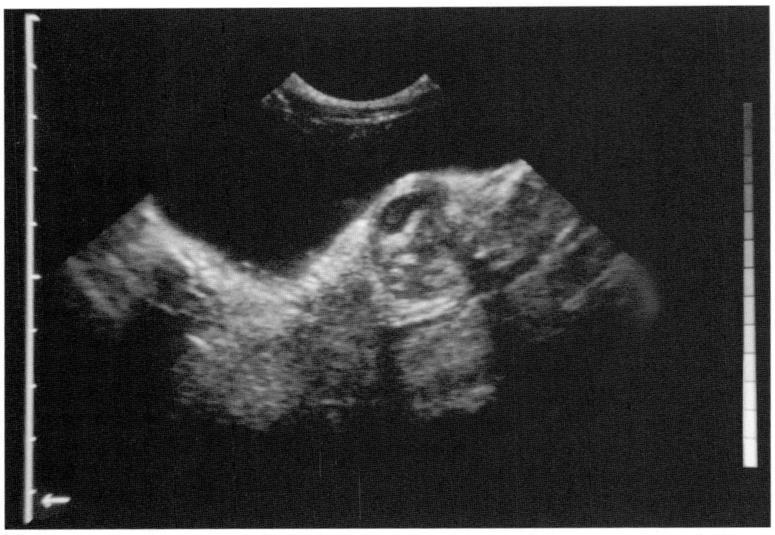

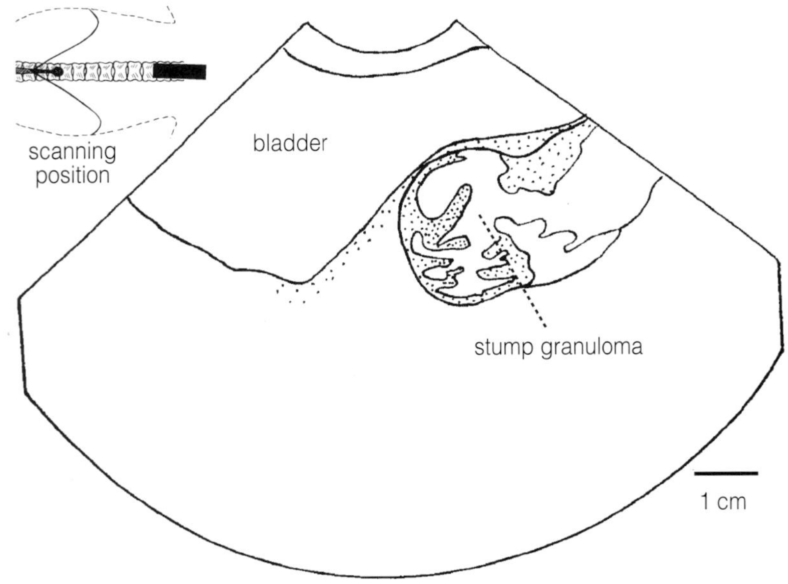

616 Stump granuloma in a dog. A round, well-demarcated complex mass is seen dorsal to the bladder, four weeks after ovariohysterectomy. Differential diagnosis includes various tumours.

617

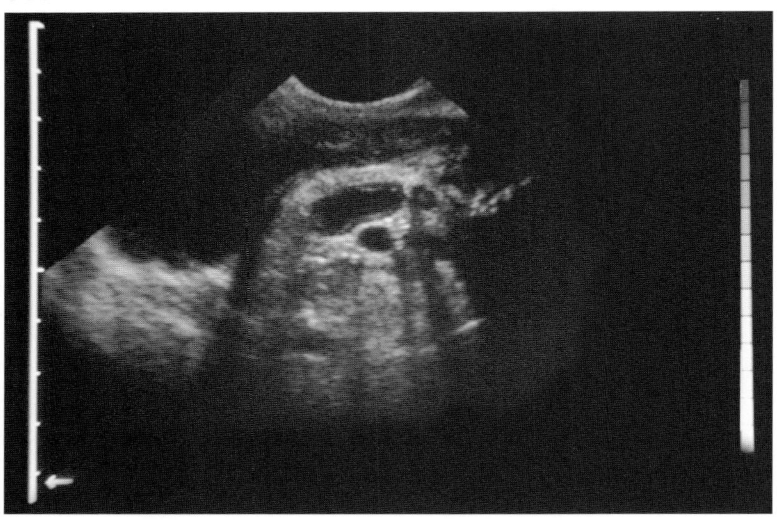

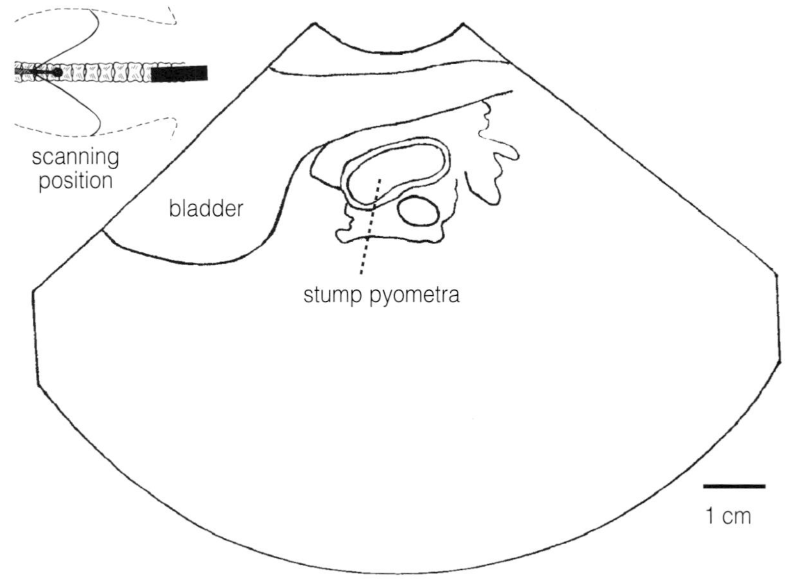

617 Stump pyometra affecting the surrounding tissue in a dog following ovariohysterectomy. Generalized hyperechogenicity is seen dorsal to the bladder neck region with anechoic vessels and a tubular structure with a distinct wall.

618

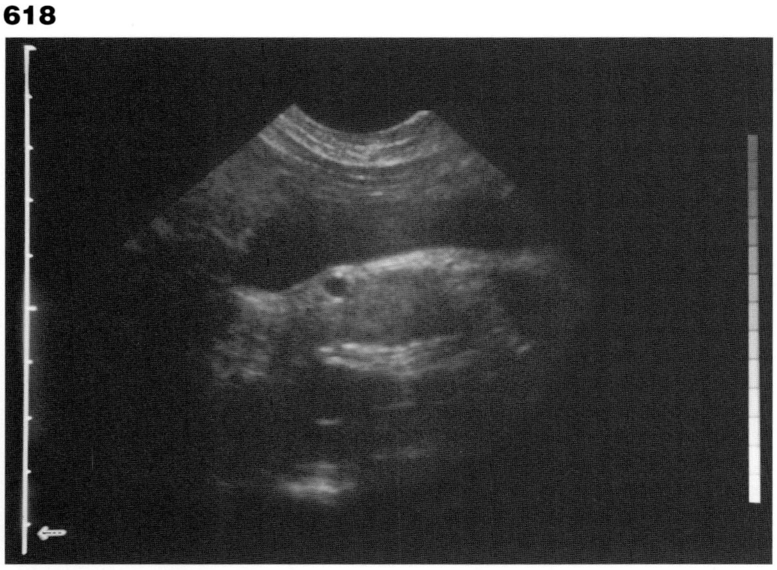

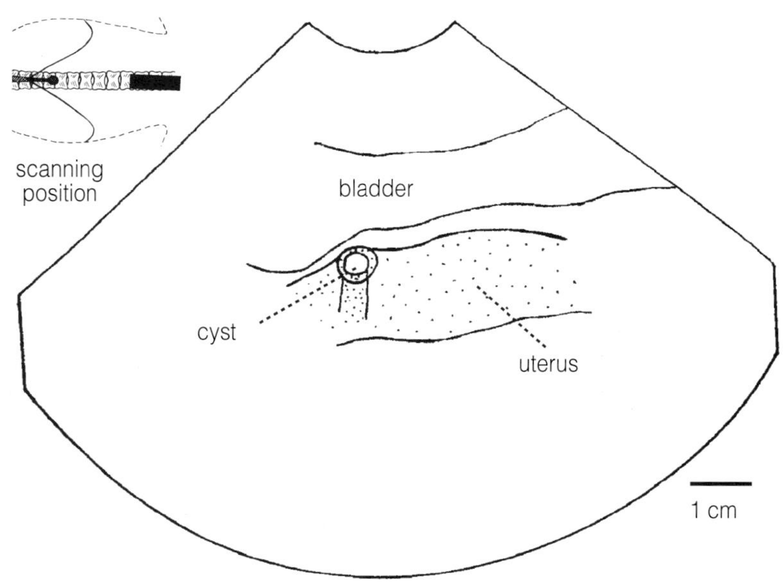

618 Solitary uterine cyst in a dog. The small cyst with distal acoustic enhancement is clearly seen in the uterine body.

619

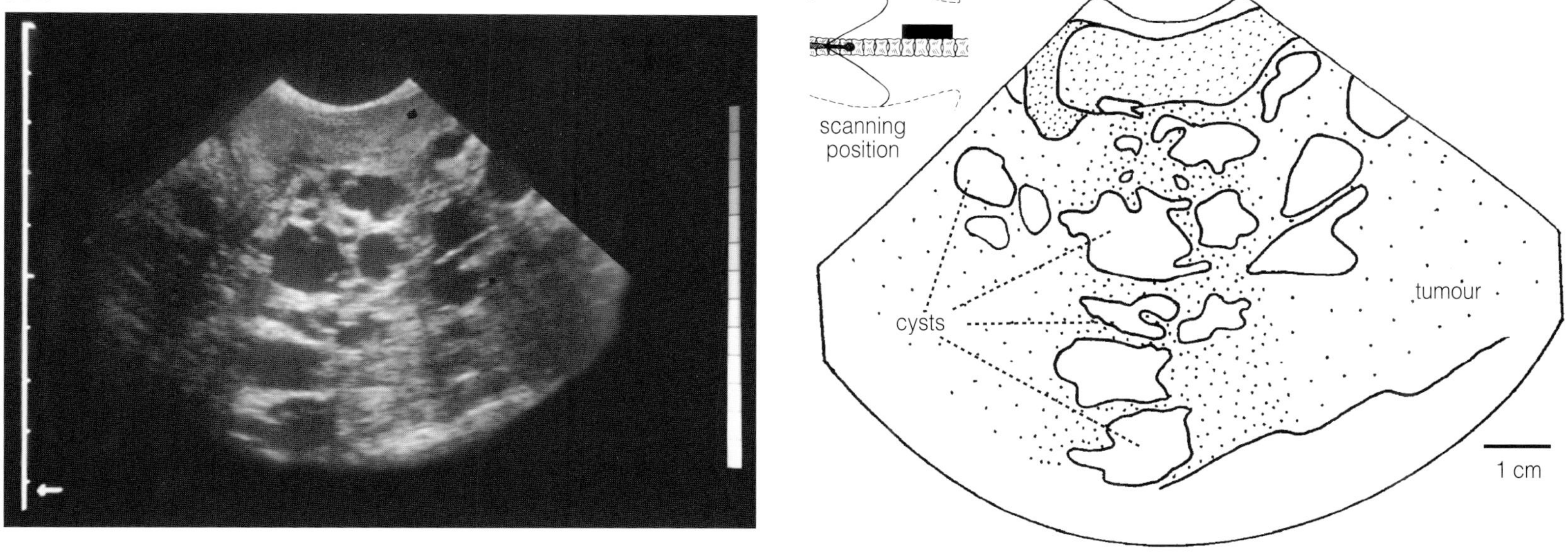

619 Two-dimensional sonogram of a large, complex uterine tumour in a dog (histopathology: cystadenocarcinoma).

620

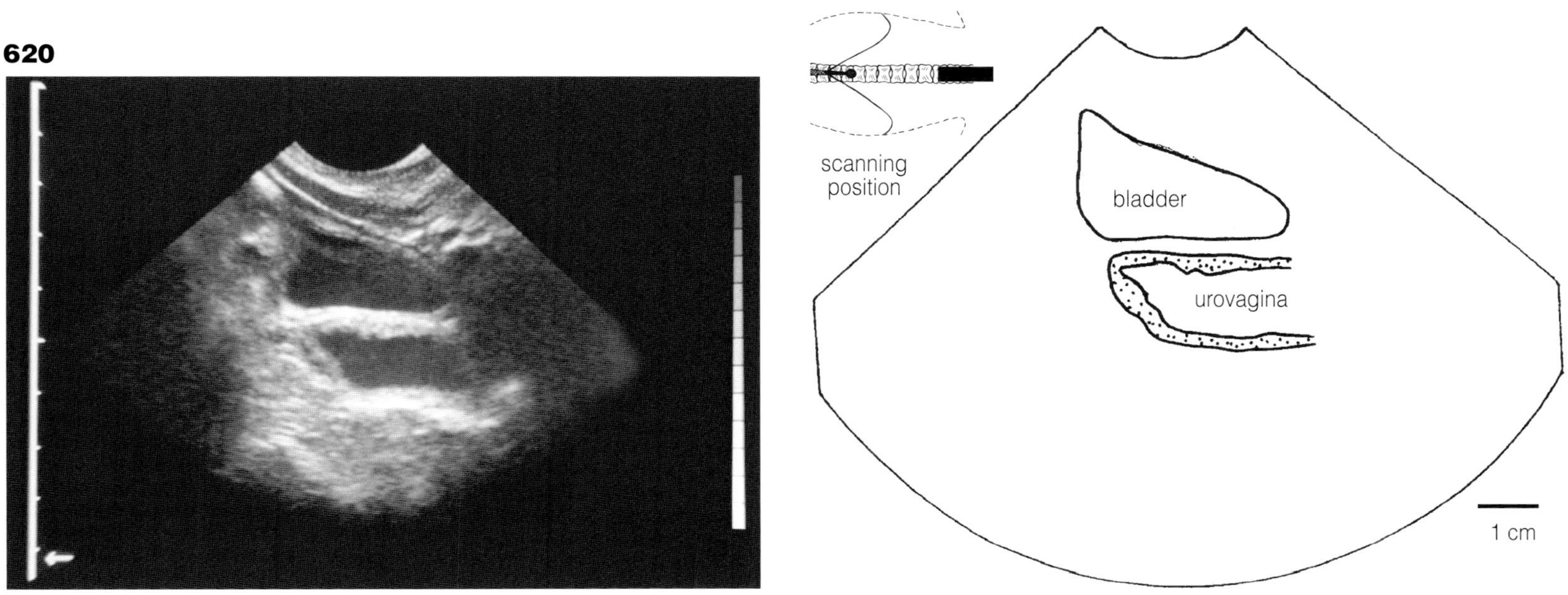

620 Urovagina in a dog. Anechoic mass dorsal to the bladder in a pseudohermaphrodite. Differential diagnosis includes a fluid-filled colon or uterus.

621

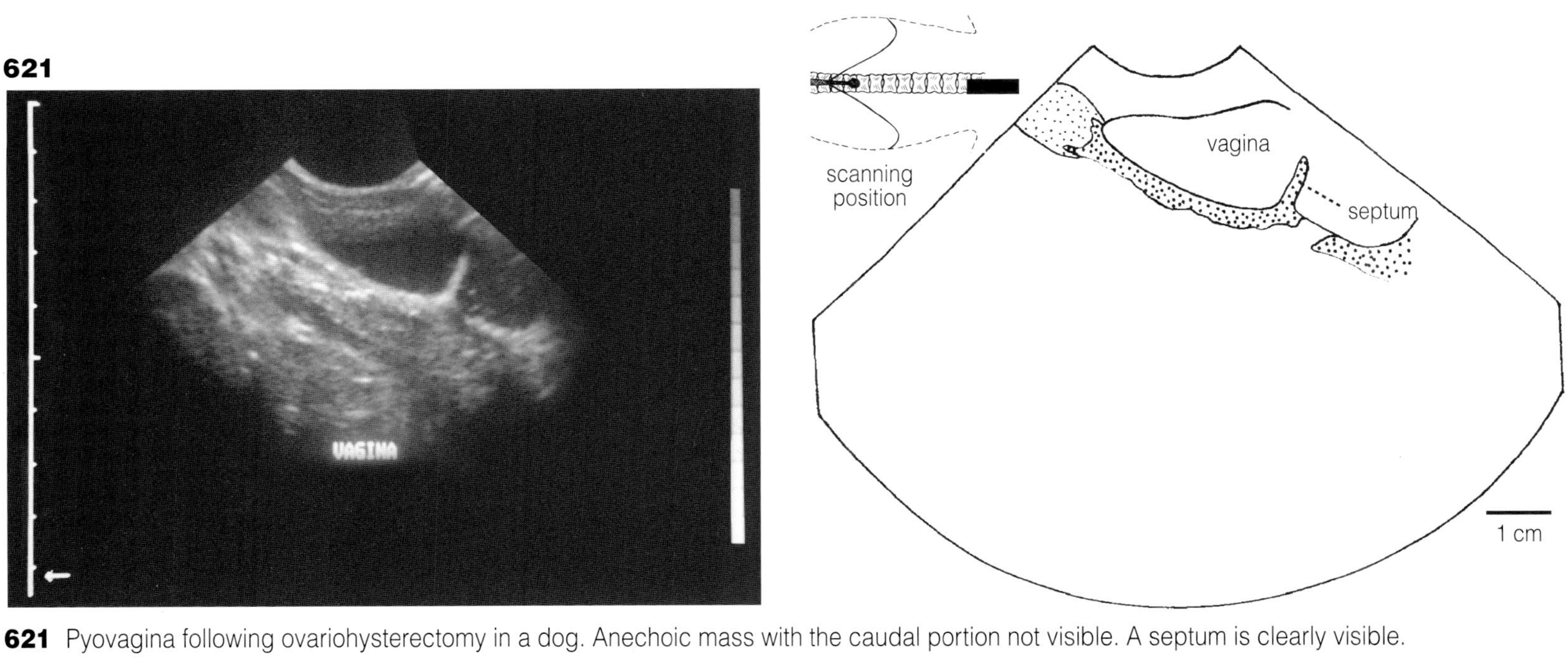

621 Pyovagina following ovariohysterectomy in a dog. Anechoic mass with the caudal portion not visible. A septum is clearly visible.

622

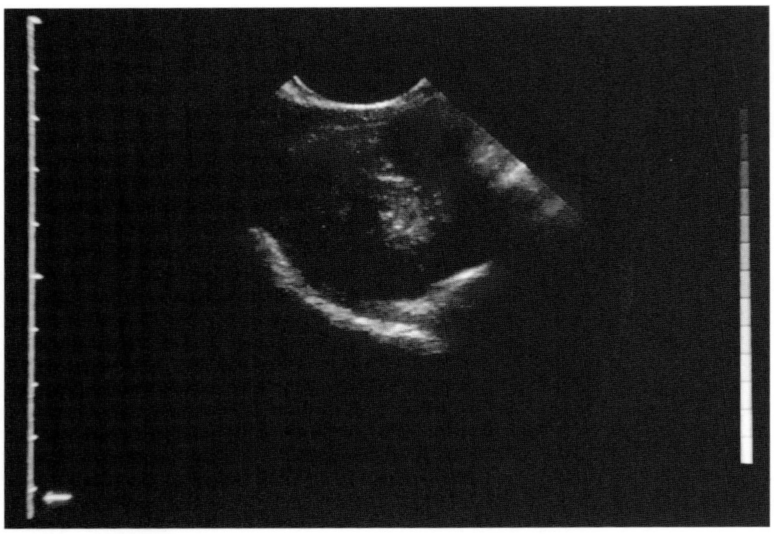

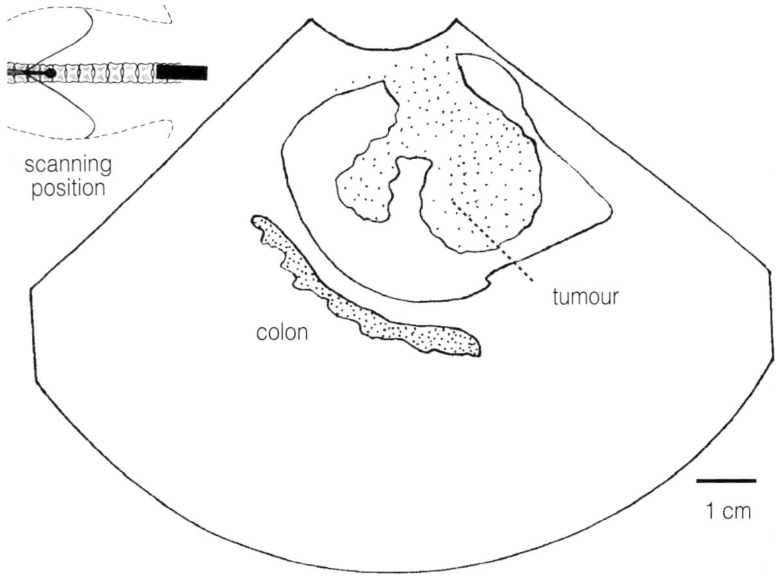

622 Vaginal tumour in a dog. Round, non-homogenous mass caudal to the bladder neck.

623

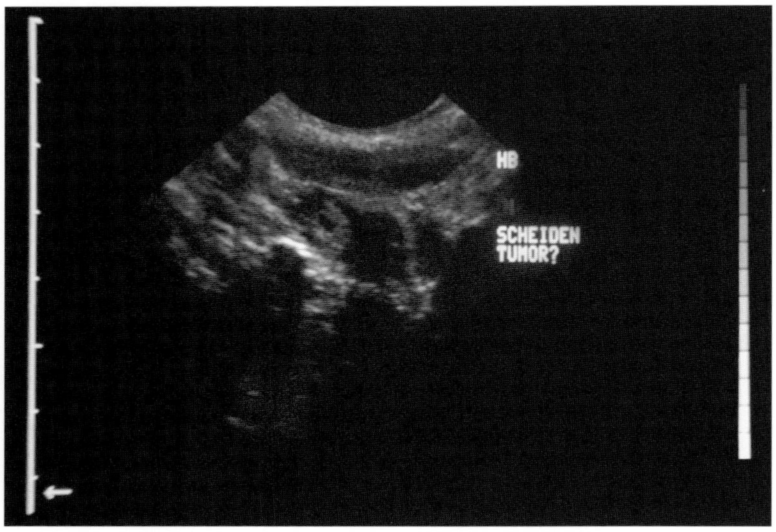

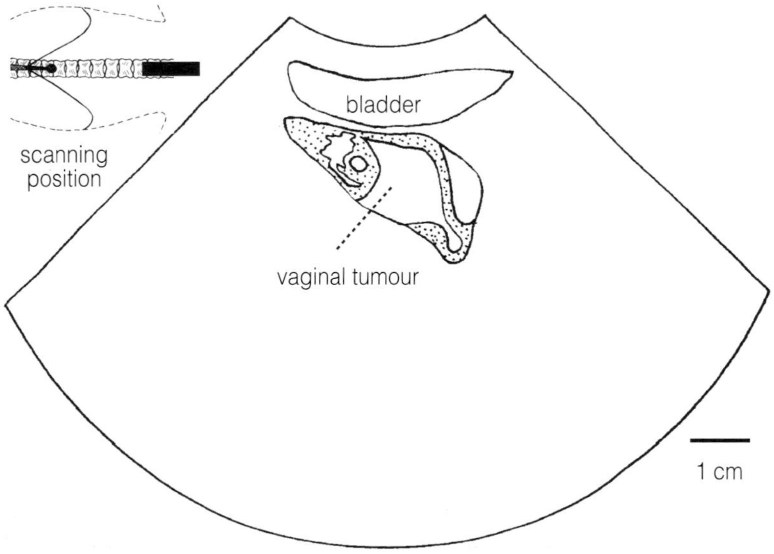

623 Vaginal tumour in a dog. Non-homogenous mass distal to the bladder neck.

Ultrasonography of Vaginal Disease

Ultrasonography of the vagina is indicated with vaginal discharge and suspected:

- Urovagina, mucovagina, pyovagina.
- Vaginal neoplasia.

A further indication is for monitoring treatment response.

Urovagina, Mucovagina and Pyovagina

Fluid accumulations in the vagina with urovagina, mucovagina or pyovagina are occasionally diagnosed. They are seen as congenital disorders in young animals (pseudohermaphrodite, vaginal septum) and in older animals following trauma (**620**). When a fluid-filled vagina is suspected, the animal should be examined in a standing position, preferably with the pelvis positioned higher.

Fluid echogenicity does not always correlate with cell contents, so a diagnosis should be made with care. A vaginal septum is rarely seen (**621**).

Vaginal Neoplasia

Vaginal tumours are seen as round, irregular, mainly hypoechoic masses near the urinary bladder neck. The ultrasonographic appearance also varies. A definitive diagnosis is made by locating the cervix cranial to the mass (**622–624**).

References

1 England GCW and Allen WE (1989) Real-time ultrasonic imaging of the ovary and uterus of the dog. *J. Reprod. Fert.* Suppl. **39**, 91–100.

2 Fayrer-Hosken RA, Mahaffey M, Miller-Liebl D and Caudle AB (1991) Early diagnosis of canine pyometra using ultrasonography. *Vet. Radiol.* **32**, 287–289.

3 Gerwing M (1993) Uterus. In: Fritsch R and Gerwing M (Eds.) *Sonographie bei Hand und Katze*. Ferdinand Enke Verlag, Stuttgart.

4 Lüerssen D (1994) Ultraschalldiagnostik des weiblichen Genitals des Handes. *Kleintierpraxis* **39**, 539–552.

5 Poffenbarger EM and Feeney DA (1986) Use of gray-scale ultrasonography in the diagnosis of reproductive disease in the bitch: 18 cases (1981–1984). *J. Am. Vet. Med. Assoc.* **189**, 90–95.

6 Schmidt S (1986) Die Ultraschalldiagnostik in der inneren and gynäkologischen Kleintierpraxis. *Berl. Münch. Tierärztl. Wschr.* **99**, 300–308.

7 Schmidt S, Schrag D and Giese B (1986) Ultraschalldiagnostik in der Gynäkologie beim Kleintier. *Tierärztl. Praxis* **14**, 123–141.

624

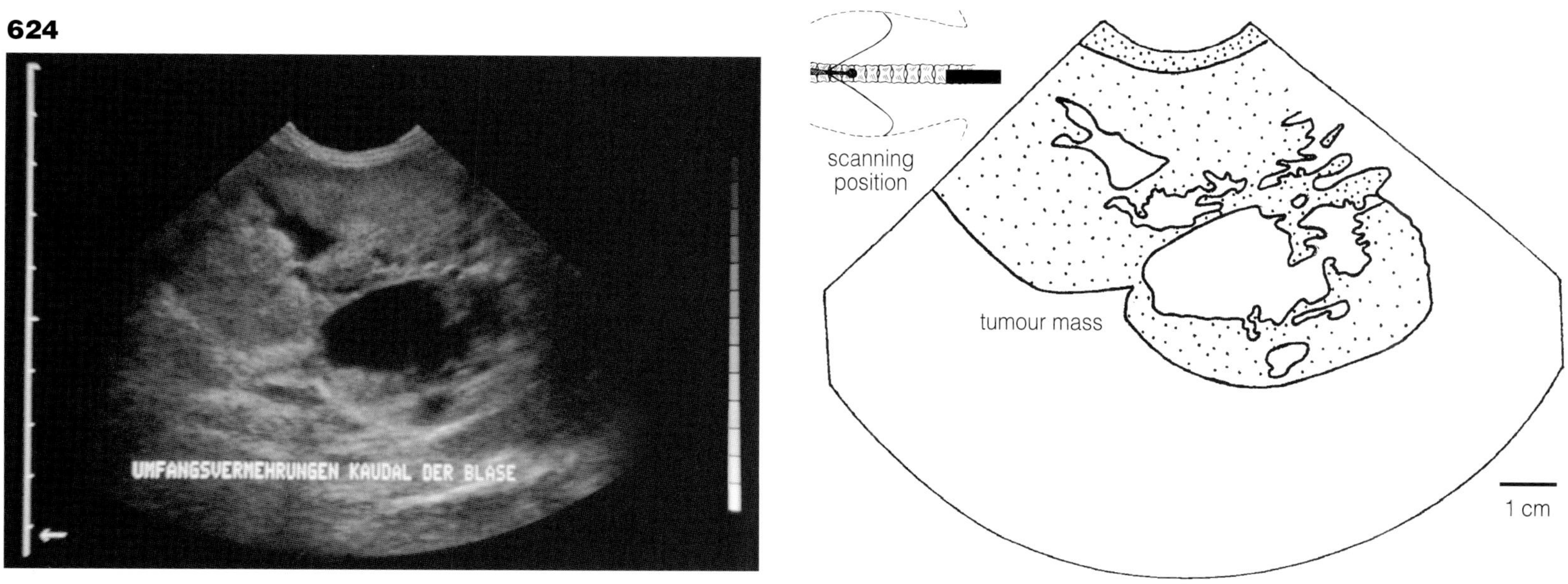

624 Vaginal tumour in a dog. Round, non-homogenous mass with anechoic foci is seen caudal to the cranially displaced urinary bladder.

8 Wrigley RH and Finn ST (1989) Ultrasonography of the canine uterus and ovary. In: Kirk RW (Ed.) *Current Veterinary Therapy X Small Animal Practice*. WB Saunders, Philadelphia, pp. 1239–1242.

Scrotum, Testes and Epididymis

Dirk Lüerssen and Martin Janthur

Instrumentation and Examination Technique

Normally descended, intrascrotal testes in the dog should be scanned with a 7.5 MHz transducer and a stand-off pad when using a sector probe. One testicle may be used as a stand-off to image the opposite one. The testis should be scanned in sagittal, transverse and longitudinal planes.

The epididymis is scanned with the testis acting as an acoustic window. Alternatively, a stand-off pad is necessary, especially when using a sector transducer.

Ultrasonography of the scrotum, testes and epididymis in the cat is more difficult than in the dog because of the smaller organ size. Since indications for testicular ultrasonography in the cat are limited, the following text refers only to ultrasonographic examinations in the dog.

Anatomy and Normal Sonographic Findings

The normal testicular parencyhma is of medium echogenicity with a homogenous, finely granulated echopattern[1]. The shape of the testis is oval with a smooth surface. The testicular parenchyma is covered by scrotal layers that appear as thin echogenic membranes and are especially hyperechoic near the septum testis. The mediastinum testis is seen as a hyperechoic central linear structure in the parenchyma on longitudinal views[3] (**625**).

625

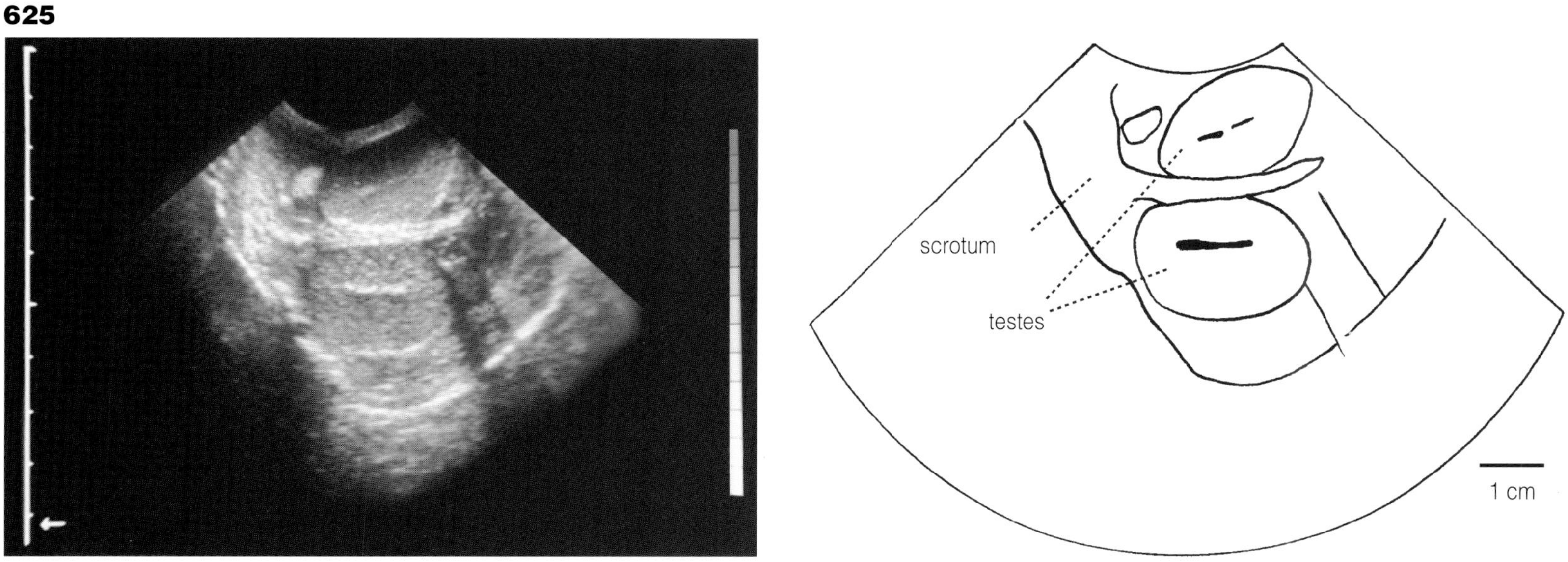

625 Normal canine testes in a sagittal view. The near testis is used as a stand-off. The distal testis is within the focal zone and is oval with a homogenous, finely textured parenchyma and a distinct, central, linear mediastinum testis. The non-homogenous scrotal layers are greatly thickened due to histologically confirmed deep pyoderma.

626

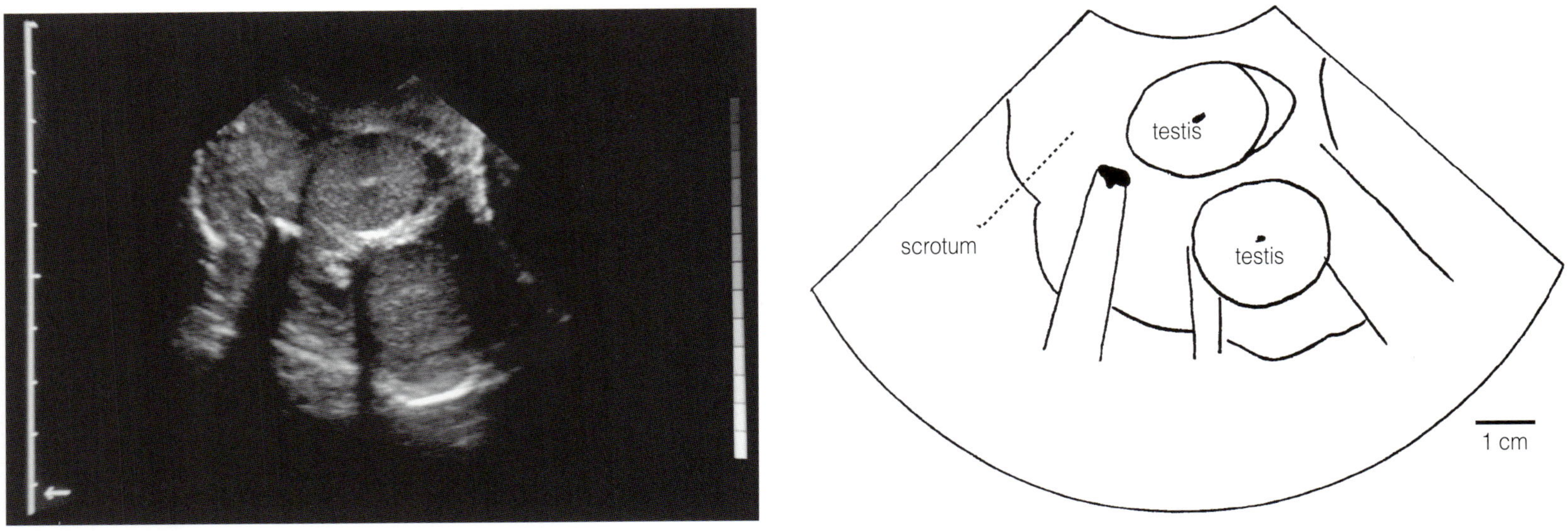

627

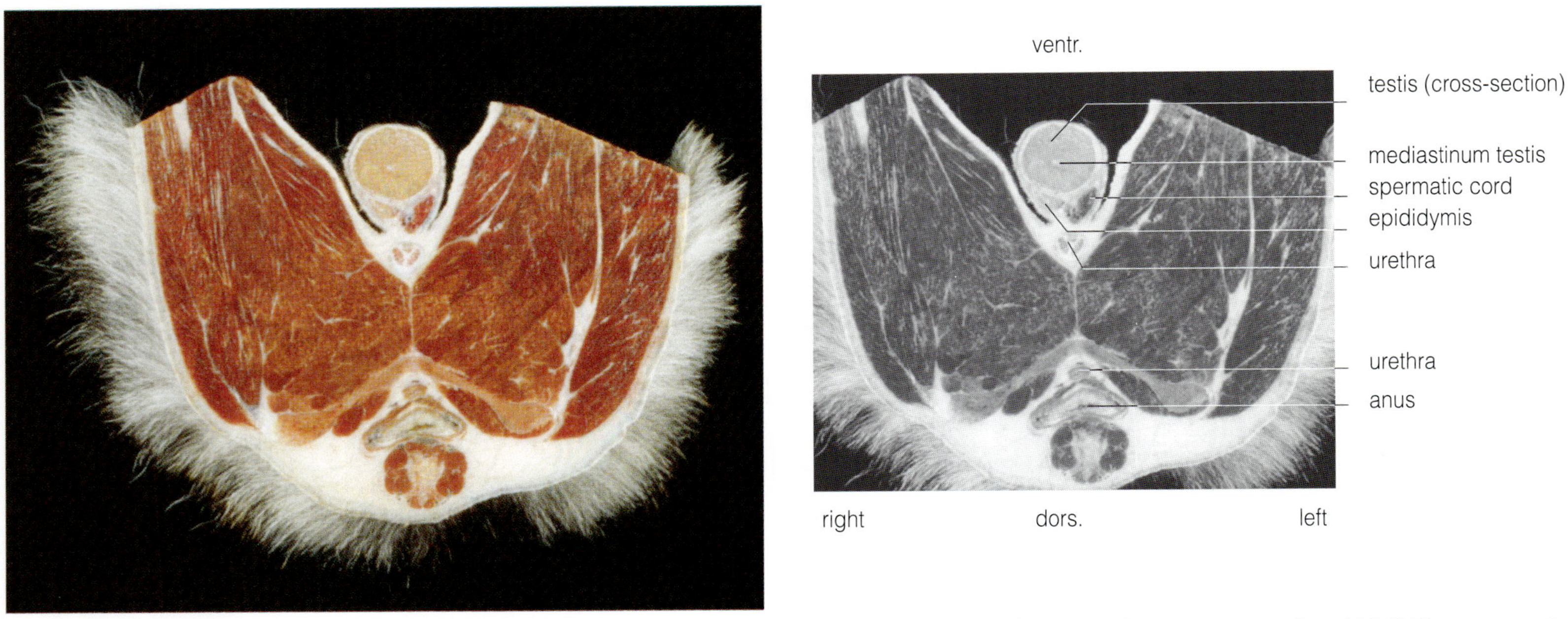

626, 627 Two-dimensional sonogram (**626**) and anatomical cross-section (**627**) of normal canine testes in a transverse view. (**626**) The near testis acts as a stand-off. The second testis is in the focal zone and shows a homogenous, finely textured parenchyma with a central, focal mediastinaum testis. The non-homogenous scrotal layers are greatly thickened due to histologically confirmed deep pyoderma.

On a transverse plane, the mediastinum testis is seen as a central focal echo (**626, 627**) (see Stand-off Pads, page 56; **99–102**). It measures approximately 2 mm in diameter[6].

The epididymis has a homogenous texture and appears less echoic than the testis (**625**). Complete evaluation is often difficult. The tail of the epididymis is larger and easier to visualize than the head or body[2].

The spermatic cord and testicular vessels are difficult to visualize ultrasonographically. Colour Doppler examinations show the tortuous testicular arteries in various colour-coded segments. PW Doppler shows uniphased, systolic, and diastolic motion. Because of the proximity of the vessel loops, blood flows towards and away from the transducer can be registered (**628–630**).

> *Indications for ultrasonography of the scrotum, testis and epididymis include all visible and palpable changes in size, consistency and location, and painful lesions with suspected:*
>
> - Testicular and epididymal inflammation including abcess formation.
> - Testicular cysts, metaplasia and neoplasia.
> - Testicular torsion and undescended testis.
>
> A further indication is for monitoring treatment response.

Ultrasonography of Scrotal, Testicular and Epididymal Disease

Normal testes should also be examined ultrasonographically when prostatic disease is present. Early forms of neoplasia may be seen within the testicular parenchyma without changes in size or consistency. Diffuse swelling of the scrotum can be divided into three diagnostic groups:

- Lesions associated with the scrotum (**625–627**).
- Scrotal lesions with fluid in the vaginal tunic and normal testis (**631**).
- Lesions of the scrotum and testis.

Determining the size of a lesion is important for deciding what treatment protocol to follow. The origin of the disease is usually unknown. The abdomen should be scanned for ascites when fluid is present within the vaginal tunic.

628

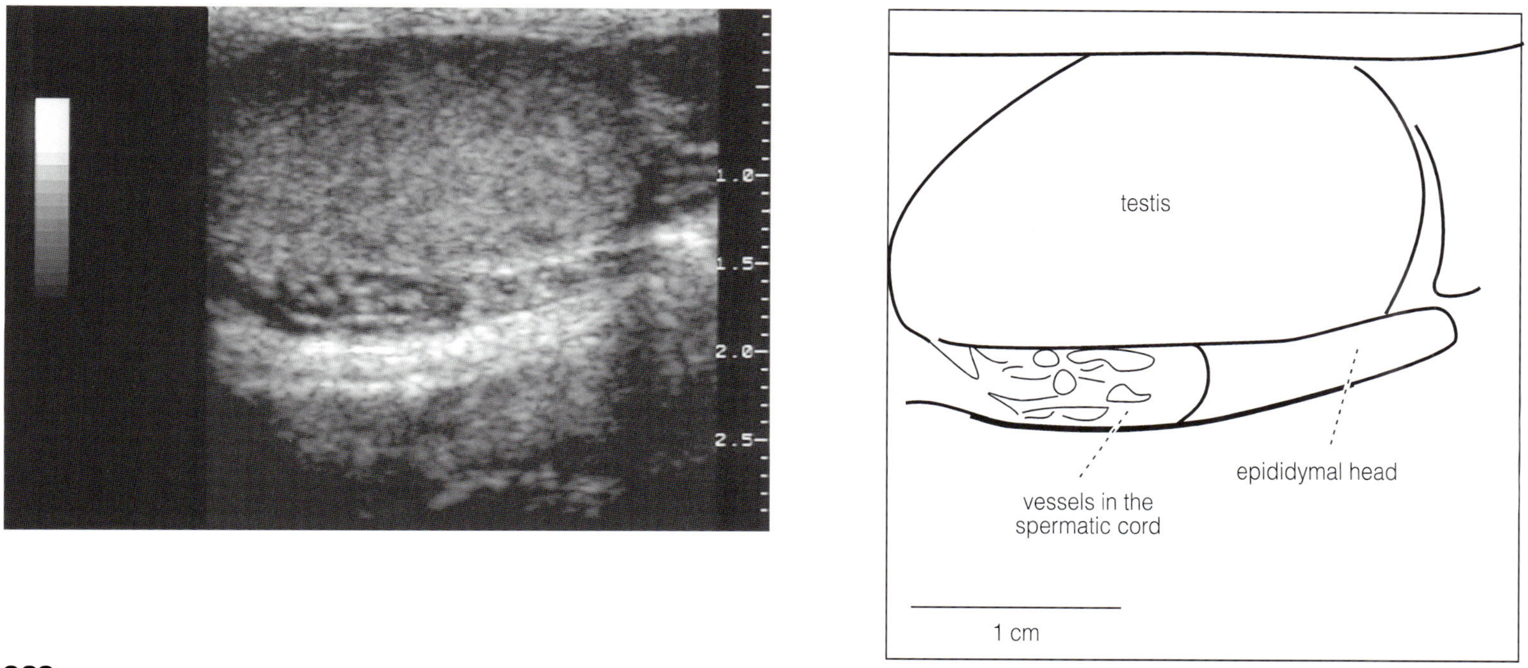

629

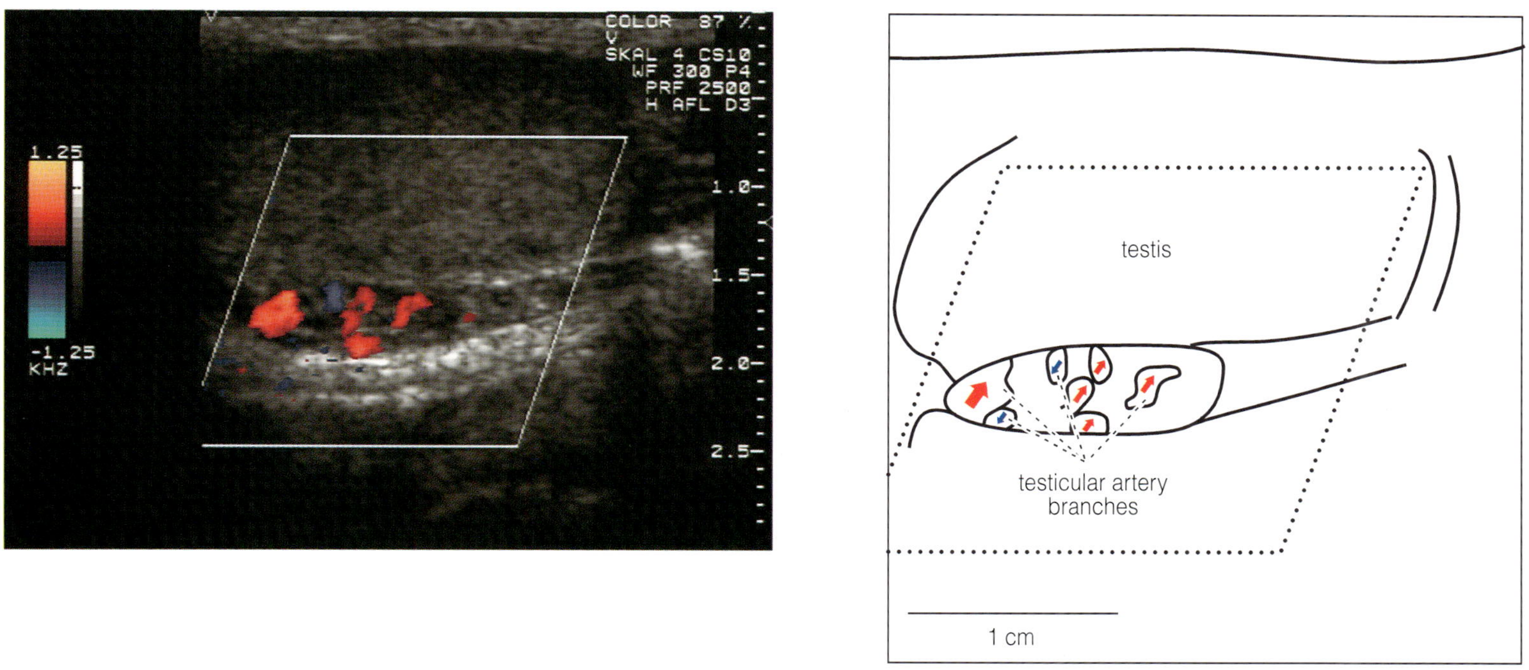

630

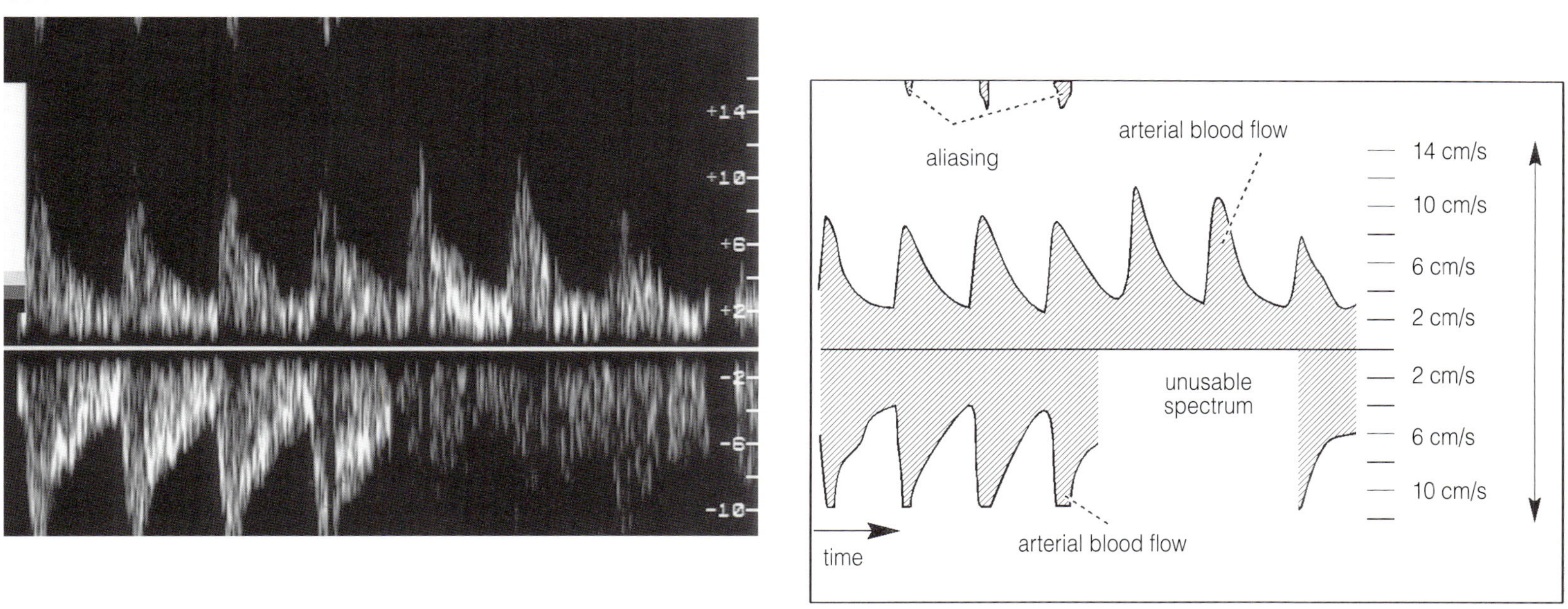

628–630 Two-dimensional sonogram (**628**), colour-coded (**629**) and PW Doppler (**630**) scan of testicular arteries.

631

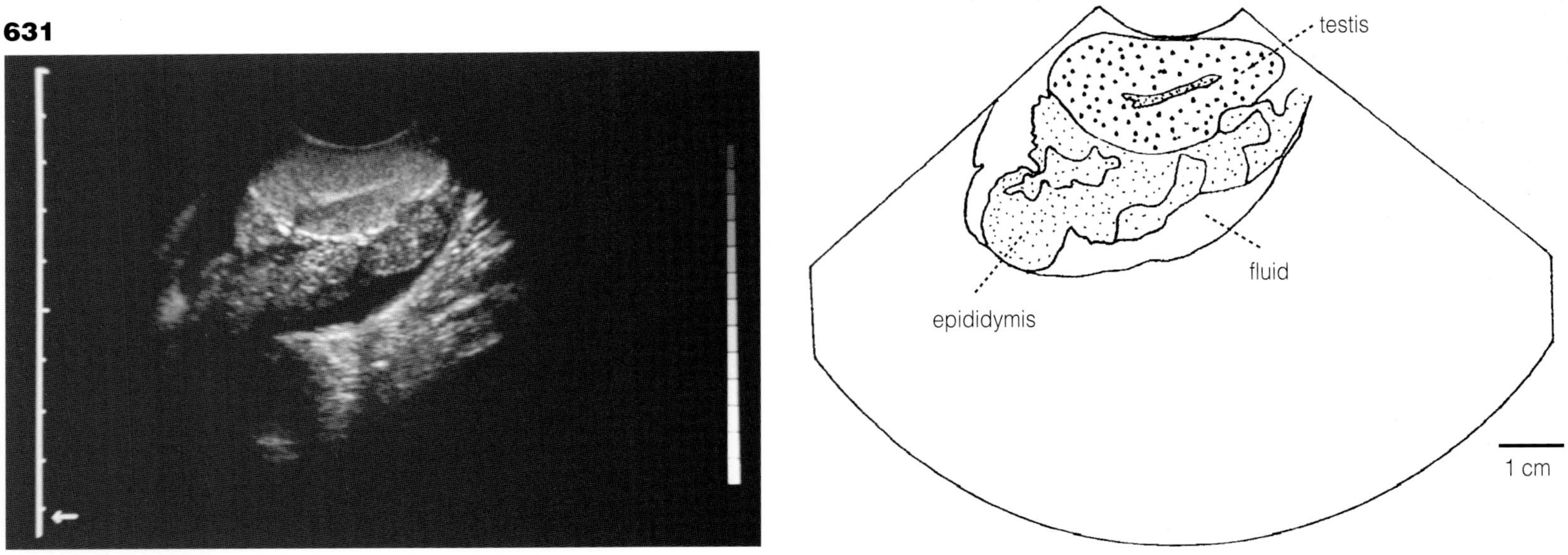

631 Anaplastic epididymal carcinoma and fluid-filled vaginal tunic in a dog. The epididymis is clearly enlarged. Ascites must be confirmed or ruled out.

632

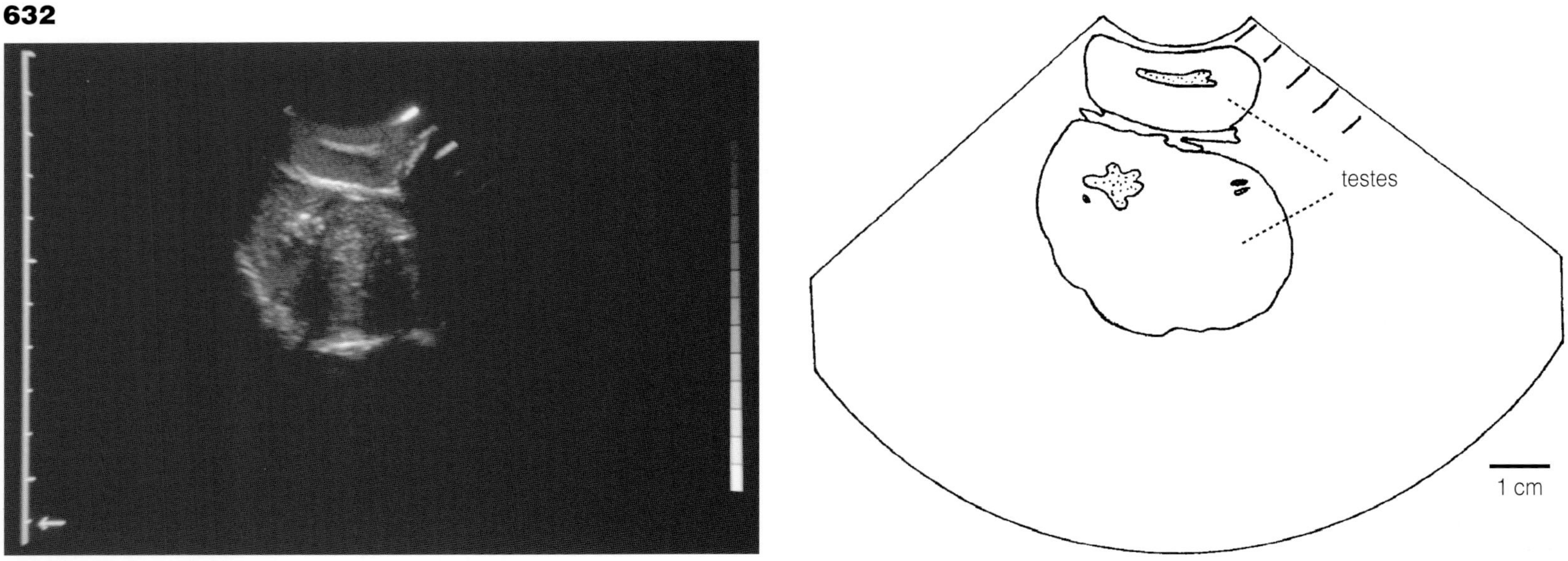

632 Orchitis in a dog. The testis is enlarged and non-homogenous. The mediastinum testis is not visible. The opposite testis is used as a stand-off.

633

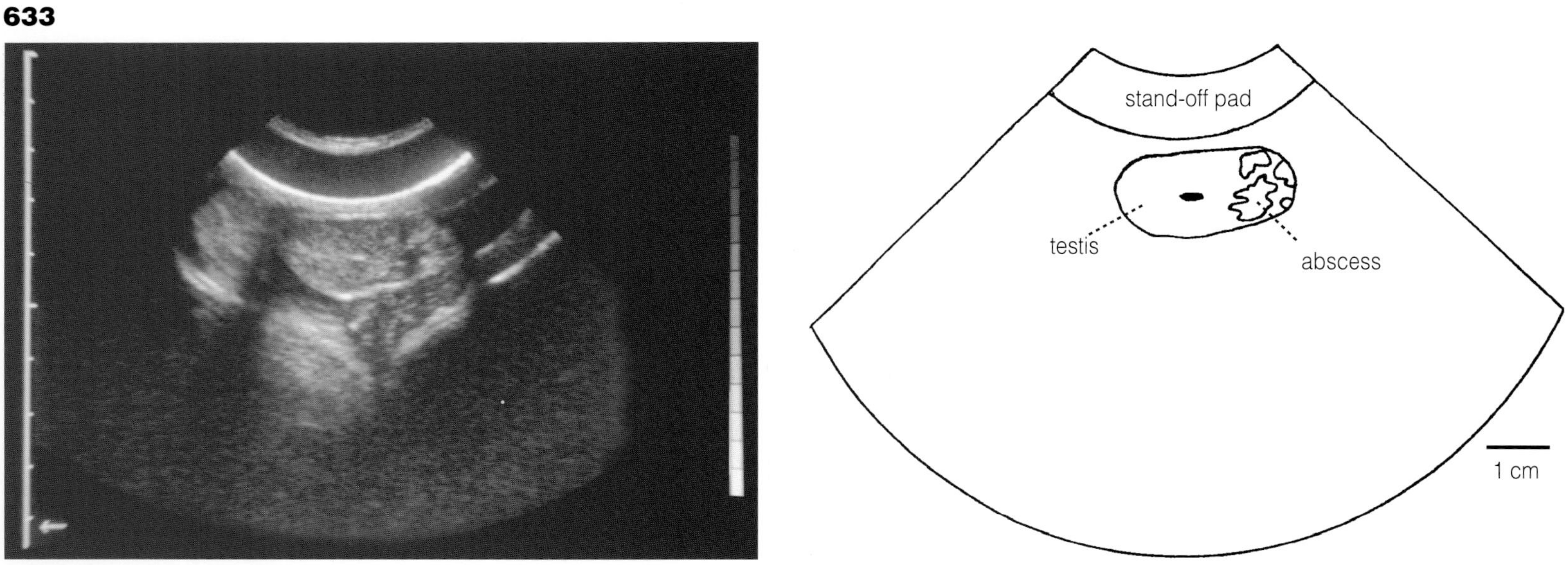

633 Abscess formation with orchitis in a dog. The longitudinal testis shows a non-homogenous texture at the distal pole and irregular, hypoechoic to anechoic areas within the parenchyma. The mediastinum testis is shortened. Irregular hypoechoic to anechoic areas are visible.

634

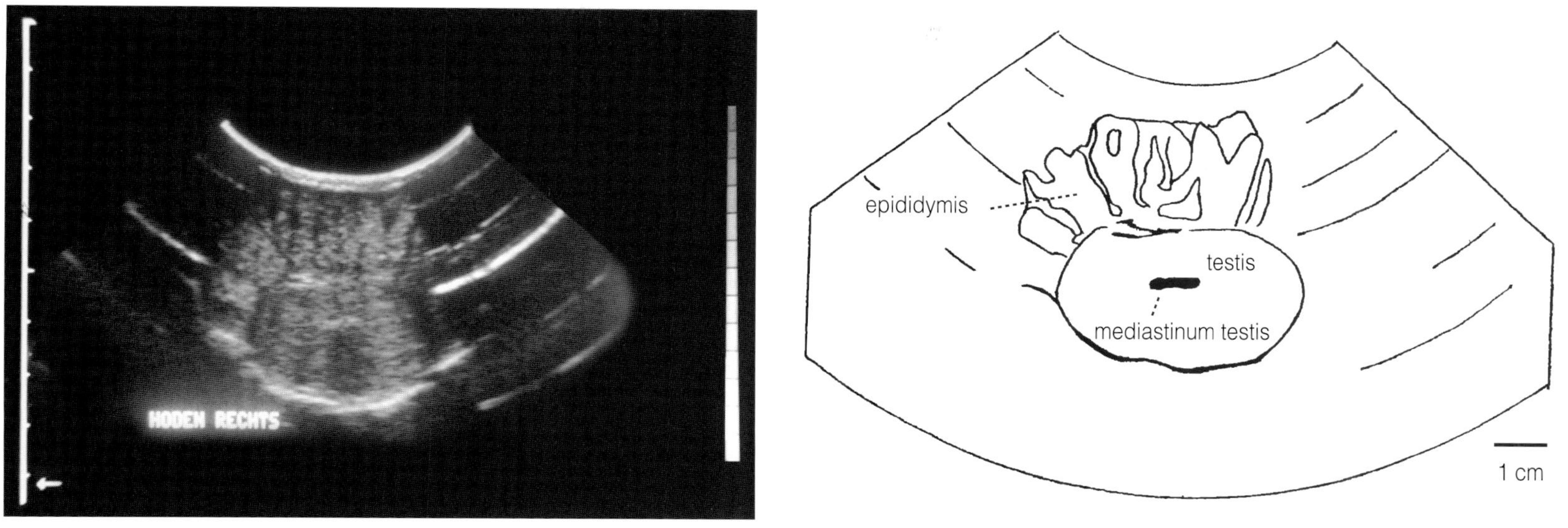

634 Epididymal enlargement in a dog with a normal testis.

635

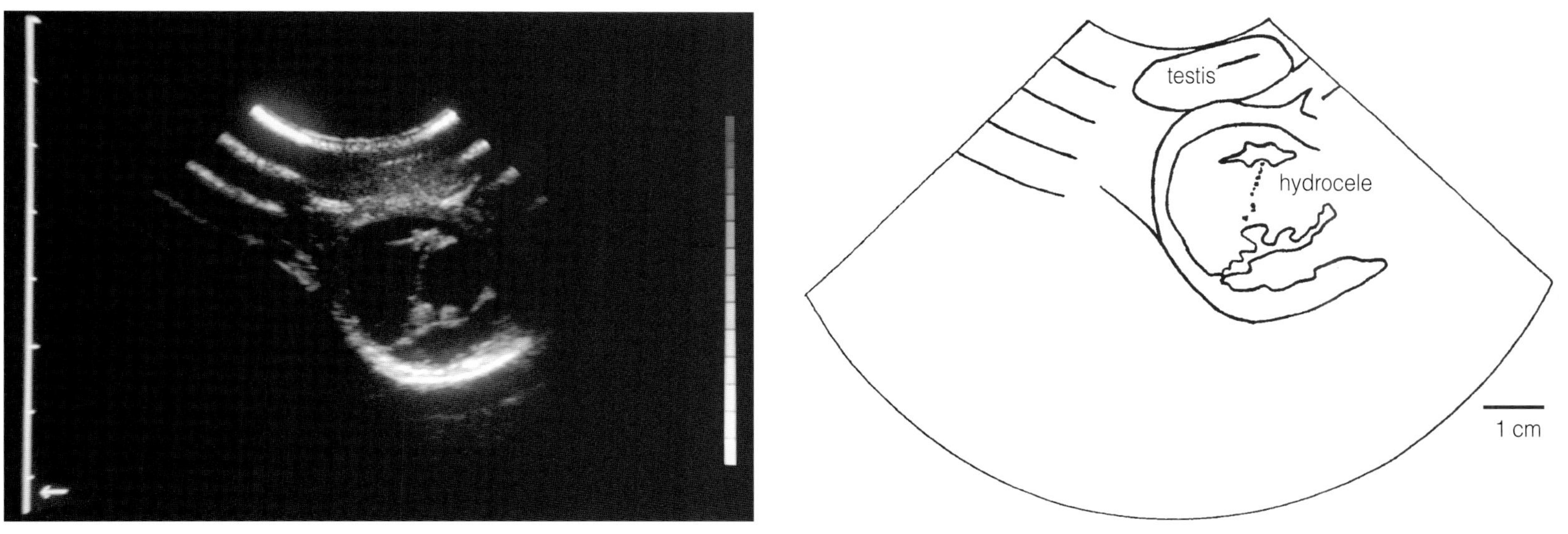

635 Hydrocele in a dog. Testicular enlargement with anechoic contents is seen. The near testis is used as a stand-off. The echogenic structures are from remaining parenchyma.

Orchitis and Epididymitis

Orchitis does not have a uniform ultrasonographic appearance. Fluid accumulation due to inflammation and oedema is usually seen within the vaginal process as an anechoic space between the testis and the scrotum. The testicular parenchyma is uniformly hypoechoic with acute infectious disease. The testes are enlarged and rounder.

As the disease progresses, the parenchyma becomes non-homogenous with more echogenic foci (**632**). Abscesses are characterized by anechoic to hypoechoic, irregular areas (**633**). Distal acoustic enhancement may be present. Pus usually has a variable ultrasonographic appearance and may even mimic homogenous parenchyma with pyogenic orchitis. Healed infections may leave metaplasia, cysts and generalized hyperechogenicity of the testicular parenchyma behind. A reduction in testicular size has been observed.

Epididymitis can occur with isolated epididymal enlargement[4] and a patchy parenchymal texture (**634**). Gas formation with echogenic foci and distal shadowing has been observed[3].

Testicular Cysts, Metaplasia and Neoplasia

Cysts (hydroceles and spermatoceles) are found as anechoic, often septated areas within or instead of testicular parenchyma (**635, 636**). Distal acoustic enhancement is always visible. Primary neoplasia is most likely the cause when there is little normal testicular parenchyma. Small cysts and metaplasia are incidental findings. Echogenic foci of 1–2 mm in diameter are usually caused by metaplasia **637**). Because these lesions often calcify, distal shadowing is observed. Metaplasia has various causes.

As well as inflammation, cysts and metaplasia, neoplasia is often found in descended testes. Tumours can be focal (**638**) or generalized (**639**). Testicular neoplasms are usually round, hyperechoic, homogenous or non-homogenous masses within the parenchyma (**638, 640–642**).

636

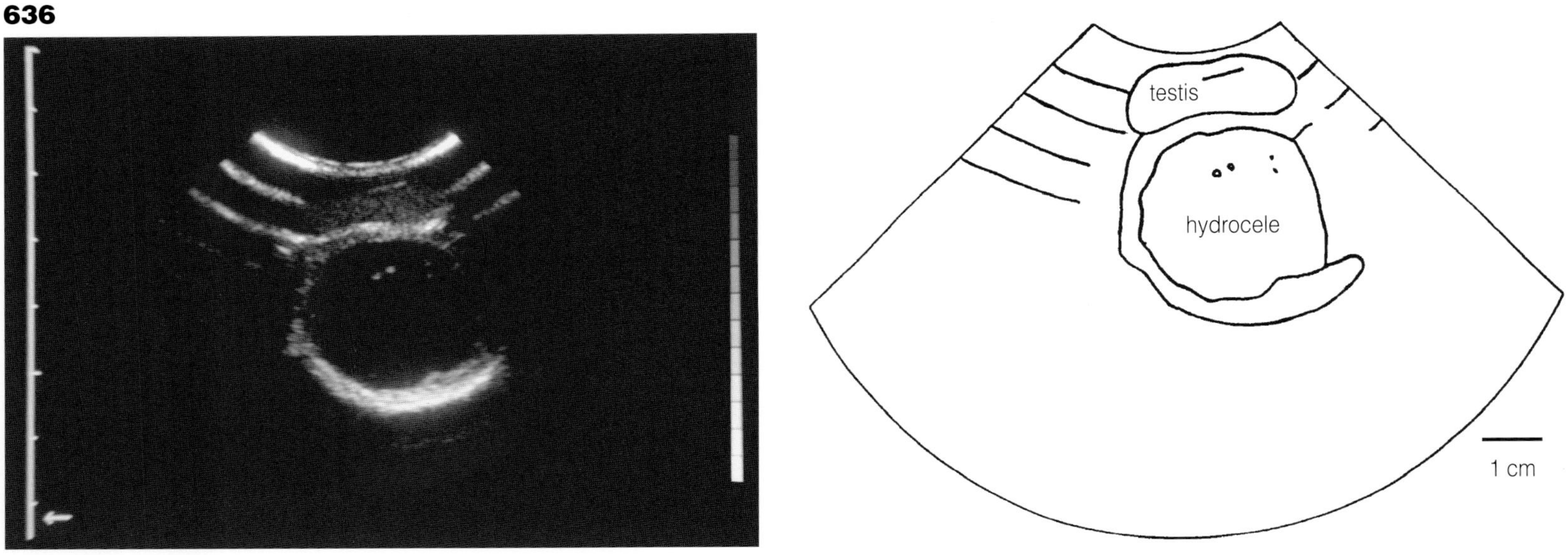

636 Hydrocele in a dog. The enlarged testis is seen in a longitudinal plane. The opposite testis is used as a stand-off. The contents of the testis are anechoic.

637

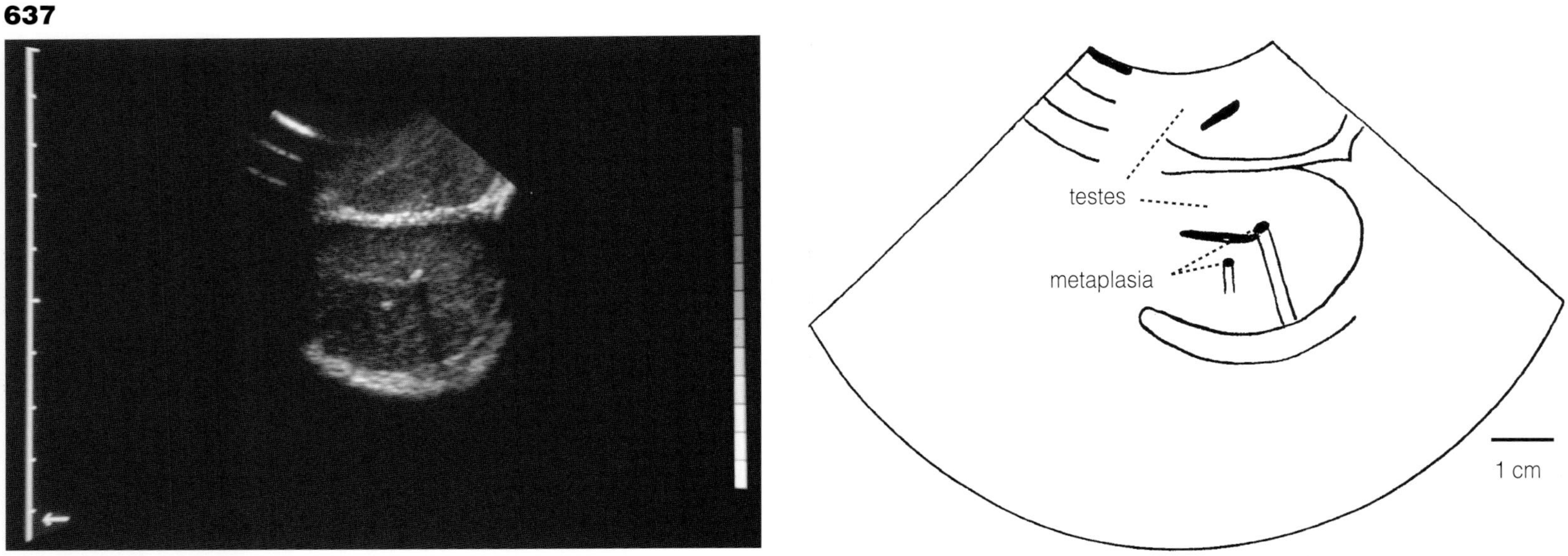

637 Metaplasia of testicular parenchyma in a dog. Two hyperechoic foci with distal shadowing are seen in this longitudinal view. The near testis is used as a stand-off. The mediastinum testis is clearly visible.

638

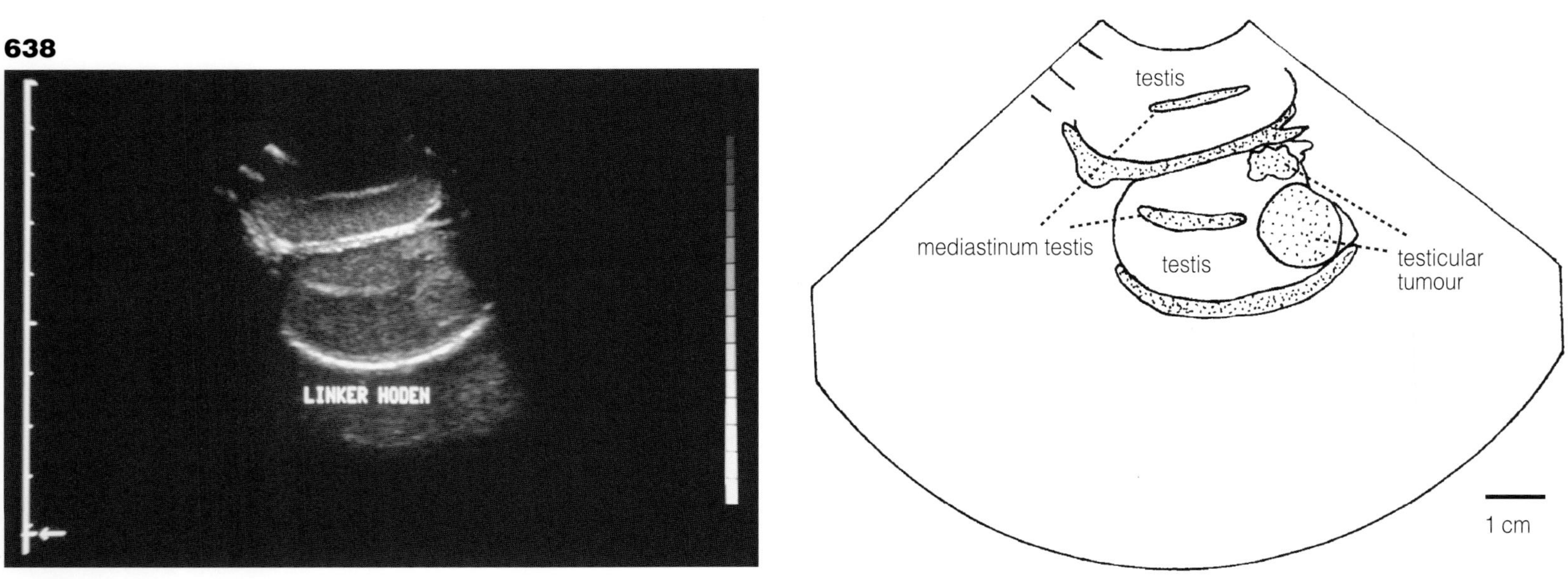

638 Testicular tumour (histopathology: Sertoli cell tumour) in a dog. The gonad shows two demarcated echogenic masses. The mediastinum testis is visible.

639

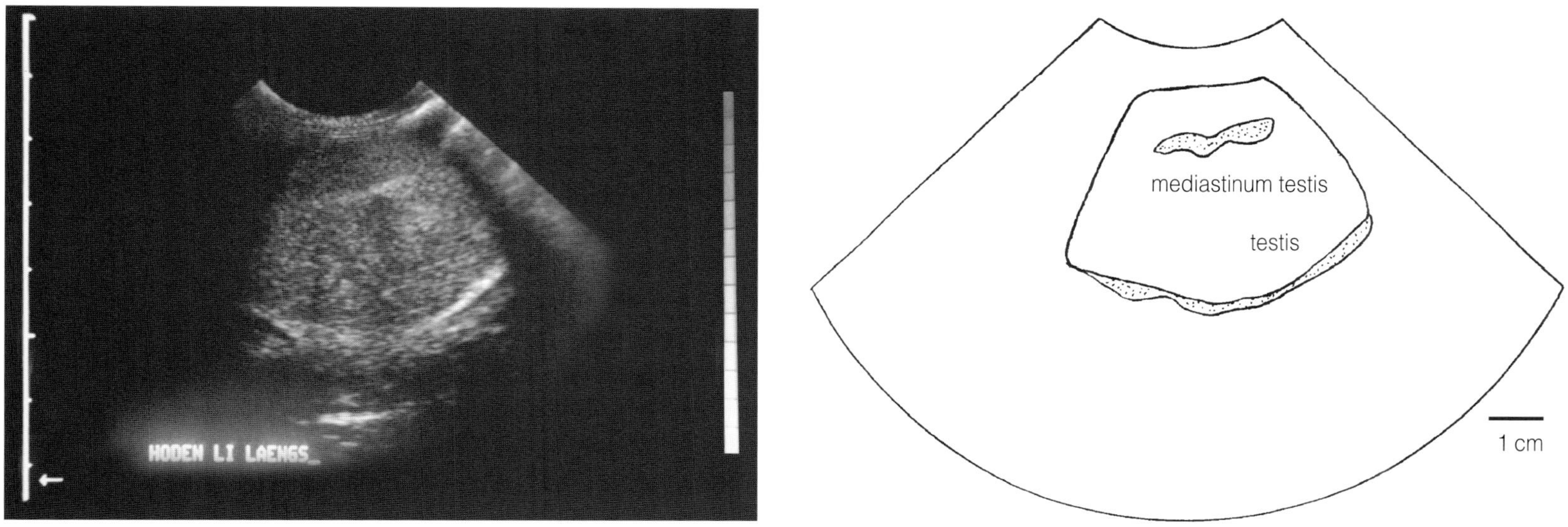

639 Testicular tumour (histopathology: seminoma) in a dog. The testis is enlarged with homogenous parenchyma. The mediastinum testis is visible but decentrally located.

640

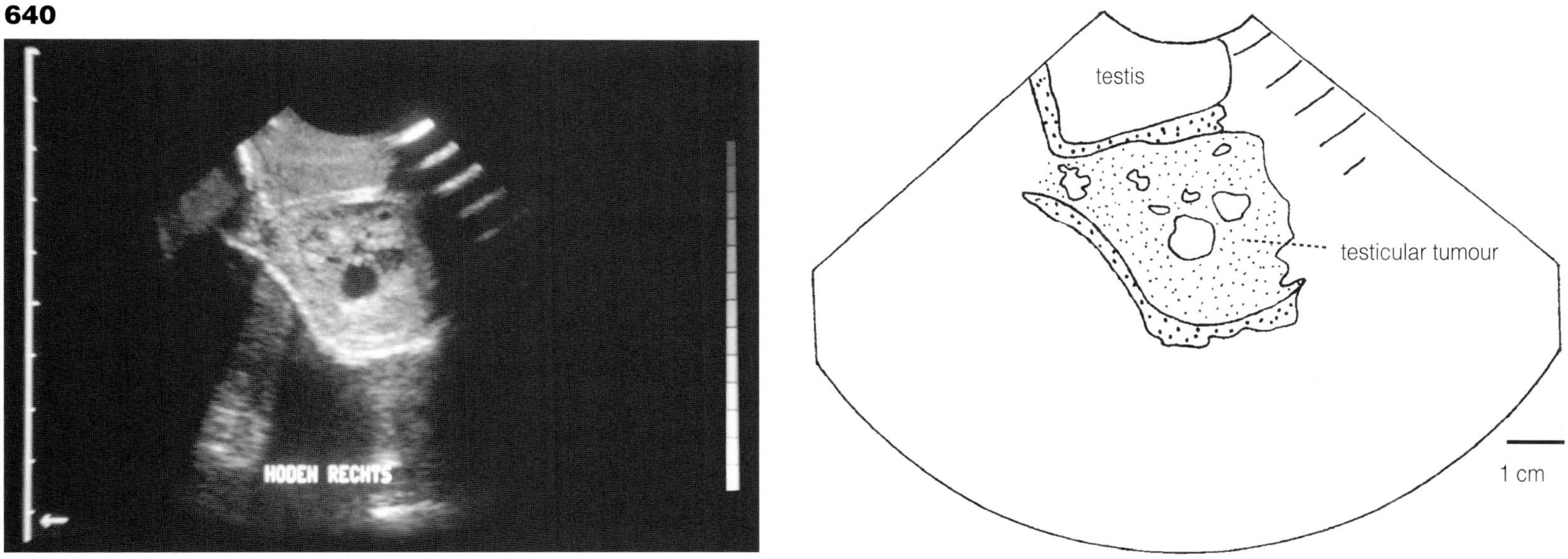

640 Testicular tumour (histopathology: interstitial cell tumour) in a dog. The enlarged testis has a mixed echo pattern and the mediastinum testis is not visible.

641

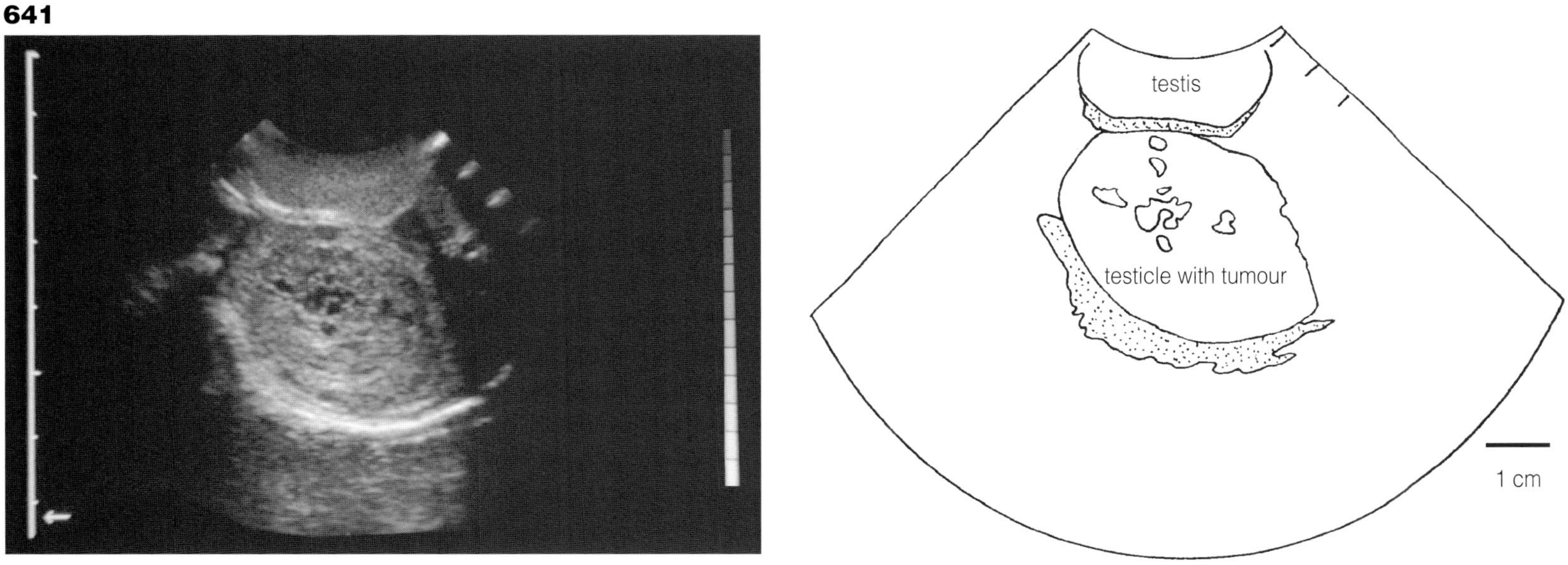

641 Testicular tumour (histopathology: Sertoli cell tumour) in a dog. The testis is enlarged with a complex echo pattern. The mediastinum testis is obliterated. Normal testicular parenchyma is not apparent.

642

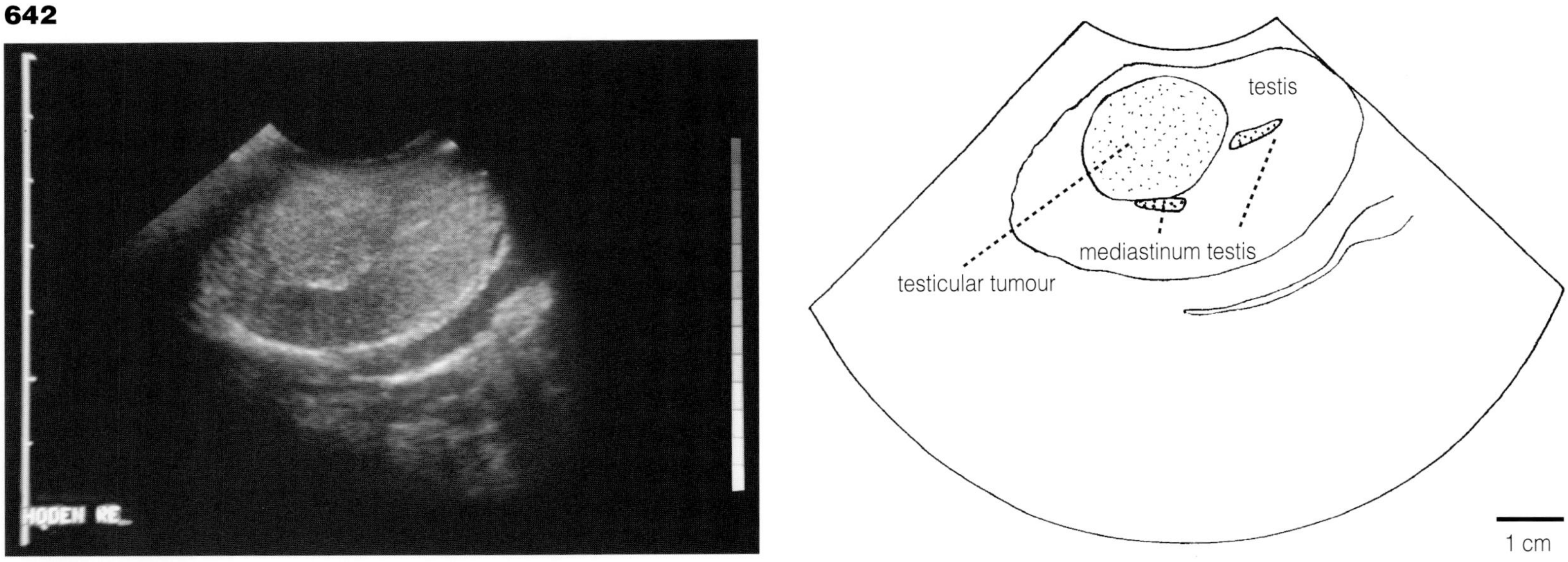

642 Testicular tumour (histopathology: Sertoli cell tumour) in a dog. The enlarged testis shows echogenic, demarcated areas. The mediastinum testis is only partially visible.

643

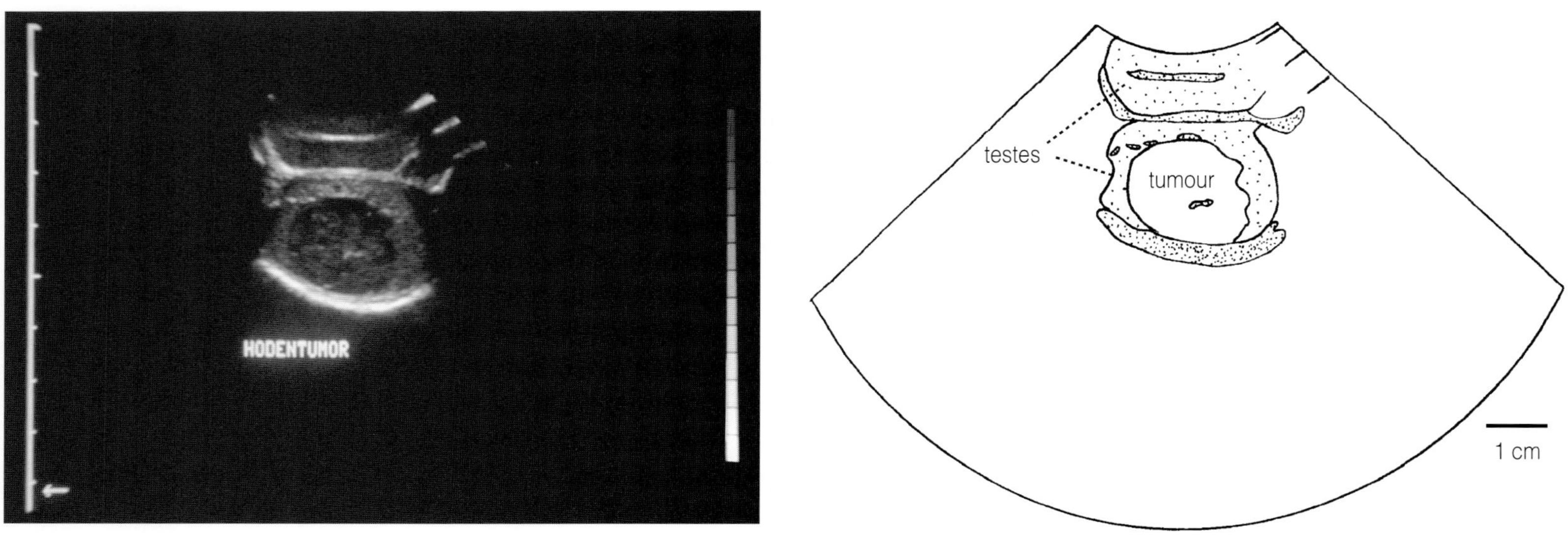

643 Testicular tumour (histopathology: seminoma) in a dog. Hypoechoic, homogenous testicular tumour. The mediastinum testis is interrupted.

644

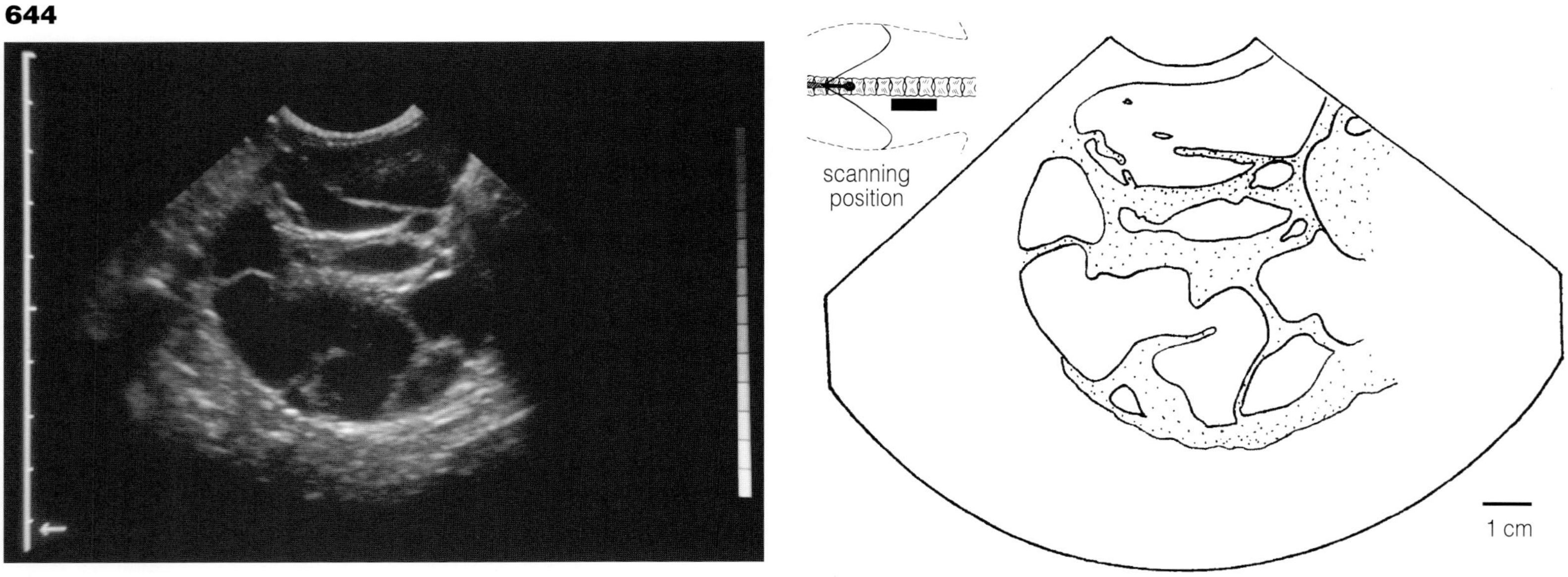

644 Two-dimensional sonogram of a tumorous abdominal testis (histopathology: seminoma) in a dog with unilateral cryptorchidism. The complex mass has anechoic cavities.

645

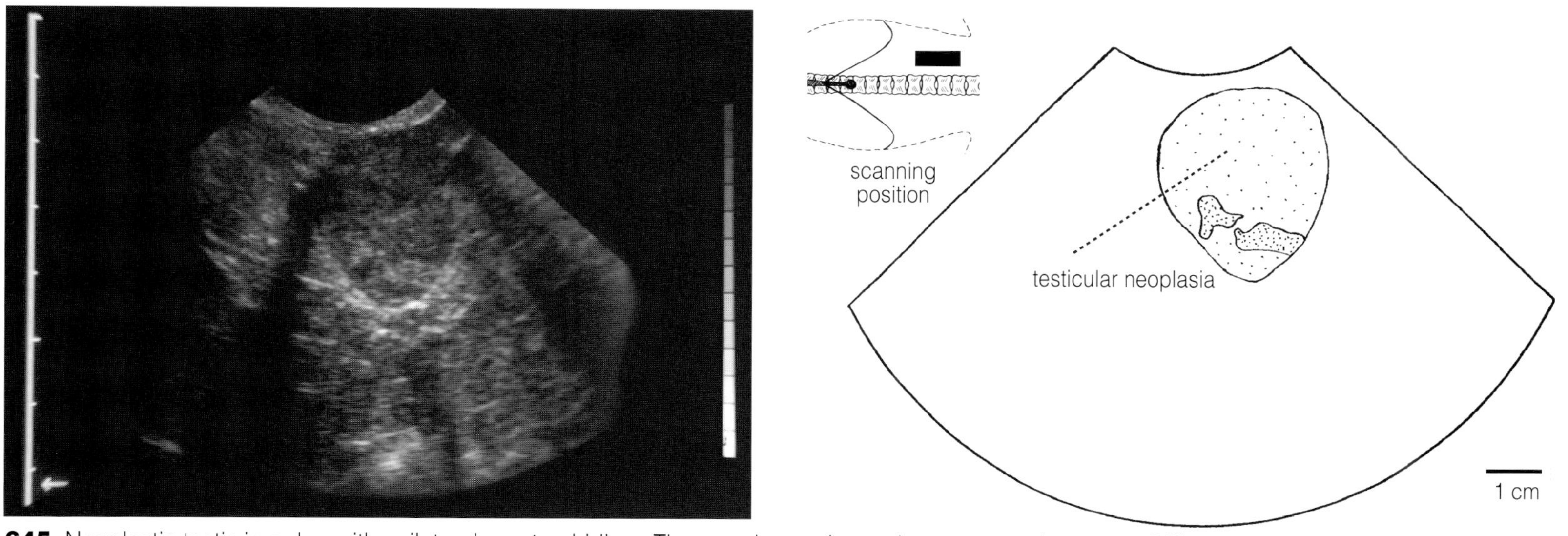

645 Neoplastic testis in a dog with unilateral cryptorchidism. The round mass is non-homogenous in texture. Differential diagnosis includes tumours of other organs, especialy enlarged lymph nodes.

646

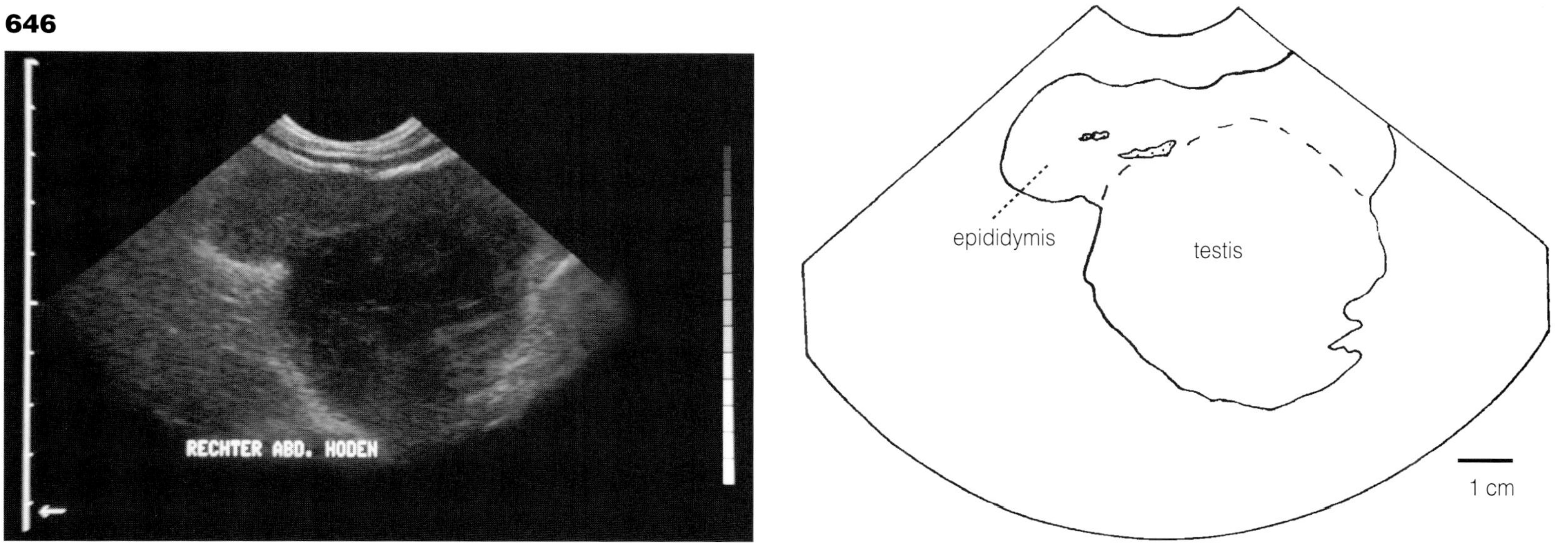

646 Testicular torsion in a dog with an enlarged but homogenous testis.

Some tumours have a normal or hypoechoic pattern (**643**). The mediastinum testis may be completely obliterated, partially missing or decentralized. This may be the only apparent indication of a testicular tumour in the otherwise homogenous, finely textured parenchyma (**639**). Tumours cannot be classified ultrasonographically. A histological examination is necessary[5].

Cryptorchid neoplastic testes may not produce any clinical symptoms and are often an incidental finding. These masses may become quite large and are usually located cranial to the urinary bladder. Their ultrasonographic appearance is that of an non-homogenous, round, complex mass (**644, 645**).

Tumours with a hypoechoic parenchymal pattern cannot be differentiated ultrasonographically from testicular torsion. The mediastinum testis is not visible. The origin of these masses cannot be determined ultrasonographically.

Testicular Torsion and Undescended Testes

Testicular and epididymal enlargement are identified with testicular torsion (**646**). In some cases, dilated vessels are observed as anechoic to hypoechoic, tubular structures distal to the torsion. Differentiation from tumours is difficult to impossi-

647

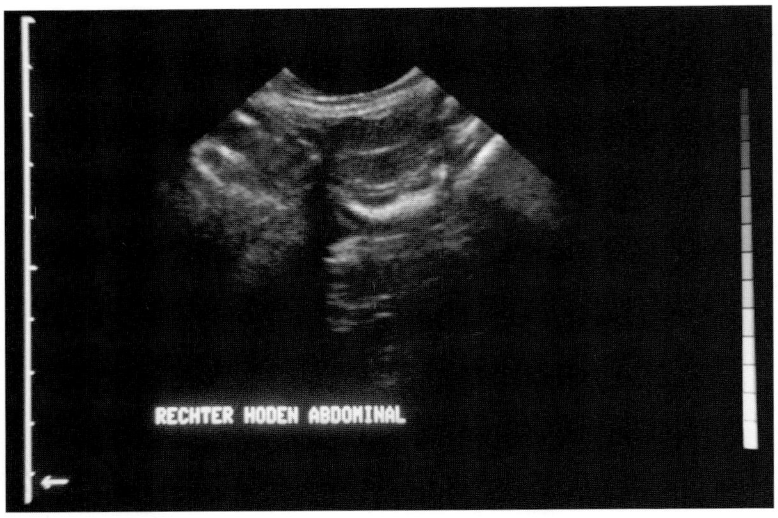

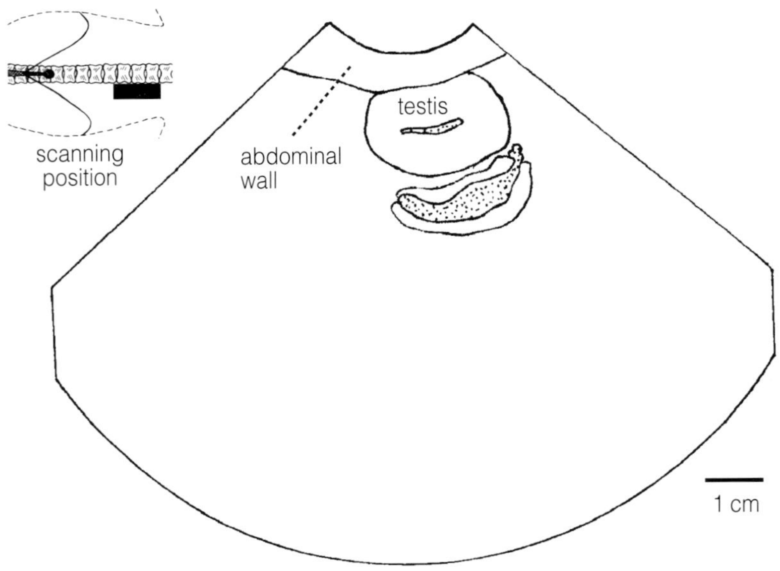

647 Abdominal testis in a dog. Testicular parenchyma is homogenous, the mediastinum testis is clearly visible. Atrophy is not extensive.

ble. Ultrasound is a non-invasive method safely to locate displaced testes. In most cases the undescended testis is found in the abdominal cavity or inguinally. Some cryptorchid testes may atrophy and are difficult to identify. The respective side should be examined from the caudal renal pole to the inguinal area.

Abdominal testes are usually oval, more hypoechoic and smaller than descended testes (**647**). They can be differentiated from lymph nodes by their proximity to the abdominal wall. The mediastinum testis may be missing in the hypoplastic cryptorchid testicle.

The normal inguinal testis usually shows a mediastinum testis. A non-apparent mediastinum in conjunction with non-homogenous parenchyma is usually indicative of neoplasia or inflammation. The inguinal testis is often atrophied and hypoechoic.

References

1 Barr FJ (1990) *Diagnostic Ultrasound in the Dog and Cat*. Blackwell Scientific Publications, Oxford.

2 England GCW (1991) Relationship between ultrasonographic appearance, testicular size, spermatozoal output and testicular lesions in the dog. *J. Small Anim.Pract.* **32**, 306–311.

3 Gerwing M (1993) Sonographie des Skrotalinhaltes – Hoden und Nebenhoden. In: Fritsch R and Gerwing M (Eds.) *Sonographie bei Hand und Katze*. Ferdinand Enke Verlag, Stuttgart.

4 Johnston GR, Feeney DA, Rivers B and Walter PA (1991) Diagnostic imaging of the male canine reproductive organs. *Vet. Clin. North Am. Small Animal Pract.* **21**, 553–589.

5 Johnston GR, Feeney DA, Johnston SD and O'Brien TD (1991) Ultrasonographic features of testicular neoplasia in dogs: 16 cases (1980–1988). *J. Am. Vet. Med. Assoc.* **198**, 1779–1784.

6 Pugh CR, Konde LJ and Park RD (1990) Testicular ultrasound in the normal dog. *Vet. Radiol.* **31**, 195–199

Prostate Gland

Adelheid Prüfer, Dirk Lüerssen and Martin Janthur

Examination Technique

The patient is generally placed in dorsal recumbency for ultrasonography of the prostate gland. Lateral recumbency or a standing position may also be used. The transducer is placed to the side of the prepuce and angled towards the pelvis to image the prostate caudal to the urinary bladder. The prostate gland should be scanned in longitudinal and transverse planes. Digital palpation may be helpful in pushing the prostate craniad.

Normal Sonographic Findings

The prostate gland is evaluated for size, shape, surface and location, as well as for parenchymal texture. In young dogs the prostate is often located within the pelvic cavity and it moves into the abdomen as the animal matures. At five years of age the prostate is situated in the abdomen[1]. Very young dogs have an almond-shaped prostate gland, while older dogs have a more oval or round shaped gland (**648**). A dorsal and ventral indentation is seen in the transverse plane (**649**). The prostatic parenchyma shows moderate echogenicity, but it is more echogenic than adjacent tissue. According to Feeney *et al.* (1989)[3] the prostatic parenchyma is more hypoechoic than its surroundings. This is true for castrated dogs but not in normal dogs, where the prostate is more echogenic. The capsule may be visualized as a thin hyperechoic rim perpendicular to the sound beam. For this reason, only small portions of the capsule covering the round prostate may be evaluated in one image. The parenchymal pattern has a fine texture in the younger dog, while older dogs show a medium to coarse texture (**650**).

The small intrapelvic prostate gland in the cat cannot be imaged transcutaneously. The large fatty deposits caudal to the bladder neck and cranial around the urethra should not be mistaken for an enlarged prostate in cats or in dogs (**651, 652**). While the fatty tissue in the dog is more non-homogenous and echogenic than the normal prostate, the feline 'bladder fat' has a lesser echogenicity.

648

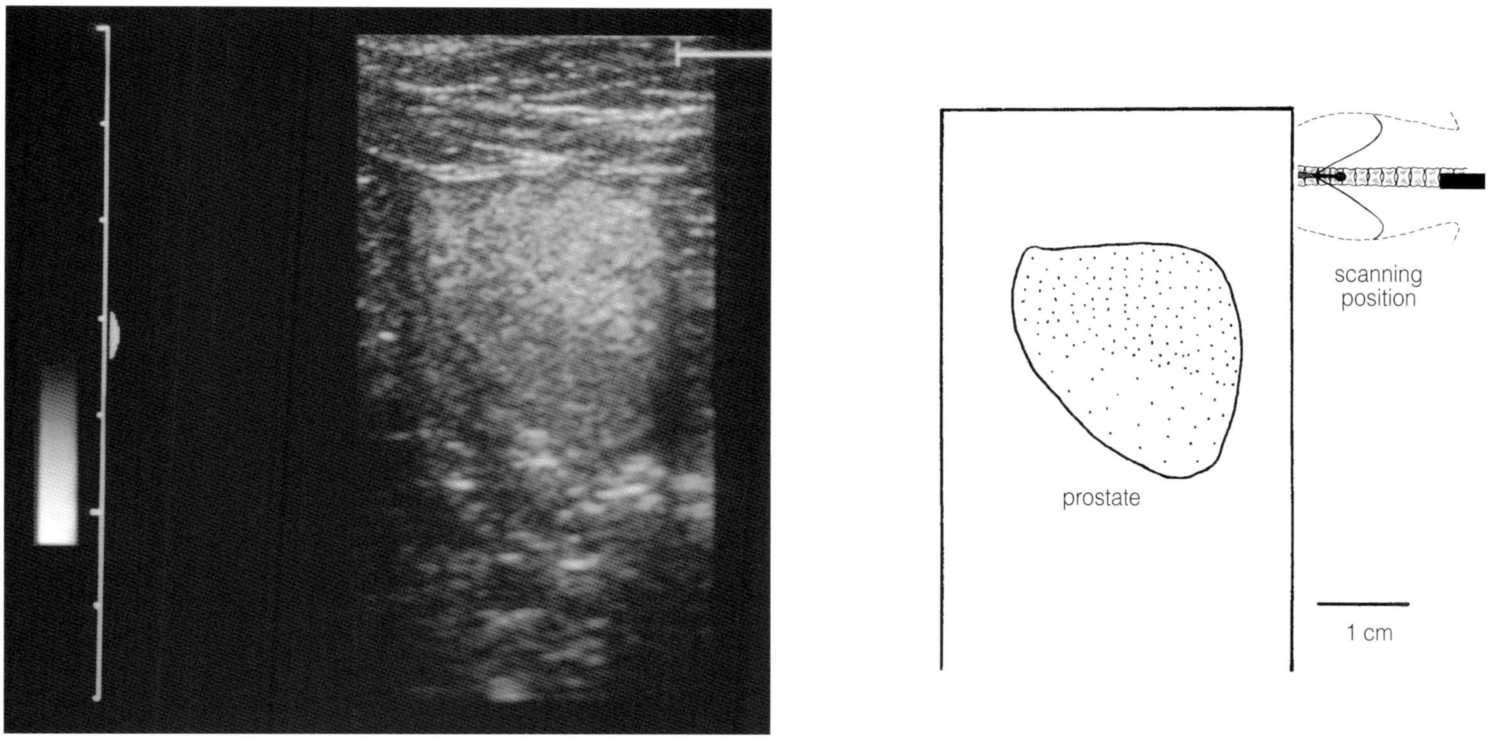

648 Normal prostate gland of a one-year-old dog in a longitudinal plane. The parenchyma is finely textured, more echogenic than the surroundings, and with smooth margins. The shape is ovoid.

649

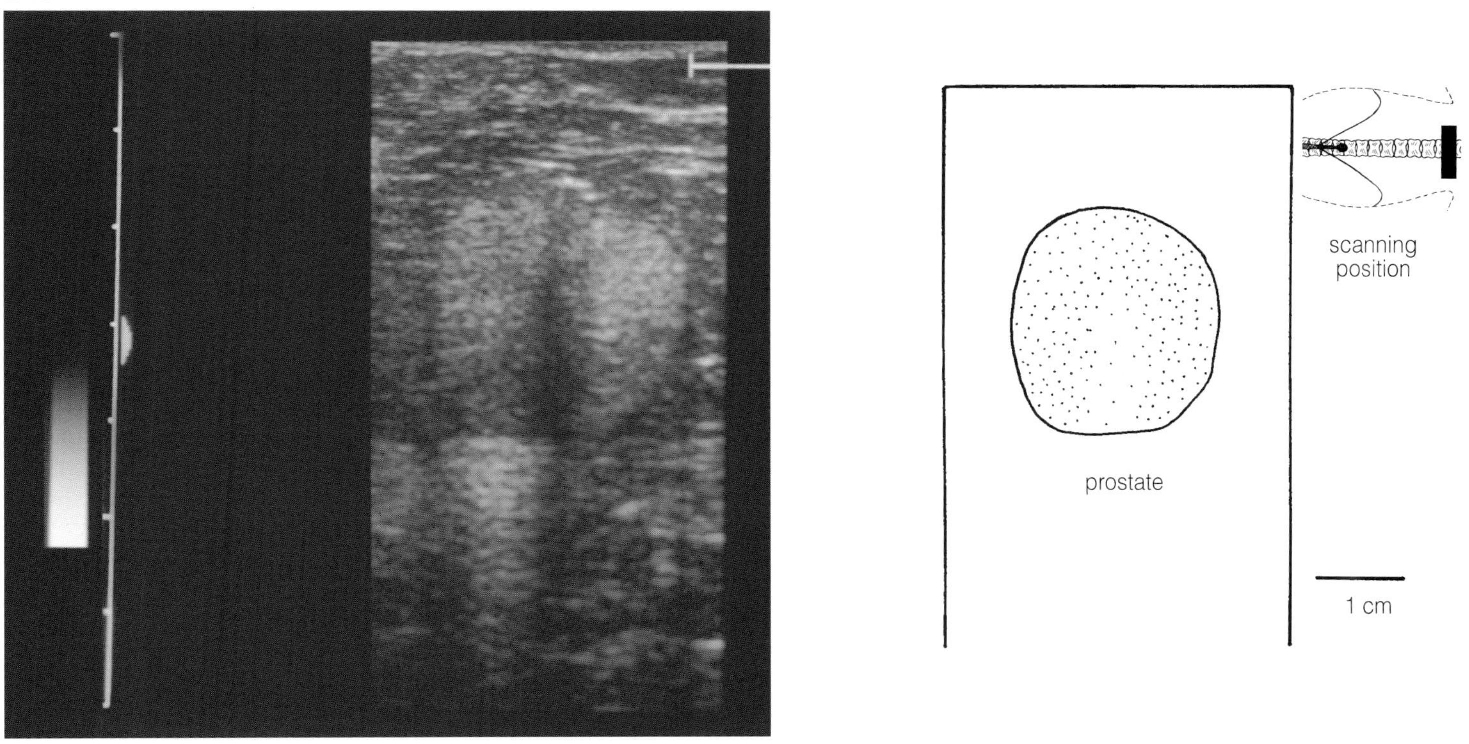

649 Normal prostate gland of a one-year-old dog in a transverse plane. The parenchyma is finely textured, more echogenic than the surroundings, and with smooth margins. The prostate is symmetric with a typical bilobar 'butterfly' shape.

Ultrasonography of Prostatic Disease

Prostatitis

Acute prostatitis is generally diagnosed clinically and on laboratory profiles, since the ultrasound examination is usually too painful for the animal. The sonogram is also non-specific with acute inflammation. The prostate gland appears hypoechoic. As the inflammation progresses, the sonographic image becomes more

Ultrasonography of the prostate gland is indicated with all problems associated with urination and defecation and suspected:

- Prostatitis.
- Prostatic hyperplasia.
- Prostatic and/or paraprostatic cysts.
- Prostatic abscesses.
- Prostatic tumours.

A further indication is for monitoring treatment response.

650

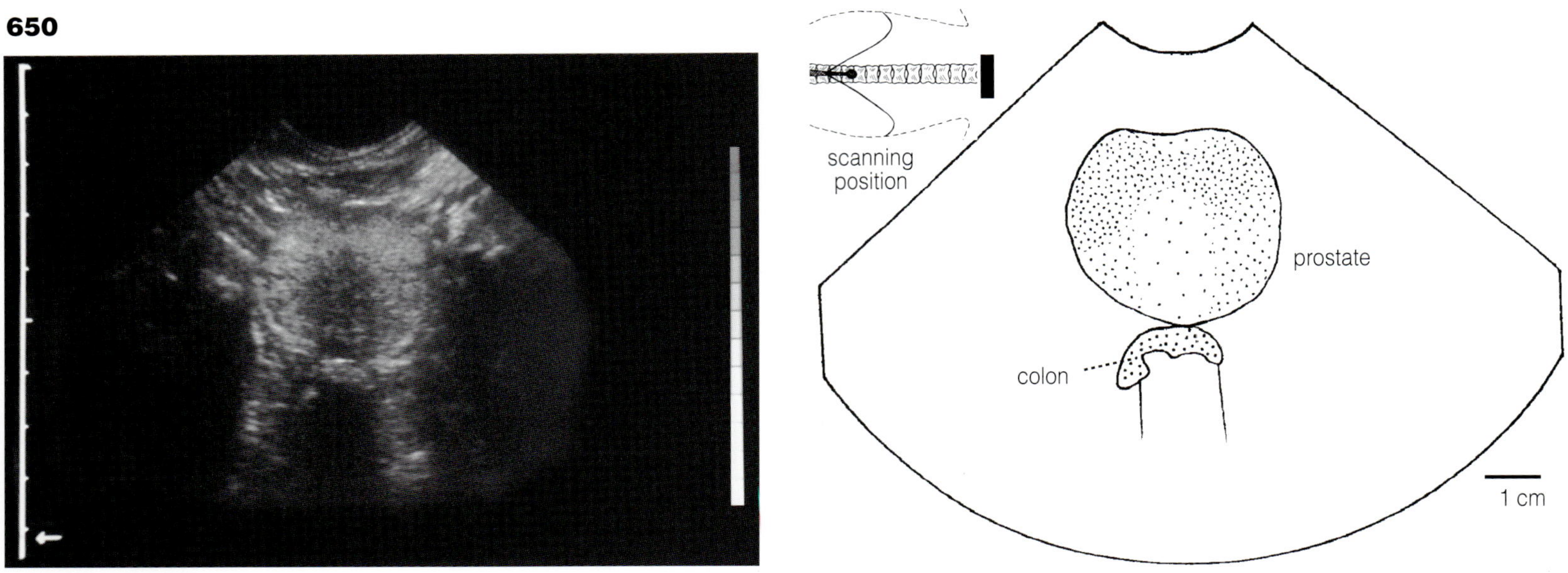

650 Normal prostate gland of a five-year-old dog in a transverse plane. The parenchyma has a coarser texture than in the younger dog and is slightly non-homogenous. The right and left lobes are nearly symmetrical.

651

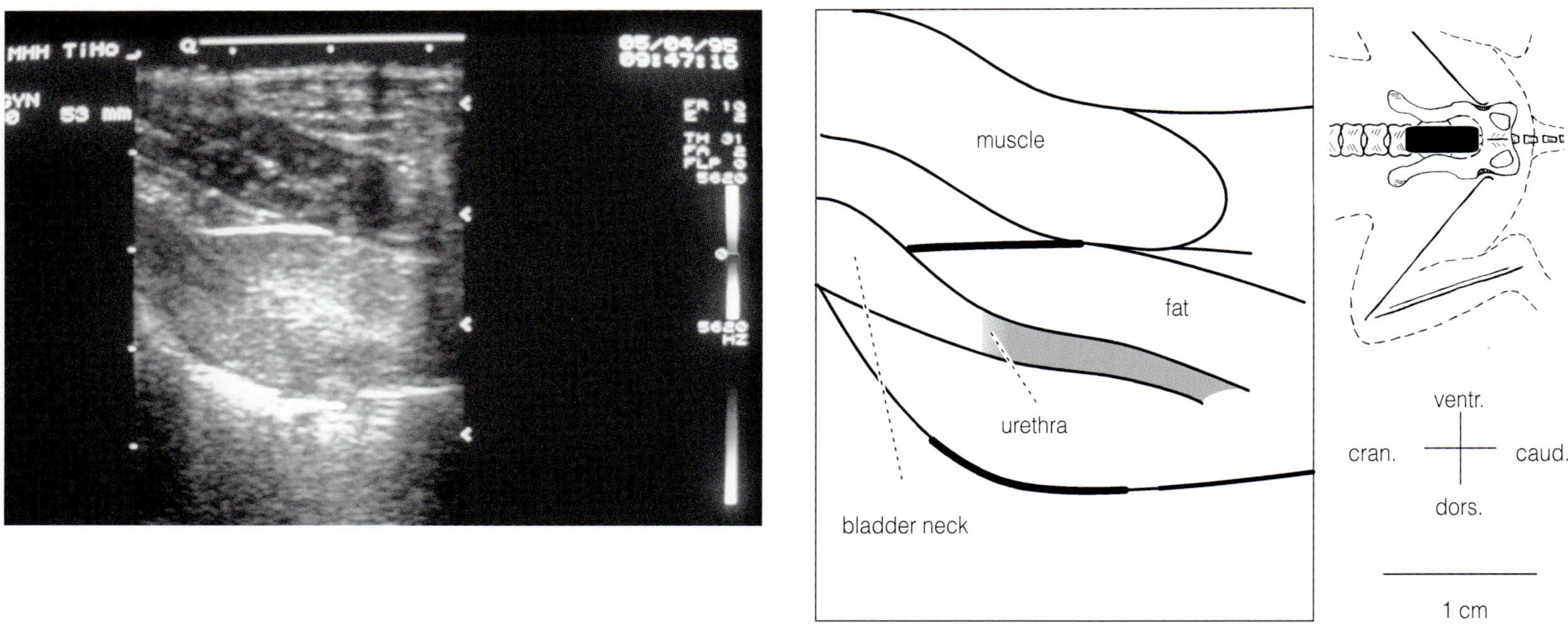

652

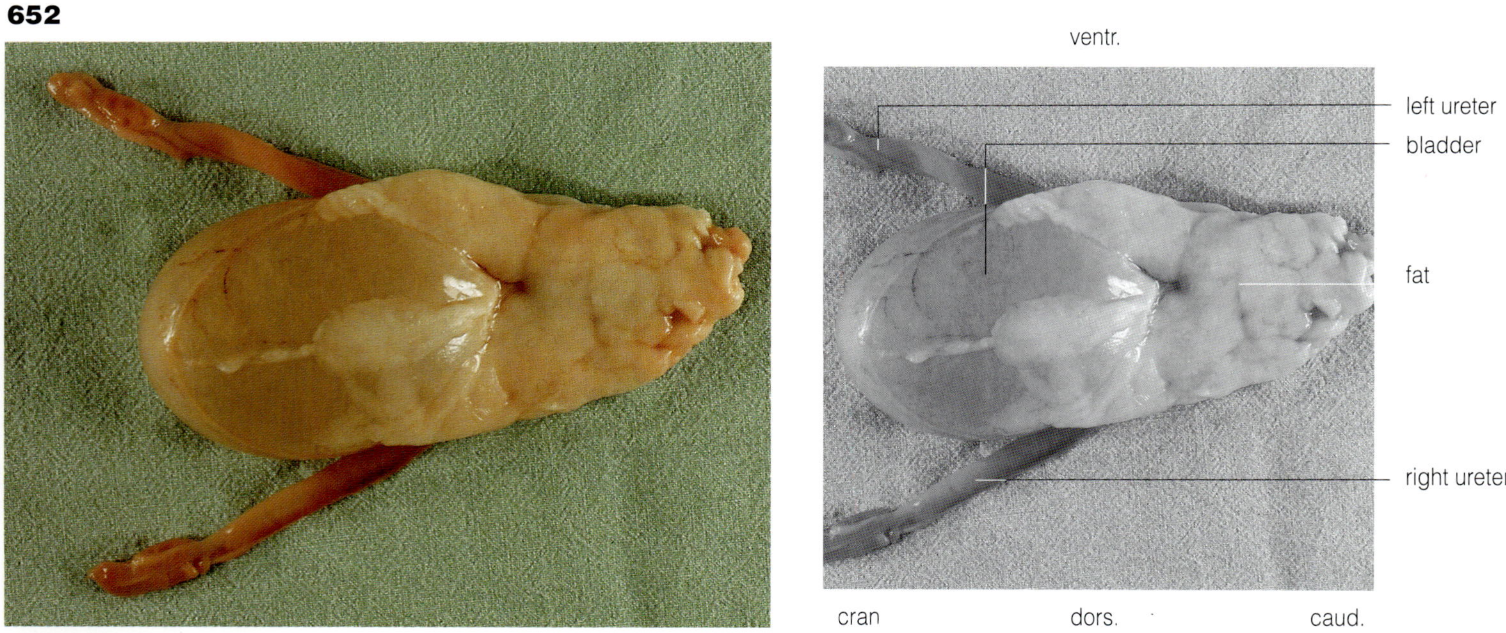

651, 652 Two-dimensional sonogram (**651**) and anatomical specimen (**652**) of fatty tissue near the bladder of a dog in a longitudinal plane. This structure should not be mistaken for an enlarged prostate gland in the sonographic image.

653

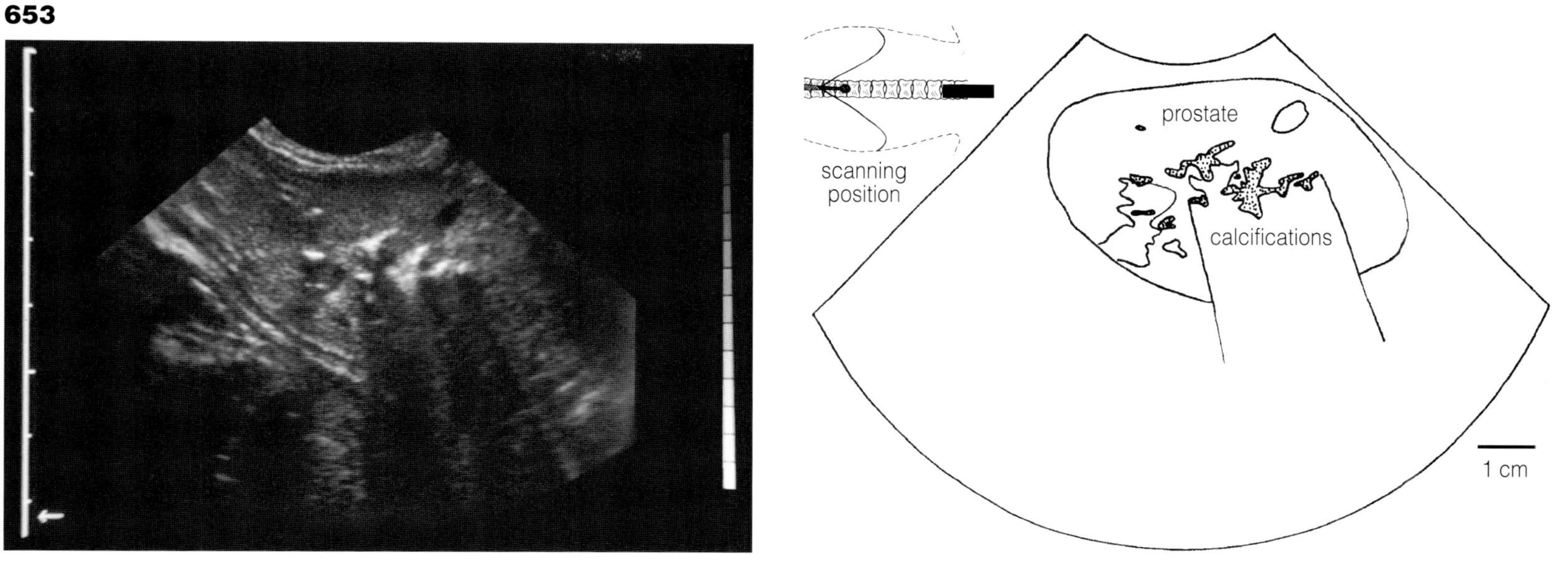

653 Chronic prostatitis in a dog with distinct, irregular calcifications and distal acoustic shadowing within the prostatic parenchyma.

654

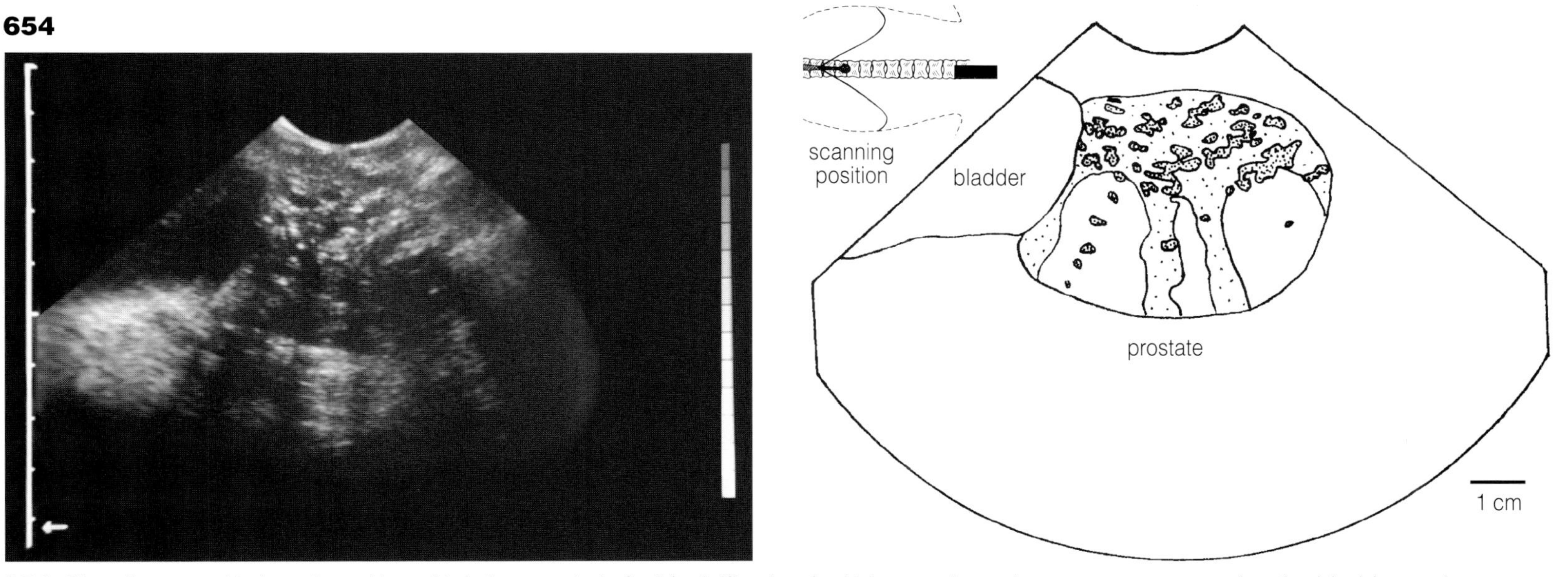

654 Chronic prostatitis in a dog with multiple hyperechoic foci (calcifications) within an enlarged prostate encompassing the bladder neck.

characteristic. The prostatic parenchyma becomes more heterogenous and echogenic. Small calcifications associated with chronic prostatitis are seen as distinct echoes with distal acoustic shadowing (**653, 654**). The gland may be asymmetric.

Chronic prostatitis cannot be differentiated from neoplasia using only ultrasonography. A definitive diagnosis can be made with ultrasound-guided biopsies and histology[4].

Prostatic Hyperplasia

Benign prostatic hyperplasia is a disease affecting older dogs. In the male dog, benign hyperplasia may also manifest itself in younger animals as glandular hyperplasia[2]. The transition from a normal to a hyperplastic prostate is confluent and ultrasonographic evaluation is often subjective. Enlargement of the prostate gland is usually noticed. This can be quantified ultrasonographically by measuring length, width and height. The echogenicity and texture may be normal. The prostate is symmetric and the margins are smooth. As the disease progresses, cysts, abscesses and metaplasia may be apparent in the parenchyma (**655**). The diagnosis, and the result of subsequent castration, can be confirmed a few weeks later by imaging a small, symmetric, hypoechoic prostate[6].

Cysts

Prostatic Cysts

Prostatic cysts of varying size occur with benign hyperplasia when small ducts are obstructed[2]. They are common in seven-year-old to ten-year-old dogs[5]. Most of these cysts are present without any

655

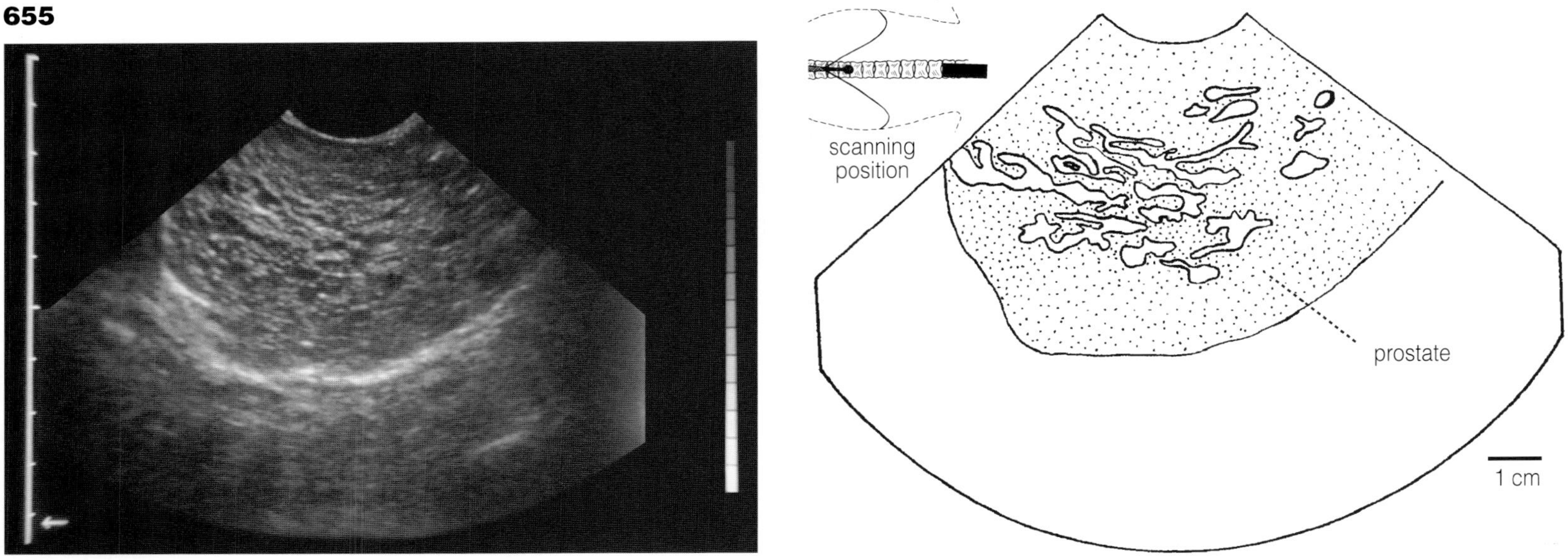

655 Prostatic enlargement and metaplasia in a dog with hypoechoic and hyperechoic areas within the entire parenchyma.

656

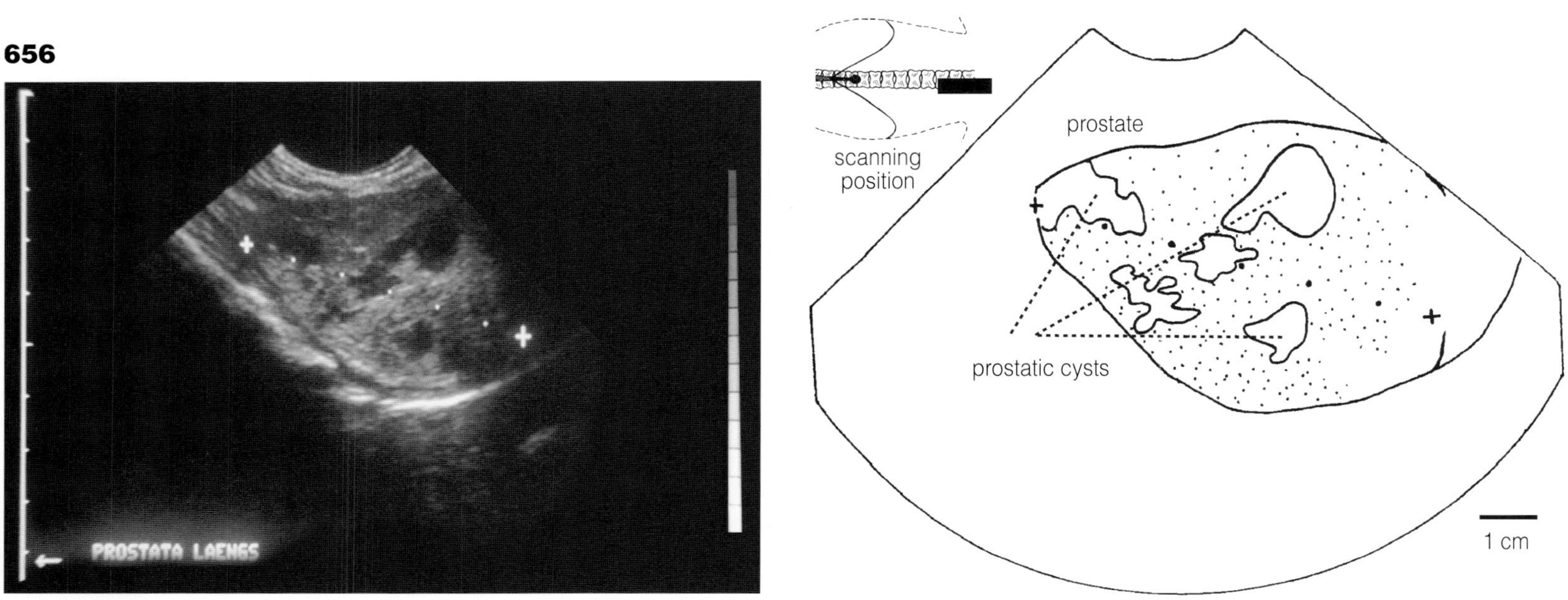

656 Numerous cysts within the prostate gland of a dog in a longitudinal plane. The anechoic areas have irregular margins. The surface of the prostate is smooth.

clinical symptoms and are incidental ultrasonographic findings. Prostatic cysts may be solitary or numerous. The anechoic cysts vary in size from a few millimetres to several centimetres. The remaining prostatic parenchyma is normal in texture. Large cysts produce an asymmetric prostate gland. Prostatic cysts are variable in number, size and echogencity (**656, 657**). For diagnostic and therapeutic purposes, the cysts may be aspirated or drained.

Paraprostatic Cysts

Cysts extending beyond the margins of the prostate are referred to as paraprostatic cysts. By definition, paraprostatic or periprostatic cysts occur through lymphatic vessel obstruction around the prostate gland[9]. Paraprostatic cysts may also be related to intraprostatic cysts and represent complications associated with cysts not recognized or treated.

These large cysts are usually located within the abdomen, cranioiateral to the urinary bladder. In rare cases they may be situated in the perineal region caudal to the bladder. These paraprostatic cysts are usually associated with a perineal hernia.

The sonographic image of paraprostatic cysts shows hypoechoic to anechoic contents. The cystic walls are smooth and thin (**658**). The attachment with the prostate may be visualized with paraprostatic cysts originating intraprostatically. In these cases, additional prostatic cysts are seen within the parenchyma[8]. The parenchymal pattern is coarse and heterogenous. Very large paraprostatic cysts are difficult to differentiate from the urinary bladder. A catheter in the bladder will show a distinct double echo within the lumen. The same method can be used to recognize the urethra.

Prostatic Abscesses

The prostatic abscess represents the most severe form of chronic prostatitis. The pus collected in the prostatic parenchyma appears as a hypoechoic area of variable size. These hypoechoic structures may extend beyond the prostatic margins. Abscesses have a thick echogenic wall and are often divided by internal septa (**659**).

657

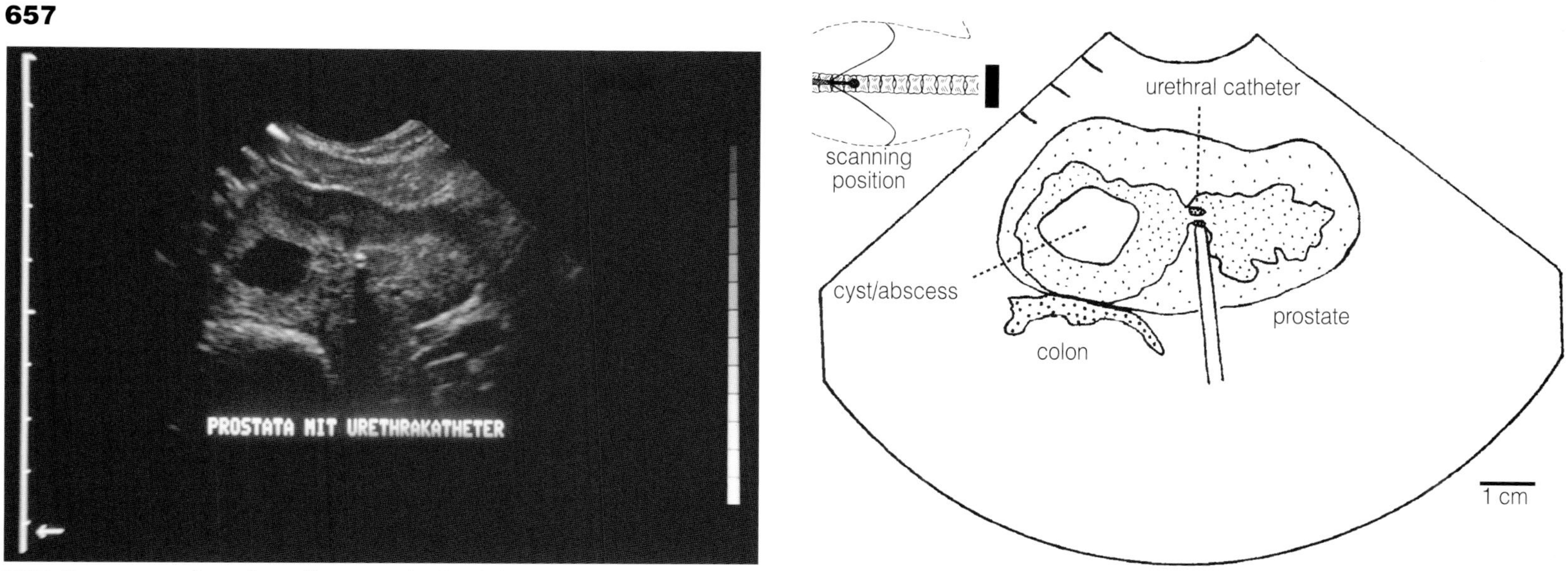

657 Transverse view of a solitary cyst in the right prostatic lobe of a dog. The prostate gland is asymmetric and heterogenous. The urethra is marked by a catheter (central double echo).

658

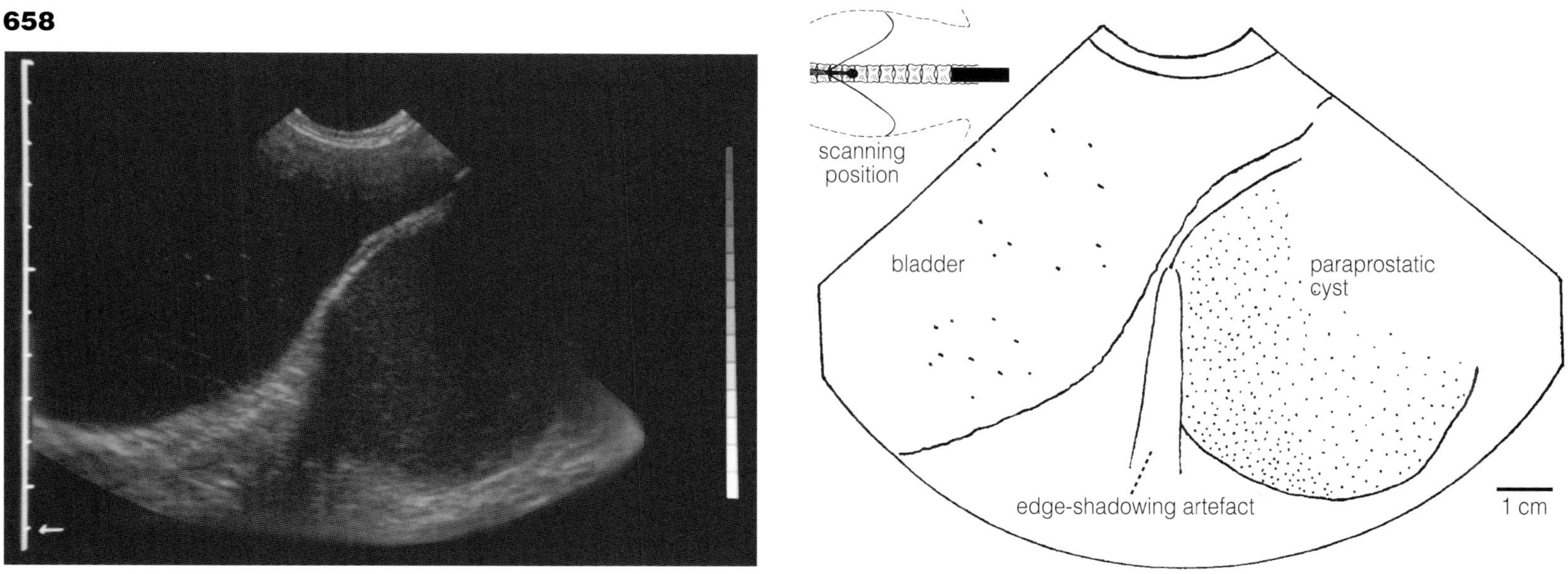

658 Paraprostatic cyst seen as a large hypoechoic mass adjacent to the urinary bladder in a dog.

659

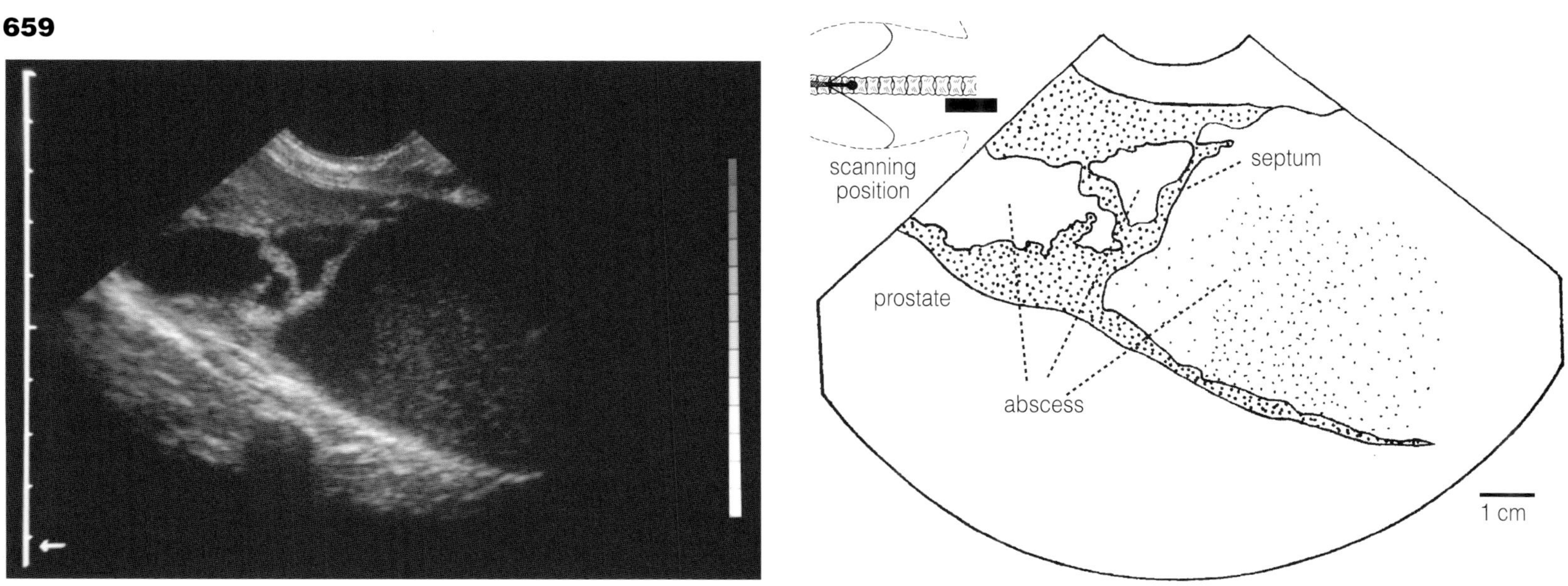

659 Prostatic abscess with internal septa and hypoechoic contents in a dog. Prostatic parenchyma is recognized peripherally.

660

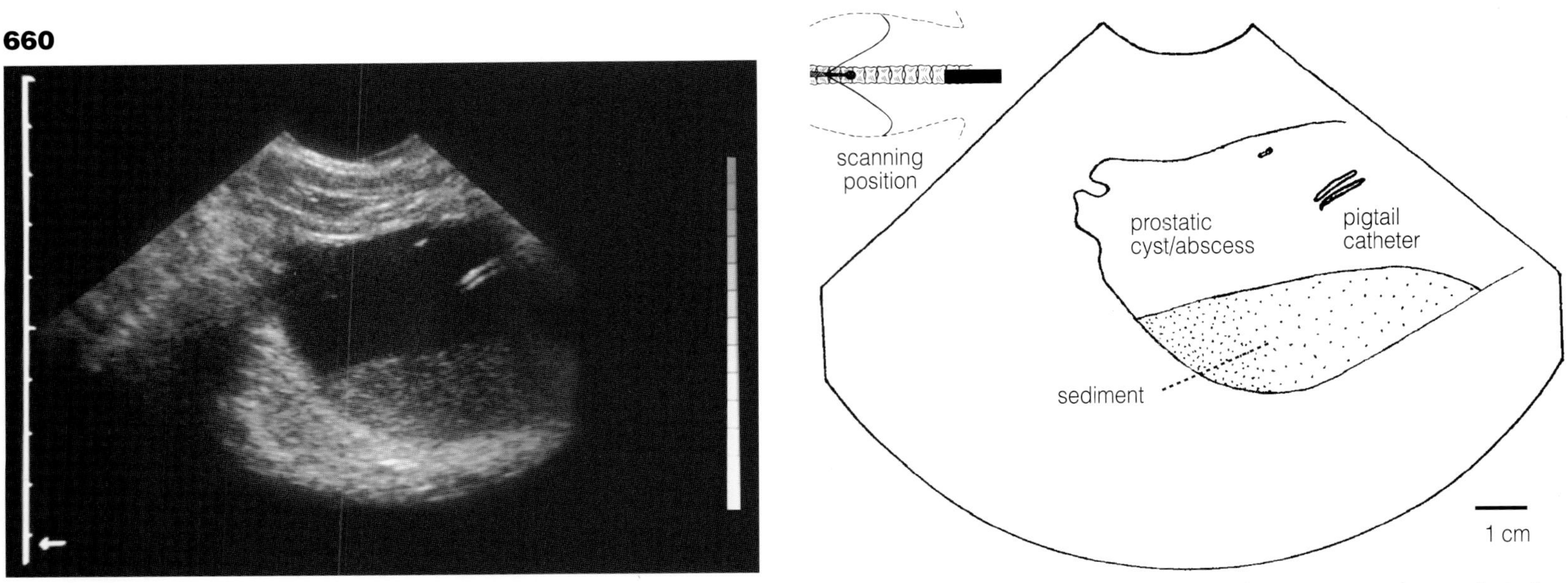

660 Prostatic abscess extending over the margins of the prostate and containing focal echogenicities in a dog. A catheter was used to aspirate the fluid.

661

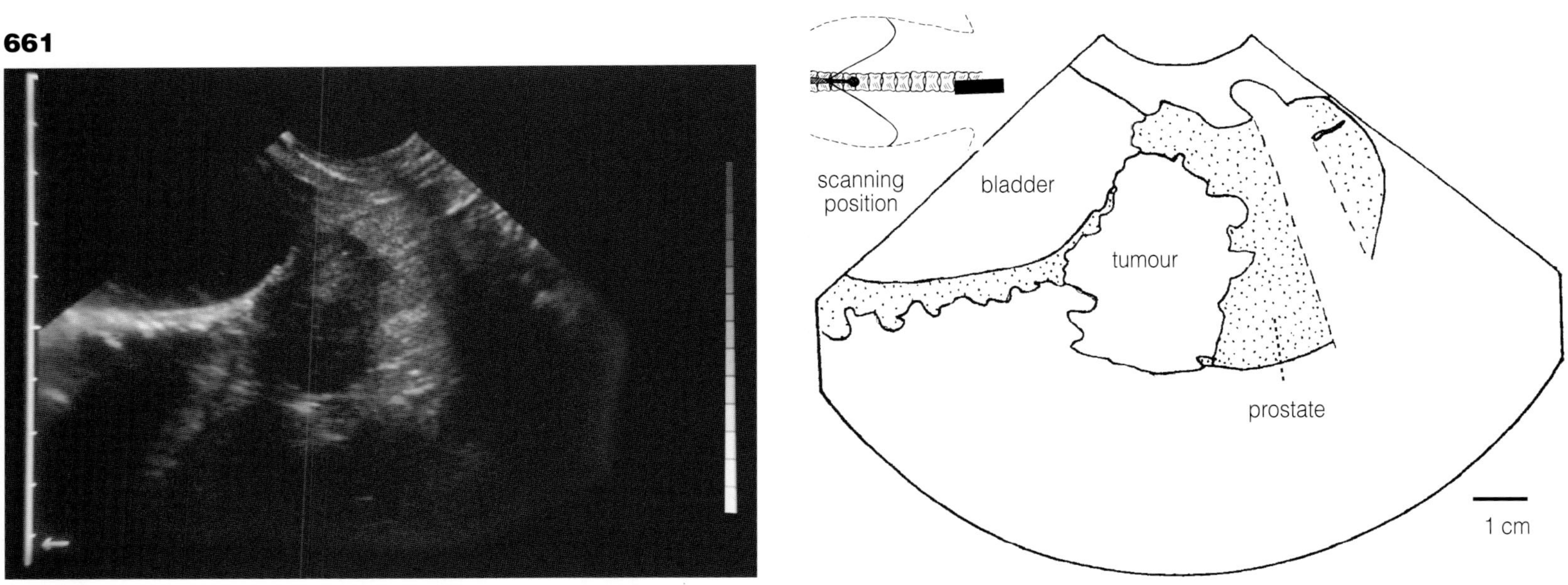

661 Focal, non-homogenous, hypoechoic mass surrounding the bladder neck and extending beyond the prostatic margins in a dog. A tumour (carcinoma) was confirmed histopathologically.

662

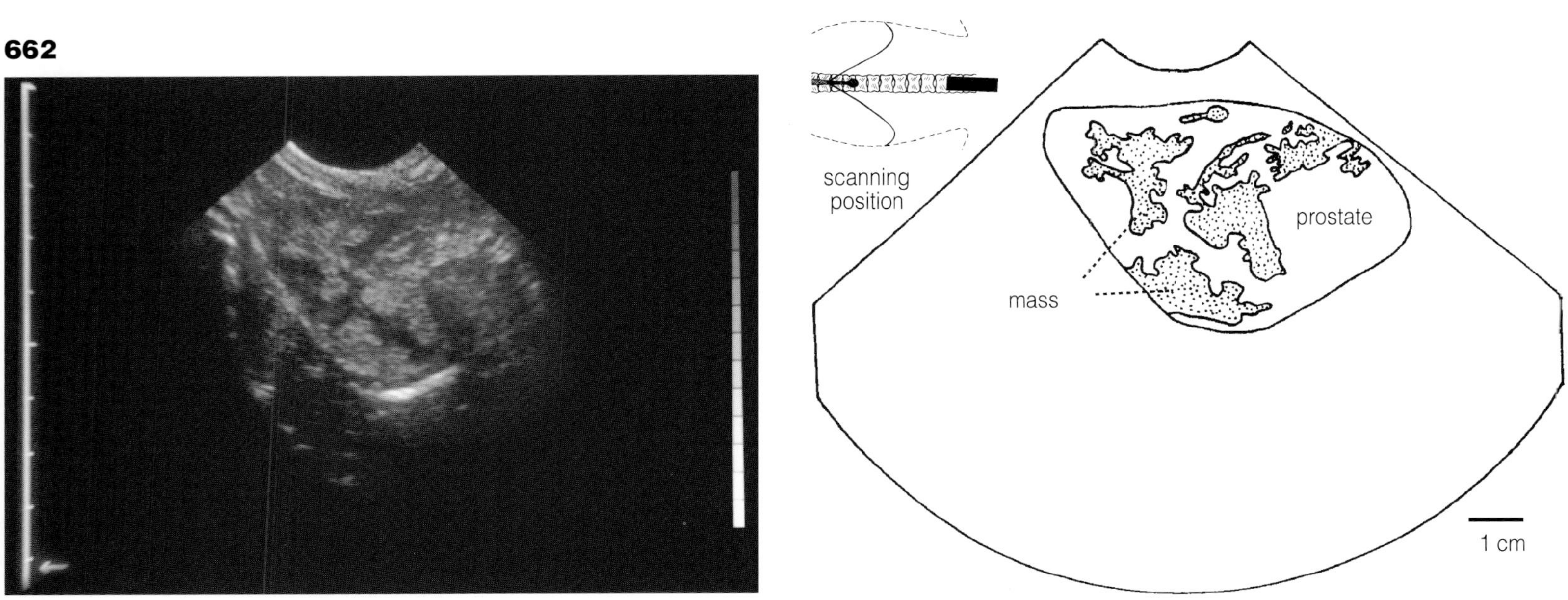

662 Hyperechoic prostatic mass with lobulated architecture in a dog. A tumour (adenoma) was confirmed histopathologically.

Focal echogenicities may be seen in the contents of the abscess. These swirling particles move to the dependent portion of the abscess (**660**). Abscesses and cysts cannot always be differentiated. Ultrasound-guided aspiration is helpful in differentiating and treating these lesions[7].

Prostatic Neoplasia

The most common prostatic tumours are adenomas and adenocarcinomas. The prostate gland is enlarged and often asymmetric. Ultrasonographic lesions are usually focal. The parenchymal texture is coarse. Focal lesions are generally more hypoechoic than the surrounding prostatic parenchyma (**661**). Hyperechoic 'white' tumours are also possible (**662**).

References

1 Dahme E and Weiss E (1983) *Grandriß der Speziellen Pathologischen Anatomie der Haustiere*. Ferdinand Enke Verlag, Stuttgart.

2 Ewing LL (1984) Testicular androgen and estrogen secretion and benign prostatic hyperplasia in the beagle. *Endocrinology* **114**, 1308–1312.

3 Feeney DA, Johnston GR and Bell FW (1989) Canine prostatic ultrasonography – 1989. *Semin. Vet. Med. Surg.* **4**, 44–57.

4 Feeney DA, Johnston GR, Klausner JS, Perman V, Linenger JR and Tomlinson MJ (1987) Canine prostatic disease – comparison of ultrasonographic appearance with morphologic and microbiologic findings: 30 cases (1981–1985). *J. Am. Vet. Med. Assoc.* **190**, 1027–1024.

5 Gerwing M (1989) *Sonographische Darstellung von Milz und Prostata des Handes unter Besonderer Berücksichtigung der Messung ihrer Lage und Größe Sowie des Sonographischen Bildes der Pathologischen Veränderungen – Das Hydroperitoneum zur Besseren Differenzierung Abdominaler Organe*. Gießen, Justus-Liebig-Univ., Veterinärmed., Diss.

6 Lamb CR (1990) Abdominal ultrasonography in small animals: intestinal tract and mesentery, kidneys, adrenal glands, uterus and prostate. *J. Small Anim.Pract.* **31**, 295–304.

7 Lüerssen D (1993) Perkutane Drainage von Prostataabszessen unter sonographischer Darstellung anhand von zwei Fallbeispielen. *Kleintierpraxis* **38**, 15–20.

8 Stowater JL and Lamb CR (1989) Ultrasonographic features of paraprostatic cysts in nine dogs. *Vet. Radiol.* **30**, 232–239.

9 Weiss E (1985) Prostata. In: Dobberstein J, Pallaske G and Stünzl H (Eds.) *Joest: Handbuch der Speziellen Pathologischen Anatomie der Haustiere. Vol. 4*. Paul Parey Verlag, Berlin, Hamburg.

11 Pregnancy and Parturition, Mammary Glands

Normal Pregnancy

General Observations

Danielle Schäffer

First reports on the successful use of ultrasonography for pregnancy diagnosis in sheep and dogs were published in the late 1960s and early 1970s[29, 37, 38]. At this time, A-mode and/or Doppler techniques were employed (see History of Diagnostic Ultrasonography, page 18; **4**). Today, two-dimensional real-time ultrasonography is almost exclusively used. This method, in conjunction with sonographic biometry, allows the estimation of gestational age and the evaluation of growth retardation or differences in fetal size within the same litter, as well as the diagnosis of deformities and abortions. PW and colour-coded Doppler ultrasonography provide additional methods of demonstrating normal or abnormal flows within the cardiovascular system of the dam and the fetus. These techniques identify decreased placental or fetal perfusion and illustrate fetal maturation.

> Ultrasonographic pregnancy diagnosis is similar in the dog and cat. Gestational age varies by a few days.

Problems with Assessing Gestational Age

Published reports on the earliest possible diagnosis of pregnancy vary from day 7 to day 28 post breeding. Much of the variation in these studies is due to differences in defining the onset of pregnancy. Authors refer to the first breeding date[5, 24, 26], the last day of breeding[10, 13] or the preovulatory LH surge in the blood[20] when determining gestational age. Variations in the canine heat cycle, such as behaviour and duration, add to these differences (see Requirements for Exact Gestational Age Determination, page 304; **699**). Gestational age is also difficult to determine because of differences in resolution of ultrasound equipment and confusing reports by dog owners.

Assessing gestational age in the cat appears to show fewer discrepancies. Breeding date and conception are closer together than in the bitch, because of induced ovulation in the cat.

The following data refer to the first successful breeding day (day 0 post breeding) or endocrinological determination of ovulation (day 0 post ovulation). Most of the following cited references are converted when possible.

Problems with Producing a Sonographic Diagnosis

A correct sonographic diagnosis not only depends on the sonographer's experience, but also on the quality or resolution of the ultrasound equipment. The choice of transducer type and frequency is therefore very important. Diagnosis of early pregnancy requires a transducer with good near-field detail. Heart movement and fetal body shapes are recognized later with low-frequency transducers (3.5 MHz) than with higher frequencies of 5.0–10 MHz (**663, 664**). In contrast, high-frequency transducers with poor penetration (7.5 and 10 MHz) may not be able to image all areas in large breed dogs during late pregnancy. Poor near-field resolution with sector transducers, compared to linear or curved-array scanners, can be improved by using a stand-off pad. The distance between transducer and skin or gestational sacs can also be increased by changing the scanning position and moving the region of interest into the focal zone (**664**).

> For extensive, two-dimensional sonographic pregnancy diagnosis, linear, curved-array and sector (with stand-off) transducers, with frequencies ranging from 5.0–7.5 MHz, represent a good compromise between resolution and penetration.

Indications for Pre- and Intranatal Sonography

Pregnancy determination, fetal number and viability can be assessed during the first half of pregnancy (day 25 to day 35 post breeding). In some cases, such as a single fetus, a breed-related higher abortion risk (e.g. Persian cats) or a history of previous problems during pregnancy, the animal should also be examined during the second half of pregnancy. The fetus should be monitored for anatomy, growth and vitality (heart and fetal motion). Intranatal sonography is helpful in assessing any problems during parturition that might indicate the need for a Caesarean section.

An exact pregnancy diagnosis can only be made with a careful and extensive sonographic examination of all gestational sacs and fetuses. This examination is time consuming. A superficial sonographic pregnancy examination can lead to a false diagnosis with reference to fetal number, development and viability, even with experienced sonographers. Congenital deformities may not be recognized during these 'quick' examinations (see Indications and Requirements, page 76).

Ultrasonography is a valuable supplementary diagnostic aid to the usual methods of palpation and hormone testing. Radiographs should be kept to a maximum of two shortly before parturition. They are useful for determining the number of fetuses and assessing fetal size in relation to the birth canal in problem breeds and single fetus pregnancies. Radiographs are usually taken on day 42 post breeding in dogs and day 38 post breeding in cats. Compared to ultrasonography, radiographs have little value in determining fetal vitality and they expose the fetus to radiation.

Patient Preparation

Dogs and cats with a long, silky hair coat do not require clipping, since the hair is easily parted after applying alcohol. Alcohol

663

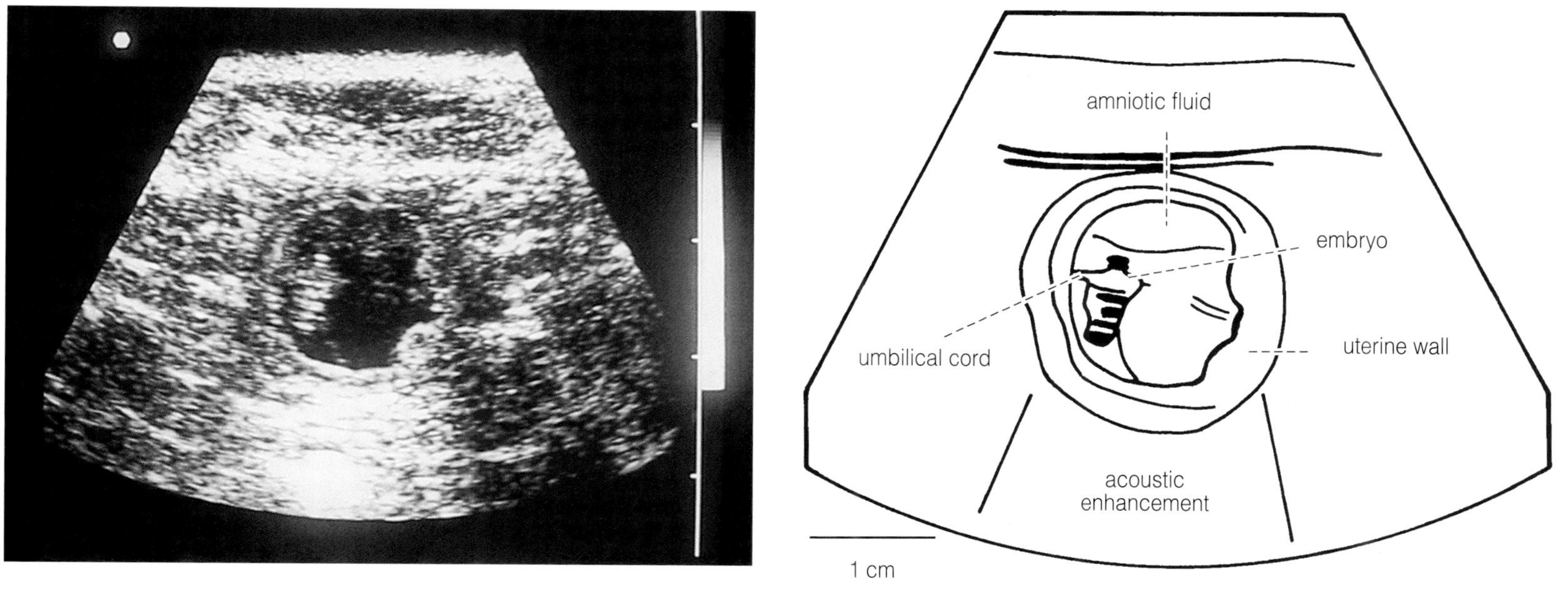

664

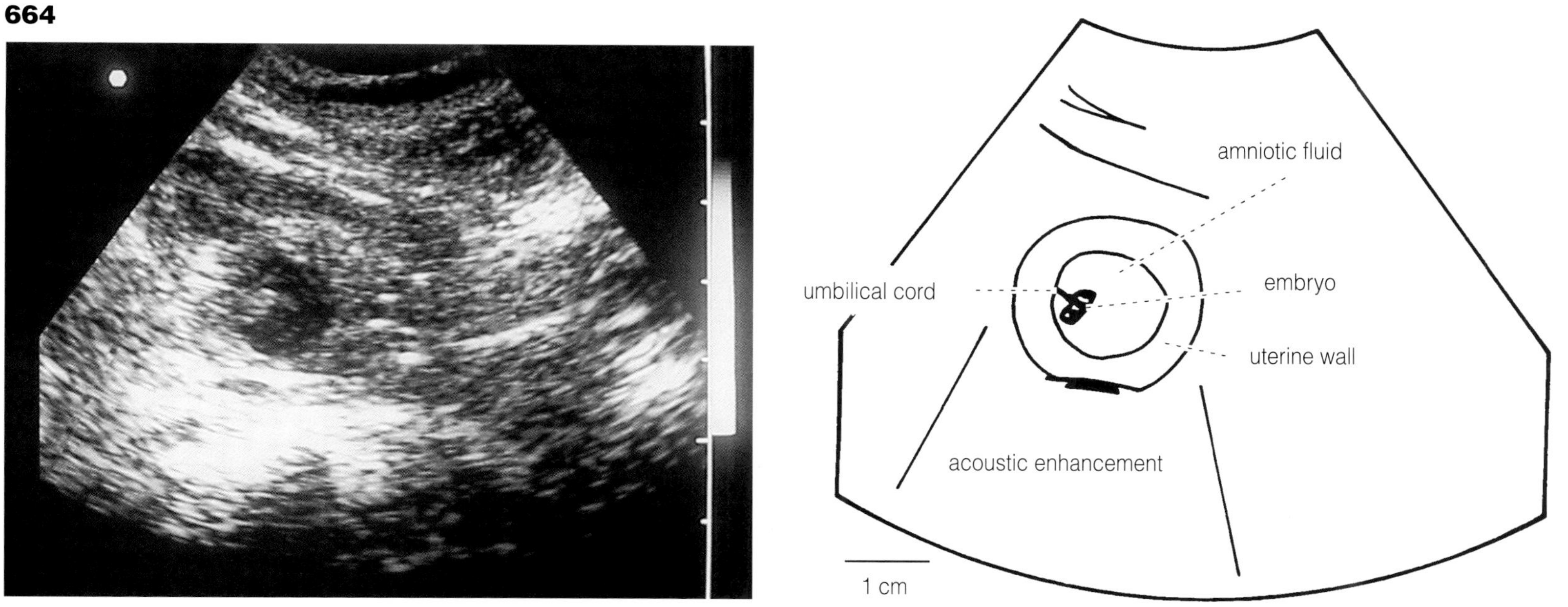

663, 664 Different frequency-dependent detail at the gestational sac wall in a cat during early pregnancy (day 18 post breeding), using a 7.5 MHz sector transducer with a built-in stand-off (**663**) and a 3.5 MHz sector transducer (**664**). The distance between the transducer and the gestational sac had to be increased with the low-frequency transducer to move the region of interest into the focal zone.

improves transducer coupling by degreasing the skin and the remaining hair.

Animals with a shorter hair coat and/or a thick undercoat should be clipped for examination in order to ensure good skin contact and improve image quality. The hair can be removed in a thin line between the mammary glands or more extensively over the entire ventral abdomen. It is important to clip the hair coat around every mammary gland, since the newborns may avoid the clipped areas. These hairless mammary glands may then develop mastitis (see Patient Preparation, page 77).

Pregnant animals should not be sedated for ultrasonographic examination.

Transcutaneous ultrasonography of the bitch should be performed with the animal in a standing position, or in lateral or dorsal recumbency, depending on the size and temperament of the animal. During late pregnancy the animals should not be placed in dorsal recumbency. Reports from human medicine have shown that excess weight on the large abdominal veins causes discomfort, queasiness and reduced placental perfusion.

Ultrasound examination in cats should be performed on the

665

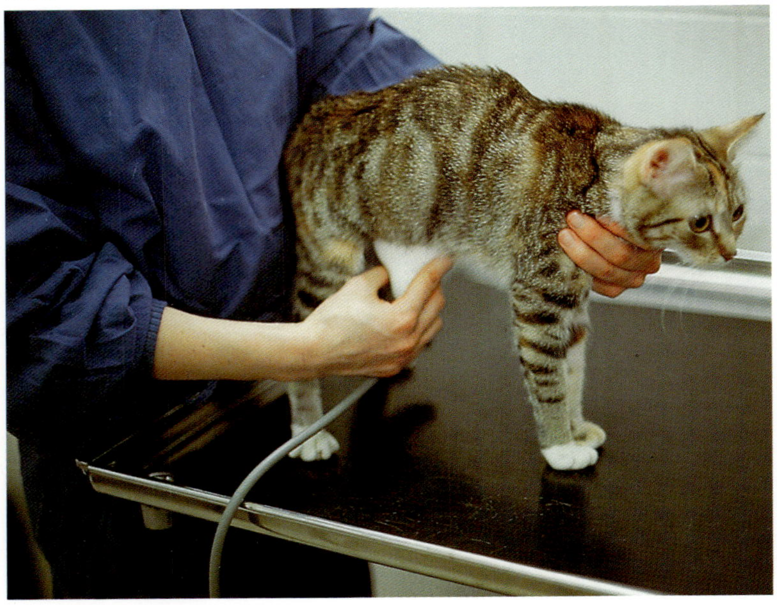

666

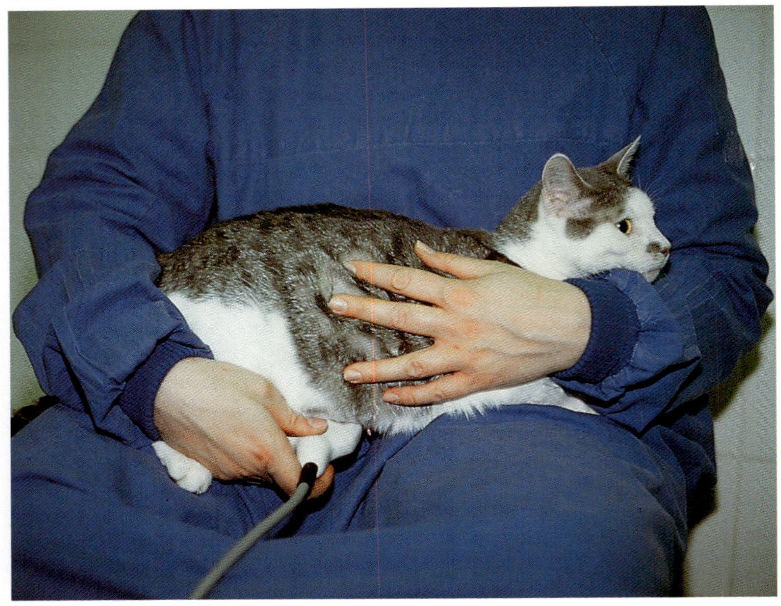

665, 666 Ultrasonographic pregnancy diagnosis in a lightly restrained standing cat (**665**) and in a cat on the sonographer's lap (**666**).

667

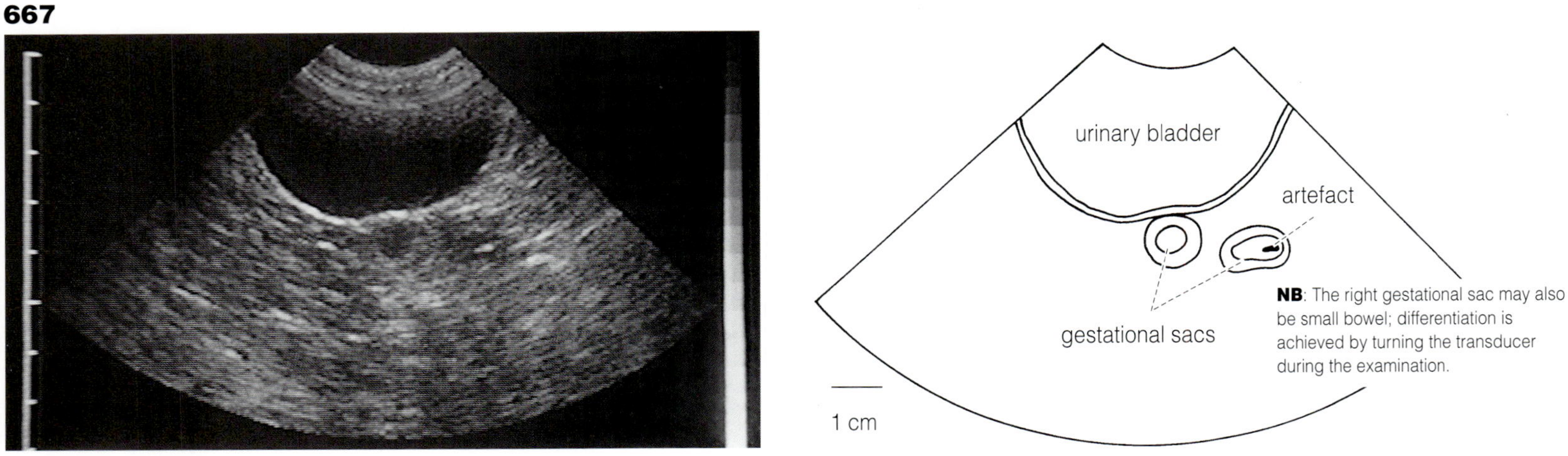

668

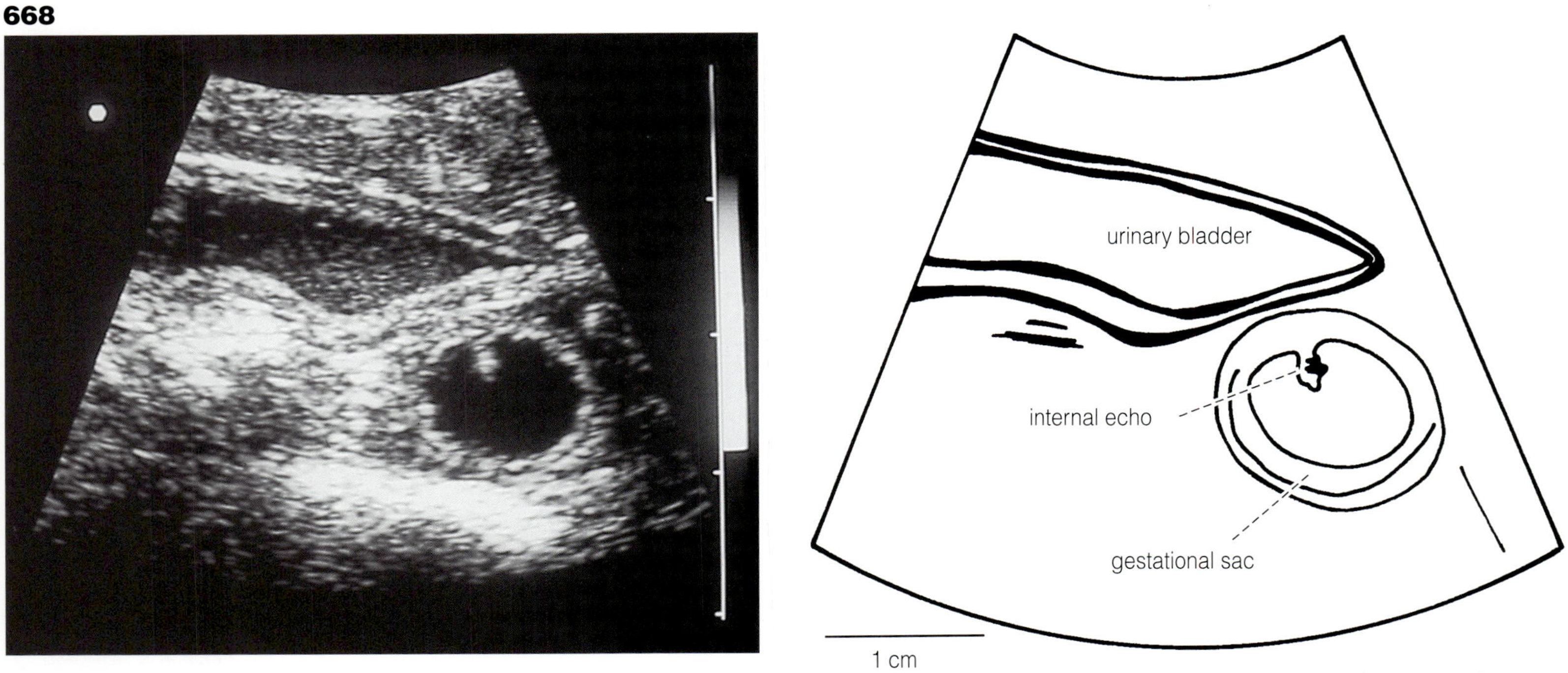

667, 668 Chorionic cavities dorsal to the urinary bladder in a cat 14 days post breeding (**667**) and 18 days post breeding (**668**). While early-stage pregnancy may be mistaken for other structures, day 18 gestational sacs (**668**) are easily identified.

669

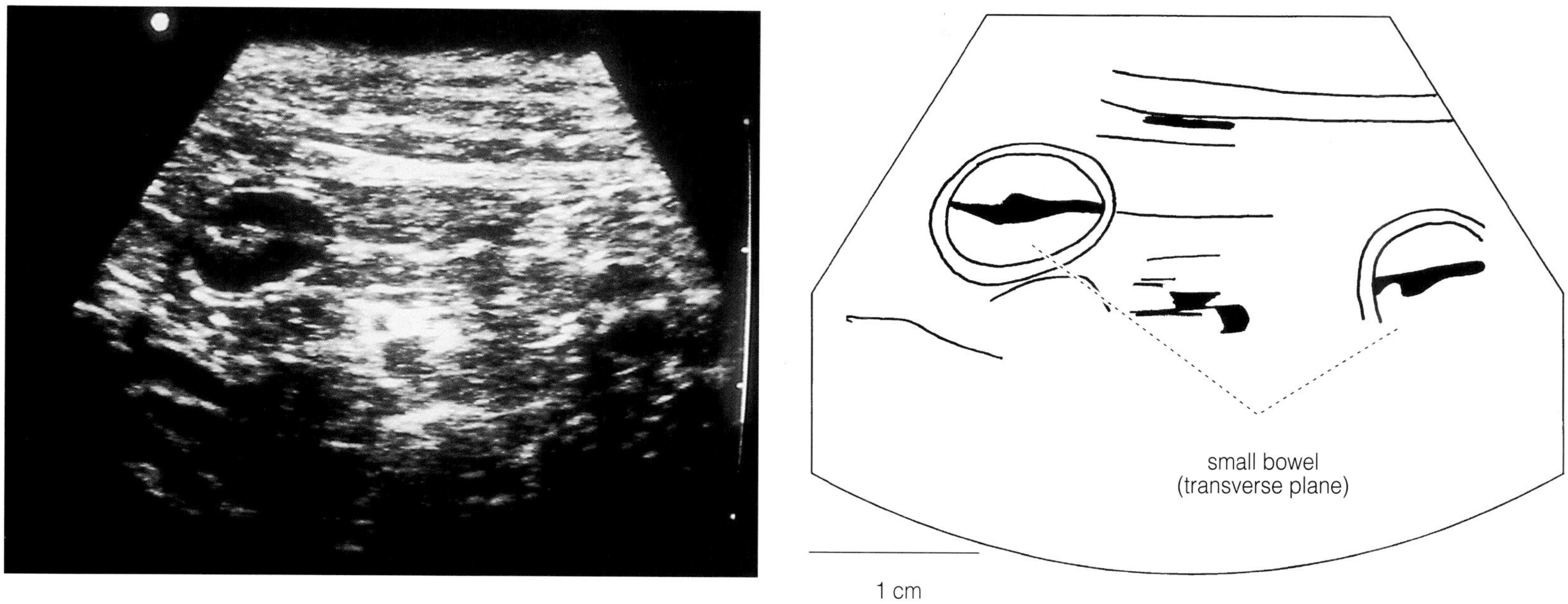

670

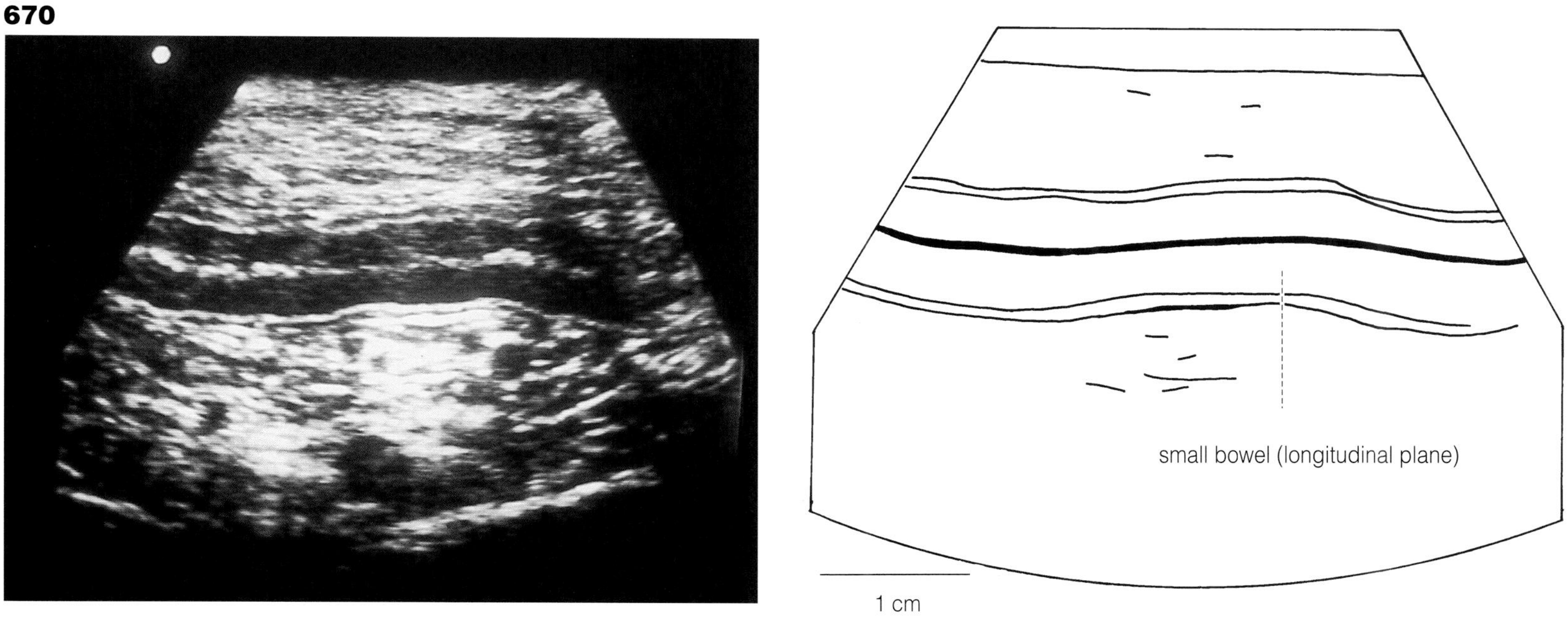

669, 670 Small bowel loops in a transverse (**669**) and a longitudinal (**670**) plane in a bitch.

standing animal, since the animals are calmer with light restraint (**665**) than in dorsal recumbency. Another practical examination technique is to place the cat over a hole in the table and scan from the ventral abdomen (see Patient Positioning, page 78; **157, 159**). Most cats can also be scanned with the sonographer holding the patient on his or her lap (**666**). This method is best if the examination is likely to take a long time, since the cat relaxes on the sonographer's lap and accepts the transducer.

The transducer is applied midline in the bladder area and moved cranially and laterally along the linea alba. By angling and turning the probe, the entire gravid uterus can be traced in various scanning planes. Gestational sacs and fetuses should be displayed and carefully assessed.

Early Pregnancy

Danielle Schäffer and Cordula Poulsen Nautrup

The first half of gestation is generally referred to as early pregnancy. Embryogenesis is the most interesting period for an ultrasound examination. This period is from day 16 to day 30 post conception in the dog[49] and from day 12 to day 24 post breeding in the cat[49]. Various structures in the echogram can be used diagnostically during embryonal development.

The first indication of pregnancy, seen between implantation and placentation, shows fluid-filled (i.e. anechoic) round structures dorsal to the urinary bladder. According to Spaulding *et al.* (1988)[56], these gestational sacs can be reliably detected on day 14 to day 16 post ovulation in the dog, while Heinze *et al.* (1994)[28] give earliest detection at day 18 post ovulation in the dog. Day 13 post breeding has been reported in the cat (**667, 668**). At this early time the gestational sacs (chorionic cavities) must be differentiated sonographically from other similar structures such as transverse bowel loops or vessels. By turning the transducer 90 degrees, bowel loops and vessels appear as elongated structures, while the gestational sacs remain round in the sonogram. The normal bowel loop has a five-layered appearance, a central hyperechoic area and peristalsis (**669, 670**) (see Normal Sonographic Findings, page 165). Arteries are charac-

> Reliable ultrasonographic pregnancy diagnosis using a 5.0 MHz transducer is possible on day 25 post breeding in the dog[24, 53, 58] and day 20 post breeding in the cat .

671

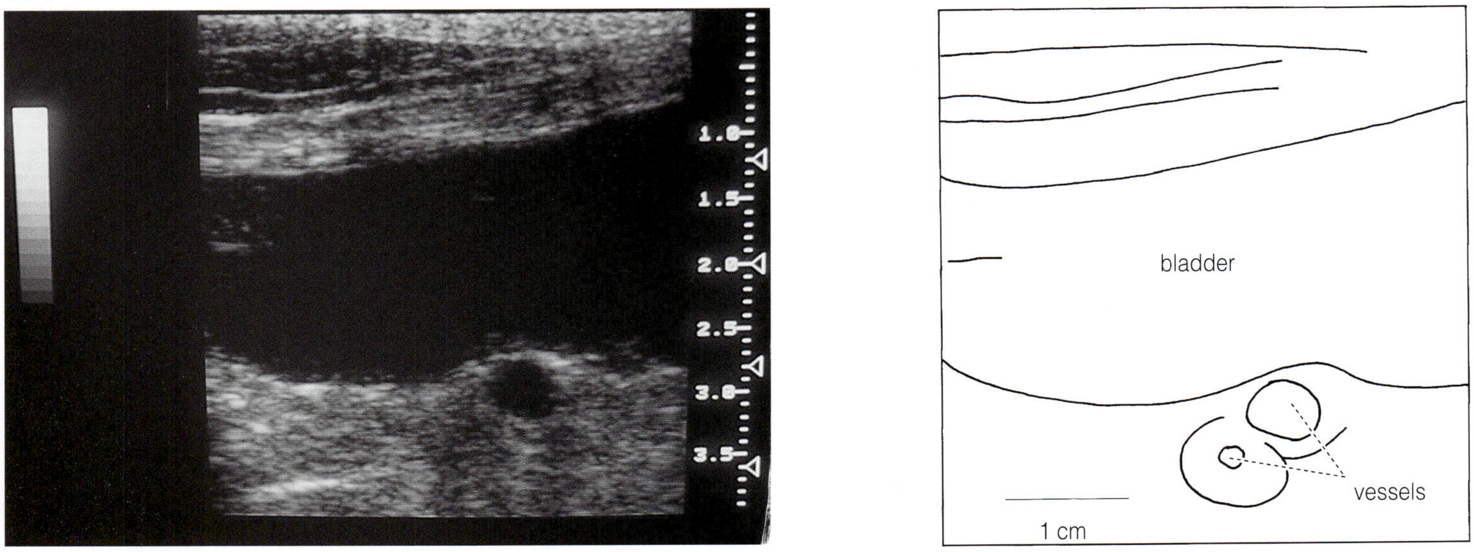

672

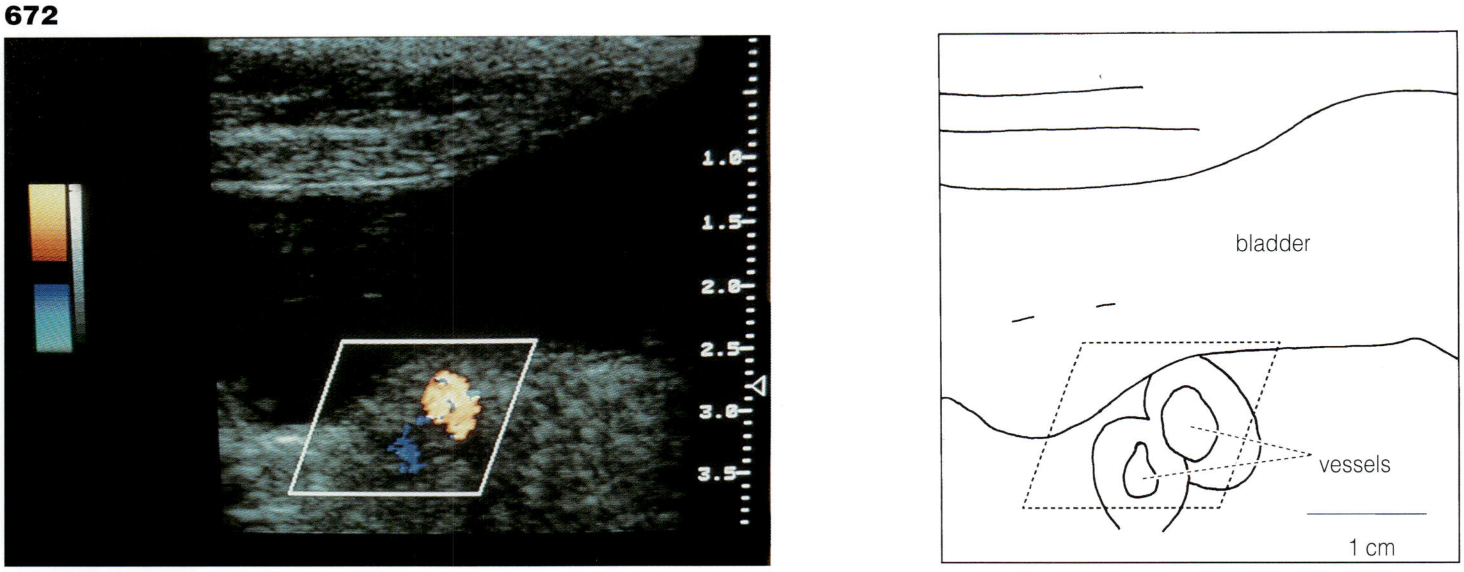

671, 672 Two-dimensional sonogram (**671**) and colour-coded Doppler (**672**) of an artery and a vein dorsal to the urinary bladder in a bitch.

673

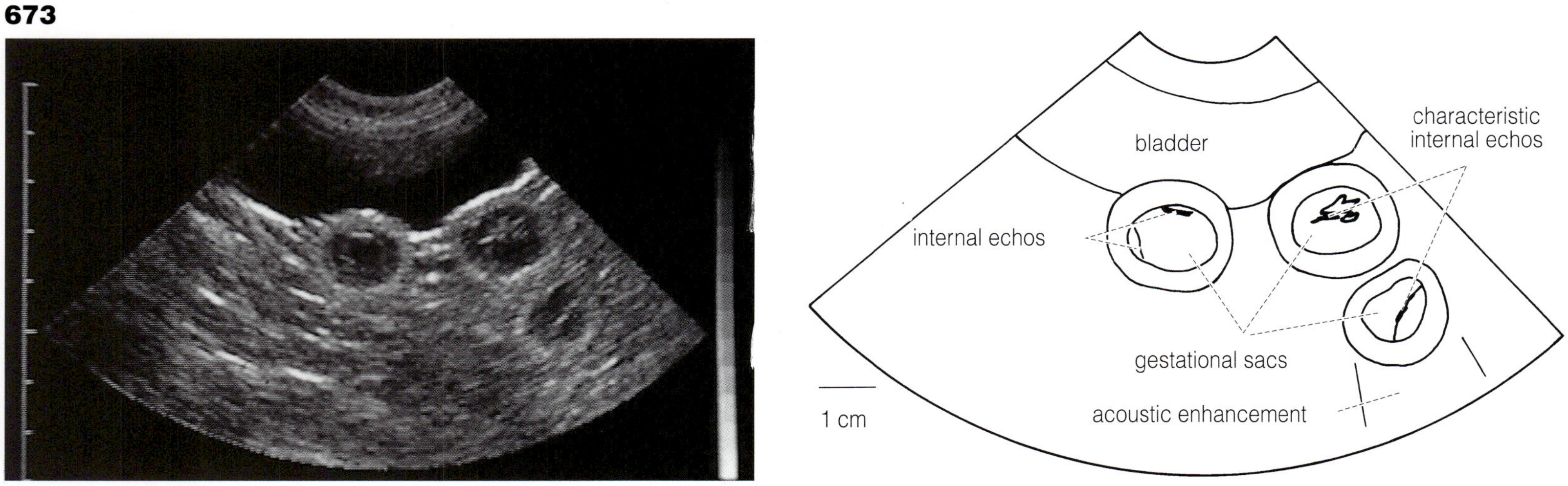

673 Three gestational sacs in a cat 19 days post breeding. The characteristic linear echo of the umbilical cord is seen within the anechoic cavities.

674

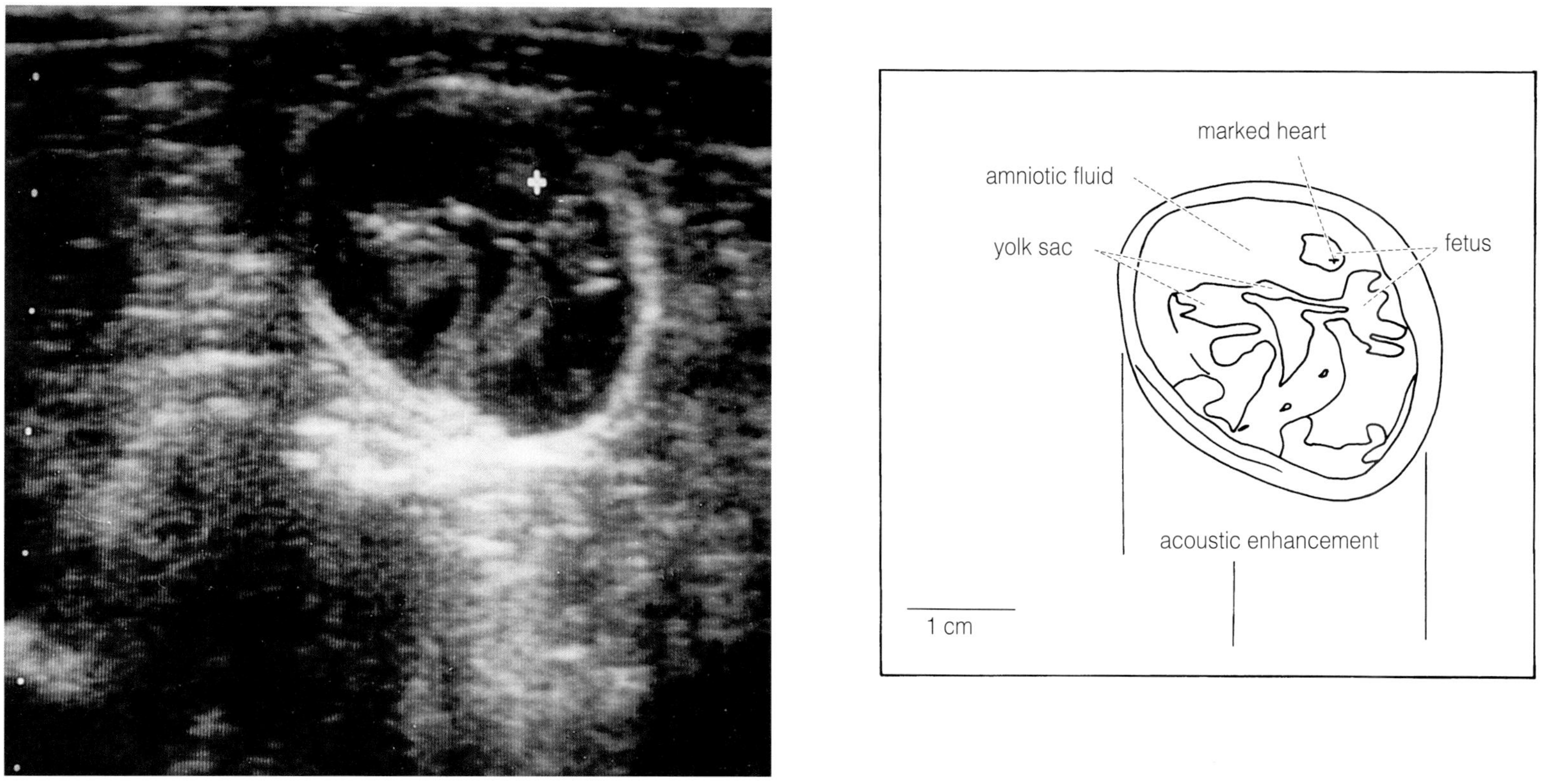

675

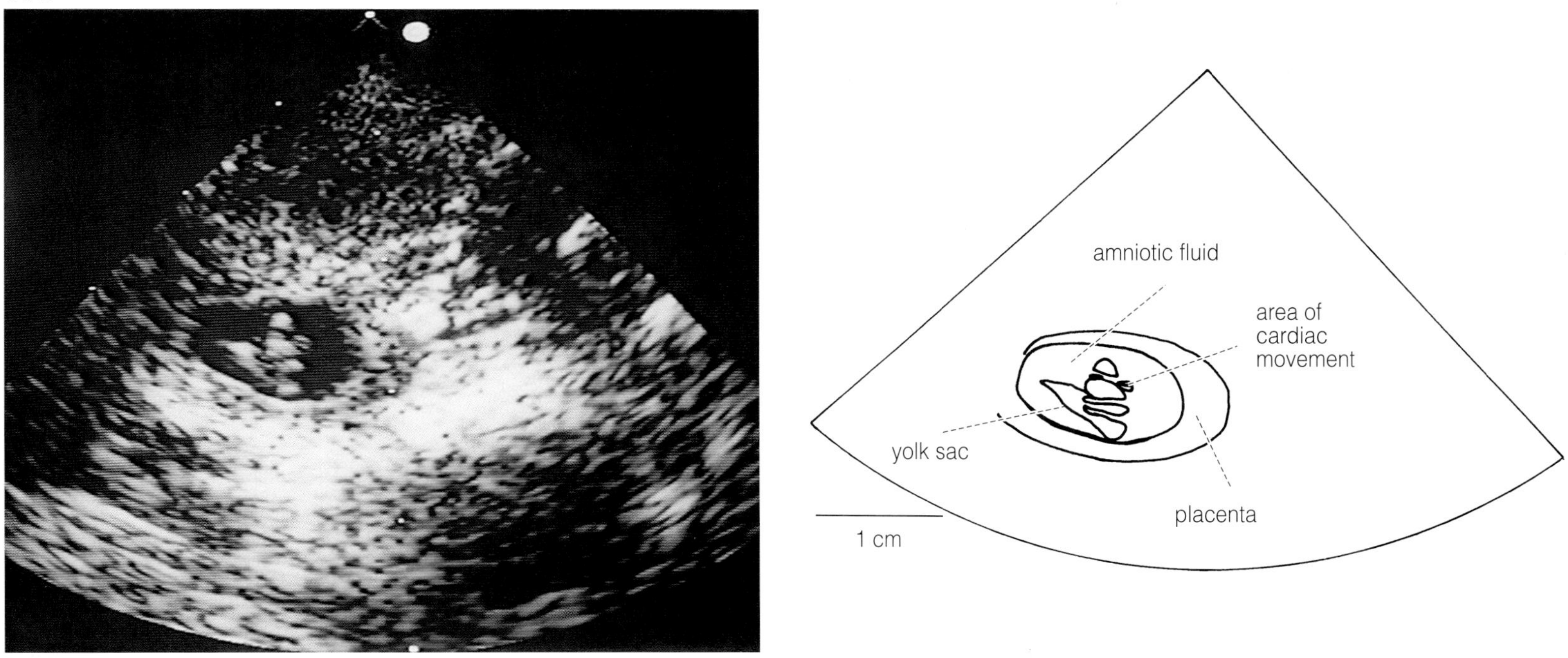

674, 675 A heart marked with a caliper in a 25 day old cat fetus (**674**) and a heart in the shape of an echogenic line in a 22 day old dog embryo (**675**). The rapid pulsations in this area are a characteristic feature of real-time ultrasonography.

terized by pulsations and veins by a thin wall. Colour-flow Doppler is also helpful in recognizing blood vessels (**671, 672**).

To avoid a false diagnosis in veterinary practice, animals should not be examined ultrasonographically on the earliest possible day.

Embryonal structures are detected within the gestational sacs from day 19 post breeding in the dog[54] and day 15 post breeding in the cat[16]. The umbilical cord is seen distinctly as a hyperechoic line (**673**). Embryo and yolk sac can be differentiated a few days later. The embryo is located and differentiated by its cardiac activity.

The first detectable embryonic vital signs are cardiac movements, seen on day 22 post ovulation in the dog[28] and day 17 post breeding in the cat. Fetal movements are observed one to two weeks later: day 28 post breeding[5] or day 34 post ovulation[28] in the dog and day 27 to day 28 post breeding in the cat.

Cardiac activity is first recognized as small fluttering linear echoes in the ultrasound image (**674, 675**).

From day 23 post breeding onwards, the embryos develop

> The number of fetuses can be determined sonographically between day 25 and day 35 post breeding in the dog[53] and day 23 to day 33 post breeding in the cat. Accurate numbers can only be given if there are few fetuses (1–4) and optimal scanning conditions of the dam.

676

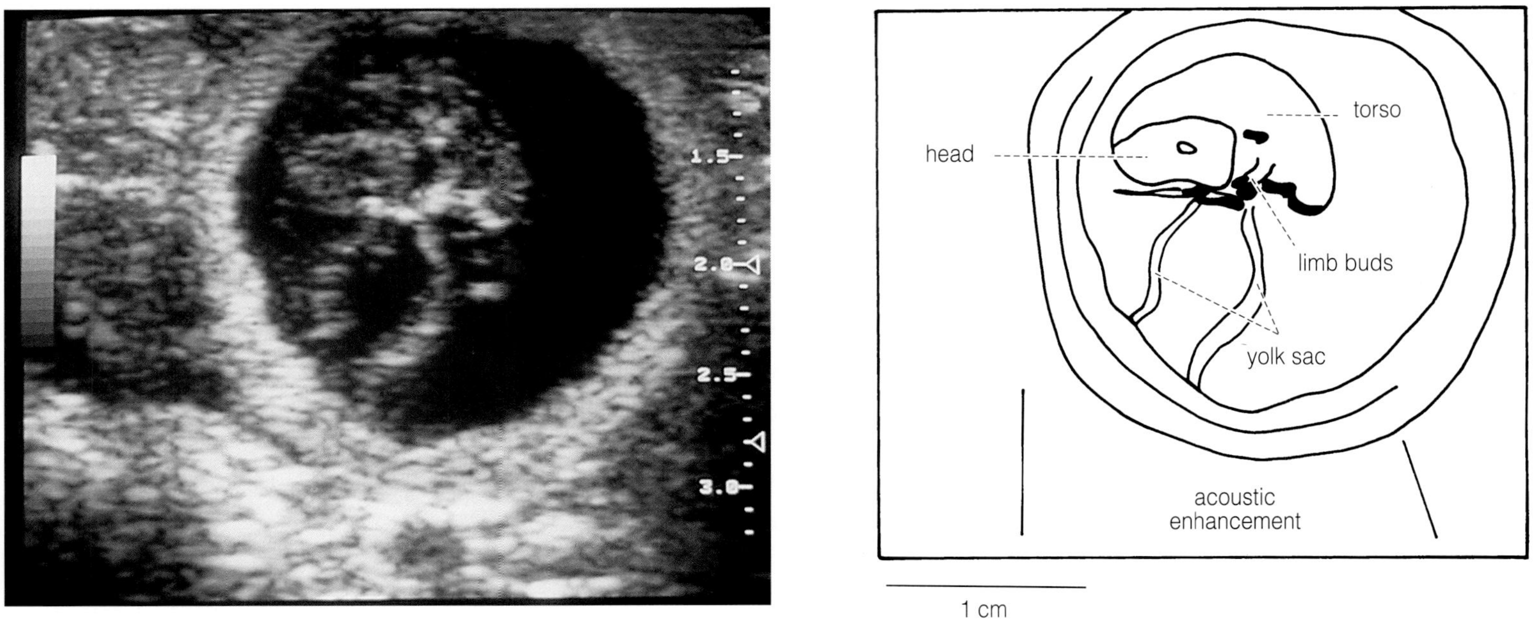

677

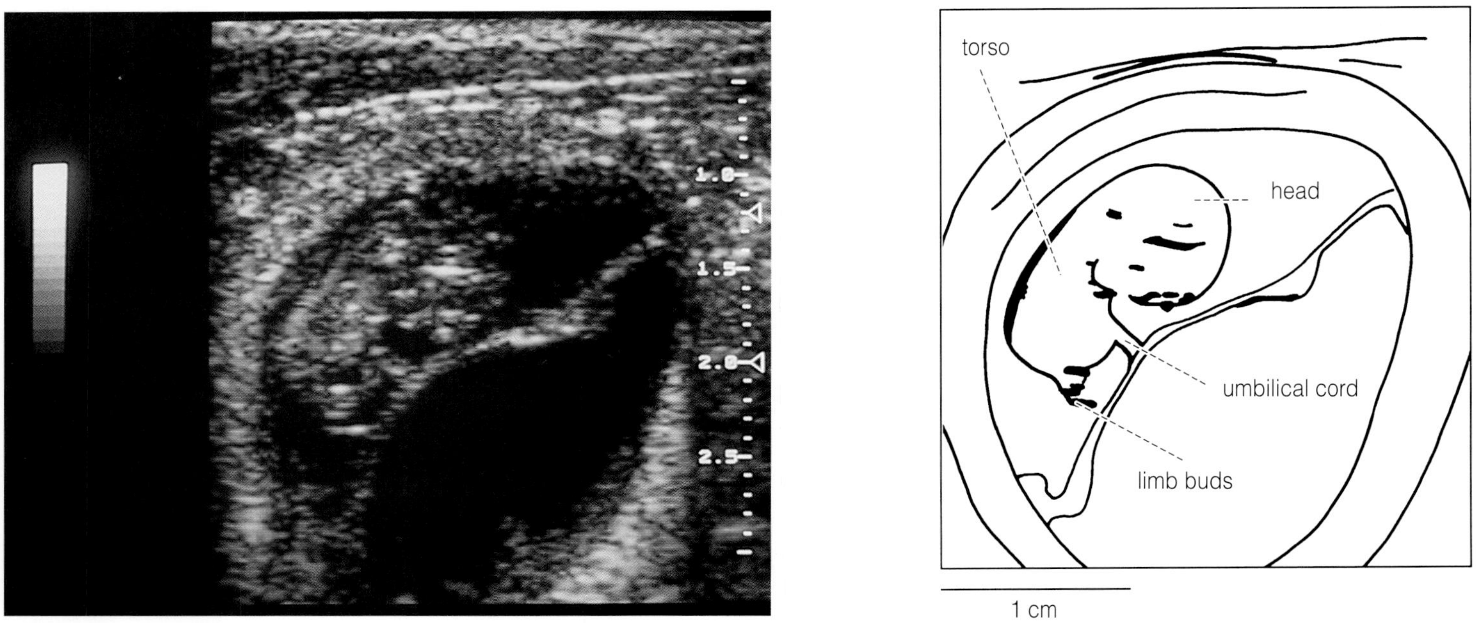

676, 677 Cat fetus 23 days post breeding (**676**) and a cat fetus 24 days post breeding (**677**) with identifiable body parts. The different parts of the body can only be recognized with high-frequency transducers (10 MHz) at this early stage.

678

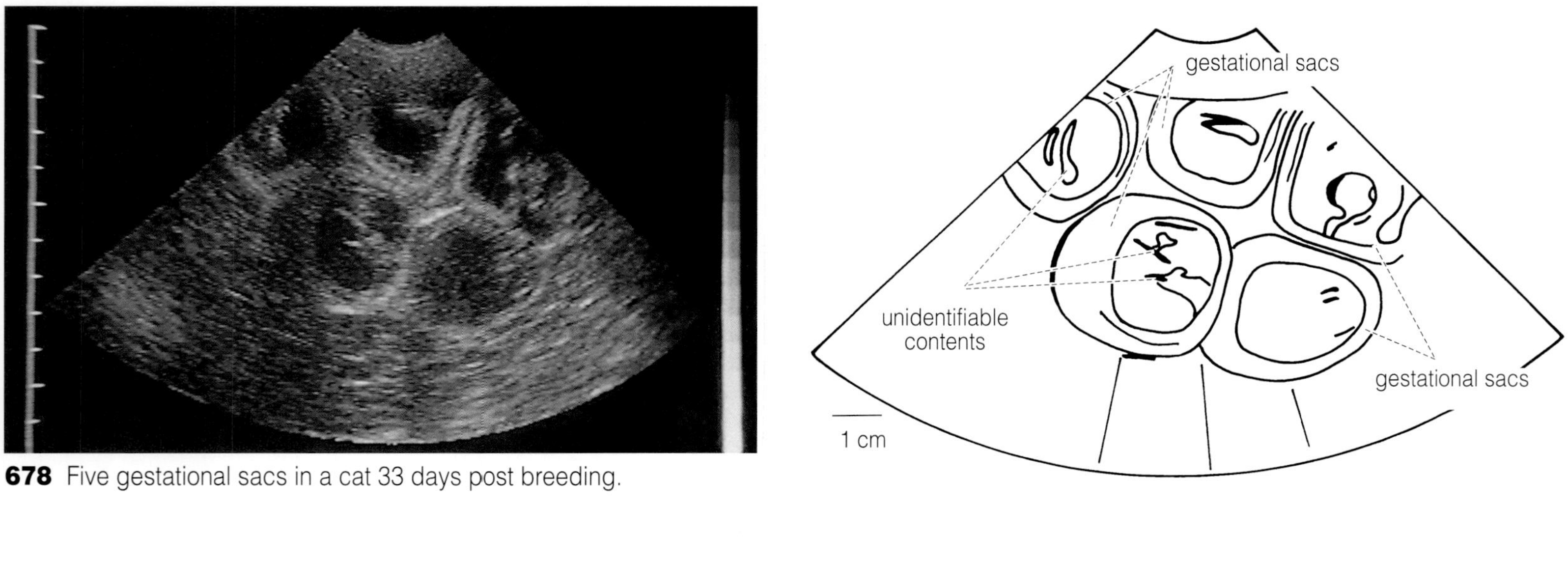

678 Five gestational sacs in a cat 33 days post breeding.

679

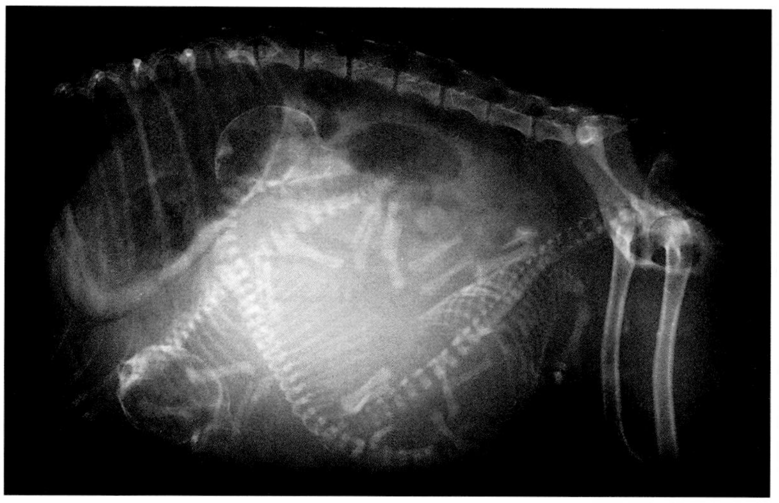

680

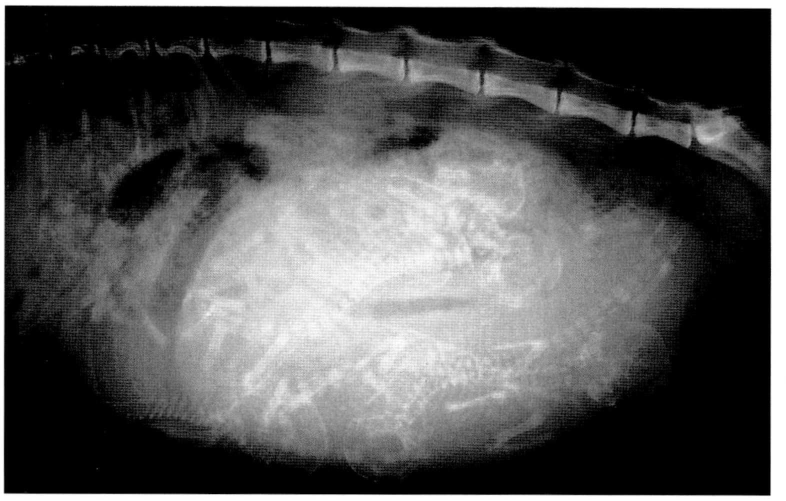

679, 680 Radiographs of two pregnant bitches with three (**679**) and six fetuses (**680**) shortly before parturition.

rapidly and are more easily recognizable. The head and body can be differentiated and the limbs appear as echogenic buds. At this point the longitudinal plane of the body is identified and the fetal crown–rump length can be measured (**676, 677**). The large amount of anechoic amniotic fluid allows optimal visualization of the fetuses at this time and until the end of the second trimester.

More than four fetuses are difficult to differentiate, even for experienced sonographers (**678**). Clients should be told that the sonographic fetal number may vary from the actual number. Fetal numbers are usually too low, since it is easier to avoid counting fetuses twice than overlooking a gestational sac[11, 53, 59]. If breeders are anxious to know the exact fetal number, the examination should be repeated twice at one week intervals. Varying fetal numbers may be due to fetal resorption.

Ultrasonographic estimations of fetal numbers in dogs are still more reliable than palpation. Cats are easier to palpate than dogs, which makes palpation more reliable than ultrasonography. The best time to determine fetal numbers by palpation in the cat is between day 18 and day 25 post breeding.

The advantage of abdominal radiographs in estimating fetal numbers is in the better overview. The disadvantage is the radiation exposure for humans and animals. Fetal bone mineralization is only recognized beyond day 42 post breeding in the dog and day 38 post breeding in the cat (**679, 680**).

Fetal Development

Danielle Schäfer and Cordula Poulsen Nautrup

Following embryonic development, the ovoid canine and round feline gestational sacs slowly become more elongated, and zonary placentation is recognized sonographically. The placenta has a three-layered, cylindrical appearance and it extends into the fetal cavity (**681–683**). These three layers of the zonary placenta demonstrate the development and structure of fetal–maternal communication. The outer hyperechoic layer is the myometrium, while the middle anechoic layer identifies the uterine crypts and deep uterine glands. The placental labyrinth makes up the inner echogenic layer.

The yolk sac takes on a tubular shape, extending over the length of the gestational sac, and becoming quite large in size (**684–686**). With the development of the allontochorion, the yolk sac placenta, typical for carnivores, becomes superfluous and recedes. The yolk sac is present until parturition, but it is more difficult to visualize ultrasonographically with fetal development and associated amniotic fluid reduction.

As already mentioned, active fetal movement is seen from day 34 post ovulation in the dog[28] and from day 27 post breeding in the cat. The motion spectrum ranges from uncontrolled, jerking movements to recognizable suckling (**687**) or grooming activity. At this time the amnion is visible, creating a hyperechoic line in the perpendicular sound beam, tightly encompassing the fetus as a thin membrane (**688**).

With cardiac development, the sonographic image changes from a pulsating echogenic line to a more or less round, echogenic, rhythmically beating organ with an anechoic cavity and a uniformly granulated myocardium of medium echogenicity. During the last trimester, the heart shows its characteristic shape of four chambers in a transverse (short-axis view, **689**) and longitudinal (long-axis view, **690**) plane. The atrioventricular valves may be visualized with a medium to high-frequency transducer and good resolution (**689**).

Fetal organs, such as lung, liver, stomach, urinary bladder and large arterial and venous vessels, as well as kidneys, may be recognized in detail during the second half of pregnancy. Early differentiation of these organs, using a 5.0–7.5 MHz transducer, is listed in *Table 37* for the dog and *Table 38* for the cat.

As mentioned earlier, the head and body can be differentiated early, while the eyes and mouth are only recognizable around day 35 post breeding (**691, 692**). The liver is visible in the cranial abdomen as a finely granulated structure of medium echogenicity and it may be differentiated from the more echogenic, cranially located lungs in the diaphragm area (**693**). The stomach is a constant indicator, seen regularly from day 34 post ovulation in the dog and from day 32 post breeding in the cat as a characteristic organ in the cranial abdomen. The stomach is filled exclusively with fluid (amniotic fluid) and it appears anechoic (**694**). The urinary bladder is recognized a few days later in the caudal abdomen as a smaller anechoic focal area (**695**).

Large blood vessels, such as the aorta, the cranial and caudal venae cavae and the ductus venosus, as well as the fetal kidneys, are seen during the last trimester under good scanning conditions (**696–698**). Smaller blood vessels, such as the umbilical arteries and veins, are not easily identified with two-dimensional ultrasonography, but they may be visualized by their blood flow using colour Doppler ultrasonography (see Duplex Ultrasonography, page 314).

681

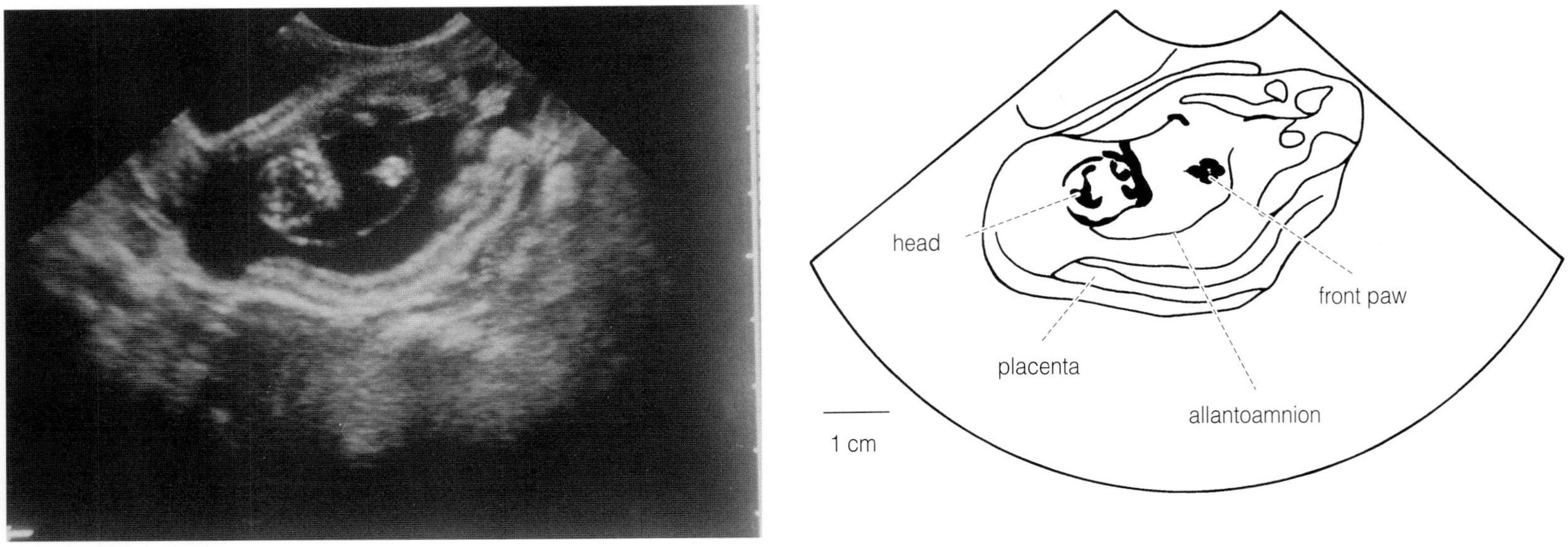

682

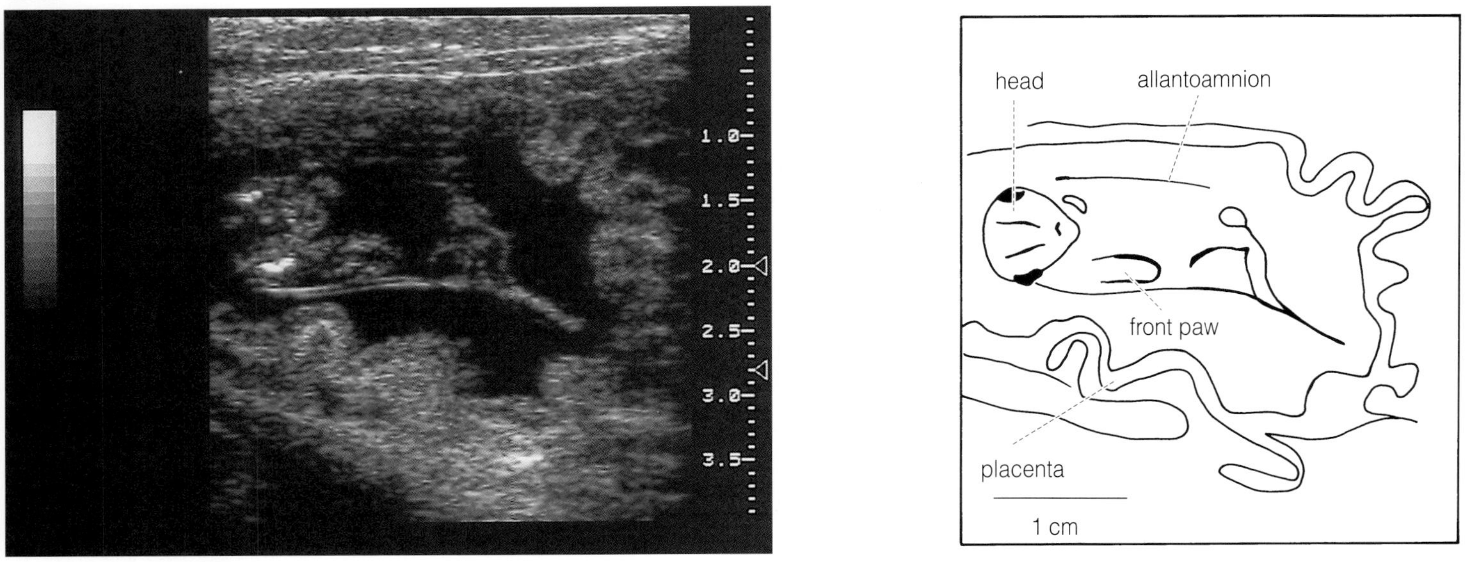

683

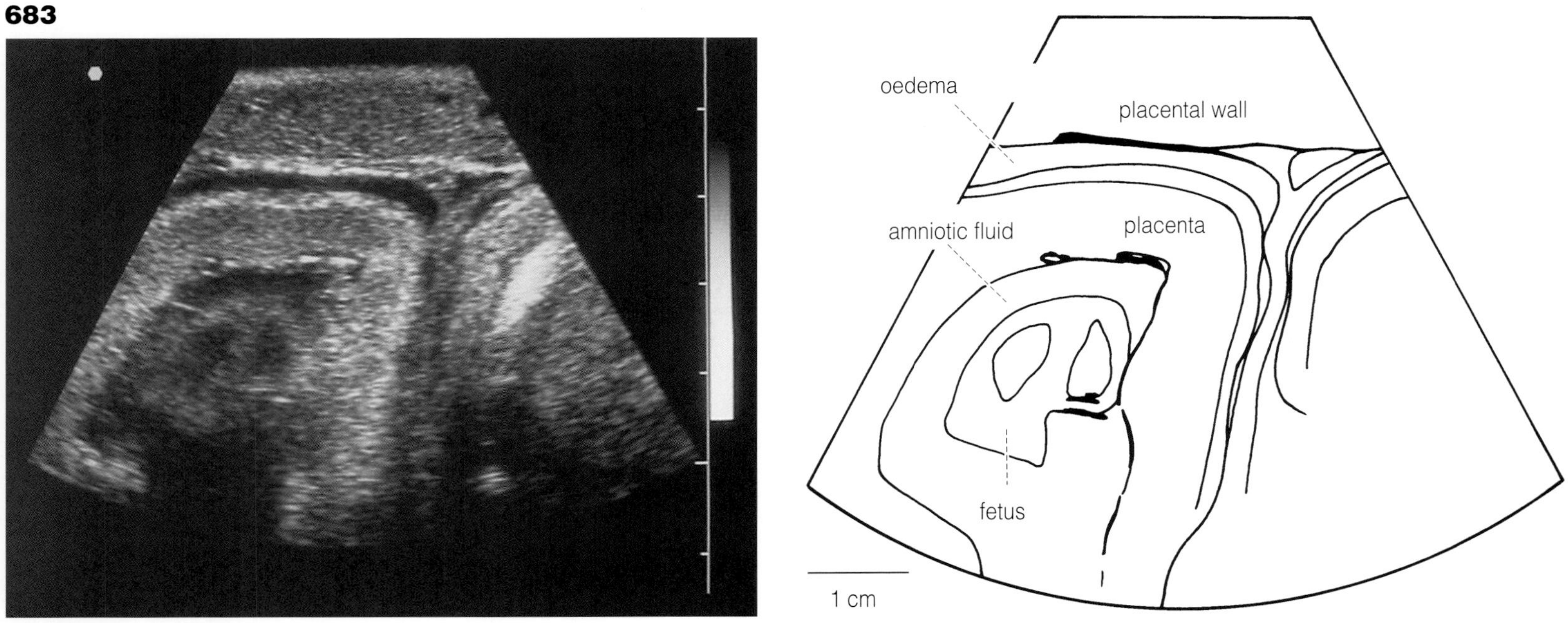

681–683 Zonary placenta in two cats on day 32 (**681**) and day 33 (**682**) post breeding, and in a dog just before parturition (**683**).

684

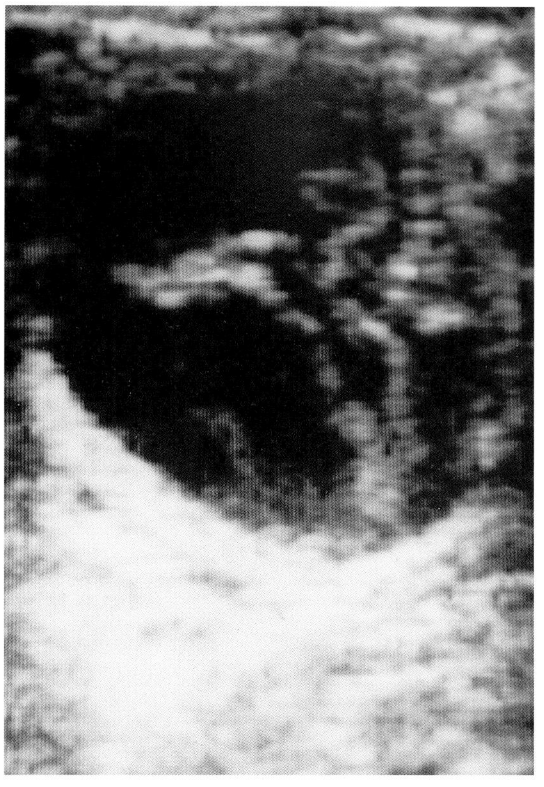

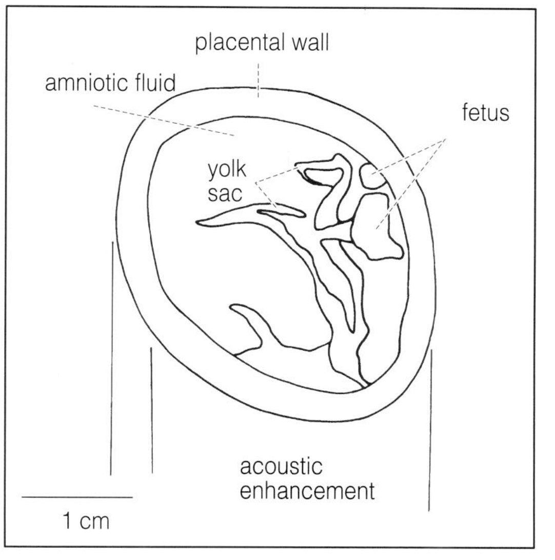

685

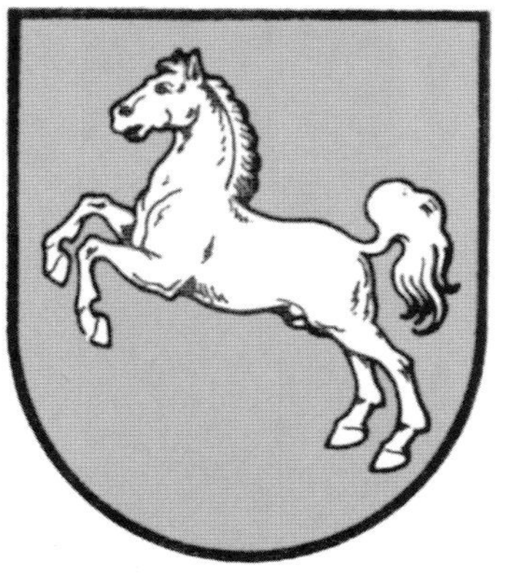

684, 685 Extended, bizarre formation of a yolk sac in a cat on day 25 post breeding (**684**). This yolk sac has the appearance of a jumping horse and is similar to the coat of arms of Lower Saxony (**685**). The examinations were performed in Hannover, the capital of Lower Saxony.

686

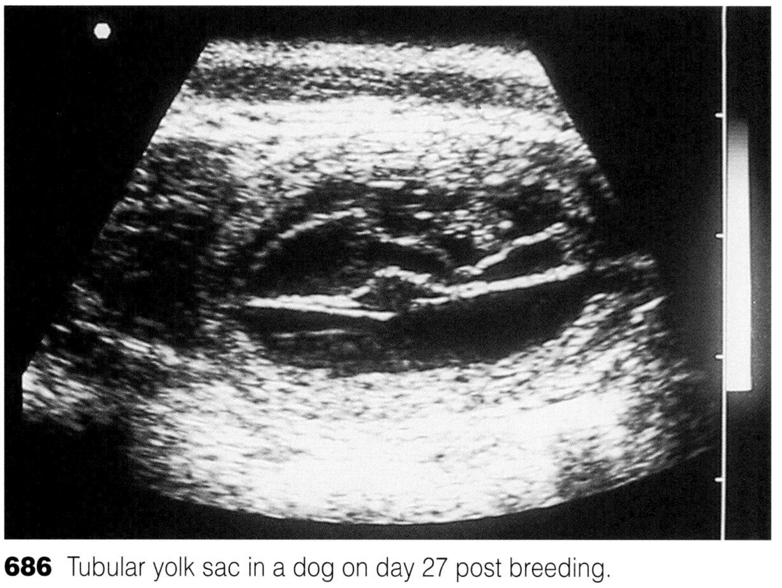

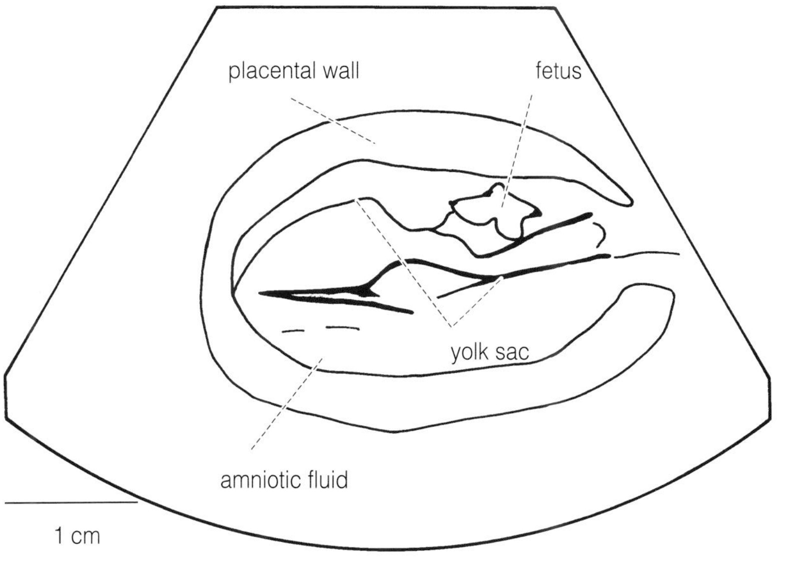

686 Tubular yolk sac in a dog on day 27 post breeding.

687

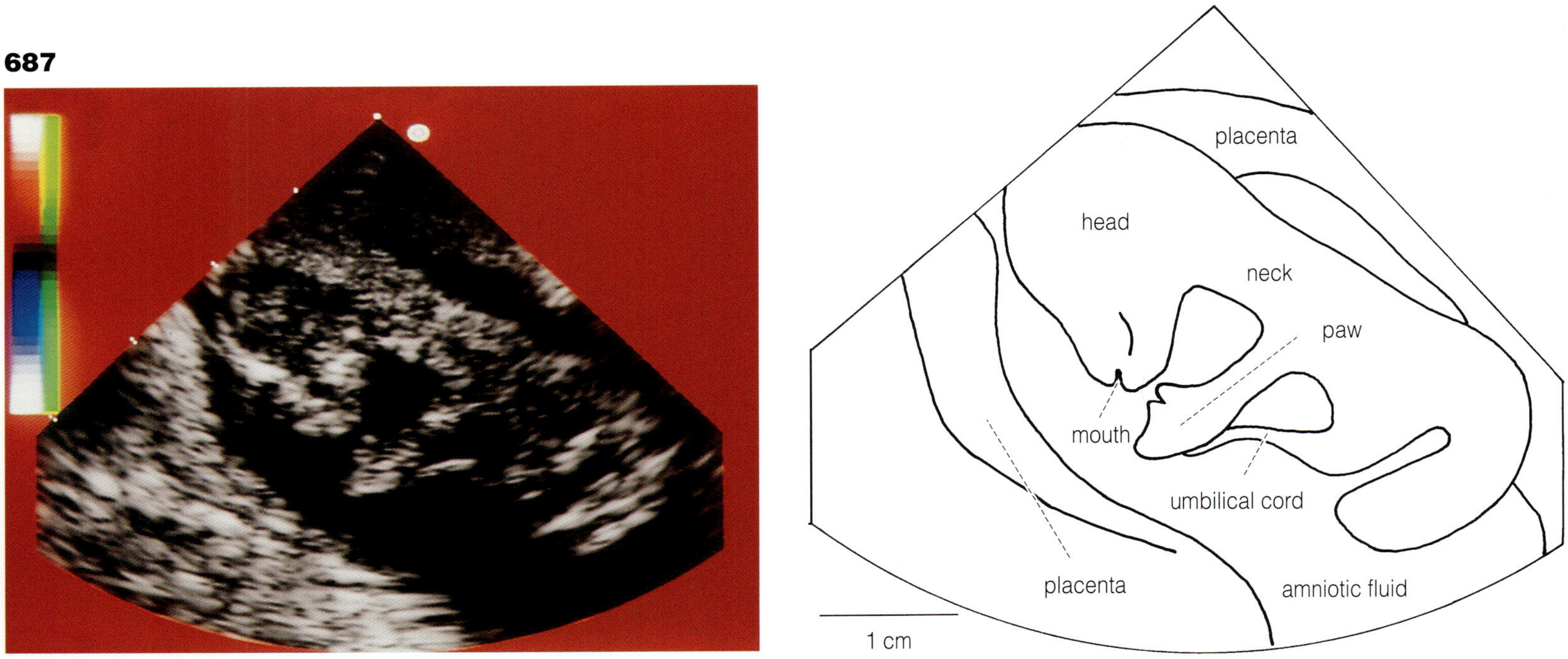

687 Dog fetus sucking his paw on day 38 post breeding.

688

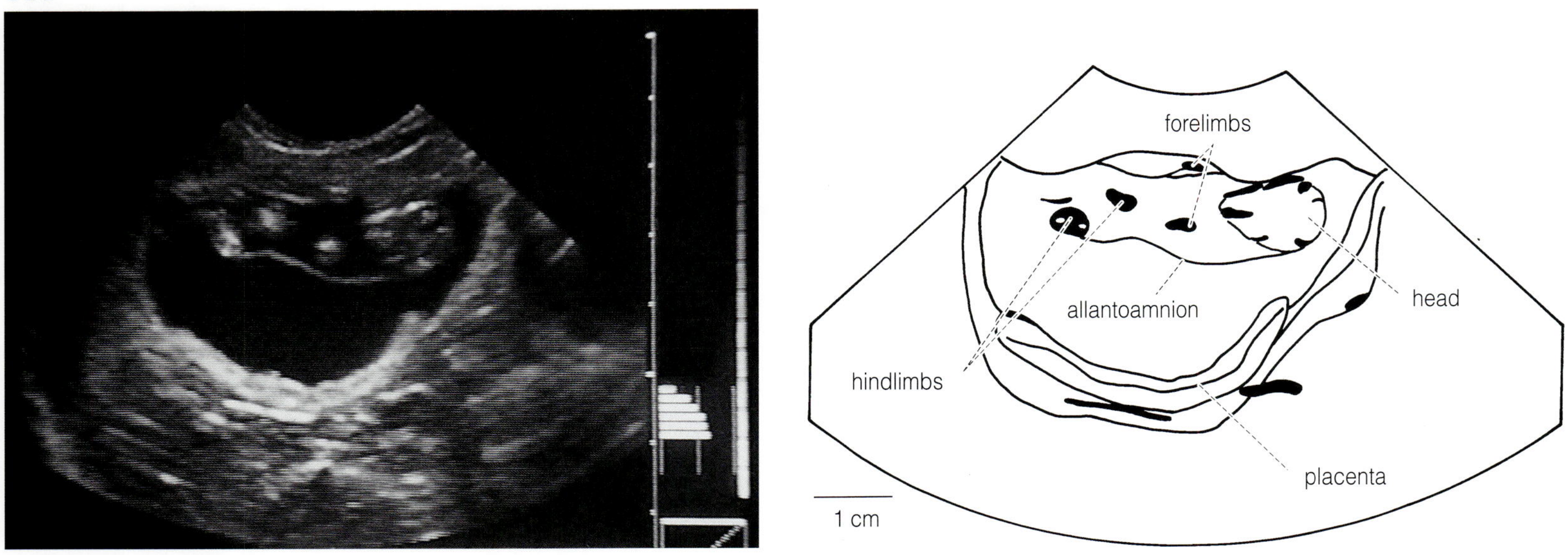

688 Cat fetus on day 33 post breeding with distinct, tightly encompassing allantoamnion.

689 Cardiac short-axis view at the level of the mitral valve in a dog fetus on day 54 post breeding. The myocardium in the left and right ventricle has the same thickness (see also **690**).

689

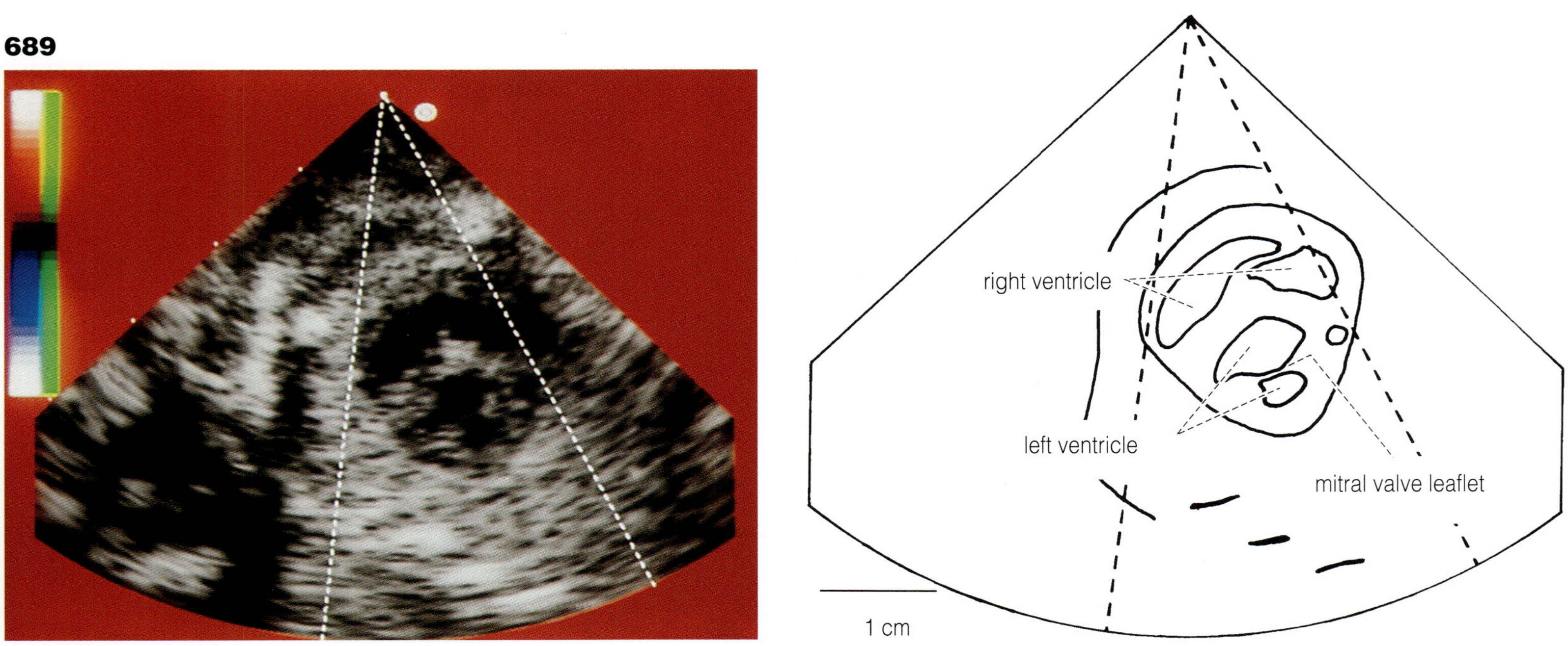

690

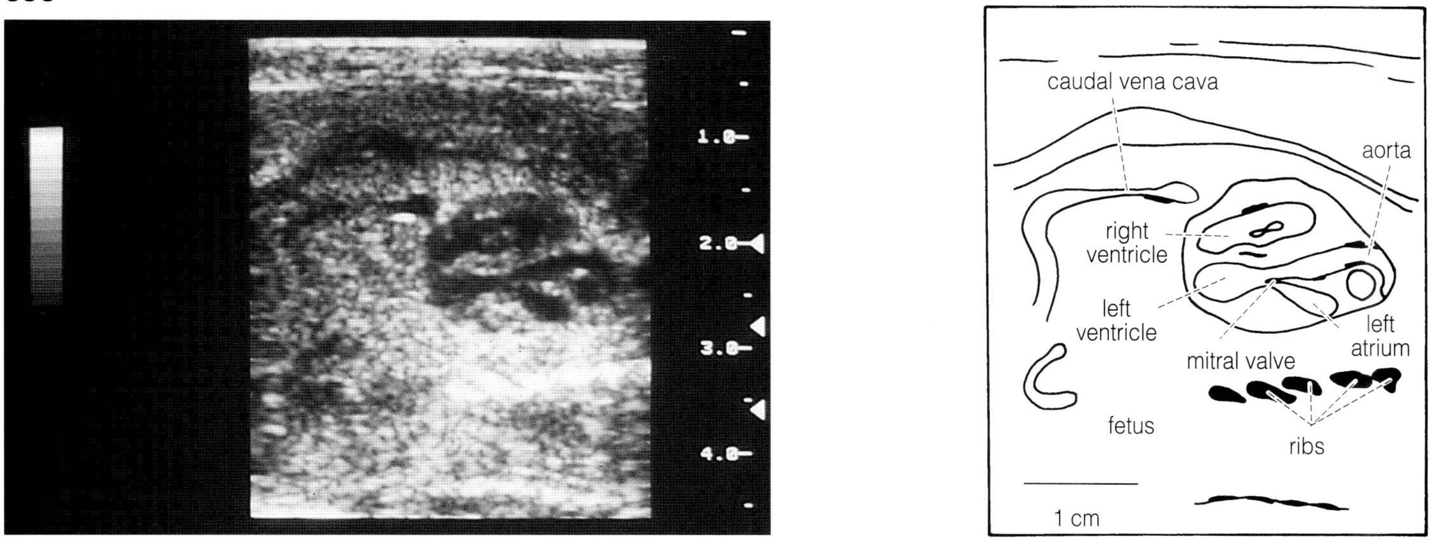

690 Cardiac long-axis view of a cat fetus on day 55 post breeding. The myocardium in the left and right ventricle has the same thickness (see also **689**).

691

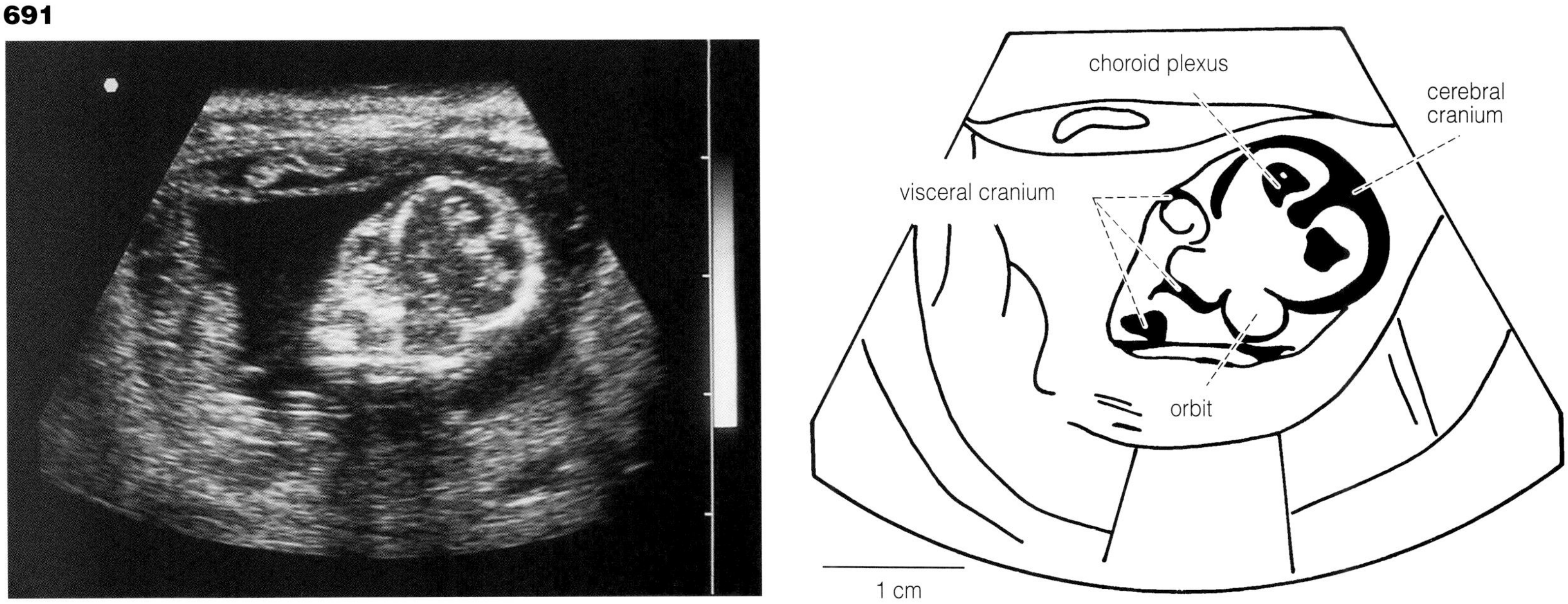

692

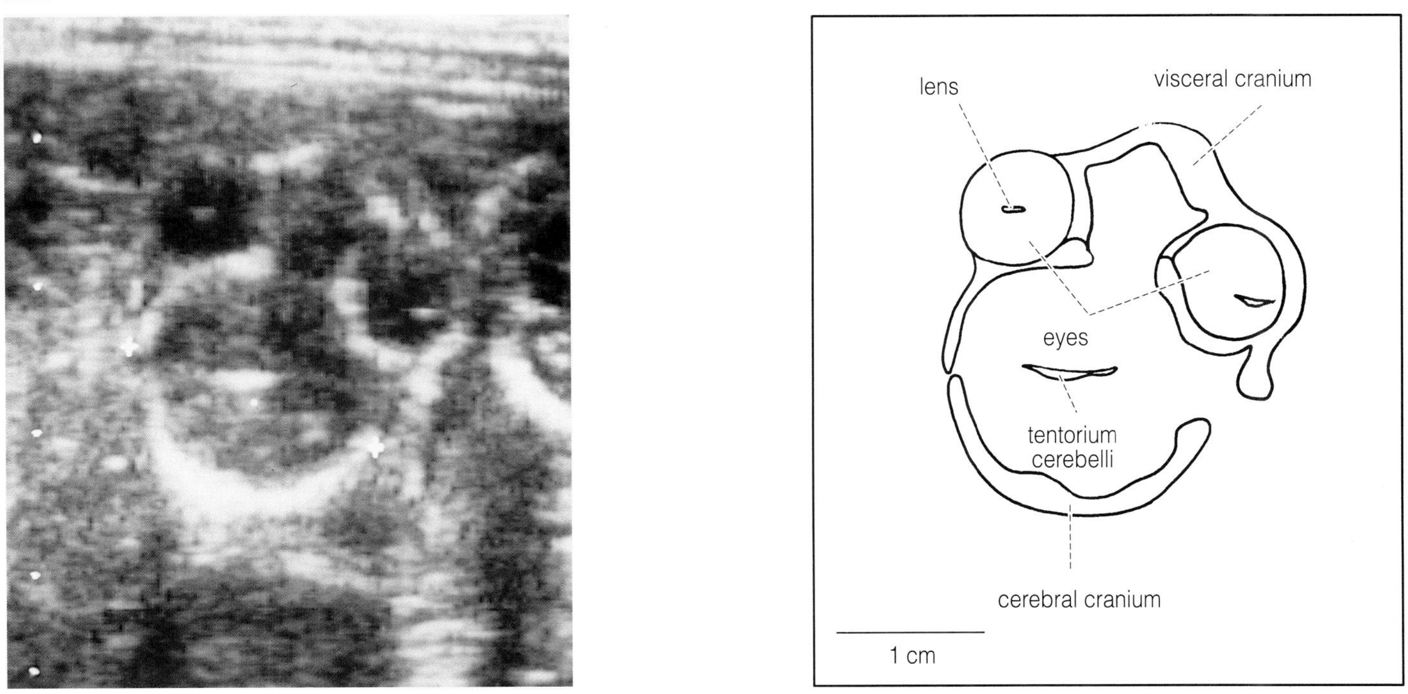

691, 692 Dorsal view of the head of a cat fetus on day 53 post breeding (**691**) and day 54 post breeding (**692**).

693

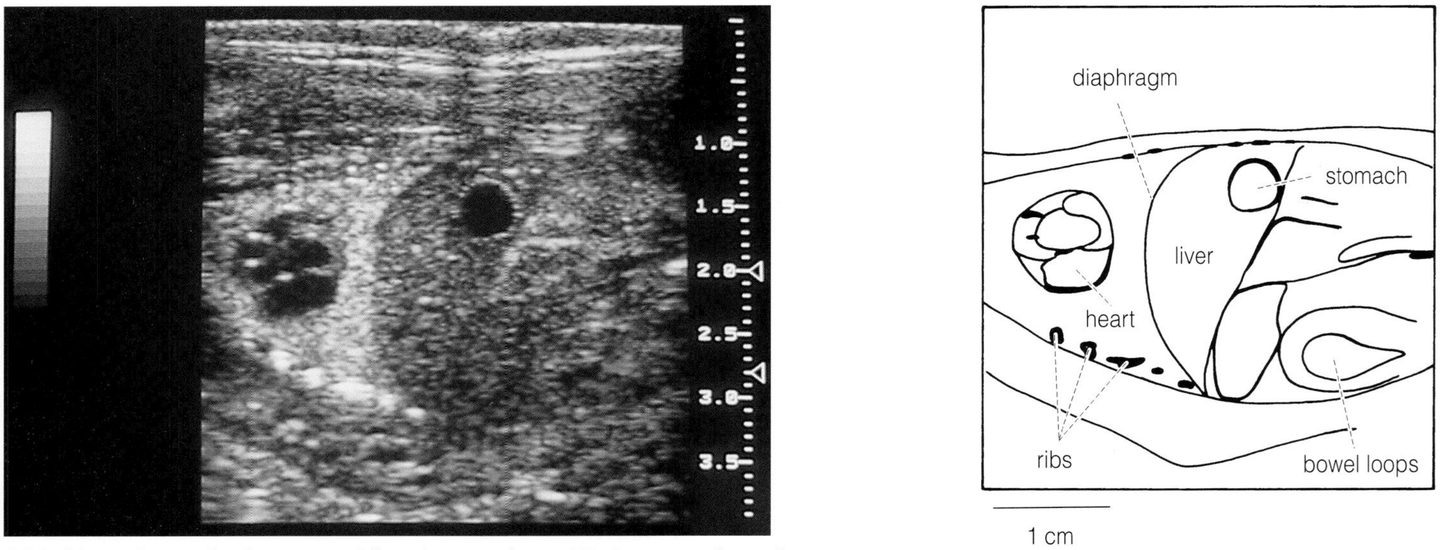

693 Heart, lung, diaphragm and liver in a cat fetus, 56 days post breeding.

694

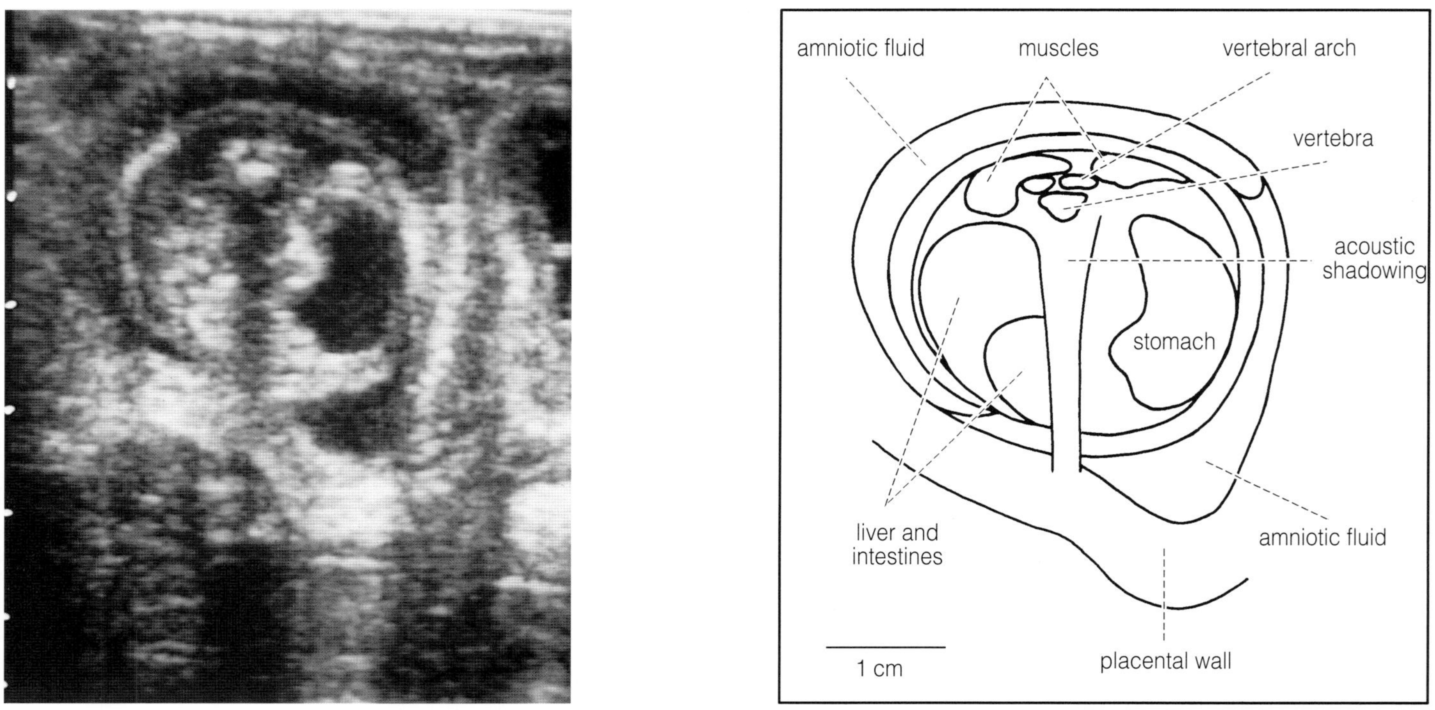

694 Spine, stomach and intestines in a cat fetus, 53 days post breeding, in a transverse view.

695

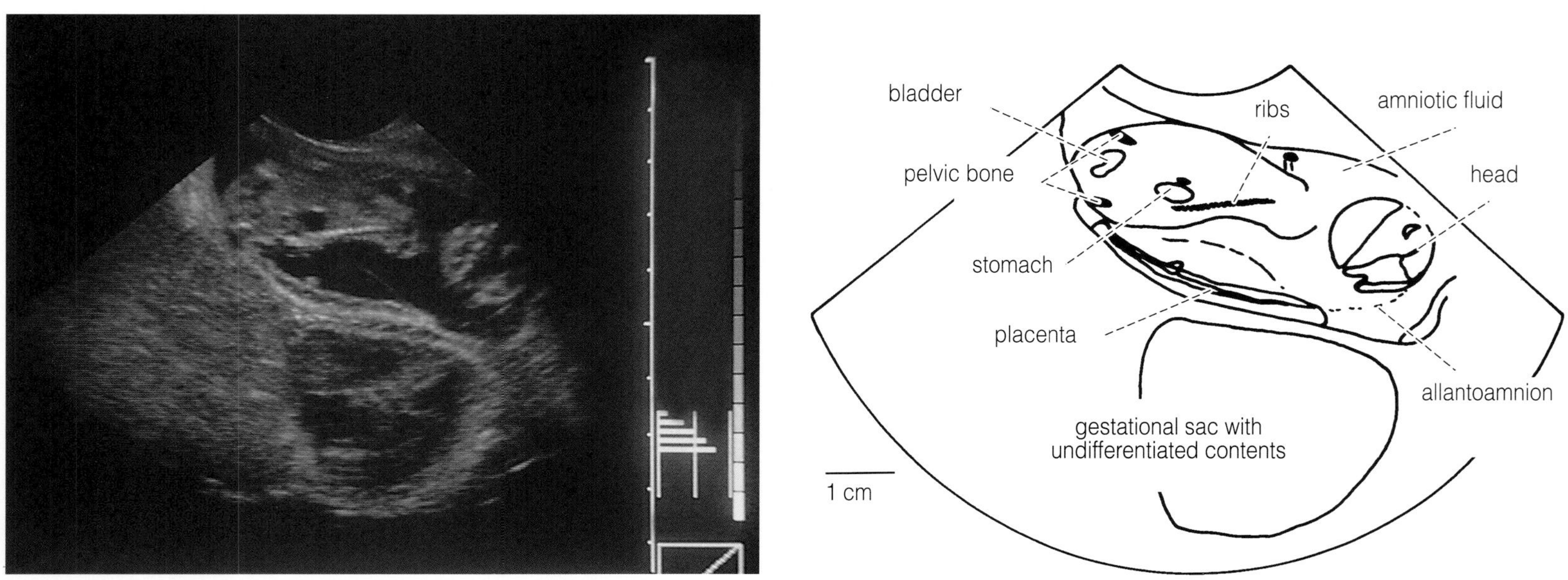

695 Urinary bladder at the pelvic bone in a cat fetus on day 38 post breeding.

696

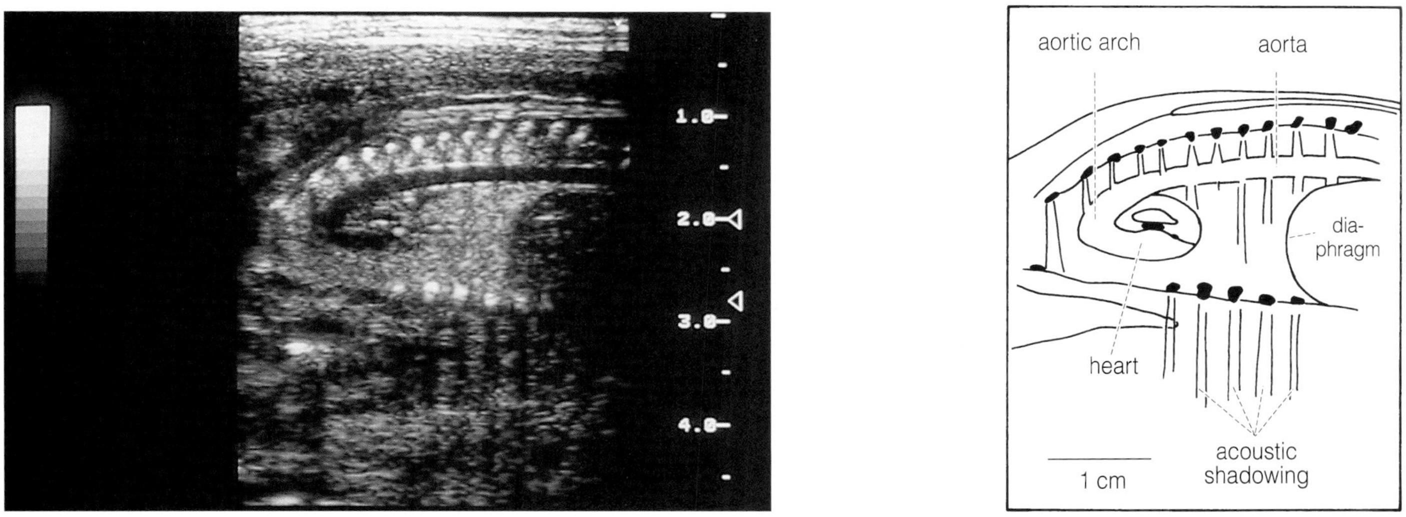

696 Aorta and ribs with distinct acoustic shadowing in a cat fetus on day 56 post breeding.

697

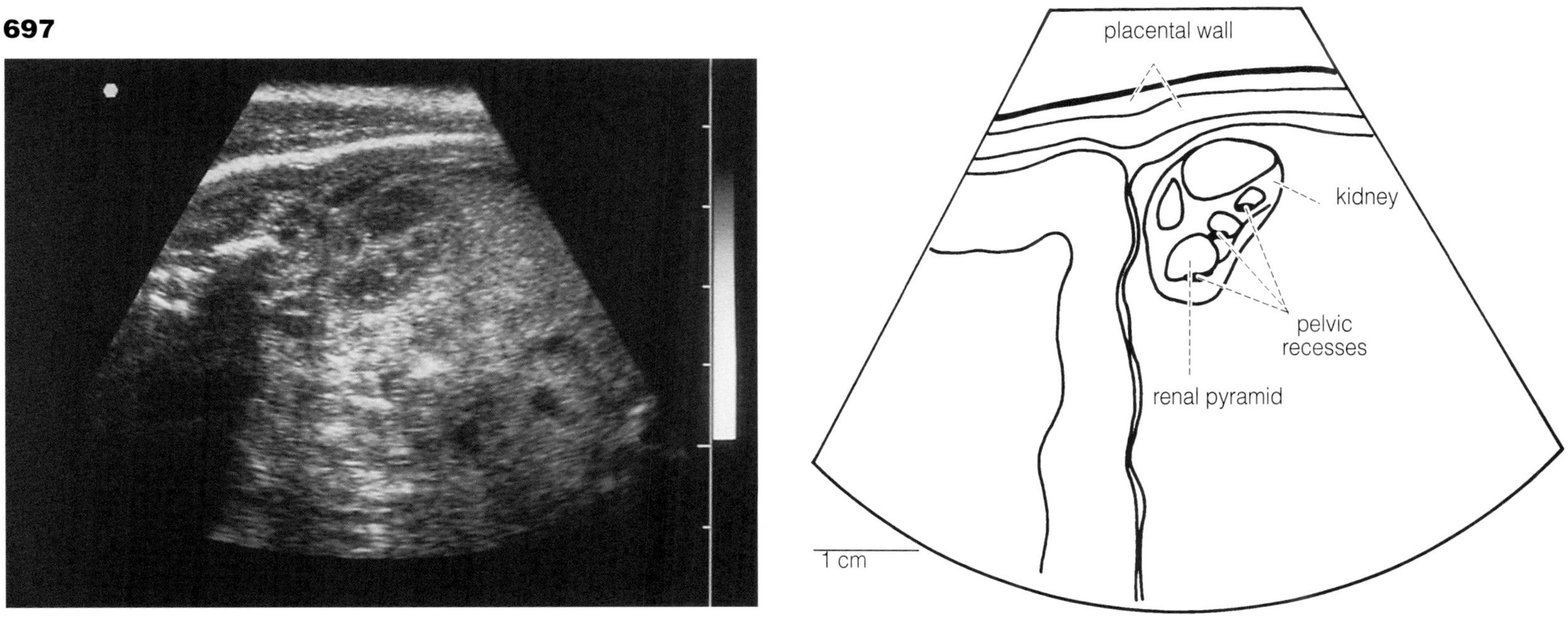

698

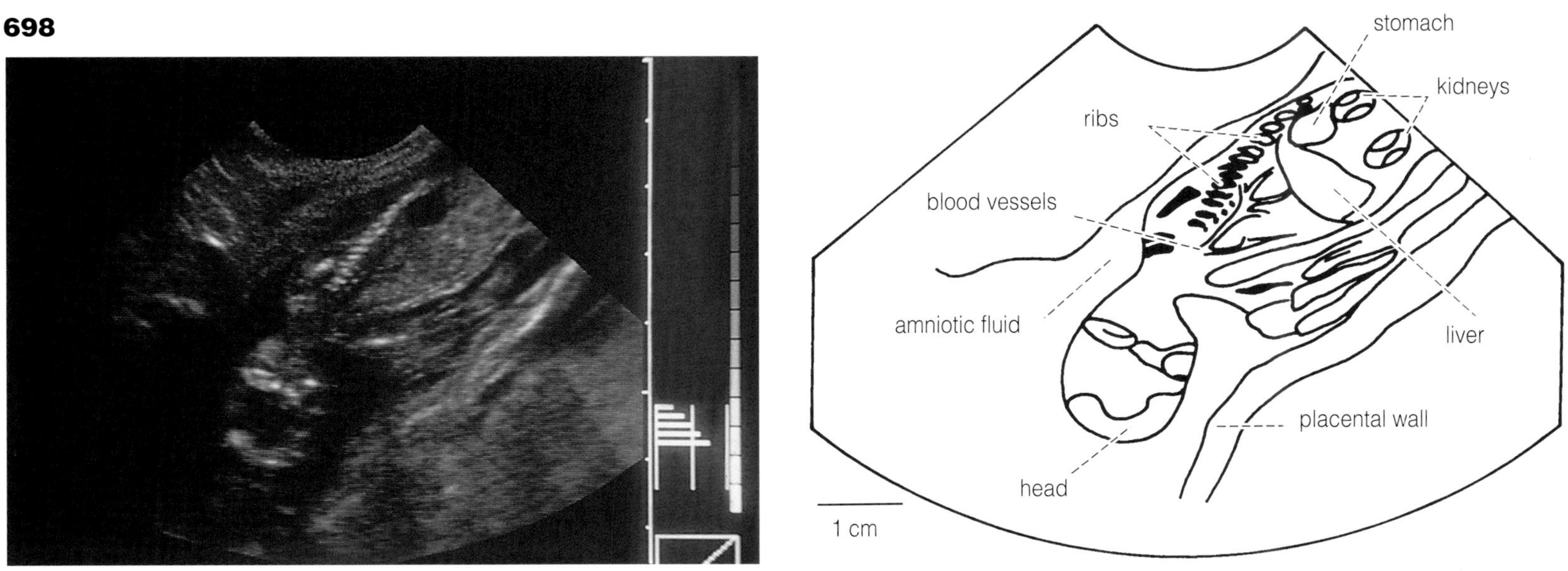

697, 698 Sagittal view of a kidney in a dog fetus, 63 days post breeding (**697**), and a dorsal view of both kidneys in a cat fetus 40 days post breeding (**698**).

Progressive bone mineralization (from day 42 to day 45 post breeding) creates acoustic shadowing, i.e. partial or total sound wave reflection at the soft tissue–bone interface, followed by absorption of ultrasound energy in the calcified tissue. The amount of shadowing depends on the size and mineralization of the bones and on the angle of the sound beam. During the last trimester, acoustic shadowing of the cranium, ribs and spine may impair imaging (**696**).

Gestational Age Estimation

Anne-Rose Günzel-Apel, Britta Heinze and Danielle Schäfer

Requirements for Exact Gestational Age Determination

An important requirement for accurately determining gestational age is the definition of the onset of pregnancy. Pregnancy (gravidity, gestation) is generally defined as the time between fertilization (conception) and parturition. The actual day of fertilization is not available for practical clinical diagnosis. For this reason, the breeding day or ovulation day is usually referred to as the beginning of pregnancy (day 0). Sonographic pregnancy diagnosis and determination of gestational age is easier in the cat, where breeding, ovulation and fertilization are within a short time period, i.e. within a maximum of 48 hours. This is not the case in the bitch, since ovulation is followed by 2–3 days of ovocyte maturation with conception taking place within the next three days[15, 31, 32, 60, 61]. Because some bitches are ready to mate several days before ovulation[14] and canine sperm is fertile for an average of 4–6 days post breeding, and even up to ten days according to Doak *et al.* (1976)[18], one servicing seven days before ovulation may still result in conception in extreme cases. For this reason, when the breeding date is referred to as day 0, gestational age may vary between 57–69 days (**699**)[14, 15].

An essential requirement for predicting gestational age in the bitch is ovulation determination as a constant, short and easily identifiable occurence during oestrus. By defining gestational age as the time interval between ovulation and examination, sonographic pregnancy diagnosis is accurate. Fetal development can be assessed. Parturition can be predicted within a time period of 3–5 days – day (61) 62 to day 64 (65) post ovulation (*Table 37*, **699**)[15, 21, 22, 28, 62, 63].

699

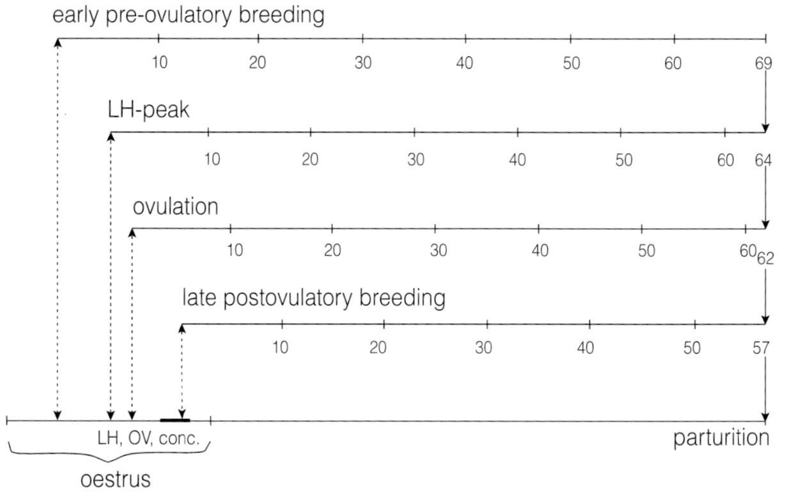

699 Pregnancy duration in a dog, depending on the breeding date. (LH: luteinizing hormone; OV: ovulation; conc.: conception)

Table 37 First sonographic visualization to characterize gestational age in the dog (from Yeager *et al.*, 1992*[63] and Heinze *et al.*, 1994**[28]). 5.0 MHz and 7.5 MHz sector transducers were used for the examinations[28].

Characteristic	Days after LH peak*	Days post ovulation**
Gestational sac	20	18–20
Uterine wall	20–23	18–20
Placenta		
thin hyperechoic layer	22–24	20–23
zonary placenta	27–30	29–31
Embryo		
oblong with wall contact	23–25	22–23
detached from uterine wall	29–33	24–27
Embryonal/fetal membranes		
yolk sac	25–28	23–25
allantoamnion	27–31	26–29
umbilical cord		28–30
Embryonal/fetal structures and characteristics		
cardiac activity	23–25	22–23
visible crown–rump length		24
head and body distinguishable	27–31	31–33
limb buds	33–35	32–33
head diameter visible	34–35	34
fetal movement	34–36	34–35
fetal skeleton	33–39	34–35
stomach	36–39	34–35
urinary bladder	35–39	34–35
lungs – more hyperechoic than liver	38–42	
liver – more hyperechoic than abdomen	39–47	
kidneys	39–47	
eyes	39–47	39–40
intestines	57–63	
placental separation		62–64
parturition	63–65	62–64

Sonographic Findings and Biometry

The earliest sonographic pregnancy diagnosis in the dog is possible between day 18 and day 20 post ovulation, a few days following nidation. Pregnancy detection in the cat is usually already possible around day 15 to day 17 post breeding. Apart from the fetal structures listed in *Tables 37* and *38* and illustrated in **686, 687, 689, 697, 700–702, 709** and **710** (dog), as well as in **667, 668, 673, 676, 677, 681–683, 688, 690** and **691–698** (cat), characteristic changes in the size of fetal and extrafetal structures can be recognized and used to predict fetal age.

Numerous sonographic measurements are applied in human medicine, such as cephalometry, thoracometry and abdominometry, as well as measuring the long limb bones[27, 45]. In veterinary medicine, determination of the crown–rump length, fetal head diameter and body diameter have proven most practical.

Most biometric parameters should be evaluated with caution. In human medicine, errors occur and are difficult to avoid. Errors can be systematic or incidental and can occur anywhere within the triad of machine, patient and sonographer[27]. Measurements are extremely dependent on the ultrasound unit used and its settings. This is especially true for older machines and transducers. False measurements in dog and cat patients are caused by the usual influences, such as image quality, bladder filling and individual growth variations, as well as 'cooperation' of dam and fetus, but they are also caused by breed-related size and shape differences. The variability in absolute measurements is greater in the dog than in the cat because of these specific breed differences. A sonographer needs a great amount of experience to reproduce biometric findings, since the areas in question must be imaged in an exact and defined plane. Another disadvantage in obstetrical ultrasonography is the time needed to measure numerous fetuses.

According to Yeager *et al.* (1992)[63], the head and body diameter are almost identical around day 32 in the dog with reference to the pre-ovulatory LH peak. Between day 36 and day 39 post ovulation the canine body diameter measures more than half the chorionic cavity diameter and increases to more than half of the outer uterine diameter between day 44 and day 46 post ovulation. After day 38 to day 40 post ovulation the dog fetus extends beyond the ends of the zonary placenta. Fetal crown–rump length (**703, 704**) can be measured from day 24 post ovulation in the dog and day 19 post breeding in the cat. It can be safely measured until day 40 post ovulation in the dog and day 45 post breeding in the cat. After this point it is not possible to image the entire fetus on the sonogram. Fetal crown–rump length is also difficult to measure because of fetal flexion and moving, agile fetuses. A large number of fetuses might also impair visualization and measurement. The findings should be evaluated with reference to the indivdual size differences of normal fetuses within a litter.

The biparietal head diameter (**705, 706**) can be used to predict gestational age in the dog and cat from day 36 to day 58 post ovulation and day 30 post breeding until parturition respectively.

Sonographic biometry can also be applied to the transverse fetal body diameter at the level of the stomach (**707, 708**). This measurement can be made between day 22 and day 58 post ovulation in the dog and from day 35 post breeding in the cat. In Beagles[63] and European domestic cats[25] the parameters mentioned show a significant correlation with gestational age (**703–708**).

Table 38 Early, late and average detection of sonographic findings to characterize gestational age in the cat (from Grof, 1992[25]). 5.0 MHz and 7.5 MHz transducers were used for the examinations.

Characteristics	Early detection (days post breeding)	Late detection (days post breeding)	Average detection (days post breeding)
Gestational sac	13	15	14
Internal echo	15	18	17
Embryonal/fetal membranes			
yolk sac	19	23	22
allantoamnion	21 (7.5 MHz) 22 (5.0 MHz)	30	27
umbilical cord	20 (7.5 MHz) 21 (5.0 MHz)	30	25
Embryonal/fetal structures and charcteristics			
cardiac activity	17	19	18
crown–rump length			19
head and body distinguishable	21	26	23
limb buds	21	26	23
head diameter visible			27
fetal movement	27	30	28
phalanges	27	34	32
ribs	30	36	34
spine	30	38	35
stomach	31	34	32
urinary bladder	33	37	35
lungs and liver distinguishable	34 (7.5 MHz) 35 (5.0 MHz)	45	40
kidneys	40 (7.5 MHz) 45 (5.0 MHz)	54	48
eyes	32	44	38
large vessels	34	48	41
heart chambers	38	42	40
acoustic shadowing of the skull	after 36		
acoustic shadowing of the spine	after 41		

700

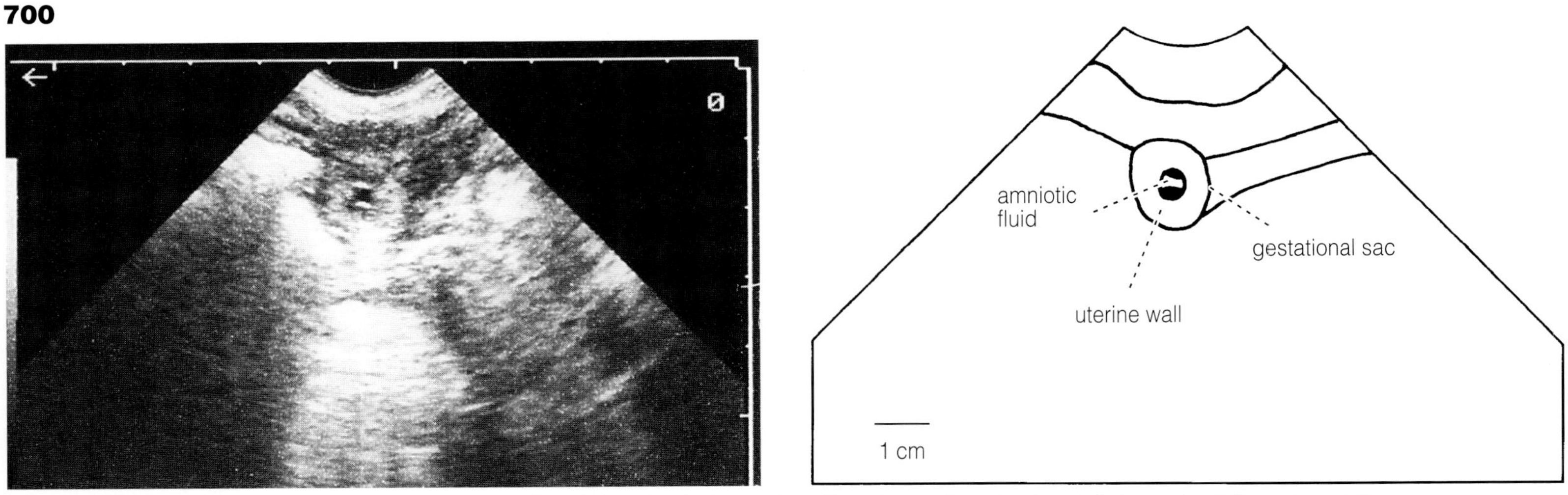

700 Gestational sac, consisting of the uterine wall and the chorionic cavity with echogenic poles in a bitch on day 20 post ovulation.

701

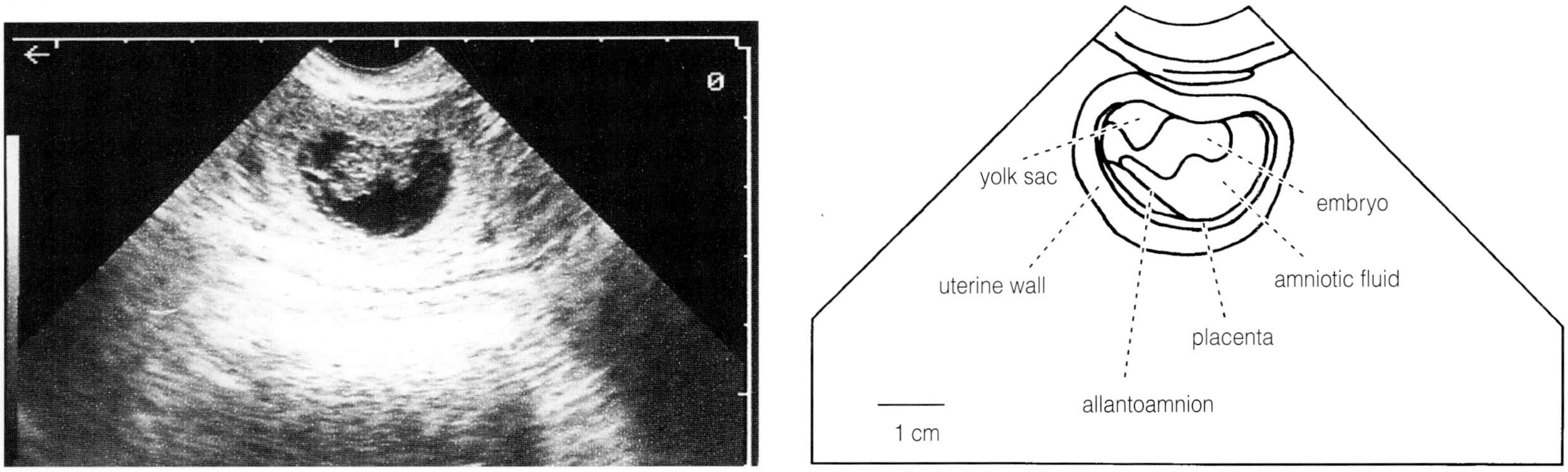

701 Gestational sac with placenta, allantoamnion, yolk sac and embryo in a bitch on day 28 post ovulation.

702

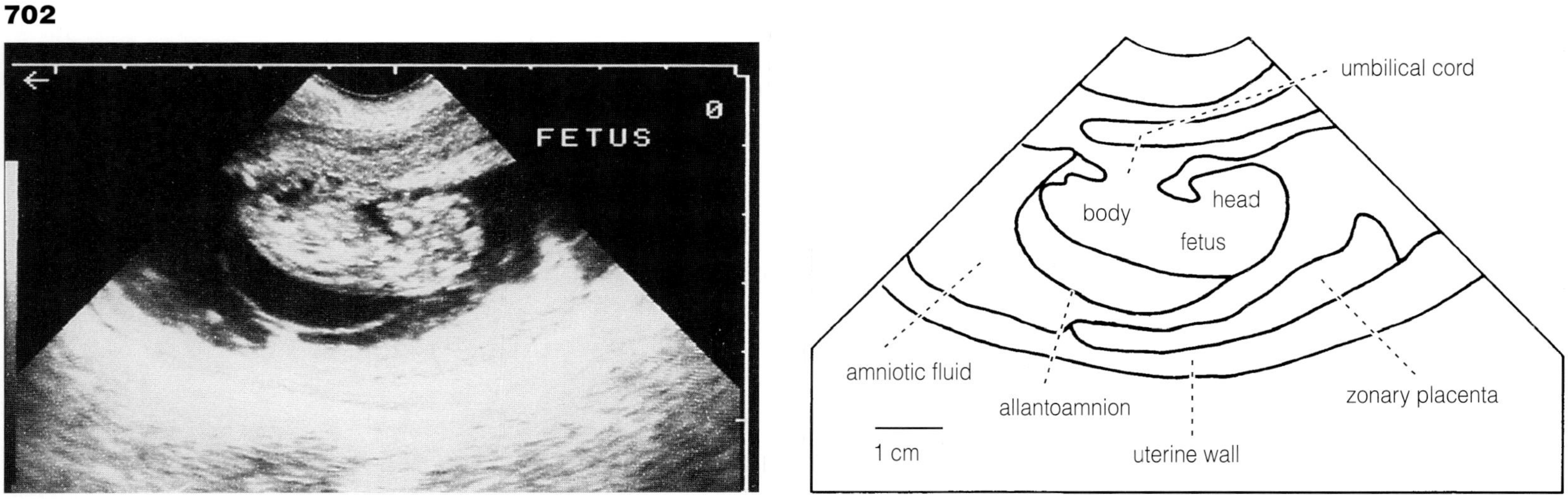

702 Gestational sac with zonary placenta, allantoamnion, umbilical cord and fetus in a bitch on day 35 post ovulation.

703

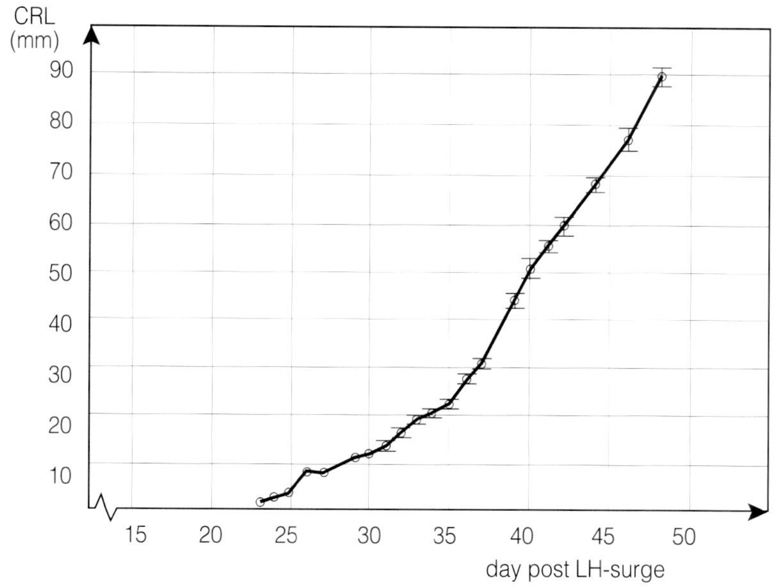

703 Graph showing increase in crown–rump length (CRL) of a Beagle fetus. (From Yeager *et al.*, 1992[63].)

704

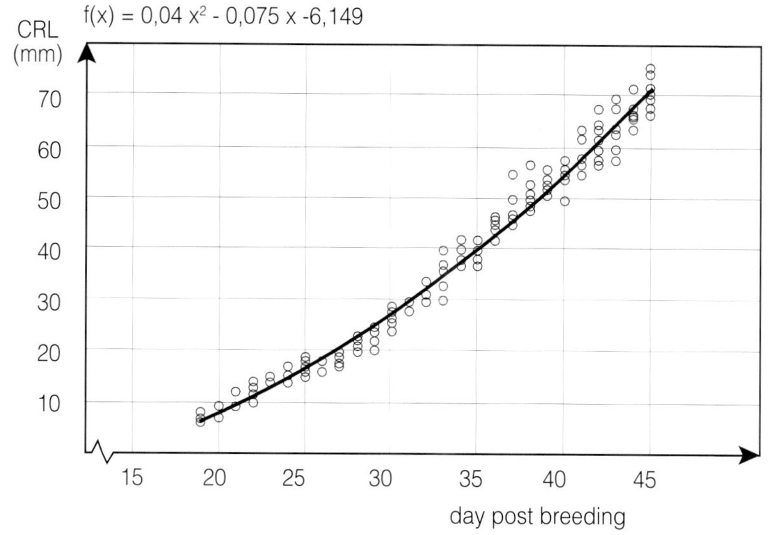

704 Graph showing increase in crown–rump length (CRL) up to day 45 of pregnancy in European domestic cat fetuses. (From Grof, 1992[25].)

705

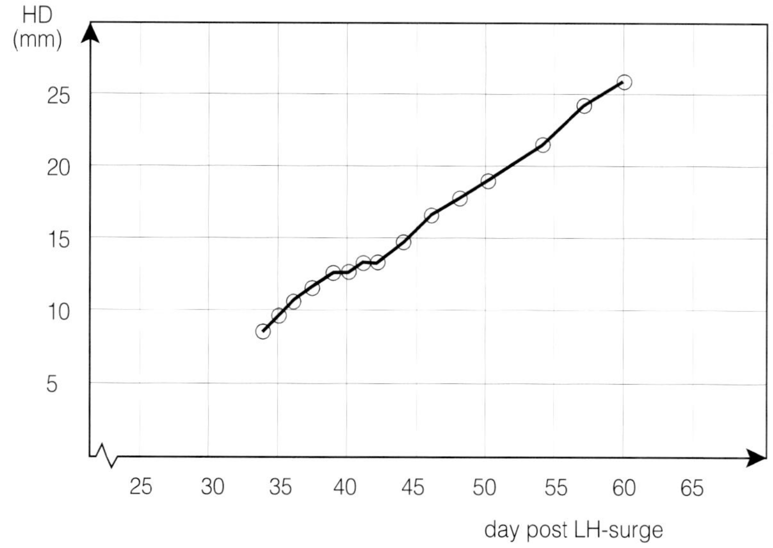

705 Graph showing increase in biparietal head diameter (HD) during pregnancy of Beagle fetuses. (From Yeager *et al.*, 1992[63].)

706

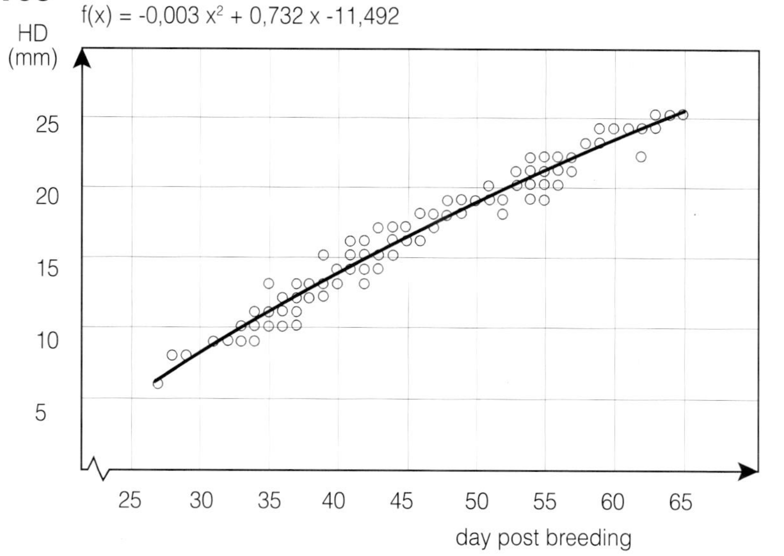

706 Graph showing increase in biparietal head diameter (HD) during pregnancy in European domestic cat fetuses. (From Grof, 1992[25].)

707

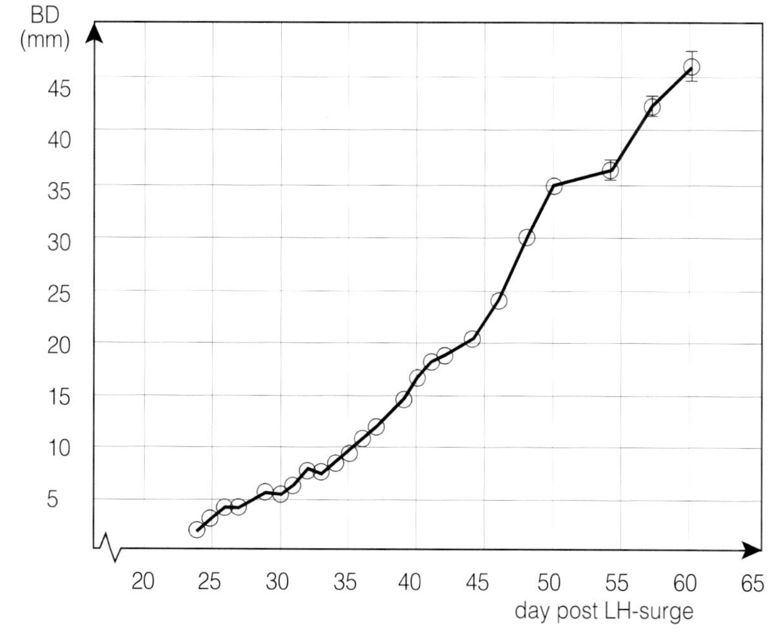

707 Graph showing increase in the transverse body diameter (BD) at the stomach level in Beagle fetuses. (From Yeager *et al.*, 1992[63].)

708

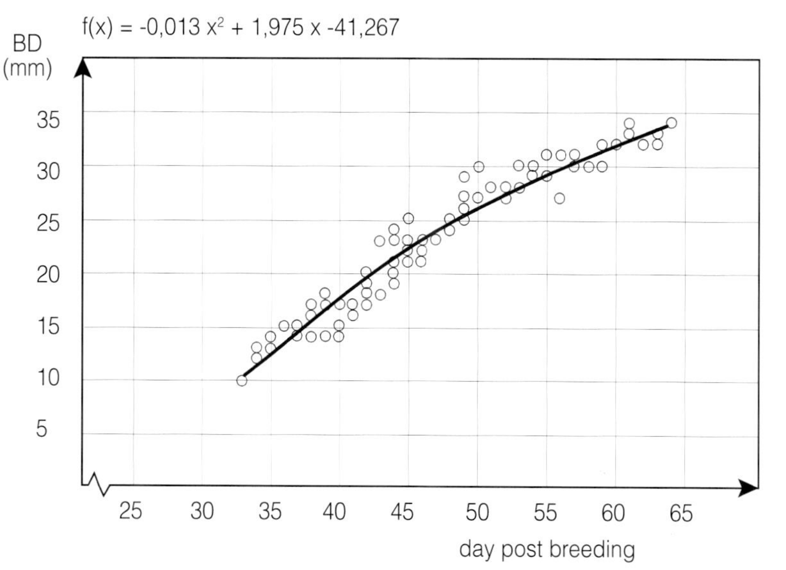

708 Graph showing increase in the transverse body diameter (BD) at the stomach level in European domestic cat fetuses. (From Grof, 1992[25].)

709

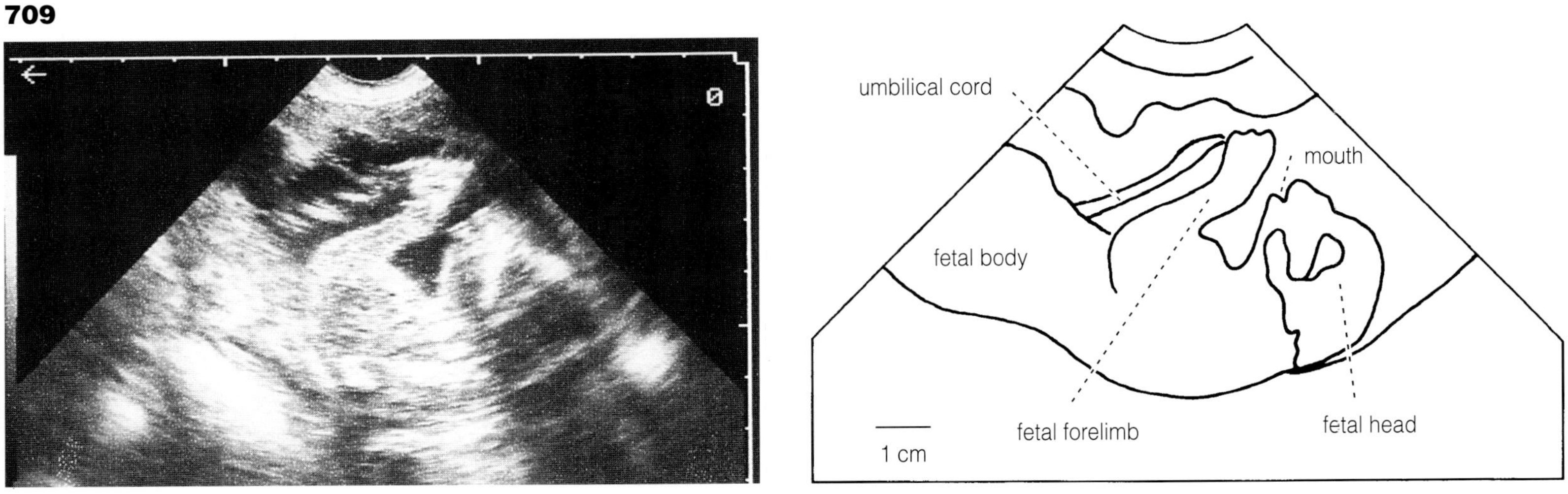

709 Head and mouth, forelimb, body and umbilical cord in a dog fetus on day 48 post ovulation.

710

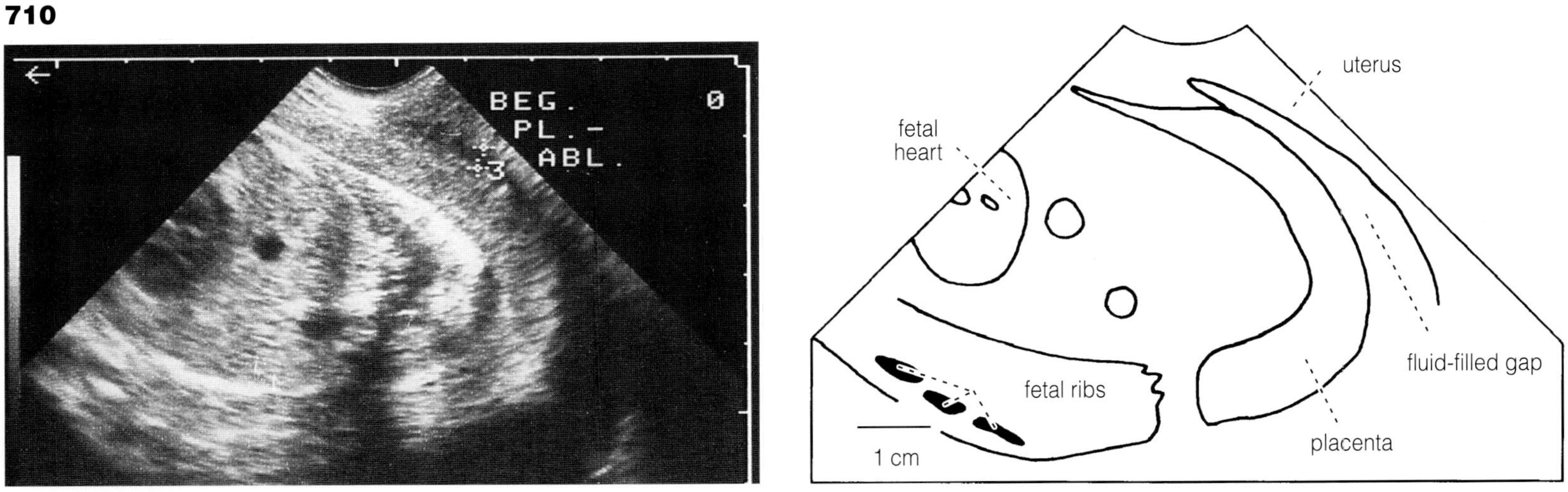

710 Placental separation before parturition with a fluid-filled gap between the placenta and the uterine wall in a bitch on day 63 post ovulation.

711

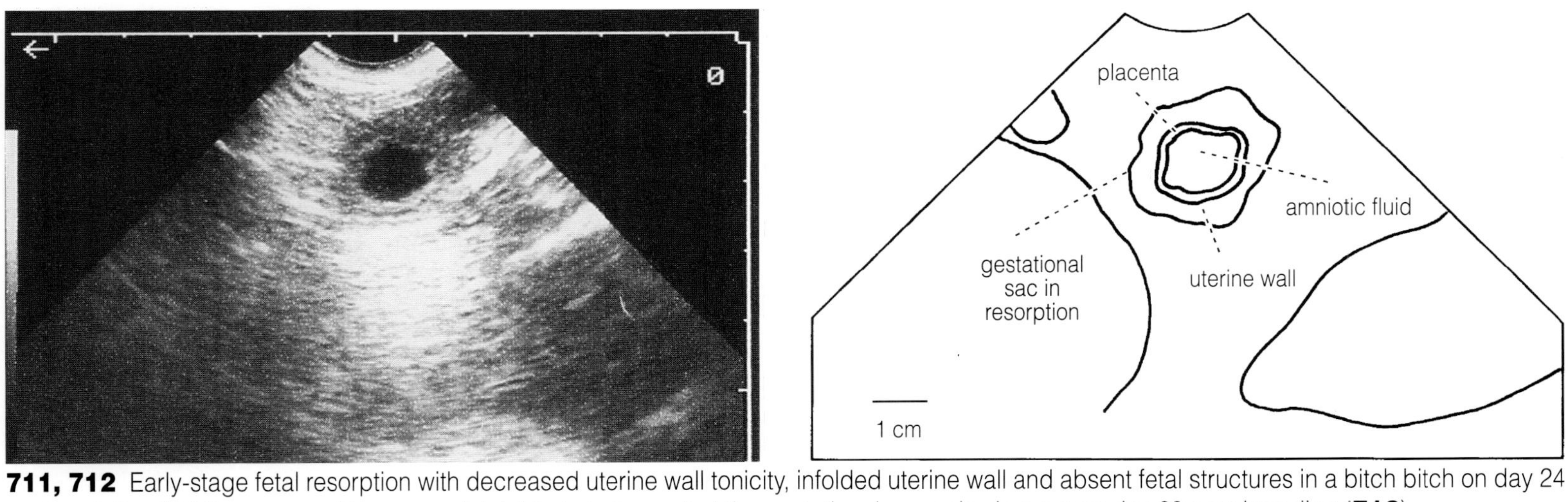

711, 712 Early-stage fetal resorption with decreased uterine wall tonicity, infolded uterine wall and absent fetal structures in a bitch bitch on day 24 post ovulation (**711**), compared to a normal, infolded uterine wall at the gestational sac poles in a cat on day 23 post breeding (**712**).

712

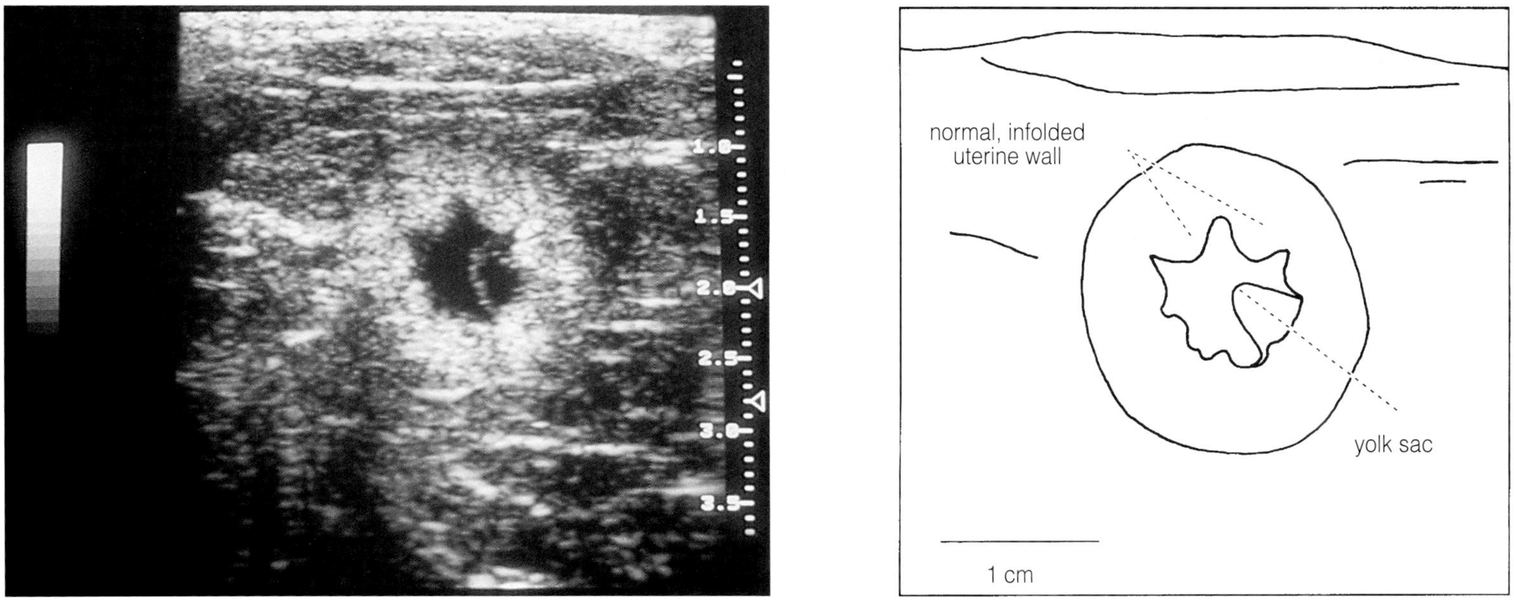

712 A normal, infolded uterine wall at the gestational sac poles in a cat on day 23 post breeding (see also **211**).

713

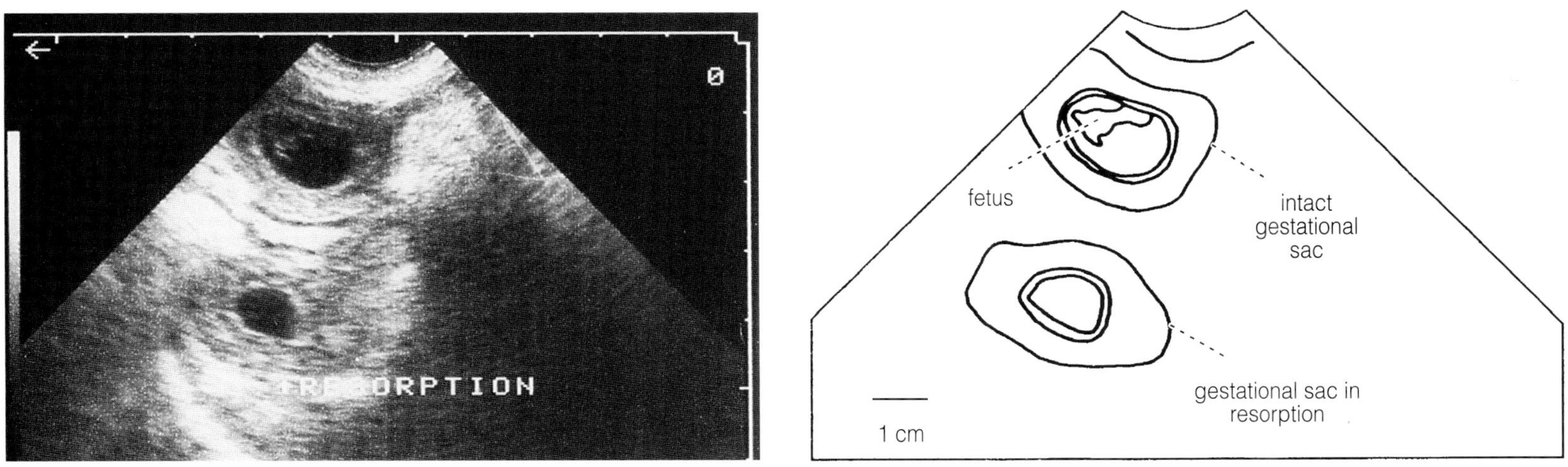

714

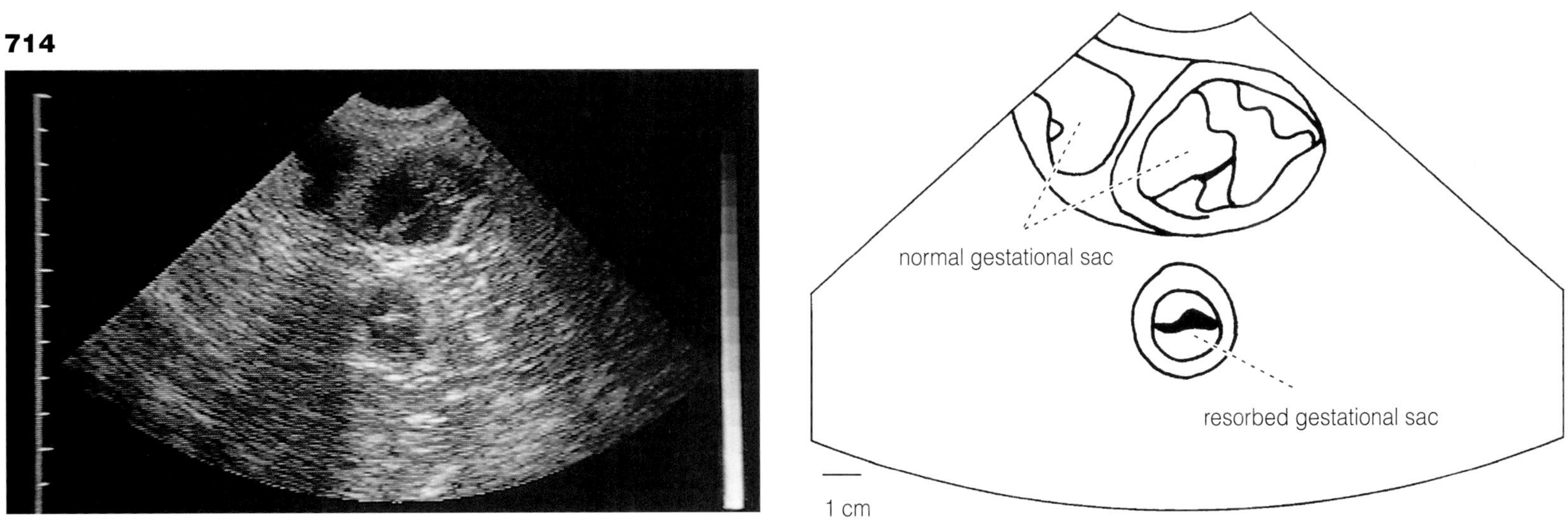

713, 714 Progressive gestational sac resorption and normally developed gestational sac with internal echos in a bitch on day 25 post ovulation (**713**). One resorbed and two normal gestational sacs in a cat on day 30 post breeding (**714**).

715

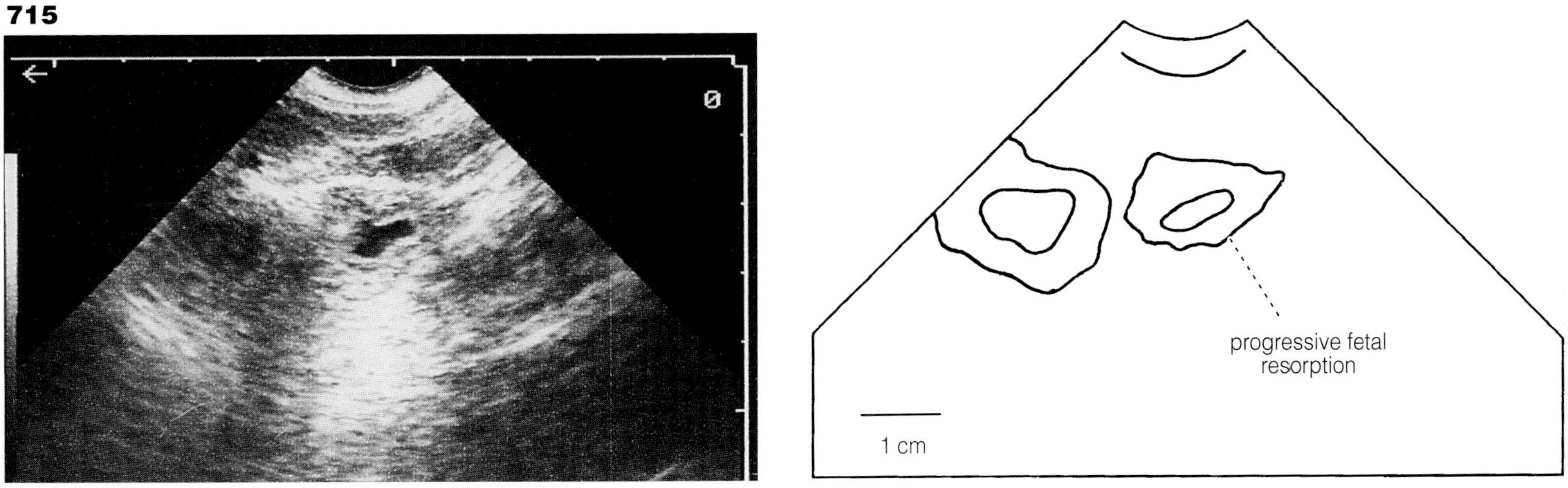

715 Progressive fetal resorption with collapsed gestational sac and decreased amount of amniotic fluid in a bitch on day 26 post ovulation.

716

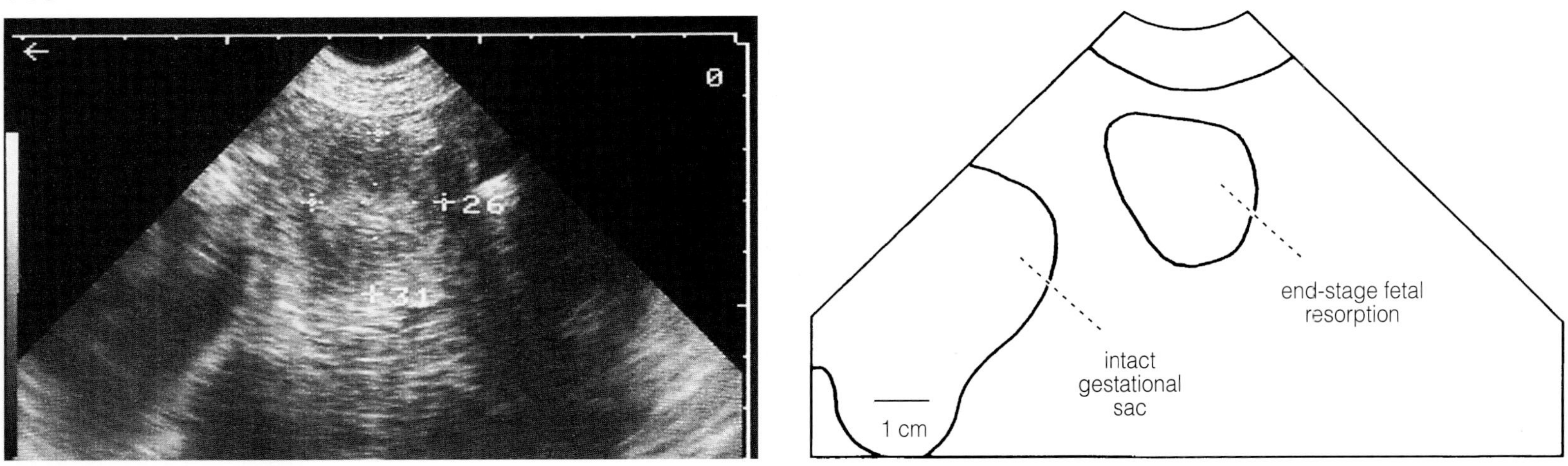

716 End-stage fetal resorption with absent amniotic fluid and marked infolding of the uterine mucosa in a bitch on day 35 post ovulation.

717

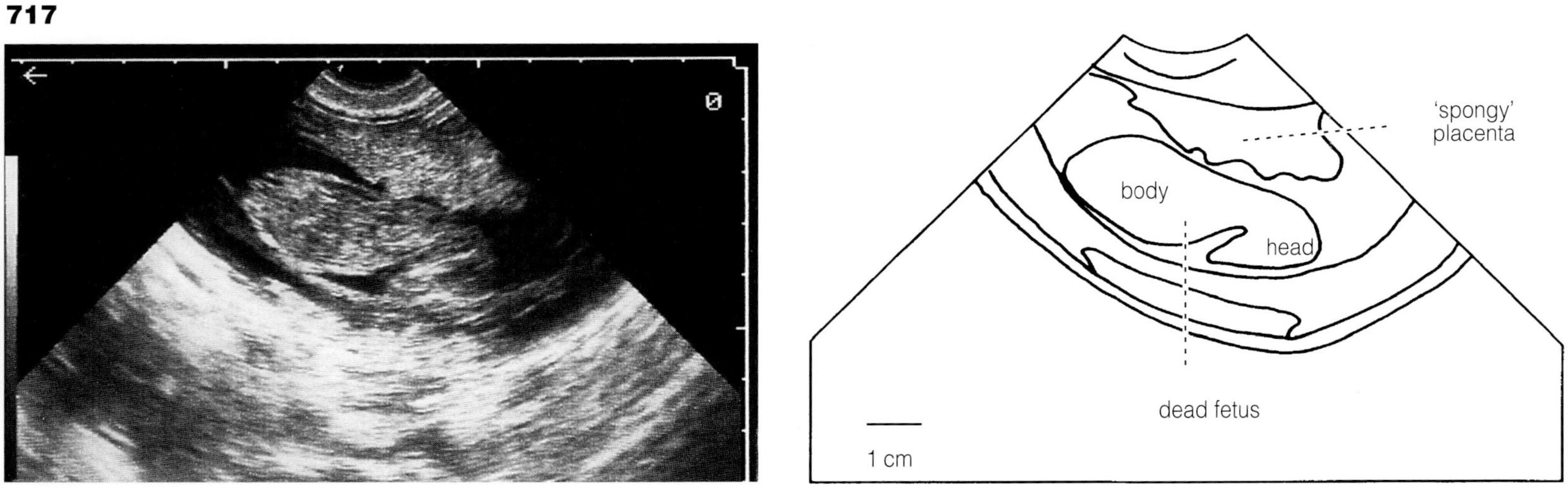

717 Abnormal fetal posture with absent cardiac activity and undefined organs in a bitch on day 40 post ovulation. The placenta appears 'spongy'.

Pathological Pregnancy

Anne-Rose Günzel-Apel and Britta Heinze

The advantage of sonographic pregnancy diagnosis is in early recognition of embryonal or fetal death, as well as fetal resorption and imminent or completed abortion. In these cases, ultrasonography is superior to the usual diagnostic methods such as palpation and radiography. Fetal resorption can be safely diagnosed 20–28 days post ovulation in the dog and 18–28 days post breeding in the cat. The precise cause of intrauterine fetal death may become apparent with sonography (see Fetal Development, page 297).

Ultrasonic determination of pathological pregnancies are possible with 5 MHz sector or linear transducers. Transducers with frequencies of 6.5, 7.5 or 10 MHz will optimize results in smaller dog breeds and in cats.

718

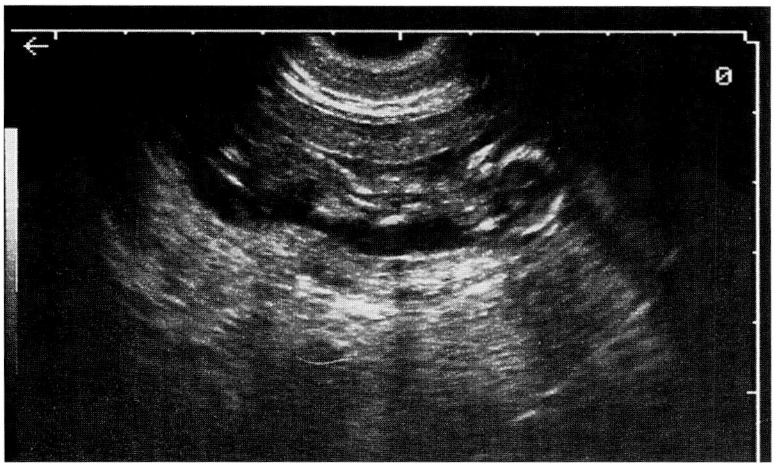

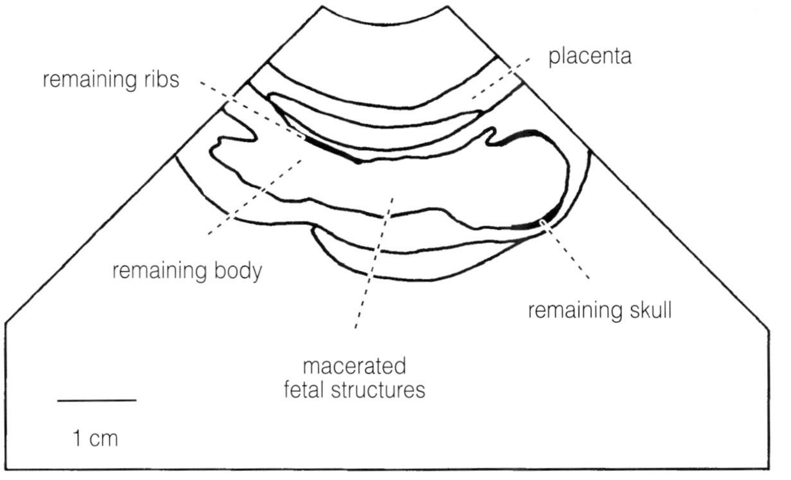

718 Early maceration with identifiable skull and spine, as well as decreased amniotic fluid, in a bitch on day 44 post ovulation.

719

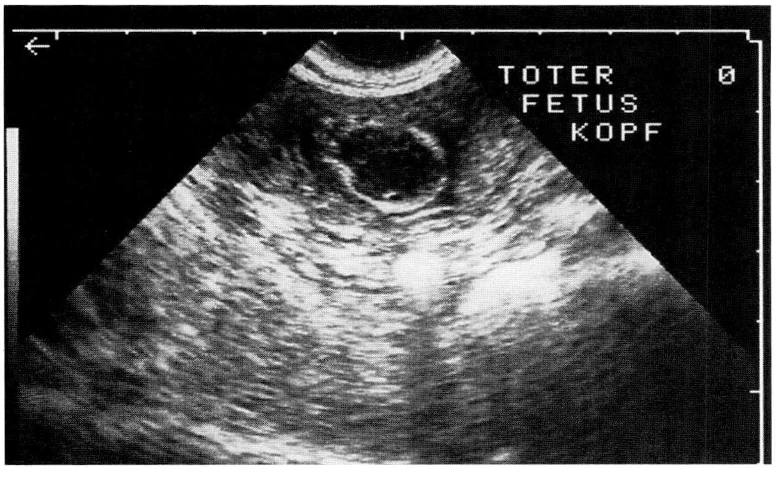

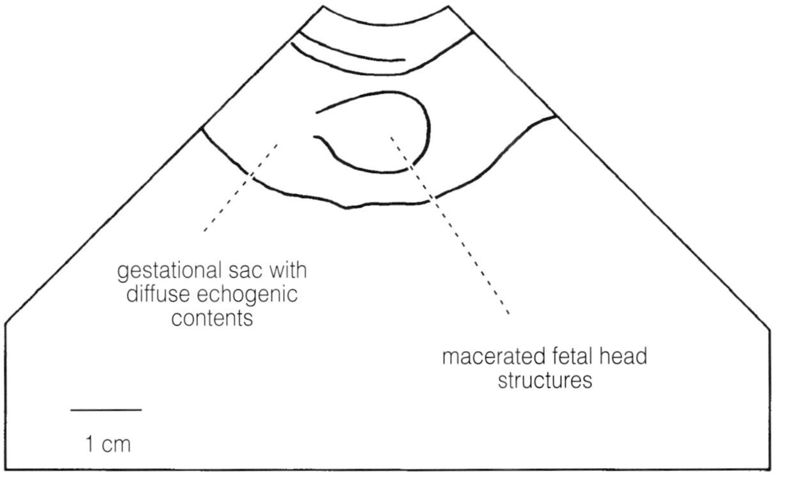

719 Macerated fetal skull, surrounded by the uterine wall, in a bitch on day 45 post ovulation.

Fetal Resorption

Fetal resorption usually occurs without any apparent clinical symptoms[46]. In most cases only one of the numerous embryos is affected. Fetal development is otherwise normal and does not indicate an abnormal pregnancy. England (1993)[19] found fetal resorption in 5% of all examined pregnant bitches, while Mueller and Arbeiter (1993)[46] described it in 12.9% of examined bitches. In a few cases, fetal resorption of all embryos has been described.

The characteristic sonographic findings with fetal resorption (*Table* 39) are smaller gestational sac size compared to other sacs (**713, 714**), infolding of the embryonic vesicle wall (**711**), decrease in amniotic fluid volume (**713–715**), disintegration of fetal structures and a collapsing fetal cavity with concurrent thickening and infolding of the vesicle wall (**711, 713–716**). The gestational sac may normally show infolding walls at both poles in the cat (**712**). The amount of amniotic fluid may also vary in each individual animal.

As fetal resorption progresses, sonographic diagnosis may be more difficult when amniotic fluid is absent. For this reason, fetal resorption cannot safely be diagnosed after day 40. End-stage resorption shows a slightly echogenic area at the former implantation site in the uterus, and the uterine mucosa is folded (**716**).

Fetal Death

Fetal death occurs during the second half of pregnancy and is often not associated with clinical symptoms, such as bloody-mucous vulvar discharge. The history occasionally refers to a sudden reduction in the size of the abdomen in the bitch. Aetiology (micobiological, serological, histopathological, hormonal) does not offer a diagnosis in most cases. These animals are able to have a normal pregnancy and parturition without complications during the following oestrus cycle, even without treatment[44].

The characteristic sonographic findings with fetal death (*Table* 40, page 312) are cardiac standstill, absent fetal movement, abnormal fetal posture, collapsed rib cage, undefined organ structure, fetal maceration, rapid decrease in amniotic fluid volume and a 'spongy' placenta[5,6] (**717–720**).

Table 39 Characteristic sonographic findings with fetal resorption.

Sonographic characteristics of fetal resorption:
• Decreased gestational sac size. • Infolded embryonal vesicle wall. • Decreased amniotic fluid volume. • Undefined or absent fetal structures. • Collapsed embryonal vesicle. • Thickening and infolding of the vesicle wall.

720

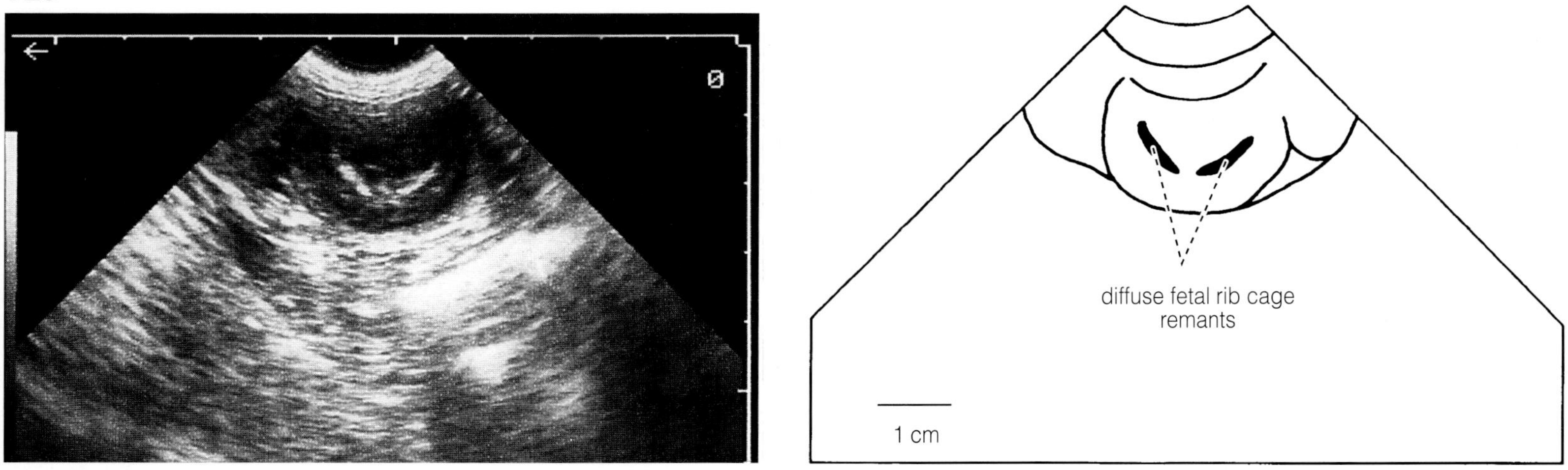

720 Fetal rib cage remnants in a bitch on day 45 post ovulation.

721

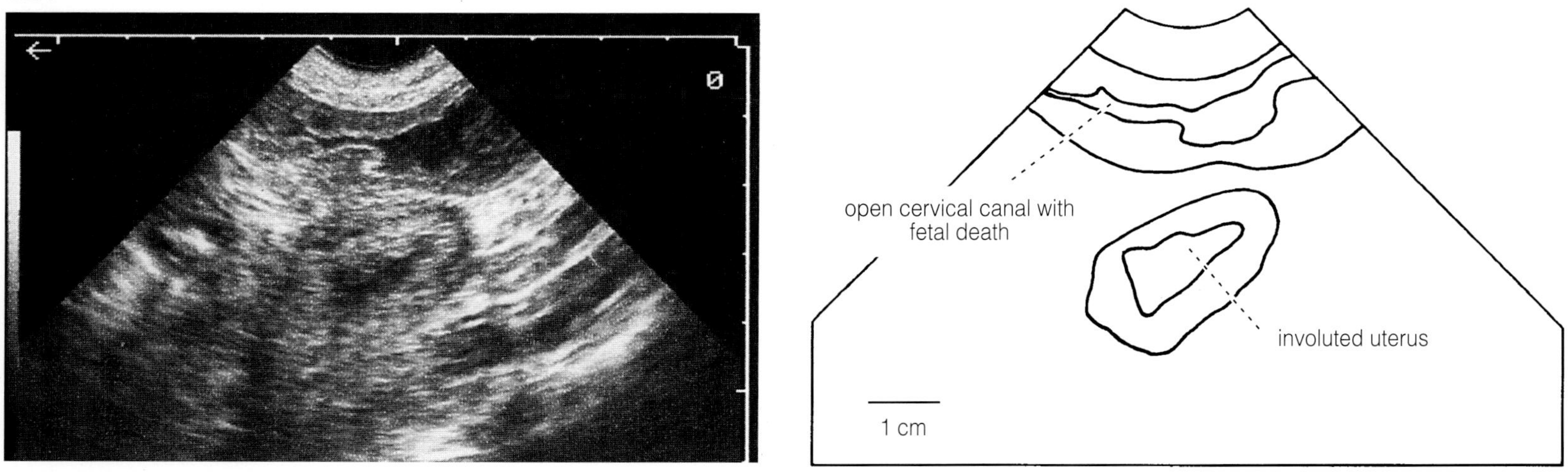

721 Open cervical canal following discharge of disintegrated fetal remnants and an involuted, empty gestational sac in a bitch on day 46 post ovulation.

Concurrently with discharged fetal remnants or aborted fetuses, the cervical canal is open and can be imaged (**721**). Placental separation can be recognized with an abortion or premature parturition (**722**) and it appears similar to a normal birth.

Fetal death towards the end of pregnancy or intra partum can be diagnosed by an absent heart rate, abnormal posture, undefined organ structures and a reduced tonicity (**723**), or by differentiation from normal live fetuses (*Table 40*).

Parturition

Danielle Schäfer and Cordula Poulsen Nautrup

Sonographic examination near parturition can be helpful in deciding whether veterinary intervention will be needed.

The examination shortly before and/or during parturition gives information on vitality, size, position and presentation of the fetus, as well as contractiliy of the uterus. This can indicate whether to wait, apply medication to induce parturition or perform a Caesarean section. When the fetuses are vital, not too large and have not entered the pelvis, the veterinarian can wait or can induce or accelerate parturition. A Caesarean section is indicated when the fetuses are deformed, dying, already dead or retained in the birth canal (**723**).

Table 40 Characteristic sonographic findings with fetal death.

Sonographic findings with fetal death:
• Cardiac standstill. • Absent fetal movements. • Abnormal fetal posture. • Collapsed rib cage. • Undefined organ structures.
Sonographic findings with fetal maceration:
• Confluent or isolated, macerated skeletal structures. • Reduction in amniotic fluid volume.

Ultrasonography is advantageous compared to radiography. With portable ultrasound machines, intrapartum examinations are easier and less stressful for the dam, as they can be examined in their own homes. Another advantage is the absolute safety for the fetus (no radiation of the gonads). Fetal vitality can also be evaluated. Prepartum radiographs are helpful in assessing the size of the fetal head in relation to the maternal pelvic bone.

722

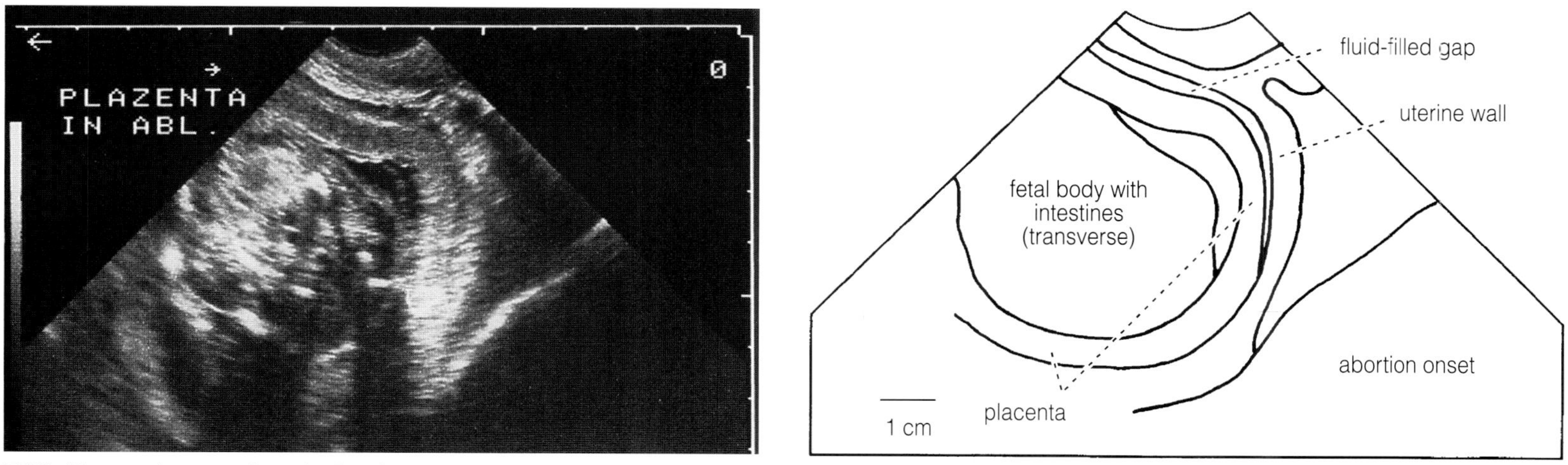

722 Placental separation of a live fetus, indicating imminent abortion in a bitch on day 54 post ovulation.

723

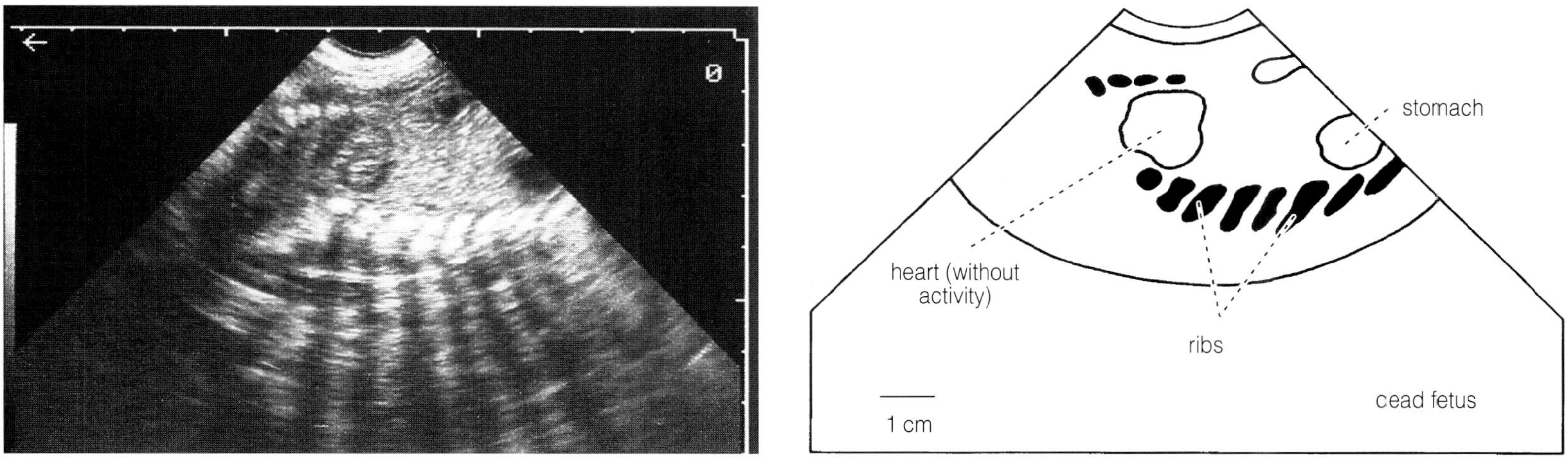

723 Fetal death intra partum of a single fetus with dystocia, cardiac standstill, deformed rib cage due to a decreased tonus and undefined organ structures in a bitch 68 days post ovulation.

724

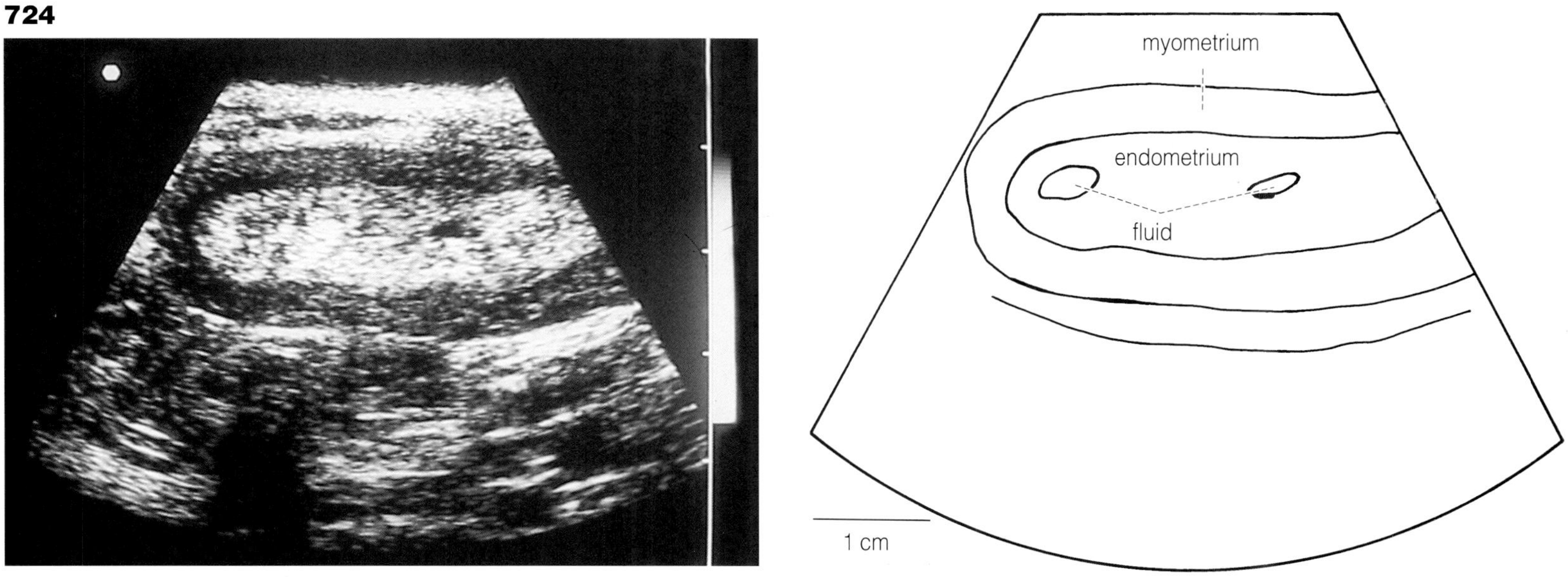

724 Normal placentation site in a longitudinal view in a bitch four days post partum.

Postpartum Uterus

Danielle Schäfer and Cordula Poulsen Nautrup

During the first week post partum, the uterus of the bitch is dilated and oedematous[1]. The placentation sites are 1.5–3 cm wide, coarse, granulated and covered with blood clots. Involution of the uterus to its normal size takes approximately 4–5 weeks in the dog[48]. During the first seven days post partum, the placentation sites of the postpartum uterus appear as granulated structures of medium echogenicity with small round anechoic areas (**724**). Luminal fluid is rarely seen[53]. While the canine uterus still measures up to one centimetre 21 days post partum, the uterus in the cat is difficult to identify. The clinical postpartum phase in the cat is usually uneventful[23]. On the day of parturition the feline uterus, with its placentation sites, is sonographically visible, similar to the dog (**725, 726**). Four days later, the involuted feline postpartum uterus is barely visible ultrasonographically.

Ultrasonography can be used to diagnose the cause of abnormal or increased lochial flow (**727**),

Duplex Ultrasonography

Cordula Poulsen Nautrup

General Observations

Duplex ultrasonography (Latin *duplex* = double) signifies concurrent imaging of macroscopic structures with two-dimensional B-mode and of blood flows using pulsed-wave (PW) or colour Doppler echography (see Doppler Mode, page 45; Pulsed-Wave Doppler (PW Doppler), page 46; Colour-Flow Doppler, page 48).

Blood flow spectrums can be evaluated using PW Doppler and are characteristic for fetal and maternal vessels, as well as for the separate pregnancy stages. Normal blood flows in the maternal uterine and placental vessels are necessary to ensure a sufficient oxygen and nutrient supply to the fetuses. This fetal nutritional situation can be monitored directly by blood flows in the fetal vessels.

In humans, duplex echography is an important diagnostic tool that complements routine two-dimensional ultrasonography during pregnancy[42]. Gynaecological and obstetrical ultrasound has been a part of most human medical literature and monographies since the late 1980s[30, 55]. Doppler ultrasonography has been used in experimental veterinary medicine to monitor pregnancy in sheep[3, 33, 34, 35, 47].

Indications for Obstetrical Duplex Ultrasonography

Duplex ultrasonography is indicated with all abnormal pregnancies. Early recognition of growth retardation, imminent fetal death or poor fetal viability is given. A complete sonographic pregnancy screening includes a Doppler examination during the first half of pregnancy with the usual diagnostics, and duplex sonography towards the end of pregnancy, i.e. the last week of pregnancy. Additional flow measurements can be made during the last weeks if necessary. Poor fetal nutrition should lead to early induction of parturition if the fetus is viable. Experience in the near future will underline the importance of this examination method, which can recognize problems early and assist in the resulting consequences.

The development of the cardiovascular system in the dog and cat is similar in duplex sonography, which is why they will be discussed together.

Two-Dimensional Ultrasonography and Colour Doppler Echography of the Embryonal and Fetal Cardiovascular System

The morphology of the developing cardiovascular system can be evaluated with two-dimensional sonography using 5–10 MHz transducers. Two-dimensional real-time ultrasound also enables evaluation of cardiovascular functions, such as cardiac activity from day 22 post ovulation (dog) or day 17 post breeding (cat) (**674, 675**). Large vessel anatomy in the dog and cat may be recognized with two-dimensional ultrasonography during the second trimester, i.e. from day 35 post ovulation or post breeding (**696, 728**). Smaller vessels are not usually identified in the sonogram (**729**). They may be visualized and differentiated by their blood flows using colour-coded Doppler echography (**730**).

Colour-coded Doppler ultrasonography is used to detect and determine the individual maternal and fetal blood vessels. Flow patterns and velocities are then recorded with PW Doppler sonography.

Pulsed-Wave Doppler Echography of Maternal and Fetal Blood Flows

The actual blood flow volume is difficult to quantify with flow velocities and vessel diameters using PW Doppler methods. The systolic/diastolic arterial blood flow ratio can be measured and calculated with the aid of PW Doppler ultrasonography. The sample volume must be placed correctly to avoid interfering with flow spectrums and a giving false diagnosis.

Pregnancy is monitored by recording blood flows in the maternal uterine and/or placental arteries, the umbilical artery, the fetal aorta, in some cases the fetal common carotid artery, a fetal cerebral vessel, and the caudal vena cava near the heart[2, 17, 36, 57].

725

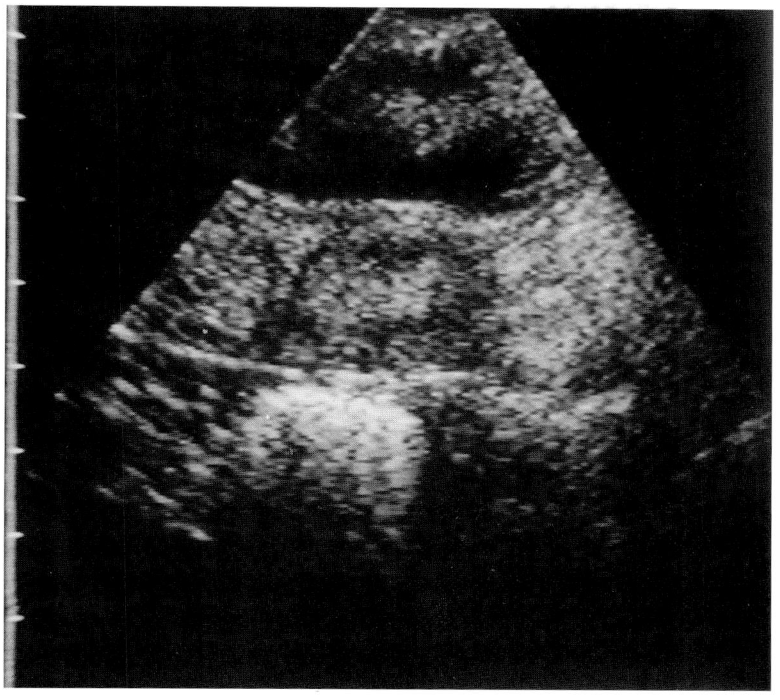

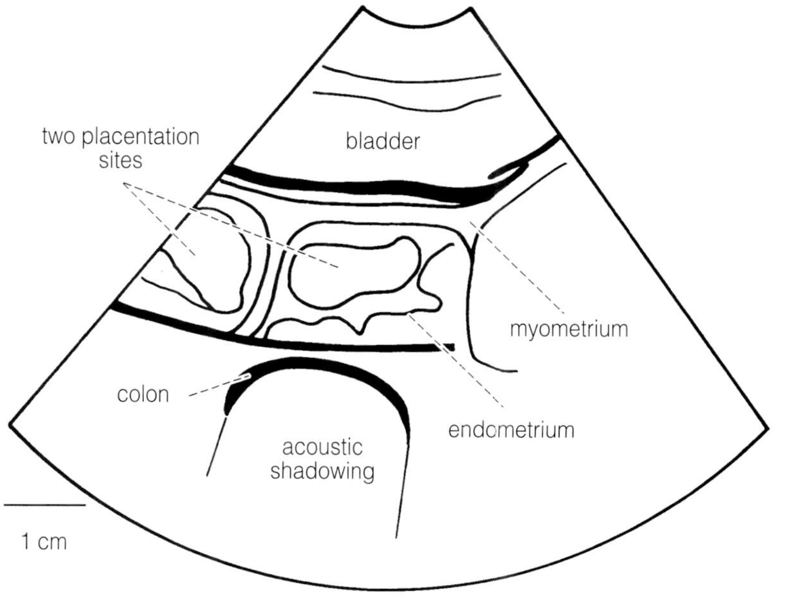

726

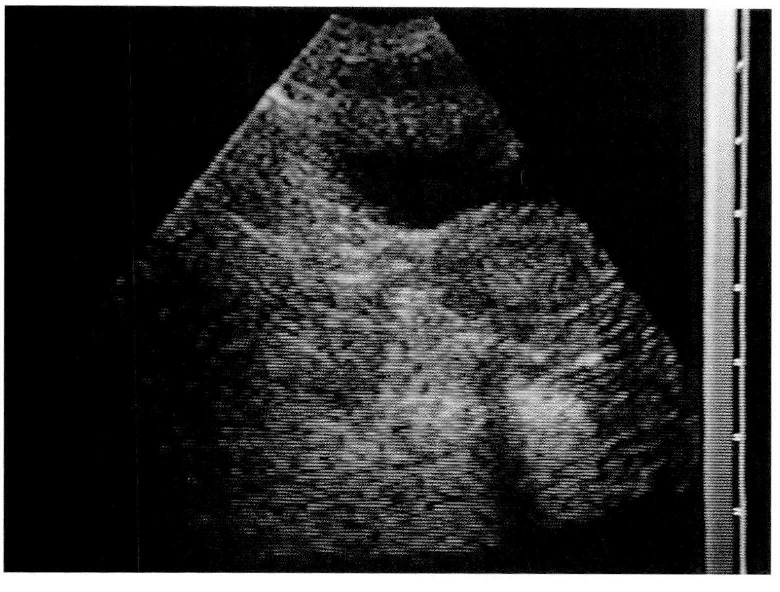

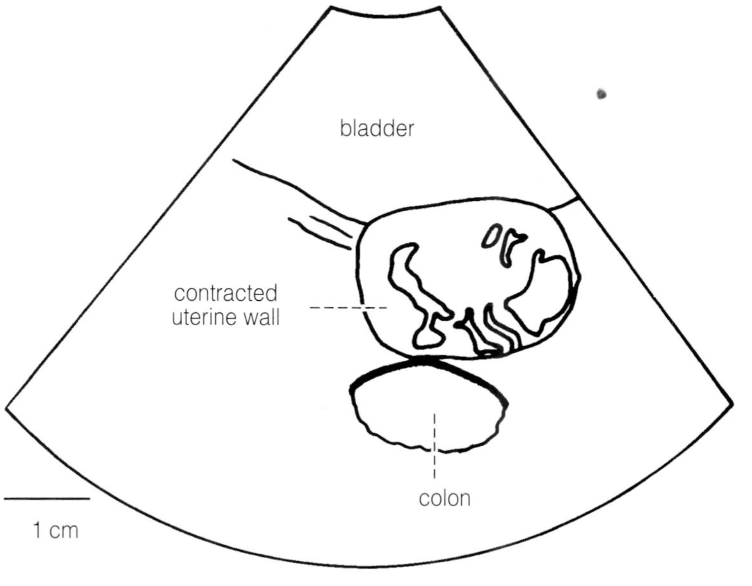

727

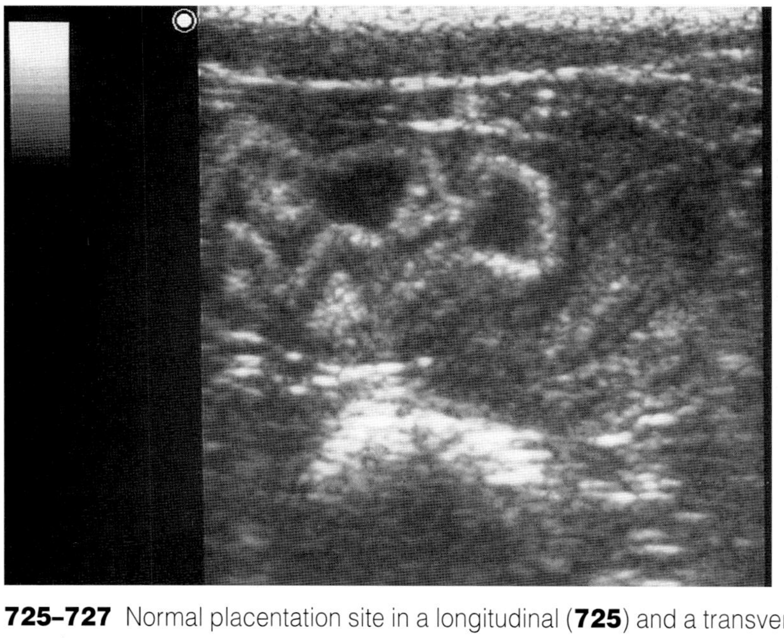

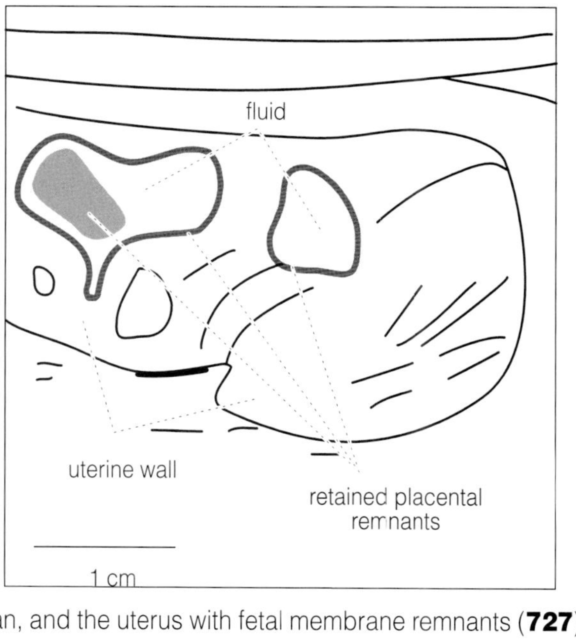

725–727 Normal placentation site in a longitudinal (**725**) and a transverse (**726**) scan, and the uterus with fetal membrane remnants (**727**) in a cat one day post partum.

728

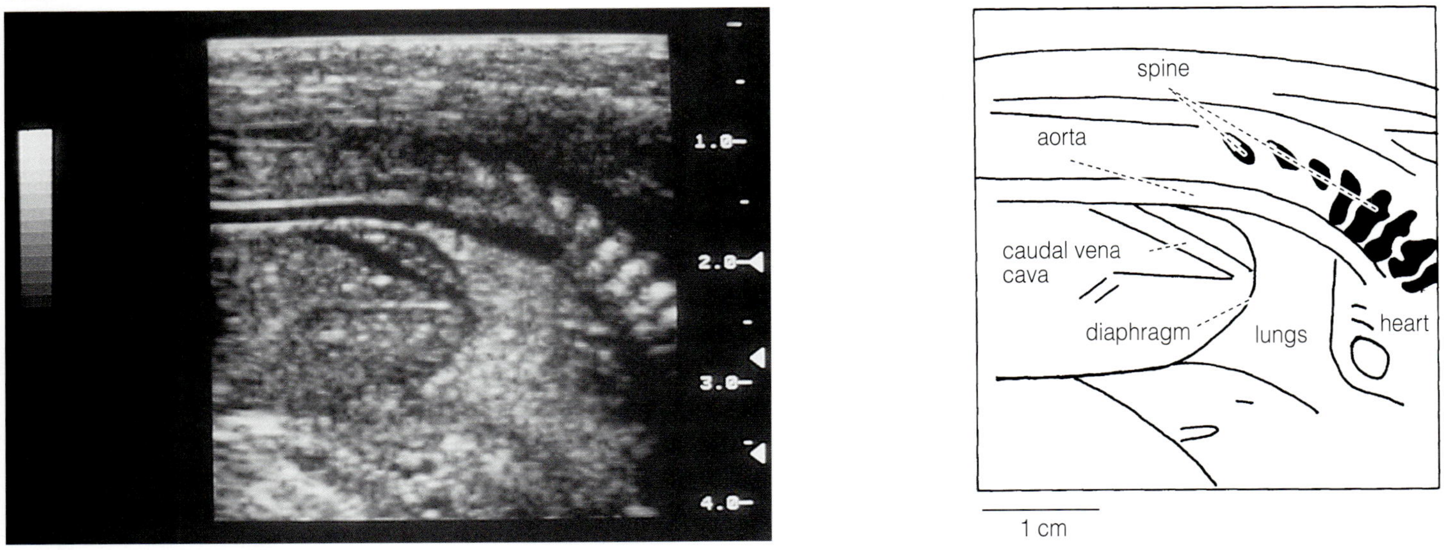

728 Two-dimensional sonogram of the aorta and caudal vena cava in a cat fetus 51 days post breeding. The sonogram was made using a 5.0 MHz linear transducer.

729

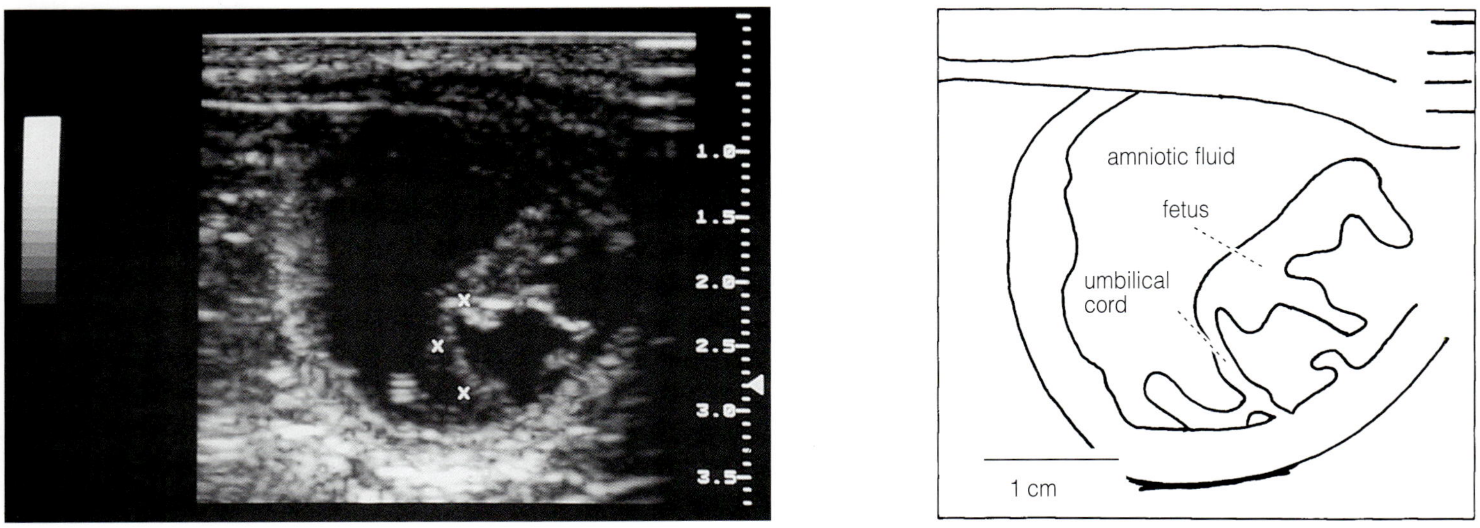

730

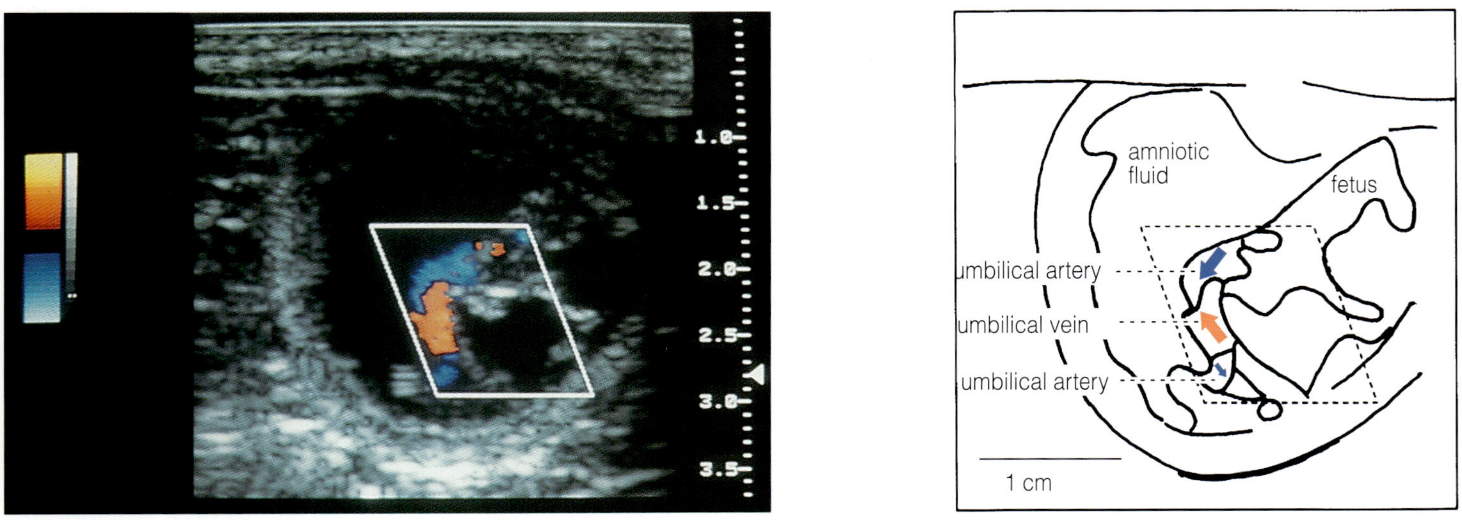

729, 730 Two-dimensional sonogram (**729**) and colour-coded Doppler image (**730**) of the umbilical cord in a cat fetus on day 26 post breeding. The two-dimensional ultrasound image does not show any vessels, while colour Doppler can differentiate between the umbilical artery (blue) and the umbilical vein (red).

731

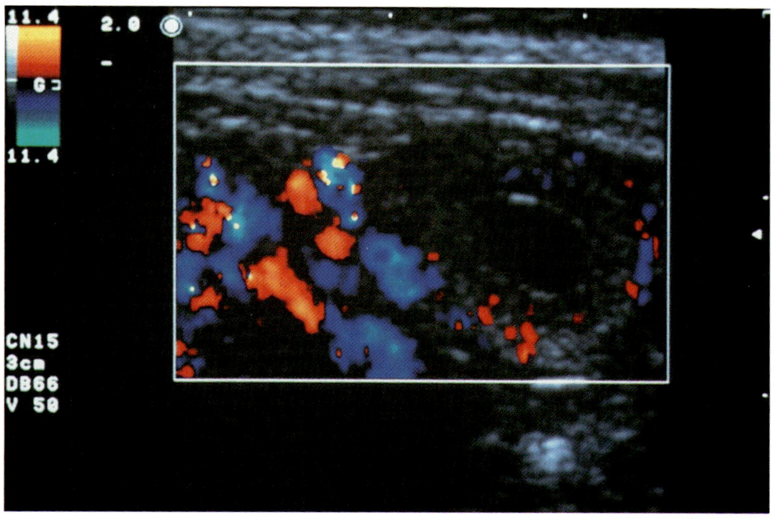

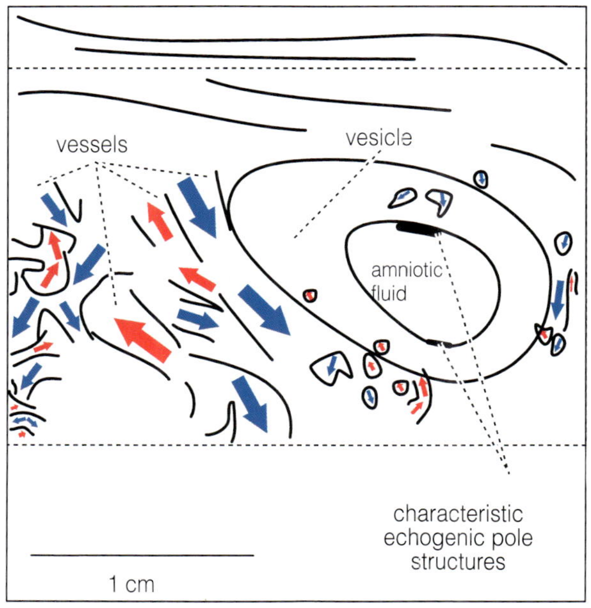

732

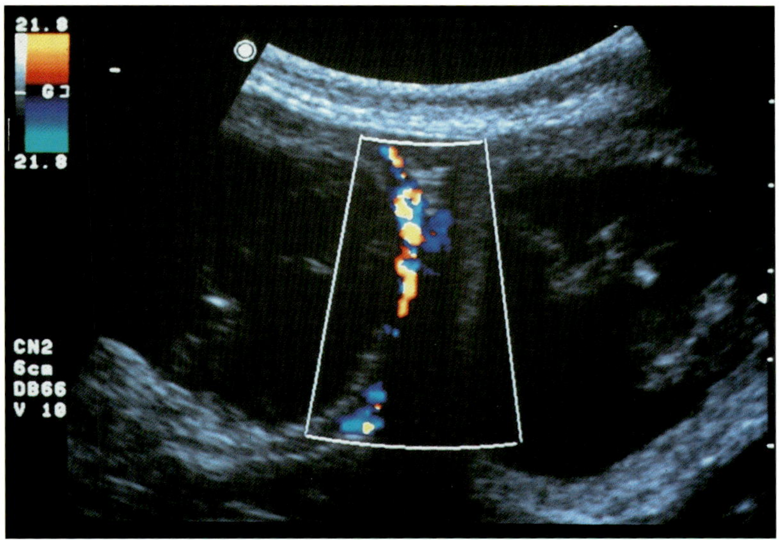

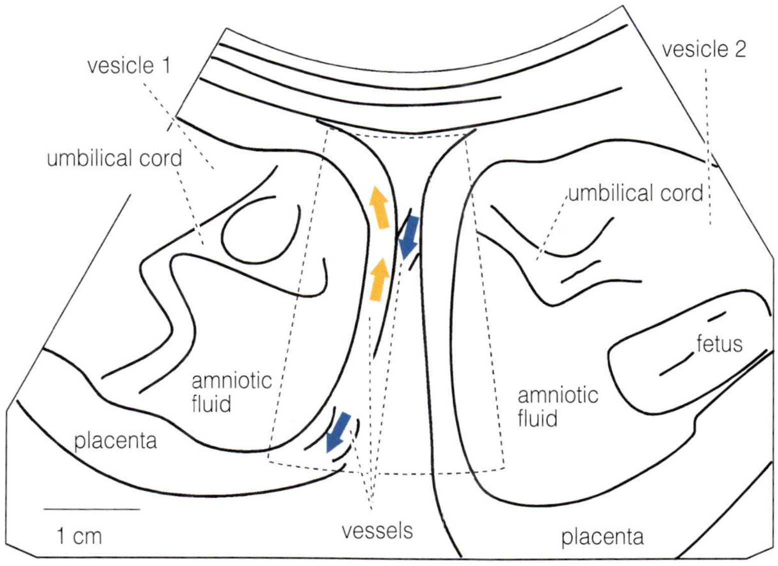

731, 732 Colour-coded Doppler sonograms of arterial blood flow in uterine wall vessels of bitches 18 days (**731**) and 48 days (**732**) post ovulation.

Maternal Vascular Blood Flows

After identifying small arteries of the maternal placenta and/or uterus with colour-coded Doppler, PW Doppler is used to record flow patterns in these vessels (**731, 732**). Characteristic blood flow patterns can already be traced in early pregnancy. These spectrums consist of a relatively fast systolic and a decreasing but forward diastolic blood flow (**732–734**). These characteristic flow tracings are seen throughout pregnancy. During the second half of pregnancy there is an increase in diastolic blood flow volume, i.e. diastolic flow velocity. This is explained by decreased resistance in the vascular bed and is due to an increase in fetal oxygen supply.

Diastolic regurgitation is not found in a normal pregnancy. An uncharacteristic pulsating flow with decreased early-diastolic velocities was found in one bitch shortly before parturition (**735**). A dead puppy was born at term.

Fetal Vascular Blood Flows

Doppler ultrasonography of fetal nutritional status should include the umbilical artery, the aorta, the common carotid artery, the cerebral vessels and the caudal vena cava (**736, 737**).

The umbilical and/or yolk sac artery an be detected 23 days post ovulation in the dog and 21 days post breeding in the cat with colour-coded Doppler ultrasonography. The flow pattern consists of a fast systolic flow with a rounded velocity peak. Diastolic flow is not present. This tracing is characteristic for the first half of pregnancy (**738**). As fetal development progresses, a diastolic flow can be detected, which shows an increase in velocity during the last weeks of pregnancy (**739, 740**).

Fetal blood flow in the aorta is measured at the level of the diaphragm. The fetal aorta also shows a forward diastolic flow. The systolic velocity is greater and shorter than in the umbilical artery (**741, 742**). The slope and peak velocity are determined by cardiac contractions. Diastolic regurgitation is seen towards the end of a normal pregnancy. Diastolic flow increase is not as great as the tracing in the umbilical artery.

The fetal common carotid artery and cerebral vessels show a discrete diastolic flow during the second half of pregnancy.

The caudal vena cava has a biphasic blood flow tracing with end-diastolic regurgitation during atrial contractions (**743A, B**).

Duplex sonography offers a complete evaluation of maternal and fetal vessels and their development. Blood flow tracings in conventional PW Doppler sonography are characteristic of certain vessels and development stages. They are similar to flow patterns found in human medicine. Abnormal flow tracings are indicative of a pathological pregnancy.

733

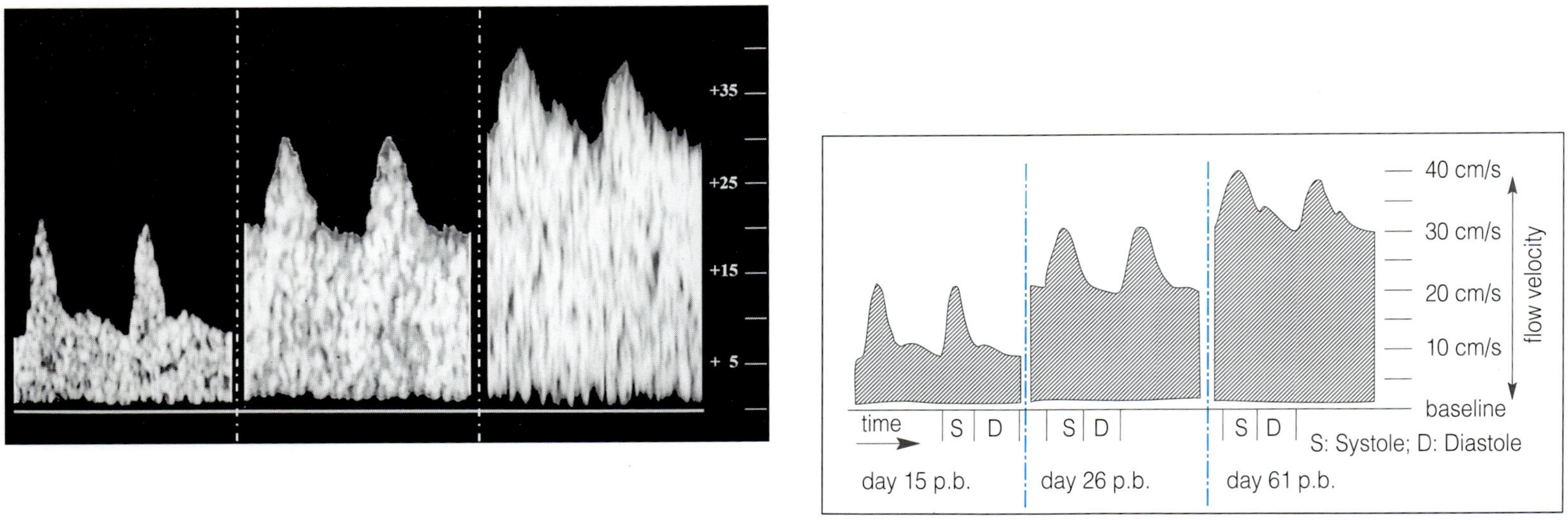

734

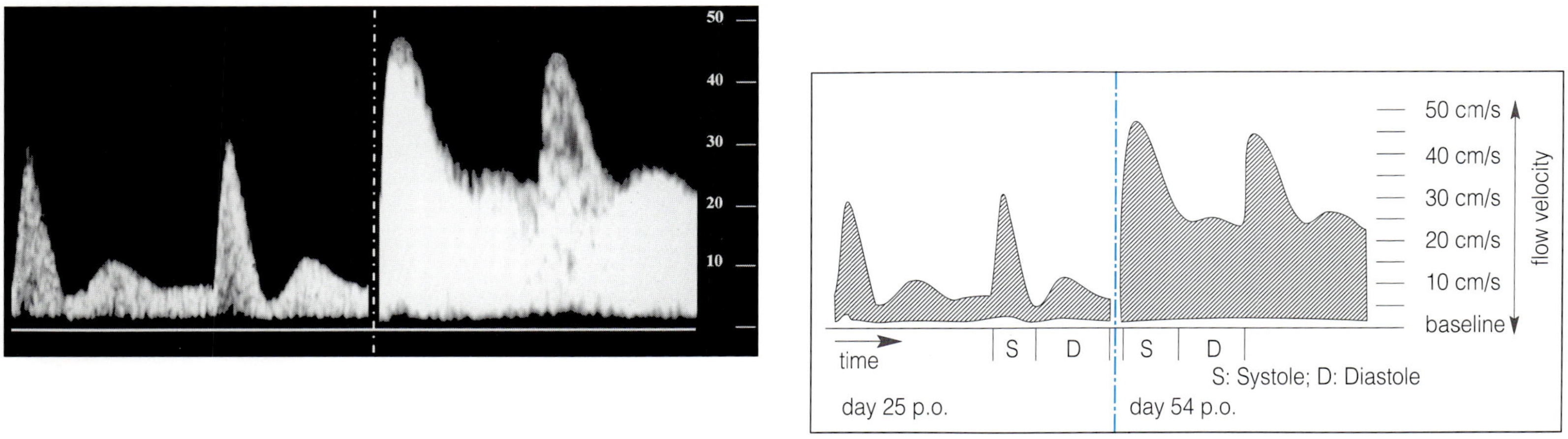

733, 734 Pulsed-wave Doppler sonograms of blood flow in uterine vessels of a cat (**733**) and a dog (**734**). Velocity increases as the pregnancy progresses.

735

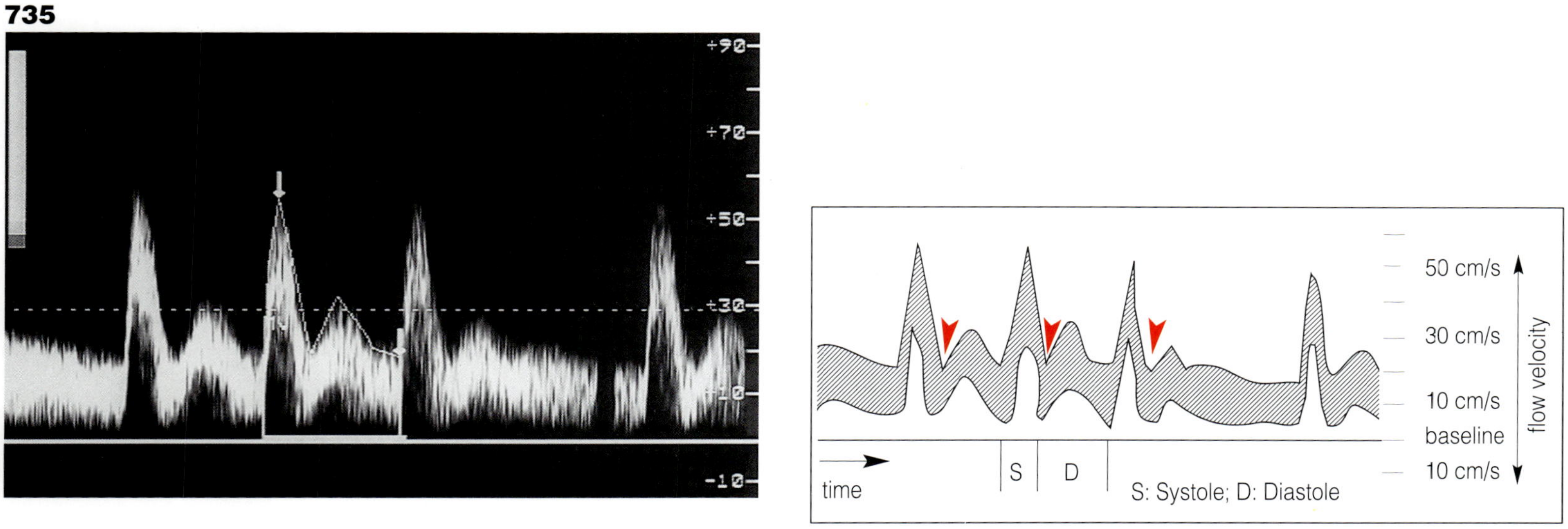

735 Blood flow measured in a uterine vessel with PW Doppler sonography of a bitch on day 58 post ovulation. The red arrow head in the diagram marks the abnormal early-diastolic velocity decrease.

736

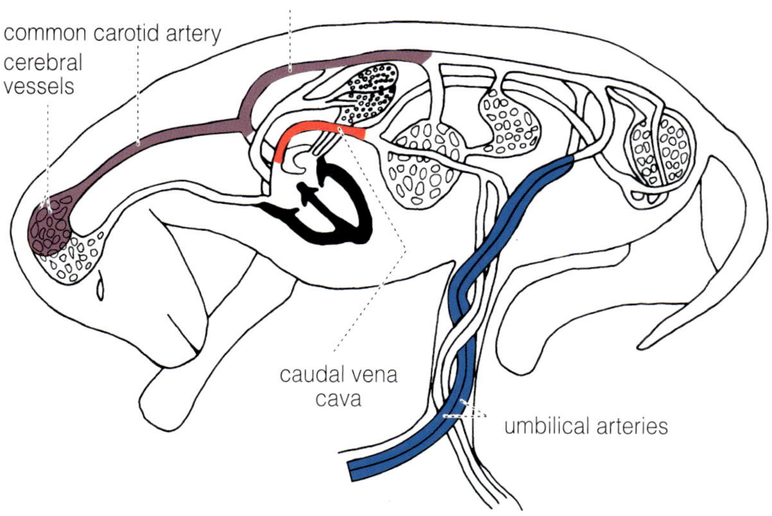

737

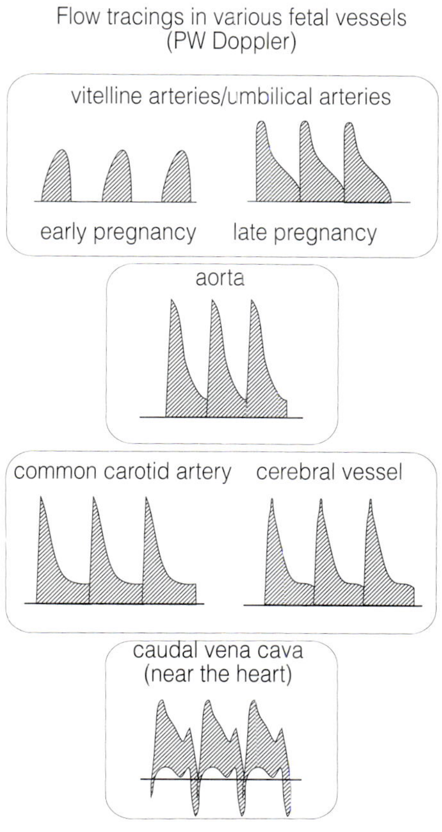

736, 737 Schematic drawing of relevant fetal vessels (**736**) and concurrent flow tracings in duplex ultrasonography (**737**).

738–740 Colour coded (**738**) and PW Doppler (**739**) echograms of the umbilical arteries and veins in a dog 36 days post ovulation (**738**) as well as at various development stages (**739**). PW Doppler echograms of arterial and venous blood flow in feline umbilical vessels (**740**, overleaf). Velocity increases are clearly noticable.

738

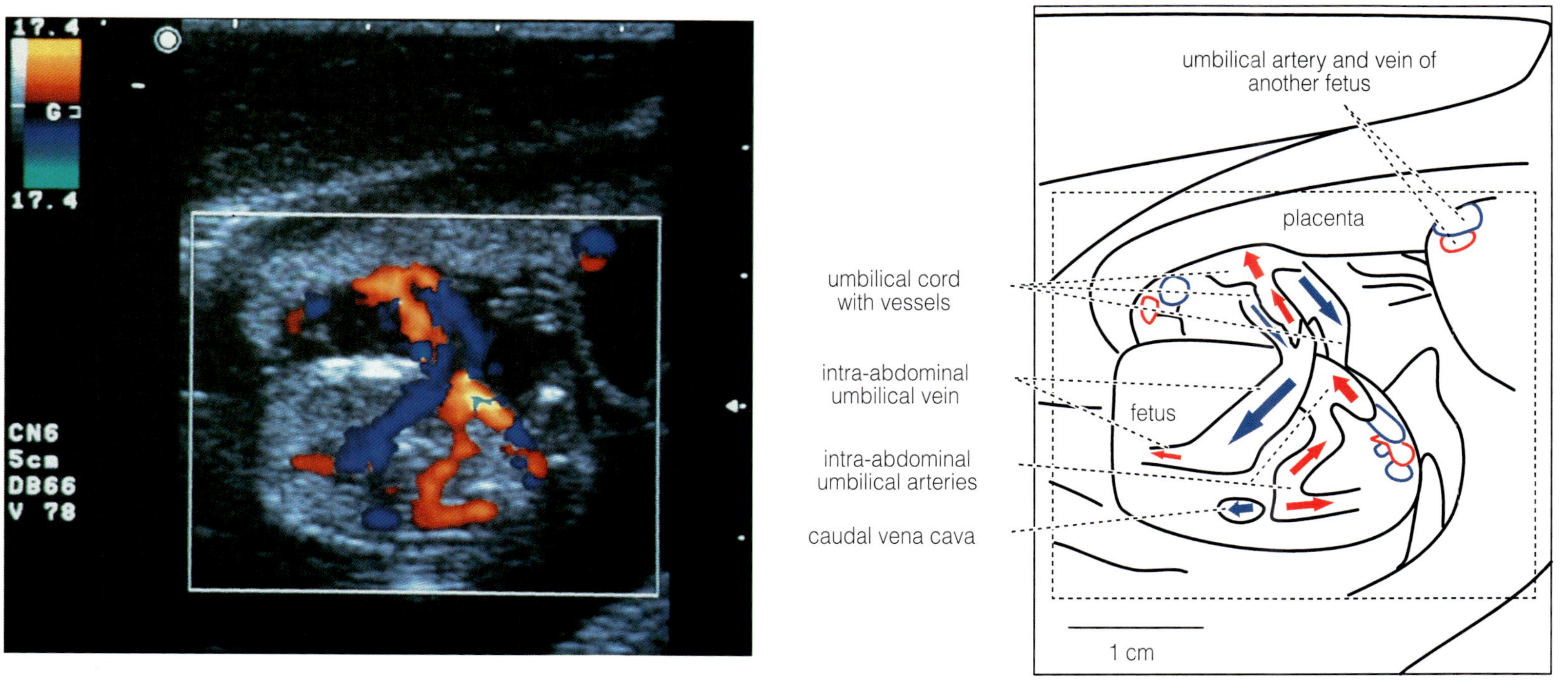

739

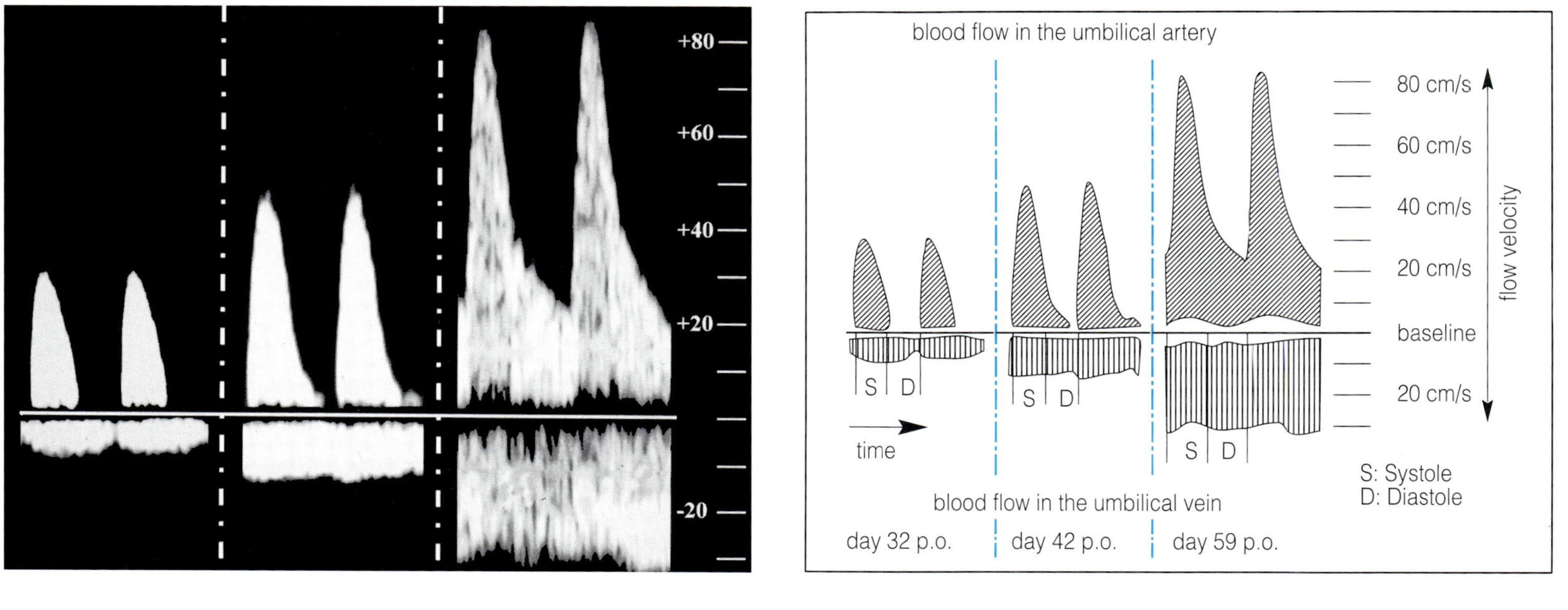

740

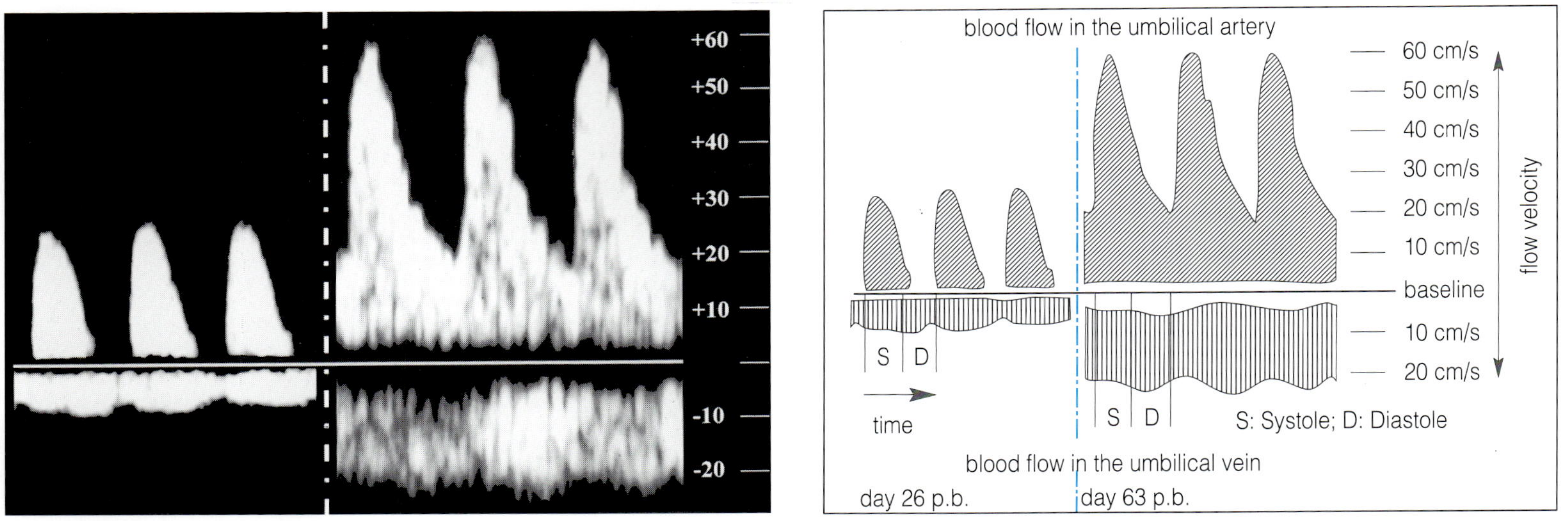

740 PW Doppler echograms of arterial and venous blood flow in feline umbilical vessels (see also **738, 739**). Velocity increases are clearly noticable.

741

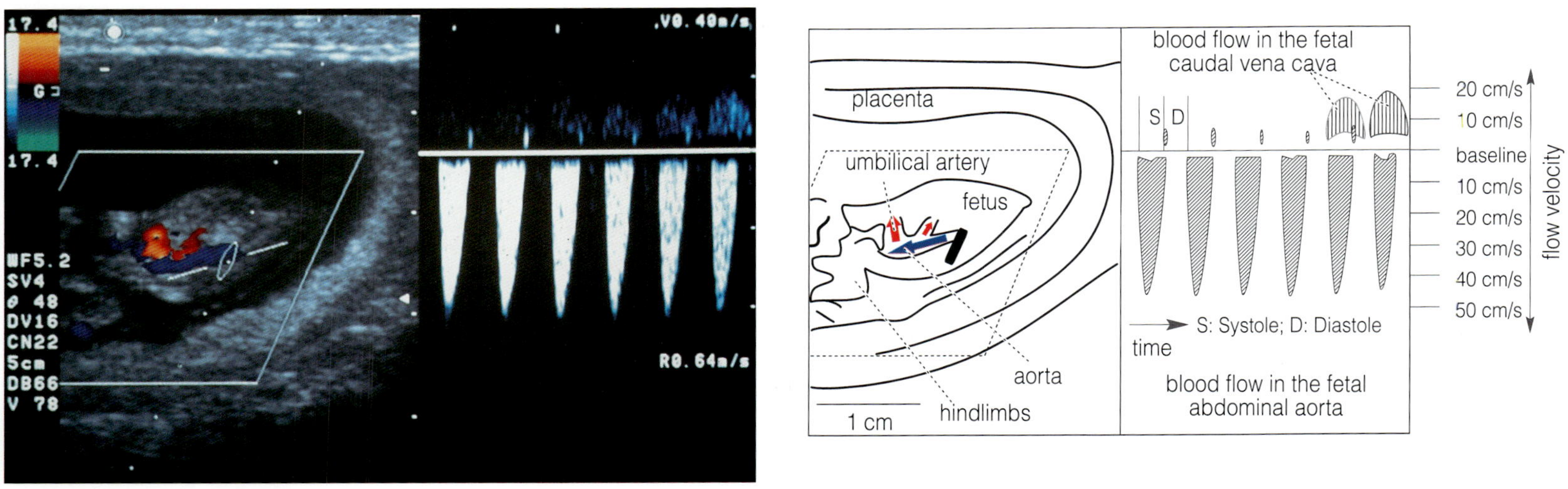

742

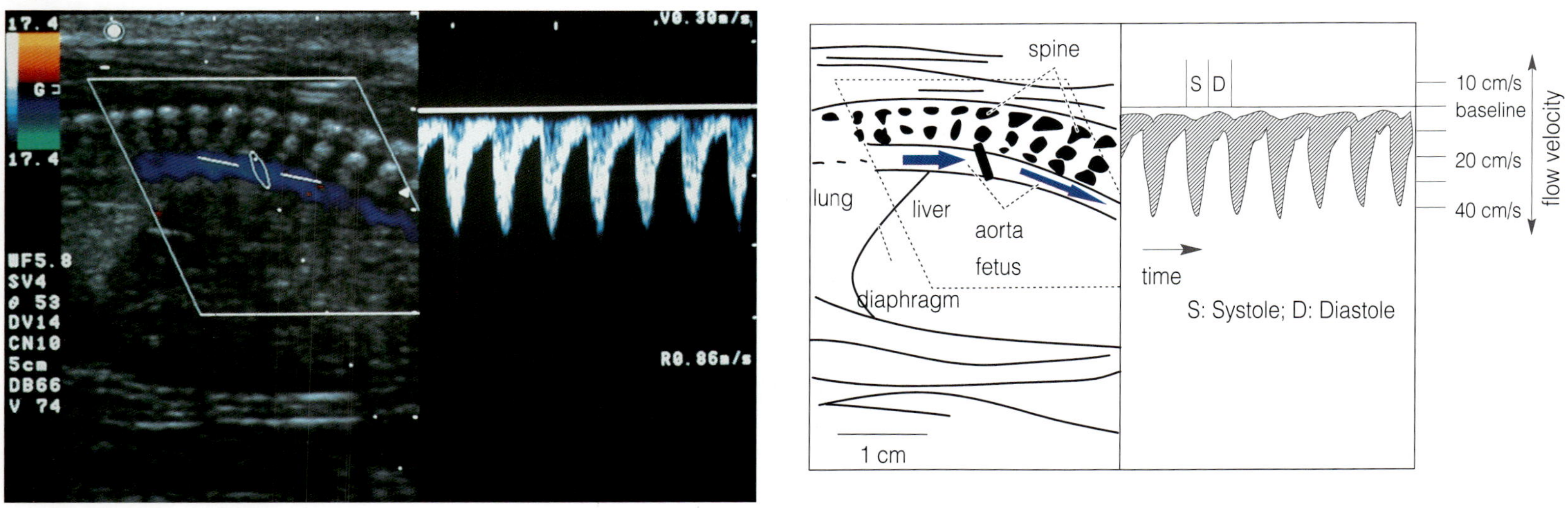

741, 742 Colour-coded and PW Doppler ultrasonography of blood flow in the fetal aorta of dog fetuses 34 days (**741**) and 52 days (**742**) post ovulation.

743

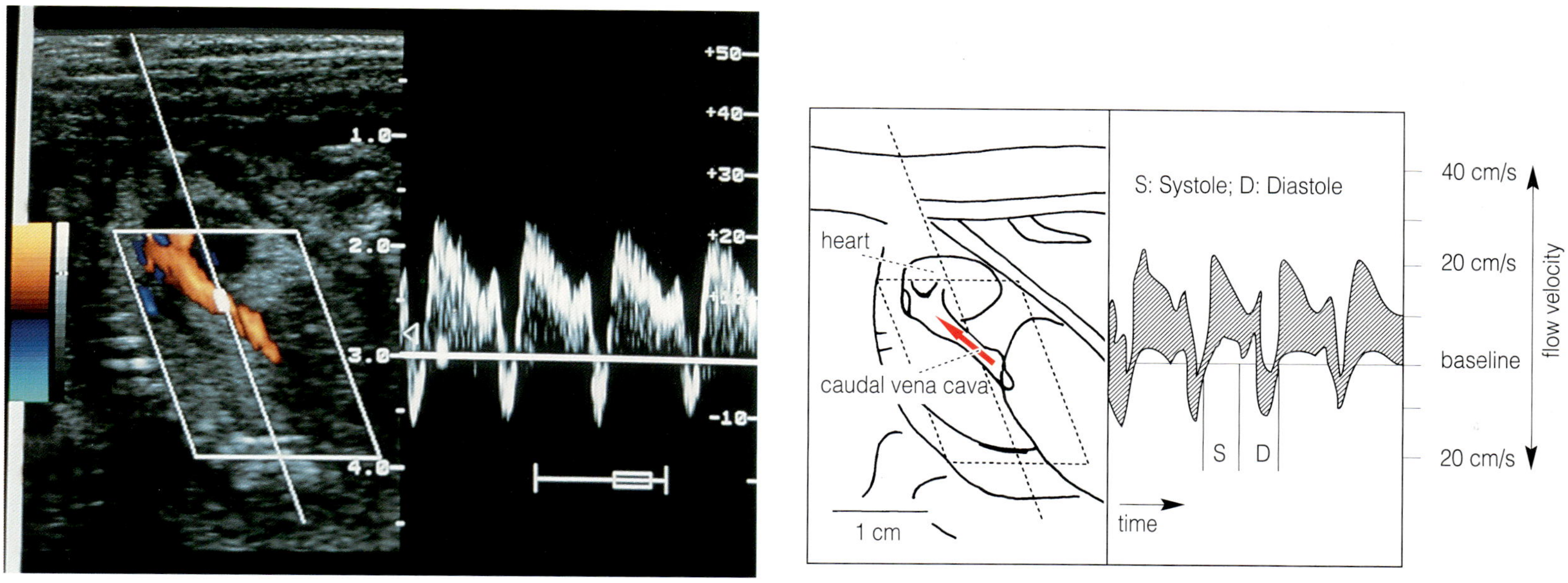

743 Colour-coded and PW Doppler ultrasonography of blood flow in the fetal caudal vena cava of a cat fetus 53 days post breeding.

744

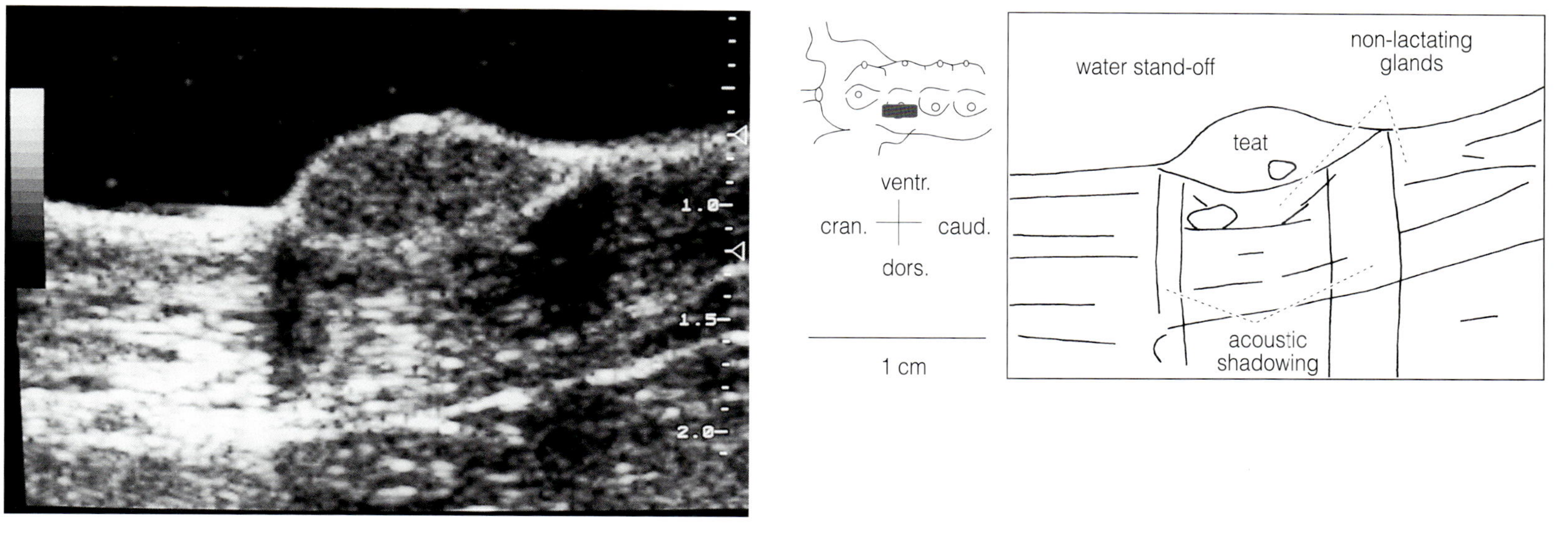

745

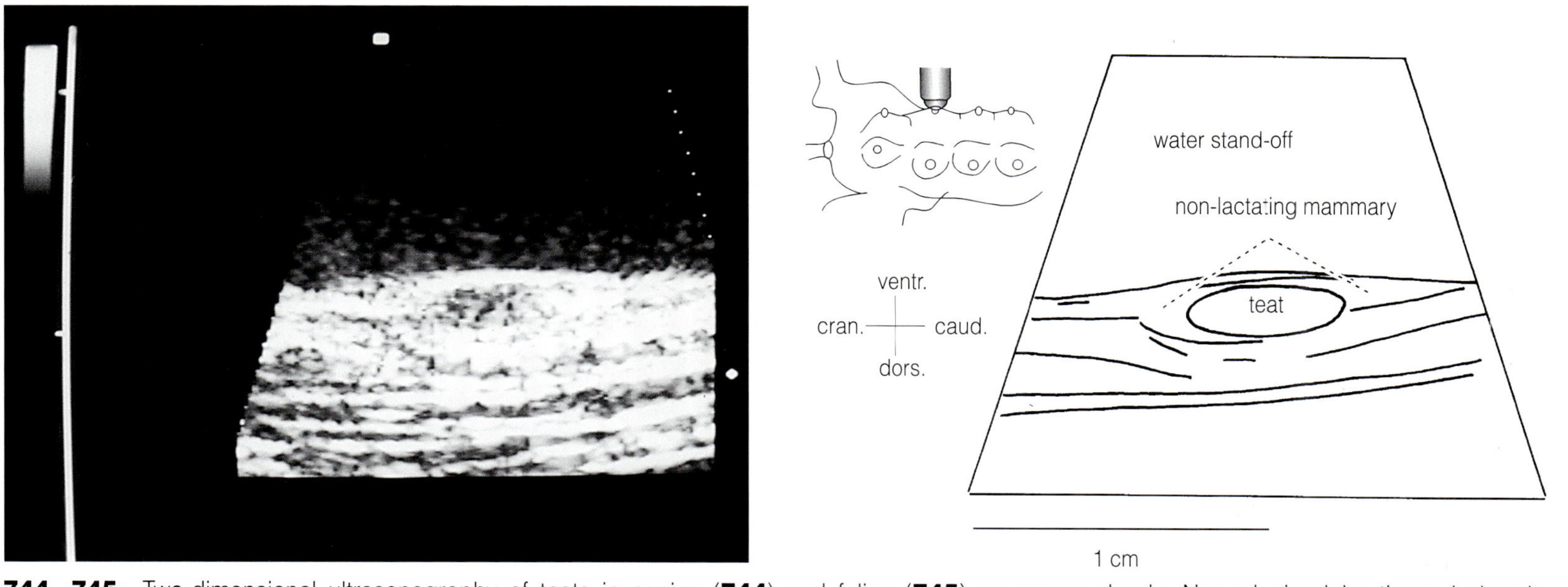

744, 745 Two-dimensional ultrasonography of teats in canine (**744**) and feline (**745**) mammary glands. Normal glandular tissue is barely recognizable.

746

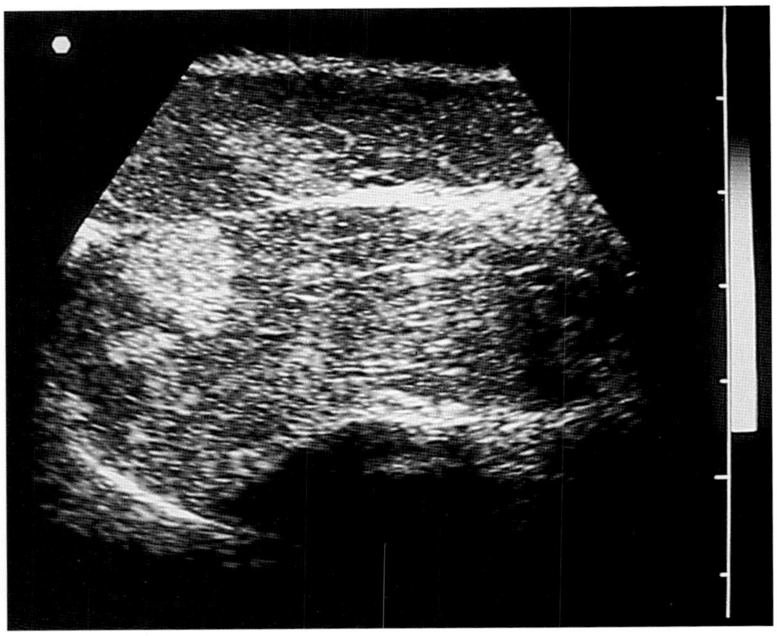

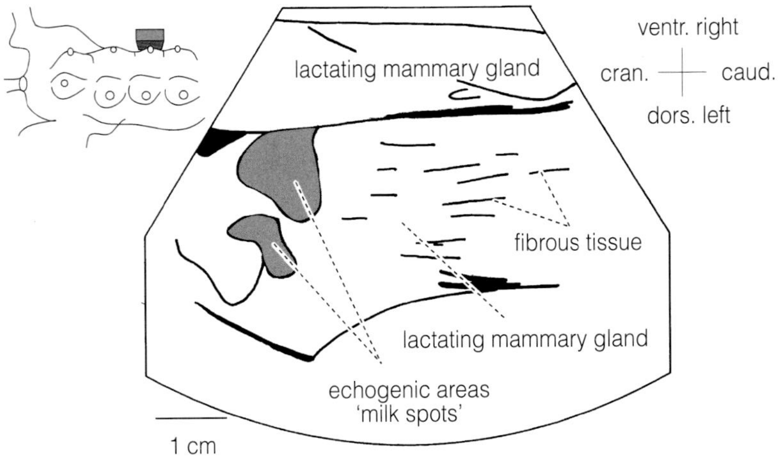

747

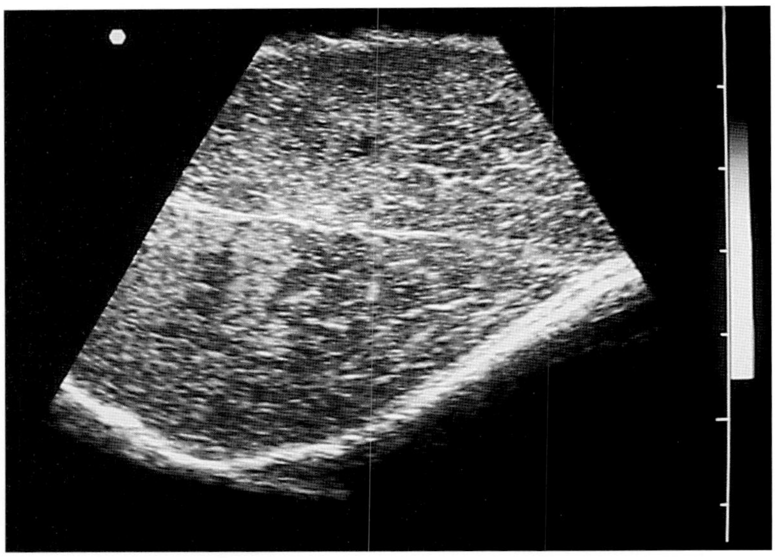

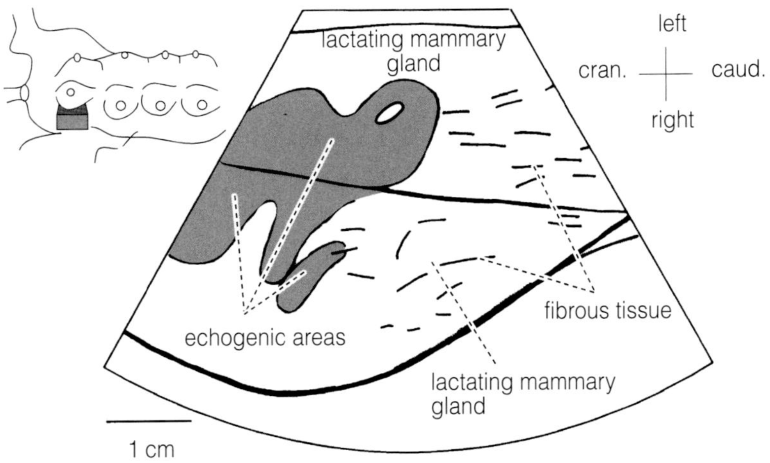

746, 747 Two-dimensional ultrasonography of two adjacent, lactating mammary glands with hyperechoic 'milk spots' (**746**) and suspensory fibrous tissue (**747**).

Mammary Glands

Cordula Poulsen Nautrup

Instrumentation and Examination Technique

Ultrasonography of the mammary glands is only possible with high-frequency transducers of at least 7.5 MHz. 10–15 MHz transducers are generally more suitable. Small linear scanners or sector scanners with built-in or adaptable stand-off pads are required to visualize the superficial mammary glands and to assure good resolution in the near field. Stand-off pads are useful to compensate for any irregularities caused by protruding teats or the uneven gland surface.

The hair covering the mammary glands should be clipped liberally and acoustic coupling gel should be applied to the skin and the transducer surface.

Normal Sonographic Findings

The non-lactating, normal mammary gland is sonographically not very impressive. The glandular tissue is homogenous with a fine texture of medium to low echogenicity. The teat is regular and moderately echogenic and shows edge shadowing (744, 745). Intraparenchymatous vessels, excretory ducts and gland, as well as teat cisterns, cannot be differentiated sonographically.

Glandular tissue shows medium echogenicity in the larger, lac-

748

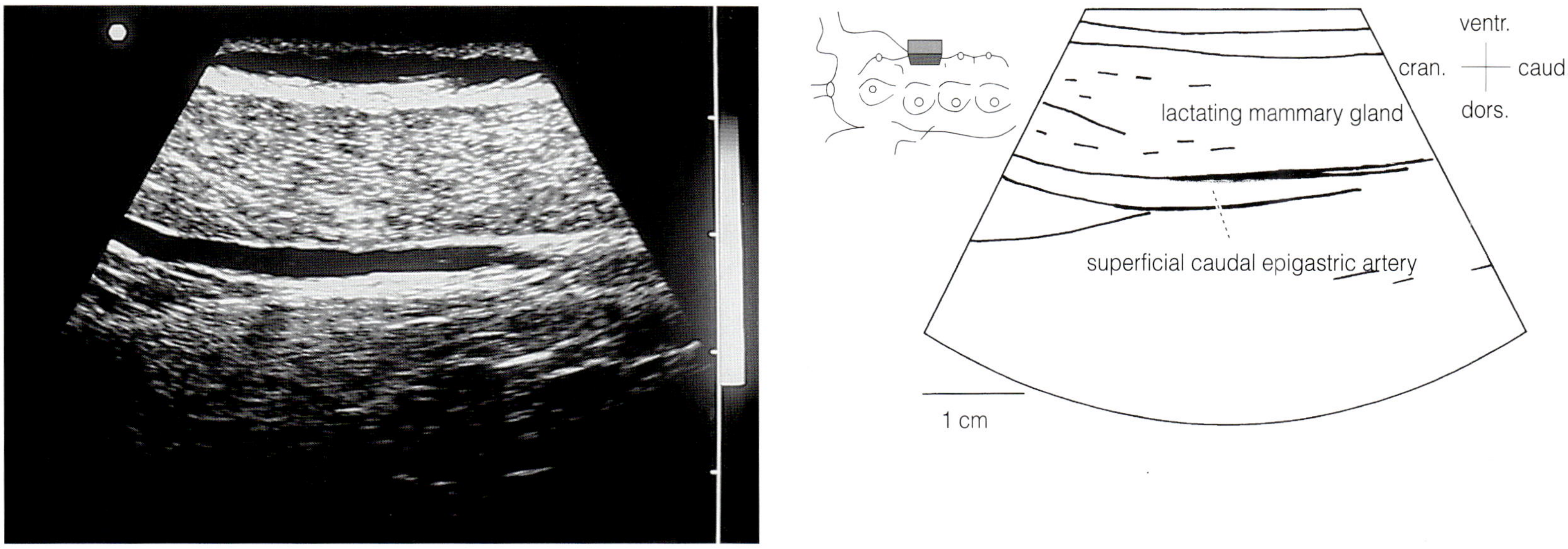

749

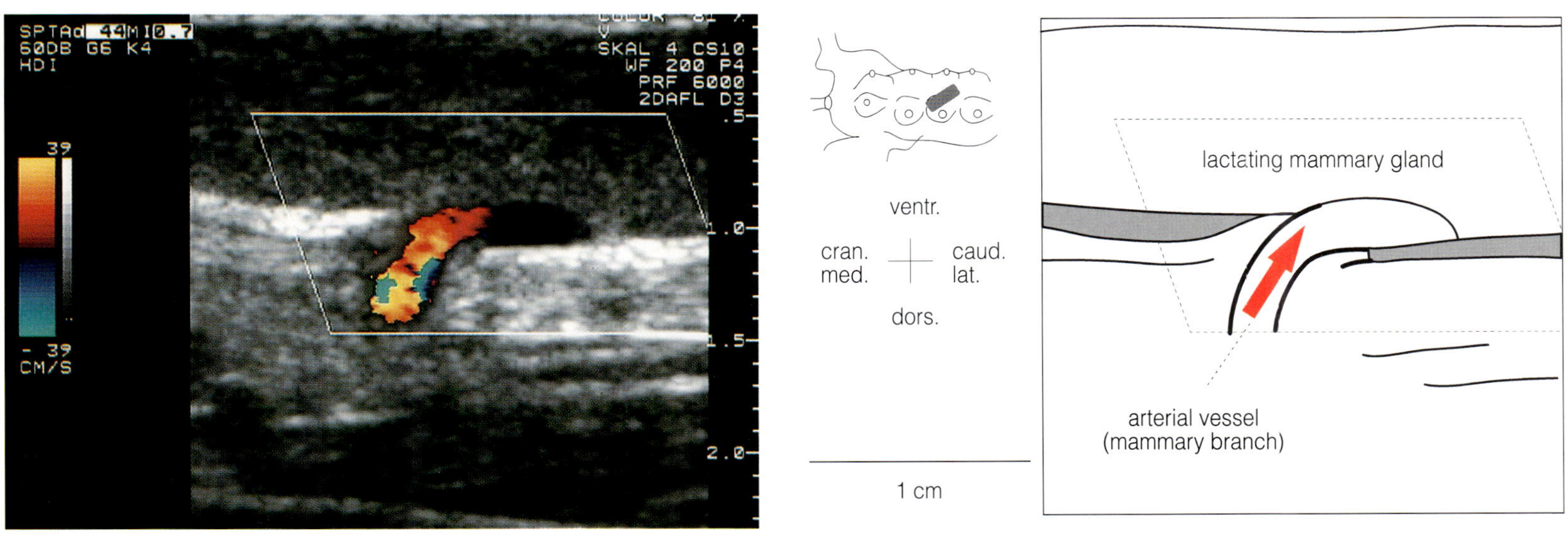

748, 749 Two-dimensional sonogram (**748**) and colour Doppler echogram (**749**) of lactating mammary glands with the deep superficial caudal epigastric artery (**748**) and large vessels entering the gland (**749**).

tating mammary gland. Characteristic echogenic areas of different shapes ('milk spots') are visible in the tissue (746). Suspensory fibrous tissue in the individual mammary glands is seen only with lactating mammary glands in the shape of thin echogenic stripes (747). Vessel branches in the mammary gland are clearly visible in the two-dimensional ultrasonogram (748) and with colour-coded Doppler (749). The epigastric arteries and veins can be identified deeper in the gland as longitudinal, anechoic, pulsating or non-pulsating structures (748).

Ultrasonography of Mammary Gland Lesions

Indications for ultrasonography of the mammary gland are follow-up examinations and treatment checks, when direct surgical intervention is not necessary or has been refused by the patient's owner. The mammary gland should also be scanned when drug treatment is ineffective.

In 1996 there were no statistical results for mammary gland diagnostics and the consequences that might follow. Sonographic findings, especially neoplastic lesions, can only be evaluted in conjunction with history and palpation. Ultrasonography can be used to follow-up false pregnancy or other hormonal dysfunctions, mastitis, abscesses, cystic lesions and, to some extent, mammary tumours.

In human medicine, ultrasonography and Doppler echography are used to ascertain, differentiate and evaluate almost all focal mammary lesions[7, 9, 39]. The malignancy of some mammary tumours are sometimes evaluated ultrasonographically[4, 8, 12, 40, 43, 51, 52].

The enlarged mammary gland during false pregnancy shows areas of higher and lower echogenicity. The sonogram is similar to

750

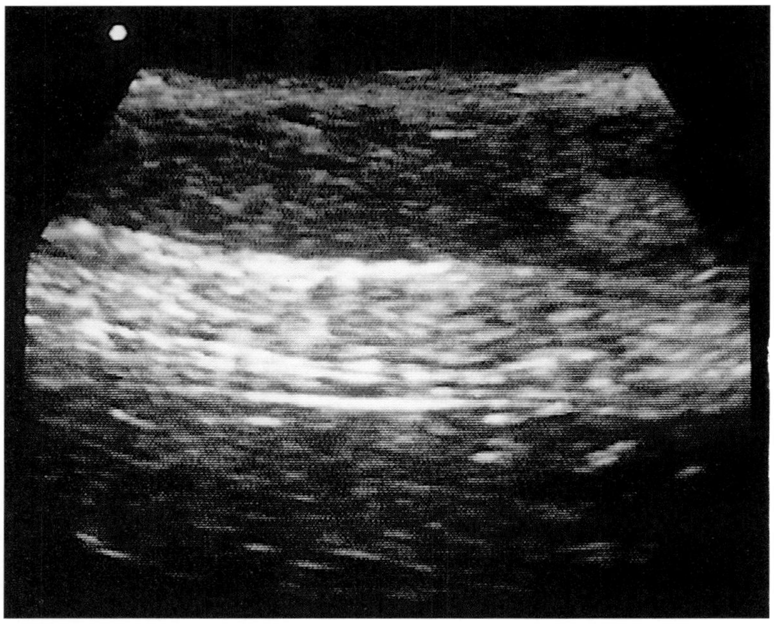

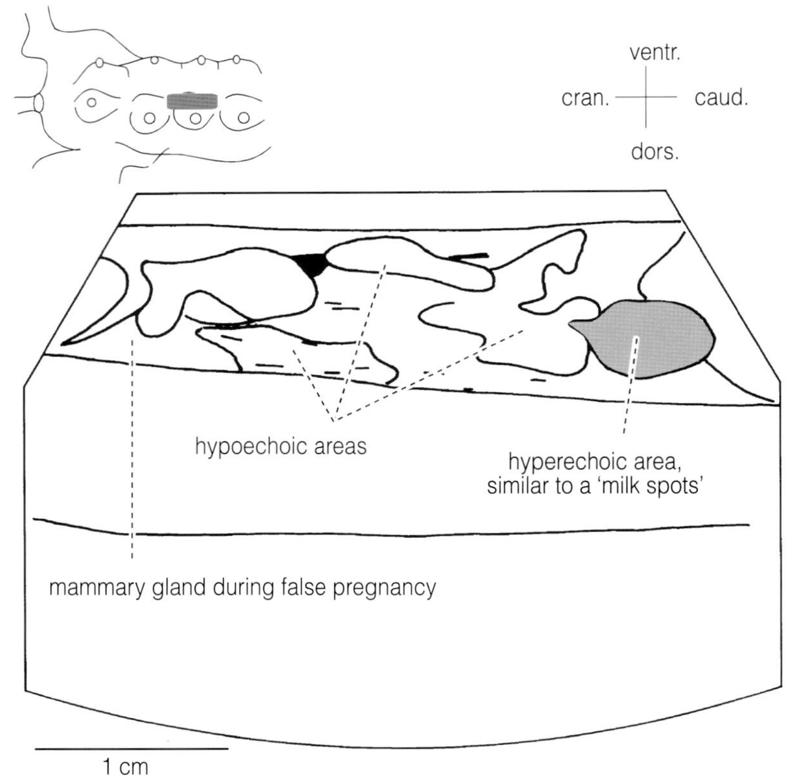

750 Two-dimensional sonogram of a bitch with a false pregnancy. Echogenic 'milk spots' are seen in the hypoechoic glandular tissue.

751

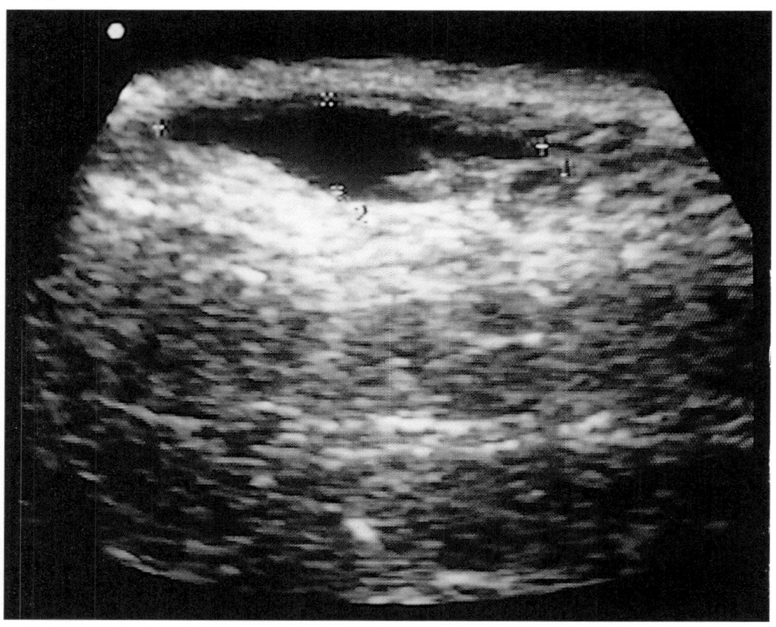

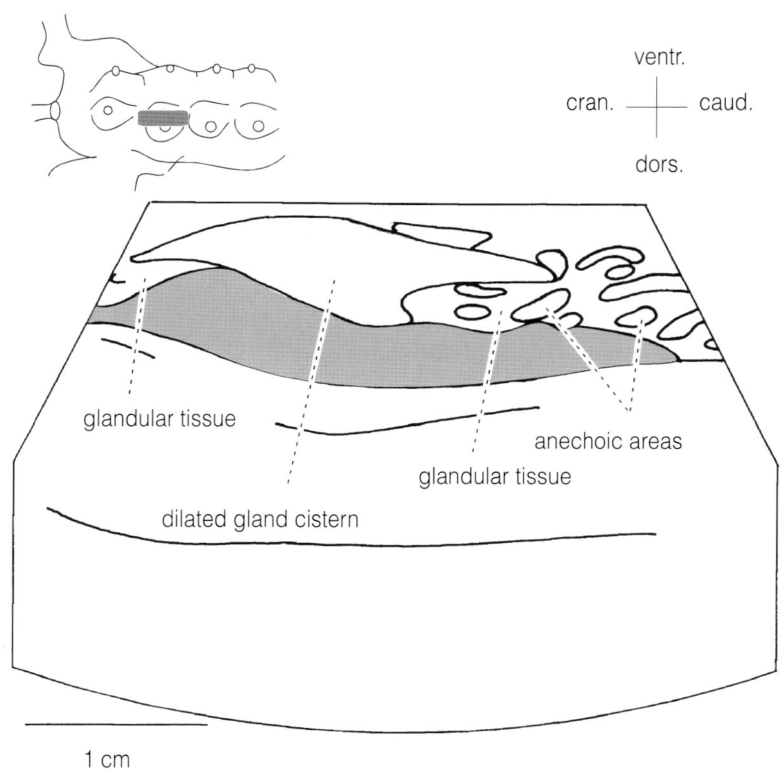

751 Two-dimensional sonogram of a six-month-old bitch with false pregnancy symptoms. Dilated, anechoic gland cisterns are visible (see also **752**).

that of a lactating mammary gland, but more hypoechoic (**750**). Anechoic, fluid-filled cavities are visible in the glands. Young bitches with hormonal dysfunctions show similar symptoms. The enlarged gland contains numerous, anechoic, fluid-filled cavities of varying size, representing the excretory ducts and the gland cisterns (**751, 752**).

Mammary gland cysts are anechoic, well-demarcated and occasionally divided by echogenic septa.

With mastitis, the gland appears non-homogenous and hypoechoic to hyperechoic, similar to a lactating mammary gland.

Mammary gland tumours show varying shapes and sonographic images (**753–757**). They range from hypoechoic to hyperechoic, and homogenous to non-nhomogenous. Echogenic, round calcified lesions with distal acoustic shadowing can be seen, as well as anechoic cavities containing secretions or necrotic tissue. Tumours may or may not be differentiatiated from normal gland tissue. Evaluation of tumour malignancy or growth is not possible with ultrasonography alone.

752

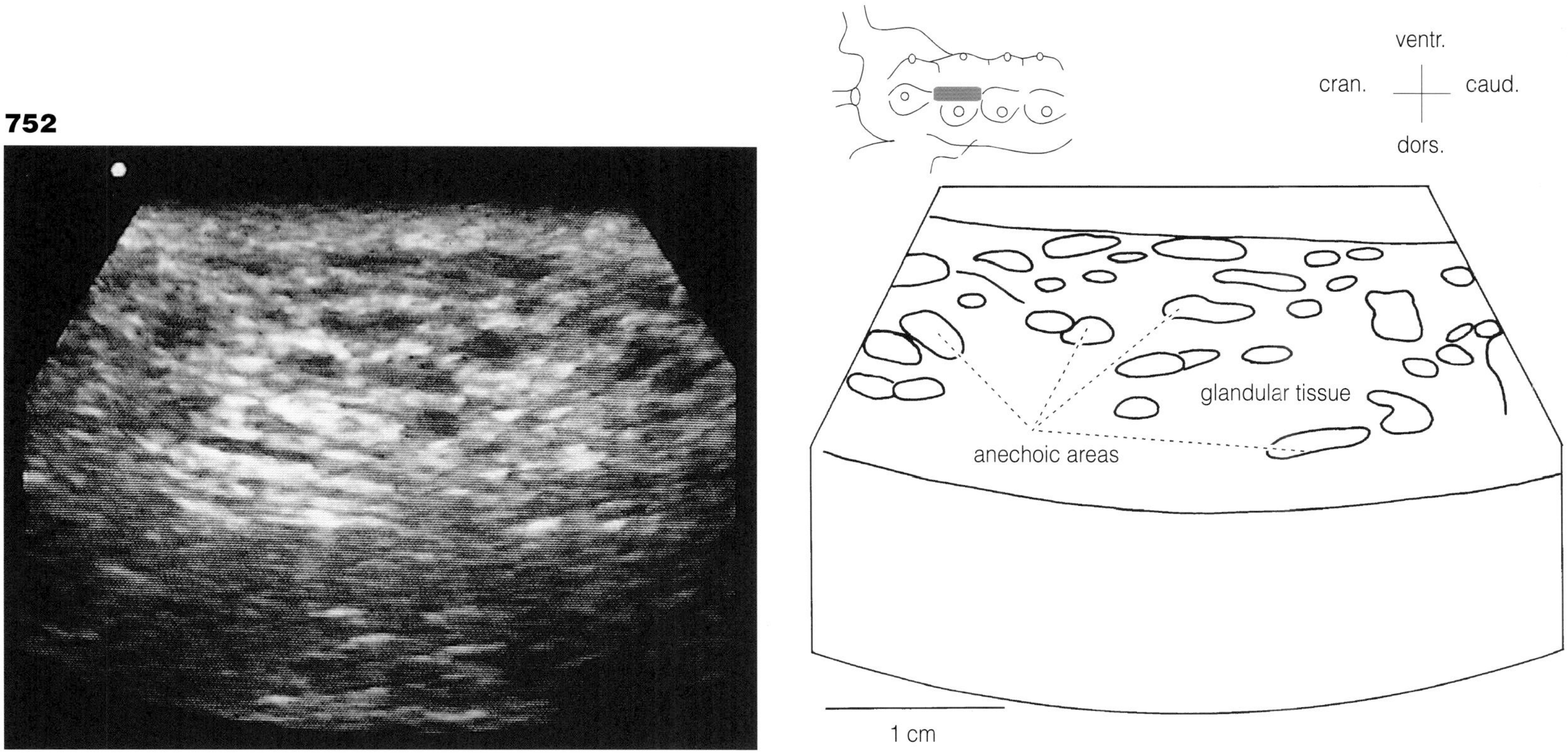

752 Two-dimensional sonogram of a six-month-old bitch with false pregnancy symptoms. Anechoic excretory ducts are visible (see also **751**).

753

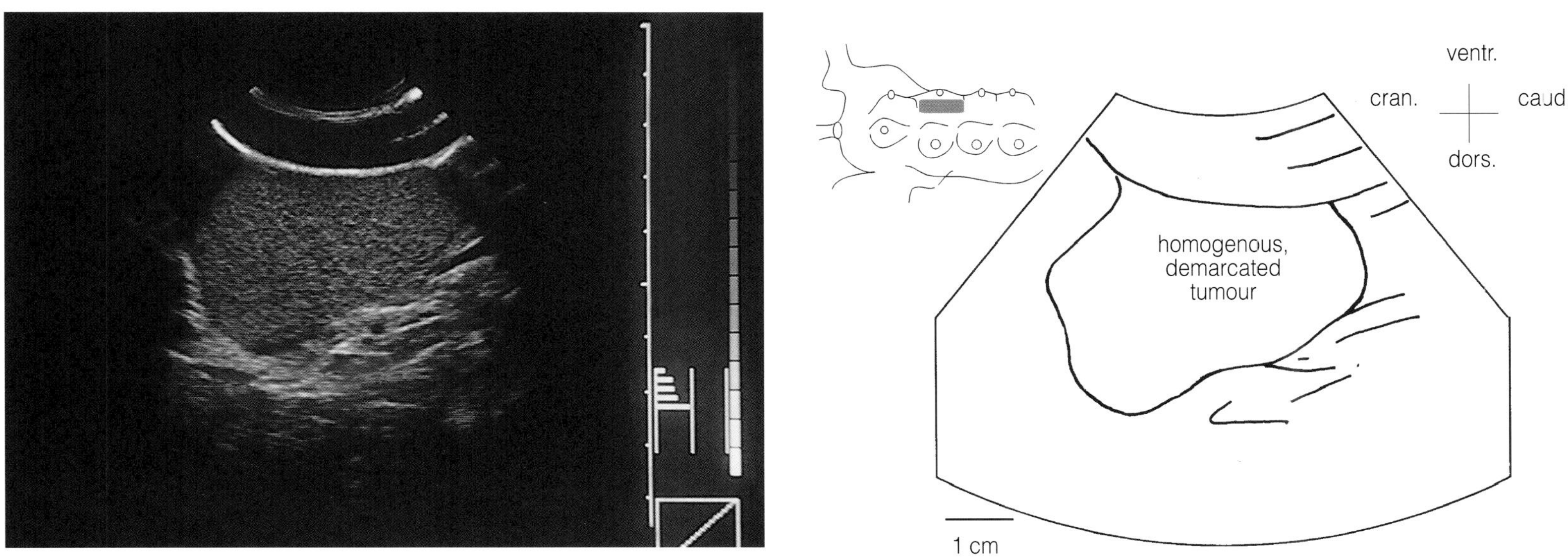

754

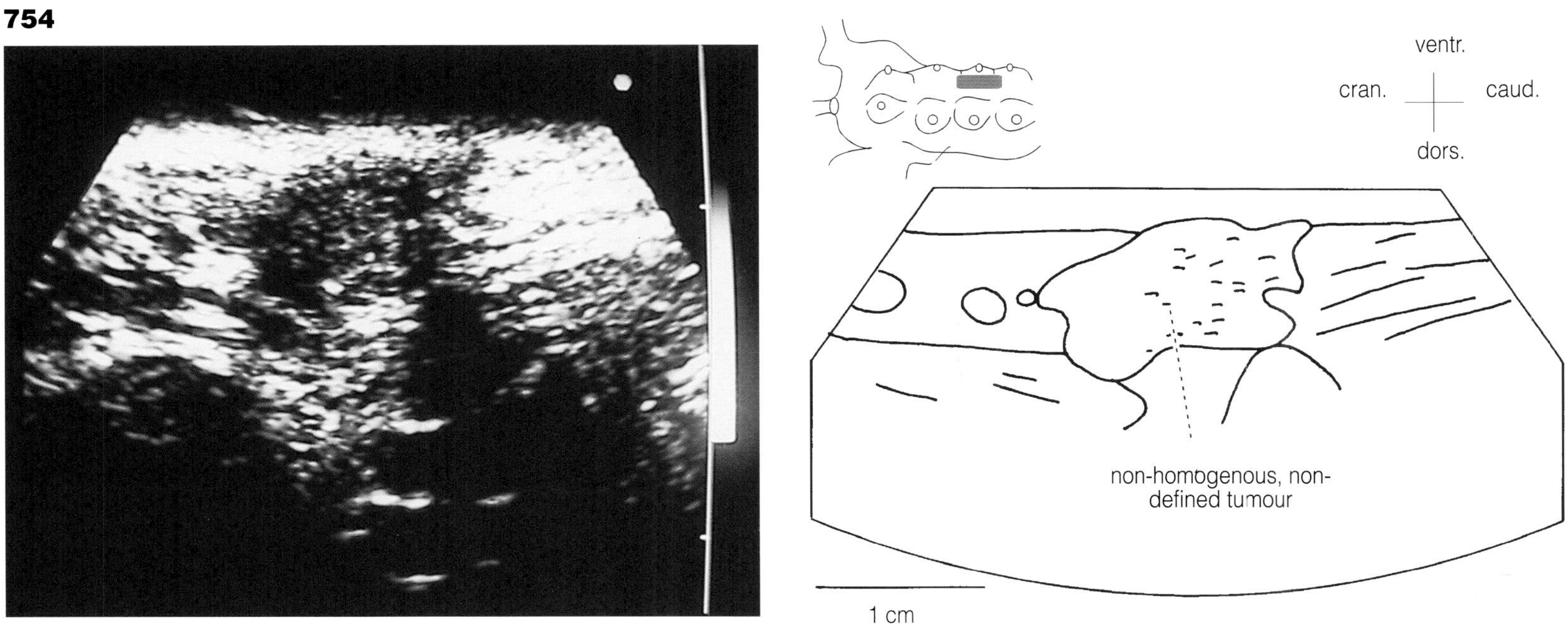

753, 754 Two-dimensional sonograms of a homogenous, demarcated (**753**) and a non-homogenous, non-defined (**754**) mammary gland carcinoma in two dogs.

755

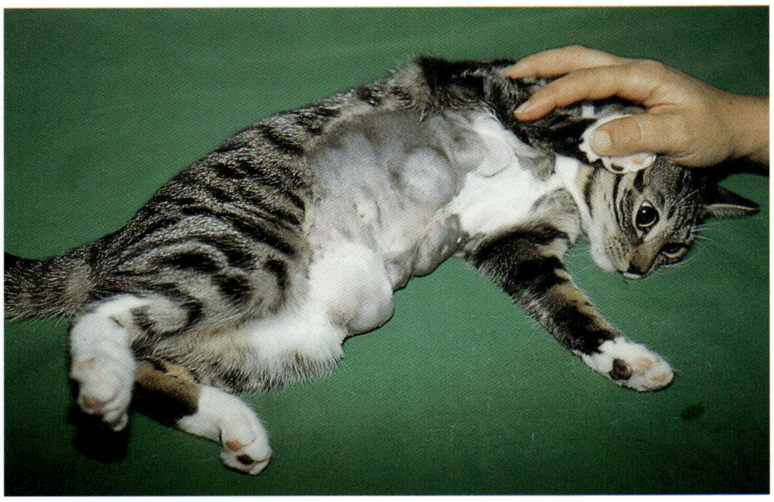

756

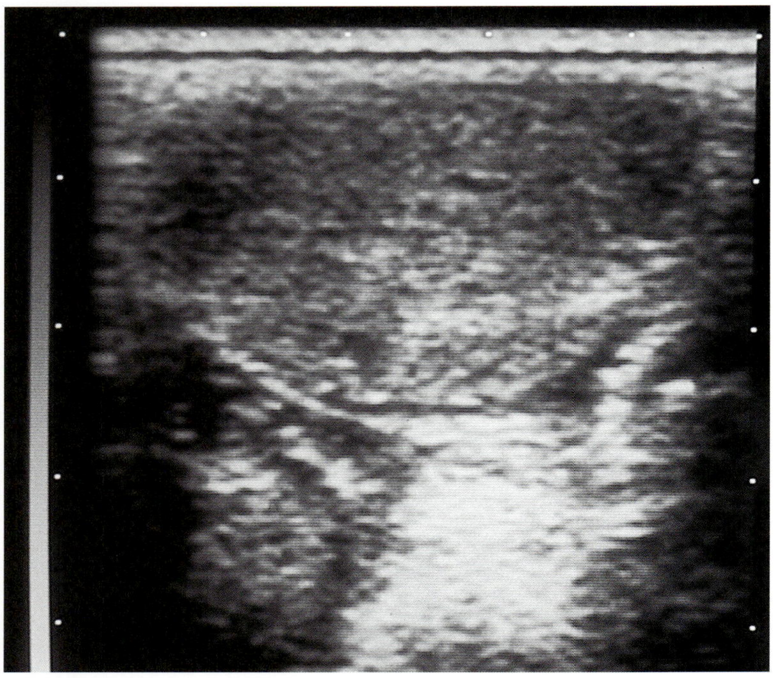

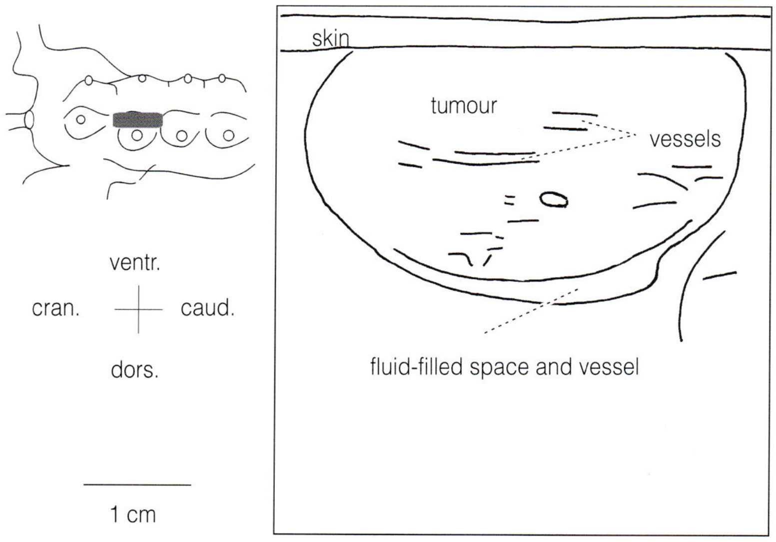

757

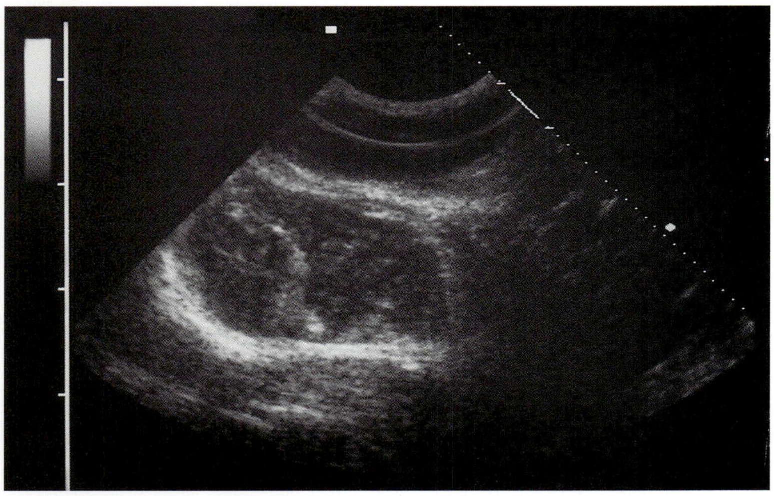

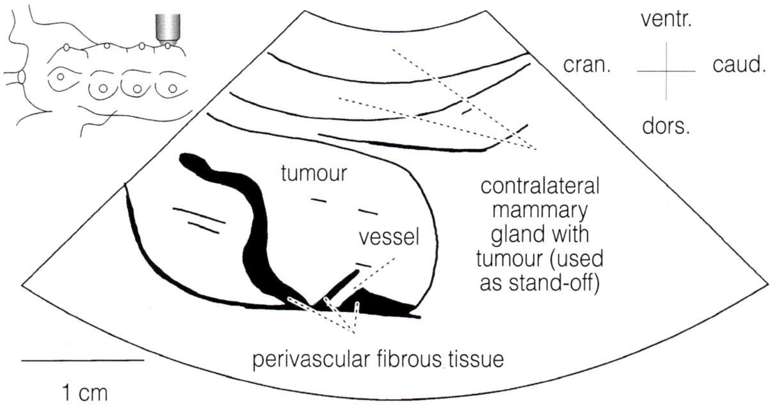

755–757 Photo (**755**) and sonograms (**756, 757**) of a feline mammary gland with a benign tumour (histopathology: fibroepithelial hyperplasia; see also Maehler *et al.*, 1994[41]). Photo (**755**) of the enlarged mammary glands. Sonograms of a well-demarcated, plum-sized homogenous mass (**756**) and a mass with hyperechoic perivascular fibrous tissue masses (**757**).

References

1 Al-Bassam MA, Thompson RG and O'Donnell L (1981) Normal postpartum involution of the uterus in the dog. *Can. J. Comp. Med. Vet. Sci.* **45**, 217–221.

2 Arabin B, Hansmann M and Weitzel HK (1992) Zerebrales Blutflußprofil beim Fetus. *Gynäkologe* **25**, 324–331.

3 Arbeille P, Fignon A, Bosc M and Bodart S (1994) Modifications des circulations utéro-placentaire et cérébrale foetales induites par la nicotine chez le foetus ovin. *J. Gynecol. Obstet. Biol. Réprod. Paris* **23**, 51–56.

4 Bade W, Bomer S, Otto WR, Degenhardt F and Schneider J (1994) Texturanalyse: ein neues Verfahren zur Beurteilung sonographisch darstellbarer Herdbefande der Mamma. *Bildgebung* **61**, 284–290.

5 Barr F J. (1988a) Pregnancy diagnosis and assessment of fetal viability in the dog: a review. *J. Small Anim.Pract.* **29**, 647–656.

6 Barr FJ (1988b) Diagnostic ultrasound in small animals. *In Practice* **Jan. 1988**, 17–25.

7 Blohmer JU, Bollmann R, Chaoui R, Kürten A and Lau HU (1994) Die Mastitis nonpuerperalis in der Real-time and Farbdoppler-Sonographie. *Geburtshilfe Frauenheilkd.* **54**, 161–166.

8 Blohmer JU, Chaoui R, Schmalisch G, Bollmann R and Lau HU (1995) Die Differentialdiagnose von Mammatumoren durch den Vergleich der Durchblutung des Tumors mit der kontralateralen Brust mittels farbkodierter, gepulster Dopplersonographie. *Geburtshilfe Frauenheilkd.* **55**, 1–6.

9 Boisserie-Lacroix M, Lafitte JJ, Sirben C, Latrabe V, Grelet P, Zeinoun R and Brun G (1993) Les lesions inflammatoires et infectieuses du sein. Contribution de l'échographie. *J. Chir. Paris* **130**, 408–415.

10 Bondestam S, Alitalo I and Kärkkäinen M (1983) Real-time ultrasound pregnancy diagnosis in the bitch. *J. Small Anim.Pract.* **24**, 145–151.

11 Bondestam S, Kärkkäinen M, Alitalo I and Forss M (1984) Evaluating the accuracy of canine pregnancy diagnosis and litter size determination using real-time ultrasound. *Acta Vet. Scand.* **25**, 327–332.

12 Brombart JC (1995) Echographie mammaire. *J. Belge. Radiol.* **78**, 34–38.

13 Cartee RE and Rowles T (1984) Preliminary study of the ultrasonographic diagnosis of pregnancy and fetal development in the dog. *Am. J. Vet. Res.* **45**, 1259–1265.

14 Concannon PW, Whaley S, Lein D and Wissler R (1983) Canine gestation length: variation related to time of mating and fertile life of sperm. *Am. J. Vet. Res.* **44**, 1819–1821.

15 Concannon PW, McCann JP and Temple M (1989) Biology and endocrinology of ovulation, pregnancy and parturition in the dog. *J. Reprod. Fert.* **Suppl. 39**, 3–25.

16 Davidson AP, Nyland TG and Tsutsui T (1986) Pregnancy diagnosis with ultrasound in the domestic cat. *Vet. Radiol.* **27**, 109–114.

17 Deutinger J (1992) Physiologie des Doppler-Flusses in maternalen Gefäßen während der Schwangerschaft. *Gynäkologe* **25**, 284–291.

18 Doak RL, Hall A and Dale HE (1967) Longevity of spermatozoa in the reproductive tract of the bitch. *J. Reprod. Fert.* **13**, 51–58.

19 England GCW (1993) Ultrasonographic imaging of spontaneous embryonic resorption in the bitch. *J. Reprod. Fert.* **Suppl. 47**, 552.

20 England GCW and Allen WE (1990) Studies on canine pregnancy using B-mode ultrasound: diagnosis of early pregnancy and the number of conceptuses. *J. Small Anim.Pract.* **31**, 321–323.

21 England GCW, Allen WE and Porte DJ (1990) Studies on canine pregnancy using B-mode ultrasound: development of the conceptus and determination of gestational age. *J. Small Anim.Pract.* **31**, 324–329.

22 England GCW and Yeager AE (1993) Ultrasonographic appearance of the ovary and uterus of the bitch during oestrus, ovulation and early pregnancy. *J. Reprod. Fert.* **Suppl. 47**, 107–117.

23 Feldman EC and Nelson RW (1987) *Canine and Feline Endocrinology and Reproduction*. WB Saunders, Philadelphia.

24 Flückiger M, Kramers P, Hirt U, Huter-Wissler K and Arnold S (1988) Früherfassung der Trächtigkeit bei der Hündin mittels Ultraschall. *J. Vet. Med. A.* **35**, 450–454.

25 Grof D (1992) *Sonographie des Graviden und Puerperalen Uterus unter Besonderer Berücksichtigung Verschiedener Stadien der Embryonalen und Fetalen Entwicklung Sowie Ultraschalldarstellung der Hoden und der Harnblase bei der Katze*. Hannover, Tierärztl. Hochsch., Diss.

26 Günzel-Apel AR and Lüning I (1983) Zur echographischen Trächtigkeitserkennung mit dem Vetoscan Ultraschallgerät. Möglichkeiten und Grenzen des Einsatzes bei der Hündin. *Dtsch. Tierärztl. Wschr.* **90**, 440–443.

27 Hansmann M, Hackelöer B-J and Staudach A (1985) *Ultraschalldiagnostik in Geburtshilfe und Gynäkologie*. Springer Verlag, Heidelberg.

28 Heinze B, Günzel-Apel AR and Hoppen H-O (1994) Ultrasonographische Darstellung des graviden und nicht graviden Uterus der Hündin unter Zuordnung der erhobenen Befande zum Ovulationstermin. *Reprod. Dom. Anim.* **29**, 262.

29 Helper LC (1970) Diagnosis of pregnancy in the bitch with an ultrasonic Doppler instrument. *J. Am. Vet. Med. Assoc.* **156**, 60–62.

30 Hill MC, Lande IM and Grossman JH (1987) Duplex evaluation of fetoplacental and uteroplacental circulation. In: Gant EG and White EM (Eds.) *Duplex Sonography*. Springer Verlag, New York, Berlin, Heidelberg, pp. 191–209.

31 Holst PA and Phemister RD (1971) The prenatal development of the dog: preimplantation events. *Biol. Reprod.* **5**, 194–206.

32 Holst PA and Phemister RD (1975) Temporal sequence of events in the estrous cycle of the bitch. *Am. J. Vet. Res.* **36**, 705–706.

33 Hüneke B and Schröder HJ (1992) Doppler-sonographische Untersuchungen des fetalen Blutstroms im Tierexperiment. *Gynäkologe* **25**, 341–351.

34 Van Huisseling H, Hassart THM, Muijsers GJIM and DeHaan J (1991) Umbilical artery pulsatility index and placental vascular resistance during acute hypoxemia in fetal lambs. *Gynecol. Obstet. Invest.* **31**, 61–66.

35 Irion GL and Clarke K-E (1990) Direct determination of the ovine fetal umbilical artery blood flow waveform. *Am. J. Obstet. Gynecol.* **162**, 541–549.

36 Künzel W (1992) Die Blutflußgeschwindigkeit und der Blutfluß in den Gefäßen der Nabelschnur and in der Aorta der Feten. *Gynäkologe* **25**, 292–296.

37 Lamm AM (1970) Ultrasound diagnosis of pregnancy in the dog. *Acta Radiol.* **Suppl. 319**, 293–294.

38 Lindahl IL (1966) Detection of pregnancy in sheep by means of ultrasound. *Nature* **212**, 642–643.

39 Madjar H, Makawiec U, Mandinger A, DuBois A, Kommoss F and Schillinger H (1994) Einsatz der hochauflösenden Sonographie zur Brustkrebsvorsorge.*Ultraschall Med.* **15**, 20–23.

40 Madjar H, Prompeler HJ, Sauerbrei W, Wolfarth R and Pfleiderer A (1994) Color Doppler flow criteria of breast lesions. *Ultrasound Med. Biol.* **20**, 849–858.

41 Mähler M, Poulsen Nautrup C and Schulze C (1994) Fibroepitheliale Hyperplasie der Mamma mit spontaner Regression bei einer Katze. *Kleintierpraxis* **39**, 869–875.

42 Marhold W and Leodolter S (1990) Terminologie beim geburtshilflichen Doppler. *Gynäkol. Randsch.* **30**, 111–114.

43 Medl M, Peters-Engl C and Leodolter S (1994) The use of color-coded Doppler sonography in the diagnosis of breast cancer. *Anticancer Res.* **14**, 2249–2251.

44 Memon MA and Mickelson WD (1993) Clinical management of bitches with vaginal discharge during pregnancy. *J. Reprod. Fert.* Suppl. **47**, 558.

45 Merz E and Goldhofer W (1989) III-6.3 Ultraschall in der Schwangerschaft. 7. Ergänzungslieferung. In: Braun B, Günther R and Schwerk W (Eds.) *Ultraschalldiagnostik. Lehrbuch und Atlas. Vol. I.* Verlag Ecomed. Landsberg, München, Zürich.

46 Müller K and Arbeiter K (1993) Ultrasonographic and clinical signs of fetal resorption in the bitch. *J. Reprod. Fert.* Suppl. **47**, 558–559.

47 Muijsers GJIM, VanHuisseling H and Hassart THM (1993) Relationship between mean arterial pressure and parameters derived from blood flow velocity waveforms in the systemic circulation of fetal sheep. *Gynecol. Obstet. Invest.* **36**, 1–7.

48 Noakes DE (1988) The normal breeding animal. In: Laing JA, Brinley WJ, Morgan WC and Wagner S (Eds.) *Fertility and Infertility in Veterinary Practice*. Baillière Tindall, London, pp. 1–38.

49 Noden DM (1986) Normal development and congenital birth defects in the cat. In: Kirk RW (Ed.) *Current Veterinary Therapy IX. Small Animal Practice*. WB Saunders, Philadelphia, pp. 1248–1257.

50 Otto RC (1993) Stellenwert des Ultraschalls in der Mammadiagnostik. *Bildgebung* **60**, 263–266.

51 Peters-Engl C, Medl M and Leodolter S (1994) Farbdopplersonographische Dignitätsbeurteilung von Mammatumoren. *Gynäkol. Geburtshilfliche Randsch.* **34**, 165–167.

52 Peters-Engl C, Medl M and Leodolter S (1994) The use of colour-coded and spectral Doppler ultrasound in the differentiation of benign and malignant breast lesions. *Br. J. Cancer* **71**, 137–139.

53 Pyczak T (1990) *Einsatzmöglichkeiten der Sonographie in der Gynäkologischen und Geburtshilflichen Diagnostik bei Hand und Katze*. München, Univ., Tierärztl. Fak., Diss.

54 Schmidt S (1986) Die Ultraschalldiagnostik in der inneren und gynäkologischen Kleintierpraxis. *Berl. Münch. Tierärztl. Wschr.* **99**, 300–308.

55 Schramm T (1989) Möglichkeiten der non-invasiven Diagnostik in der Beschreibung des fetalen Zustands. In: Schramm T and Gloning K-P. (Eds.) *Pränatale und Gynäkologische Sonographie*. Enke Verlag. Stuttgart, pp. 188–197.

56 Spaulding KA, Whitcare MD and Van Camp SD (1988) Sonographic

pregnancy diagnosis in the bitch. *Annual Meeting of the American College of Veterinary Radiology and Ultrasonography. Symposium, 20th–22nd October 1988.* Washington D.C.

57 Stuart B, Drumm J, Fitzgerald DE and Duignen NM (1980) Fetal blood velocity waveforms in normal pregnancy. *Br. J. Obstet. Gynecol.* **87**, 780–785.

58 Taverne MAM, Okkens AC and Van Oord R (1985) Pregnancy diagnosis in the dog: a comparison between abdominal palpation and linear-array real-time echography. *Vet. Quart* **7**, 249–255.

59 Toal RL, Walker LA and Henry GA (1986) A comparison of real-time ultrasound, palpation and radiography in pregnancy detection and litter size determination in the bitch. *Vet. Radiol.* **27**, 102–108.

60 Tsutsui T (1989) Gamete physiology and timing of ovulation and fertilization in the dog. *J. Reprod. Fert.* **Suppl. 39**, 169–175.

61 Tsutsui T and Shimizu T (1975) Studies on the physiology of reproduction in the dog. V: On the fertile period of ovum after ovulation. *Jap. J. Anim. Reprod.* **21**, 65–69.

62 Yeager AE and Concanon PW (1990) Association between the preovulatory luteinizing hormone surge and the early ultrasonographic detection of pregnancy and fetal heartbeats in beagle dogs. *Theriogenology* **34**, 655–665.

63 Yeager AE, Mohammed HO, Meyers-Wallen V, Vannerson L and Concanon PW (1992) Ultrasonographic appearance of the uterus, placenta, fetus, and fetal membranes throughout accurately timed pregnancy in beagles. *Am. J. Vet. Res.* **53**, 342–351.

12 Limbs and Spine

Requirements

Andreas Engelke and Gabriele Gassner

General Indications

Ultrasonography is helpful in imaging soft tissues of the locomotor system. In this way, ultrasonography complements radiography, which evaluates only bony structures.

Ultrasonography is indicated for imaging muscle, tendon and ligament lesions. Information on the physiological and pathological morphology of these structures is gained.

Technical Requirements

A high-frequency transducer (7.5–10 MHz) is needed to obtain good resolution in the near field with depth penetration of up to 5 cms. The longitudinal structures require a linear scanner or sector transducer with a built-in stand-off. Small sector probes produce a 'key-hole' image and are useful only for certain examinations such as the stifle or shoulder joints. These transducers have a tendency to create artefacts at other scanning sites. Linear transducers have a parallel sound beam with a good overview and the necessary near-field resolution. Irregularities at the limb surface, resulting in poor skin contact, can be compensated with a stand-off pad[46] (see Stand-Off Pads, page 56). At the same time, the distance between the transducer and the skin surface is increased, which moves the region of interest into the focal zone. This increase in distance may be necessary to image superficial tendons[25]. The stand-off should be firmly attached to the transducer to ensure easy manipulation.

Ultrasound unit adjustments should be made according to the individual scanning site. Soft tissue examinations with fine structural detail should be performed with a wide grey scale and low contrast. With joint ultrasonography, the image should be high in contrast to accentuate contours[27].

Patient Preparation

A successful examination requires good patient positioning and calm handling of the animal. Sedation is only necessary when the examination is painful and the animal is uncooperative (*Table 41*). Hair should always be removed from the scanning site.

Examination Technique

Real-time mode offers a dynamic evaluation of musculoskeletal functions as well as dysfunctions. This means that the joints and tendons should be imaged in real-time by passive movement of the limb[15, 37]. Small lesions are detected by comparing images of the diseased limb with those of the opposite normal limb[25].

Documentation

Sonographic findings should primarily be recorded on video devices and, additionally, with video printers (see Instrumentation and Documentation, page 51). Image orientation or labelling makes follow-up examinations of sonographic lesions easier. These markings and labels indicate the scan site and can be reproduced at later examinations (see Image Orientation and Documentation, page 81).

Image orientation of the patient with longitudinal planes shows proximal to the left and distal to the right of the screen. Orientation on transverse views is generally more difficult to define.

Muscles

Andreas Engelke and Gabriele Gassner

Ultrasonography of Normal Muscle

Muscles are easy to image ultrasonographically (*Table 42* lists the sonographic characteristics of normal muscle). Indications for muscle ultrasonography include inflammatory, degenerative or traumatic lesions.

Muscles should be displayed longitudinally and transversely to

Table 41 Drugs to sedate patients for an orthopaedic ultrasound examination.

Dog:	
• Propofol (Rapinovet®)	5–6 mg/kg body weight i/v as needed
• Diazepam (Valium®)	1–2 mg/kg body weight i/v
• Acepromazine (Vetranquil®)	0.01-0–1 mg/kg body weight i/m or i/v
• Medetomidine (Domitor®)	20–40 µg/kg body weight i/v
Cat:	
• Ketamine + Xylazine	10 mg/kg + 1 mg/kg body weight i/m
• (Ketavet® + Rompun®)	

Table 42 Sonographic characteristics of normal muscles.

Sonographic morphology of normal muscles:
• Separated by echogenic fascia and septa.
• Typical longitudinal pattern.
• Homogenous hypoechoic muscle tissue between the septa
• Anechoic, well-demarcated vessels that pulsate (arteries) or are compressible (veins).

758

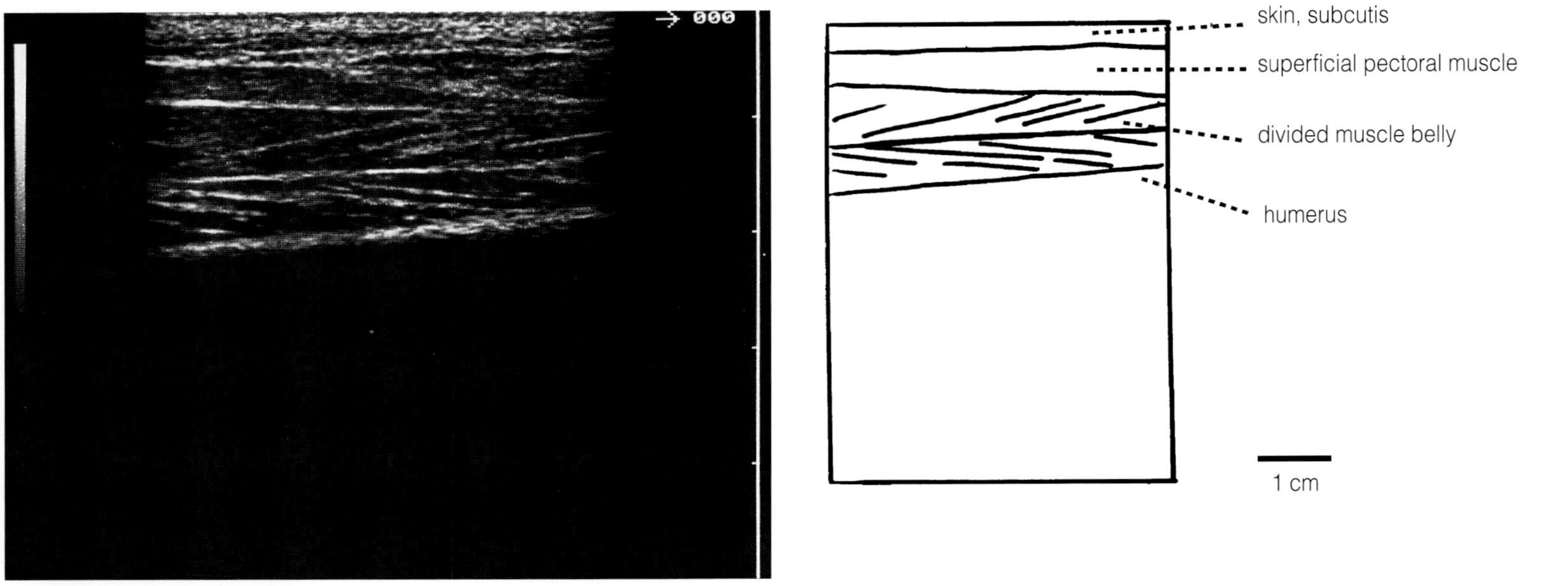

758 Normal muscle in a longitudinal plane, exemplified by the biceps brachii muscle of a dog.

759

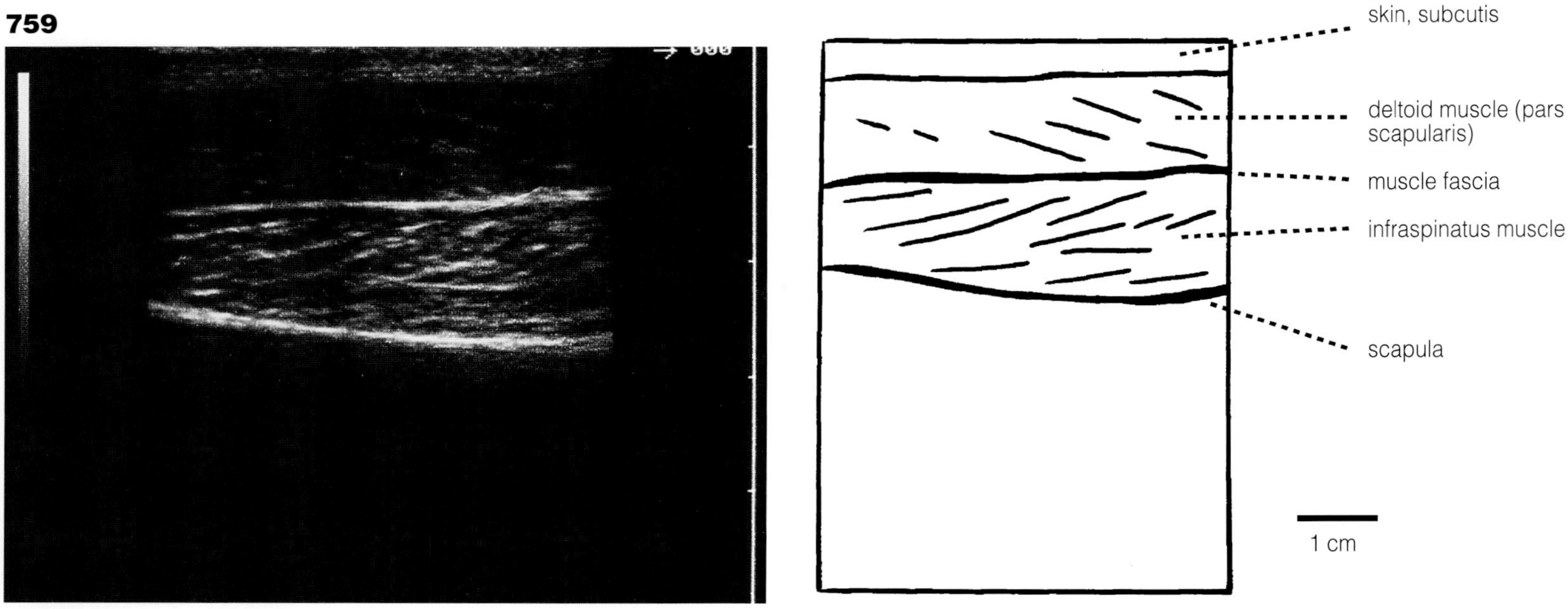

759 Normal muscle in a longitudinal plane exemplified by the infraspinatus muscle of a dog.

the course of the fibres. Normal muscle is hypoechoic with a characteristic echogenic reticular pattern. Longitudinal scans of some muscles have characteristic fibre patterns, e.g. the biceps muscle with a typical 'fish-bone pattern'[23] (**758**) or the infraspinatus muscle with a one-sided, dorsal muscle fibre appearance (**759**).

The characteristic muscle sonogram shows organized muscle fibres with primary and secondary muscle bundles, including fibrous septa and fascia. The fascia are seen as smooth, hyperechoic lines (**760, 762**). These internal echoes are focal in the transverse plane[6, 7, 22, 23] (**761, 762**). The echogenicity of the muscle layers varies and depends on the course of the fibres in relation to the scanning direction. The smallest recognizable structures are the secondary muscle bundles, surrounded by perimysium.

An optimal scan direction should be chosen for each individual muscle. Muscles tend to be dependent on the incident angle of the sound beam, because of the strong reflections of the echogenic fibrous tissue. A slightly oblique sound wave angle produces an artefactual hypoechoic image, which mimics a mass in the muscle tissue.

Table 43 Sonographic characteristics of muscle lesions.

Sonographic evaluation of muscle lesions by:
• Location, size, shape. • Distribution pattern of the lesions (diffuse or focal). • Demarcation to surrounding tissue. • Echogenicity (hypoechoic to hyperechoic). • Echo distribution (homogenous to non-homogenous).

Ultrasonography of Muscle Lesions

Several criteria used to evaluate muscle lesions are summarized in *Table 43*.

Space-Occupying Lesions

Sonographic diagnosis of space-occupying lesions in the limb area is very sensitive, but rather non-specific. The masses can be differentiated as solid or fluid-filled lesions (see *Table 44*, page 335). Space-occupying lesions include haematomas, abscesses and tumours (**763–768**). Determination of the masses according to their echogenicity is not possible or at least limited. Echo distribution gives a slight indication of the disease.

760

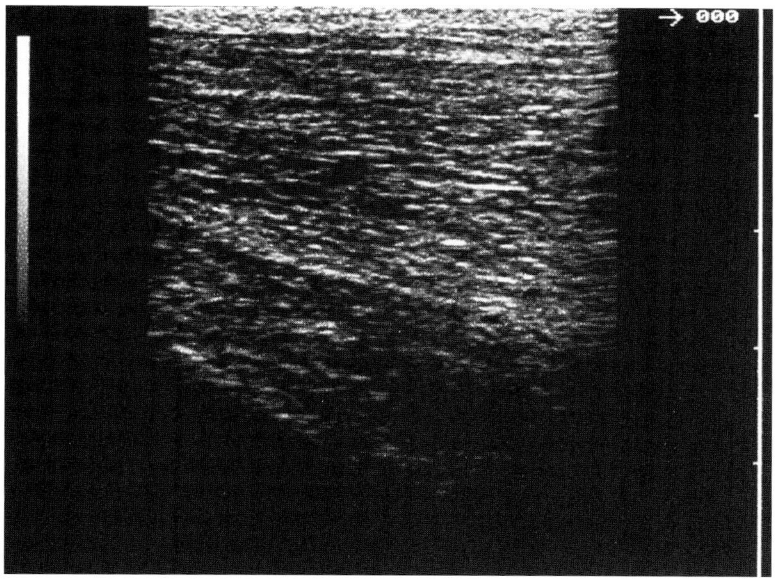

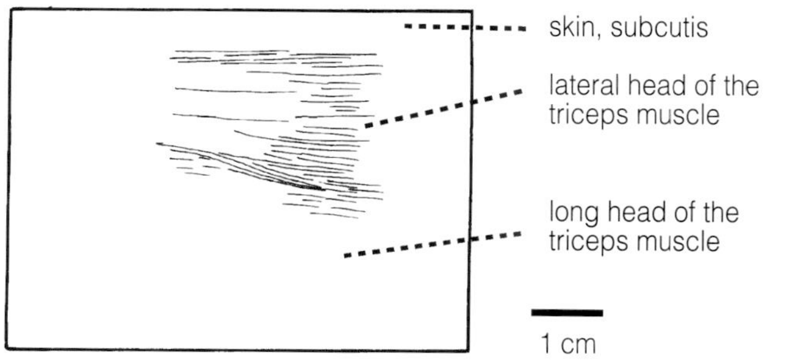

761

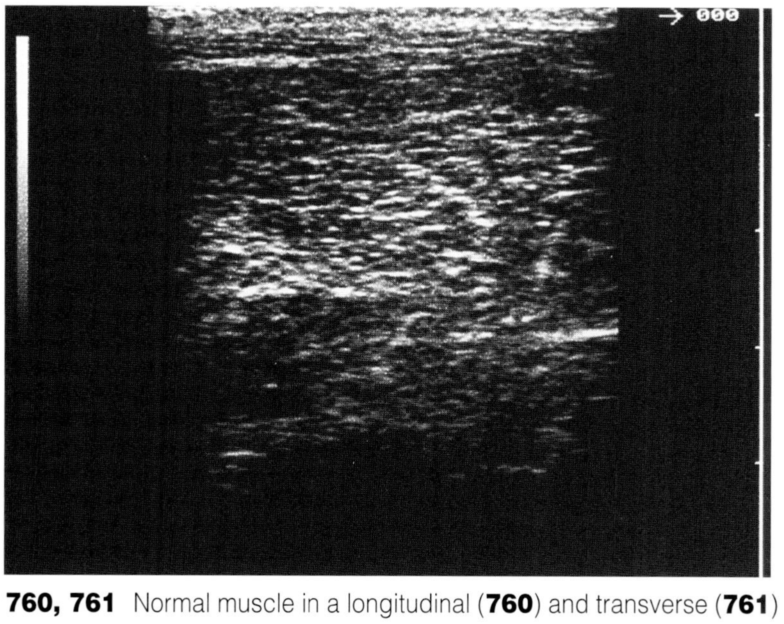

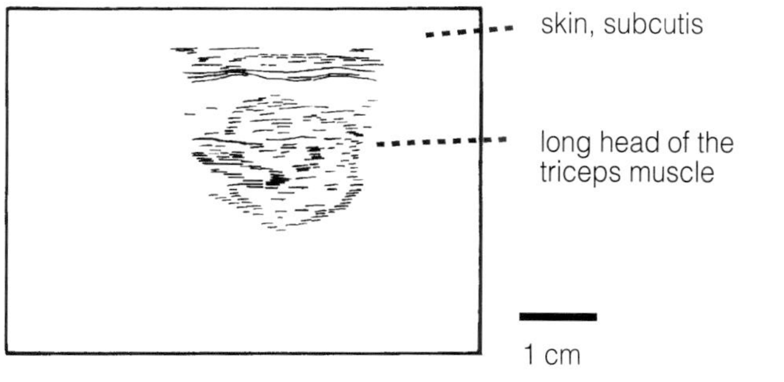

760, 761 Normal muscle in a longitudinal (**760**) and transverse (**761**) plane exemplified by the triceps muscle of a dog.

762

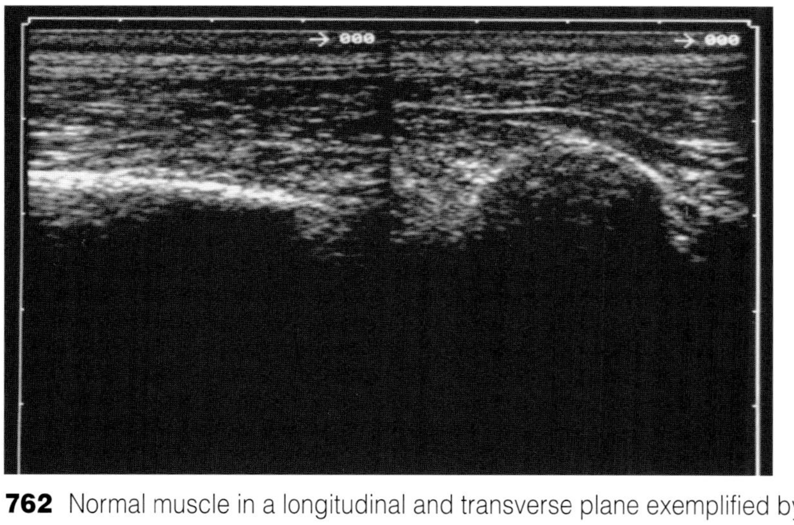

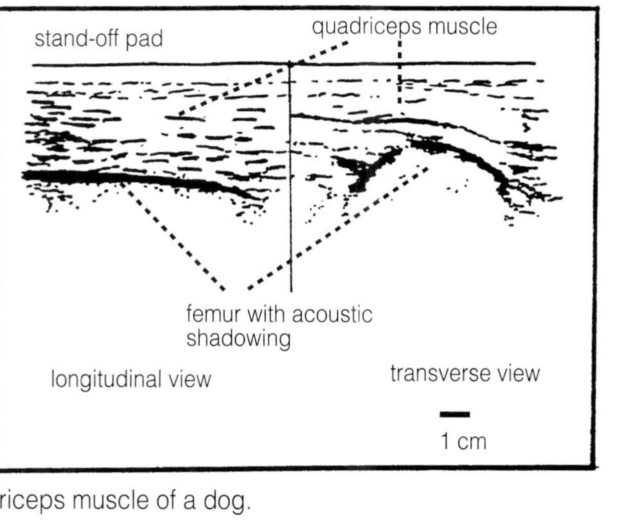

762 Normal muscle in a longitudinal and transverse plane exemplified by the quadriceps muscle of a dog.

763

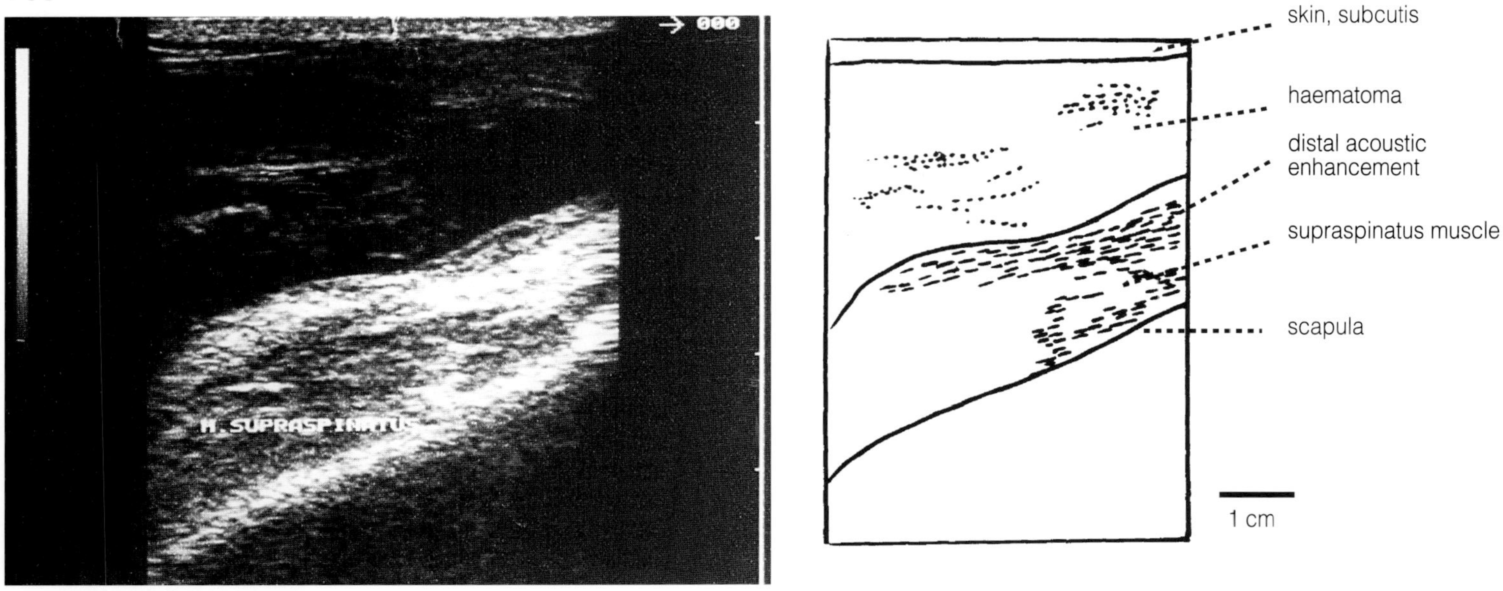

763 Longitudinal view of an intramuscular haematoma in the supraspinatus muscle of a dog.

764

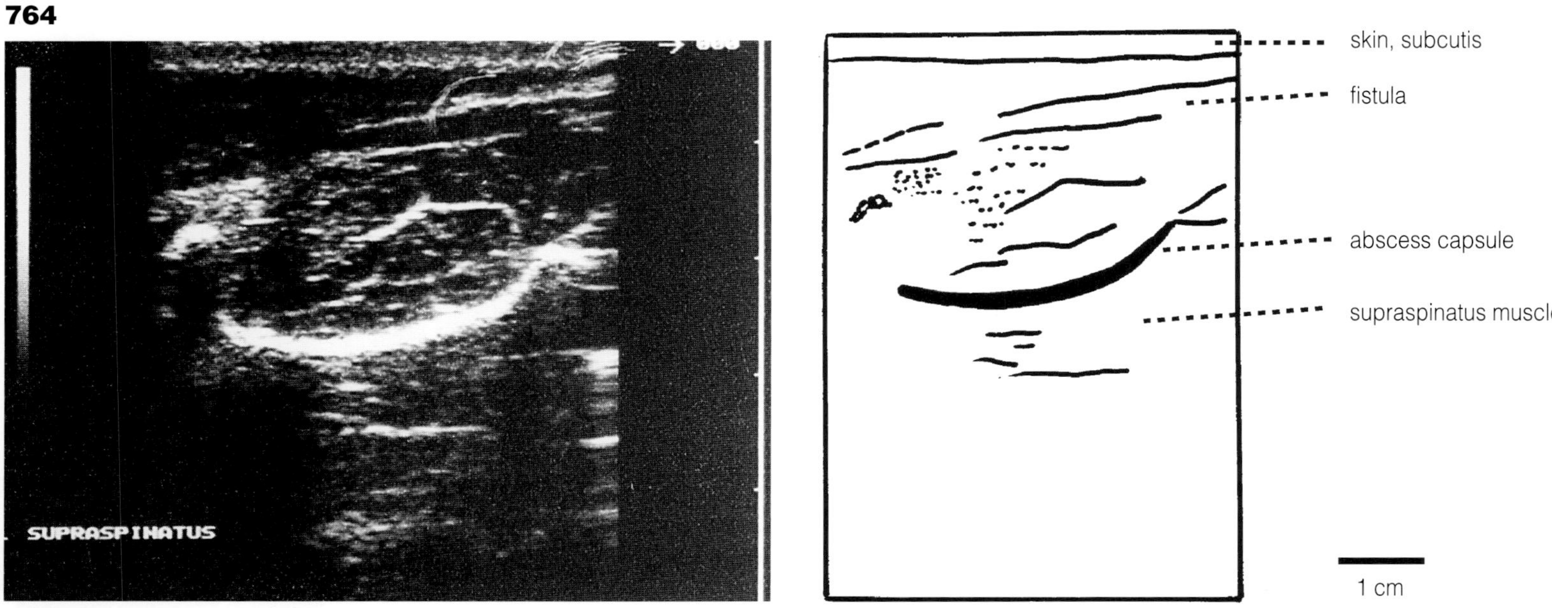

764 Longitudinal view of a cavitated abscess with fistulas in the supraspinatus muscle of a dog.

765

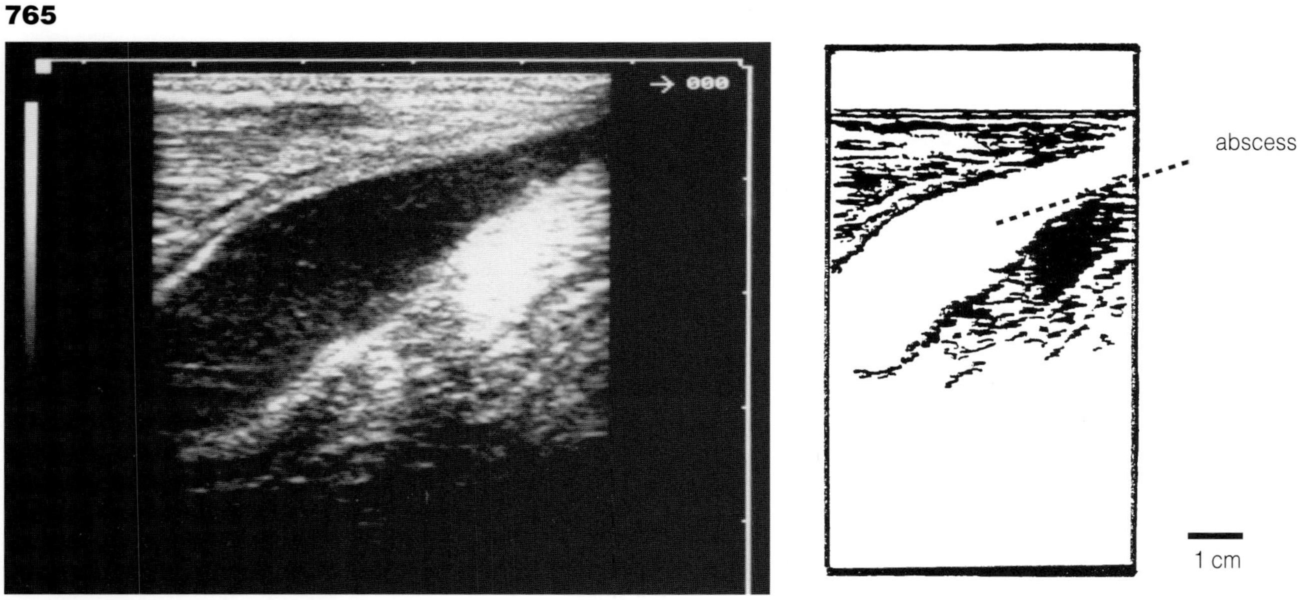

765 Abscess in the popliteal fossa of a dog.

766

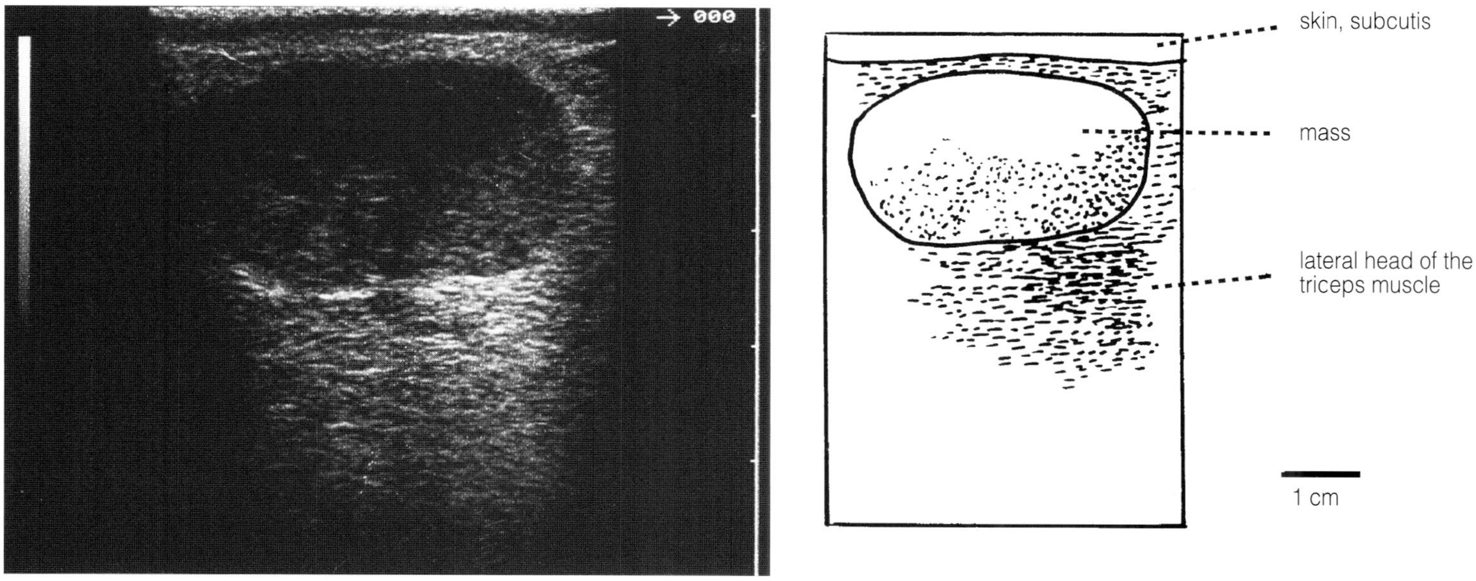

766 Transverse view of a mass (histopathology: haemangiosarcoma) in the triceps muscle area of a dog.

767

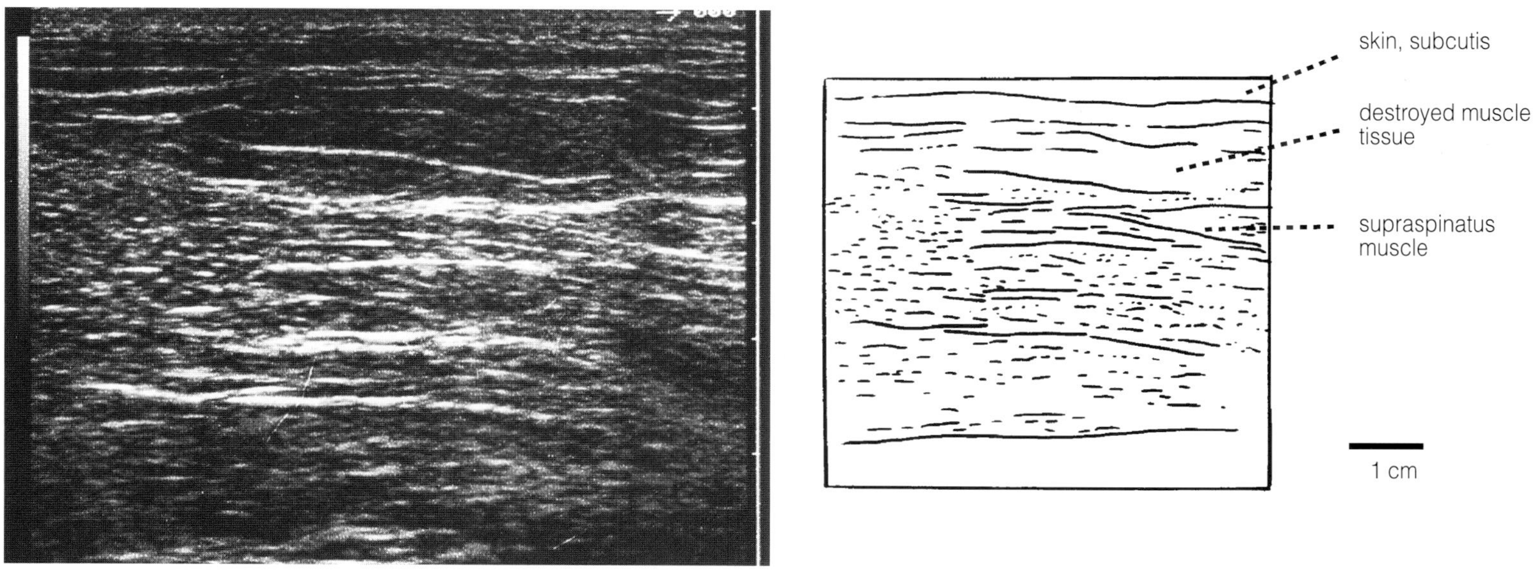

767 Longitudinal view of an intramuscular lipoma in the supraspinatus muscle of a dog.

768

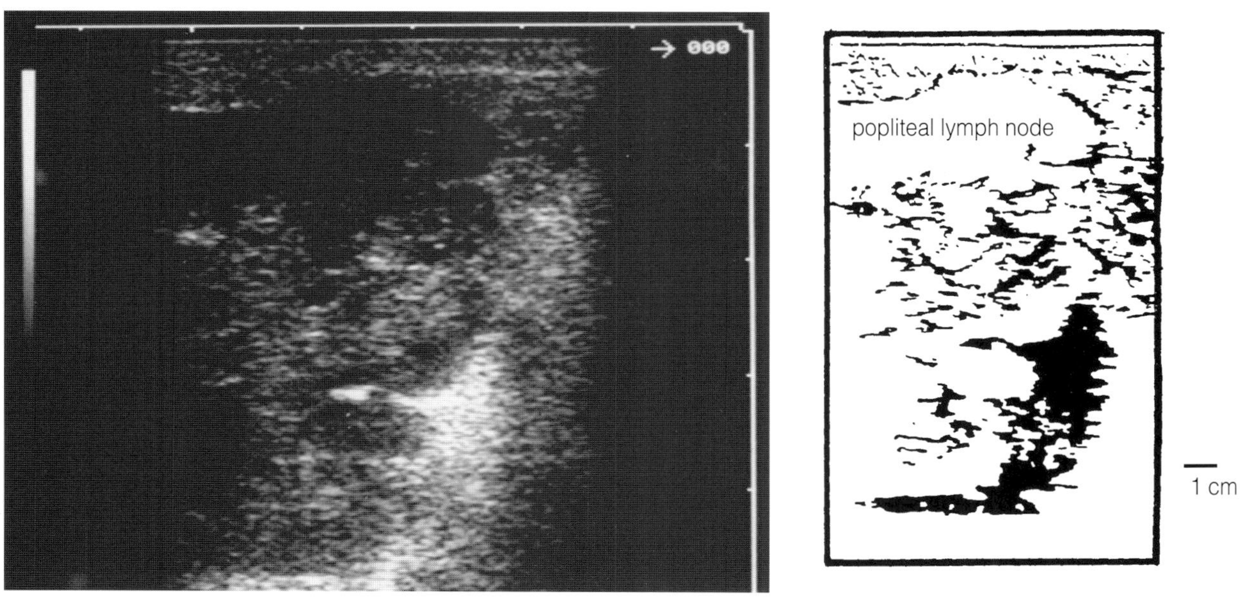

768 Popliteal lymph node enlargement (histopathology: lymphosarcoma) in a dog.

769

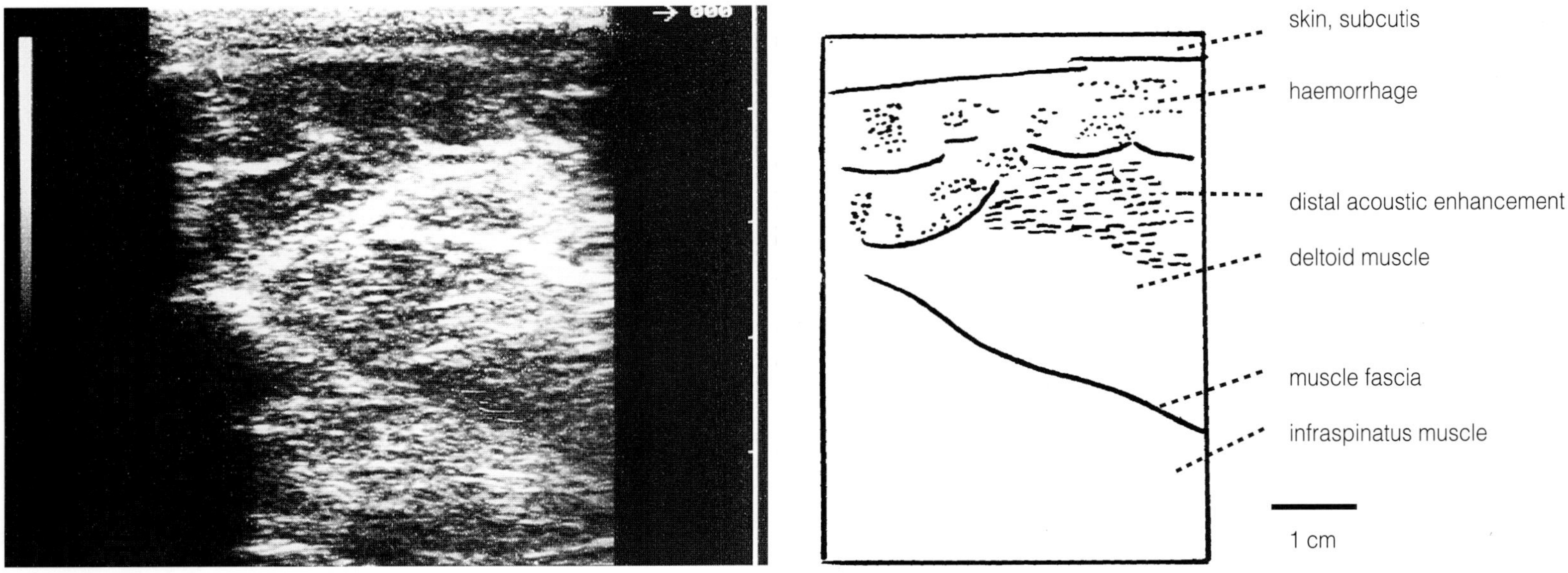

769 Longitudinal view of a deltoid muscle tear in a dog.

770

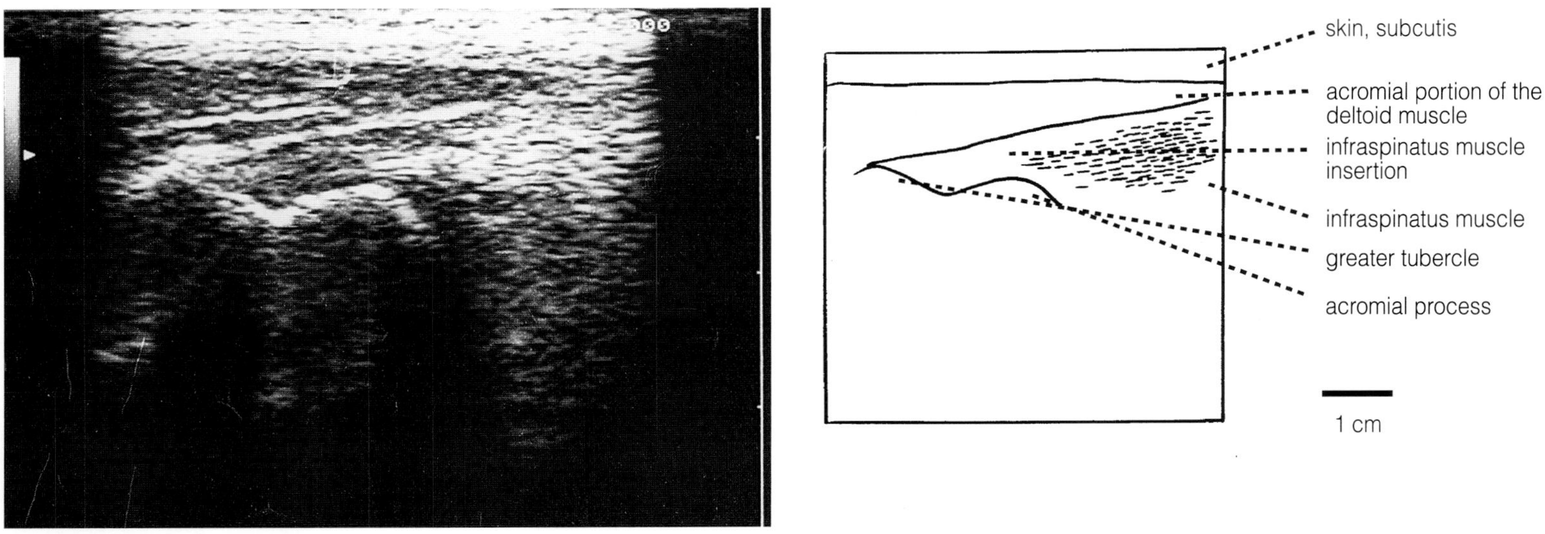

771

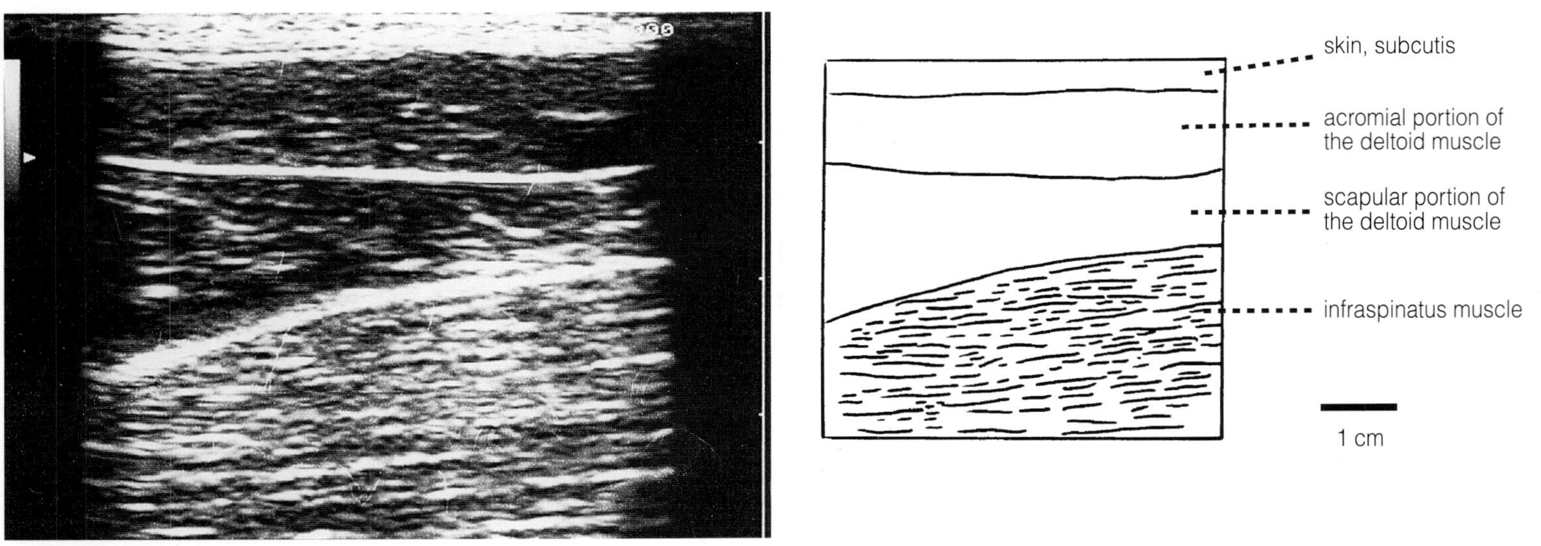

770, 771 Longitudinal view of infraspinatus muscle contracture at the myotendinous junction (**770**) and at the level of the muscle belly (**771**) in a dog.

772

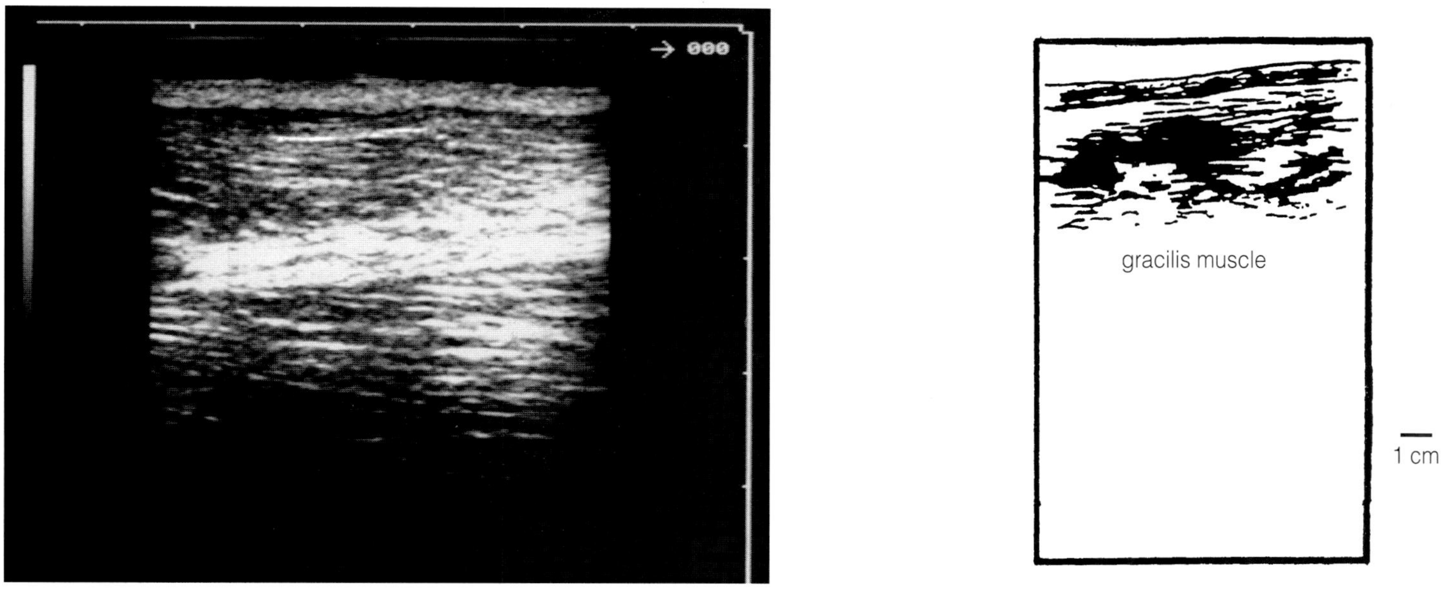

772 Longitudinal view of a gracilis muscle contracture in a dog.

Table 44 Sonographic differentiation of space-occupying muscle lesions.

Space-occupying lesion	Echogenicity and echo distribution	Characteristics
Seroma	anechoic, homogenous, well-demarcated	distal acoustic enhancement
Haematoma	hypoechoic (acute) to hyperechoic (organized), homogenous to non-homogenous, relatively well-demarcated	possible floating particles (fibrin), occasionally septated
Abscess	hypoechoic (acute) to hyperechoic (organized), homogenous to non-homogenous, well-demarcated	fistula, granulation tissue, trapped air, calcification
Tumour	anechoic to hyperechoic, homogenous to non-homogenous, defined to infiltrative	not compressible with a solid, echogenic structure, calcification, well vascularized (seen with colour Doppler), no diagnosis of type or malignancy
Calcification	hyperechoic with distal acoustic shadowing	

Sonographic characterization of masses is possible by[6, 38]:

- The compressibility of the mass.
- Mobile, swirling echoes within the structure.
- Septation and vascular supply.

The location of the lesion in relation to the surrounding tissue offers additional important information. Clinical findings, such as painfulness, fever or known trauma, help to differentiate some lesions. An ultrasound-guided fine-needle aspiration or biopsy, followed by a histological examination, provides a final diagnosis (see Ultrasound-Guided Biopsy, page 366). Ultrasound examinations are useful for planning further procedures and providing the surgeon with information about the size and shape of the mass. Treatment can be monitored with ultrasonography.

Muscle Tears

Muscle tears or strains with fibre rupture are seen sonographically in a longitudinal plane (**769**). The typical muscle texture is destroyed at the rupture site. A haematoma is usually present. In the acute stage, haematomas have a hypoechoic appearance, surrounded by muscle fascia. Functional examinations show that the torn muscle ends with a clubbed appearance. With passive movement, the torn margins move apart[6, 10, 13, 24, 25]. Clot organization causes the sonogram to become more echogenic, non-homogenous and occasionally septated[6, 7, 8, 13].

Muscle Contractures

Muscle contractures of the infraspinatus, supraspinatus, gracilis, semimembranosus and quadriceps muscles produce characteristic lamenesses, and they are distinguished sonographically (**770–772**). The ultrasound image shows echogenic muscular structures or hyperechoic bands, which are caused by a change in muscle tissue. This image is similar to that seen with tendons. The characteristic muscle pattern is lost through fibrosis[43].

Infraspinatus muscle contractures are seen frequently in hunting dogs. The characteristic fibrous induration between the muscle and the insertion site is visible sonographically at the level of the acromion[3]. The spine of the scapula assists orientation in longitudinal and transverse views. Further distal, the bone echo of the greater tubercle indicates the scan site in a longitudinal plane. The longitudinal scanning position gives a good overview of the non-homogenous, echogenic lesions (**770, 771**). The transducer is angled craniodistal along the muscle fibres and moved from the infraspinatus fossa over the shoulder joint. To visualize the tendon insertion and fibrosis between muscle and tendon, the scanner should be held caudoproximal to the joint[23, 26]. A stand-off pad is useful.

773

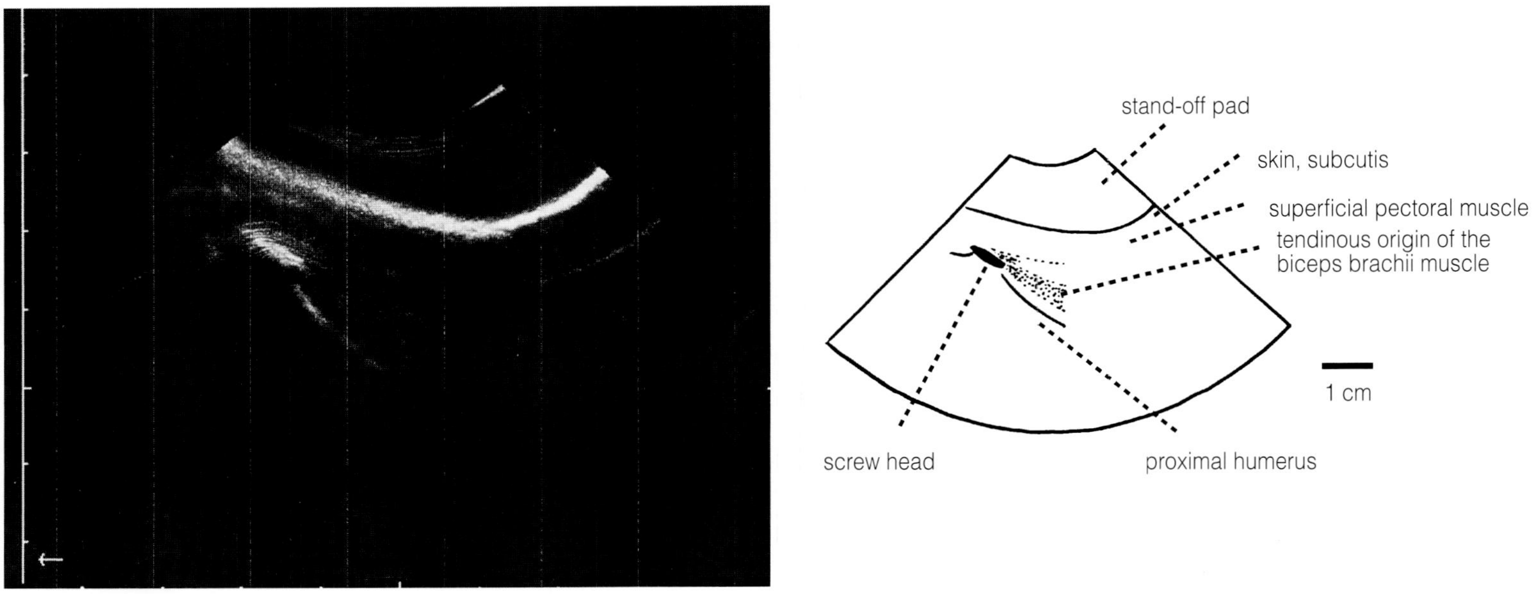

773 Implant (screw head) on the humerus following transposition and fixation of the tendinous origin of the biceps brachii muscle in a dog.

Foreign Bodies

Ultrasonography can be used to find radiolucent, intramuscular foreign bodies, e.g. wood splinters, glass, tooth fragments or suture material[7, 8, 13]. Implants and metallic foreign bodies are distinguishable as highly reflective structures[13] (**773**). Secondary abscessation and fistulas may be detected and evaluated. Muscles should be scanned in at least two planes at the site in question to identify small foreign bodies.

Tendons

Gabriele Gassner and Andreas Engelke

Ultrasonography of Normal Tendon

The tendon in a healthy patient is displayed as an evenly defined, relatively hyperechoic band in a longitudinal plane (*Table* 45). Echoes are produced by sound wave reflection at interfaces between the endotenon and collagen fibre bundles. They appear in the shape of slightly wavy, longitudinal echoes. This characteristic tendon structure is seen only in a perpendicular sound beam. A slightly angled sound beam gives the tendon a more hypoechoic appearance[6, 7, 13, 22, 23]. Tendon sheaths, i.e. wall echoes, appear as an echogenic line. Real-time examination shows the tendon gliding within the sheath.

Because of the varying pathogenesis of tendon lesions, individual tendons will be discussed separately and be limited to the most important tendons.

Table 45 Sonographic characteristics of the normal tendon.

Sonographic morphology of normal tendon in a longitudinal view with perpendicular sound waves:
• Uniformly defined hyperechoic band. • Slightly wavy, longitudinal internal echoes. • Gliding tendon in real-time examination.

Bicipital Tendon

Ultrasonography of the Normal Bicipital Tendon

The tendon of the biceps brachii muscle has a curved path and should be displayed in a number of separate views to ensure a perpendicular image of each region. The joint should be extended and rotated maximally to the outside for the examination[23].

In a long-axis view the supraglenoid tubercle acts as a bony marker and is located proximal to the intertubercular groove and the head of the humerus. The tendon is surrounded by an echogenic tendon sheath and it runs in a curved path around the head of the humerus[23, 26] (**774**).

In a transverse view the greater and lesser tubercles, located to the left and right of the intertubercular groove, represent more or less distinct markers. The lesser tubercle in large breed dogs is seen only as a small slope of the echogenic bone surface, while it is not visualized at all in medium to small breed dogs.

The characteristic 'fried egg' image appears in a transverse view. The tendon itself produces a round to oval, hyperechoic central structure, surrounded by a synovial 'tendon sheath' which, in this case, represents the joint capsule sac (**775**).

Ultrasonography of Bicipital Tendon Lesions

Tendonitis

Tendonitis lesions are usually associated with tenosynouitis. In cross-section the biceps tendon is surrounded by a wide hypoechoic rim[10]. Fluid accumulation alone in the 'tendon sheath' cannot be diagnosed as a sign of tendinitis, since the sheath is openly connected to the shoulder joint[6, 36].

Tendinitis characteristically appears with oedematous fibre tissue and an increase in tendon volume. The more hypoechoic appearance, even in a perpendicular sound beam, is caused by disintegration and/or oedema of fibre texture, as well as loss of the parallel structure of collagen fibrils[6, 10, 18, 20]. In most cases there is a distinct alteration in echogenicity between diseased and normal tendon tissue (**776**).

774

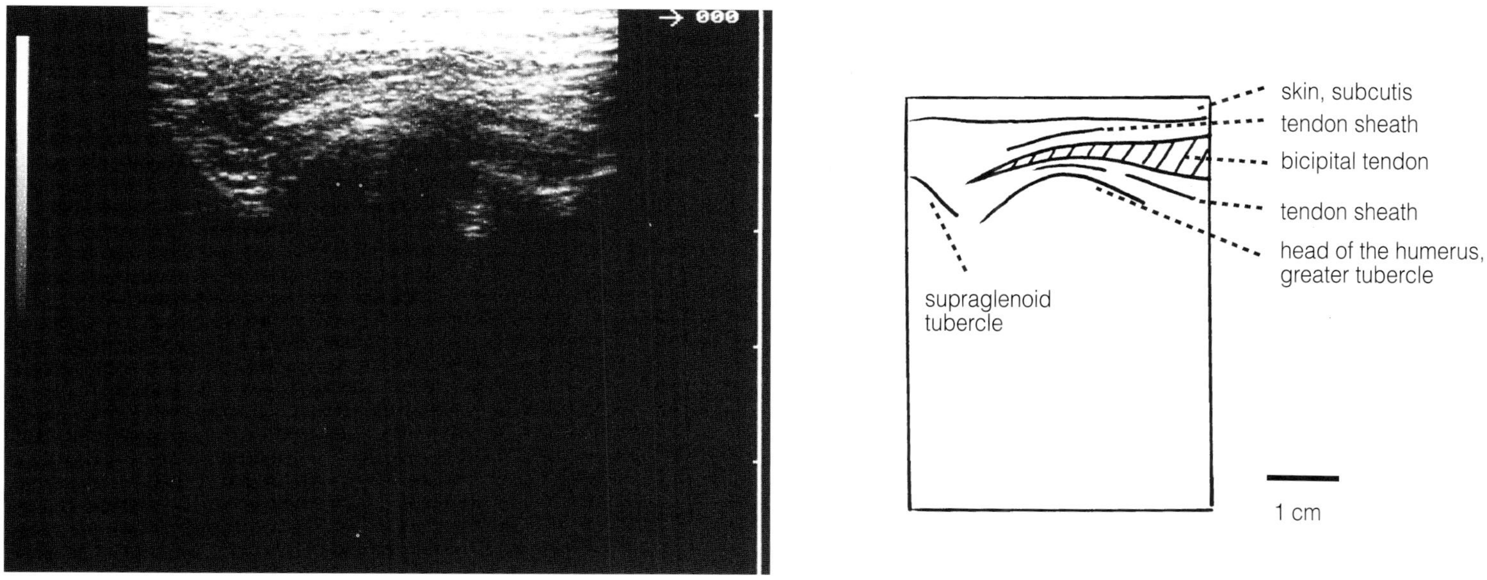

775

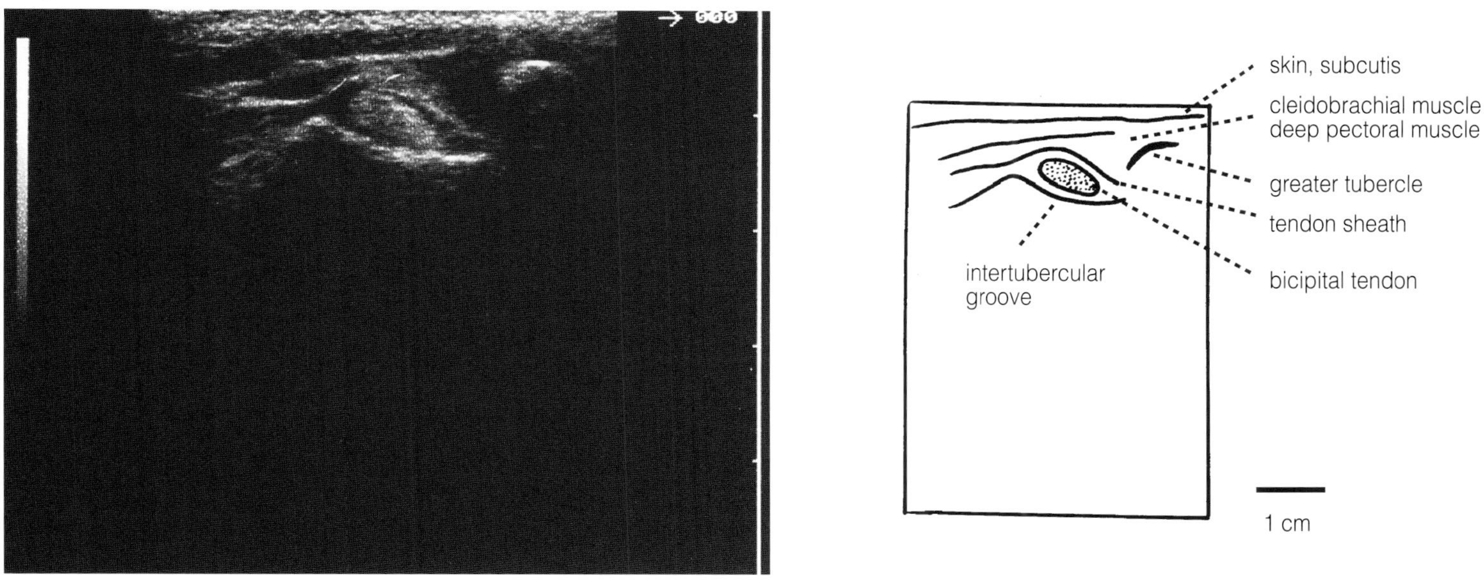

774, 775 Longitudinal (**774**) and transverse (**775**) views of a normal bicipital tendon in a dog.

776

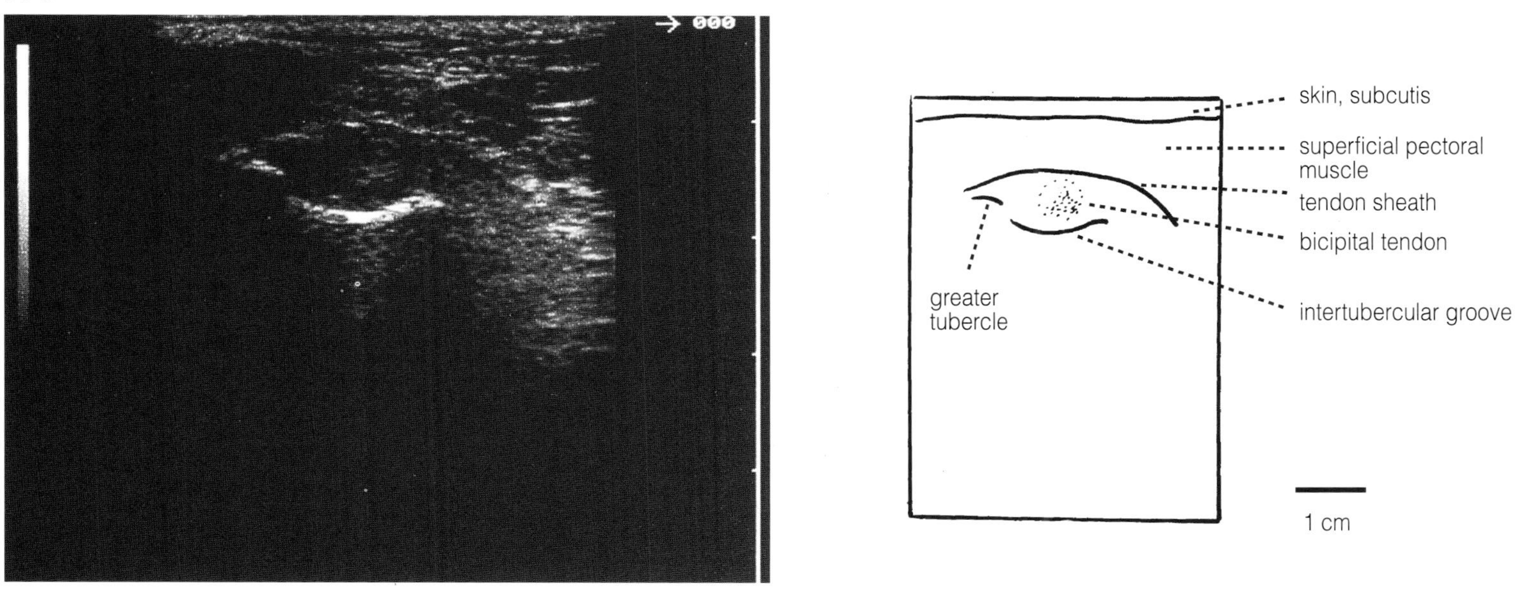

776 Transverse view of tendon degeneration caused by chronic inflammation of the bicipital tendon of a dog.

777

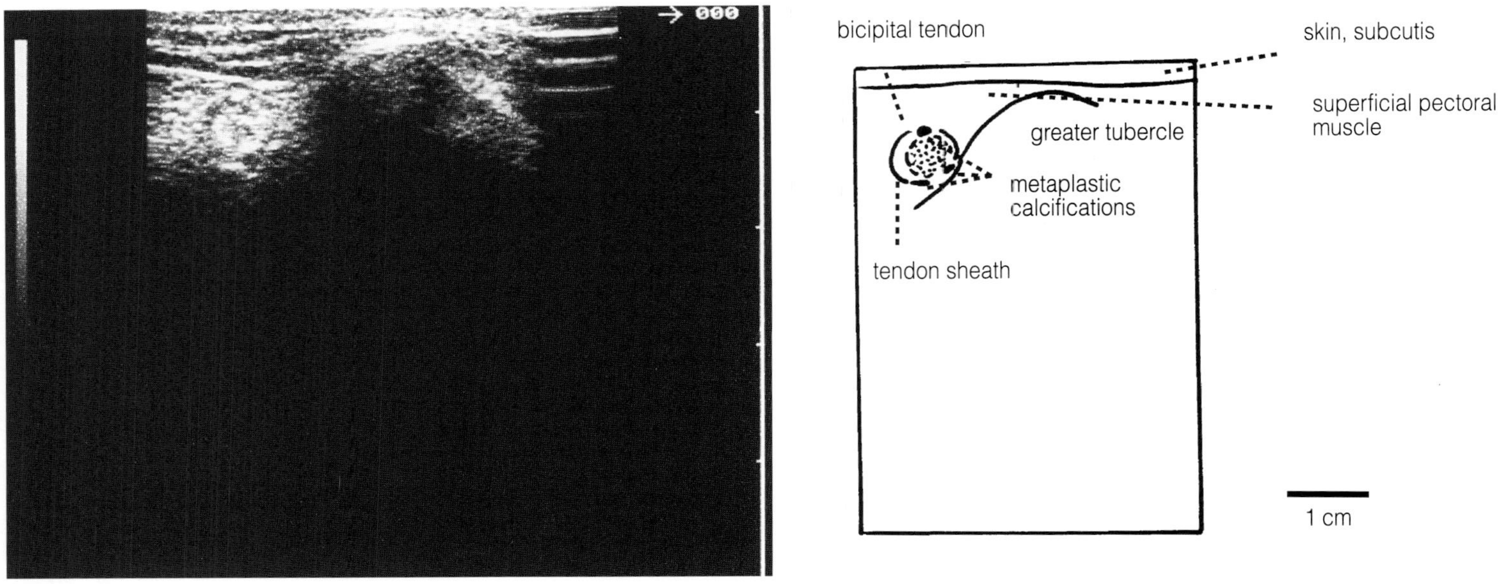

777 Transverse view of calcified tendinitis of the biceps tendon in a dog.

778

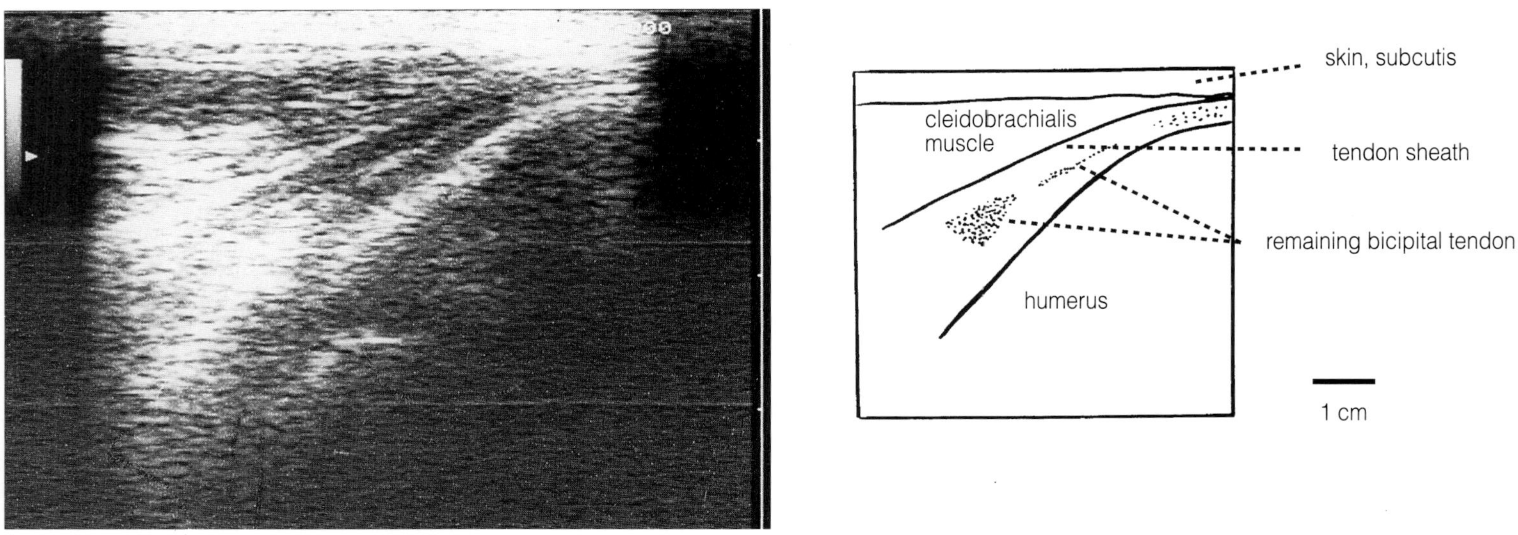

779

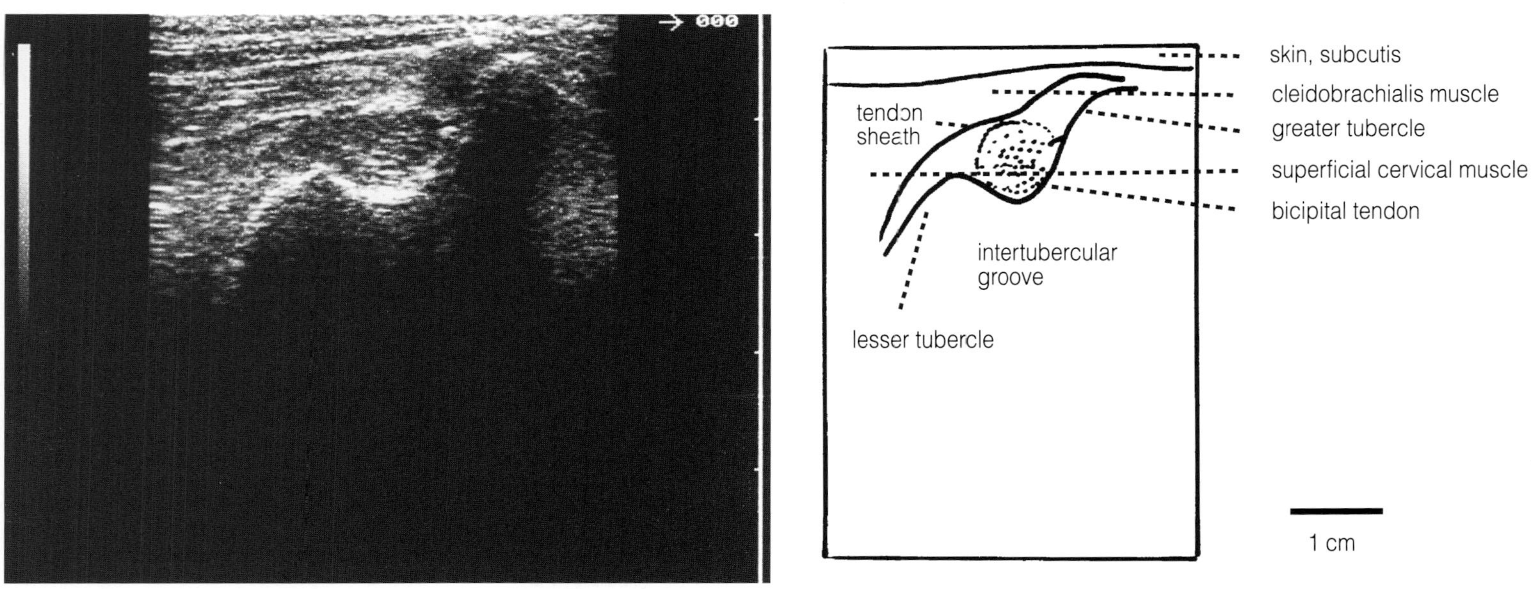

778, 779 Longitudinal (**778**) and transverse (**779**) scans of a partial bicipital tendon rupture in a dog.

780

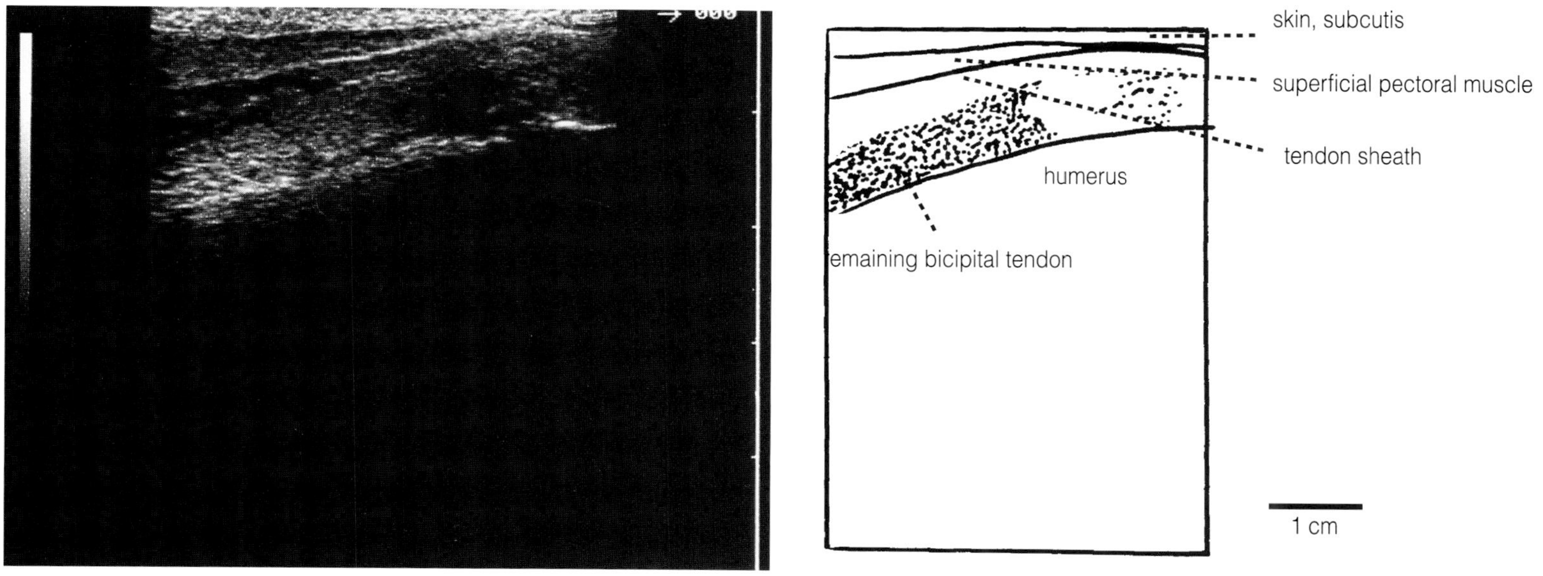

781

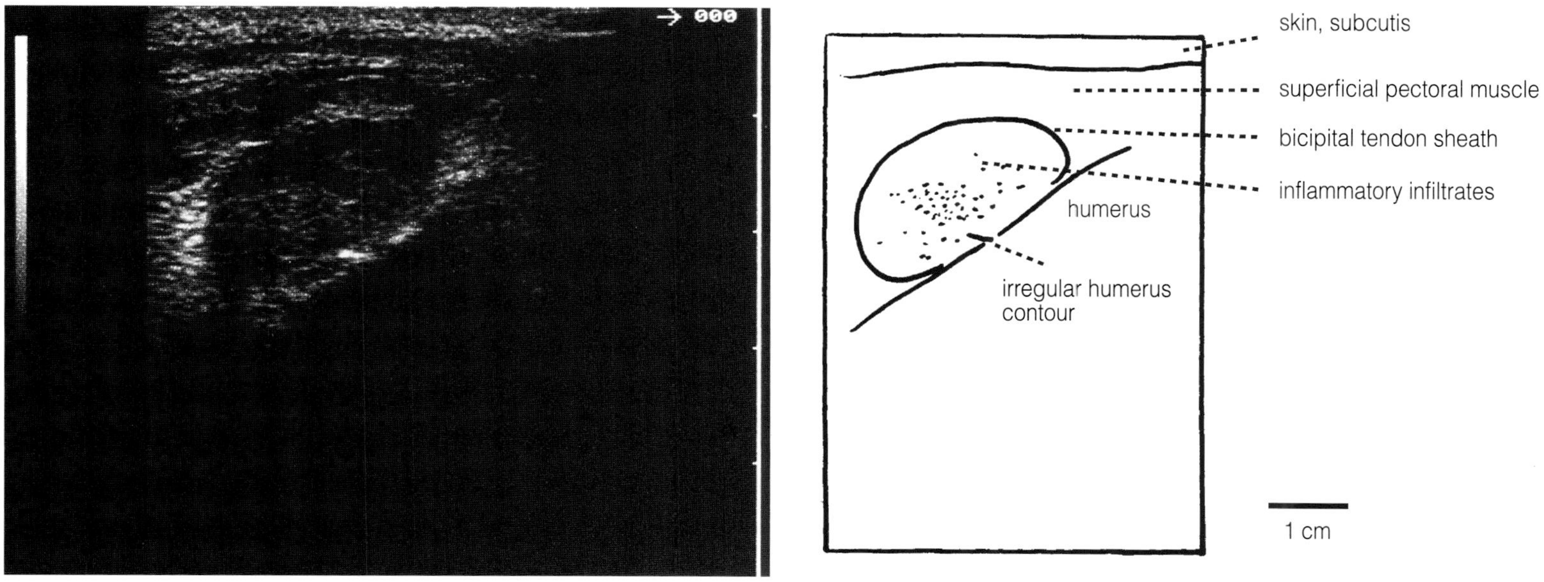

780, 781 Longitudinal (**780**) and transverse (**781**) scans of a complete bicipital tendon rupture in a dog.

Well-defined regenerative areas with cell accumulation show high echogenicity. Metaplastic changes with resulting calcification are also hyperechoic. Larger calcifications with calcified tendinitis are easily recognized as hyperechoic areas with distal acoustic shadowing[13] (**777**). Amorphous calcifications with low density and crumbly consistency often do not have surface echoes or shadowing[6]. Calcifications are usually aligned parallel to the tendon fibres[39]. In the acute stage they are always concurrent with oedema. Echogenic, intratendinous infiltrations may be diffuse or focal and they have no distal acoustic shadowing[34].

Complete and Partial Bicipital Tendon Rupture

Sonographic images of acute ruptures show a hypoechoic to anechoic tendon, caused by haemorrhaging (**778, 779**). The retracted tendon fragments appear hyperechoic and slightly thickened[10] (**780, 781**). A real-time examination of an acute rupture shows the club-like tendon fragments or borders moving apart .

The intertubercular groove appears empty in conjunction with complete tendon rupture[6, 19]. In a long-axis view the paratendon and tendon sheath may mimic an intact tendon. This may also be true for hyperechoic granulation tissue in this area (**782**).

782

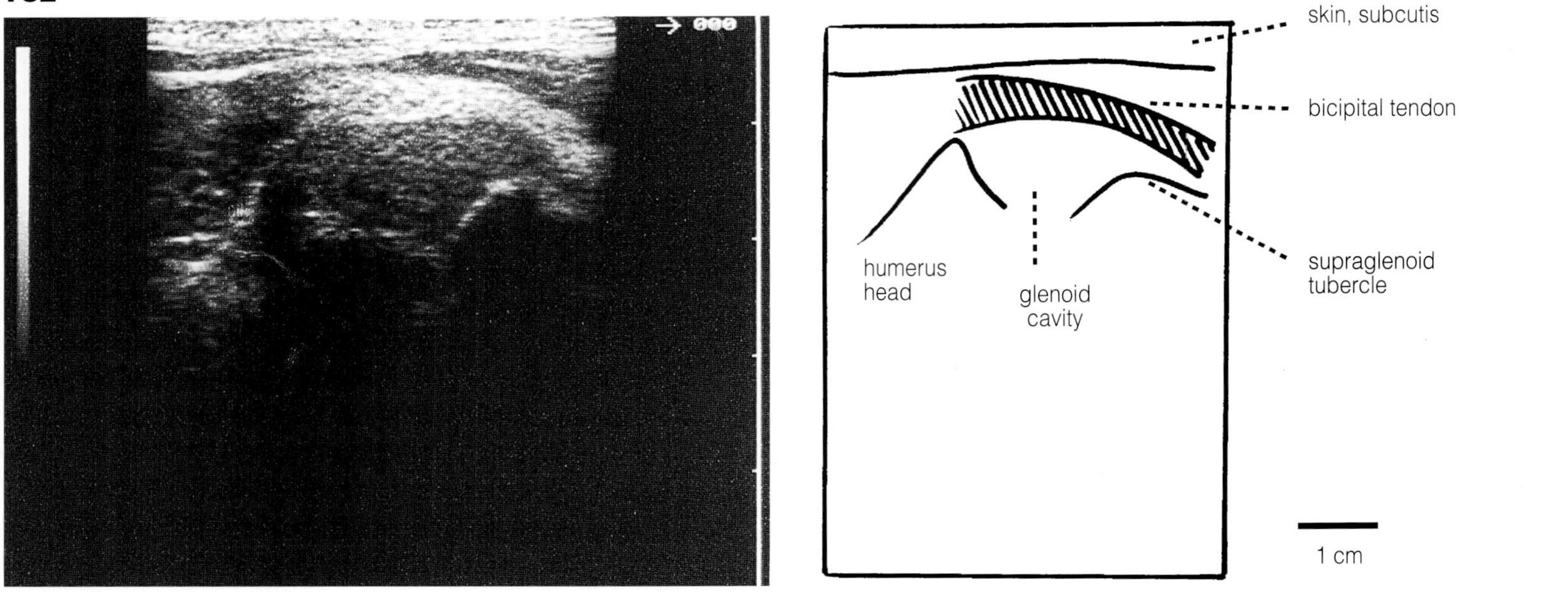

782 Longitudinal scan of an older bicipital tendon rupture in a dog.

783

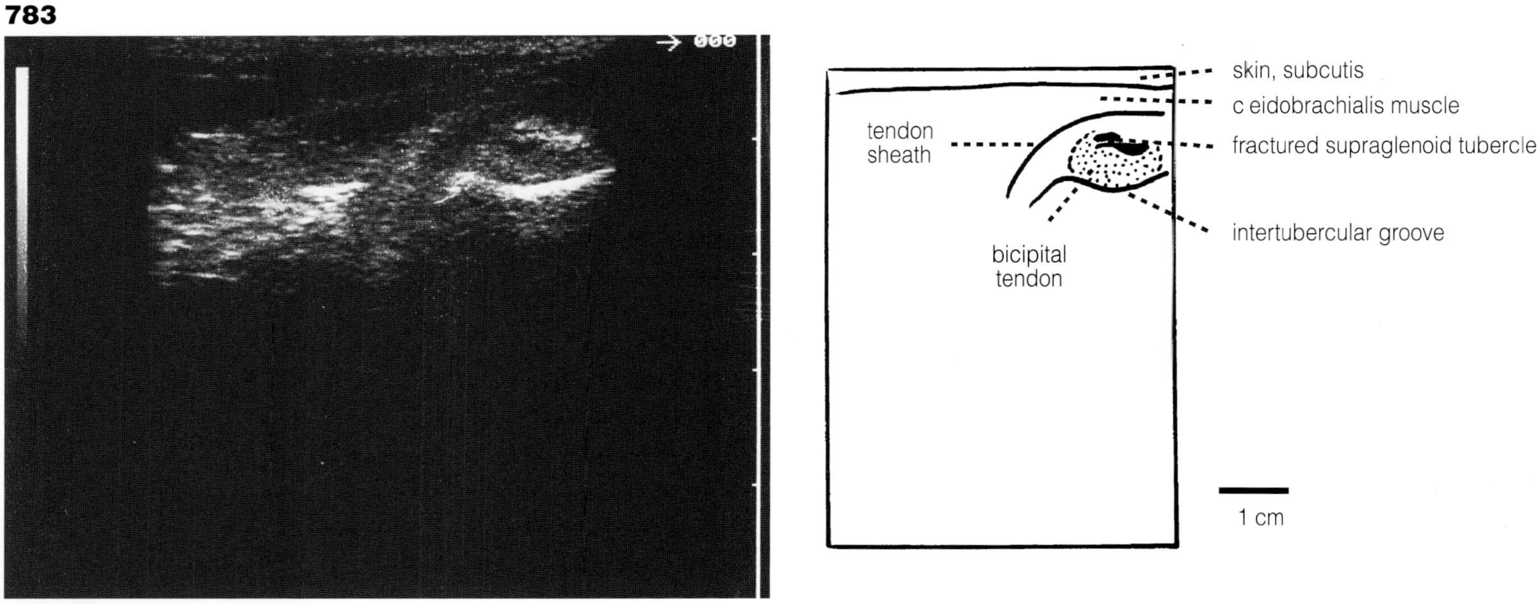

783 Transverse scan of a bicipital tendon avulsion fracture in a dog.

784

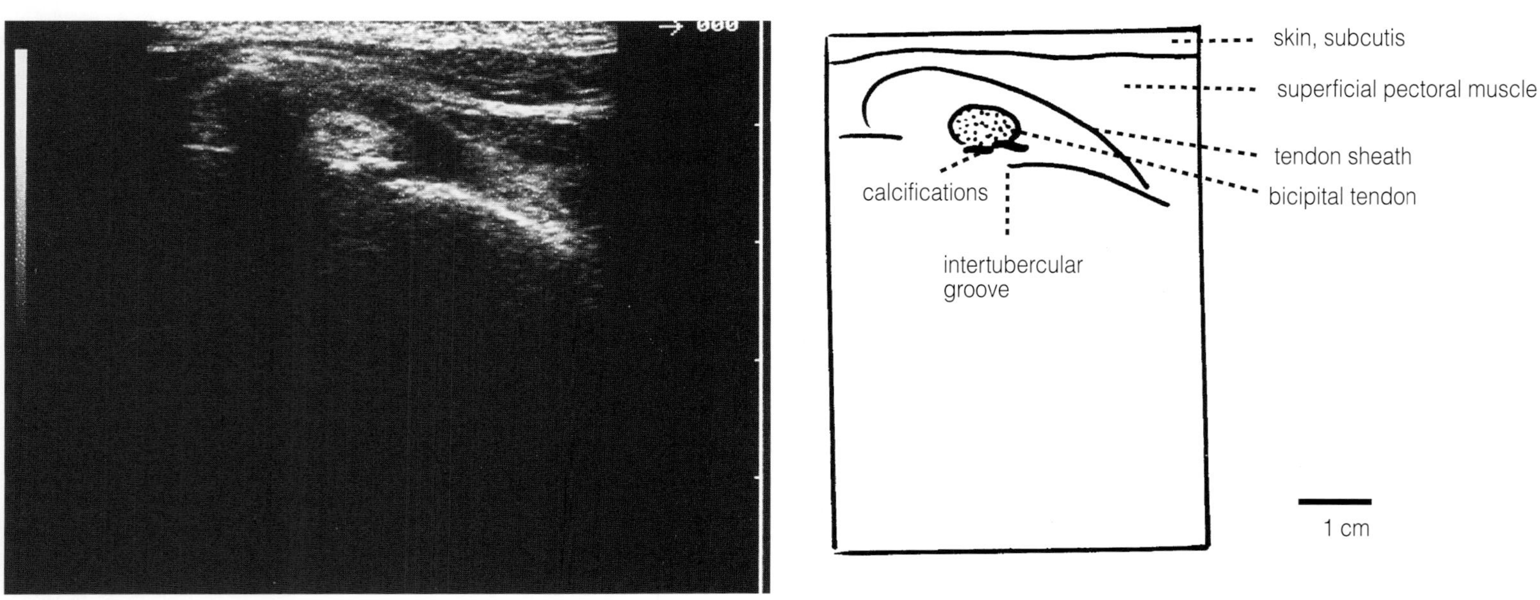

785

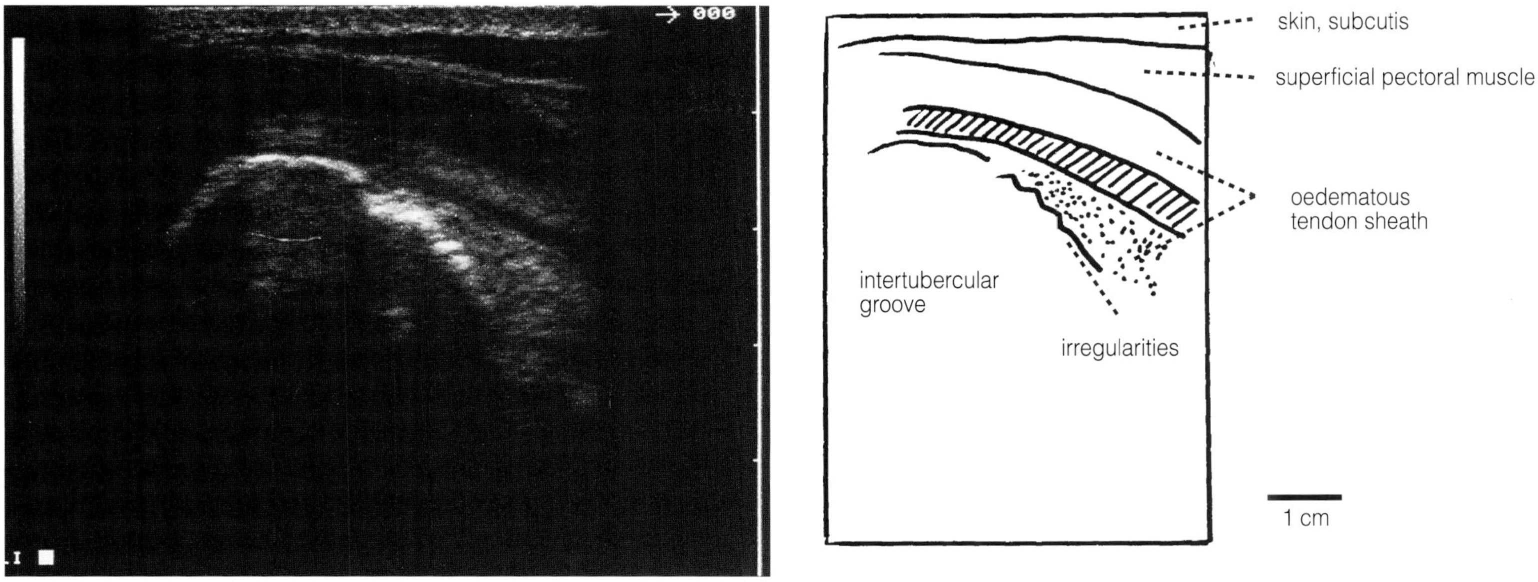

784, 785 Longitudinal (**784**) and transverse (**785**) scans of groove osteophytes in the bicipital tendon area of a dog.

786

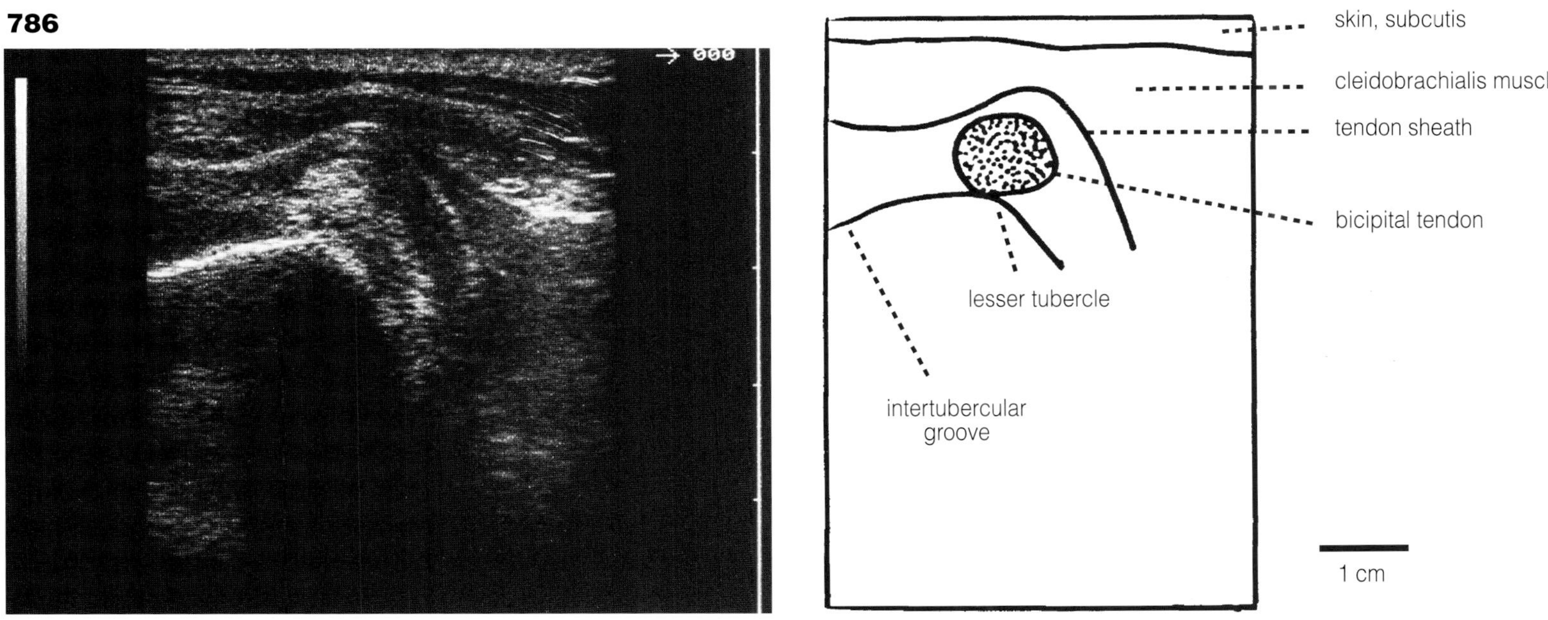

786 Transverse scan of habitual bicipital tendon luxation in a dog.

Tendon Avulsion Fractures

Dislocated tendon avulsion fractures at the apophysis show decreased echogenicity because of oedema or haemorrhaging. Displacement and a change of position are characteristic for avulsion fractures[30] (783). Bone fragments are often identified within the tendon[8].

Instability and movement of the fractured apophysis are recognized during a real-time examination[30]. A haematoma is often seen under the detached periosteum in the acute fracture area. A break in the cortex and the normal hyperechoic, linear bone surface is characteristic for these lesions. The spongiosa does not cause the same acoustic shadowing as the cortex.

Bicipital Groove Osteophytes

Osteophytes are often the cause of bicipital tenopathy. They are produced by degenerative lesions, calcifications or calculi in the intertubercular groove. In a transverse view the groove appears less rounded, with the edges of the tubercles falling off into the groove and producing shadowing[13] (784). Fluid accumulation is usually associated with acute lesions. In a longitudinal view the uniform surface of the humerus changes into a more irregular, wavy cortex (785). Instead of characteristic total reflection, several areas of varying echogenicity are displayed.

Tendon Luxation

Dislocated tendons following intertubercular transverse ligament ruptures are detected in real-time ultrasonography by the tendon being displaced from the groove in a transverse scan[10] (786). The intertubercular transverse ligament itself cannot be identified[10, 23]. An empty intertubercular groove indicates tendon luxation[36]. The tendon rides on the groove edge or on the lesser tubercle[34].

Tenosynovitis

Tenosynovitis may be distinguished in a transverse scan by echogenic foci floating within the tendon sheath and surrounding the bicipital tendon. In a longitudinal scan the intertubercular groove shows bony irregularities[42].

787

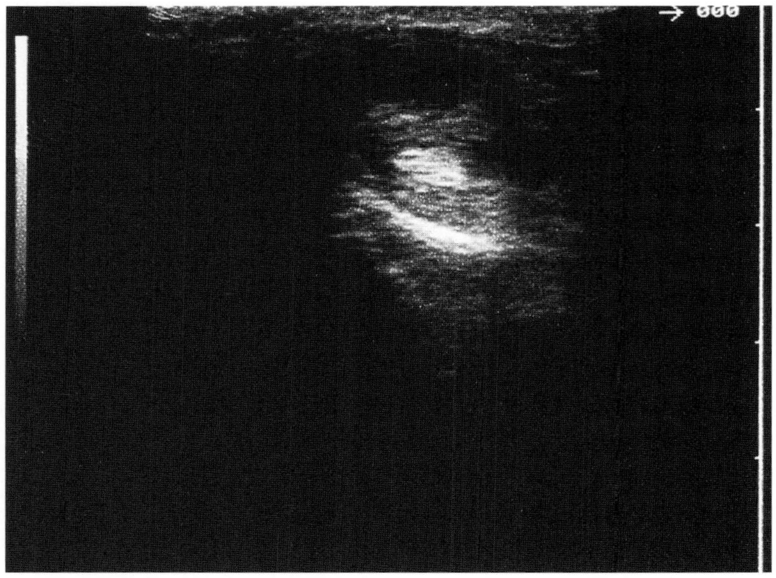

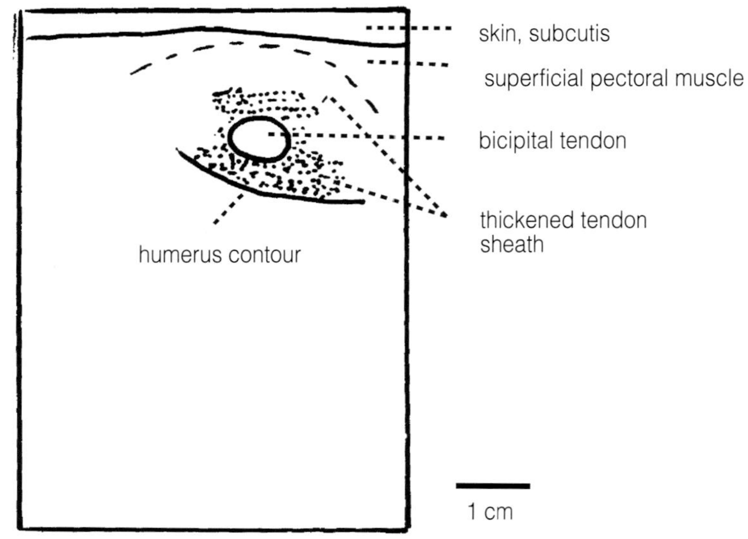

787 Transverse scan of bicipital tendon sheath degeneration in a dog.

788

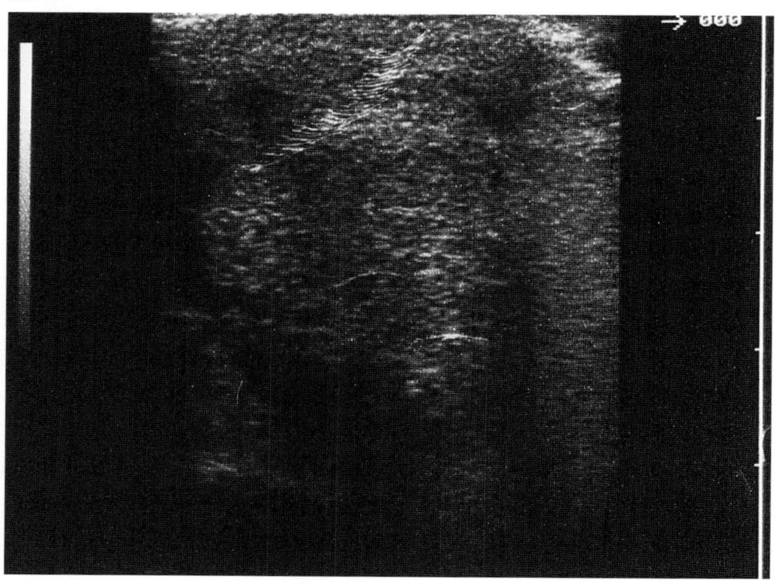

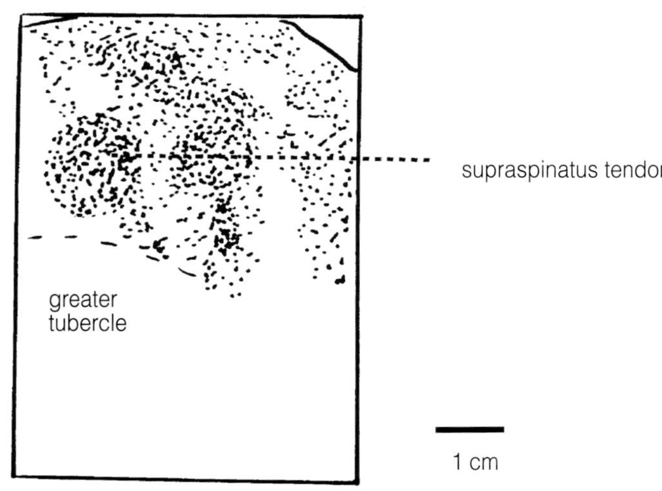

788 Transverse scan of a supraspinatus tendon tumour in a dog.

Degenerative tendon sheath lesions show thickened and oedematous sheaths. The tendon sheath has a similar echogenicity as the tendon itself and it has increased volume (**787**).

Tendon Sheath Effusion

Increased joint effusions affecting the tendon sheath also show a wide anechoic rim around the tendon[34, 35].

Tendon and Tendon Sheath Tumours

Tendon and tendon sheath tumours lead to loss of soft tissue structures in the sonographic image. Echo distribution is nonhomogenous and the size may vary (**788**). Hyperechoic areas representing calcifications may be present.

Common Calcanean Tendon *(Tendo calcaneus communis)*

Anatomy

The common calcanean tendon, often falsely referred to as the Achilles tendon, is composed of the actual Achilles tendon (gastrocnemius tendon), the superficial digital flexor tendon, the triceps sura, the biceps femoris and the semitendinosus tendons. The actual Achilles tendon is comprised of tendons of the gastrocnemius and soleus muscle and it inserts at the calcaneal tuberosity. It is joined by the curved superficial flexor tendon, creating a wide band over the calcaneus. The subtendinous calcaneal bursa is located under this cap.

Ultrasonography of the Normal Common Calcanean Tendon

Due to its length and straight course, the common calcanean tendon is easily examined ultrasonographically (**789, 790**). A stand-off pad is necessary to visualize this superficial tendon. A hypoechoic area is seen directly proximal to the calcaneal tuberosity when scanning the common calcanean tendon, since the inserting tendons are not met by perpendicular sound waves. By changing the scanning angle, these tendon portions also become echogenic[25]. The separate portions of the common calcanean tendon are occasionally differentiated by their course.

The subcutaneous and calcaneal bursae are recognized ultrasonographically only when they are enlarged. Fatty tissue between

789

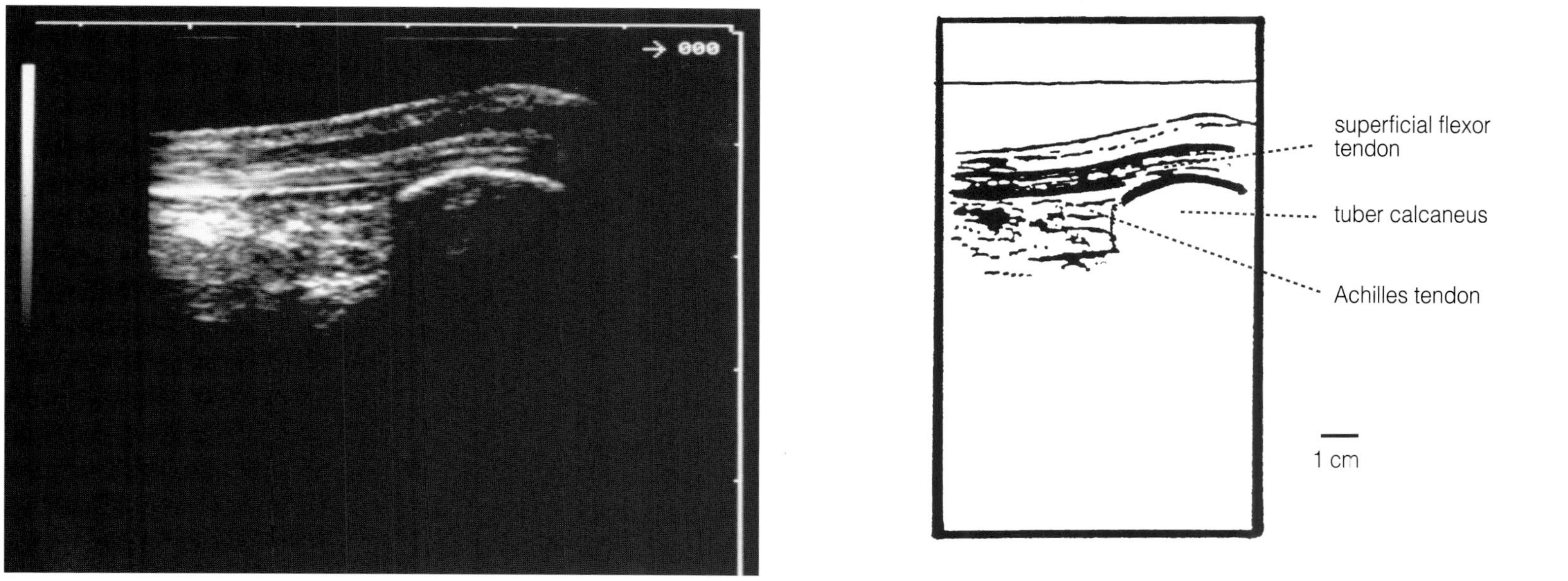

790

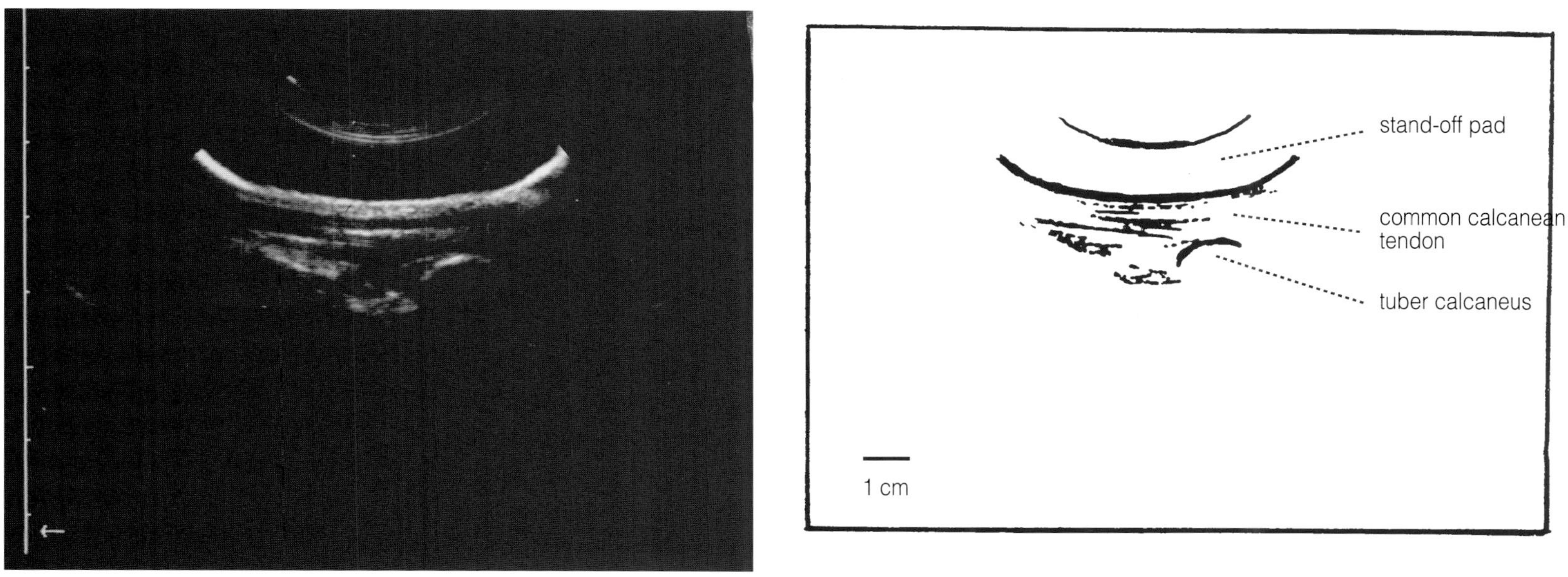

789, 790 Linear (**789**) and sector (**790**) sonograms of a normal common calcanean tendon of a dog in longitudinal views.

791

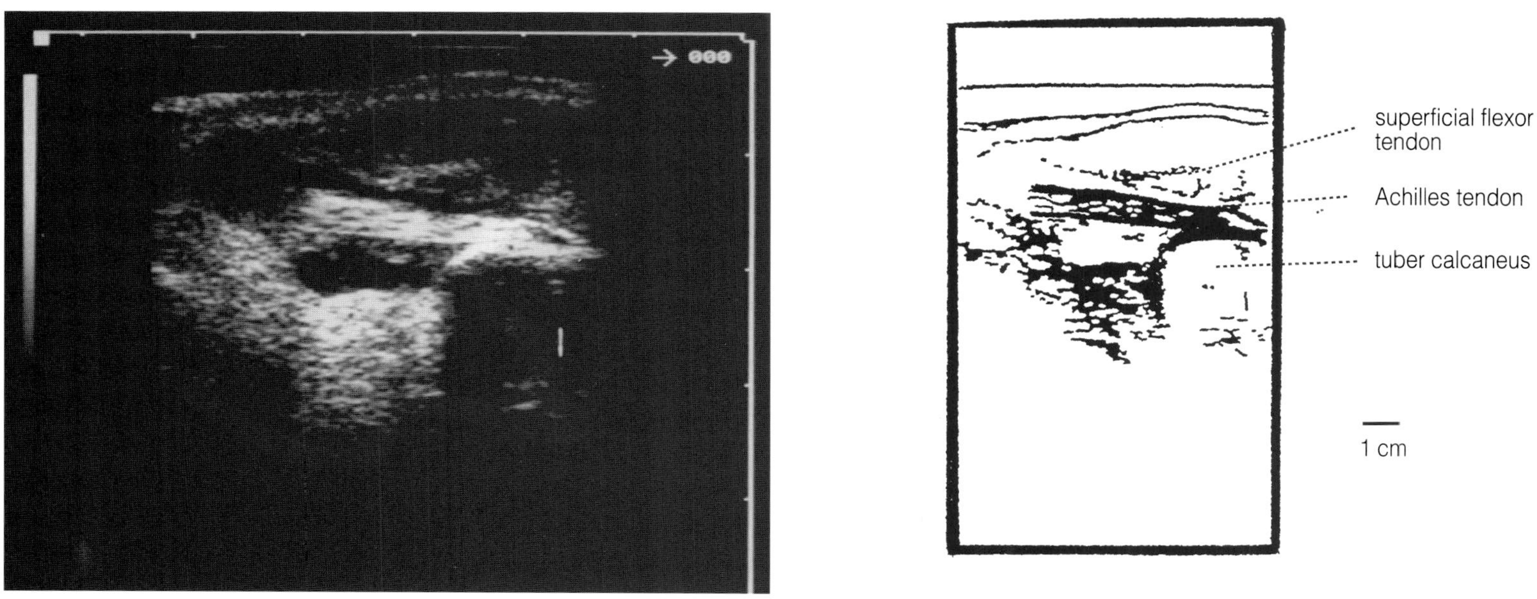

791 Longitudinal view of an elongated superficial flexor tendon with a ruptured Achilles tendon in a dog.

792

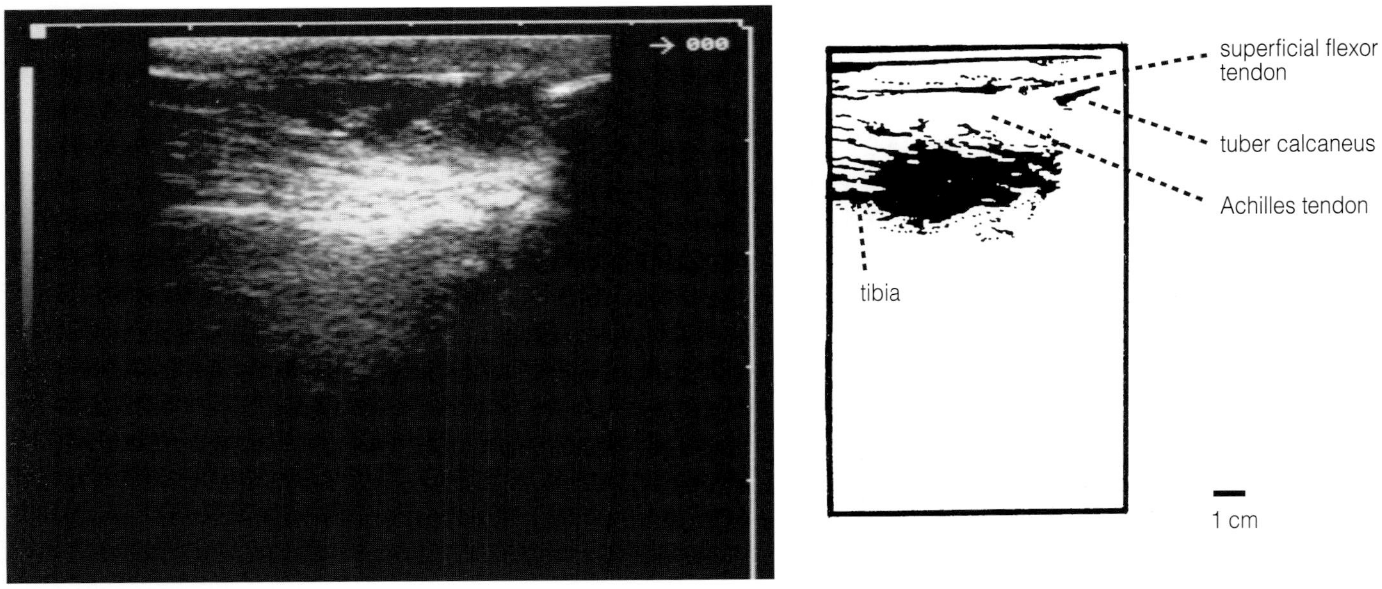

792 Longitudinal scan of a ruptured Achilles tendon with intact superficial flexor tendon in a cat.

793

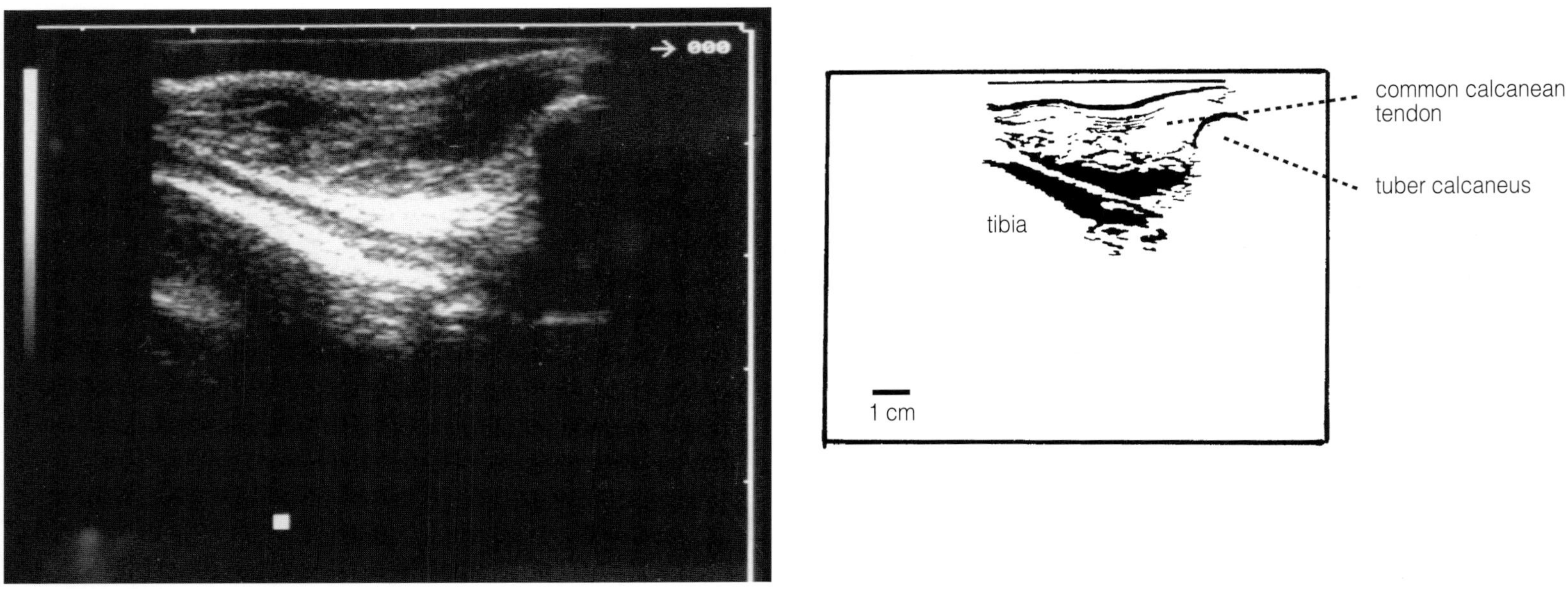

793 Normal healing process following a rupture of the common calcanean tendon in a dog.

the common calcanean tendon, the calcaneus and the tibia is hypoechoic and irregular. Bone surfaces of the tibia, talus and calcaneus are seen as hyperechoic linear structures with distal acoustic shadowing.

Ultrasonography of Complete and Partial Common Calcanean Tendon Rupture

Complete tendon tears show typical clinical symptoms as well as a characteristic sonogram of the tendon fragments. The fragments move apart within the intact tendon sheath in a real-time image. The space in between is filled with hypoechoic fluid (**791**). The parallel echogenic fibre structure is disrupted. Haematoma is present in subacute cases.

Ultrasonography is helpful in diagnosing partial ruptures. The echogenicity of the tendon is decreased with a loss of the parallel structure (**792**). Echo distribution is non-homogenous. The tendon is thickened in this area. A hypoechoic rim surrounds the tendon with effusion in the tendon sheath. Tendon fragments are club-like and shaggy[9, 25].

Ultrasonography is useful for planning and monitoring treatment. A healing tendon becomes thickened with a swollen spindly appearance (**793**). Haematoma is resorbed, which changes the echogenicity during the healing period. Granulation tissue with fibrosis and scarring is seen during this time. Suture material in the shape of hyperechoic reflexes is evident following surgery. A normal longitudinal fibre structure is apparent after six weeks. This structure is less distinct than in a normal tendon[25]. Increased tendon sheath fluid is easily recognized and is seen with peritendinous inflammation.

Bone

Gabriele Gassner and Andreas Engelke

(See also Monitoring Bone Healing with B-Mode Ultrasonography, page 371; Ultrasonographic Usefulness and Limitations in Monitoring Secondary Fracture Healing, page 377.)

794

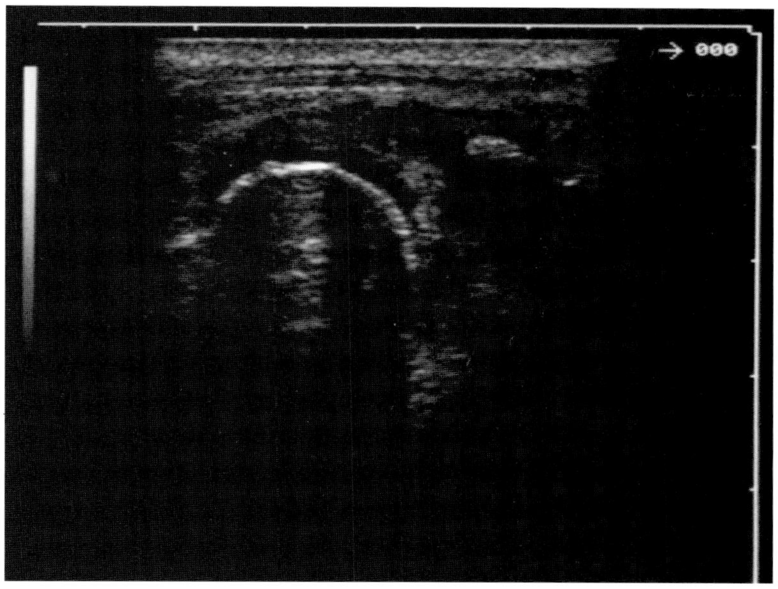

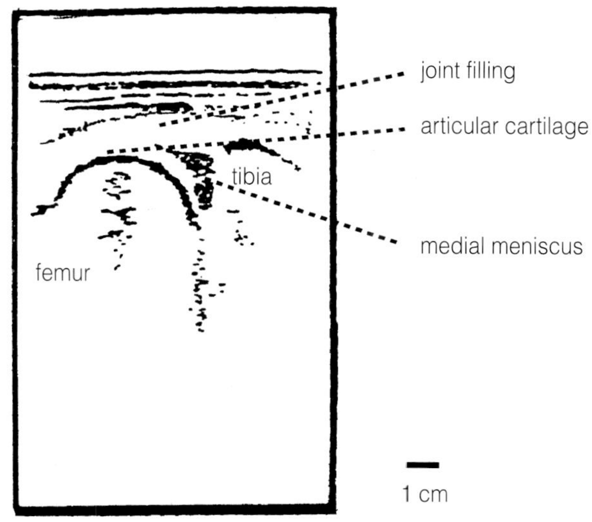

794 Normal femoral condyles in a dog.

795

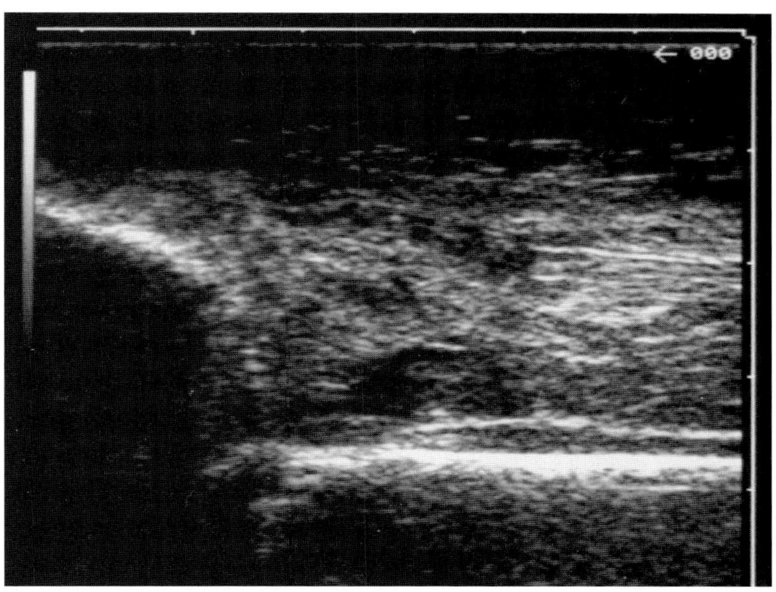

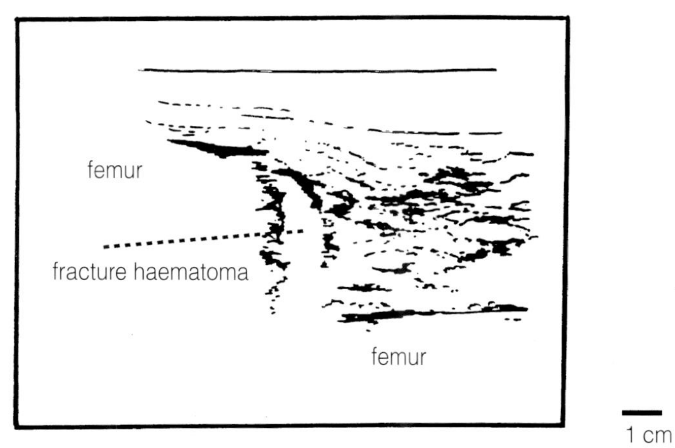

795 Longitudinal scan of a fractured femoral bone in a dog.

Table 46 Ultrasonographic characteristics of bones.

Ultrasonographic bone morphology:
• Hyperechoic line at the interface of muscle, periosteum and cortex with distal acoustic shadowing. • No evaluation of inner structure. • Frequent reverberation artefacts.

Ultrasonography of Normal Bone

The inner structure of bones cannot be visualized because of sound wave reflection and absorption (see *Table 46*). Evaluation of the bone surface is only possible in an exact perpendicular sou... beam. Oblique or slanted bone surfaces, such as the femoral condyles, produce poorly defined, hypoechoic reflections (**794**). Artefacts may mimic structural defects.

Ultrasonography of Bone Lesions

Fractures

Fractures, especially of long bones, may be distinguished ultrasonographically (**795**). Ultrasonography does not replace radiography, but it offers additional information on soft tissue trauma, haemorrhaging within the fracture site, periosteal detachment, and granulation tissue with older fractures. Ultrasonography is superior to radiography in detecting some bone fractures, such as fractures in the sternum (see Monitoring Bone Healing with B-Mode Ultrasonography, page 371). Complications associated with fractures, such as infections or osteomyelitis, may be diagnosed sonographically by their secondary lesions in muscles and periosteum, and by the presence of haematomas.

796

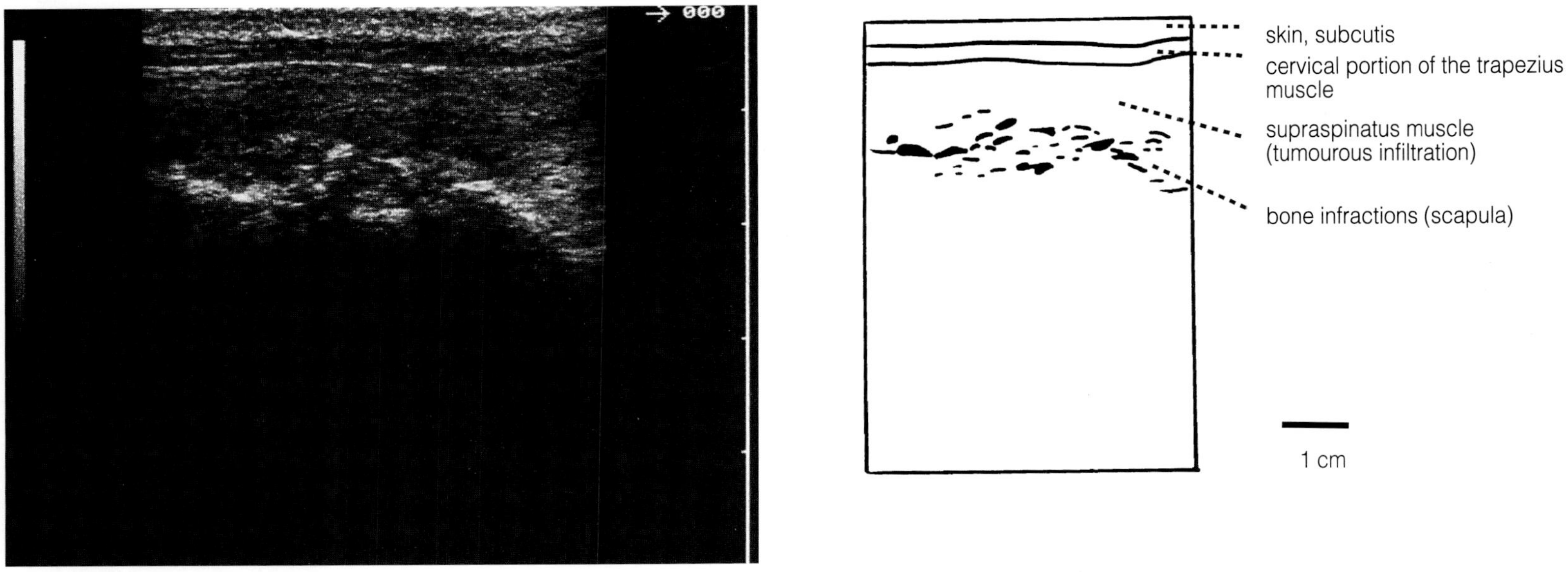

796 Longitudinal view of a bone tumour in the scapula of a dog.

797

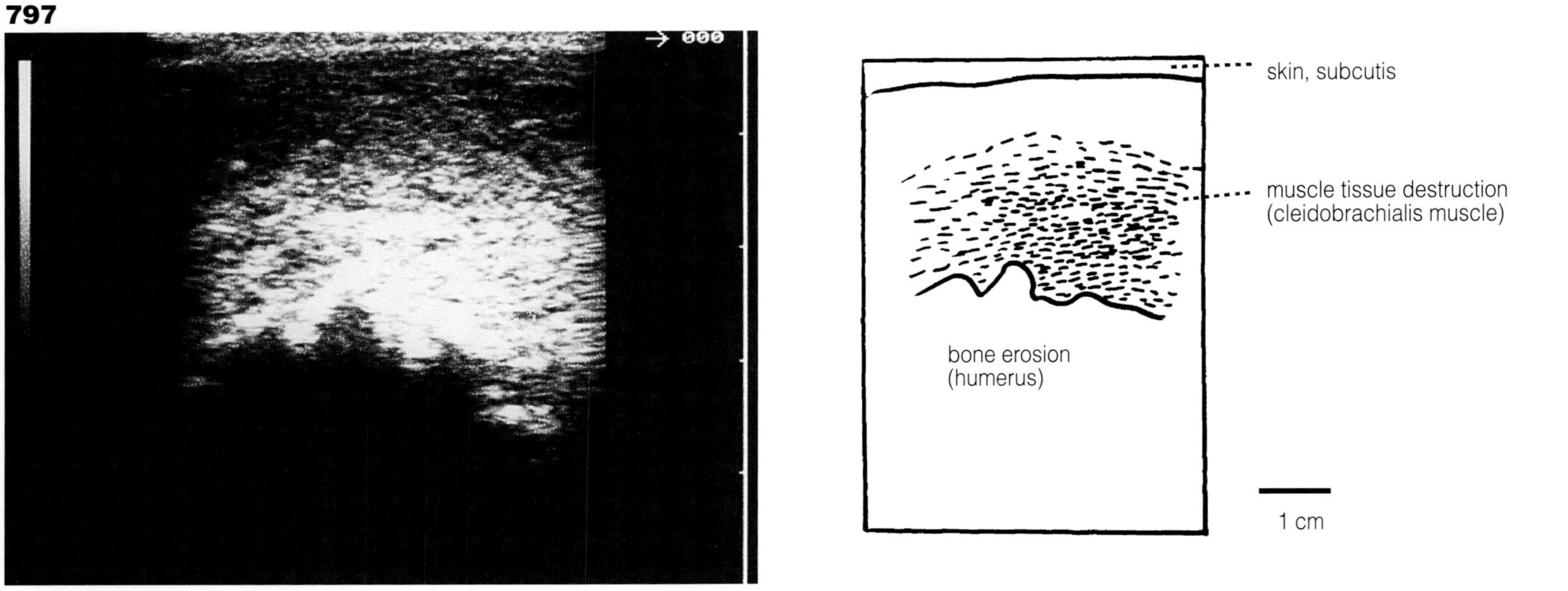

797 Longitudinal view of a bone tumour in the humerus of a dog.

Tumours

Bone tumours are usually detected on radiographs, although information on associated soft tissue masses cannot be gained with this imaging method. Ultrasonography is advantageous in this area. Apart from the superficial, rubble-like, destructive bone lesions with cortical infractions, ultrasonography is able to distinguish soft tissue lesions (**796, 797**). Osteolysis allows visualization of the spongiosa. Ultrasonography cannot differentiate the finer structure of a tumour, but it assists in determining treatment and prognosis.

Joints

Basic Joint Ultrasonography

Andreas Engelke, Gabriele Gassner, Carolyn Döhner and Jan-Gerd Kresken

Ultrasonography visualizes all non-bony structures in the joint area, including the joint cavity and capsule and the ligaments, as well as the surrounding muscles and tendons. The difficulty is in finding the optimal scanning angle. The small size of these struc-

798

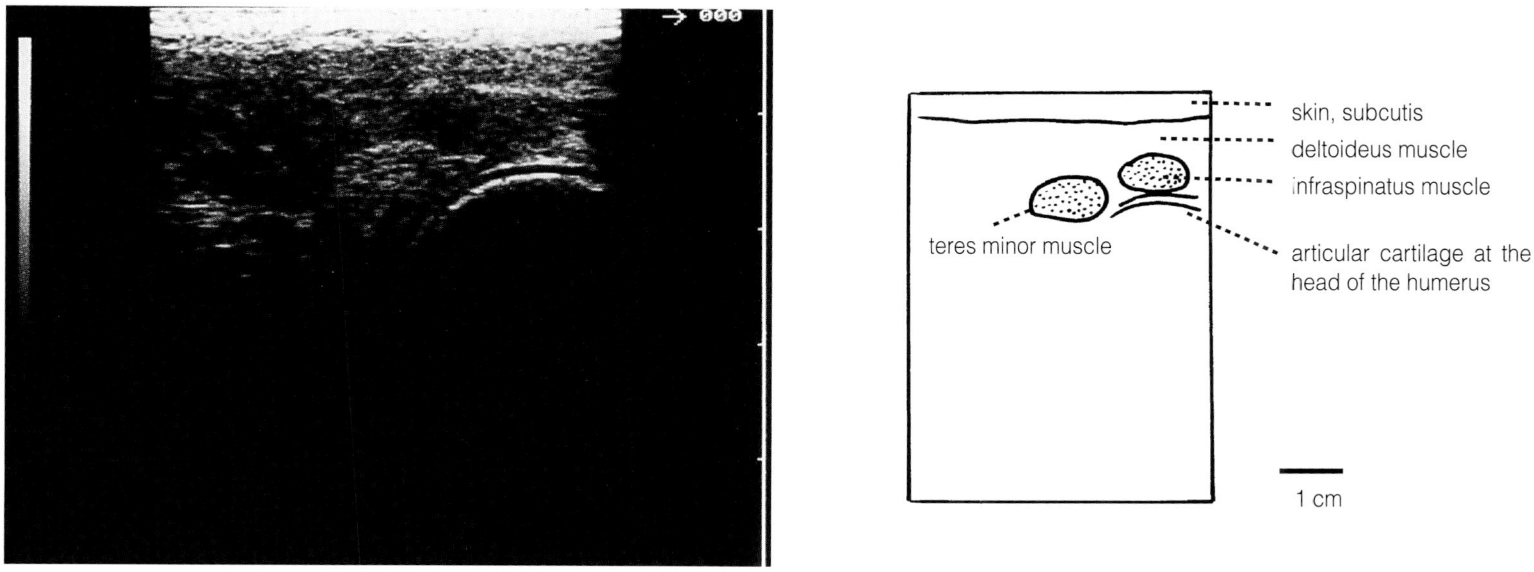

798 Normal shoulder joint in a dog.

tures, their proximity to bones and the choice of transducer limit their visualization.A definite indication for arthrosonography is thickened joints without clear radiological findings.

Joint evaluation must be made with the sound beam perpendicular to the bone surface; this is seen as an echogenic line and distal shadowing. Rounded bone surfaces, such as the femoral condyles, produce irregular echoes (**794**). The hyaline articular cartilage with its fluid contents forms a thin hypoechoic rim superficial to the bone. Evaluation of cartilage surface and thickness is also only possible in a perpendicular sound beam. Cartilage defects may be seen on the humerus head or femoral condyles in the form of osteochondritis dissecans. The acoustic window must be adequate for a good image, which is often difficult. Fibrous cartilage appears more echogenic than hyaline cartilage, because of its histological structure[17]. Joint effusions are easily detected as anechoic to hypoechoic areas in the joint cavity. Haematogenous or purulent joint effusions contain cells, which produce more or less echogenic reflections.

Shoulder Joint *(Articulatio humeri)*

Gabriele Gassner

Ultrasonography of the Normal Shoulder Joint

The shoulder is surrounded and stabilized by several muscles and tendons. Tendons of the supraspinatus, infraspinatus and deltoid muscles are found laterally. Insertions of the subscapularis and teres minor muscles are medial, while the biceps tendon is cranial.

The joint may be visualized from a lateral scanning position with the transducer angled craniodistal. The acromion acts as an orientation point. The transducer is applied distal to this area. The contour of the humerus head appears as a half-circle, with a convex, echogenic, smoothly contoured line and distal shadowing. A double lamella is often seen at the surface of the humerus head, enclosing a hypoechoic layer, which represents the articular cartilage (**798**). The diagnostically important caudal areas of the humerus head can be visualized by passive rotation and adduction of the shoulder joint, while keeping the transducer in place.

Scanning the shoulder joint from a cranial position is difficult because of limited transducer application, caused by the protruding greater tubercle. A caudal scanning position is not possible, due to limited space. Ultrasonography of the shoulder joint from the medial aspect is also impossible because of the close fibromuscular attachment of the scapula to the thoracic wall[23].

Ultrasonography of Shoulder Joint Lesions

Ultrasonography allows early detection of osteochondritis dissecans. With this disease the normally echogenic, rounded and smooth humeral head shows irregularities in the caudal portion. As the disease progresses, infractions of the contour of the humeral head appear (**799**). Detached cartilage may be seen as hyperechoic, irregular corpora libera within the joint. Distal acoustic shadowing is present with calcification. Reactive thickening of the capsule and joint effusion are distinguished ultrasonographically[7, 8].

Elbow Joint *(Articulatio cubiti)*

Carolyn Döhner

Anatomy

The canine elbow joint is a congruent hinge joint, composed of the humeral condyles and the proximal portions of the radius and ulna[47] (**800**). The medial portion of the humeral condyle, the trochlea humeri, articulates with the ulna, while the lateral condyle, the capitulum humeri, articulates with the radius[4]. The ulna bears only a small portion of the weight compared to the radius[1]. The olecranon of the ulna protrudes above the radius and is thickened proximally at the tuber olecrani. The anconeal

799

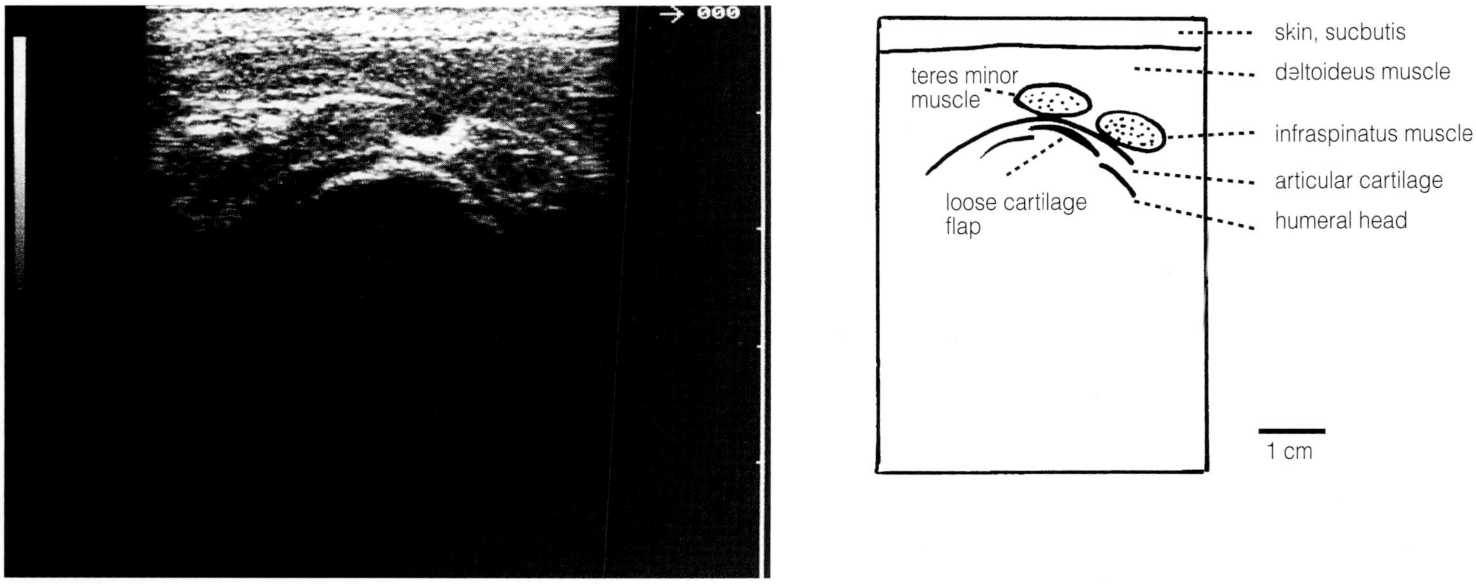

799 Osteochondritis dissecans of the shoulder joint in a dog.

800

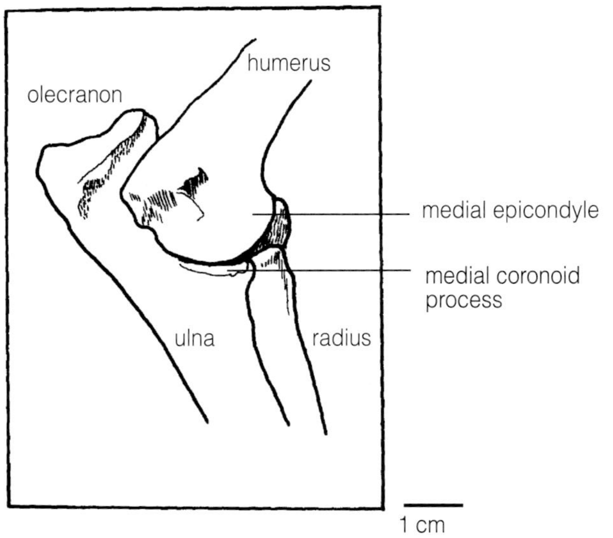

800 Schematic drawing of the elbow joint with a craniomedial scanning position.

process is located cranially, with the trochlear notch distal. The concave ulnar surface articulates with the humerus. The articular surface of the radius extends craniodistal to the bilateral coronoid processes. The medial coronoid process is more prominent than the lateral one[2]. The coronoid processes increase the surface area of the joint with the humerus and take up 20–25% of the weight from the humerus[5].

The elbow joint consists of the humeroradialis joint, the humeroulnaris joint and the proximal radioulnaris joint[4].

Ultrasonography of the Normal Elbow Joint

A 7.5 MHz linear transducer is necessary for ultrasound of the medial portion of the elbow joint. A stand-off pad allows the probe to be applied on an even surface, especially in smaller dogs. The dog lies on the limb to be examined, which should be slightly flexed. The joint is visualized from the medial aspect. Two scanning positions are sufficient to image the elbow joint:

The transducer is placed craniomedial to the joint, using ample amounts of ultrasound gel. A longitudinal plane is produced, corresponding with the axis of the joint. The medial portion of the humeral condyle, consisting of the humeral trochlea and the epicondyle, assists orientation (**800**). The articular space is displayed as an anechoic narrowing between the trochlea and the medial coronoid process in the sonogram. Bony structures appear as highly echogenic lines. Reverberation artefacts are often helpful in identifying the intra-articular space. Bones are covered by the superficial digital flexor muscle, partially by the flexor carpi radialis muscle and by the humeral head of the deep digital flexor muscle.

Examination of the anconeal process is performed by placing the transducer caudally on the flexed joint. The probe is parallel to the humerus. A caudodistal view of the joint is obtained with this technique.

Ultrasonography of Elbow Joint Lesions

Lesions diagnosed with the help of ultrasonography include osteochondritis dissecans of the humeral trochlea, fragmented coronoid process and ununited or fragmented anconeal process, as well as nutrition-dependent diseases of the elbow joint. Elbow joint lesions are usually recognized by secondary changes such as synovitis and osseous destruction.

Fragmented Coronoid Process

The medial coronoid process is displayed in a craniomedial longitudinal scan. Because of insufficient resolution using a 7.5 MHz transducer, a fissure or thin fracture line that is suspected radiographically may remain undetected. Sonographic secondary lesions, such as joint effusion, may confirm radiographic findings. Joint effusion causes the articular space to appear wider and more visible than the normal side. The annular ligament, which may show oedematous swelling with joint lesions, is often difficult to distinguish (**801**). Ultrasonography is useful in evaluating surrounding soft tissue, which is not seen on radiographs.

Ununited or Fragmented Anconeal Process

The fracture line is easier to visualize ultrasonographically when it is not too close to the joint. The transducer is placed caudal to the joint and parallel to the humerus. The echogenic line of the olecranon with the tuber olecrani is seen. A fracture line is also recognizable. The ununited or fragmented anconeal process often presents with exostoses (**802, 803**). The surrounding soft tissue with the tendinous triceps muscle can also be evaluated.

801

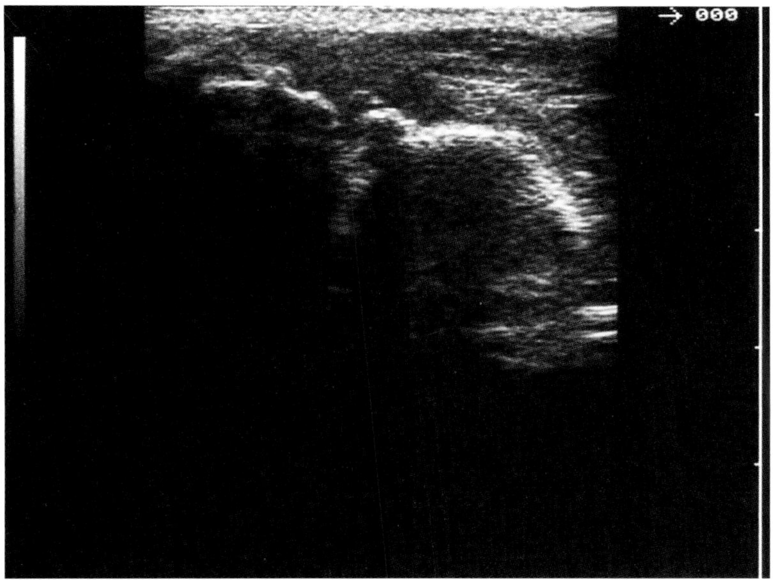

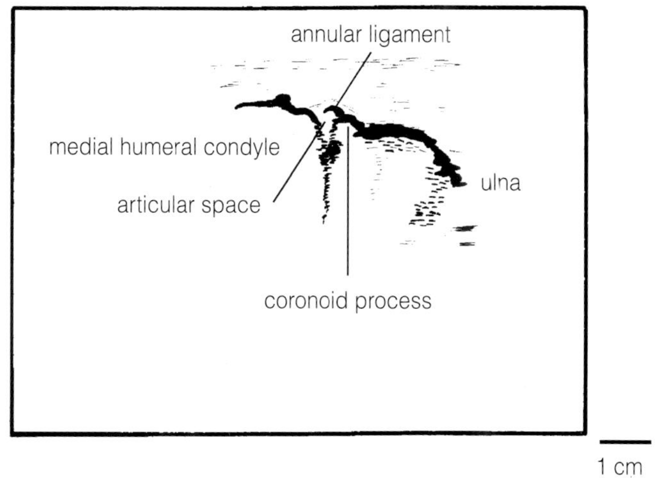

801 Fragmented medial coronoid process in a dog.

802

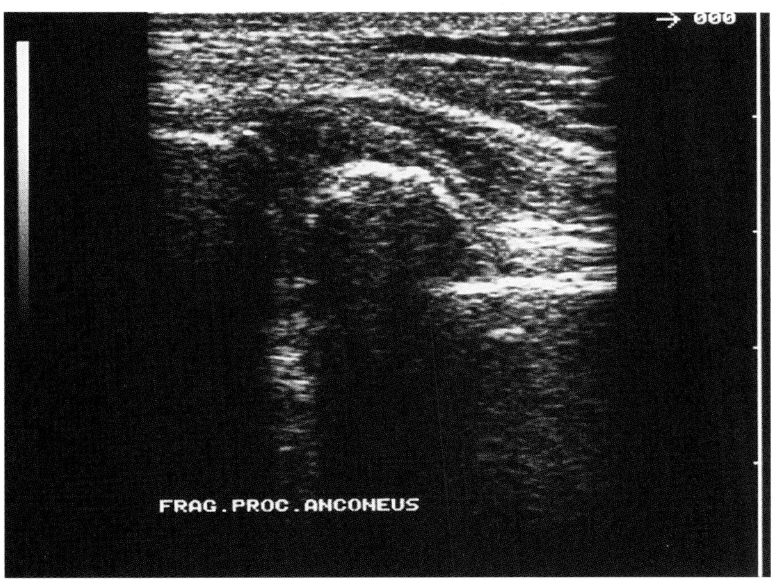

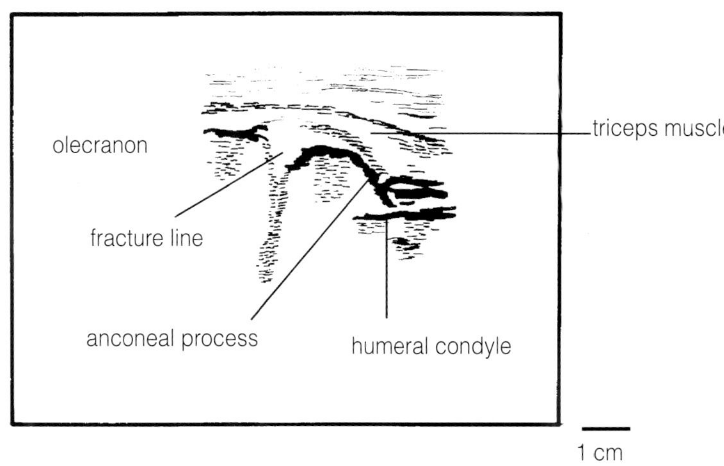

803

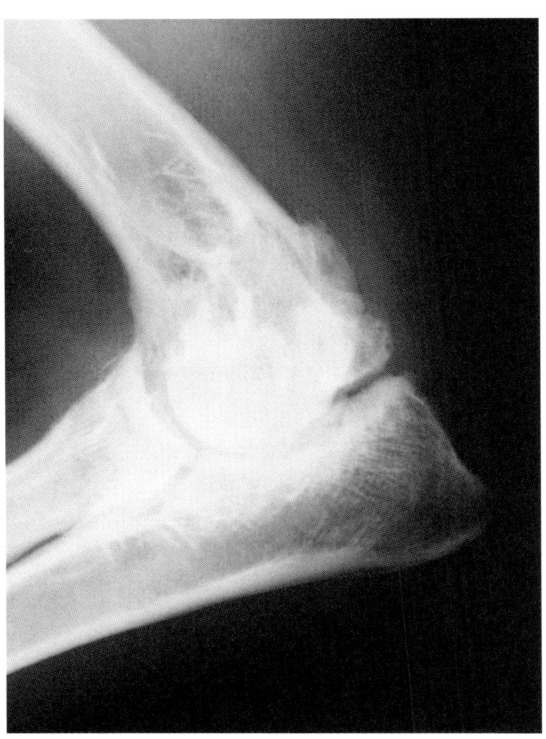

802, 803 Two-dimensional sonogram (**802**) and radiograph (**803**) of an ununited anconeal process in the elbow joint of a dog.

Cubital Bursitis

Inflammation of the olecranon bursa causes exudative swelling of this area. The effusion appears anechoic to hypoechoic in the sonogram. Fibrinous contents with cellular debris are echogenic with possible acoustic shadowing. By compressing the joint, these structures will show movement.

Hip Joint *(Articulatio coxae)*

Jan-Gerd Kresken

In human medicine, ultrasonographic diagnosis of hip dysplasia and luxation in infants, as well as determination of intra-articular effusion, is widely recognized and is the non-invasive method of choice[11, 12, 16, 50]. The canine hip joint is easily accessible with ultrasound because of the large natural stand-off (muscles, fat, etc.), similar to the shoulder joint. Visualization and evaluation of the canine hip joint is therefore possible.

Hip joint diseases are similar in animals and man. Ultrasonographic visualization of the hip joint in dogs is possible at any age. Articular cartilage on the femoral head or acetabulum may be seen up to week 16 in young animals[27].

804

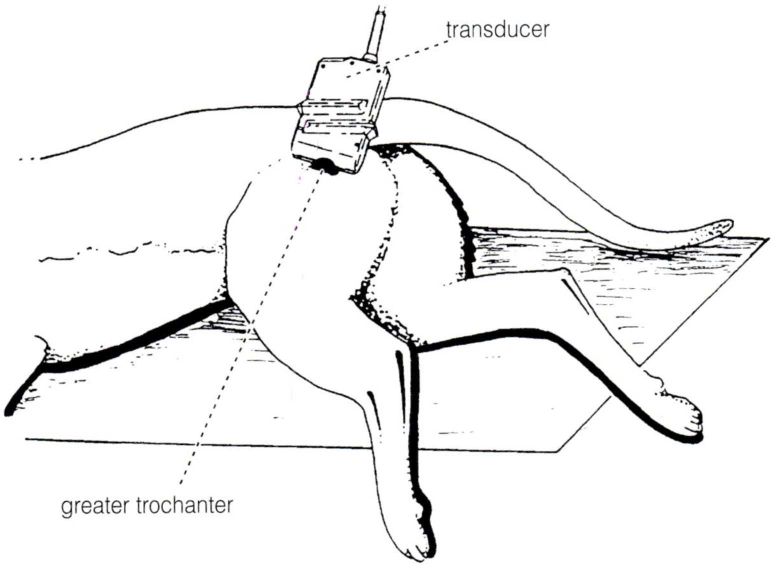

804 Schematic drawing of position I with patient positioning and transducer application.

805

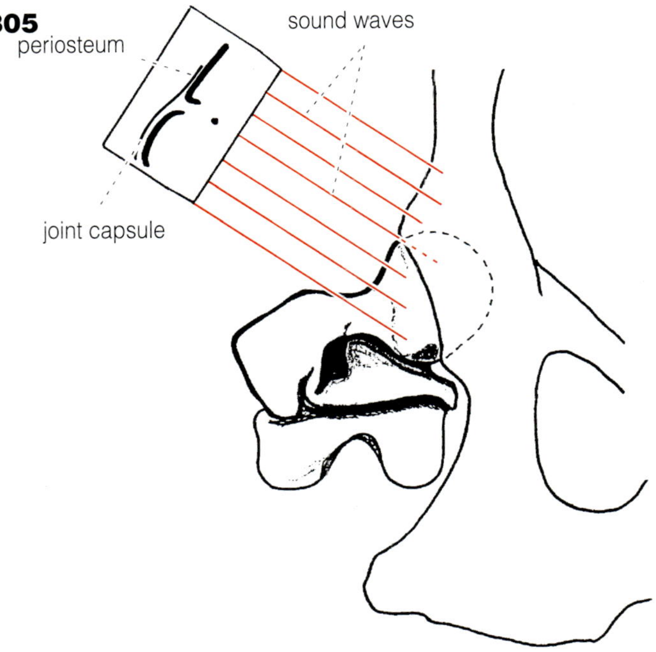

805 Schematic drawing of the anatomical structures and corresponding sonogram with the patient in position I.

806

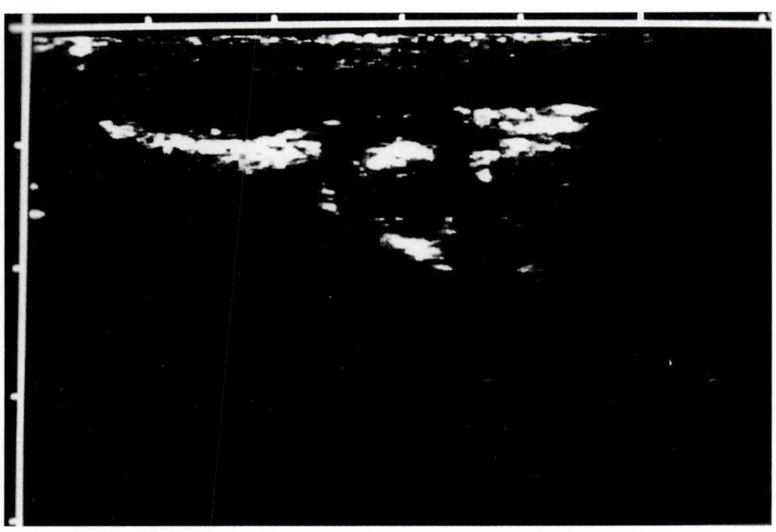

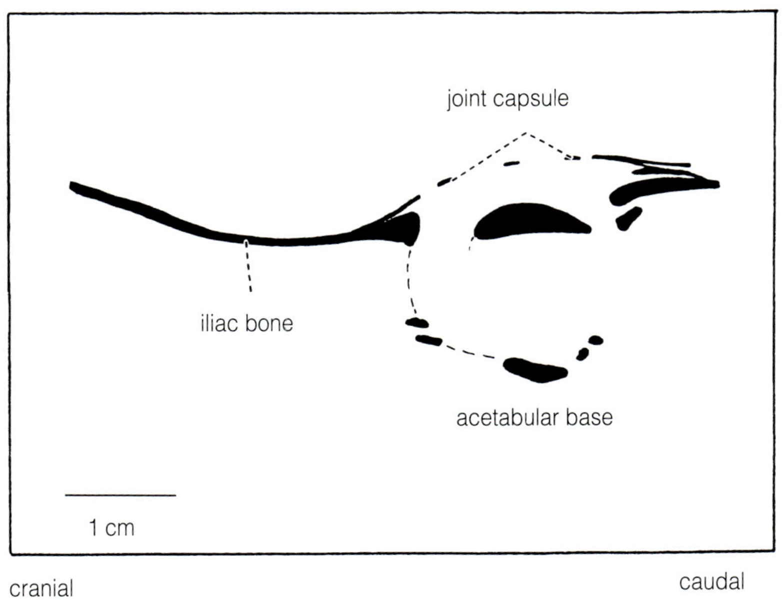

Ultrasonography of the Normal Hip Joint

The hip joint can be scanned from three different patient and transducer positions.

Position I for a lateral scan

The dog is positioned in right lateral recumbency to scan the left hip joint. The limb angle in the hip joint corresponds with that of the normal standing extremity and is 108 ± 8 degrees[35]. The tibia is parallel to the table surface. The lower limb is pulled behind the upper one (804).

The middle of the transducer is placed proximal to the greater trochanter on the clipped skin surface, using coupling gel. The long axis of the transducer is angled in a craniodorsal direction to the iliac bone. The transducer is also angled 45 degrees vertical to the table surface, towards the sagittal plane of the animal. In this scanning position the iliac cortex, as well as the rounded femoral head silhouette, are displayed (805–807).

The skin and subcutis are seen as a thin echogenic line parallel to the top of the image (807). Next, the sound beam passes through the distal portion of the superficial gluteal muscle, transverse to the fibres. The middle gluteal muscle is located deeper, with its fascia and intramuscular tendinous fibres appearing as

807

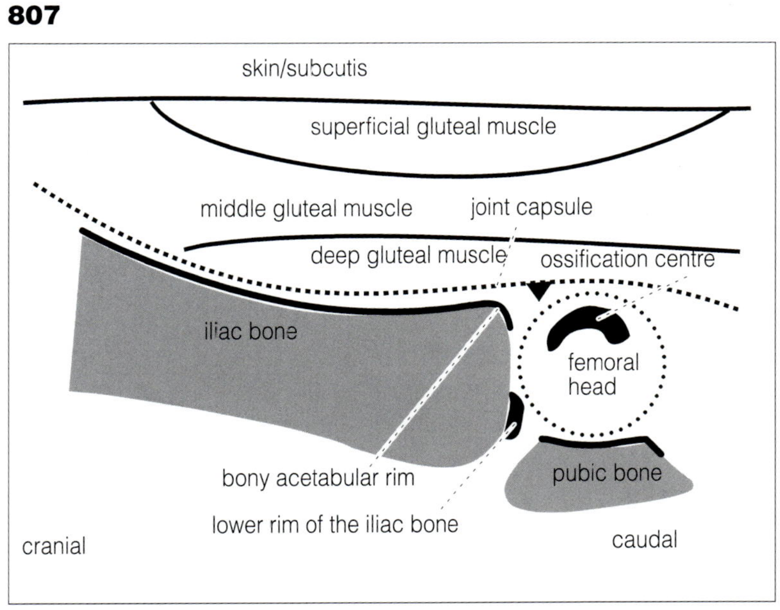

806, 807 Sonogram (**806**) and schematic drawing (**807**) of the right hip joint of a five-week-old dog in a lateral scan.

808

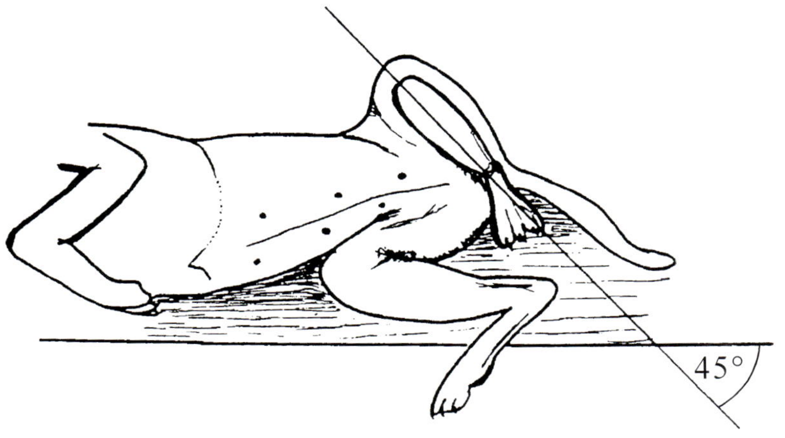

808 Schematic drawing of patient positioning in position II.

809

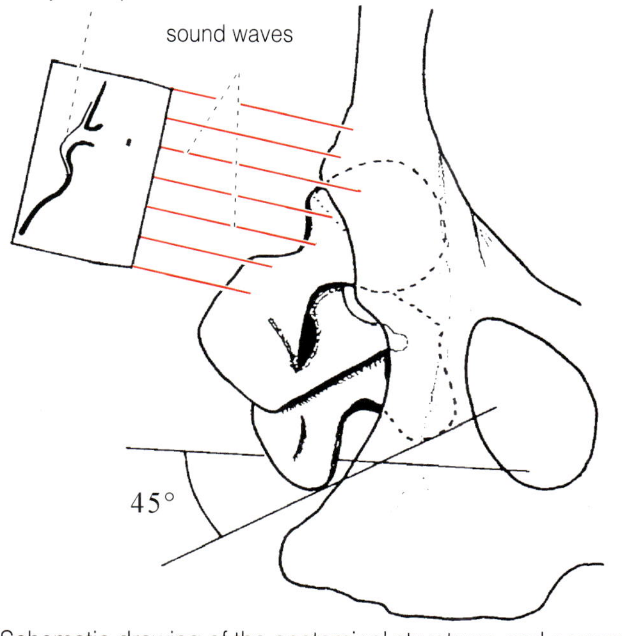

809 Schematic drawing of the anatomical structures and corresponding sonogram with the patient in position II.

810

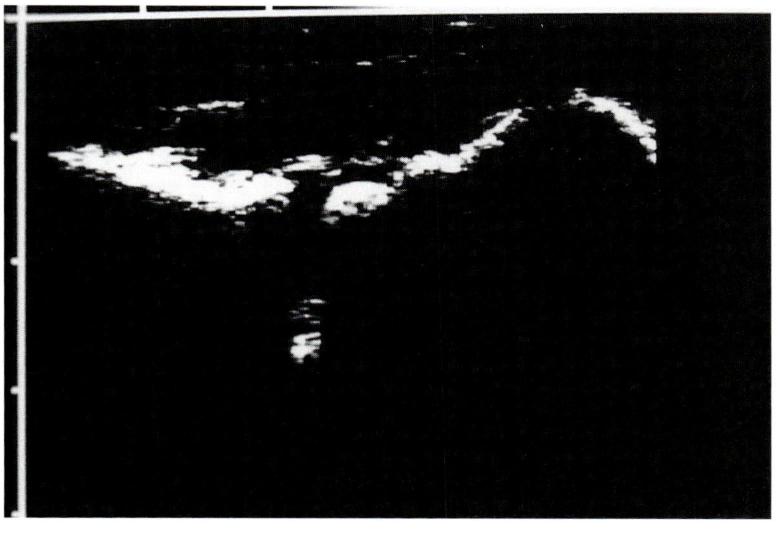

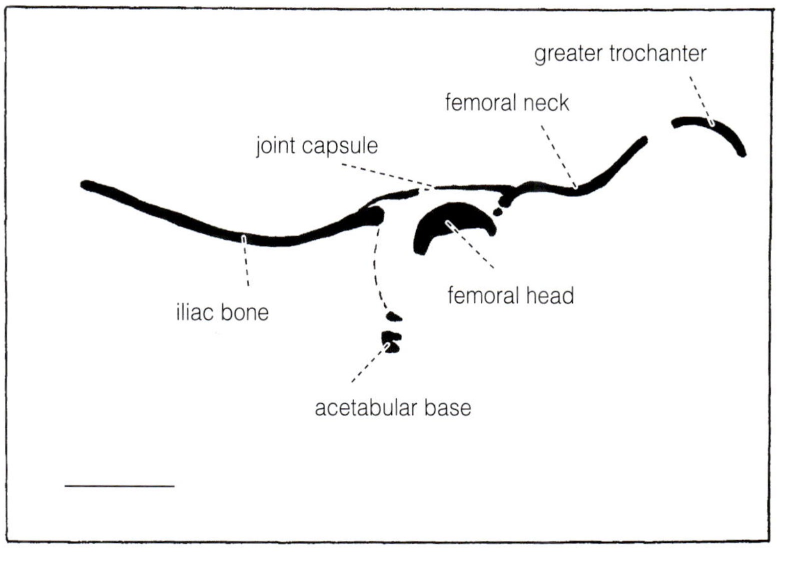

811

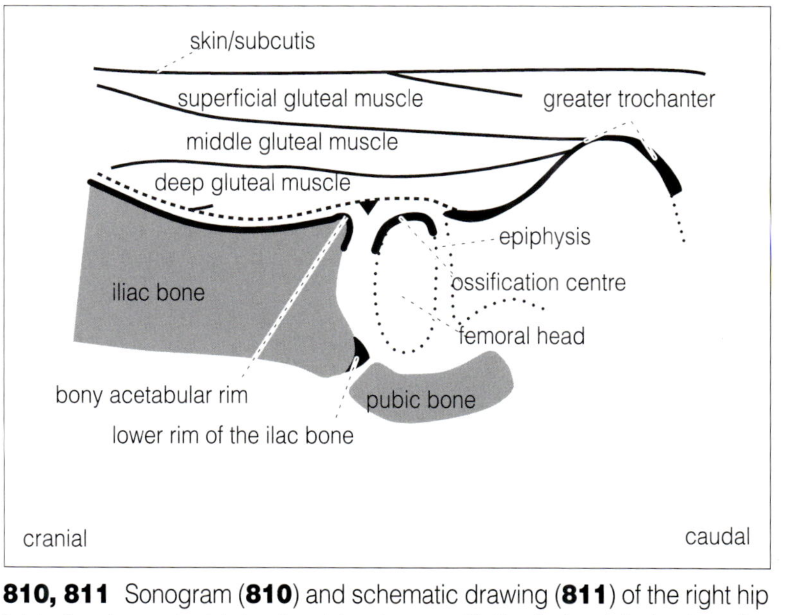

810, 811 Sonogram (**810**) and schematic drawing (**811**) of the right hip joint of a six-week-old dog in a lateral scan with the limb rotated outwards.

parallel echogenic lines running caudally. Muscle fibres are almost horizontal to the direction of the sound beam. Fine echoes, produced by the muscle bellies, are filtered out to give a better view of the joint. The deep gluteal muscle is located medial to the middle gluteal muscle and distally in the image (807). The cranial portion of this muscle lies directly on the slightly concave iliac bone. Caudally, the ischiadic spine portion of the deep gluteal muscle pushes between the middle gluteal muscle and the joint capsule in the direction of the greater trochanter. Two-thirds of the iliac bone length are seen in this image. It shows a regular concave surface with a straight line at the bottom. A wide echogenic band represents the outer cortex and it is already seen in young dogs. This echo also includes periosteum, which acts as an insertion site for the iliac portion of the deep gluteal muscle and continues into the joint capsule. The iliac bone is slightly rounded at the caudal margin. A hypoechoic area also continues into the joint capsule. This area represents the cartilaginous, preformed portion of the iliac bone, which later becomes a major part of the acetabular roof (807). A small, polygonal, echogenic structure is seen deeper to this area (806, 807) and this is the lower rim of the iliac bone. The sound waves pass through the fluid-filled joint space, as well as the hyaline cartilage of the femoral head, and thereby produce

812

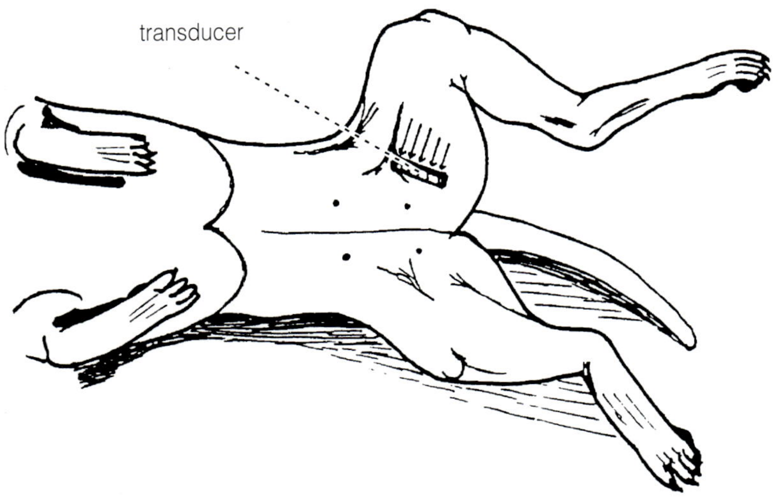

812 Schematic drawing of position III with patient positioning and transducer application.

813

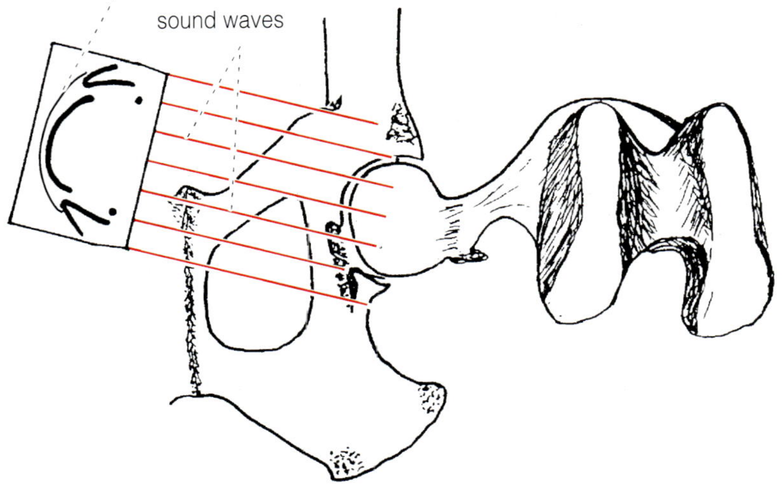

813 Schematic drawing of the anatomical structures and corresponding sonogram with the patient in position III.

a good image of the bottom of the acetabulum, which belongs to the pubic bone. The joint capsule is seen as a slightly convex, echogenic line which continues caudally from the caudal rim of the cartilaginous, preformed acetabular roof. A small, distinct echo is seen at the junction of the hypoechoic area and the joint capsule, also producing a stronger echo than the capsule. This structure represents the acetabular labrum (807).

Ultrasonography of the hip joint is possible in the first week of life. In the first eight weeks the entire acetabulum is easily visualized because of its cartilaginous consistency. With progressive age and calcification, imaging of the acetabulum becomes more difficult. After fourth months of age, the base of the acetubulum can only be distinguished through a narrow articular space.

Position II for a lateral scan with outward rotation

Patient positioning and transducer application are identical to position I, except that the normally angled limb is rotated outwards. The sonographer holds the stifle of the upper limb, so that the tibia is retroverted (turned backwards) in a 45 degree angle to the table surface (808). The greater trochanter is then slightly abducted and turned into the scan area (809).

The concave femoral neck leads into the silhouette of the convex, protruding greater trochanter (810, 811). Decreased contrast settings allow visualization of muscle fascia and septa to their insertion on the lesser trochanter. This is seen especially well if the limb is moved during the examination.

The femoral head is recognized ultrasonographically by the disc-like shape of its ossified epiphyseal centre. Ossification has progressed relatively far by the sixth week, leaving only an image of the outer curve of the epiphysis (810). This echo is not directly connected to any of the surrounding structures. Cranially, the articular space separates the femoral head from the acetabulum. The femoral head contour is separated dorsally from the joint capsule by articular fluid. Caudally, the bone contour shows a hypoechoic interruption, which represents the cartilaginous epiphyseal disc. Smaller calcified areas may be seen deep within the cartilage.

Position III for an inguinal scan

The dog is placed in dorsal recumbency. At the same time the examined limb is abducted at an angle of 45 degrees (812). The anterior part of the transducer is placed transversely to the palpable femoral canal in the direction of the stifle skin fold.

The sound waves pass medially through the skin and muscles, including the gracilis muscle and the pectineus et adductor longus muscle, as well as the adductor muscles (814, 815). The outer cortex of the iliac bone is seen as an echo leading dorsally in the cranial part of the image. The iliopsoas muscle is located directly above the iliac bone.

In this position the iliac and ischiadic bones appear as part of the acetabulum (813). The lower rim of the iliac bone leads into the lower ischiadic rim, with one interruption. This interruption is at the growth suture between the two bones (815). The acetabular area of the ischiadic bone does not surround the femoral head as far laterally as the iliac bone (814). The joint capsule is always seen as a distinct convex, band-like echo in the ultrasound image. In this position the transverse deep femoral artery and the longitudinal medial circumflexa femoris artery assist the sonographer in setting standardized examination planes (815).

The scanning plane and resulting sonogram are demonstrated by projecting the ultrasound image on a radiograph on a scale of 1:1. The silhouette on the radiograph in a ventrodorsal view is comparable to the sonogram in position II. Generally, projections of ultrasound images on radiographs, producing a summation image, are problematic but they should help in understanding the scan. In this example the hip joint structures are congruent (816). The contours of the iliac bone and the femoral head and neck, as well as the greater trochanter, are nearly identical.

The three scanning positions described are helpful in diagnosing pathological changes of hip joints in young and adult dogs.

Ultrasonography of Hip Joint Disease

Examples of common hip joint lesions found ultrasonographically are hip joint luxation, arthritis and Legg-Calvé-Pérthes disease.

Traumatic Coxofemoral Luxation

With cranial coxofemoral luxation the completely dislocated femoral head lies in the surrounding muscles. Corresponding with its shape, the femoral head appears as a half-circle above (lateral to) the iliac bone (817). By rotating the limb during the examination, movement of the femoral head is seen within the ruptured muscles.

814

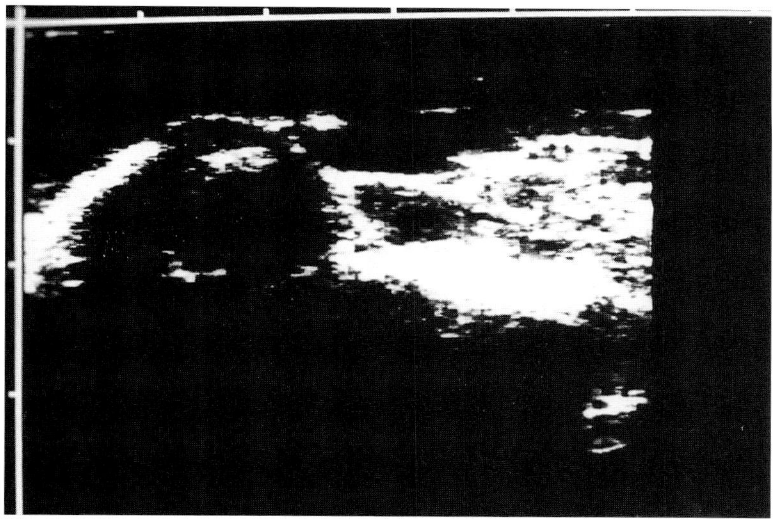

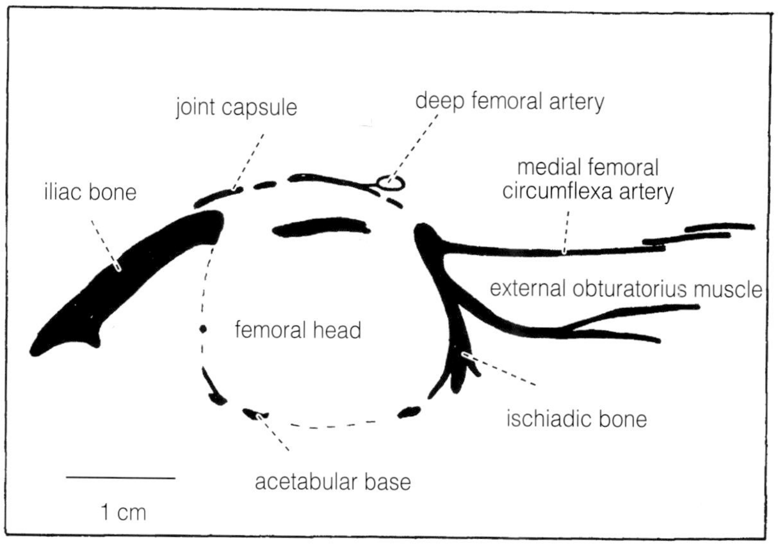

815

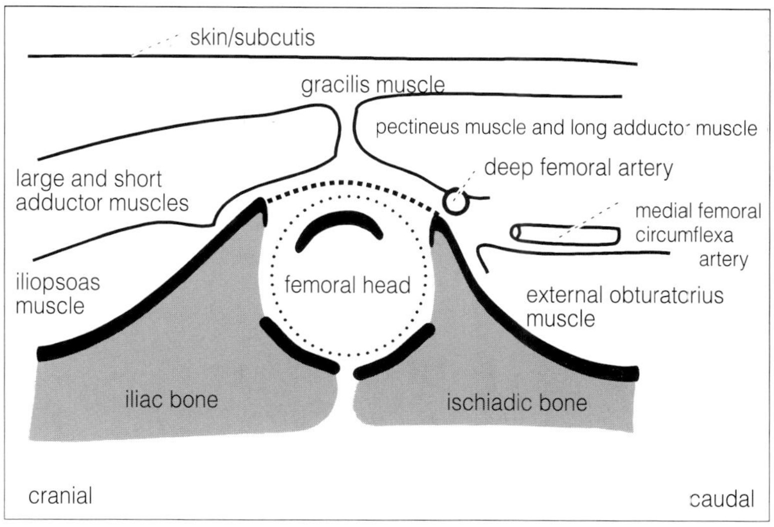

814, 815 Sonogram (**814**) and schematic drawing (**815**) of the right hip joint of a six-week-old dog in an inguinal view.

816

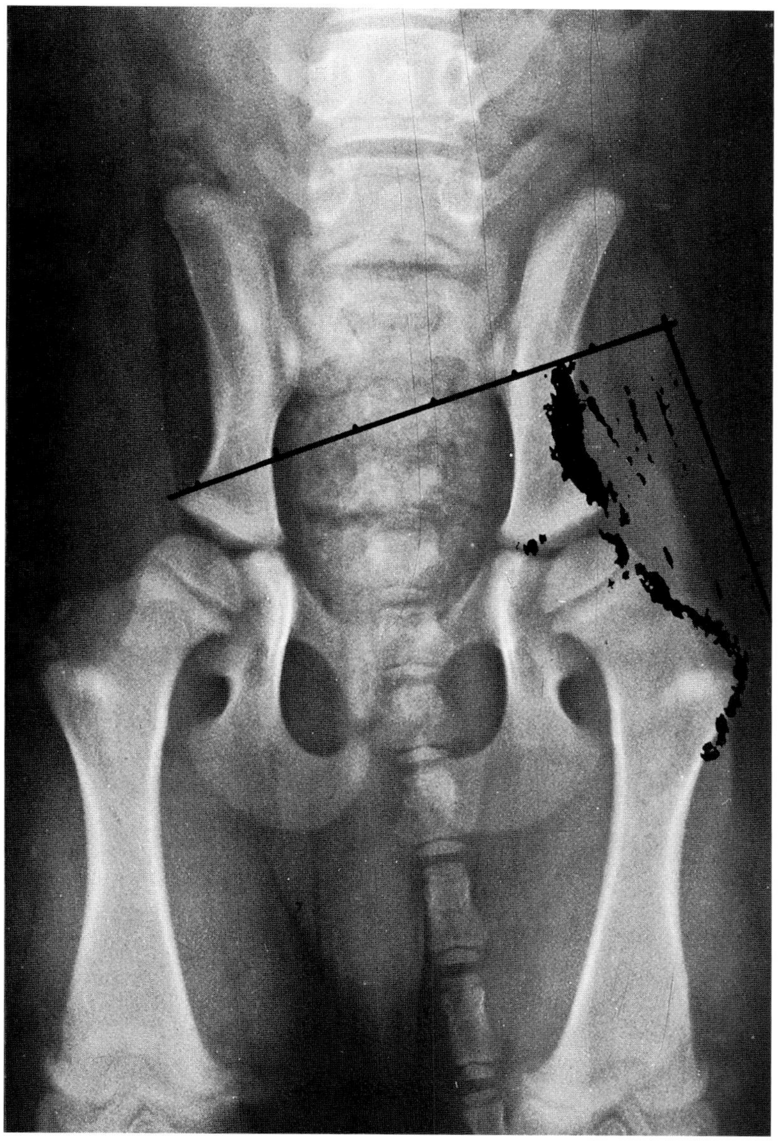

816 Sonogram superimposed on a hip radiograph of an eight-month-old dog.

Degenerative Joint Disease with Hip Dysplasia in Adult Dogs

Degenerative hip joint disease in the adult dog, with changes of the acetabulum, femur and joint capsule, are always visible.

With severe degenerative hip joint disease the acetabulum appears flat (**818**) with an uneven craniodorsal rim and an irregular femoral head. The joint capsule shows no contact with the femoral head and it appears thickened. Joint effusion is usually present (**819**)[49]. Severe arthrosis leads to unstable movement of the animal.

Standardized measurements are described to determine joint capsule thickness[29]. By comparing both hip joints, quantification of joint effusion is possible[27]. Early diagnosis of hip dysplasia in puppies is possible using modified measurements from human medicine. Statistical data on follow-up examinations are not available, which still makes early diagnosis of hip dysplasia difficult[14, 28].

Legg-Calvé-Pérthes Disease

Legg-Calvé-Pérthes disease causes hip joint degeneration. The disease mainly affects the femoral head, which may become necrotic as the disease progresses[33]. Femoral head osteochondrosis is a juvenile disease, appearing in dogs between 3–13 months of age, most often in the 6th and 7th month [32].

During the early stage of the disease, hyperaemia of the surrounding soft tissue may be noticed. The joint capsule becomes thickened and the femoral head is irregular due to pathological fractures of subchondral bone cavities[31]. The contour of the femoral head changes progressively as granulation tissue fills the defects and is then surrounded by bone and causes a deformed femoral head[21, 48].

817

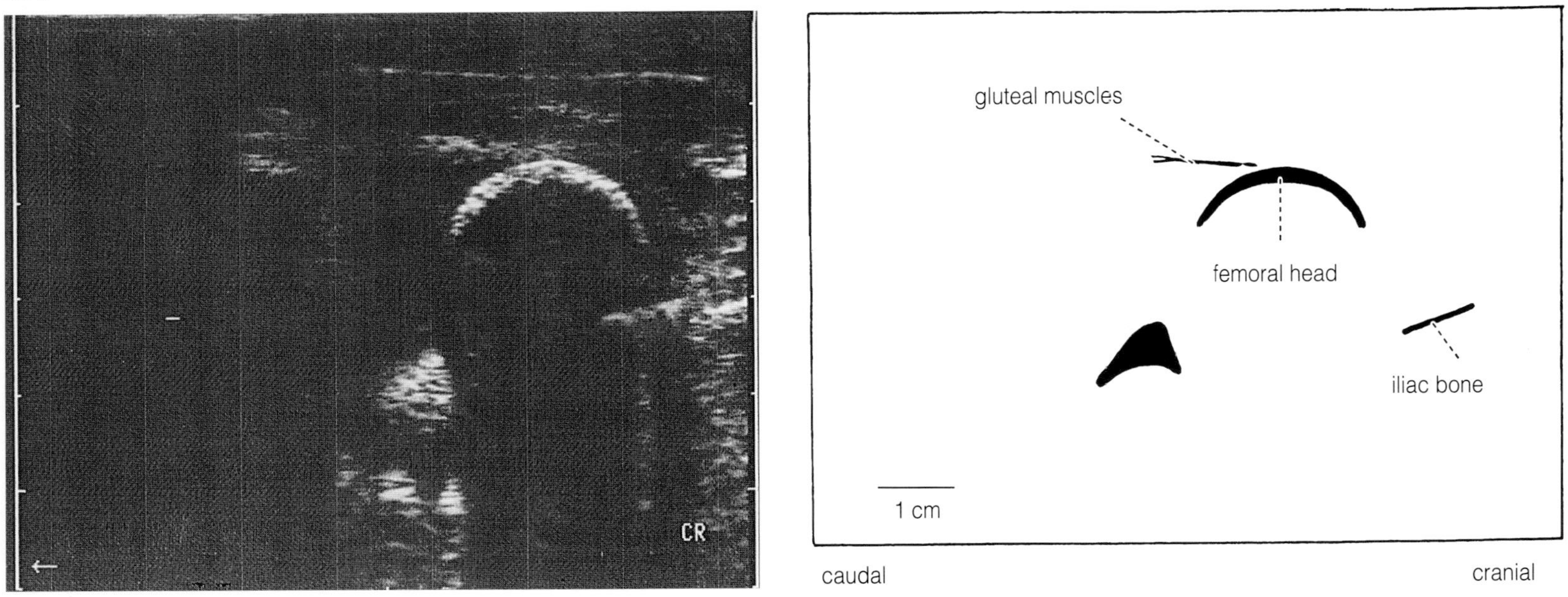

817 Cranial coxofemoral luxation in a dog.

818

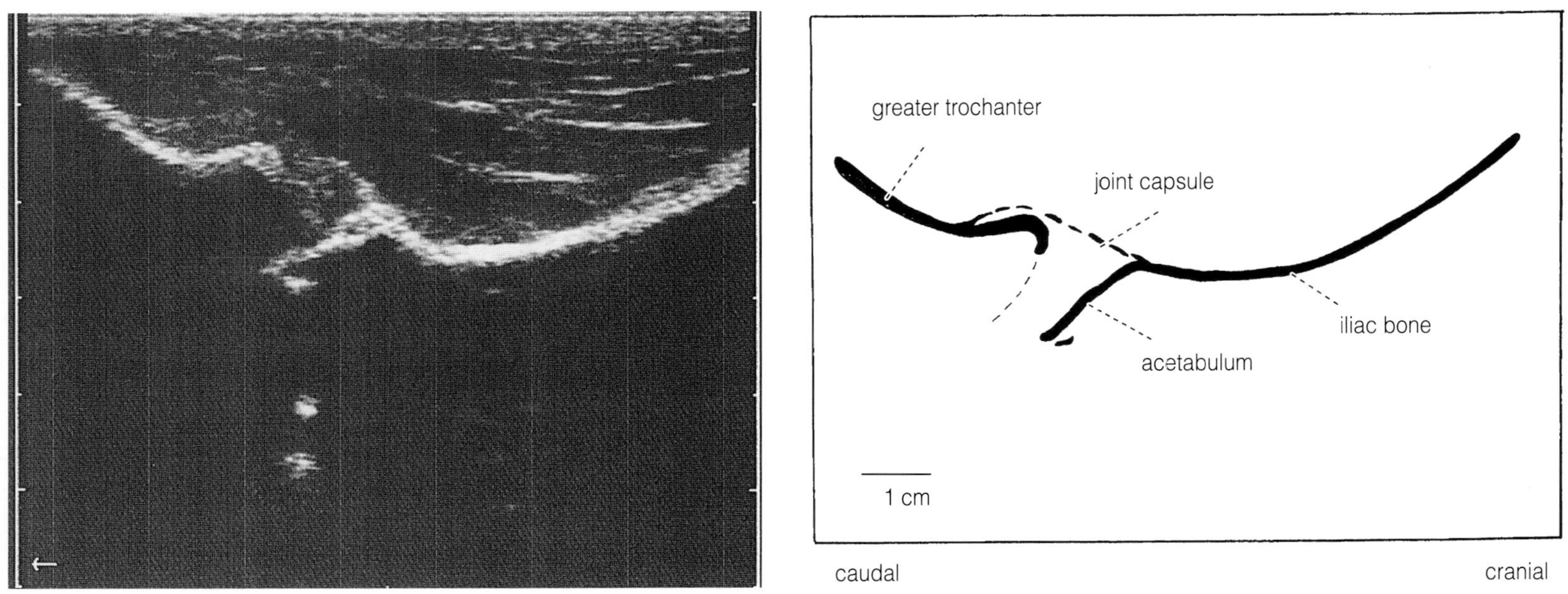

819

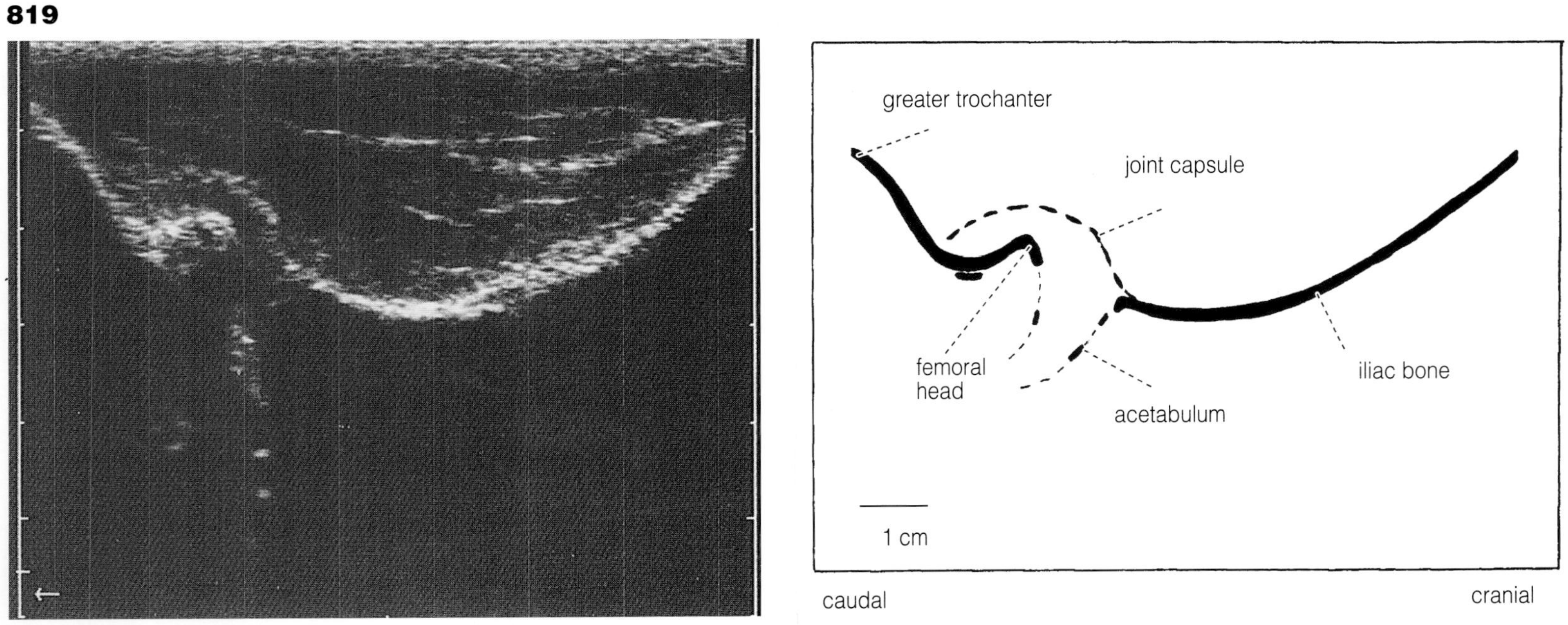

818, 819 Hip joint dysplasia in an adult dog with outward (**818**) and inward (**819**) rotation of the femoral head.

820

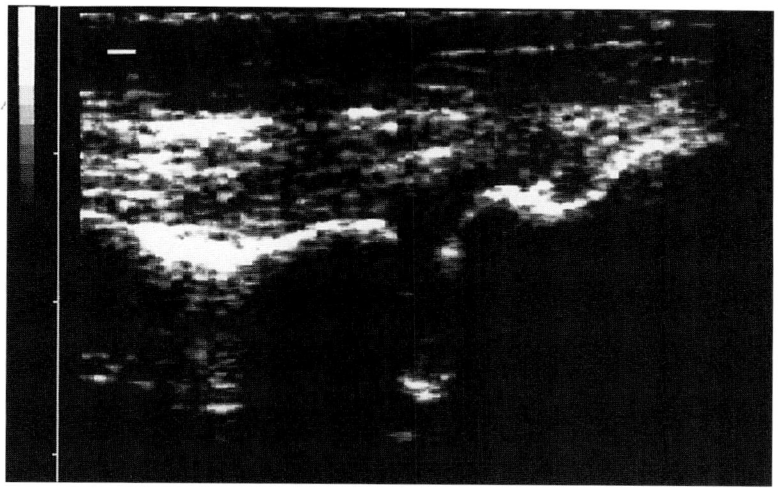

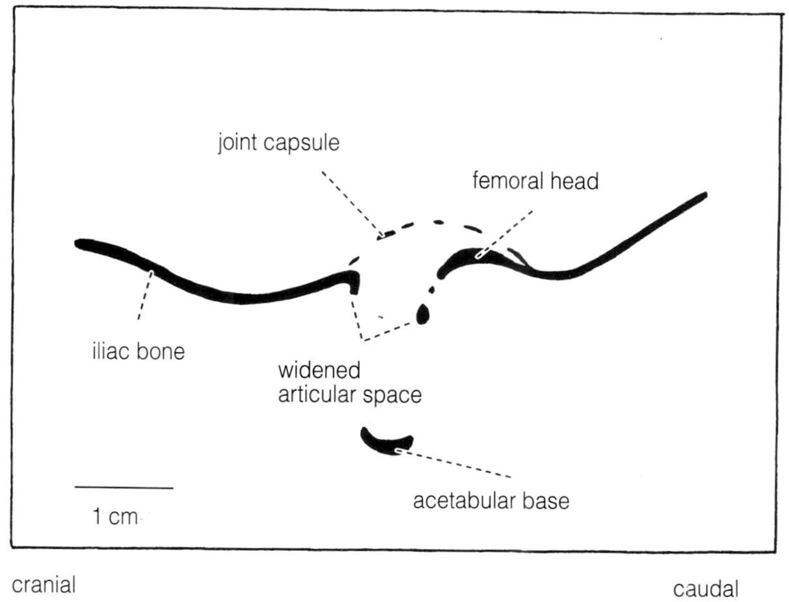

820 Stage II of Legg-Calvé-Pérthes disease (from Lundgren, 1967[33]) with widening of the articular space and a 'moth-eaten' femoral head surface in a dog.

821

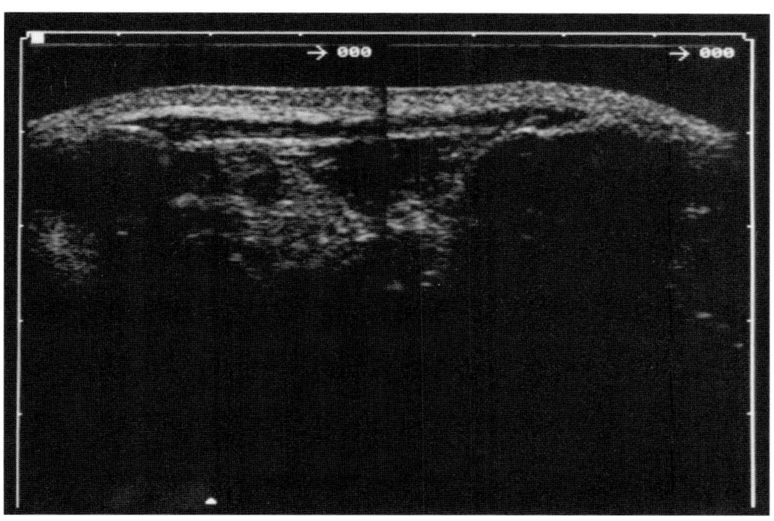

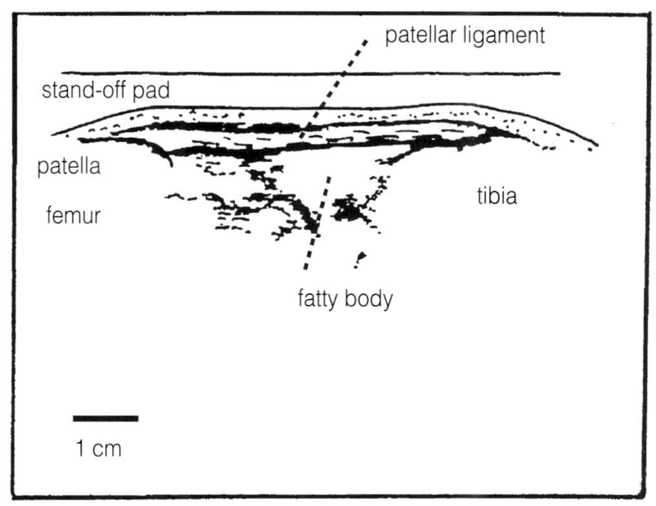

821 Infrapatellar long-axis view of a normal patellar ligament in a dog.

Secondary lesions associated with Legg-Calvé-Pérthes disease and visible on the sonogram include a wider articular space, joint effusion and defects in the femoral head contour (**820**).

***Stifle Joint** (Articulatio genus)*

Andreas Engelke

Anatomy

The stifle joint in the dog and cat, together with the popliteal and patellar joint regions, consists of three basic bony structures: the femur, the tibia and the fibula. Other bony structures in the stifle area include the sesamoid bones (patella in the quadriceps femoris tendon, both gastrocnemius sesamoid bones and various forms of popliteal bones, etc.).

Soft tissue includes the respective muscles, the joint capsule and the joint ligaments with the collateral and cruciate ligaments. The patellar joint includes the patellar ligament and the quadriceps tendon with the embedded patella. The ligament inserts at the tibial tuberosity. Both half moon-shaped articular menisci compensate for the incongruence between the femoral condyles and the tibia plateau and act as a buffer. The menisci also have their respective fixation ligaments. Many pathological disorders are usually apparent within the joint cavity. This cavity is difficult to display ultrasonographically.

Ultrasonography of the Normal and Diseased Stifle Joint

Examination of the stifle joint should follow the method used by Galanski and Milbradt (1990)[6]. The joint is divided into six areas with standardized scanning planes.

1. Infrapatellar area

This plane displays the distal pole of the patella, the patellar ligament, the insertion site at the tibial tuberosity, the infrapatellar fatty body (Hoffa fatty body) between the patellar ligament, the distal infrapatellar bursa, and the joint capsule, as well as the articular cartilage on the femoral condyles (**821–825**).

822

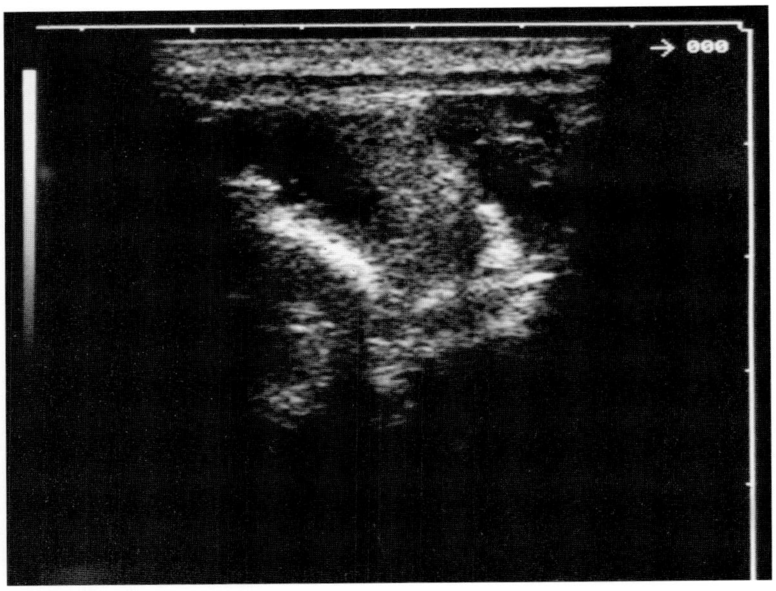

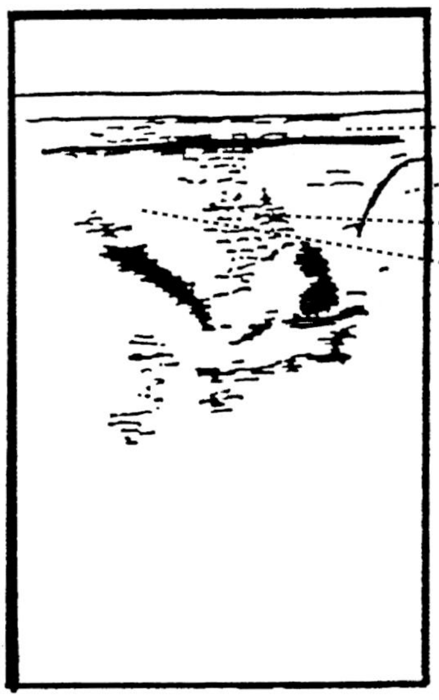

823

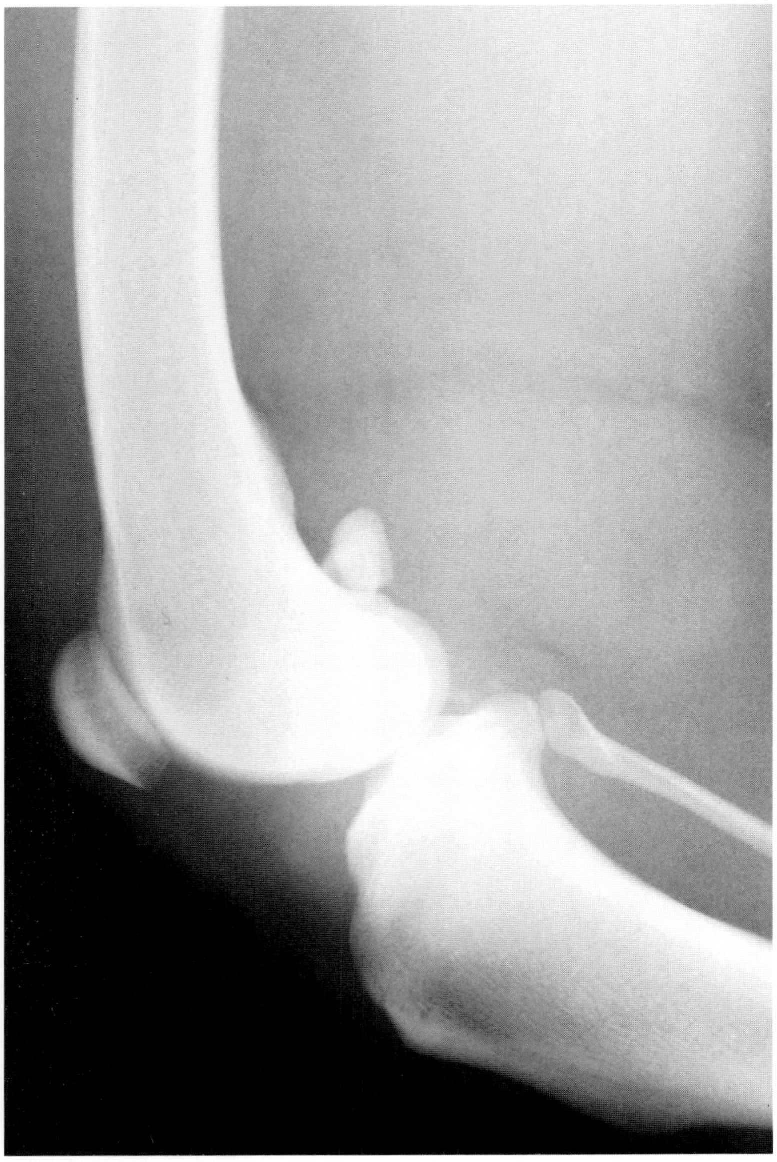

822, 823 Sonogram (**822**) of the patellar ligament in an infrapatellar long-axis view, and lateral radiograph (**823**) of the stifle joint in a dog with a ruptured cruciate ligament.

824

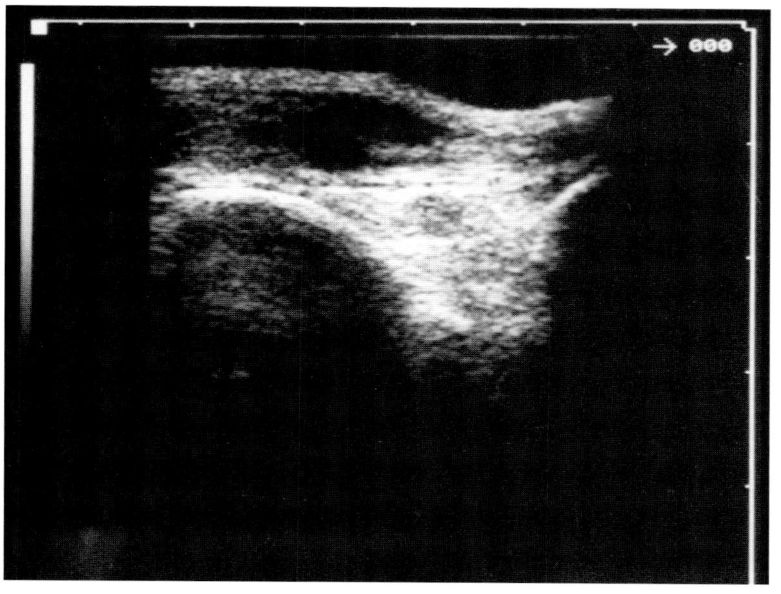

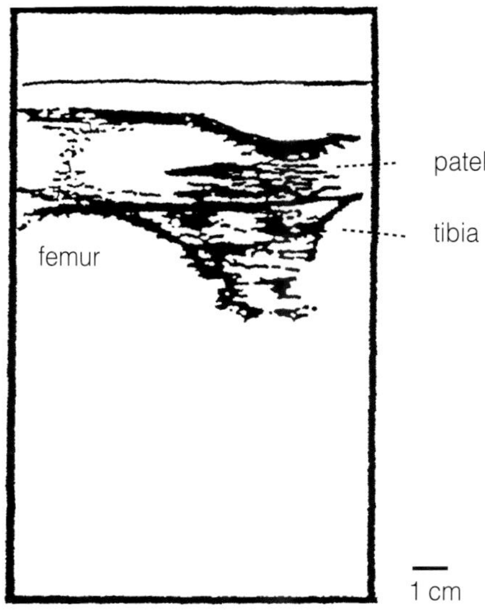

825

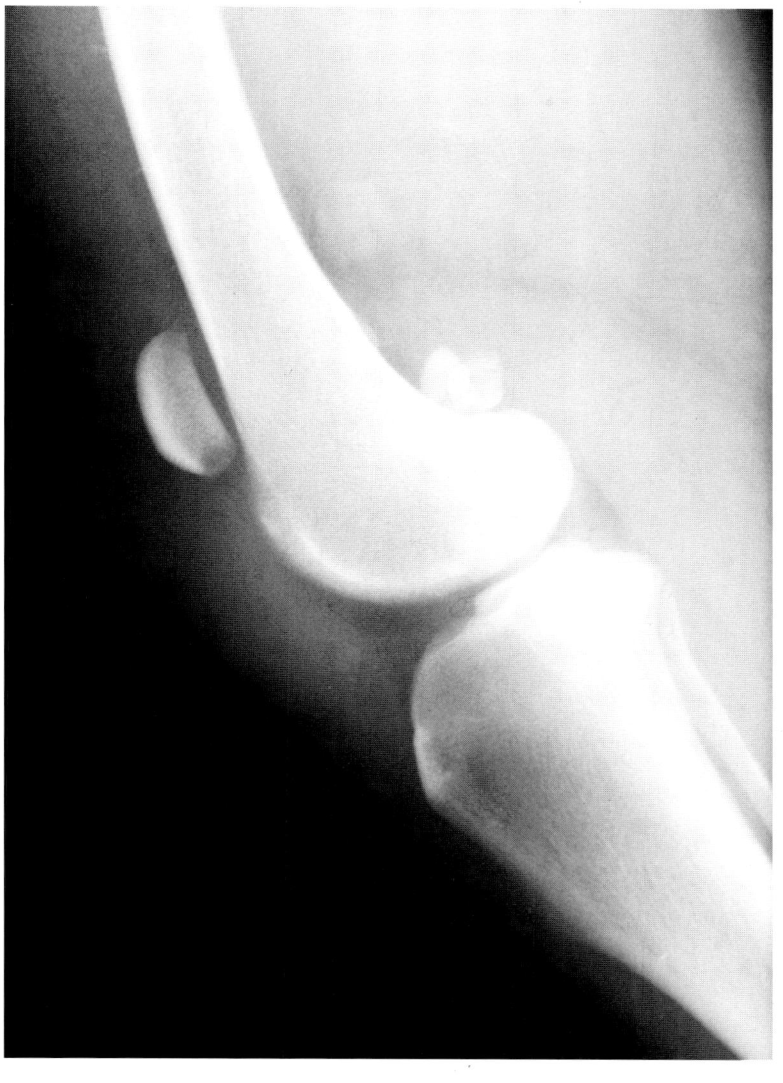

824, 825 Sonogram (**824**) of a ruptured patellar ligament in an infrapatellar long-axis view, and lateral radiograph (**825**) of the stifle joint with patella alta in a dog.

826

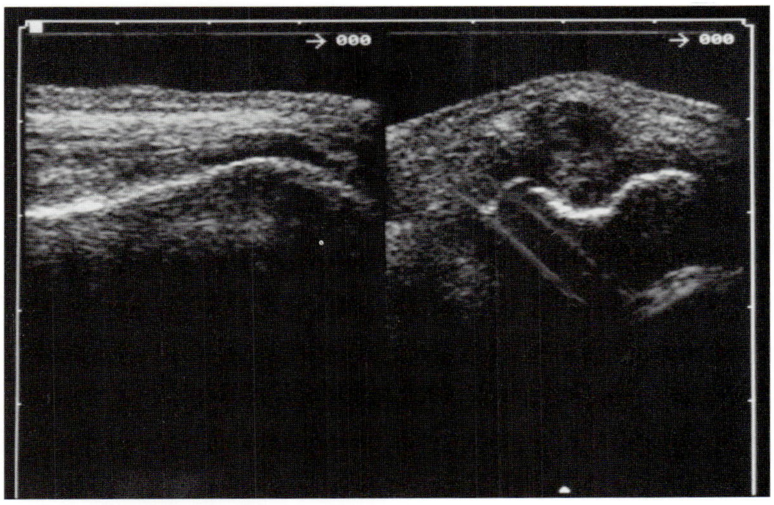

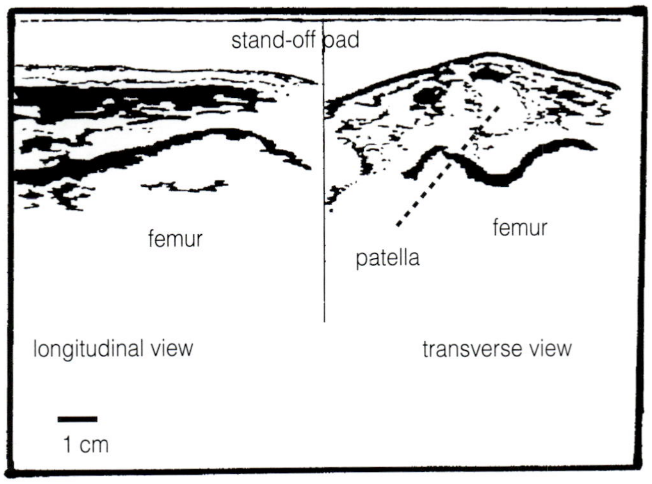

826 Suprapatellar longitudinal and transverse views of normal articular cartilage on the femoral trochlea in a dog.

827

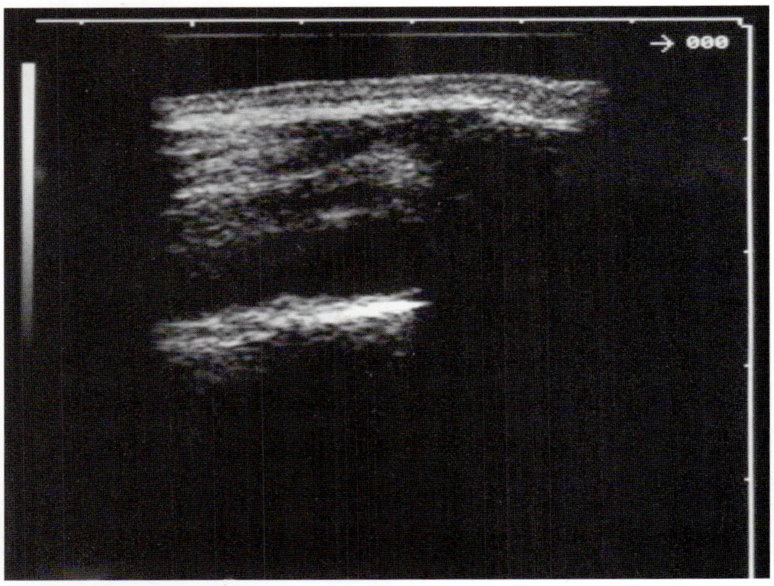

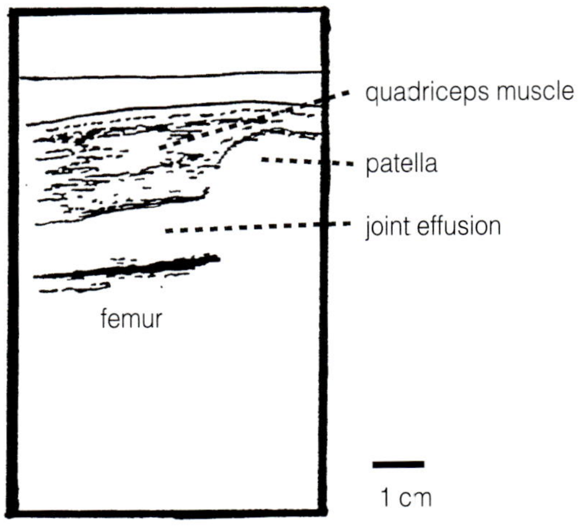

827 Suprapatellar long-axis view of joint effusion in a dog.

828

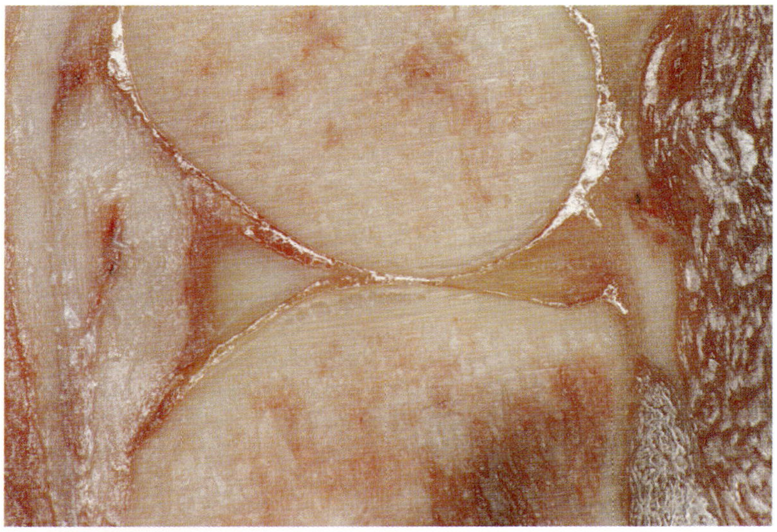

828 Anatomical cross-section of the stifle joint.

2. Suprapatellar area

This plane evaluates the junction between the quadriceps femoris muscle and the straight patellar ligament, with the patella as its sesamoid bone. In a transverse view, joint cartilage of the femoral trochlea is visible. It represents the thin hypoechoic rim on the echogenic bone cortex (**826**). The dorsal recess of the joint capsule reaches further proximal, which enables sonographic diagnosis of joint effusion (**827**).

3. Medial/lateral area

The lateral ligaments are imaged in this plane (**828–830**). It is often impossible to differentiate these ligaments from subcutaneus tissue. Joint effusion is recognized medially and laterally.

4. Popliteal area

Portions of the popliteal artery and vein, with branches, help orientation in this area. The vessels are surrounded by fatty tissue. Articular cartilage on the femoral condyles is partly seen in a perpendicular sound beam (**831**). The tibial plateau is not seen, since the sound waves of a linear transducer are almost parallel to the bone.

829

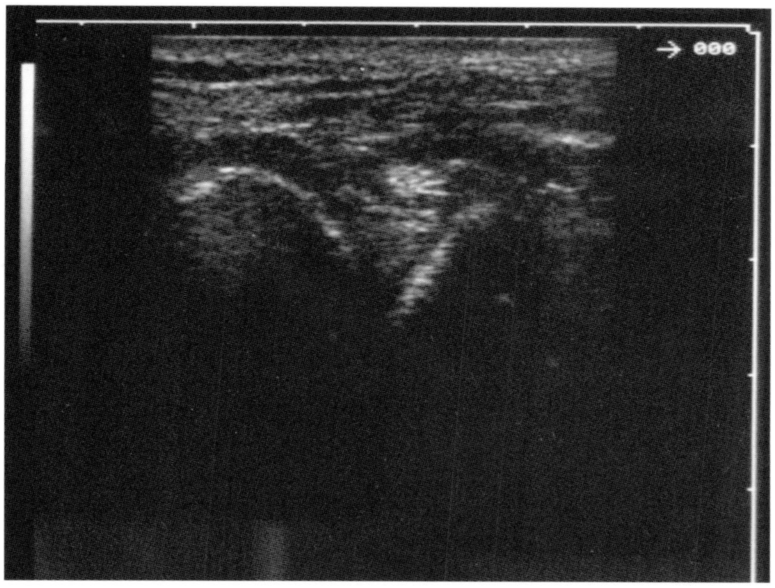

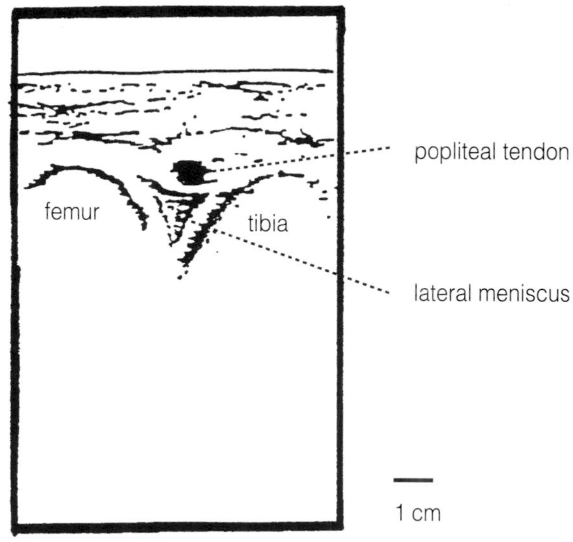

830

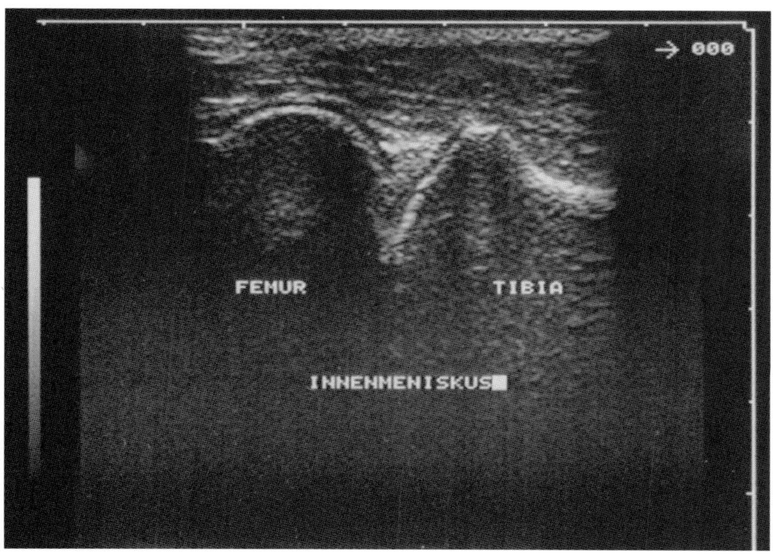

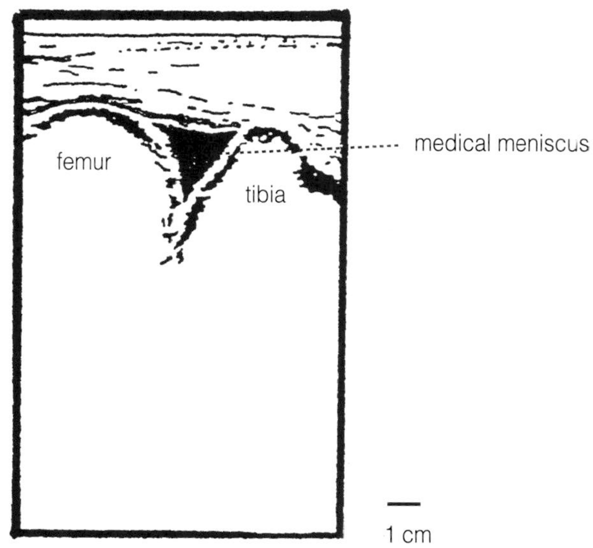

829, 830 Normal canine stifle joint in a lateral (**829**) and medial (**830**) view.

831

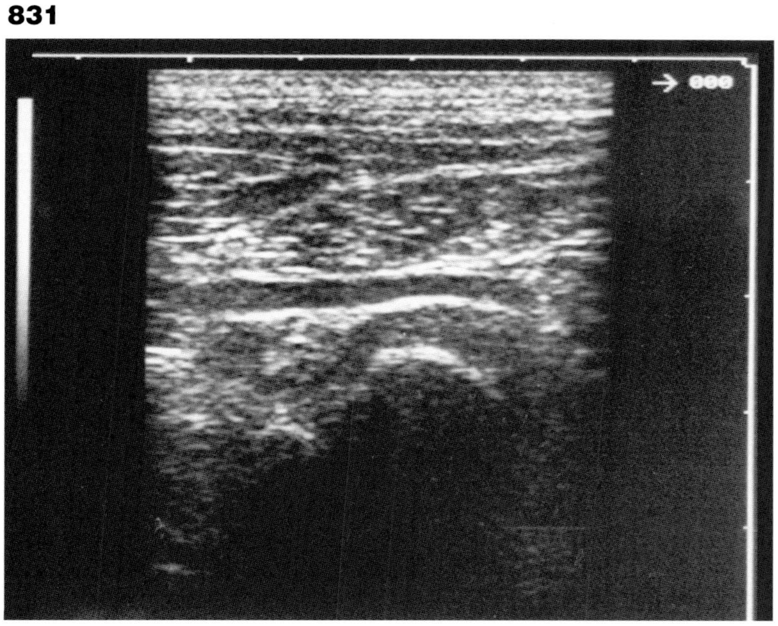

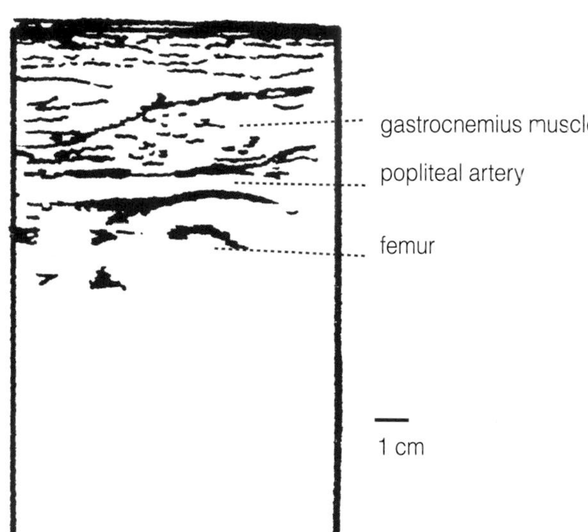

831 Popliteal view of a normal canine stifle joint.

832

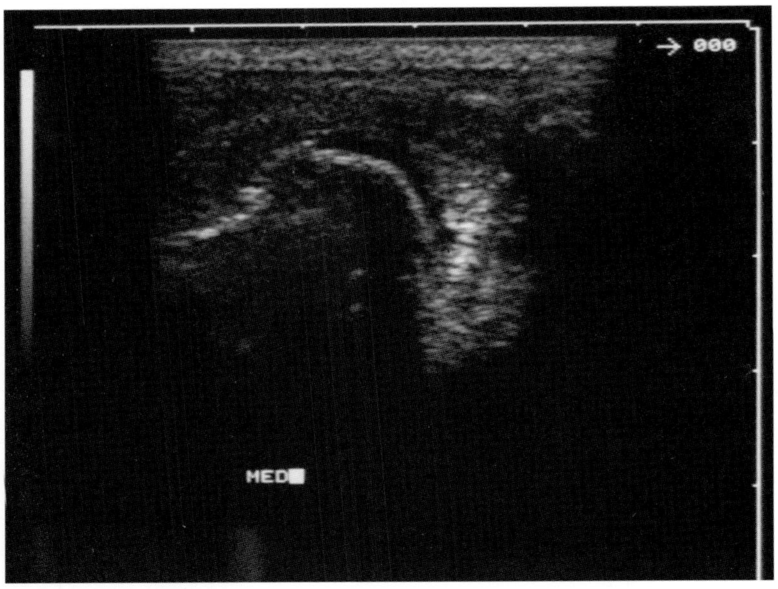

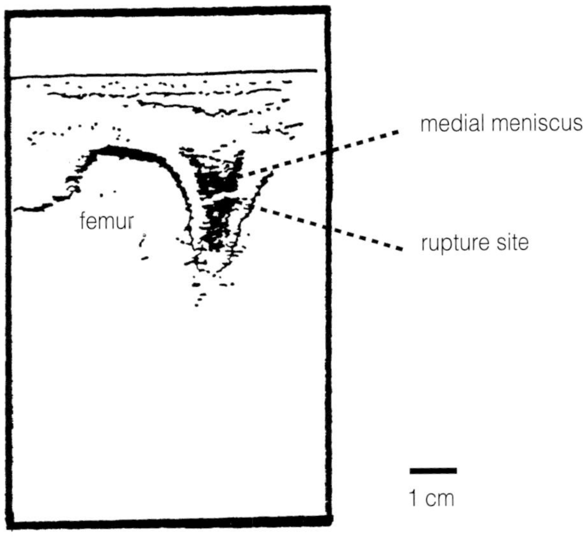

832 Longitudinal view of a 'basket handle' rupture of the medial meniscus of a dog.

5. Cruciate ligament area

The cruciate ligaments are located deep within the joint cavity. The anatomy of these structures does not allow diagnostic imaging, because the ligaments cannot be imaged in a perpendicular sound beam.

6. Articular menisci area

Menisci consist of fibrous cartilage with uniform medium echogenicity and a triangular shape in the longitudinal view. The base of the triangle is at the joint capsule. The medial meniscus is attached to the capsule peripherally. The lateral meniscus is more mobile. Each meniscus should be scanned from the anterior horn over the intermediate portion to the posterior horn. A sector transducer may be helpful with diverging sound waves and concurrent depth penetration into the narrow joint space.

Meniscal lesions produce additional interfaces, which are identified as echogenic lines. Tears located transverse to the sound beam are easily recognized[15, 44]. 'Basket handle' tears are detected when scanning the circumference of the menisci (832). Frequently, the posterior horn of the medial meniscus may become detached from the joint capsule, especially with ruptured anterior cruciate ligaments. The cranial portion of the meniscus may turn under, depending on the size of the detached area. This process can be visualized ultrasonographically. These findings are more recognizable with joint effusion[40, 41].

Meniscus evaluation often leads to a false diagnosis. Numerous artefacts, such as reverberation, are produced at the highly reflective bone interfaces. This diagnostic method should be interpreted carefully.

Carpal and Tarsal Joints *(Articulationes carpi et tarsi)*

Ultrasonography of the carpal and tarsal joint requires extremely high resolution and a great amount of experience to differentiate small superficial structures. A tentative diagnosis of joint lesions can be made when haematomas and effusion are present.

833

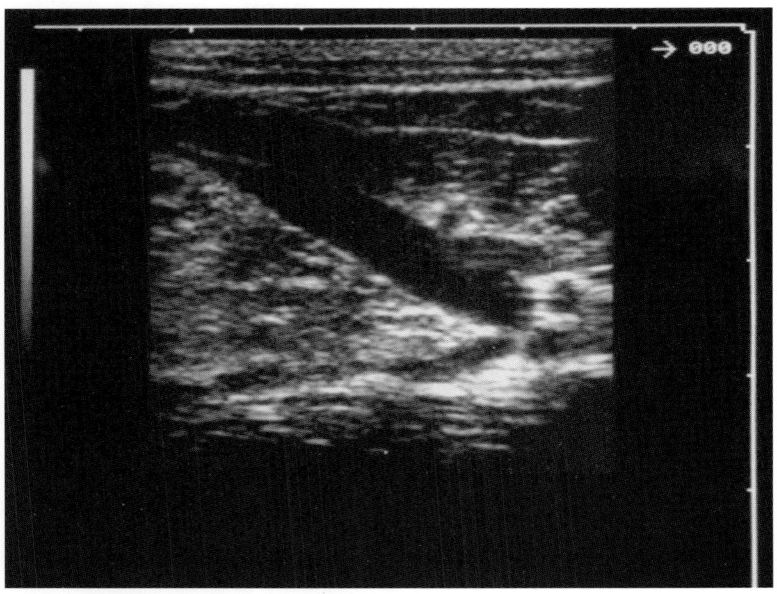

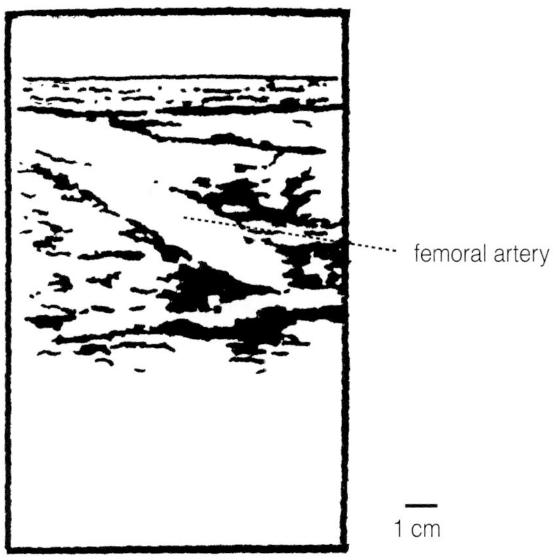

833 Two-dimensional sonogram of the femoral artery in a dog.

834

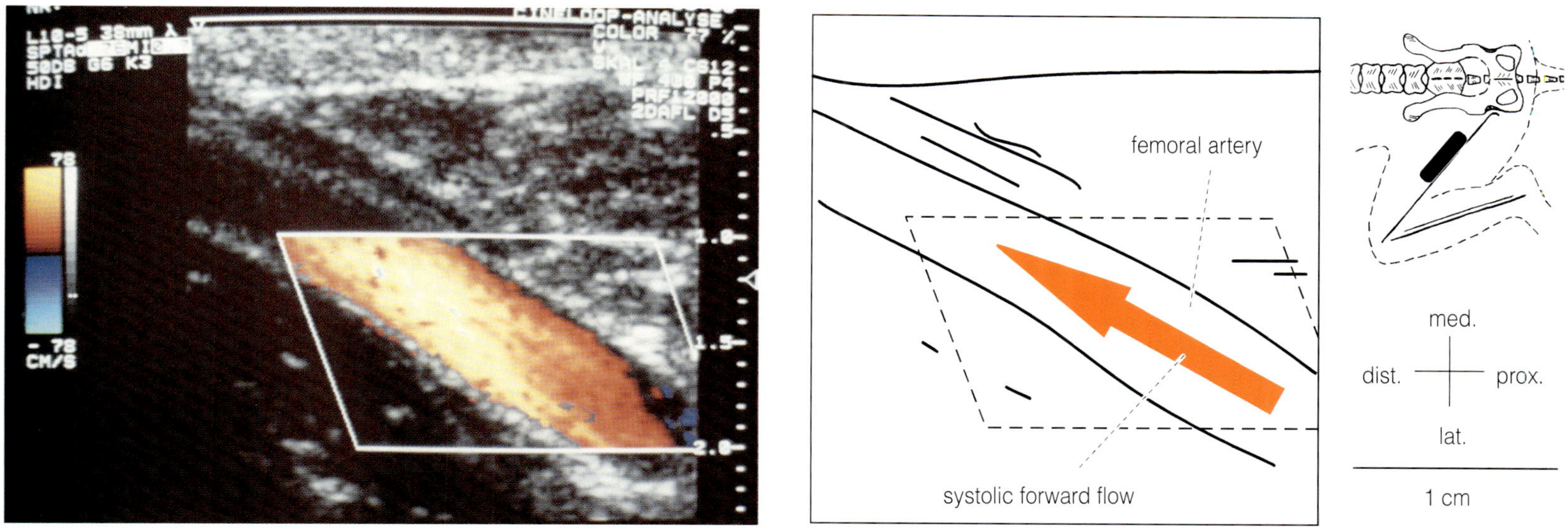

835

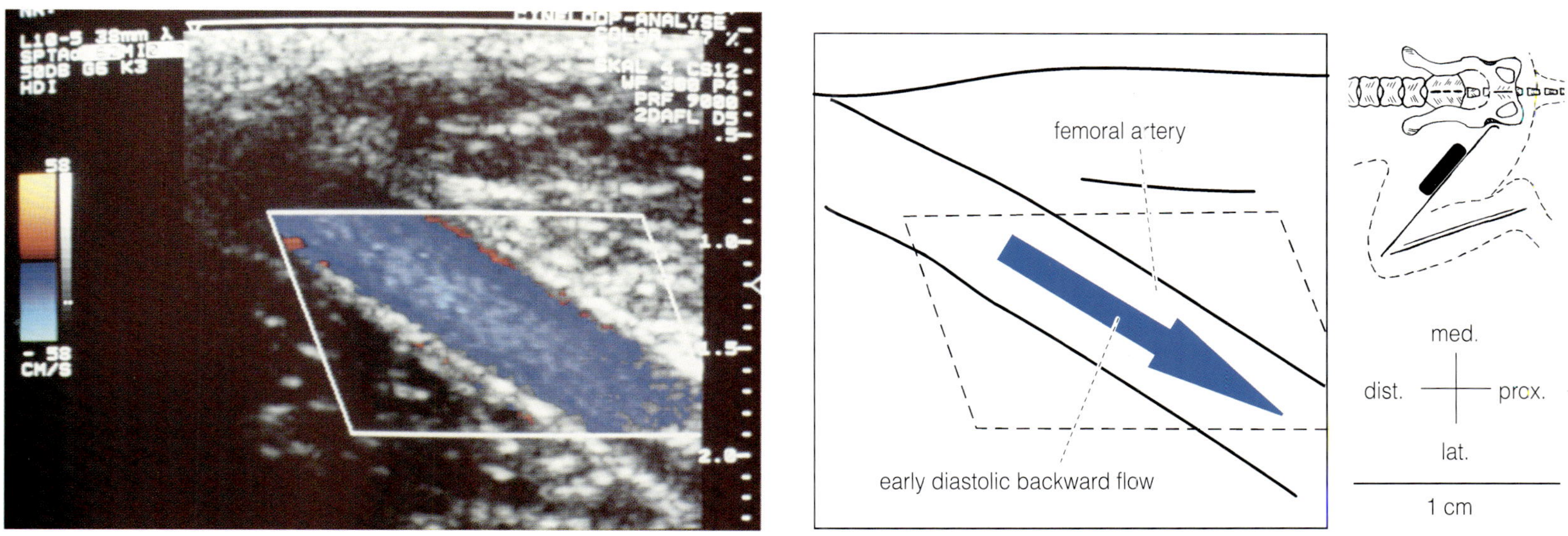

836

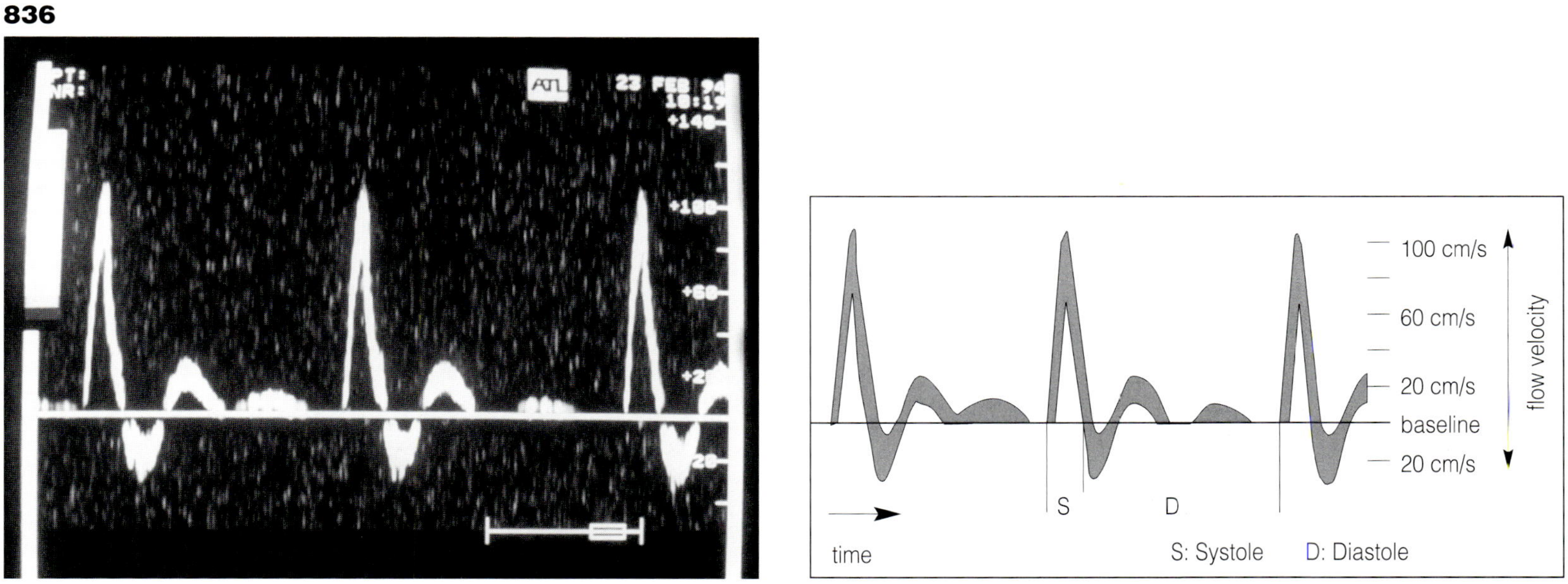

834–836 Colour-coded Doppler sonograms (**834, 835**) and a PW Doppler (**836**) of normal blood flows in the femoral artery of a dog.

Vessels and Nerves

Andreas Engelke and Gabriele Gassner

Vessels

Large vessels are easily located on the two-dimensional sonogram and they help with orientation (833). Arteries are recognized by their pulsations. Veins can be compressed with slight transducer pressure. In some cases, and with technically high resolution, venous valves are visible. Additional examinations should be made using Doppler sonography (834–838) or intravasally (see Interventional Ultrasonography, page 390). Colour-coded Doppler ultrasonography is useful in finding stenoses of the vessels.

837

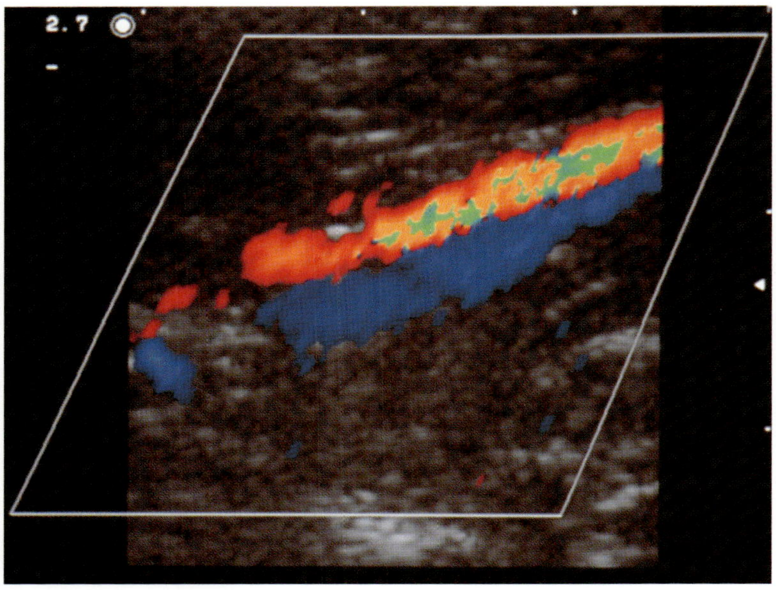

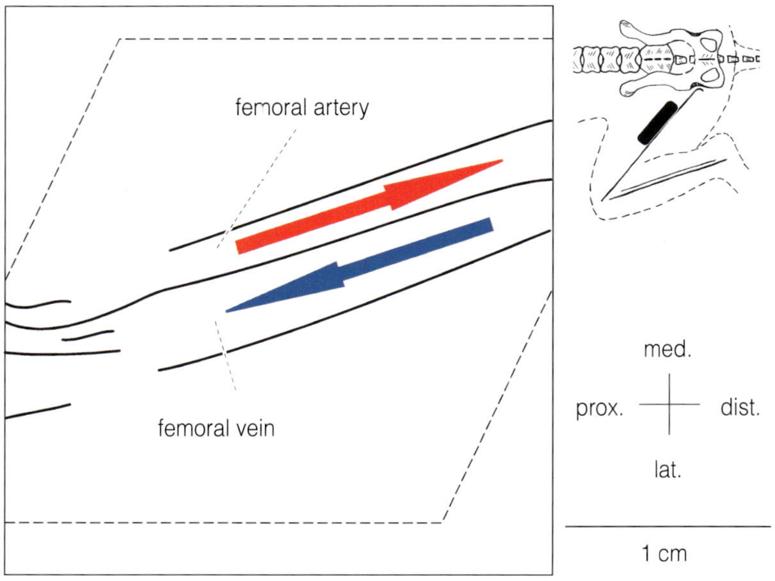

838

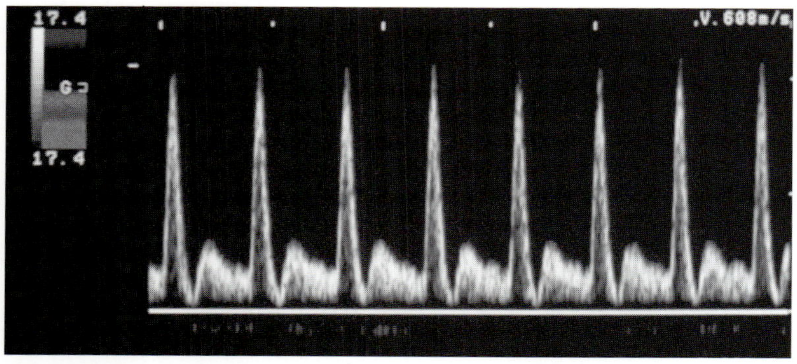

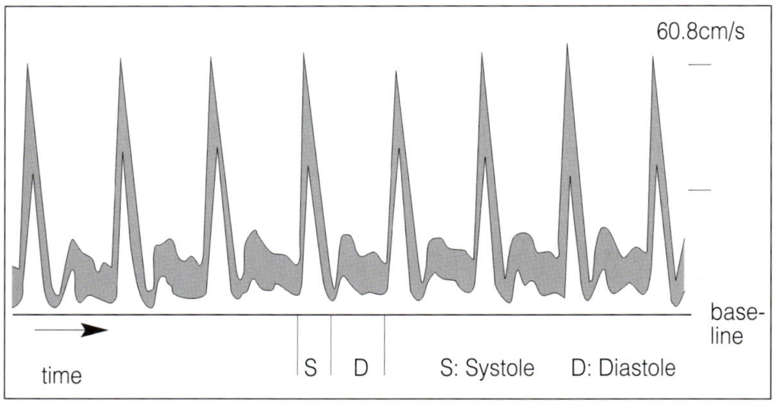

837, 838 Colour-coded Doppler sonogram (**837**) and PW Doppler (**838**) of normal blood flows in the femoral artery of a cat. (Printed with permission from Frank Goeddenhenrich; Hannover].

Nerves

Ultrasonography of normal nerves is usually an incidental finding. Large tumours of the brachial plexus are safely diagnosed ultrasonographically by recognizing disorganized nerves as well as by showing numerous vessels[10, 25] (839).

839

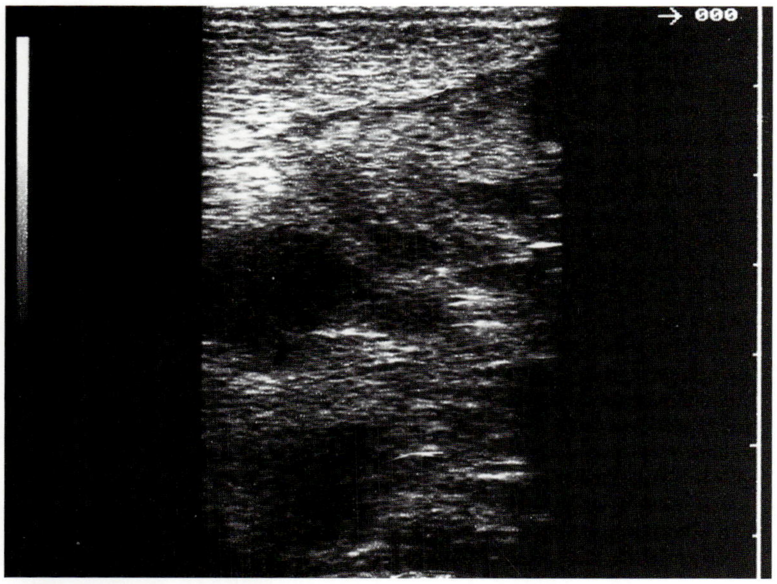

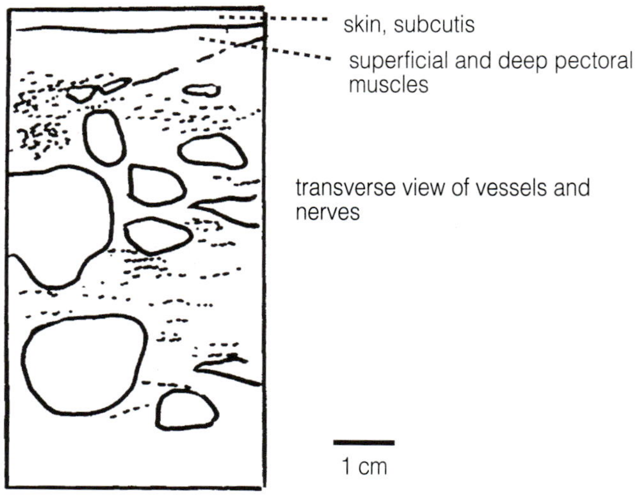

839 Transverse scan of a tumorous brachial plexus in a dog.

840

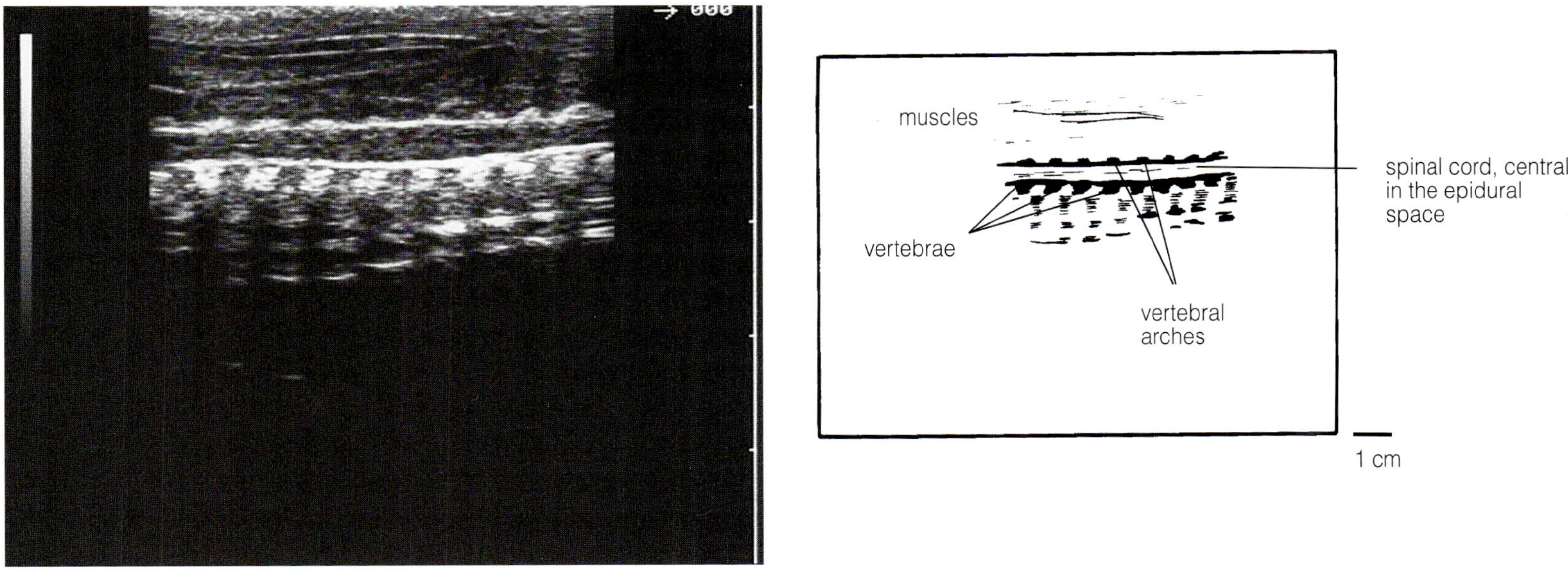

840 Longitudinal view of a normal spinal cord in a puppy (day 1 post partum).

841

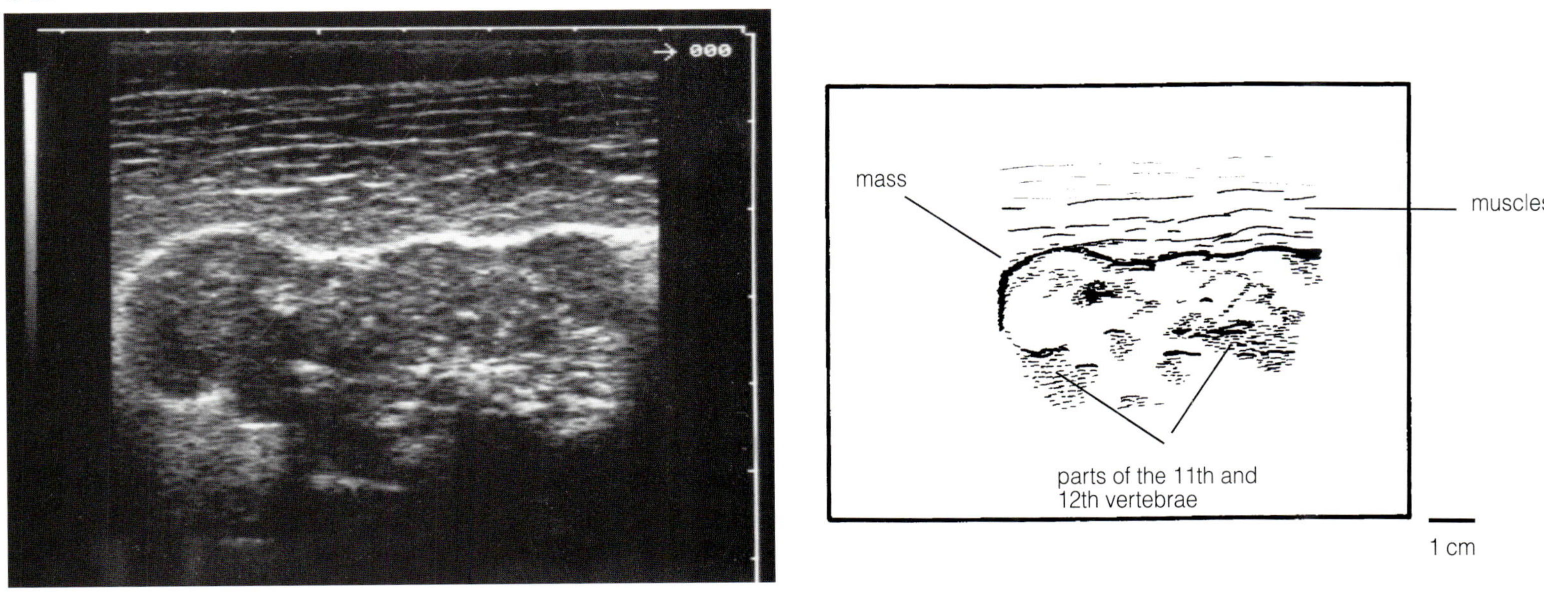

842

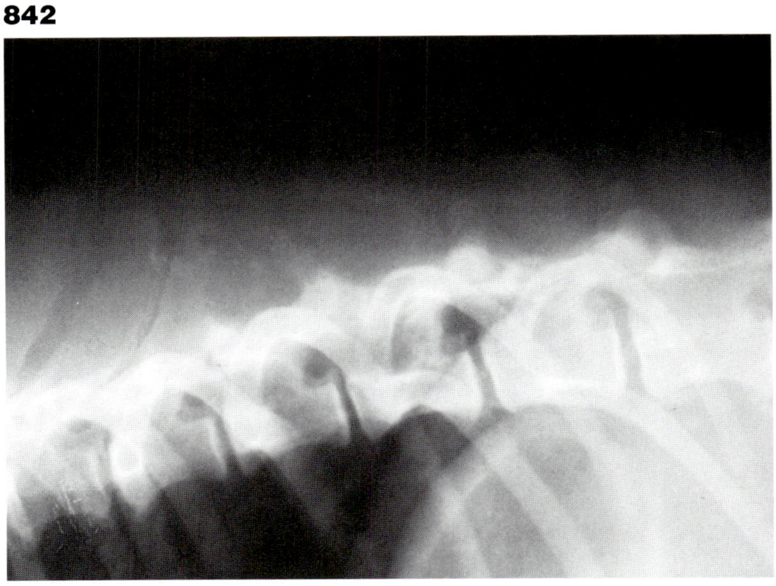

843

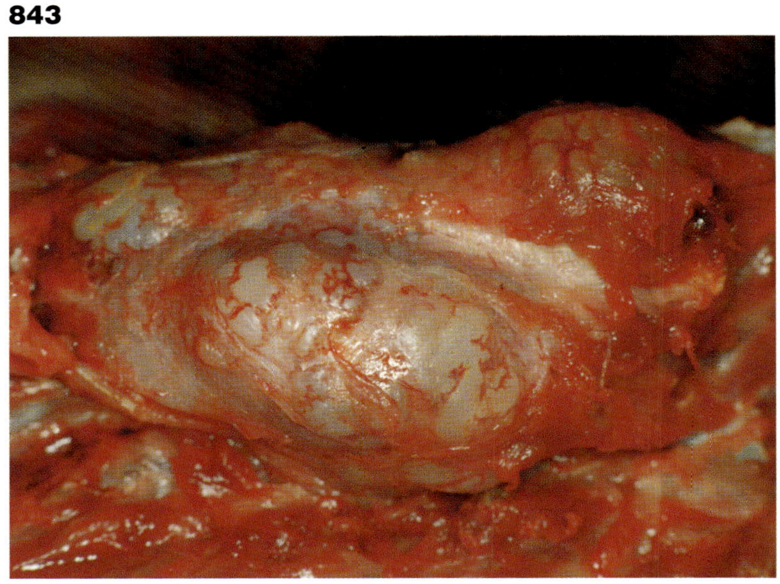

841–843 Two-dimensional sonogram (**841**), radiograph (**842**) and photo (**843**) of a well-demarcated, hyperechoic mass (histopathology: chondrosarcoma) of the 11th and 12th vertebrae in a dog.

844

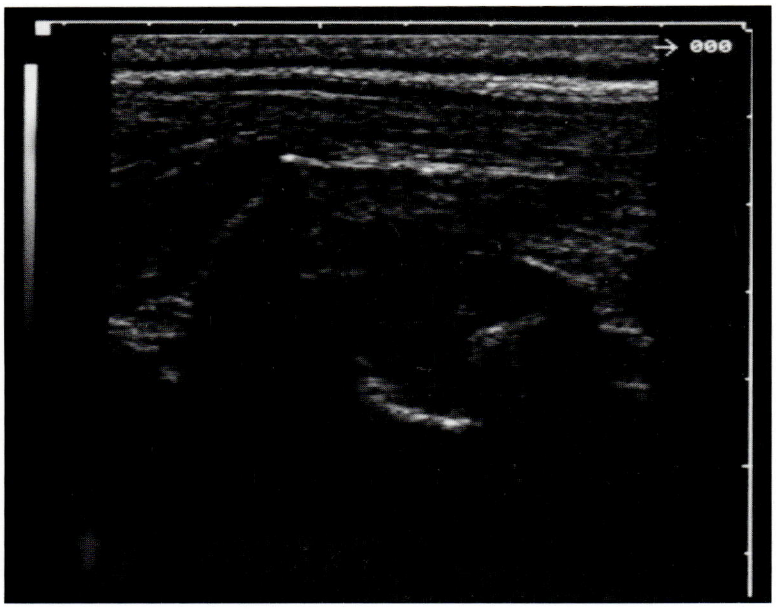

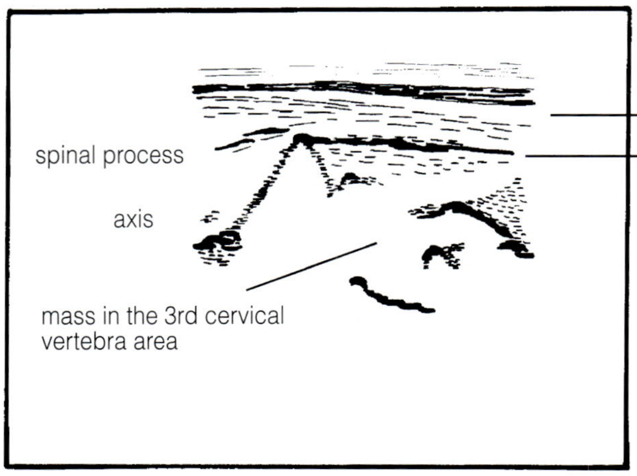

845

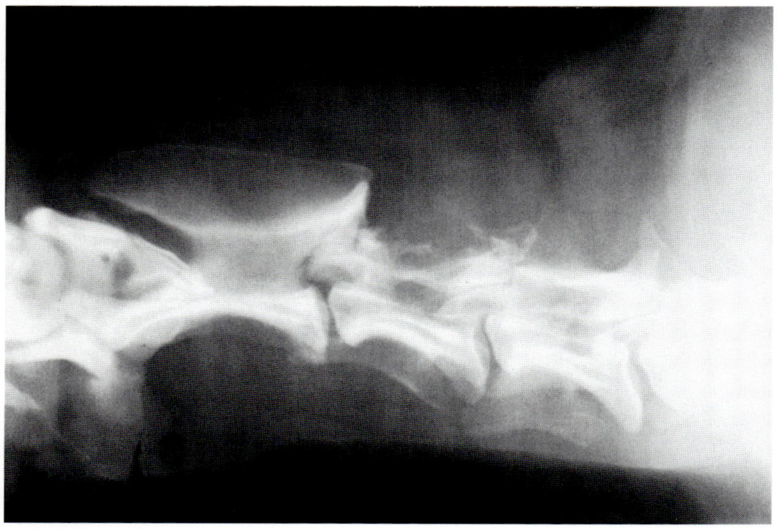

846

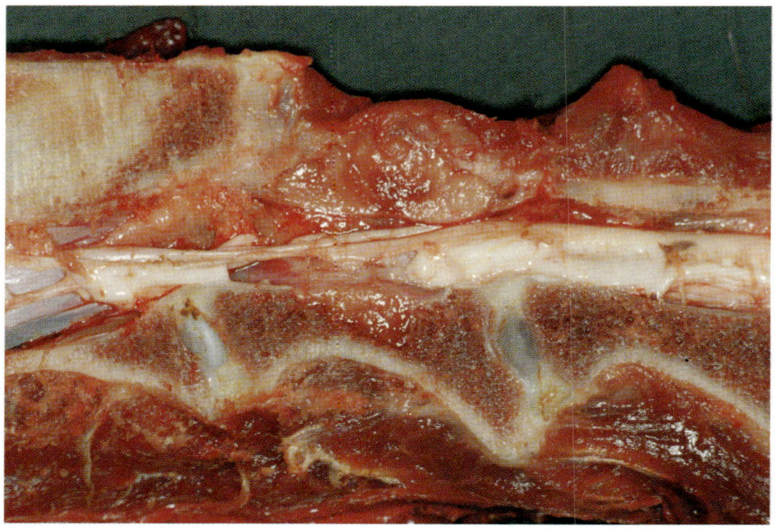

844–846 Two-dimensional sonogram (**844**), radiograph (**845**) and photo (**846**) of an undemarcated, non-homogenous mass (histopathology: non-keratinized squamous cell carcinoma) at the third cervical vertebra in a dog.

Spine

Carolyn Döhner

Ultrasonography of the Normal Spine

The spinal cord and the spinal canal can be scanned in young animals with incomplete ossification of the spinal arch and the spinous processes. A high frequency transducer of at least 7.5 MHz is required for this examination. Linear transducers or sector scanners with stand-offs offer good resolution in the near field.

In older and adult animals the ossified vertebral arches prevent sound waves from penetrating. Transabdominal spinal ultrasonography, used in human medicine, is possible but difficult due to the short space between the separate vertebrae and the relatively great distance between the abdominal wall and back. The areas dorsal and lateral to the spine are easily accessible.

The spinal canal is visualized with the patient in sternal recumbency. The course of the spine should be straight. In young animals the incompletely ossified spinal arches and the hypoechoic spinal cord, including the echogenic central canal, are identifiable (840).

Ultrasonography of Spinal Lesions

Indications for ultrasonography of the spinal canal include all soft tissue masses with suspected infiltration of the spinal canal and/or the spinal cord. Radiographic findings of vertebral lesions, especially spinal dysraphia and possible meningocele or meningomyelocele, should always be followed by an ultrasonographic examination.

Ultrasonography may be helpful in determining demarcation with the surrounding tissue and soft tissue involvement of masses near the spine showing osteolytic lesions on radiographs (841–846).

Finally, the authors would like to stress the importance of clinical examination, radiography and, possibly, scintigraphy in orthopaedics. The value of ultrasonographic findings is limited because of the numerous artefacts and the experience of the sonographer.

References

1 Berzon JL and Quick CB (1980) Fragmented coronoid process: anatomical, clinical, and radiographic considerations with case analysis. *J. Am. Anim. Hosp. Assoc.* **16**, 241–251.

2 Bienz HA (1985) *Klinische und Radiologische Untersuchungen über den Fragmentierten Processus Coronoideus Medialis im Ellbogengelenk des Berner Sennenhandes und Anderen Sennenhande-Rassen.* Zürich, Univ., Veterinärmed. Fak., Diss.

3 Brunnberg L, Waibl H and Nakasala-Situma J (1981) Zur Kontraktur des Musculus infraspinatus beim Hand. *Kleintierpraxis* **26**, 197–264.

4 Ellenberger W and Baum H (1943) *Handbuch der vergleichenden Anatomie der Haussäugetiere.* 18th Edn. Springer Verlag, Berlin, Heidelberg, New York.

5 Fox SM, Bloomberg S and Bright RM (1983) Developmental anomalies of the canine ellbow. *J. Am. Anim. Hosp. Assoc.* **19**, 605–615.

6 Galanski M and Milbradt H (1990) *Sonographie des Stütz- und Bewegungsapparates.* Byk Gulden Pharmazeutika, Schnetztor-Verlag GmbH Konstanz.

7 Gerwing M and Kramer M (1991) Sonographie in der Orthopädie. *XVI. WSAVA-Weltkongreß, 02.-05.10.1991, Wien*, pp. 407–408.

8 Gerwing M and Kramer M (1991) Neue Anwendungsgebiete der Sonographie beim Kleintier. *37. Jahrestagung der DVG-Fachgruppe "Kleintierkrankheiten" vom 31.10.– 02.11.1991, Fellbach*, pp. 51–54

9 Gerwing M and Kramer M (1993) Die Sonographie der Achillessehne beim Hand. *Tierärztl. Prax. Sonderheft*, 40–41.

10 Gerwing M and Kramer M (1994) Die Sonographie des Schultergelenkes and seiner umgebenden Weichteile beim Hand. Teil B: Sonographische Diagnostik von Erkrankungen im Bereich des Schultergelenkes. *Kleintierpraxis* **39**, 141–156.

11 Graf R (1984) Classification of hip joint dysplasia by means of sonography. *Arch. Orthop. Trauma. Surg.* **102**, 248–255.

12 Graf R (1987) Die sonographische Diagnose von Hüftreifestörungen. Prinzipien, Fehlerquellen und Konsequenzen. *Ultraschall* **8**, 2–8.

13 Graf R and Schuler P (1988) *Sonographie am Stütz- und Bewegungsapparat bei Erwachsenen und Kindern.* Edition Medizin, VCH Verlagsgesellschaft mbH, Weinheim.

14 Greshake JG and Ackerman N (1992) Ultrasound evaluation of the coxofemoral joints of the canine neonate. *Vet. Radiol. Ultrasound* **33**, 99–104.

15 Grifka J and Richter J (1992) *Meniskussonographie.* Enke Verlag, Stuttgart.

16 Harland U (1986) Sonographische Befande an Hüftgelenken von Kindern, Jugendlichen und Erwachsenen. In: Henche HR and Hey W (Eds.) *Sonographie in der Orthopädie und Sportmedizin.* ML Uelzen, pp. 47–53.

17 Harland U and Sattler H (1991) *Ultraschallfibel. Orthopädie, Traumatologie, Rheumatologie.* Springer Verlag, Berlin.

18 Hedtmann A and Fett H (1988) *Atlas und Lehrbuch der Schultersonographie.* Ferdinand Enke Verlag, Stuttgart.

19 Hedtmann A and Fett H (1990) Schultersonographie. In: Hedtmann A (Ed.) *Degenerative Schultererkrankungen.* Ferdinand Enke Verlag, Stuttgart.

20 Hedtmann A and Fett H (1991) *Atlas und Lehrbuch der Schultersonographie.* 2nd Edn. Ferdinand Enke Verlag, Stuttgart.

21 Hulth A, Norberg I and Olsson SE (1962) Coxa plana in the dog. *J. Bone Jt. Surg.* **44**, 918–930.

22 Kramer M (1991) Sonographische Anatomie des Schultergelenkes beim Hand. *37. Jahrestagung der DVG-Fachgruppe 'Kleintierkrankheiten' vom 31.10.-02.11.1991, Fellbach.*

23 Kramer M (1992) *Die sonographische Anatomie des Schultergelenkes und seines Weichteilmantels beim erwachsenen Hand.* Gießen, Justus-Liebig-Univ., Veterinärmed. Fak., Diss.

24 Kramer M, Gerwing M and Fritsch R (1993) *Die Sonographie des Schultergelenkes beim Hand.* Tierärztl. Prax., Sonderheft, p. 39.

25 Kramer M, Gerwing M und Schimke E (1993) Diagnostik und Therapie ausgewählter Sehnen- and Muskelerkrankungen beim Hand. *Kleintierpraxis* **38**, 703–711.

26 Kramer M and Gerwing M (1994) Die Sonographie des Schultergelenkes and seiner umgebenden Weichteile beim Hand. Teil A: Die sonographische Anatomie des Schultergelenkes und seines Weichteilmantels. *Kleintierpraxis* **39**, 71–80.

27 Kresken JG (1991) *Zur Ultraschalluntersuchung des Hüftgelenkes beim Handewelpen.* München, Univ., Tierärztl. Fak., Diss.

28 Kresken JG and Köstlin RG (1992) The ultrasonic examination of the hip joint in young dogs. *IVRA Meeting 1992,Veldhoven, Netherlands.*

29 Kresken JG (1993) *Die Untersuchung des Hüftgelenkes mit Ultraschall beim Hand.* Tierärztl. Prax. Sonderheft, pp. 39–40.

30 Lazovic D and Wegner U (1992) Sind Apophysenverletzungen sonographisch darstellbar? Ultraschalldiagnostik 1992, 16. Drei-Länder-Treffen, Karlsruhe, 21.10.-24.10.1992. In: Bartels H, Erbel R, Hansmann M und Otto R (Eds.) *Ultraschall in Klinik and Praxis.* **7 (3)**, Verlag Springer, p. 223.

31 Lee T (1970) A study of the radiographic and histological change occuring in Legg-Calve-Perthes disease in the dog. *J. Small Anim.Pract.* **11**, 621–638.

32 Lee T and Fry PD (1969) Some observations on the occurence of Legg-Calve-Perthes disease in the dog, and evaluation of excision arthroplasty as a method of treatment. *J. Small Anim.Pract.* **10**, 309–317.

33 Ljunggren G (1967) Legg-Perthes disease in the dog. *Acta Orthop. Scand. Suppl.* **95**, 1–79.

34 Löffler L (1989) *Ultraschalldiagnostik am Bewegungsapparat.* Georg Thieme Verlag, Stuttgart.

35 Mann FA, Wagner-Mann C and Tangner CH (1988) Manual goniometric measurement of the canine pelvic limb. *J. Am. Anim. Hosp. Assoc.* **24**, 189–194.

36 Middleton WD, Reinus WR, Totty WG, Melson GL and Murphy WA (1985) Ultrasound of the biceps tendon apparatus. *Radiol.* **157**, 211–215.

37 Milbradt H, Reimer P and Thermann H (1988) Die Sonomorphologie der normalen Achillessehne und Muster pathologischer Veränderungen. *Radiologe* **28**, 330–333.

38 Neuberth M, Stefansson P and Hertsch B (1990) Die sonographische Untersuchung als Methode zur Diagnosestellung von Hämatomen und Abszessen im proximalen Abschnitt des Bewegungsapparates des Pferdes. *Pferdeheilkande* **6**, 237–244.

39 Patten RM, Mack LA, Wang KY and Lingel J (1992) Nondisplaced fractures of greater tuberosity of the humerus. Sonographic detection. *Radiol.* **182**, 201–204.

40 Reimer P, Taubert K, Milbradt H and Lobehoffer P (1989) Sonoanatomie, Sonopathologie und diagnostische Möglichkeiten der Kniegelenkssonographie. *Röntgenpraxis* **42**, 11–16.

41 Röhr E (1991) *Kniegelenkssonographie.* Georg Thieme Verlag, Stuttgart.

42 Rivers B, Wallace L and Johnston GR (1992) Biceps tenosynovitis in the dog: radiographic and sonographic findings. *Vet. Comp. Orthop. Traumatol.* **5**, 51–57.

43 Schimke E, Kramer M, Gerwing M and Schachenmayer W (1992) Musculus-gracilis-Kontraktur. In: *38. Jahrestagung der Fachgruppe Kleintiere der DVG.* Bonn, 1992, pp. 404–405.

44 Sohn C and Casser HR (1988) *Meniskussonographie.* Springer Verlag, Berlin.

45 Stahl C, Konermann H and Kuck W (1986) Sonographie bei Periarthropathia humeroscapularis. *Orthop. Praxis* **9**, 662–669.

46 Van Schie HTM (1989) Diagnostische Sonographie an der Gliedmaße des Pferdes. *Tierärztl. Prax.* **Suppl. 4**, 47–55.

47 Vollmerhaus B, Schebitz H, Roos H, Brunnberg L and Waibl H (1983) Anatomische Grandlagen und funktionelle Betrachtungen zur Olecranonfraktur beim Hand. *Kleintierprax.* **28**, 5–15.

48 Warren DV and Dingwall JS (1972) Legg-Perthes disease in the dog: a review. *Can. Vet. J.* **13**, 135–137.

49 Wilson DJ, Green DJ and McLarnon JC (1984) Arthroscopy of the painful hip. *Clin. Radiol.* **35**, 15–17.

50 Wingstrand H (1986) Transient synovitis of the hip in the child. *Acta Orthop. Scand. Suppl.* **219**, 57–59.

13 Specific Diagnostic Ultrasound Procedures

Ultrasound-Guided Biopsy

Angelika Hörauf and Susanne Thamke

Percutaneous ultrasound-guided biopsy procedures have been used in human medicine since the early 1970s[1]. After ultrasonography had been introduced to veterinary medicine in the early 1980s[3], Hager *et al.* (1985)[2] and Smith (1985)[5] first reported on ultrasound-guided biopsies in animals.

Indications for a biopsy, followed by histology, cytology or bacteriology, include diagnosis and evaluation of tumours, as well as lesions of parenchymatous organs, which could not be verified by clinical, radiographic and laboratory examination.

The advantages of an ultrasound-guided biopsy, compared to a blind biopsy, are as follows:

- Location, size and parenchymal structure of the tissue in question can be evaluated before the biopsy procedure.
- The position of the biopsy needle is visible with hand-free biopsies. Exact placement of the needles is achieved with biopsy guides.
- Potential complications, such as haemorrhaging, are easily detected following the biopsy.

Three biopsy methods are used:
Tissue-core biopsy: tissue samples for histology
Fine-needle aspiration biopsy: tissue samples for cytology
Aspiration: of fluids (urine, fluid in body cavities)

Tissue-Core Biopsy

Tissue-core biopsy is used to obtain larger tissue samples for histology. Biopsy guides should always be used with this technique (847). This technique is used for kidney and liver biopsies.

847

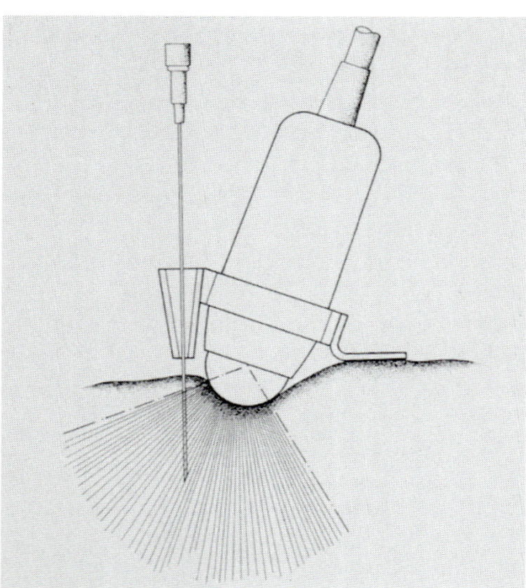

847 Schematic drawing of a biopsy procedure, using a special puncture guide – ultrasound-guided biopsy. (From Otto RC and Wellauer J (1985) *Ultrasound-Guided Biopsy.* Springer Verlag, Berlin[4]).

848

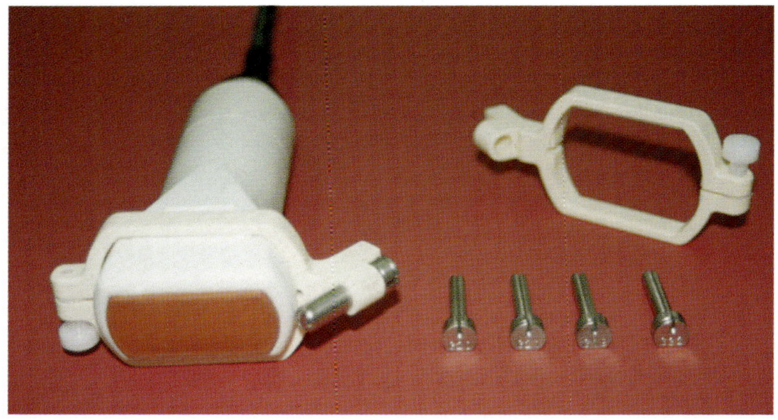

849

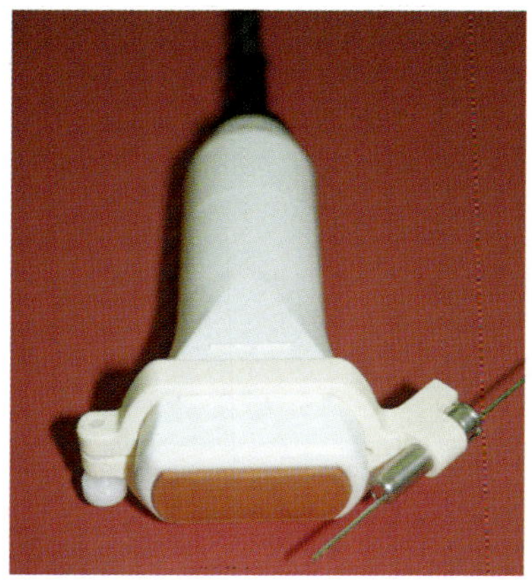

848, 849 Equipment for an ultrasound-guided biopsy. (**848**) Biopsy kit containing needle guides of different sizes (bottom right) and a transducer collar (top right). (**849**) Transducer with attached biopsy guide system and inserted needle.

850

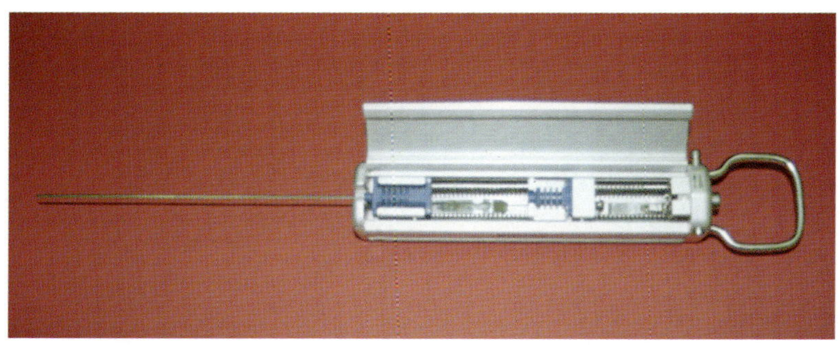

850 Disposable biopsy needle (Biopty-Cut® and Biopty® gun for a semi-automated, tissue-core biopsy (Radiplast AB, Uppsala, Sweden).

Equipment

Ultrasound-guided biopsies are possible with biopsy guides attached to the transducer. These guides have a groove to insert the needle and direct the path of the needle. For exact guidance, the grooves must have different sizes to accommodate different needle sizes (848–850).

Patient Preparation

Before the biopsy, the patient should be thoroughly examined with regard to history, physical examination and laboratory work-up. Screening tests for coagulopathies should rule out the risk of post-operative bleeding.

851

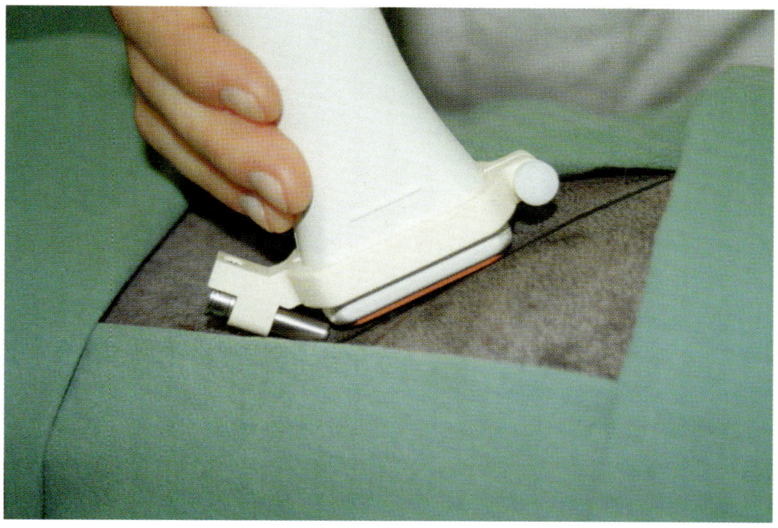

852

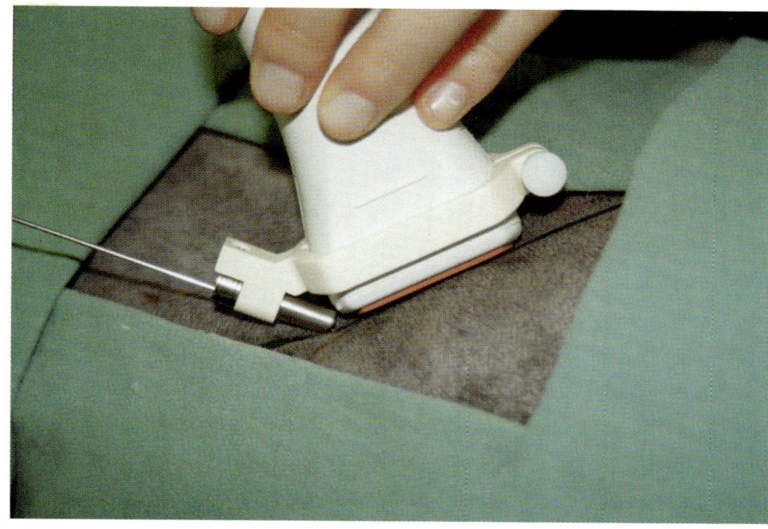

851, 852 Tissue-core biopsy of the left kidney. (**851**) Transducer application caudolateral to the rib cage. (**852**) Needle insertion through the biopsy guide into the abdominal cavity.

853

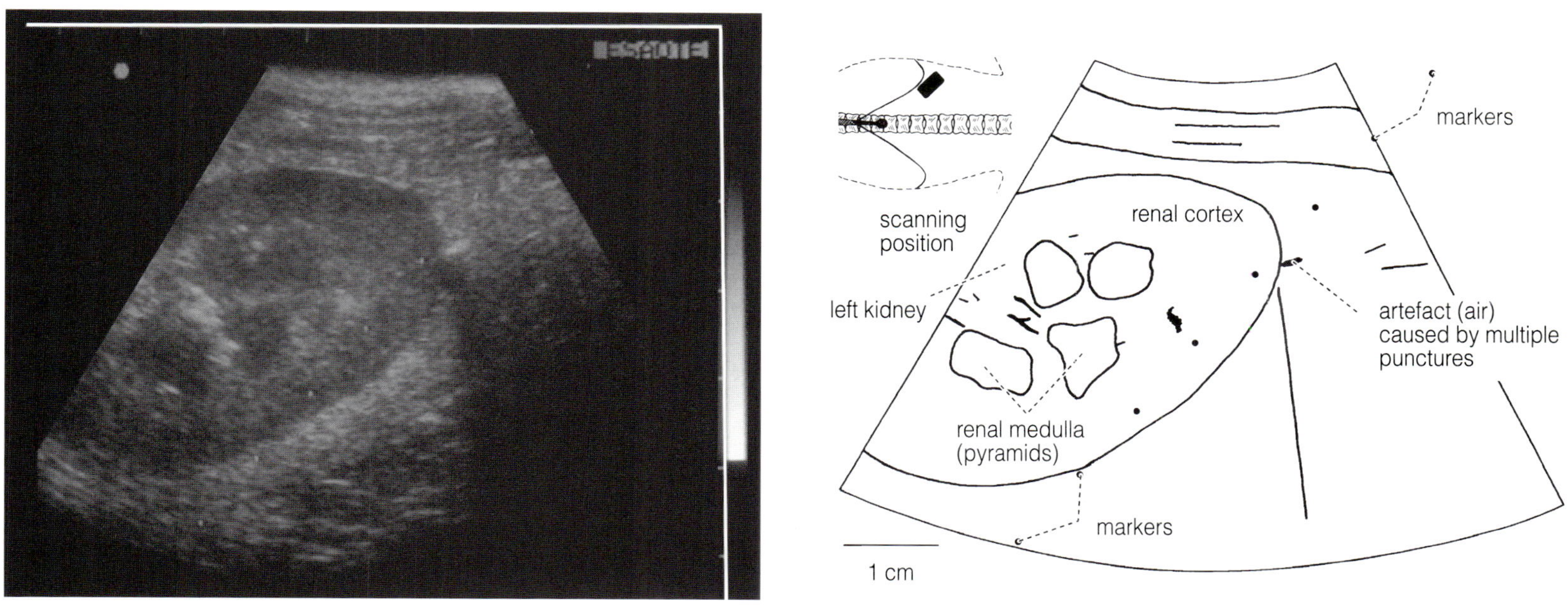

854

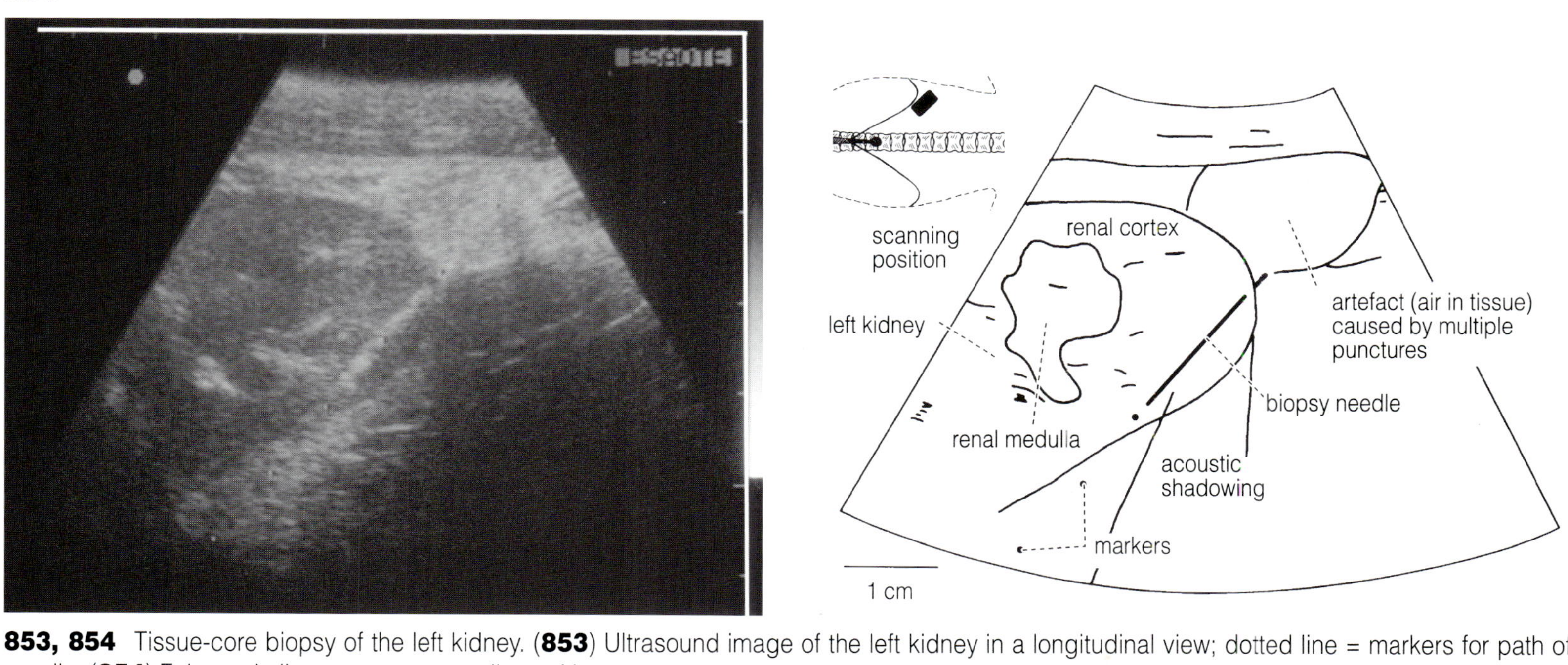

853, 854 Tissue-core biopsy of the left kidney. (**853**) Ultrasound image of the left kidney in a longitudinal view; dotted line = markers for path of needle. (**854**) Echogenic line represents needle position.

855

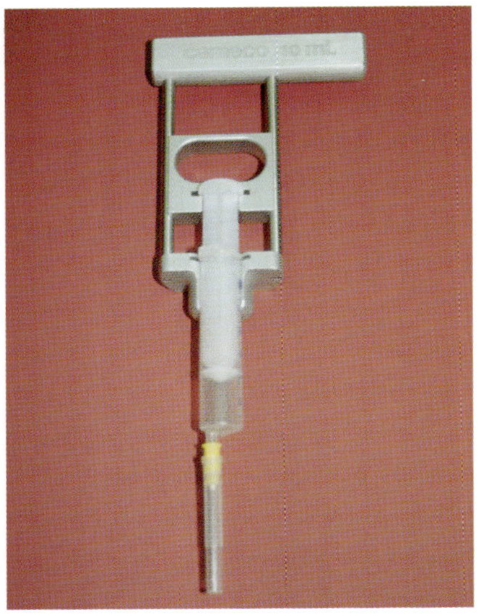

855 Syringe suction device for fine-needle aspiration biopsies.

856

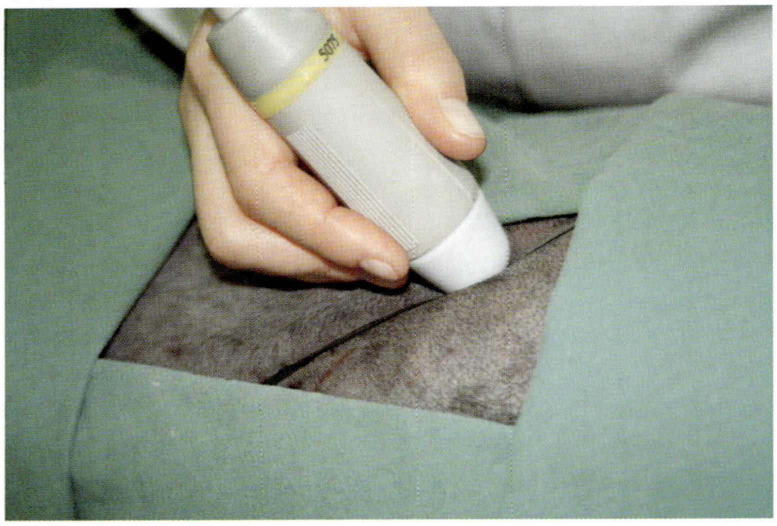

857

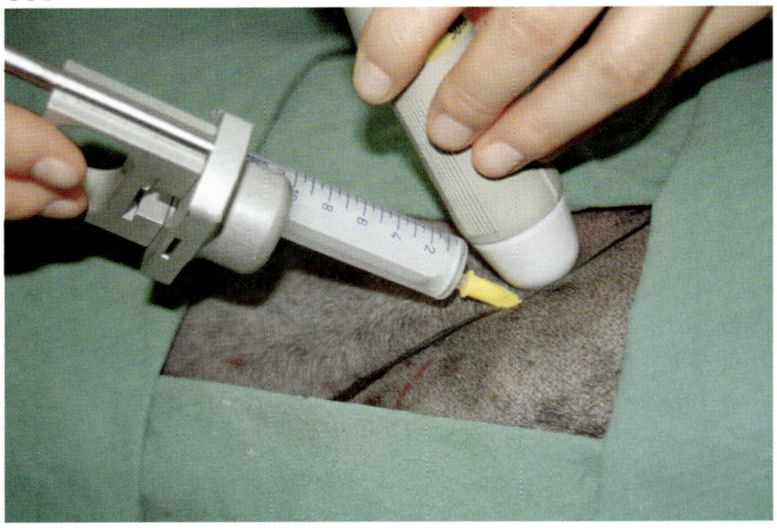

856, 857 Fine-needle aspiration biopsy of the liver. (**856**) Transducer placement caudal to the rib cage. (**857**) 'Hand-free' puncture of the liver with ultrasound guidance.

Technique – Demonstrated on a Kidney Biopsy

The kidney should be biopsied at the renal cortex to obtain useful tissue samples and to avoid postoperative complications. The biopsy needle should not penetrate the corticomedullary junction, since the vascular network of arcuate arteries and veins is located in this area and haemorrhaging is likely. For this reason, kidney biopsies must be performed on anaesthetized animals. Biopsies of other abdominal organs (liver, spleen, prostate) and masses may be obtained without general anaesthesia in cooperative patients.

Kidney biopsies are performed with the dog in right lateral recumbency. The biopsy site is prepared surgically. Transducer–skin contact is achieved with disinfectant agents and sterile ultrasound gel. (Ample amounts of alcohol are usually sufficient when sterile gel is not available.)

The transducer is placed caudal to the rib cage, and the caudal pole of the kidney is localized (851). After the biopsy markers have indicated the expected path of the needle and are directed to the renal cortex (853), the needle is advanced through the biopsy guide into the abdominal cavity (852) and guided ultrasonographically to the renal capsule. When using a semi-automated Biopty® gun (850), the needle is shot into the renal cortex (854), removed immediately from the organ, and the tissue sample placed in a fixative solution.

Potential haemorrhaging should be ruled out with postbiopsy scans of the kidney and bladder.

Patient Management Following Biopsy

Following a biopsy procedure, the patient should have cage rest for 24–48 hours and monitored for postbiopsy haemorrhage. A continuous intravenous drip is recommended to prevent blood clots in the renal pelvis. Abdominal palpation should be avoided. Antibiotic prophylaxis is usually not necessary, but is helpful in weakened patients.

Fine-Needle Aspiration Biopsy

Ultrasound-guided, fine-needle aspiration biopsies, followed by cytology, are used to obtain information an tumorous masses in the abdominal cavity. They are usually performed as 'hand-free' biopsies.

Equipment

Disposable syringes with 0.6–0.9 mm needles are used for fine-needle aspiration biopsies. Suction syringe devices are recommended (855).

Technique – Demonstrated on a Liver Puncture

Samples of diffuse parenchymal lesions are taken from the left liver lobe to avoid complications involving the gallbladder on the right side. Focal lesions must be biopsied at their location.

General anaesthesia is necessary only in uncooperative patients. The dog is placed in dorsal recumbency, the biopsy site prepared surgically, sterile ultrasound gel applied and the transducer placed caudal to the rib cage (856). After imaging the left liver lobe in a longitudinal plane (858), the needle is advanced into the abdominal cavity (857) and the needle position monitored by its tip echo

858

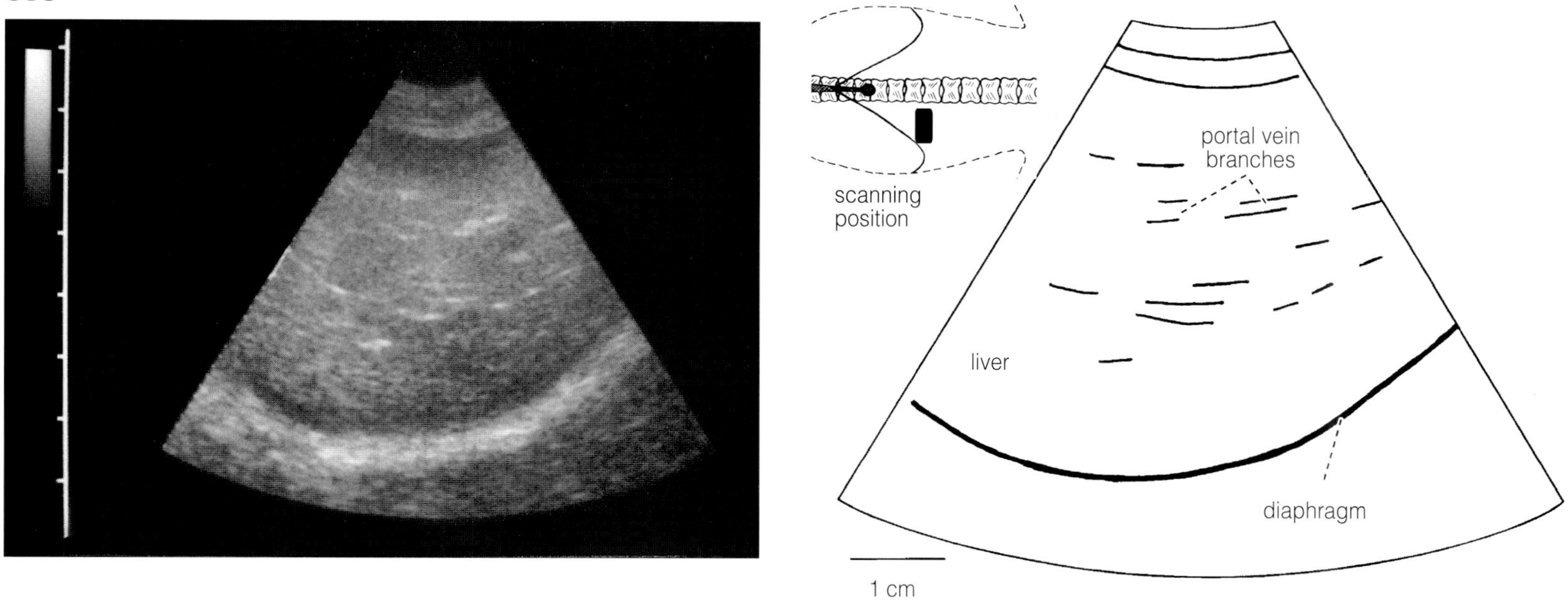

859

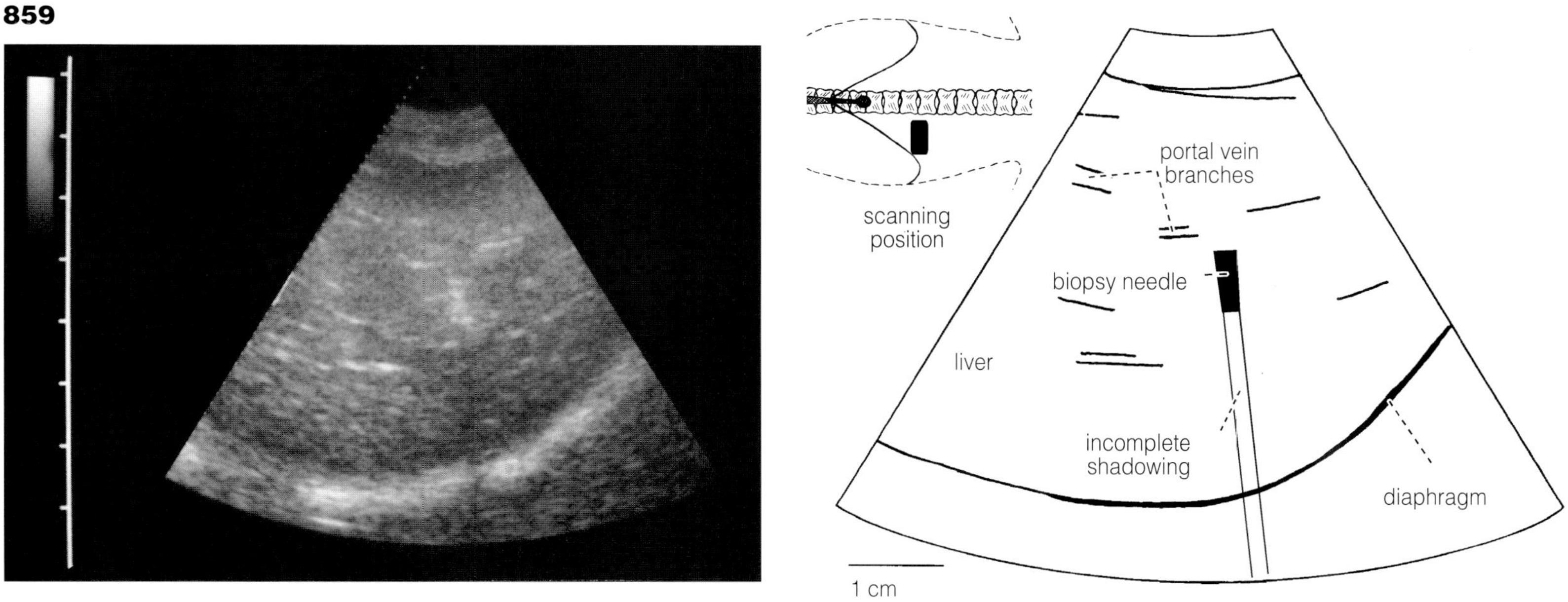

858, 859 Fine-needle aspiration biopsy of the liver. (**858**) Ultrasound image of the liver. (**859**) Distinct needle tip echo.

(859). Cell samples are obtained by frequent aspirations. These samples are then smeared onto a slide, fixated and stained.

Postbiopsy complications with fine-needle aspirations are uncommon.

Fluid Aspiration

Ultrasound examination allows aspiration of small amounts of fluid from the body cavities and the pericardium. Guided aspirations reduce the risks of this procedure.

Ultrasound-guided cystocentesis is also advantageous. Urine samples are not contaminated with bacteria, cells and cellular debris from the urogenital tract. The risk of iatrogenic bacterial contamination is also reduced.

Equipment

Aspiration is done with the help of disposable syringes and needles not exceeding 0.7 mm in size. Other body fluids may require thicker needles, depending on fluid viscosity.

860

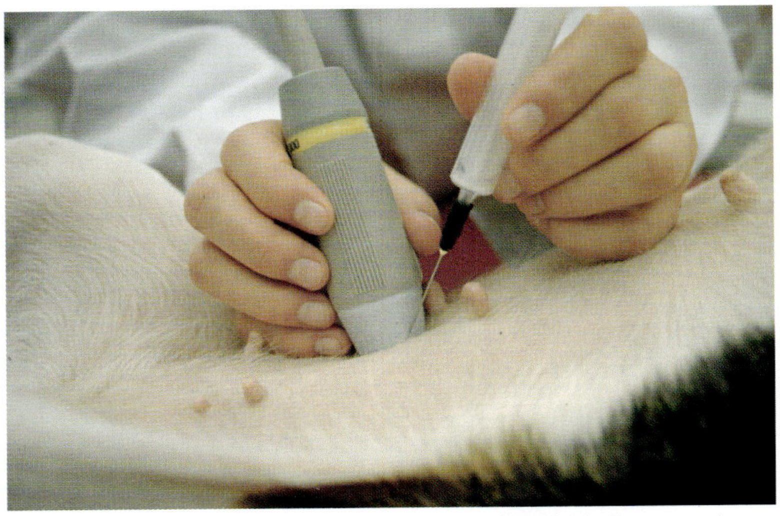

861

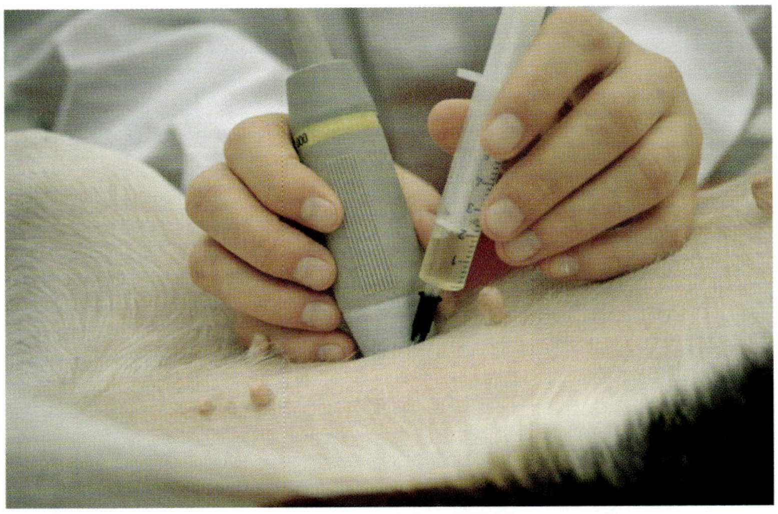

860, 861 Urine sample from cystocentesis. (**860**) Median transducer placement, caudodorsal needle insertion. (**861**) Urine sample.

862

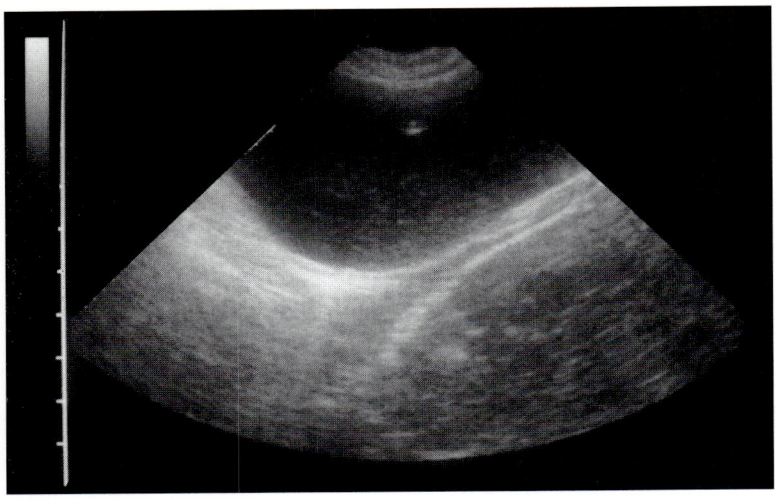

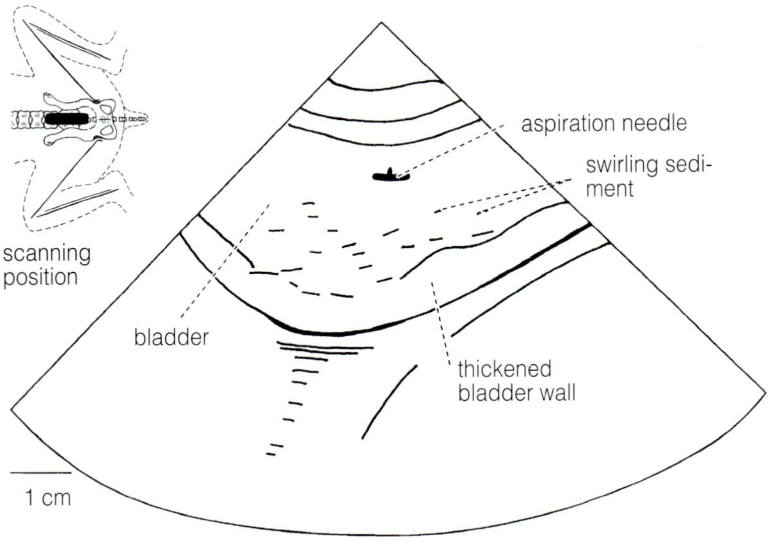

862 Urine sample from cystocentesis. Ultrasound image of the bladder with the visible needle tip.

Technique – Demonstrated by Cystocentesis

The animal is placed in dorsal recumbency, the caudal abdomen clipped and the skin cleaned. Ample amounts of alcohol allow good transducer–skin contact.

The transducer is placed cranial to the pubic symphysis (**860**). The urinary bladder is located and evaluated for location and size. The needle is inserted in a caudodorsal direction (**861**). Because the needle tip echo is visible in the filled bladder (**862**), its position can be monitored during the procedure.

References

Cited References

1 Bahlmann J and Otto P (1972) Perkutane Nierenbiopsie mit Ultraschall-Lokalisation. *Dtsch. Med. Wochenschr.* **97**, 840–842.

2 Hager DA, Nyland TG and Fisher P (1985) Ultrasound-guided biopsy of the canine liver, kidney, and prostate. *Radiol.* **26**, 82–88.

3 Nyland TG, Park RD, Latimer JC, Lebel JL and Miller CW (1991) Gray-scale ultrasonography of the canine abdomen. *Vet. Radiol.* **22**, 220–227.

4 Otto RC and Wellauer J (1985) *Ultraschallgeführte Biopsie*. Springer Verlag, Berlin, Heidelberg, New York.

5 Smith S (1985) Ultrasound-guided biopsy. *Vet. Clin. North Am. Small Anim. Pract.* **15**, 1249–1262.

Additional Reading

Höauf A and Lechner J (1991) Die Zystozentese bei Hand und Katze. *Tierärztl. Praxis* **19**, 535–538.

Jeraj KA, Osborne CA and Stevens JB (1982) Evaluation of renal biopsy in 197 dogs and cats. *J. Am. Vet. Med. Assoc.* **181**, 267–369.

Nash AS, Boyd JS, Minto AW and Wright NG (1983) Renal biopsy in the normal cat: an examination of the effects of a single needle biopsy. *Res. Vet. Sci.* **34**, 347–356.

Osborne CA, Finco DR, Low DG and Perman V (1967) Percutaneous renal biopsy in the dog and cat. *J. Am. Vet. Med. Assoc.* **151**, 1474–1480.

Osborne CA and Low DG (1971) Iatrogenic lesions in serial renal biopsy samples. *J. Urol.* **106**, 805–809.

Osborne CA and Low DG (1971) Size, adequacy, and artefacts of canine renal biopsy samples. *Am. J. Vet. Res.* **32**, 1865–1871.

Osborne CA (1971) Clinical evaluation of needle biopsy in the kidney and its complications in the dog and cat. *J. Am. Vet. Med. Assoc.* **158**, 1213–1228.

Osborne CA, Stevens JB and Perman V (1974) Kidney biopsy. *Vet. Clin. North Am. Small Anim. Pract.* **4**, 351–365.

Osborne CA, Johnston GR and Schenk MP (1977) Cystocentesis: indications, contraindications, technique and complications. *Minn. Vet.* **17**, 9–14.

Wise LA, Allen TA and Cartwright M (1989) Comparison of renal biopsy techniques in dogs. *J. Am. Vet. Med. Assoc.* **195**, 935–939.

863

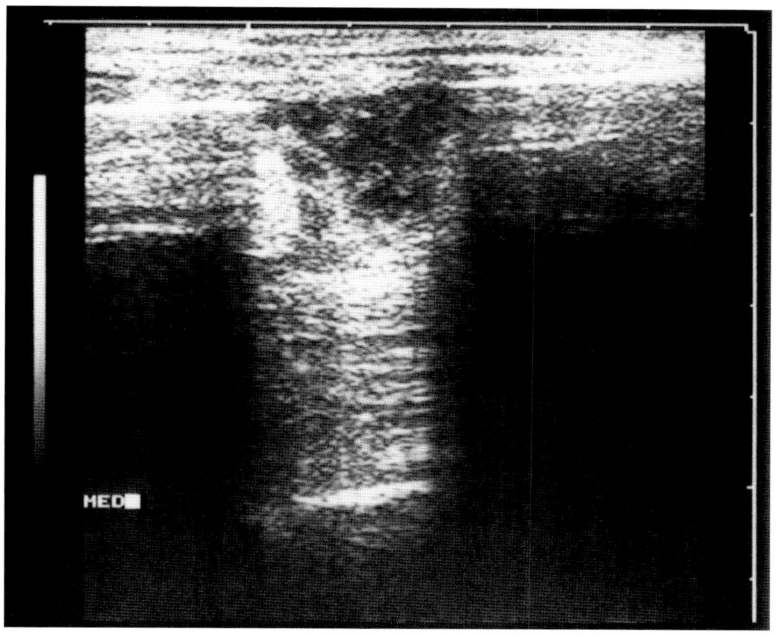

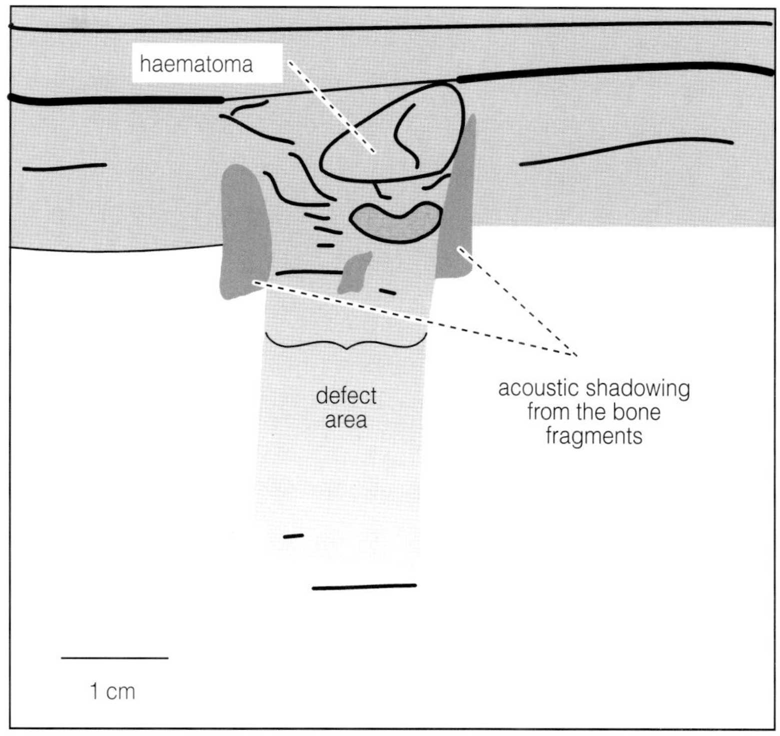

864

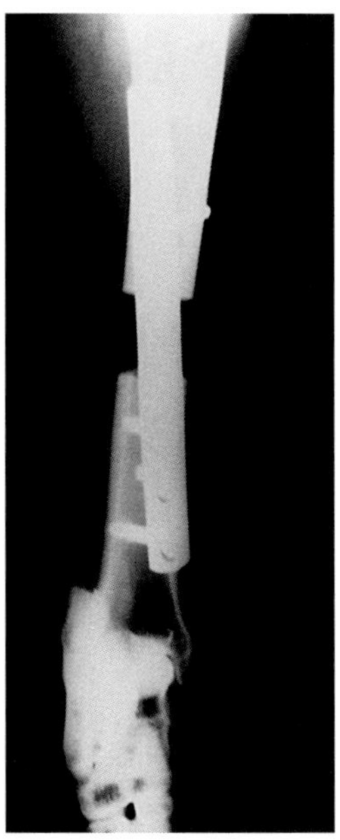

863, 864 Two-dimensional sonogram (**863**) and radiograph (**864**) of an open defect one week post surgery. Echogenic bone with regular surface contours is recognizable. The segmental defect is visible as a deep echo, marginated sharply by the bone fragments. The hypoechoic structures above the echogenic line represent haematomas.

Monitoring Bone Healing with B-Mode Ultrasonography

Burkhard Wippermann and Jörg Wefer

Research in ultrasonography of the musculoskeletal system includes visualization of ligaments and joints with associated lesions and also direct imaging of bones and their defects. Ultrasound was used successfully to diagnose fractures as early as 1958[2]. Over the following decades, the usefulness of ultrasonography, even with regard to standard radiography, was proven in images of stress fractures[5], obscured fractures[3], osteomyelitis[1, 6], skeletal metastasis[4] and other bone lesions.

In human medicine, ultrasonography has almost replaced radiography in displaying fractures in children and fractures of the sternum[7]. In some hospitals, ultrasound examinations are usually undertaken first in cases of provisional fracture diagnosis in children. Radiographs are only taken when there are uncertain ultrasound findings, e.g. long spiral fractures without displacement.

When interpreting ultrasonographic bone images, the following points must be considered:

- Since ultrasound waves cannot penetrate bone, the bone can only be evaluated for its surface shape and consistency.
- When scanning the bone in longitudinal planes, the transducer must be positioned until a regular echogenic line appears, resulting from a perpendicular sound beam.
- Each structure seen distal to this echogenic line must be considered an artefact.

To reconstruct the two standard radiographic views, four scanning planes should be imaged.

In this chapter the use of B-mode ultrasonography to monitor bone healing in a segmental defect of a sheep tibia is demonstrated. This animal experiment compares radiographic to ultrasonographic findings. The following images are from observations on the course of healing. Conventional radiographs in two planes and ultrasonographic long-axis views of all four tibial sides (cranial, caudal, medial, lateral), using a 7.5 MHz linear transducer, were produced (863–875). The sheep showed a 2 cm segmental defect in the middle of the tibial diaphysis. In seven animals the defect was left open; in eight sheep it was filled with autogenous spongiosa from pelvic bone. The defect

865

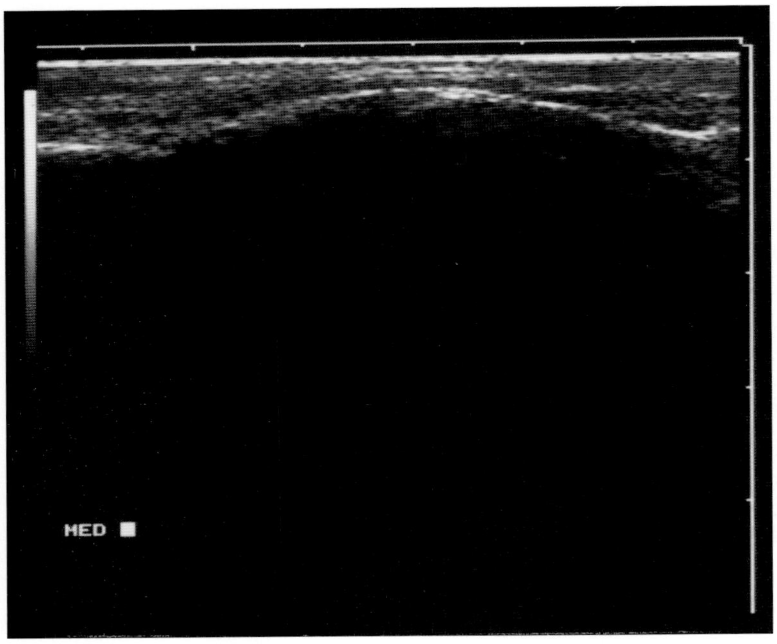

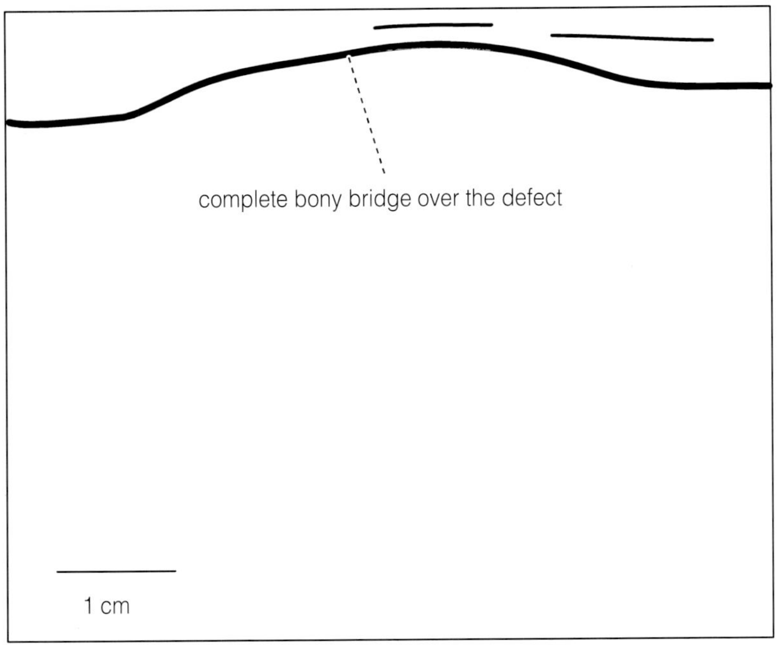

866

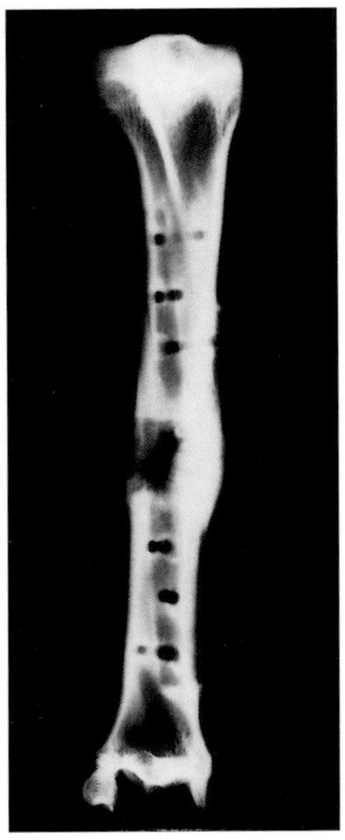

865, 866 Two-dimensional sonogram (**865**) and radiograph (**866**) of an open defect after sufficient ossification of the defect, twelve weeks post surgery. The ossified defect is almost identical to the adjacent tibial bone; the contours are smooth. There is no recognizable dehiscence between tibial bone and the newly formed bone.

was stabilized with an osteosynthesis plate. The animals were monitored for 12 weeks. Radiographs were made on the day of surgery. One week later, radiographic as well as ultrasonographic examinations were carried out and then repeated two, four, eight and 12 weeks post surgery.

Some references describe bone healing in sheep to be similar to that in dogs and cats[8].

The group with the open defect showed a pseudoarthrosis on radiographs and on plate removal. Six out of the seven cases were recognized as pseudoarthrosis on ultrasound examination. A cone-shaped gap was seen ultrasonographically. In the group with the spongiosa-filled defect, all animals showed a cortex-like structure ('corticalization') in the defect area, representing bony consolidation. Radiographic and macroscopic findings coincided with the sonographic findings in all eight animals.

In human medicine, 'corticalization' is used as a criterium in bone healing, e.g. femoral fractures in children. Fractures are considered healed when three of the four scanning planes show corticalization. Ultrasonography is therefore a reliable method for monitoring bone healing, especially healing of spongiosa grafts.

References

1 Abiri MM, Kirpekar M and Ablow RC (1989) Osteomyelitis: detection with ultrasound. *Radiol.* **172**, 509–511.

2 Anast T, Fields T and Siegel IM (1958) Ultrasonic technique for the evaluation of bone fractures. *Am. J. Phys. Med.* **37**, 157–159.

3 Graf M, Stahl-Kent V, Ben-Ami T, Strauss S, Amit Y and Itzchak Y (1988) Sonographic detection of occult bone fractures. *Pediatric Radiol.* **18**, 383–385.

4 Mende U, Rieden K, Braun A, Weischedel U and Zum Winkel K (1986) Die real-time-Sonographie – Ein wichtiges bildgebendes Verfahren bei Diagnostik und Therapieplanung von Skelettmetastasen. *Rö. Fo.* **145**, 373–378.

5 Moss A and Mowatt AG (1983) Ultrasonic assessment of stress fractures. *Br. Med. J.* **286**, 1479–1480.

6 Williamson SL, Seibert JJ, Glasier CM, Leithiser RE and Aronson J (1991) Ultrasound in advanced pediatric osteomyelitis. *Pediatric Radiol.* **21**, 288–290.

7 Wippermann BW (1993) Sonographie der Frakturen. *Hefte zu der Unfallchirurgie* **232**, 678–283.

8 Wissing H, Stürmer KM and Breidenstein G (1990) Die Wertigkeit verschiedener Tierspezies für experimentelle Untersuchungen am Knochen. *Hefte zur Unfallheilkande* **212**, 479–488.

867

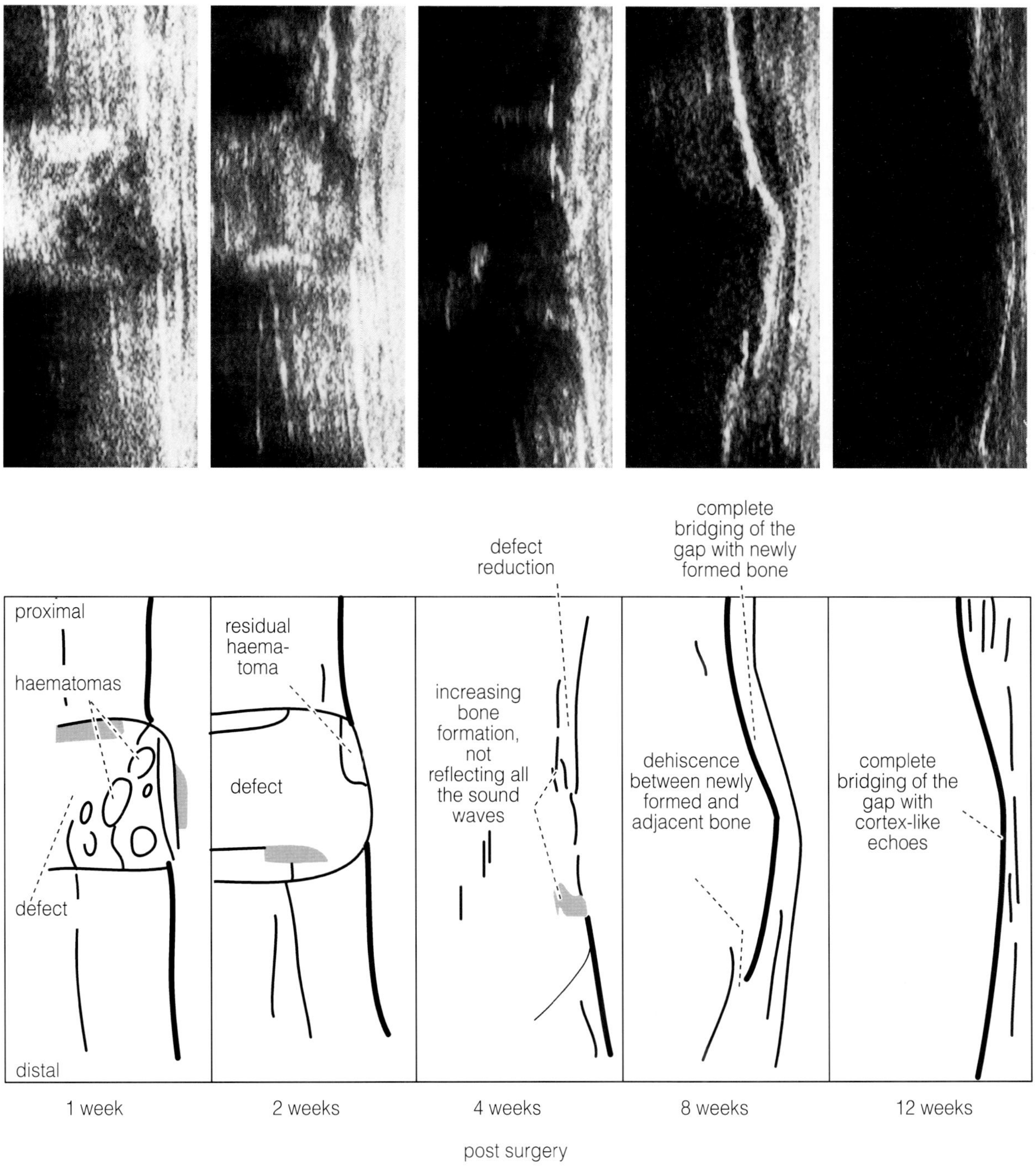

867 Two-dimensional sonograms of sufficient healing of the bone defect. The gap becomes progressively smaller. This represents callus formation at the defect margins. Depending on callus formation deeper in the defect, the size of the echo appears smaller. The surface of the defect becomes more regular and echogenic, coinciding with increasing bone mineralization.

868

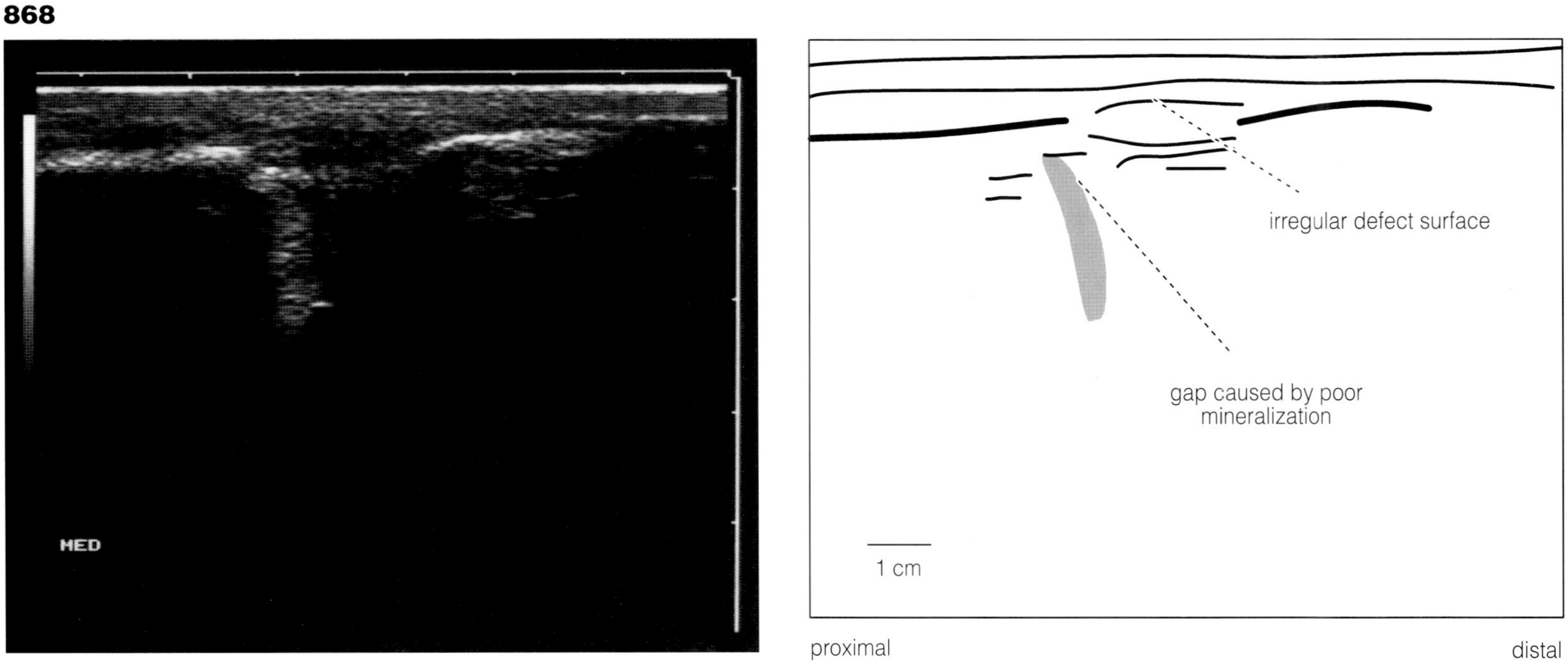

869

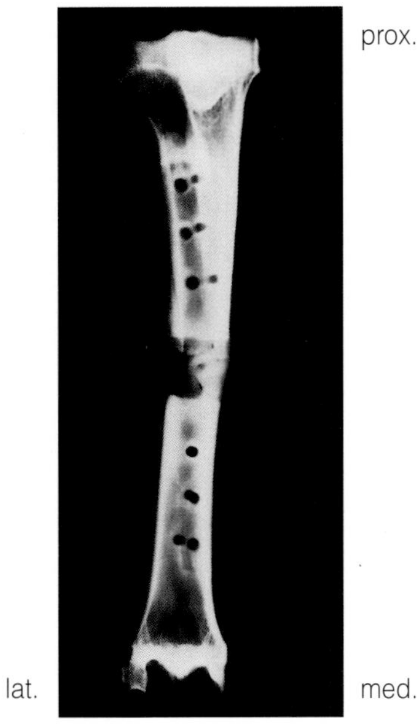

868, 869 Two-dimensional sonogram (**868**) and radiograph (**869**) of an incomplete union of the fracture ends, twelve weeks post surgery. The defect appears narrower and sound penetration deep to the defect is clearly reduced. The defect surface is not as echogenic as the adjacent bone. Differentiation between the defect itself and the original bone is still possible. Acoustic enhancement is produced by the poorly mineralized gap, which is also seen medially on the radiograph.

870

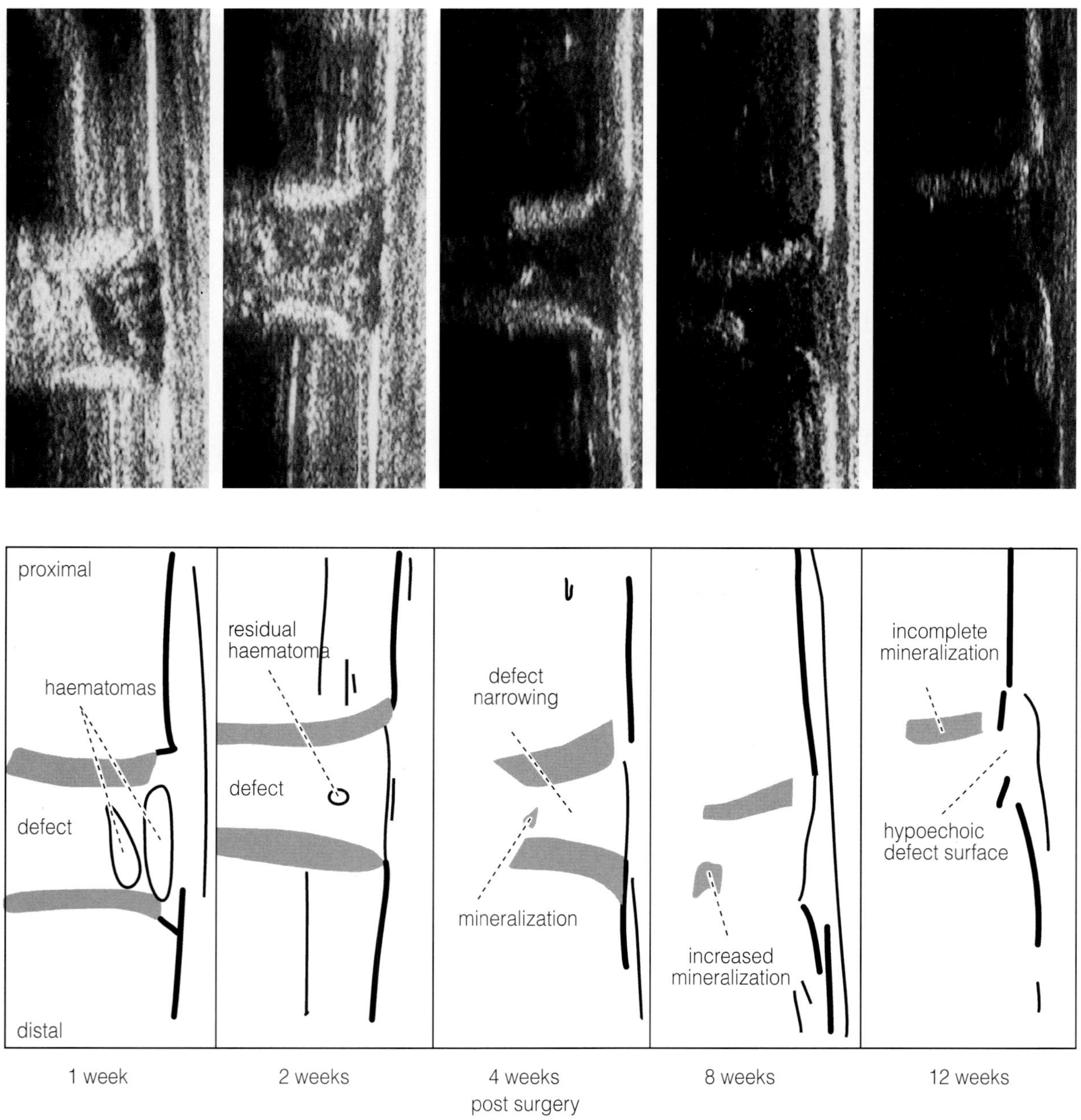

870 Two-dimensional sonograms, showing non-union of the bone defect. The gap is somewhat smaller, although the surface does not show the cortex-like echoes characteristic for union of the defect. Acoustic enhancement represents the gap.

871

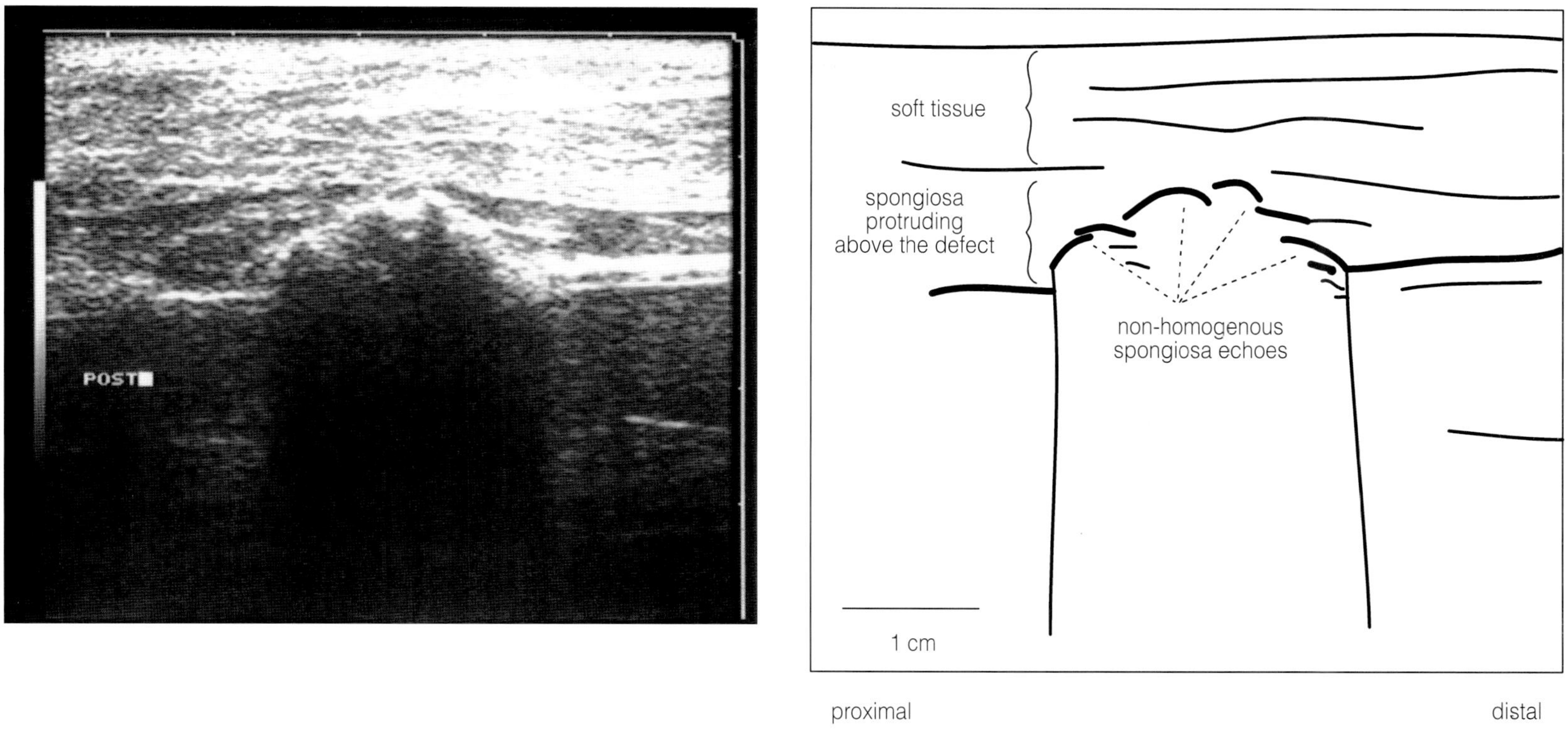

872

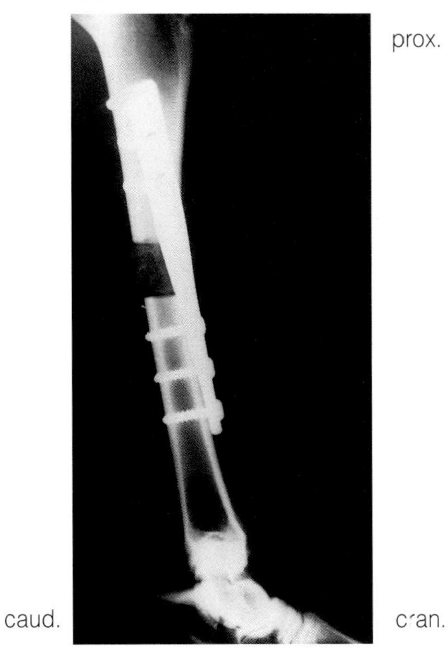

871, 872 Two-dimensional sonogram (**871**) and radiograph (**872**) of a spongiosa transplant, one week post surgery. The spongiosa-filled defect, i.e. the spongiosa material, appears less echogenic and regular than the surrounding bone. Both the sonogram and the radiograph show the spongiosa transplant protruding above the defect.

873, 874 Two-dimensional sonogram (**873**) and radiograph (**874**) of a spongiosa transplant twelve weeks post surgery, with complete ossification and integration of the spongiosa within the tibia. The original defect is not clearly visible. The bone surface has a regular, total reflection, without dehiscence between the original and newly-formed bone.

873

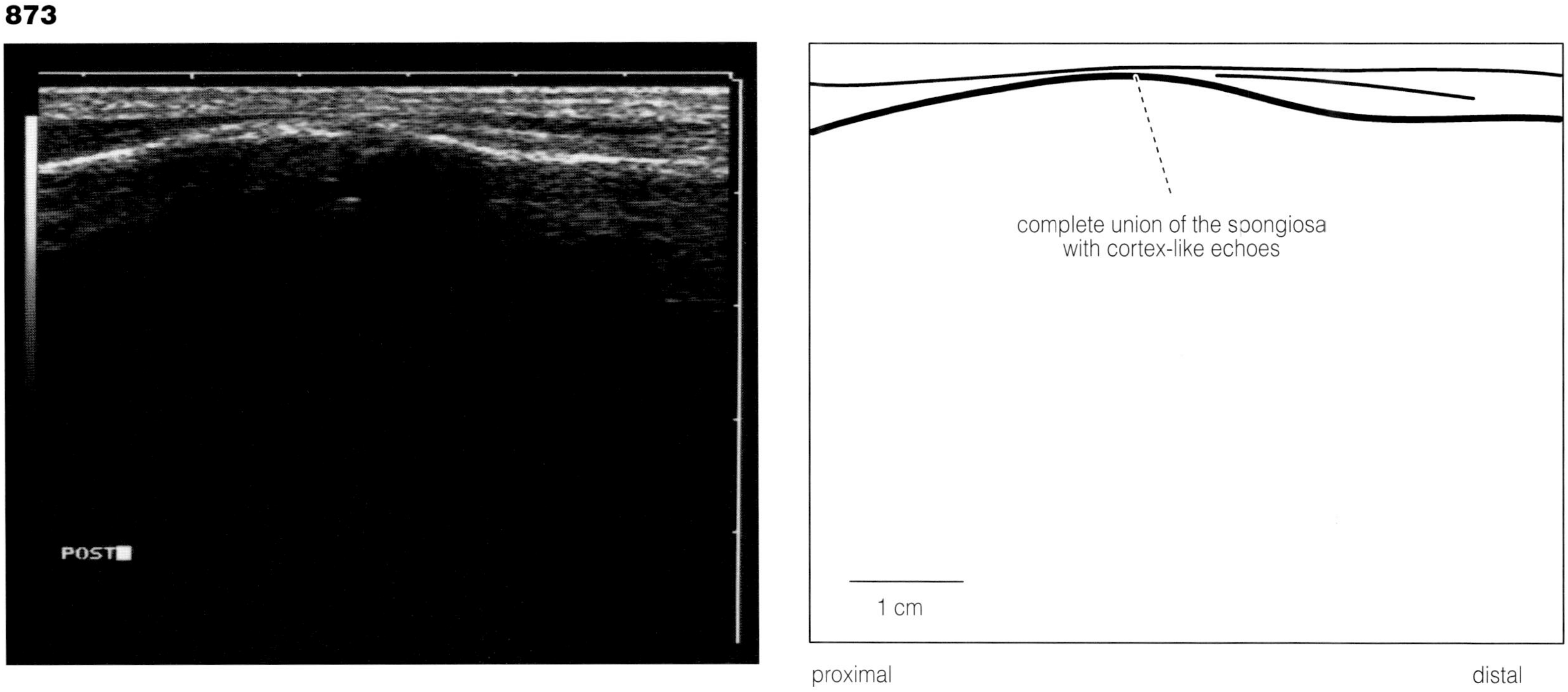

874

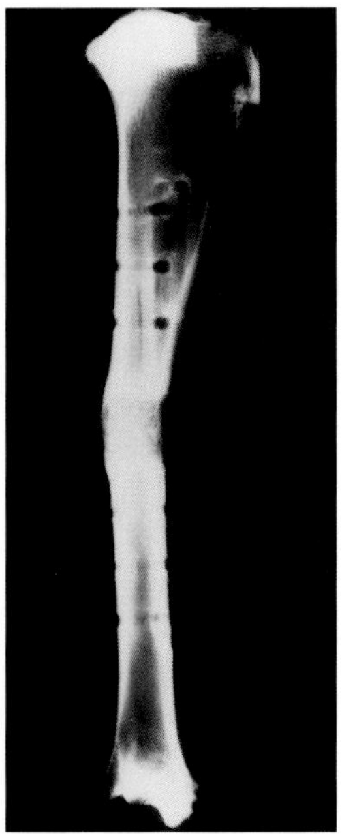

874 Radiograph of a spongiosa transplant twelve weeks post surgery, with complete ossification and integration of the spongiosa within the tibia (see also **873**).

875

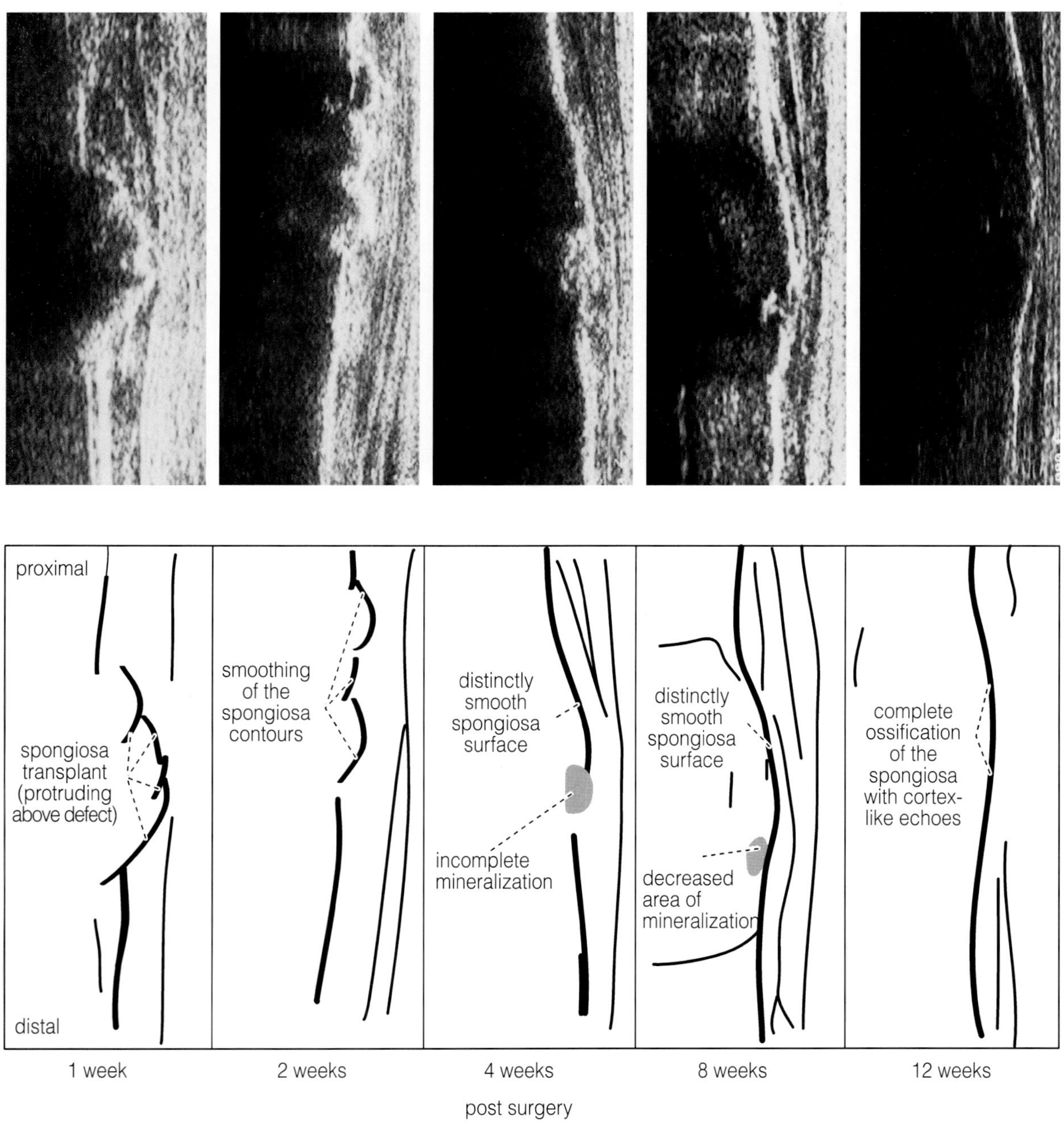

875 Two-dimensional sonograms showing union of a spongiosa transplant. Mineralization and ossification of the spongiosa produce a more homogenous and echogenic defect surface. The surface structure and echogenicity appear similar to the adjacent bone.

Ultrasonographic Usefulness and Limitations in Monitoring Secondary Fracture Healing

Julia Henke, Barbara Güssregen and Martin Köhle

General Observations

Veterinary traumatology and orthopaedics requires an easy and non-invasive method for early postoperative monitoring of periosteal callus formation with fracture healing. Repeated radiographs are problematic, because of radiation exposure to the animal, owner and veterinary personnel. Furthermore, radiographic methods display only the inorganic callus components, while disregarding the organic constituents influencing stability. Summation artefacts in radiographs and scintigraphy often mask numerous clinical complications, such as fissures and pseudoarthrosis, that are important to recognize and treat early in the healing process. Nuclear medicine examinations e.g. magnetic resonance imaging, are limited to larger clinics, because of the technical equipment requirements and cost. Ultrasonography offers a non-invasive method to monitor continuously fracture healing in all planes.

Instrumentation and Examination Technique

A 7.5 MHz transducer (sector scanner) with a built-in stand-off pad is useful for evaluating the surface structure in long bones of the dog. The extremity does not have to be clipped, since the area in question has usually been prepared surgically. **NB:** In the first weeks post surgery, the scanning site should be chosen carefully to avoid non-removed or non-resorbable suture material. The same is true for plates, screws and cerclages not placed intramedullary.

After applying coupling gel, the region of interest should be scanned in its entirety. It is important to scan longitudinally to the anatomy of the long bone, and to chose the axial plane. From experience, this is easiest along the diaphysis. This area allows the best transducer positioning (**876A[1]**). Then move it over craniolaterally to a cranial position (**876A[2]**), and over caudolaterally to a caudal position (**876A[3]**). Finally, an evaluation from the medial aspect should follow (**876B[4]**). Mediocranial and mediocaudal regions in the femoral area are not usually visible because of muscle topography.

With cranial and caudal transducer positions, closeness to the bone should be considered. Slight transducer pressure will displace some of the muscles.

Ultrasonographic Evaluation Criteria in Clinical Use

During secondary fracture healing, a continuous increase in echogenicity is seen ultrasonographically in the area of periosteal callus formation. This is caused by progressive transformation of the fracture haemotoma to fibrous bone. Other critera include structural non-homogenicity and development of a border lamella. Differentiation of varying mineralization stages helps to evaluate maturation of the newly formed bone. This is usually seen about four weeks earlier than on radiographs. Mineralization does not provide information on biomechanical qualities of the bone. Ultrasonography is also important in detecting pseudoarthrosis and differentiating between atrophic and hypertrophic forms when monitoring fracture healing.

876

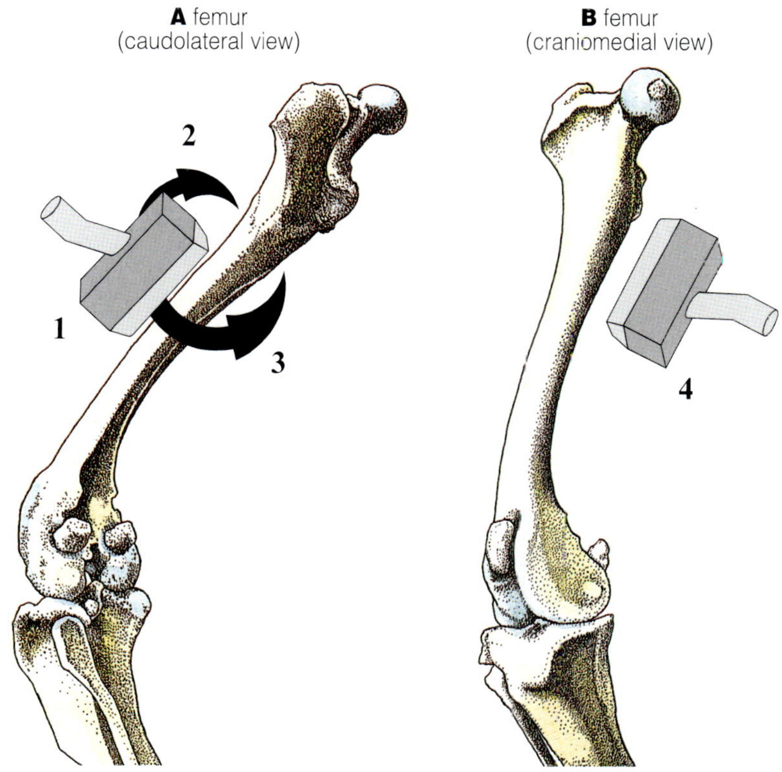

876 Transducer positioning on the femur. (Reprinted with kind permission of Prof. Dr. K.-D. Budras, Berlin from Budras K-D, Fricke W and Richter R (1996) *Atlas der Anantomie des Hundes.* 5th ed. Schluetersche Verlagsanstalt und Druckerei, Hannover.)

Ultrasonography is also very useful in monitoring bone traction osteogenesis in orthopaedics, such as bone axis misalignments following premature epiphyseal closure or after tumour surgery to fill in the bone defect. This non-invasive method monitors callus formation.

Ultrasonographic characteristics of secondary fracture healing are listed in *Table 47*.

Table 47 Ultrasonographic characteristics of secondary fracture healing.

Ultrasonographic characteristics:
• Displacement or gap in the fracture or osteotomy area. • Early focal ossification. • Periosteal callus formation. • Bony bridging and consolidation of the fracture or osteotomy. • Transformation of bone transplants.

Case Study of Normal Fracture Healing (877–882)

877

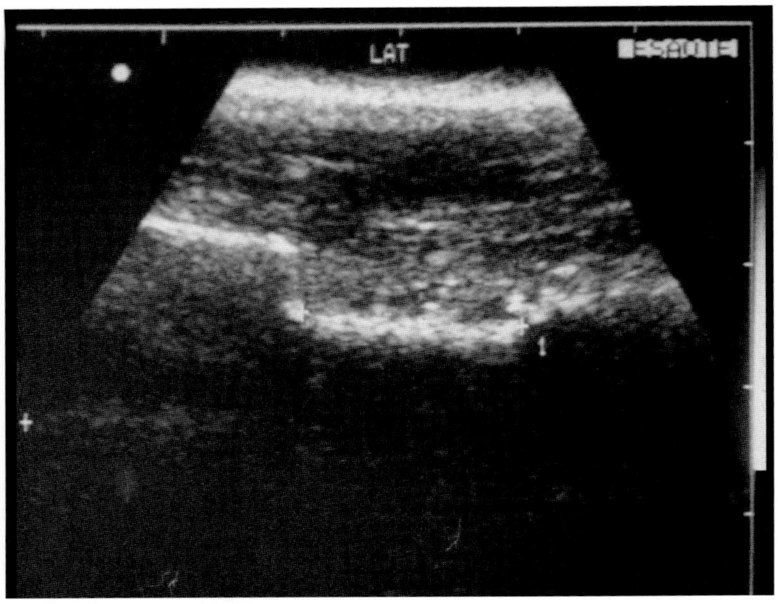

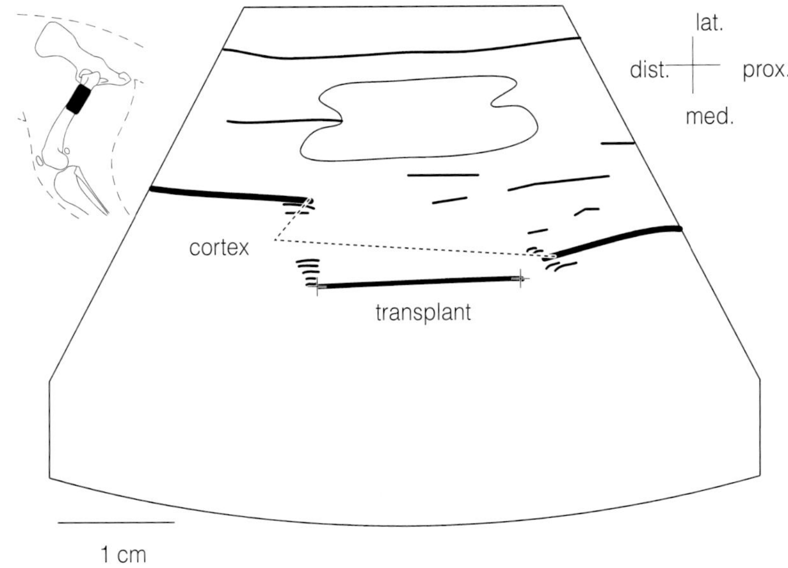

878

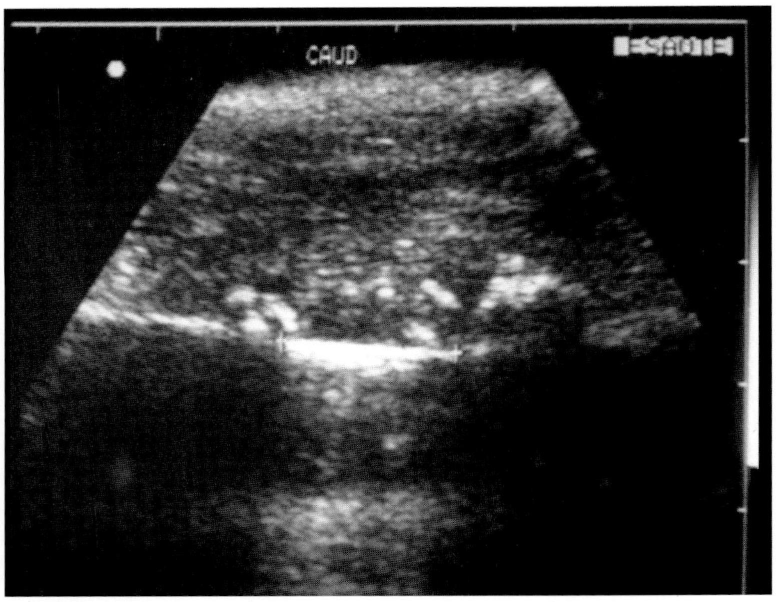

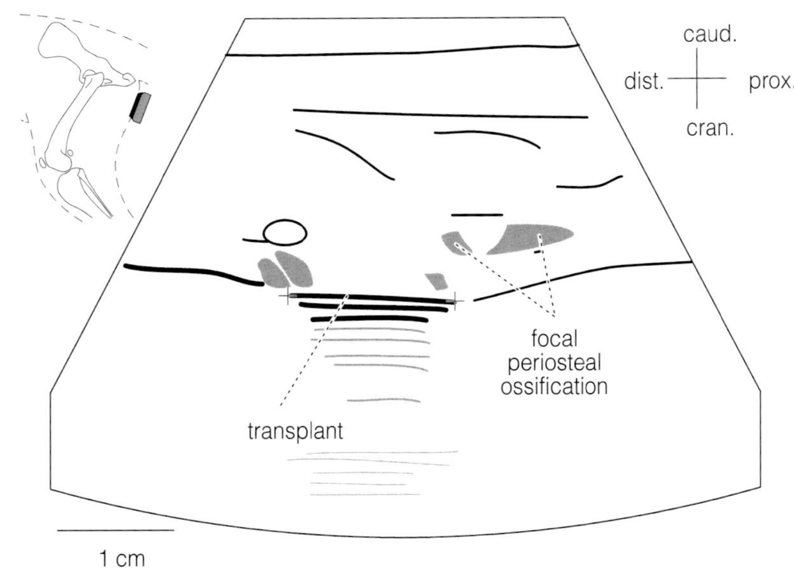

877, 878 Two-dimensional sonogram four weeks post surgery. (**877**) Lateral view: cortex reflections with medial acoustic shadowing in the transplant area (calipers) and non-homogenous, hypoechoic callus structure. (**878**) Caudal view: decreased echogenicity of the transplant and focal periosteal ossification.

879

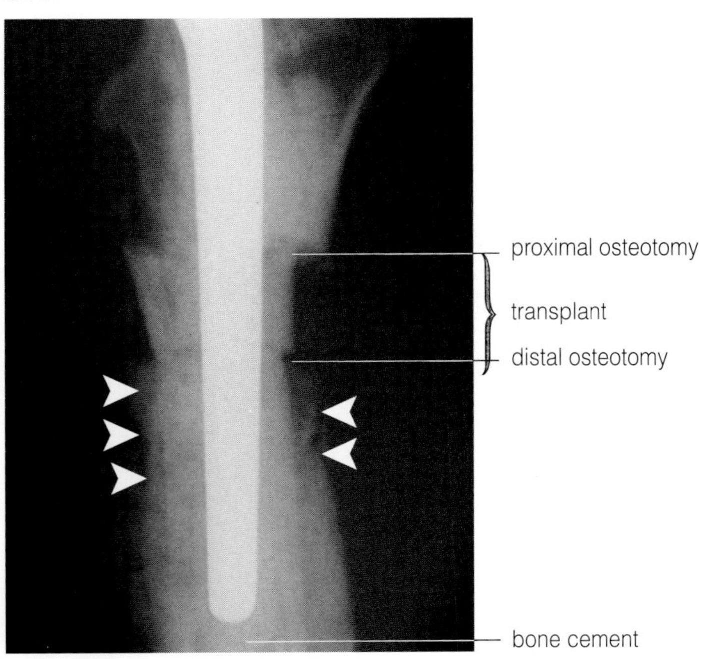

879 Radiograph in a mediolateral plane eight weeks post surgery. Slight periosteal bone apposition (arrowheads).

880

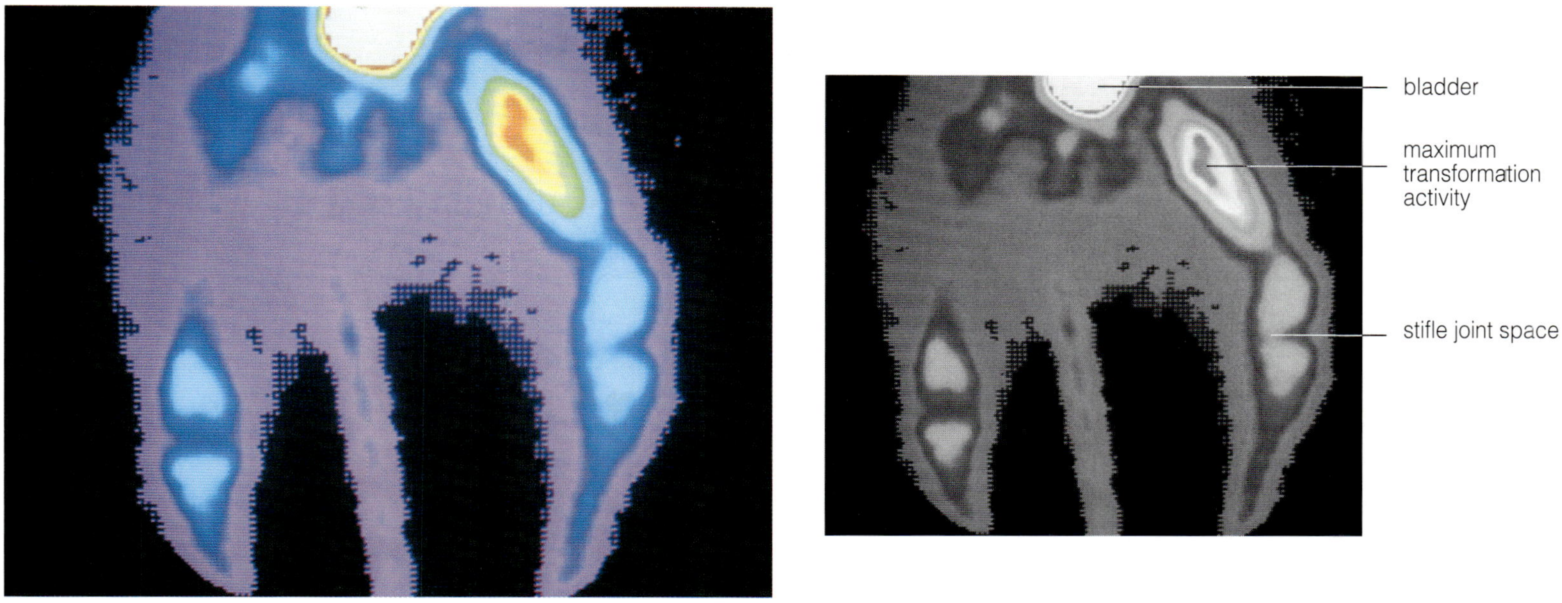

880 Late static bone scintigram (Tc99m - diphosphate) 12 weeks post surgery. Maximum transformation activity.

881

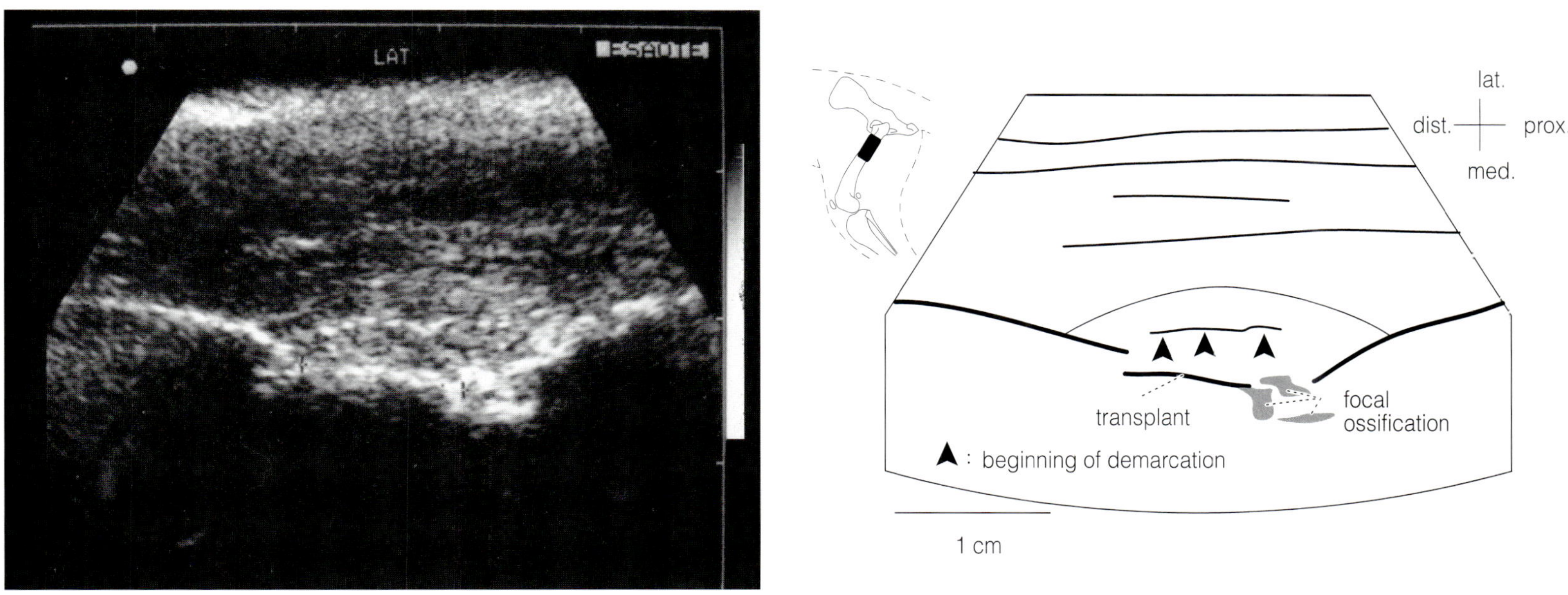

881 Two-dimensional sonogram 18 weeks post surgery. Beginning of demarcation of the border lamella (arrowheads).

882

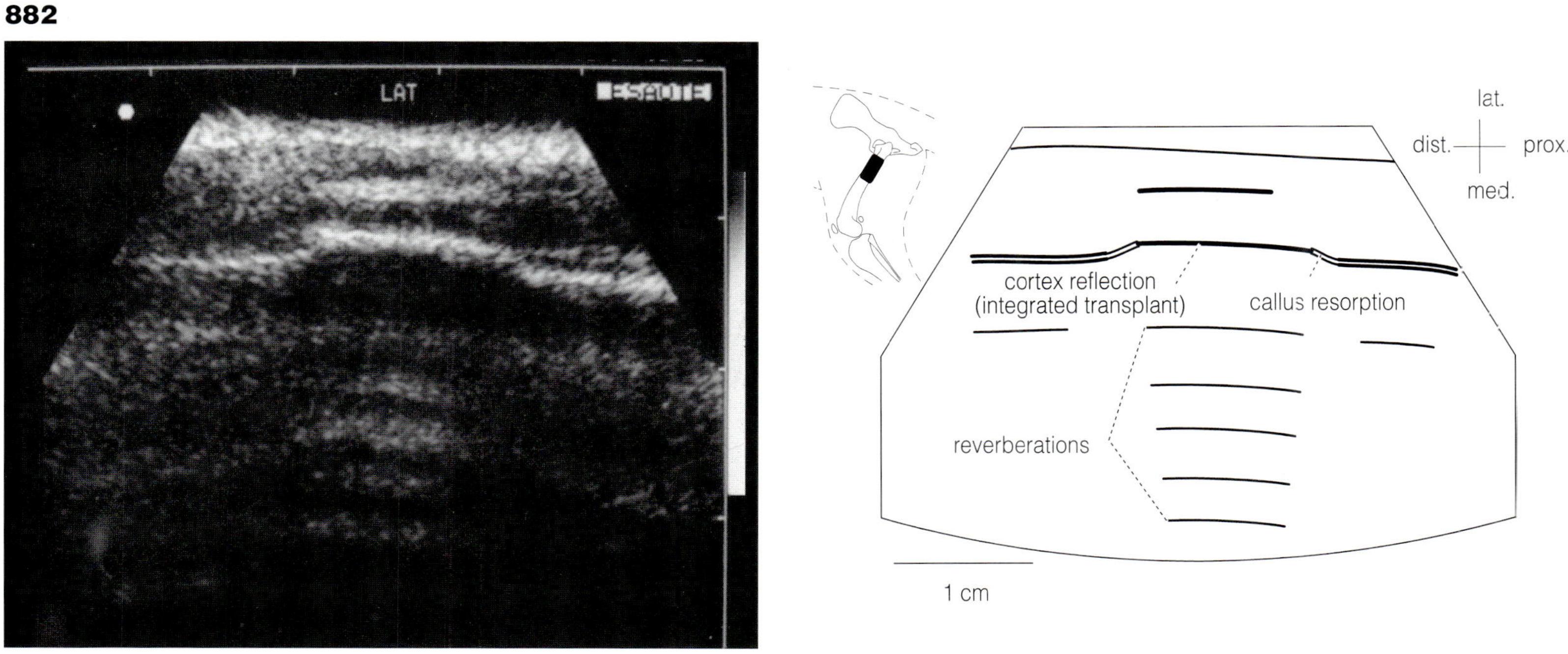

882 Two-dimensional sonogram 36 weeks post surgery. Cortex reflection with reverberations, representing bony integration of the transplant.

Case Study of Delayed Fracture Union (883–885)

883

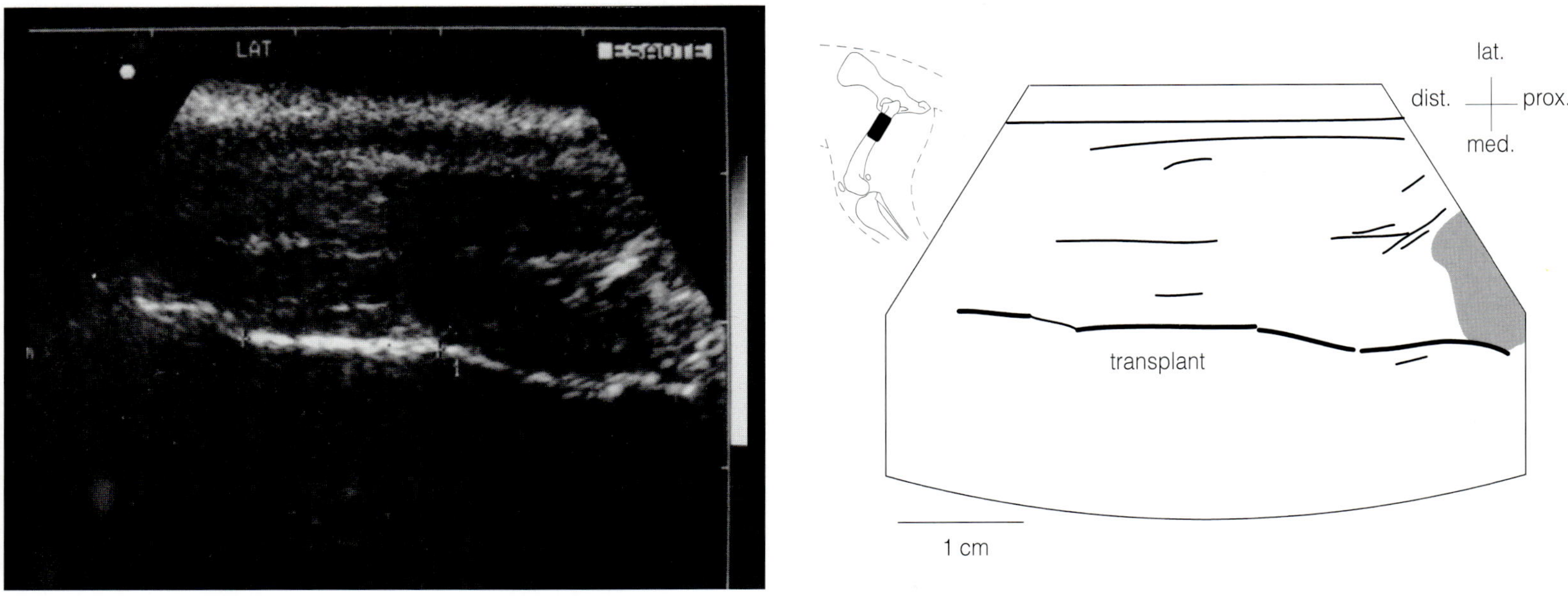

884

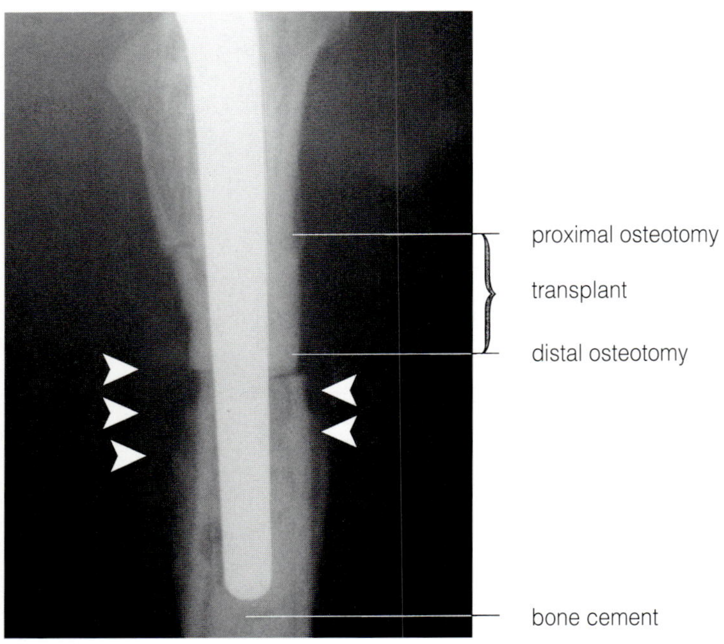

883, 884 Two-dimensional sonogram (**883**) and radiograph in a mediolateral view (**884**) eight weeks post surgery. (**883**) Cortex reflection with medial acoustic shadowing. (**884**) No apparent periosteal bone apposition with distinct osteotomy site (arrowheads).

885

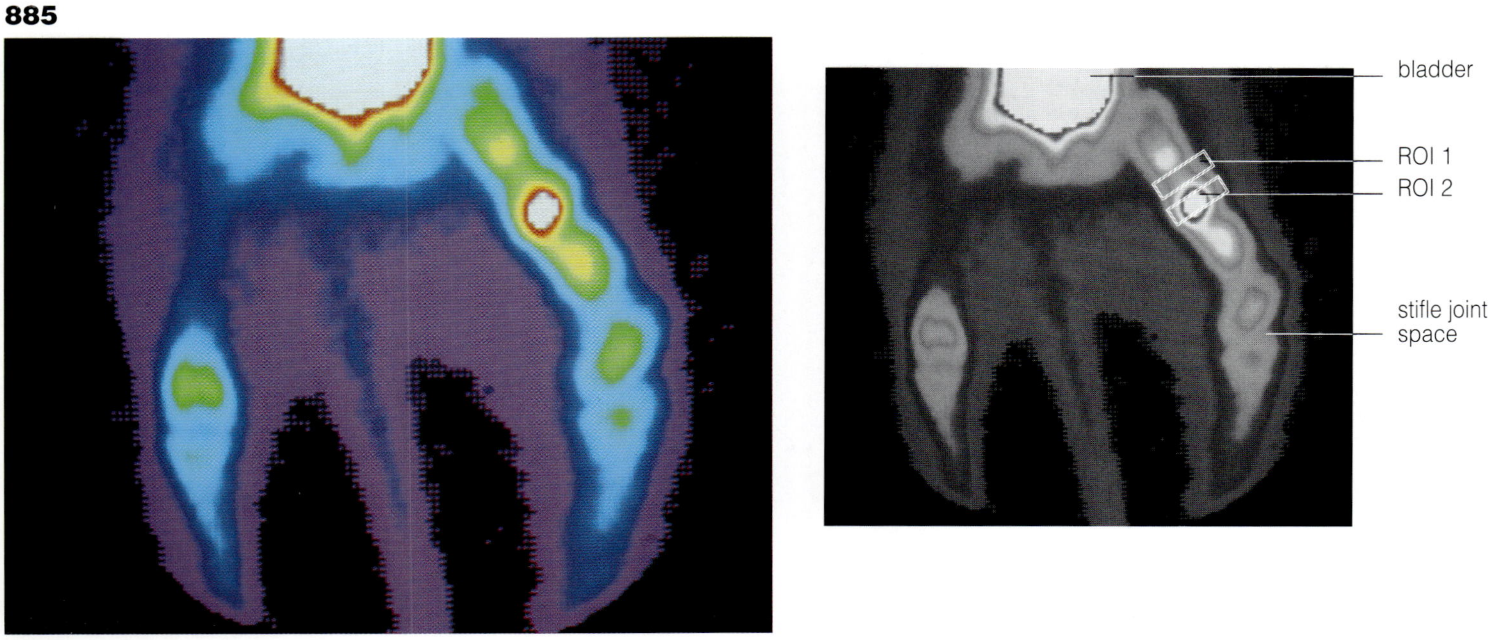

885 Scintigraphy 12 weeks post surgery. No nuclide accumulation in the transplant area (ROI 1 = region of interest 1: 'cold lesion') and activity accumulation in the adjacent diaphysis (ROI 2 = region of interest 2).

Comparing Imaging Methods

Compared to radiographic techniques, ultrasonography offers the following advantages when evaluating fracture healing phases:

- General advantages of ultrasonography over radiation exposure methods (quick, easy, cheap, repeatable).
- Easy handling and management of the unsedated patient; ultrasonography can be used earlier post surgery.
- Evaluation of the bone surface in its entire circumference.
- Higher sensitivity in detecting focal ossification and therefore earlier detection of organic callus substances influencing stability (about four weeks earlier than radiography).

The following disadvantages limit the use of ultrasonography in traumatology and orthopaedics:

- General disadvantages of ultrasonography, e.g. experience of the sonographer and relatively time consuming.
- Identical measurements require the same sonographer, control settings, measuring site.
- Thick muscles in some areas prevent scanning of certain structures.
- Osteosynthesis materials interfere with evaluation.
- With completely mineralized bone, total sound reflection off the cortex allows evaluation of the surface only.
- Quantification of periosteal callus formation is not possible.
- Complex fractures lead to difficulty in anatomical orientation.

Ultrasonography offers additional information about bone healing processes, compared to standardized radiological methods such as skeletal scintigraphy and radiography. Although ultrasonography is complementary to these methods, it can never replace the radiograph because of the limitations of its methodology.

References

Dickens JR, Bray DE and Palmer RH (1994) An ultrasonic attenuation parameter for investigating the holding power of non-threaded fixation pins (*in vitro*). *Ultrasonics* **32**, 65–70.

De Lutio di Castelguidone E, di Maggo B and di Gaeta S (1993) Echography in the monitoring of bone callus in fractures treated with external fixation. *Radio. Med. Torino* **85**, 579–582.

Eyres KS, Bell MJ and Kanis JA (1993) Methods of assessing new bone formation during limb lengthening. *J. Bone Joint Surg.* **75-B**, 358–364.

Fery-Lemonnier E, Roux C, Hazebroucq V, Legmann P and Viens-Bitkern C (1993) Value of techniques of measurement of bone. Radiological methods and constribution of ultrasonics. *J. Radiol.* **74**, 305–310.

Friedrich RE and Volkenstein RJ (1991) The value of ultrasonography in the diagnosis of zygomatic arch fractures. *Dtsch. Z. Mand Kiefer Gesichtschir.* **15**, 472–479.

Mafulli N, Hughes T and Fixsen JA (1992) Ultrasonographic monitoring of limb lengthening. *J. Bone Joint Surg.* **74-B**, 130–132.

Hamanishi C, Yosii T and Tanaka S (1994) Maturation of the distracted callus. Sonographic observations in rabbits applied to patients. *Acta Orthop. Scand.* **65**, 335–338.

Markel MD and Chao EY (1993) Noninvasive monitoring techniques for quantitative description of callus mineral content and mechanical properties. *Clin. Orthop.* **293**, 37–45.

Ricciardi L, Perissinotto A and Dabala M (1992) External callus development on ultrasound and its mechanical correlation. *Ital. J. Orthop. Traumatol.* **18**, 223–229.

Ricciardi L, Perissinotto A and Dabala M (1993) Mechanical monitoring of fracture healing using ultrasound imaging. *Clin. Orthop.* **293**, 71–76.

Stewart A, Reid DM and Porter RW (1994) Broad band ultrasound attenuation and dual energy X-ray absorptiometry in patients with hip fractures: which techniques determinates fracture risk. *Calcif. Tissue Int.* **54**, 466–469.

We dedicate this section posthumously with thanks to University Professor Dr. med. G. Bluemel.

Three-Dimensional Ultrasonography

Cordula Poulsen Nautrup

One of the disadvantages of two-dimensional ultrasonography lies in the visualization of separate scanning planes, which show a great variability – any plane is possible – and are therefore difficult to interpret and reproduce. Some lesions, such as cysts or neoplasia, often cannot be linked to a certain organ. The involvement of other structures with these lesions, such as abscesses, is often overlooked.

Since the late 1980s, human medicine has tried to solve this problem by reconstructing sonographic findings three-dimensionally[1, 8, 9].

Requirements for Three-Dimensional Scanning

Computer-based reconstruction of a spatial structure from separate two-dimensional images is only successful when numerous planes are available as basic material and their location to each other is exactly, i.e. mathematically, defined.

This type of 'coordinated slice sequence'[7] is produced in computed tomography (CT) and magnetic resonance tomography (imaging) (MRT/MRI) by a parallel image shift at a defined distance.

In conventional real-time ultrasonography, this parallel sequence shift is prevented by uneven body surfaces and the necessary firm application of the transducer on the skin. Every sideways movement of the transducer, in conjunction with irregularities and impressability of the skin, leads to a slight, but unavoidable, angulation in the scanning plane (**886**). In ultrasonography the defined cross-sectional sequences are achieved by rotating the scanning plane on a vertical or horizontal axis without changing the probe position. The 'coordinated ultrasono-

886

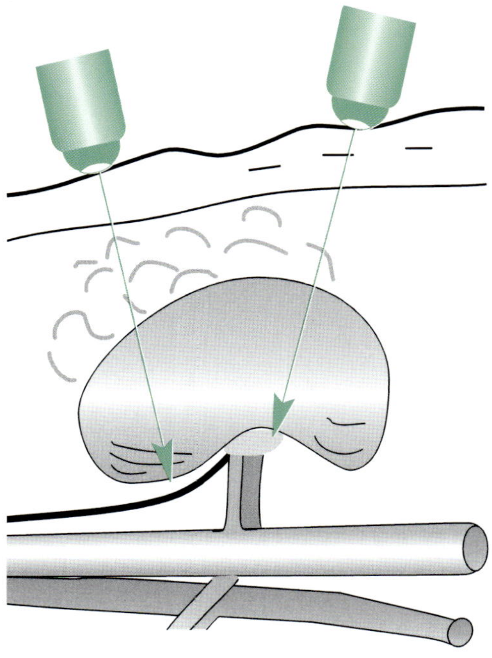

887

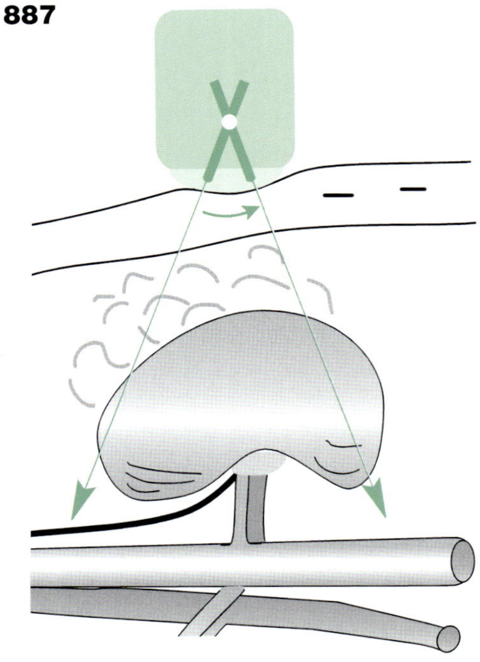

886, 887 Schematic drawings showing the impossibility of an angle-free shift of the transducer (**886**) and a defined horizontal rotation (**887**) to produce parallel scanning planes. (Modified from Sohn and Bastert, 1994[7]).

888

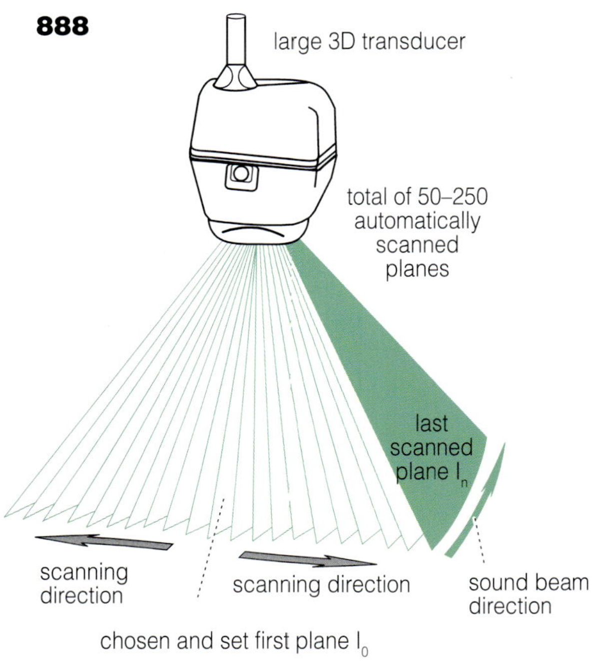

888 Schematic drawing of a horizontal rotation in a sector plane to produce a coordinated, i.e. defined, cross-sectional sequence.

graphic cross-sectional sequence'[7] is usually produced by horizontal rotation (**887, 888**).

At the present time (beginning of 1996), most commercially available ultrasound systems for 'real' three-dimensional scanning work by this principle (e.g. Combison 530 with 5.0, 7.5 and 10 MHz transducers, by Kretztechnik, Austria). This unit uses characteristic sector transducers with an additional mechanism which allows the scanning plane to be angled or rotated horizontally. Because of these technical features, the transducers are extremely large and difficult to handle (**889, 890**). Some companies also manufacture commercially available 3D guides, that allow defined transducer movements and thereby an exact shift or rotation of the scanning plane (TOMTEC, Imaging Systems, Unterschleissheim).

Apart from 'real' three-dimensional ultrasonography, 'pseudo-3D sonography' also provides subsequent spatial reconstruction. The basic materials for this procedure are multiple, not necessarily adjacent, conventional ultrasound planes. This method can be applied, for example, on the heart or with vessels. The different characteristic or simple anatomical structures produce relatively well-defined images.

889

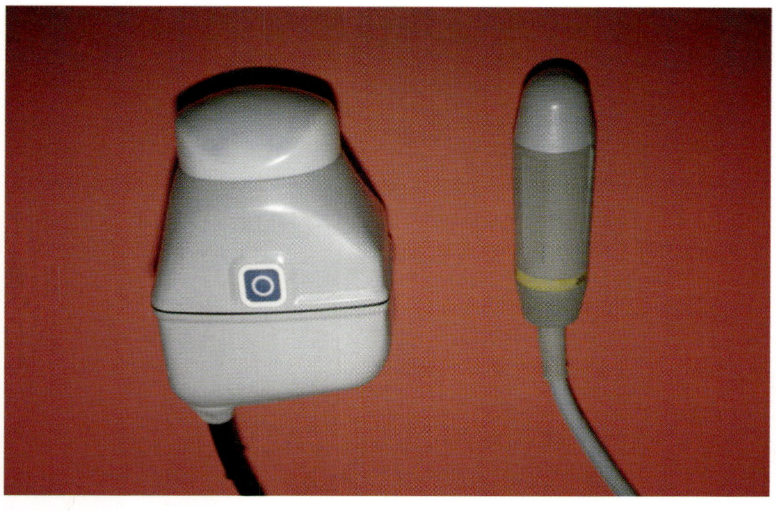

890

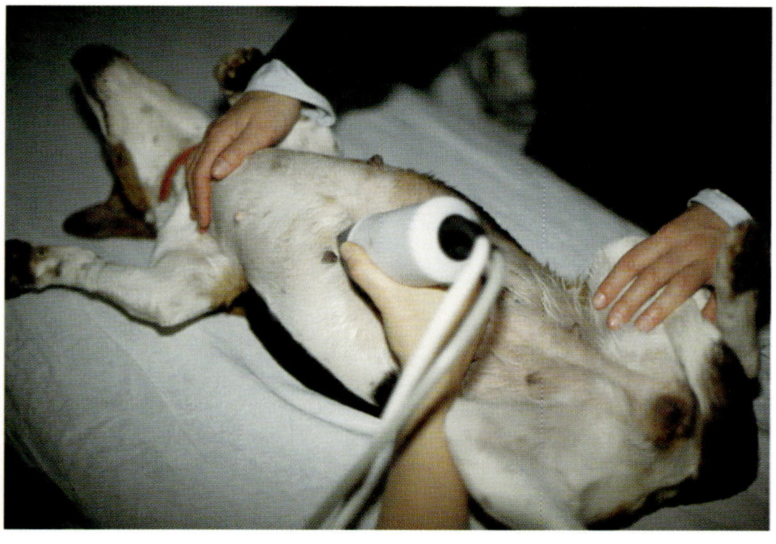

889, 890 Sector (**889** – left) and curved-array (**890**) transducer for three-dimensional reconstruction compared with a conventional sector probe (**889** -right). (**890**) Curved-array transducer used for a 3D scan of the liver in a medium-sized dog.

891

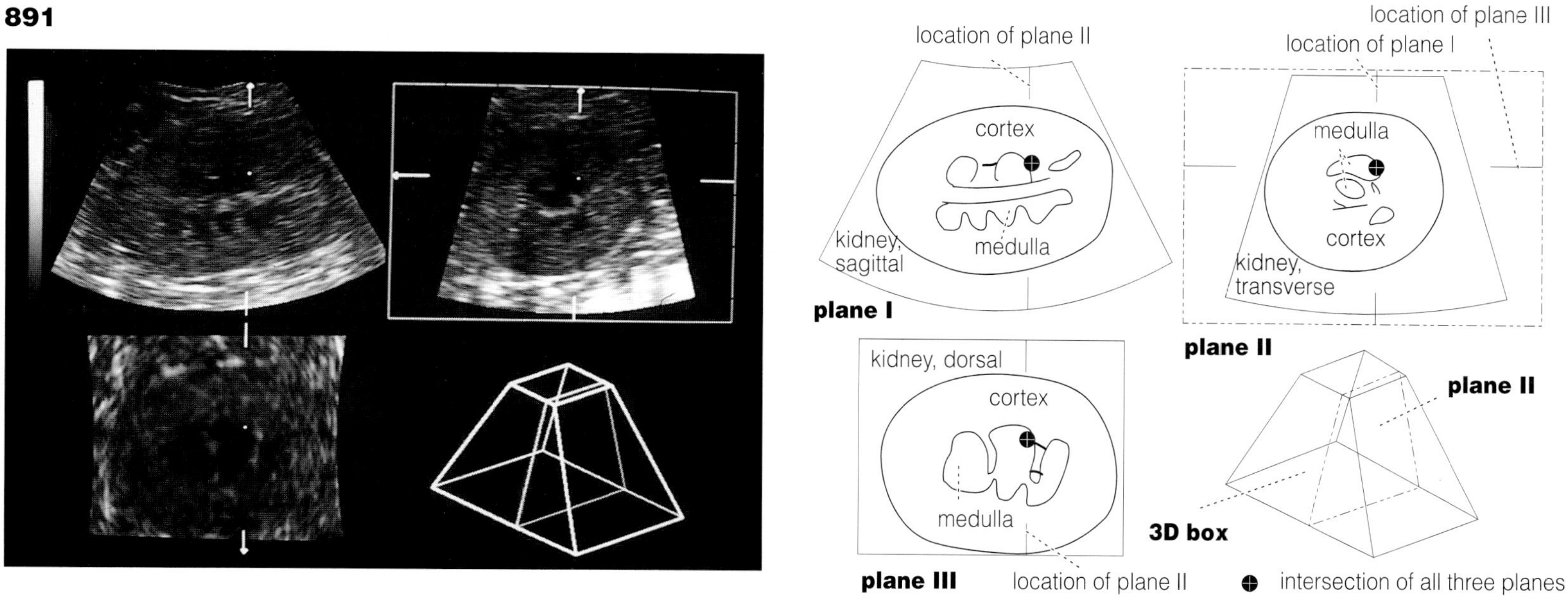

891 Normal left kidney of a dog in dorsal (I: scanned first plane), transverse (II: second plane) and sagittal (III: third plane) views. The three planes are perpendicular to each other. The location of each plane relative to the others is marked by the lines on the side. The dot marks the same structure in each image.

892

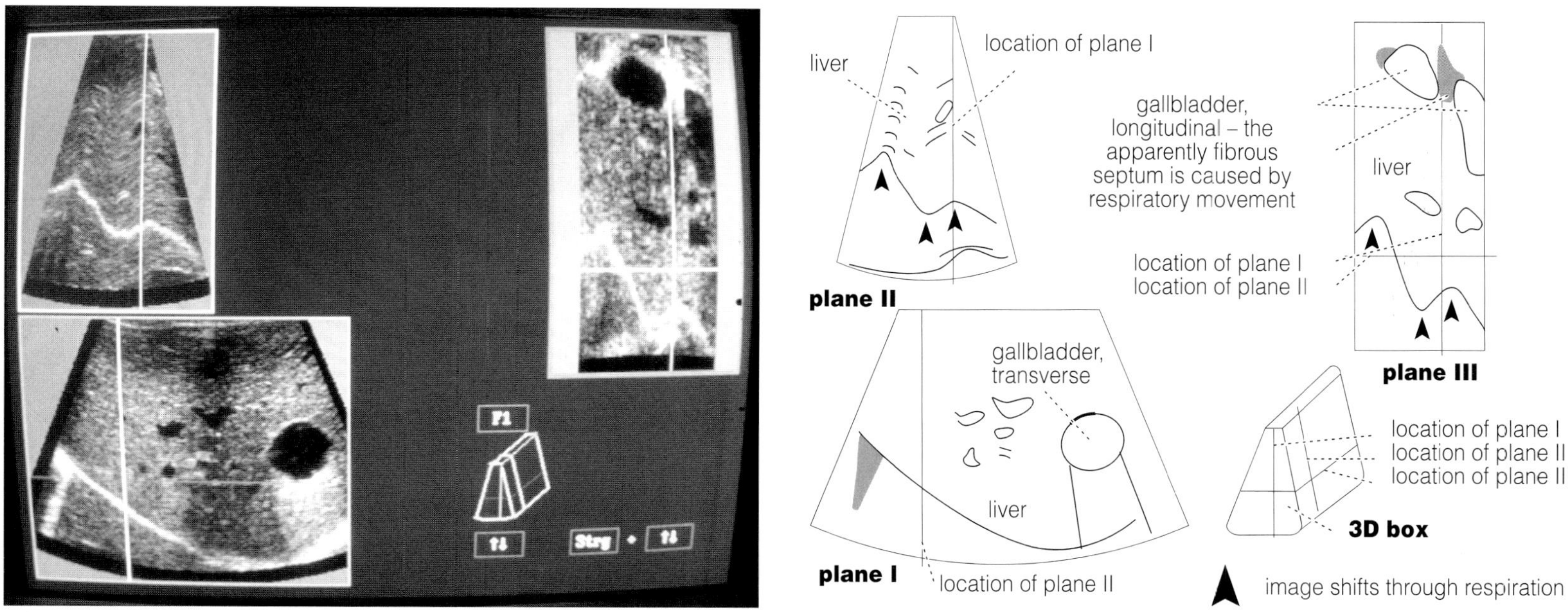

892 Normal canine liver in the actual first scan (plane I) and the perpendicular second (plane II) and third (plane III) view. In the last two images, organ movement caused by respiration is noticeable by the image shifts (arrowheads).

Ultrasonographic Imaging of the Three Planes

In conventional two-dimensional ultrasonography the transducer is rotated 90 degrees from the first plane to the perpendicular second plane. This rotation inevitably leads to a slight angulation of the probe. To produce a third plane the transducer must be placed differently. Many organs, such as the thyroids or kidneys, can be imaged in these three planes (see Image Orientation and Documentation, page 81, **165–170**; and Anatomy and Normal Sonographic Findings, page 210, **466–482**). These images in three planes, produced by transducer rotation and placement, are never exactly perpendicular to each other and they show different sections. The region of interest can only be localized to a certain extent. Visualization of the third plane in some organs, such as the prostate or pancreas, is not possible, due to surrounding bone or an overlying gas-filled gastrointestinal tract. When using a three-dimensional ultrasound unit, every structure can be exactly localized and viewed in all three orthogonal planes (**891**).

The number of scanned, adjacent ultrasound images determines the size and resolution of the 'volume scan' or 'three-dimensional box'. Twelve to twenty images can be scanned in one second. During the scanning procedure the patient should not move and the transducer must be held absolutely still. The main factors limiting the number of images and the scanning time are the patient's cooperation and the examination site. For example, a larger number of planes can be scanned in bladder or prostate ultrasonography than in liver ultrasonography. Respiratory movement of most organs results in blurring or 'image shifts'. For this reason the patient's nose and mouth must be held closed during scanning to achieve clear image planes (**892**). Sedation is usually not necessary in the dog and cat. Contractions of the heart pre-

893

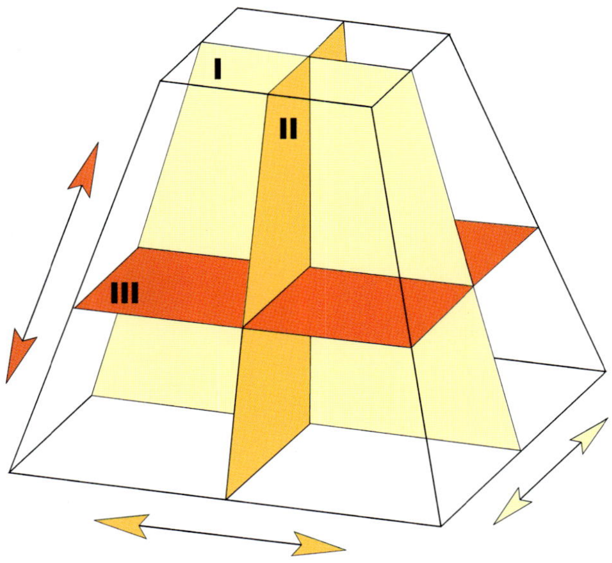

894

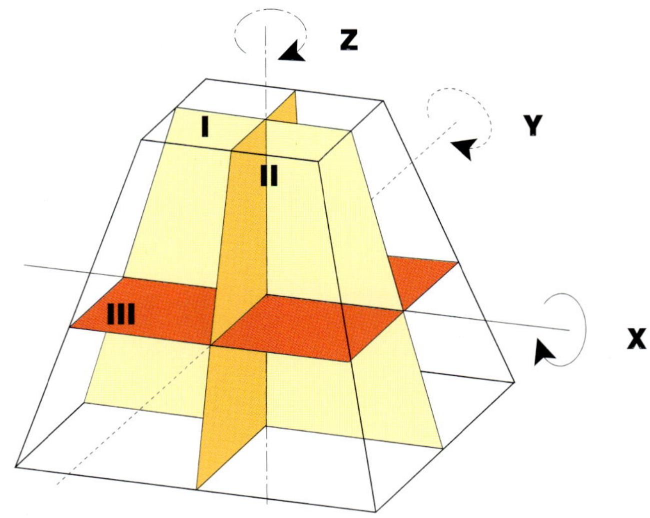

893, 894 Schematic drawings of possible movement (**893**: displacement; **894**: rotation) of the separate planes in a 3D scan.

vent three-dimensional echocardiography as described. Three-dimensional ultrasonography of cardiac structures requires ECG or respiratory triggering of the scanning procedure.

When recording the three-dimensional box, an individual compromise between scanning as many planes as possible and the time involved must be found. In abdominal ultrasonography of the dog and cat, recording approximately 60–120 planes in 2–5 seconds has proven useful.

Of the actual scanned planes, the computer calculates the perpendicular second and third planes. In this way, every region in the three-dimensional scan is defined. Every plane in the three-dimensional box can be shifted and rotated (**893–899**). Each structure within the scanned body can be viewed in three orthogonal planes and, additionally, in every oblique view. Within the three-dimensional scan, each visible dot can be allocated within space and to its surroundings. This form of imaging is not possible with conventional methods and subsequent 'pseudo-3D' calculations.

The disadvantage of three-dimensional ultrasonography is the time-consuming procedure to evaluate the recorded and digitally stored 3D scans. The actual ultrasound examination is barely longer than conventional two-dimensional ultrasonography. One positive aspect is the fact that the sonographer is forced to re-evaluate the diagnostic findings. This avoids dangerous 'quick' ultrasound examinations, which almost always lead to a false diagnosis.

Three-dimensional reconstruction of a region on a two-dimensional medium is problematic. At the present time, various methods for spatial display are in use:

- Exclusive surface imaging, e.g. in the shape of ring structure images used in 3D reconstruction of computed tomograms.
- Complete image of all planes within the 3D scan in the shape of a transparent, glass-like quader (**900, 901**).

In the first case the surface can evaluated, while the second method also displays all inside structures compared to their surroundings. A combination of both methods is possible. The objects are rotated to achieve a spatial impression when viewing the images on a flat monitor. The disadvantage of both methods is the poor image resolution. These methods are not suited for hard-copy documentation. A compromise to the almost spatial image of the orthogonal planes is the so-called topographic image, a graphic perspective representation (**902, 903**).

The major advantage of three-dimensional ultrasonography lies in better evaluation of complex anatomical and pathological structures (**904–907**). Definition, demarcation and allocation of focal lesions in particular, such as cysts (**895–899**), abscesses and neoplasia (**906, 907**), are better in three-dimensional ultrasonography than in the two-dimensional image[5, 12, 13]. The difference between demarcated as opposed to infiltrative tumour growth is apparent on the three-dimensional image by viewing the entire mass. With the help of three-dimensional ultrasonography, malignant mammary tumours in women can be relatively easily determined by their irregularity[6].

While three-dimensional ultrasonography plays an important role in human prenatal diagnostics in determining fetal integrity[4, 10, 11], its use in canine and feline pregnancy monitoring is problematic. The minimal restlessness of the mother animal, and the number of fetuses and their vitality make three-dimensional pregnancy monitoring difficult, especially in the dog (**908, 909**).

Apart from prenatal and abdominal examinations, three-dimensional ultrasonography is also used for joint diagnostics in human medicine[2, 3].

In summary, three-dimensional ultrasonography is a good supplement to two-dimensional imaging. Because of the high cost of '3D ultrasound systems', which is similar to colour Doppler units, this imaging method is limited to large practices and clinics.

895

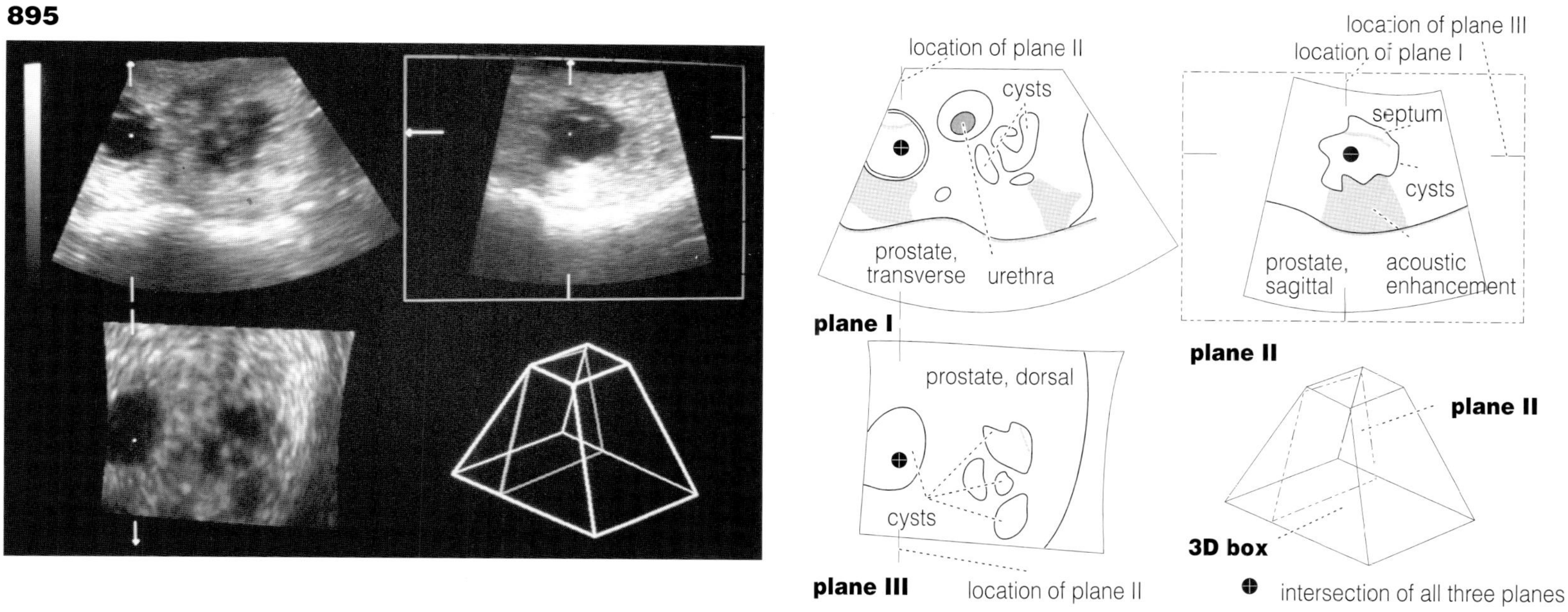

896

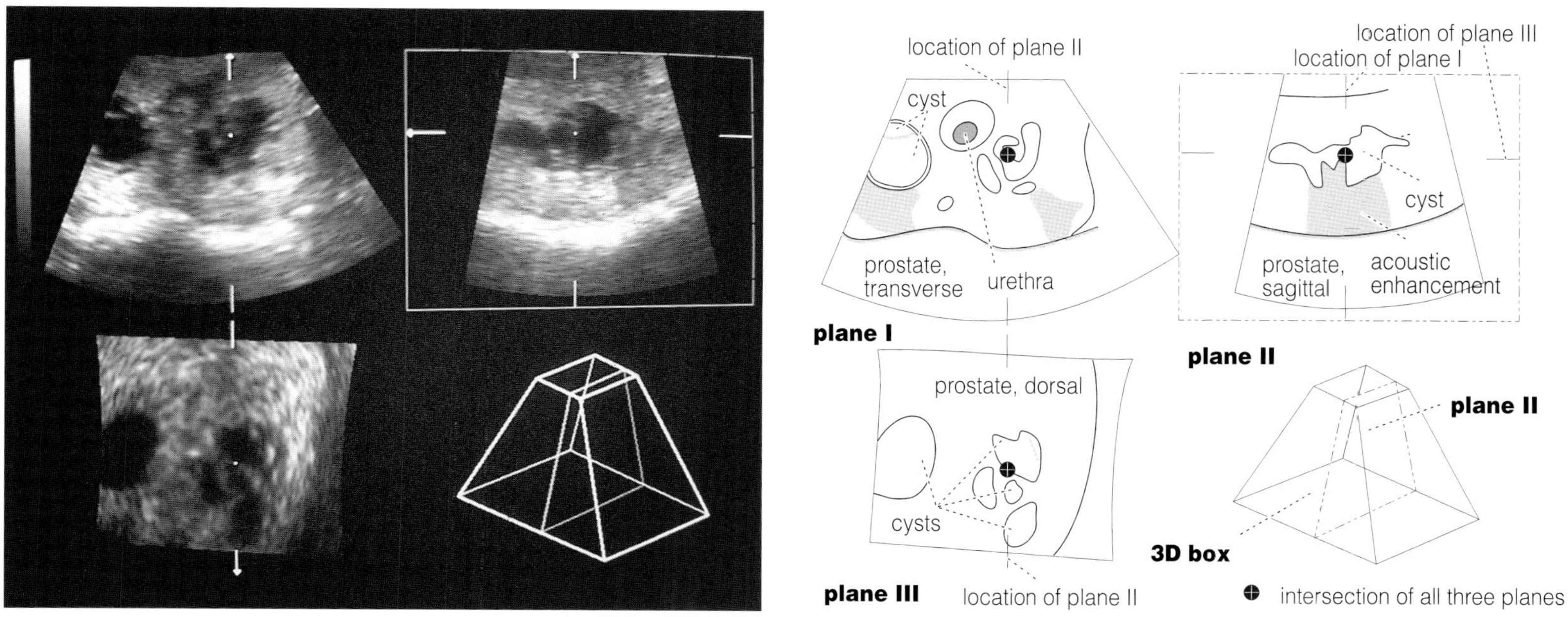

897

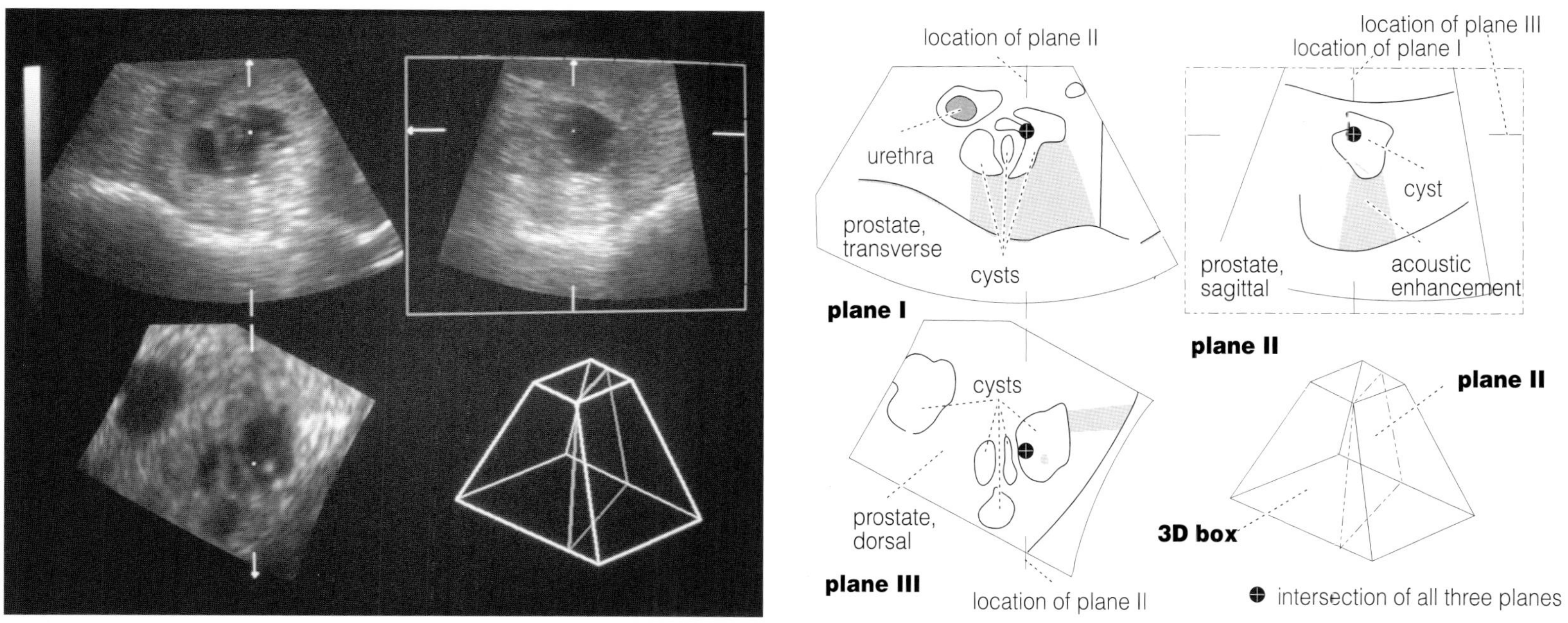

895–899 'Three-dimensional sonograms' of a cystic prostate in a dog. Within the 3D scan, each separate plane can be displaced (**895, 896**) and rotated (**897–899**). Adaptation of the planes, perpendicular to the manually changed one, is automatic. In this case the second plane of a cyst in the right prostate lobe (**895**) was placed into an anechoic structure in the left lobe (**896**). This view was then rotated (**897**) and the respective position changes of the first (**898**) and third (**899**) plane observed.

898

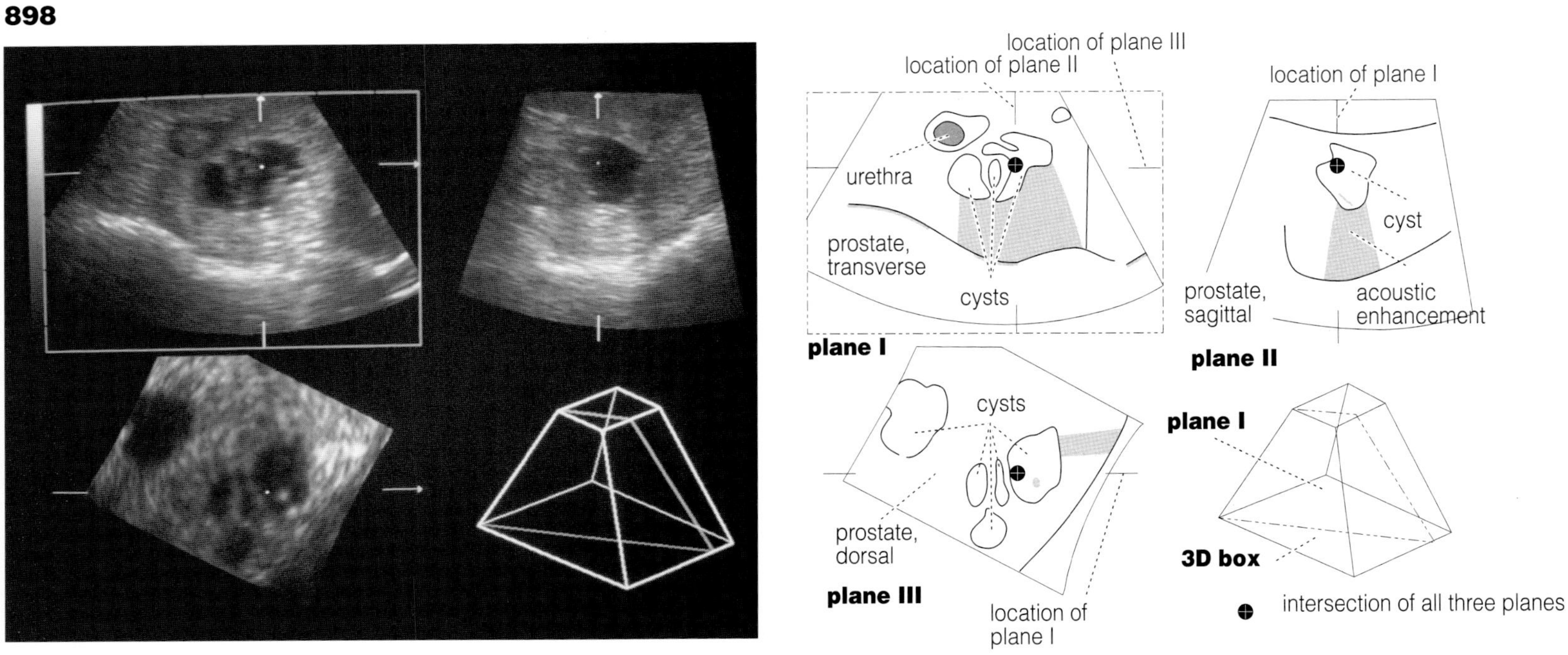

899

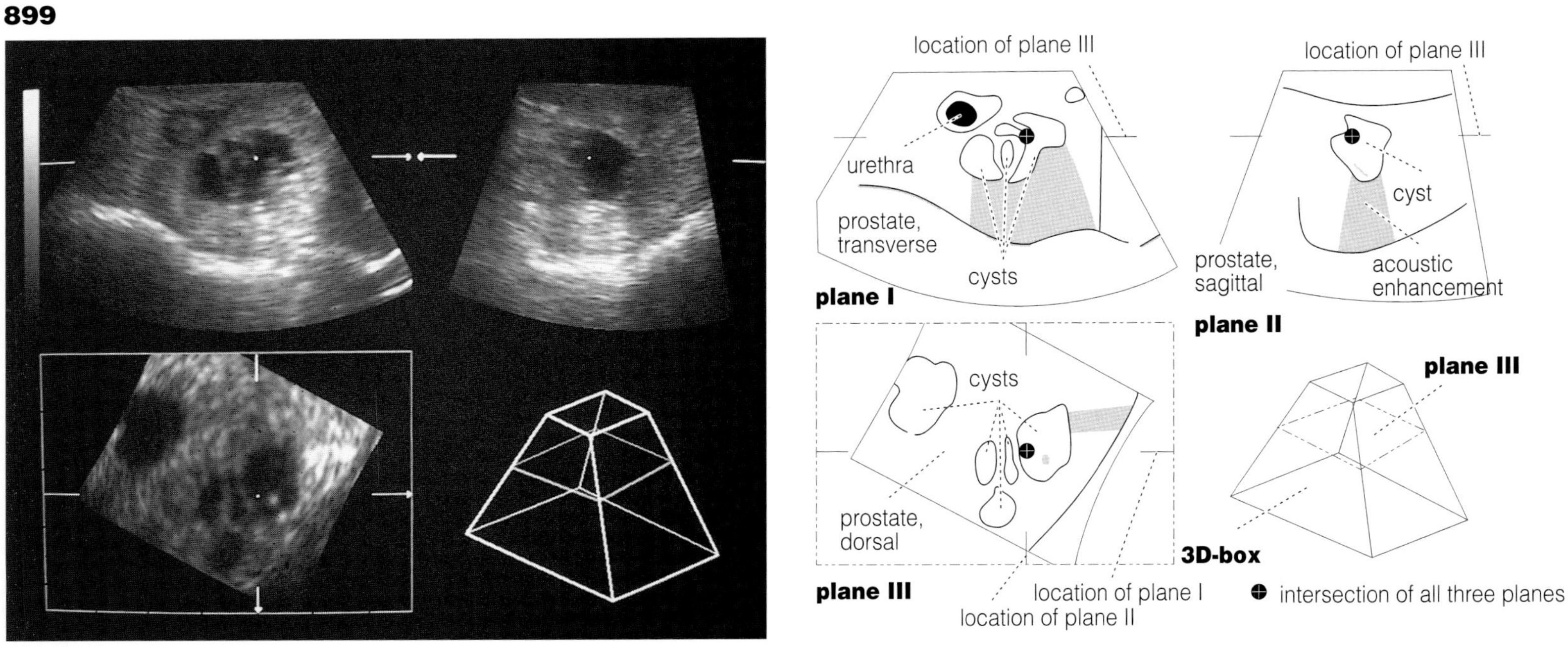

898, 899 'Three-dimensional sonograms' of a cystic prostate in a dog (see **895–897**).

900–903 Transparent spatial displays (**900, 901**) and topographic images (**902, 903**) of cystic lesions in a canine prostate.

900

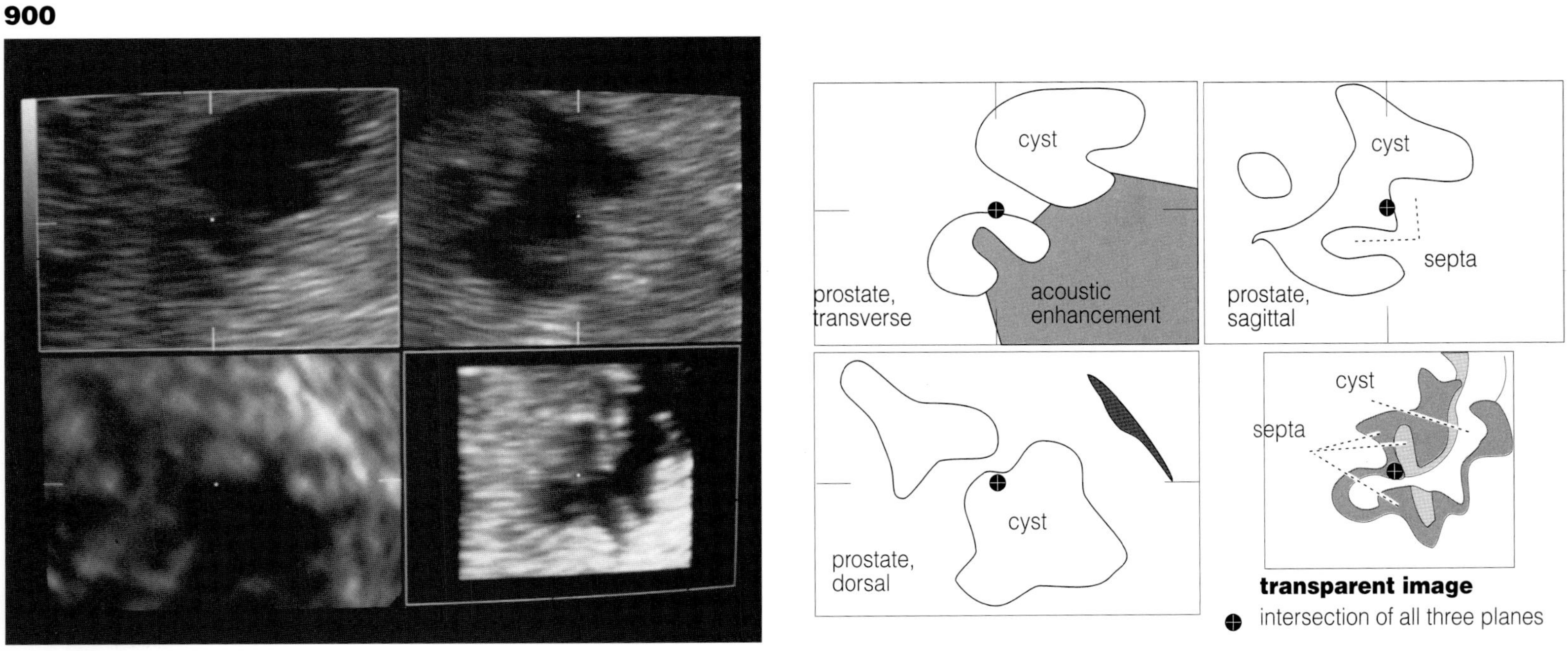

901

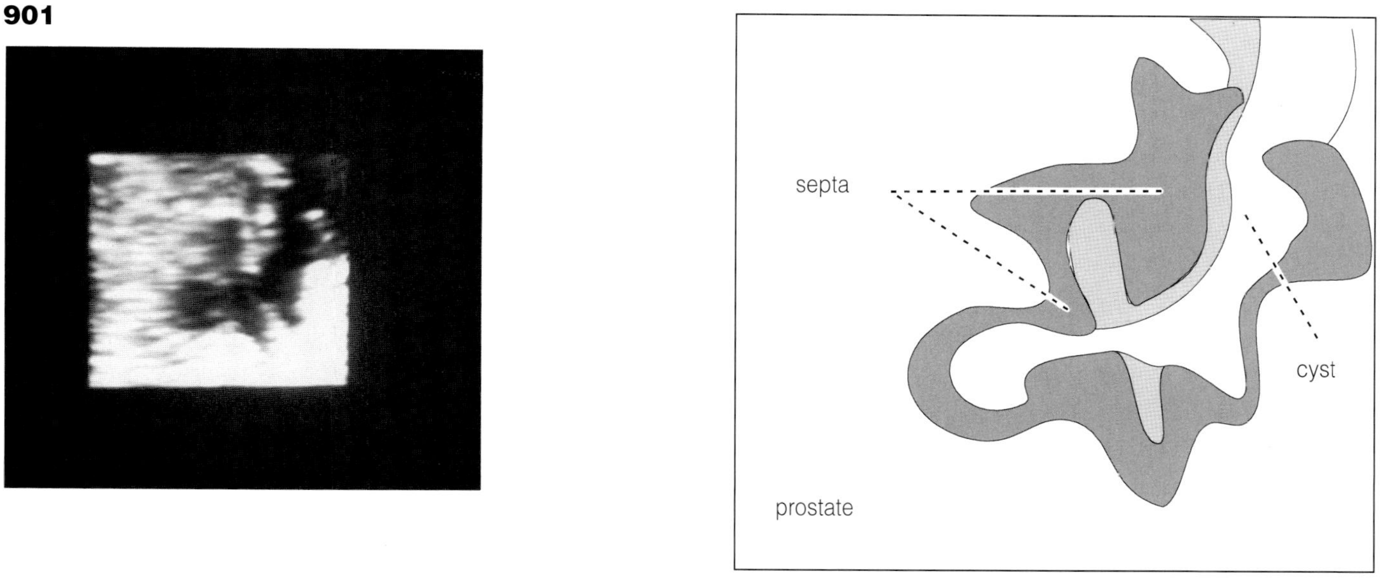

transparent image

902

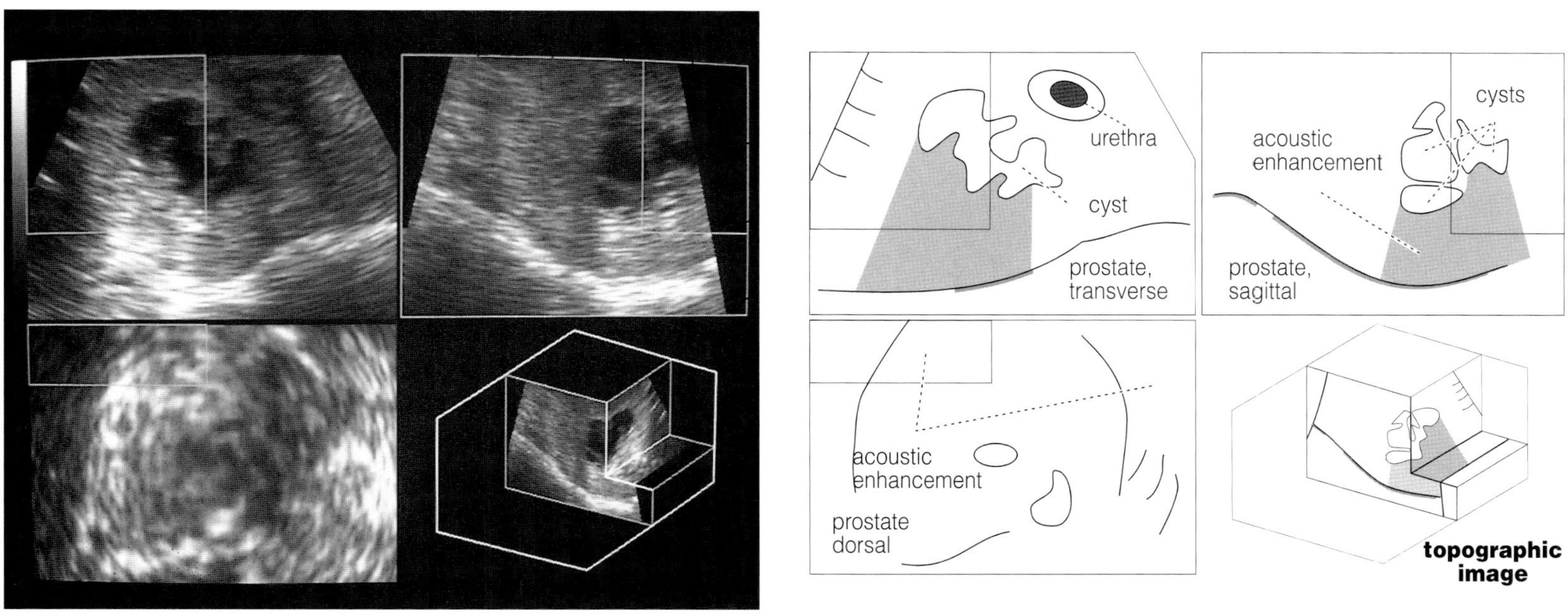

topographic image

903

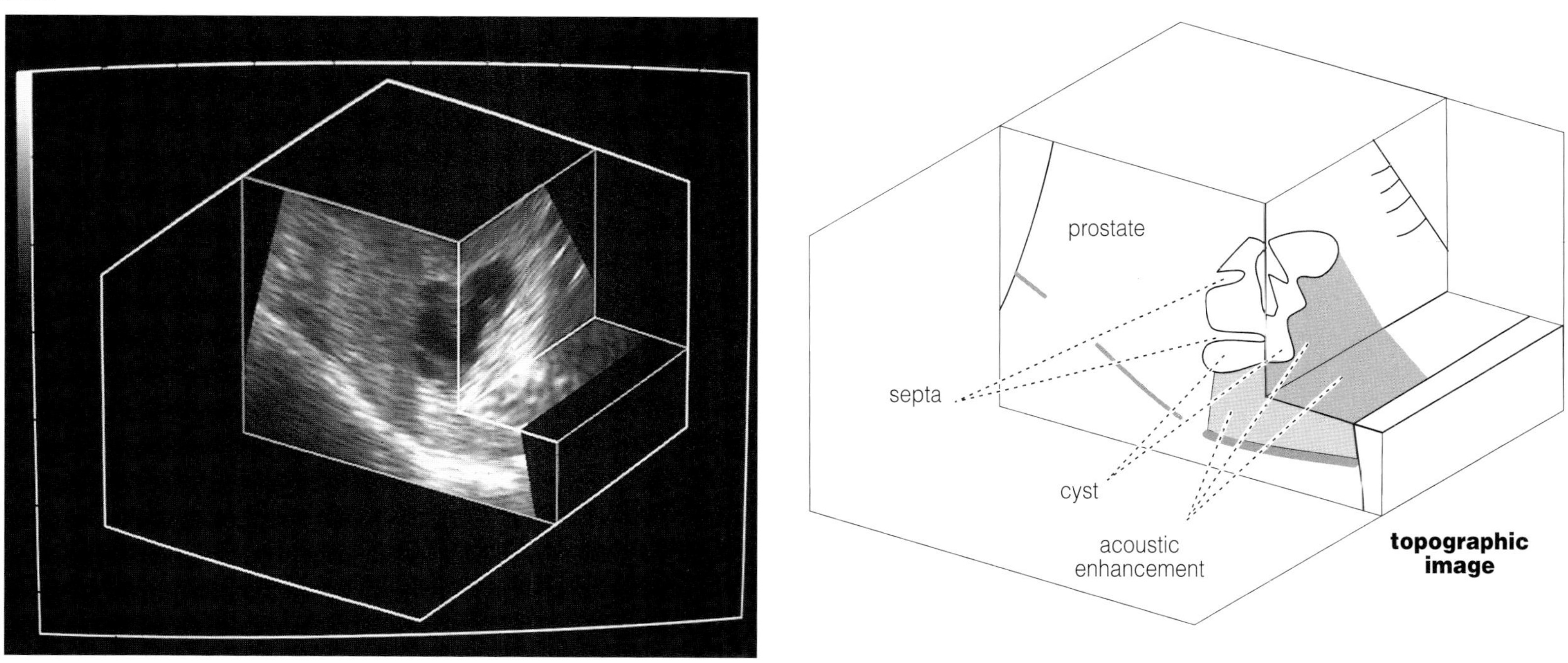

topographic image

904

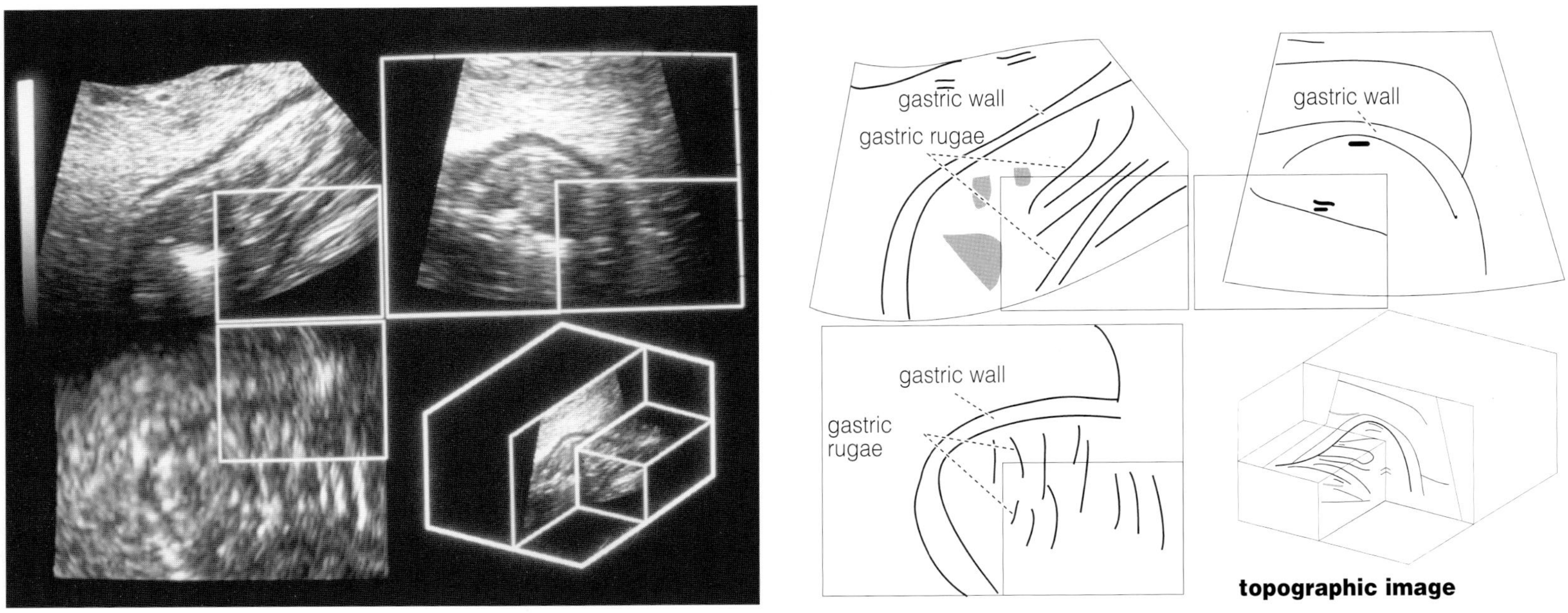

905

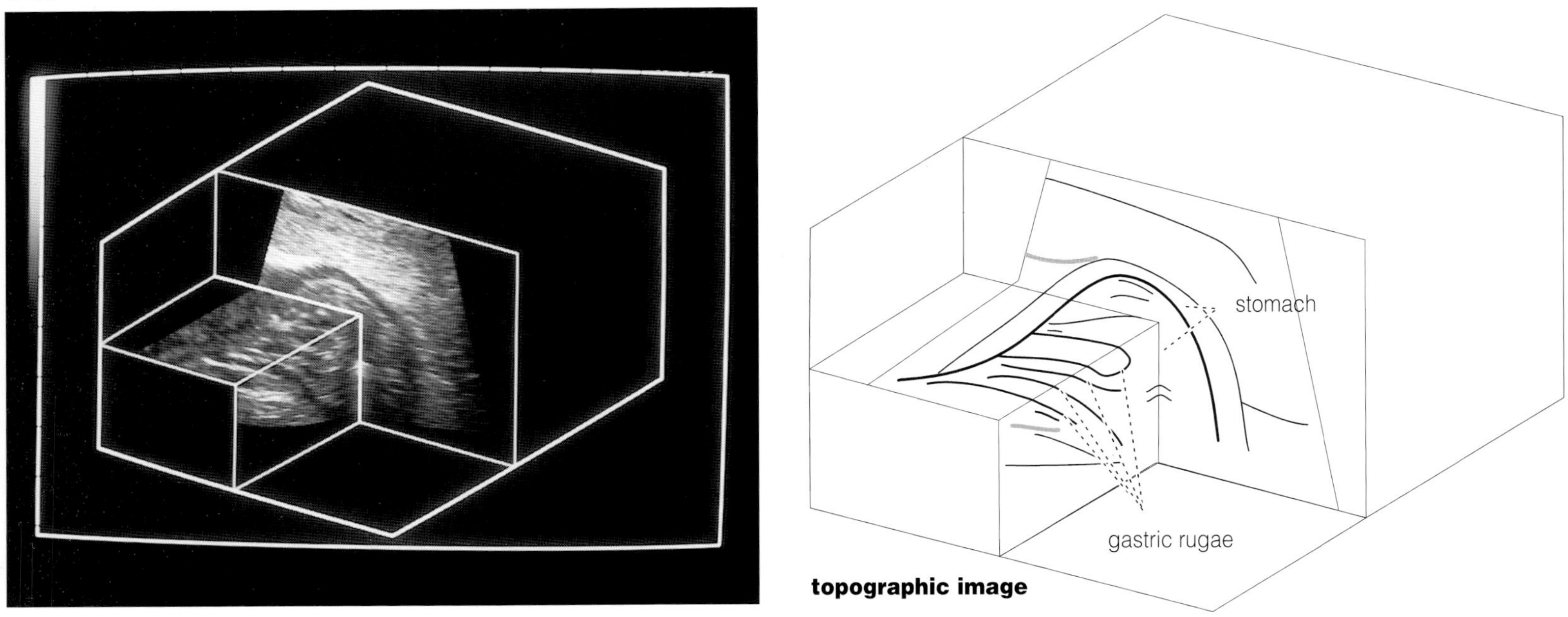

904, 905 Orthogonal planes (**904**) and topographic image (**905**) of a normal, almost empty stomach in a dog.

906 Orthogonal planes of perivascular splenic infiltration in a dog (see also **907**).

906

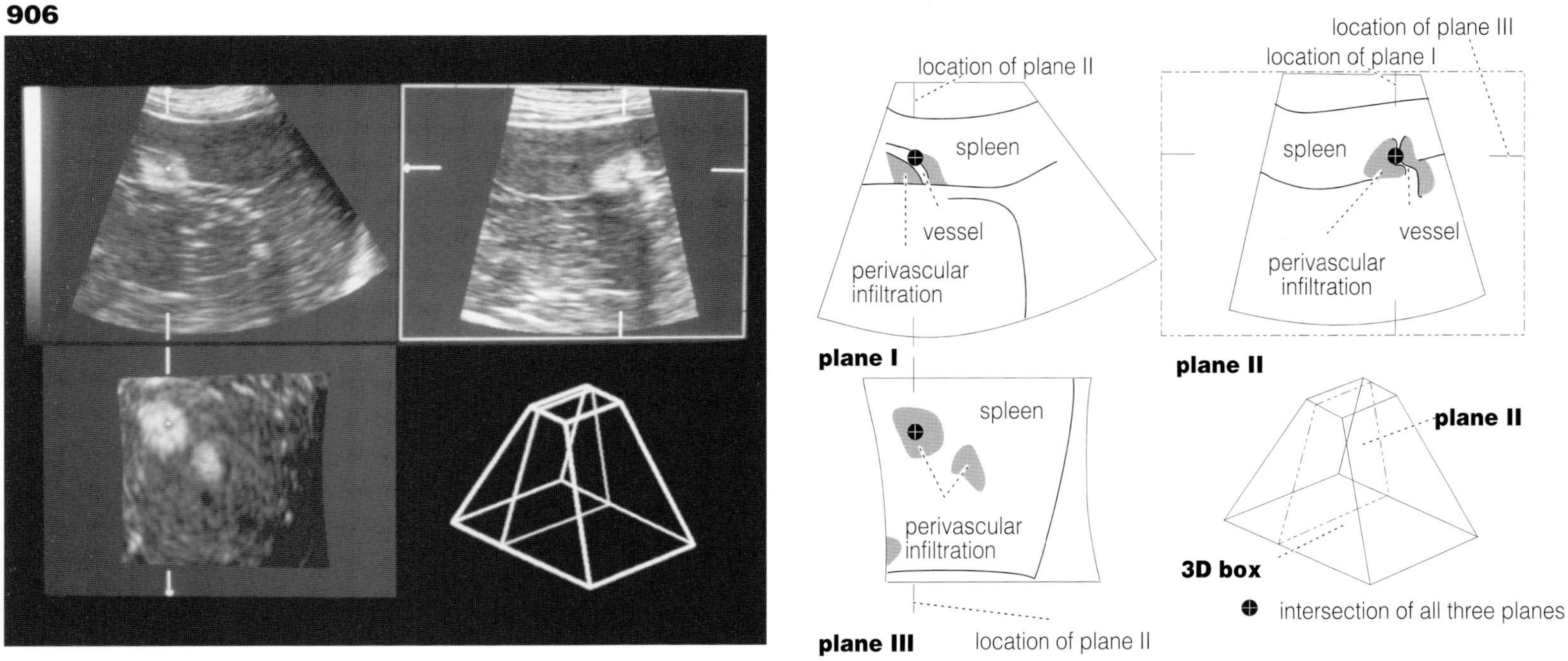

907

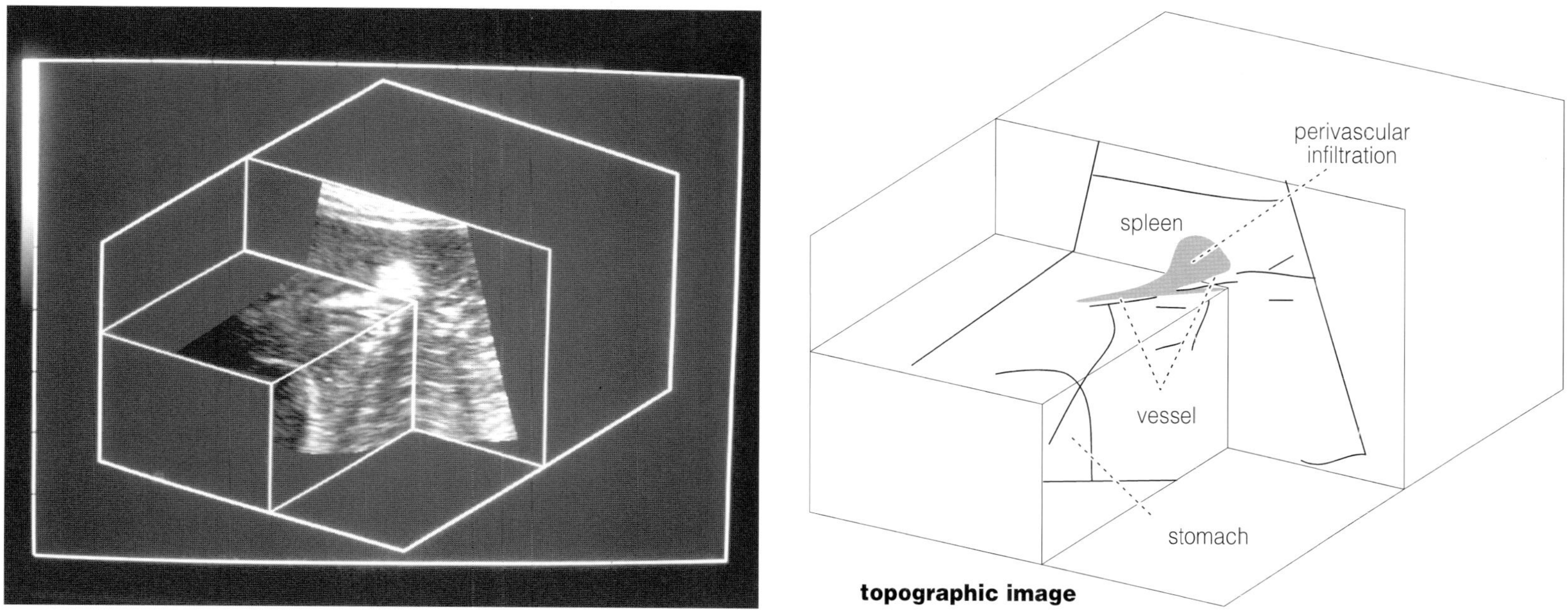

907 Topographic image of perivascular splenic infiltration in a dog (see also **906**).

908

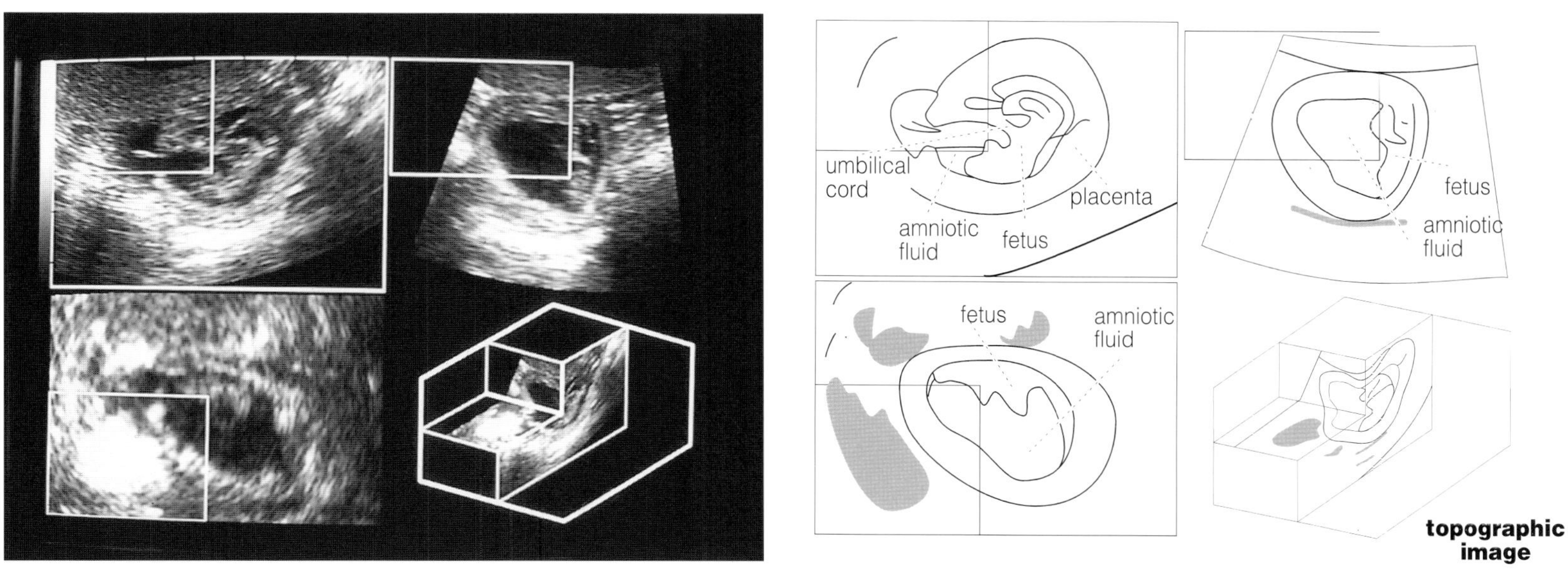

909

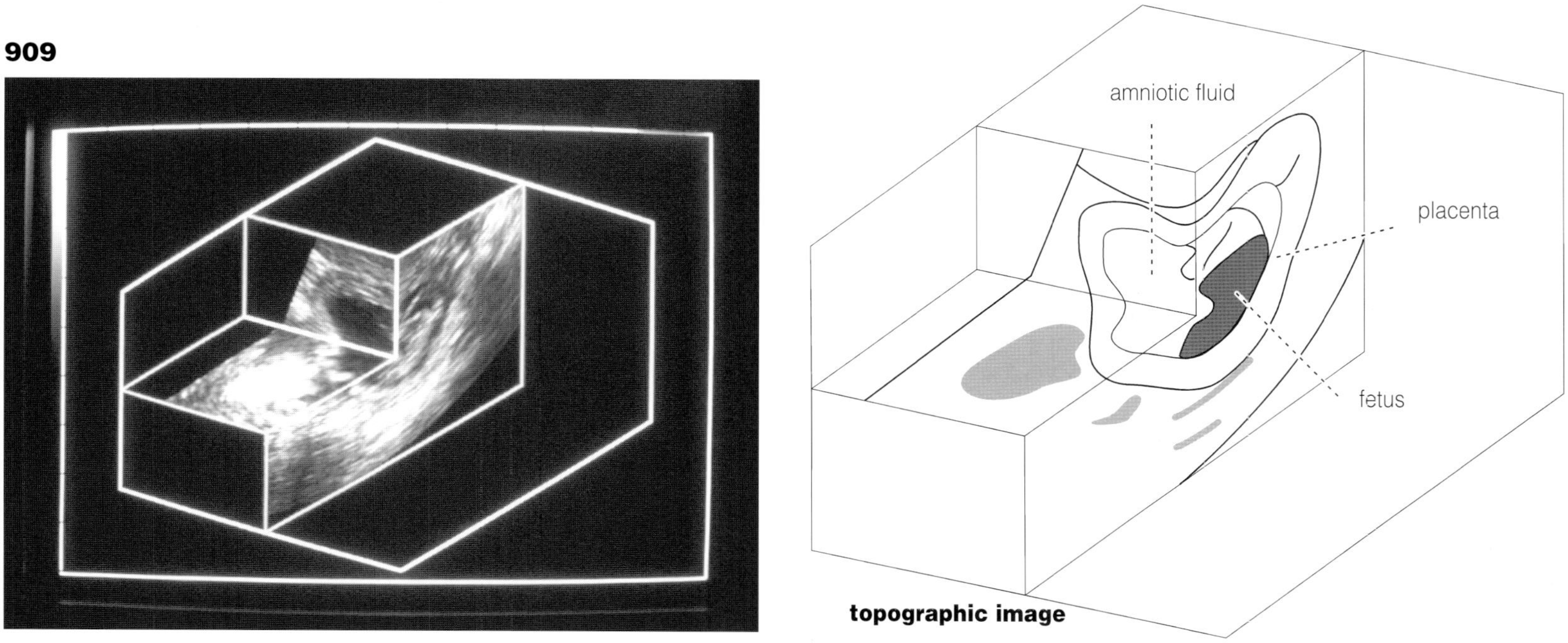

908, 909 Orthogonal planes (**908**) and topographic image (**909**) of a dog fetus, 23 days post breeding.

References

1 Baba K, Satch K, Sakamoto S, Okal T and Shiego I (1989) Development of an ultrasonic system for three-dimensional reconstruction of the fetus. *J. Perinat. Med.* **17**, 19–24.

2 Böhm K and Niethard FU (1994) Dreidimensionale Ultraschalldarstellung der Säuglingshüfte. *Bildgebung* **61**, 126–129.

3 Kellner H, Liess H and Zoller WG (1994) 3D-Sonographie an Weichteilen and Gelenken. *Bildgebung* **61**, 130–134.

4 Merz E, Bahlamm F and Weber G (1995) Volume scanning in the evaluation of fetal malformations: a new dimension in prenatal diagnosis. *Ultrasound Obstet. Gynecol.* **5**, 222–227.

5 Sackmann M, Pauletzki J, Zwiebel FM and Holl J (1994) Three-dimensional ultrasonography in hepatobiliary and pancreatic diseases. *Bildgebung* **61**, 100–103.

6 Sohn C (1994) Die Vorteile der räumlichen, dreidimensionalen Ultraschalldarstellung in der klinischen Anwendung. *Bildgebung* **61**, 87–94.

7 Sohn C and Bastert G (1994) *Die Dreidimensionale Ultraschalldiagnostik.* Springer Verlag, Berlin, Heidelberg, New York.

8 Sohn C, Grotepass J., Schneider W, Sohn G, Funk A, Jensch P, Fendel H, Ameling W and Jung H (1988a) Dreidimensionale Darstellung in der Ultraschalldiagnostik. Erste Ergebnisse. *Dtsch. Med. Wochenschr.* **113**, 1743–1747.

9 Sohn C, Grotepass J, Schneider W, Funk A, Sohn G, Jensch P, Ameling W and Jung H (1988b) Erste Untersuchungen zur dreidimensionalen Darstellung mittels Ultraschall. *Z. Geburtshilfe Perinatol.* **192**, 241–248.

10 Steiner H, Staudach A, Spitzer D, Graf AH and Wienerroither H (1993) Bietet die 3D-Sonographie neue Perspektiven in der Gynäkologie and Geburtshilfe? *Geburtshilfe Frauenheilkand.* **53**, 779–782.

11 Steiner H, Staudach A, Spitzer D and Schaffer H (1994) Three-dimensional ultrasound in obstetrics and gynaecology: technique, possibilities and limitations. *Hum. Reprod.* **9**, 1773–1778.

12 Wagner S, Gebel M, Bleck JS and Manns MP (1994) Clinical application of three-dimensional sonography in hepatobiliary disease. *Bildgebung* **61** 104–109.

13 Zoller WG and Liess H (1994) 3D-Sonographie in der Gastroenterologie. *Bildgebung* **61**, 95–99.

910

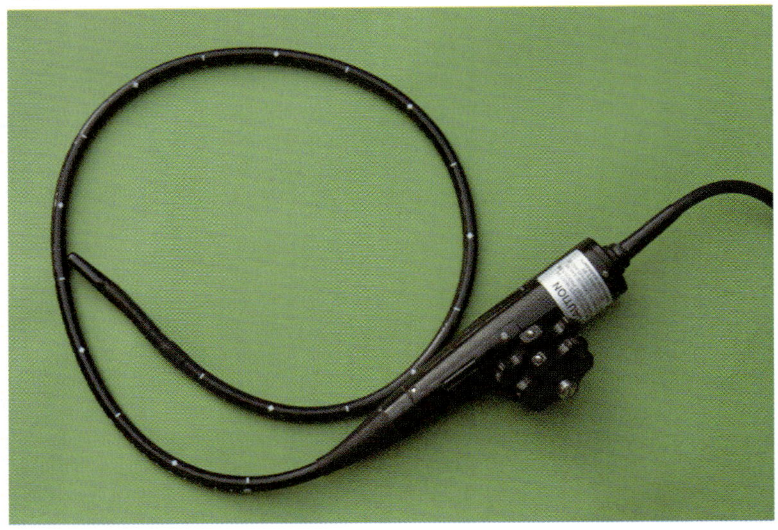

911

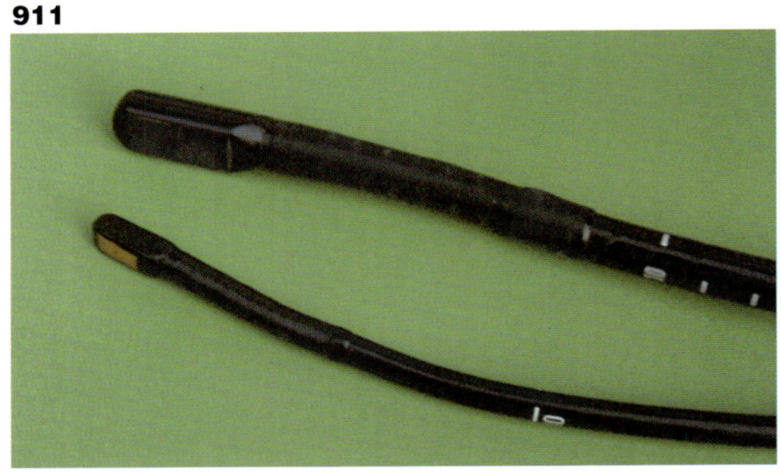

912

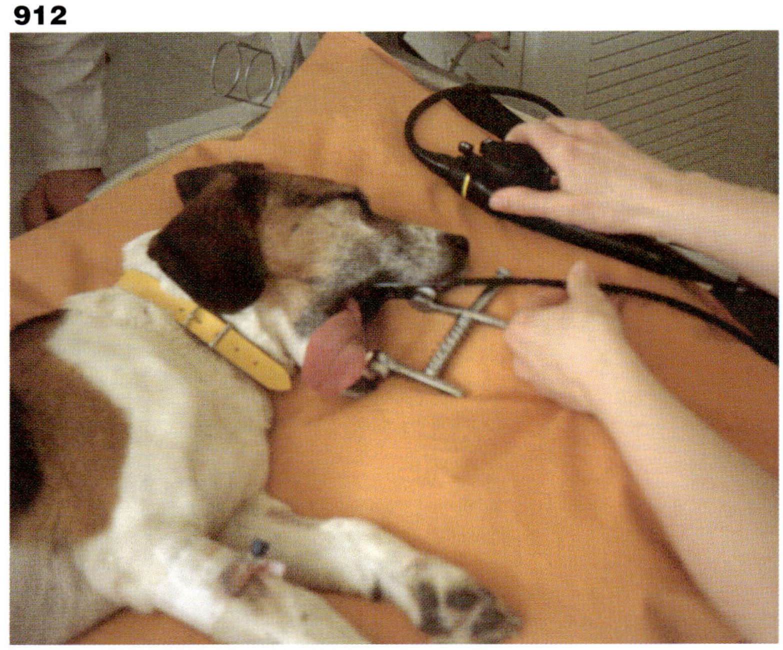

910–912 Transducer for transoesophageal echocardiography with control unit and centimetre markings (**910**). End-pieces of two different sized TEE probes for canine and feline transoesophageal echocardiography as used in human adult and paediatric cardiology (**911**). Inserted probe in an anaesthetized dog (**912**).

Interventional Ultrasonography

Cordula Poulsen Nautrup

Interventional ultrasonography, including transoesophageal, transrectal, transvaginal and intravascular examination, is widely used in human medicine. Transrectal ultrasonography is also a standard method used in large animal gynaecology and obstetrics.

The other listed ultrasound methods are rarely used in small animal practice. Apart from technical problems pertaining to small patient size, especially small dogs and cats, financial aspects also play a role in the acceptance of these methods. Additionally, the relatively easy, extensive and high quality transcutaneous sonographic examinations in small animals with medium to high resolution, 5–10 MHz transducers limit the use of endosonography. Some diagnostic indications do justify the use of interventional ultrasonography in animals, with the result that these methods will be more widespread in the future.

Semi-invasive transoesophageal and fully invasive intravascular ultrasound examinations should be performed with the animal owner's written agreement. Patients should be fasted for all interventional examinations.

Transoesophageal Ultrasonography

The probe for transoesophageal echocardiography (TEE) consists of a fully flexible endoscope, similar to a gastroscope (910). The stiff end-piece contains the 5 or 7.5 MHz transducer (911). In addition to one- and two-dimensional imaging methods, colour-coded, pulsed-wave (PW) and also continuous-wave (CW) Doppler techniques are possible. For TEE in most dogs (912), the same transducers used in human medicine are applicable, while cats require thinner endoscopes with a diameter of

913

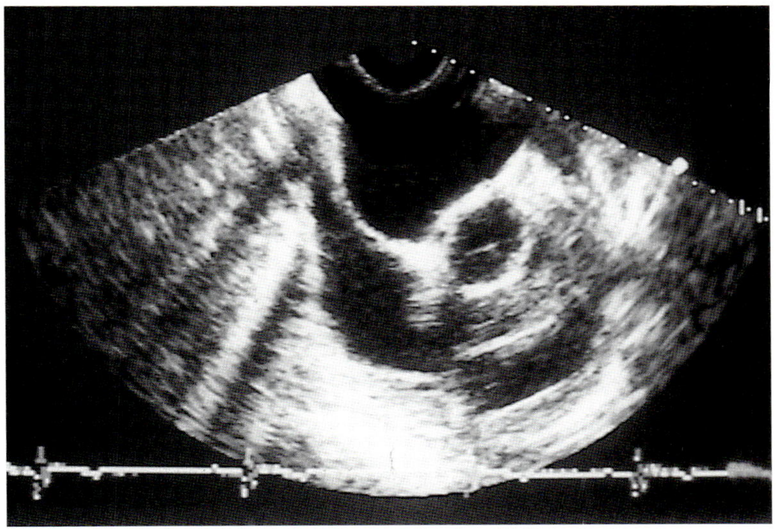

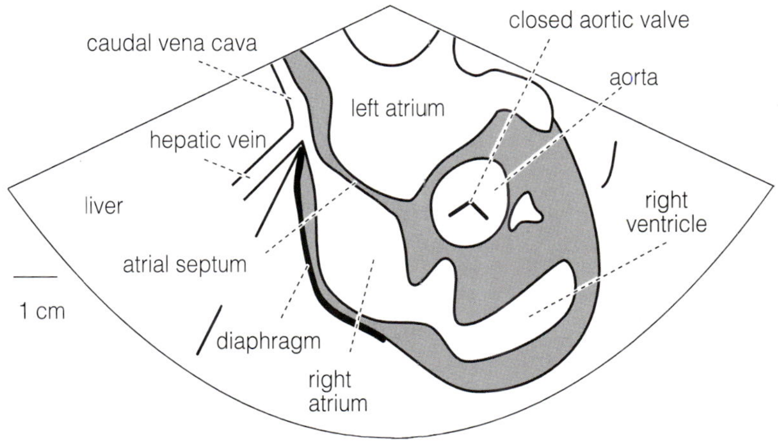

913, 914 Transoesophageal echocardiogram of the left and right atrium, right ventricle and caudal vena cava in a transverse view (**913**). The caudal scanning position is taken from Loyer and Thomas[3] (**914**).

914

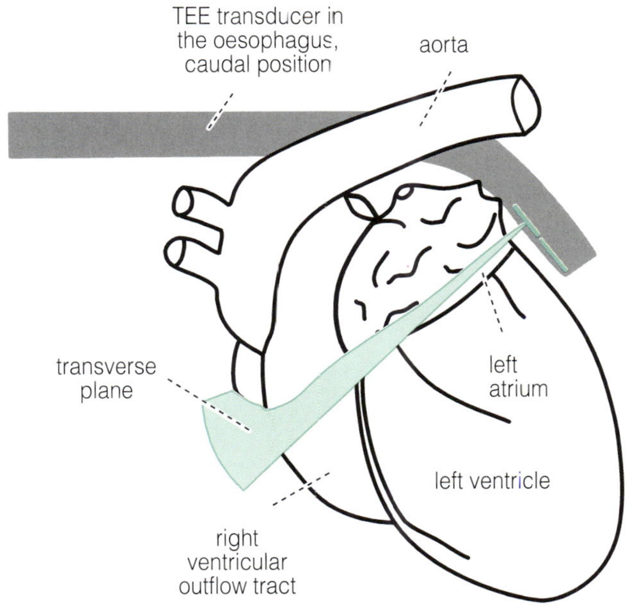

under 10 mm, as used in paediatric cardiology (**911**). The sedated animal is positioned in lateral recumbency for the examination, the jaws are kept open with a mouth wedge or retractor, and the probe is passed into the stomach and pulled back slowly. Good echocardiographic planes are achieved by sliding the probe back and forth, rotating to the left and right, as well as angling the tip. The scanning planes can be turned 90 degrees with biplanar transducers and 360 degrees with multiplanar probes. In this way, transverse and longitudinal or multiple views are produced.

All the important cardiac regions, including the valves, can be more or less visualized from a cranial, medial and caudal position. A limiting factor for high quality echocardiograms is the position of the trachea between the oesophagus containing the probe and the heart[3].

Indications for TEE include poor visualization of the heart due to extremely air-filled lungs as a result of lung oedema or bronchopulmonary diseases. Thoracic deformities or rib lesions after trauma also make transcutaneous echocardiography more difficult and require transoesophageal imaging for an accurate diagnosis. During inhalation anaesthesia, imaging of the heart is best performed with the help of a TEE probe[5]. Even with good transcutaneous imaging, some cardiac regions are imaged better with transoesophageal ultrasonography. These structures include the atrial septum and the right atrium and auricle with the cranial and caudal venae cavae (**913, 914**)[5], as well as the left atrium and auricle. Evaluation of the latter structures is particularly important in cases of suspected arterial thromboembolism in cats with hypertrophic cardiomyopathy. In human medicine, 2–5% of all echocardiography patients in the cardiology department are evaluated with transoesophageal echocardiography[1].

915

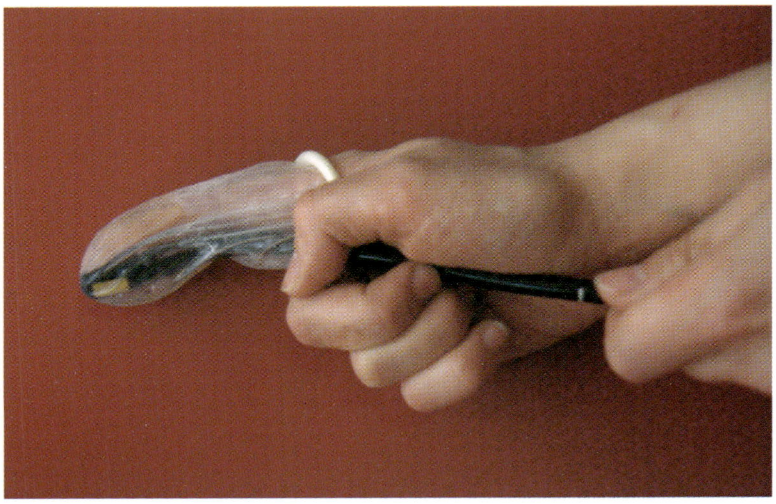

916

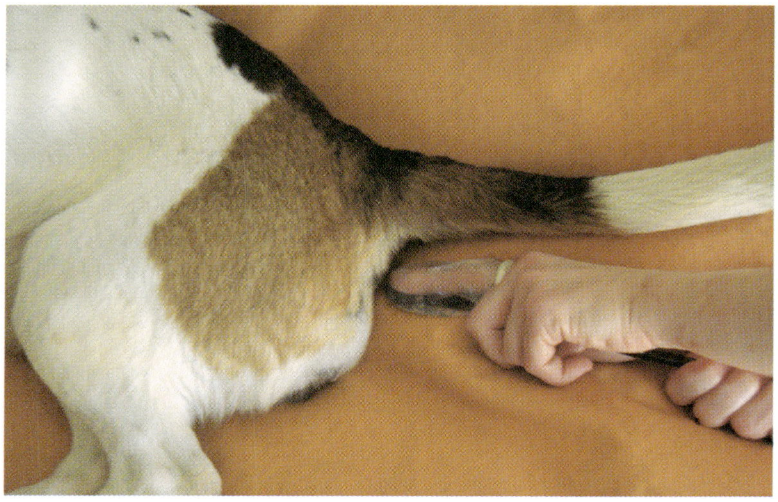

917

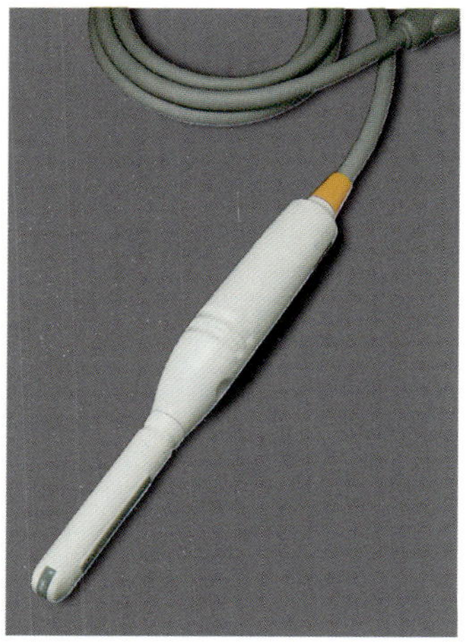

915–917 Finger with small TEE probe (**915**) for 'digital' transrectal ultrasonography in the dog (**916**). Endorectal transducer with a diameter of 22 mm from human medicine (**917**).

Transrectal and Transvaginal Ultrasonography

Ultrasound gastroscopes and some TEE probes are suitable for transrectal ultrasonography in cats and small dogs (**915**). In medium-sized to large dogs, all the endorectal probes used in human medicine are acceptable (**917**). The disadvantage of TEE probes lies in their poor near-field resolution, since they are sector transducers. Small transducers, in conjunction with a wide anus and rectum, can be inserted and guided rectally using the sonographer's finger (**916**). To preserve the transducer, a latex covering (so-called medical condom) filled with ample amounts of ultrasound gel is pulled over the instrument and possibly over the finger.

Sedation of most dogs and cats is not necessary. The animals remain standing and are supported ventrally. After emptying the bowels – in most cases normal defecation prior to the examination is sufficient – the probe is inserted rectally and pushed cranially as far as possible. Faeces may prevent coupling with the intestinal wall and this produces useless images.

Indications for transrectal ultrasonography include all unclear findings in the area of the anus, rectum, urinary bladder, urethra (**918–921**), prostate, root of the penis, uterus, vagina and perineum, especially perineal hernias. By imaging not only the visible cavity surfaces, ultrasonography enables more in-depth visualization of the extent of a lesion and the inclusion of other structures. Transrectal ultrasonography of prostatic disease in the male dog provides additional information. Lesions of the capsule with infiltrative tumours may be more clearly visible transrectally than transabdominally[4].

Transvaginal examinations can be performed in most dogs with the same probes used in human medicine. The main indication for endovaginal ultrasonography in humans is gynaecological and obstetrical examinations, especially during early pregnancy. These examinations are not carried out in cats and dogs where there are multiple pregancies and a bicornuate uterus.

918

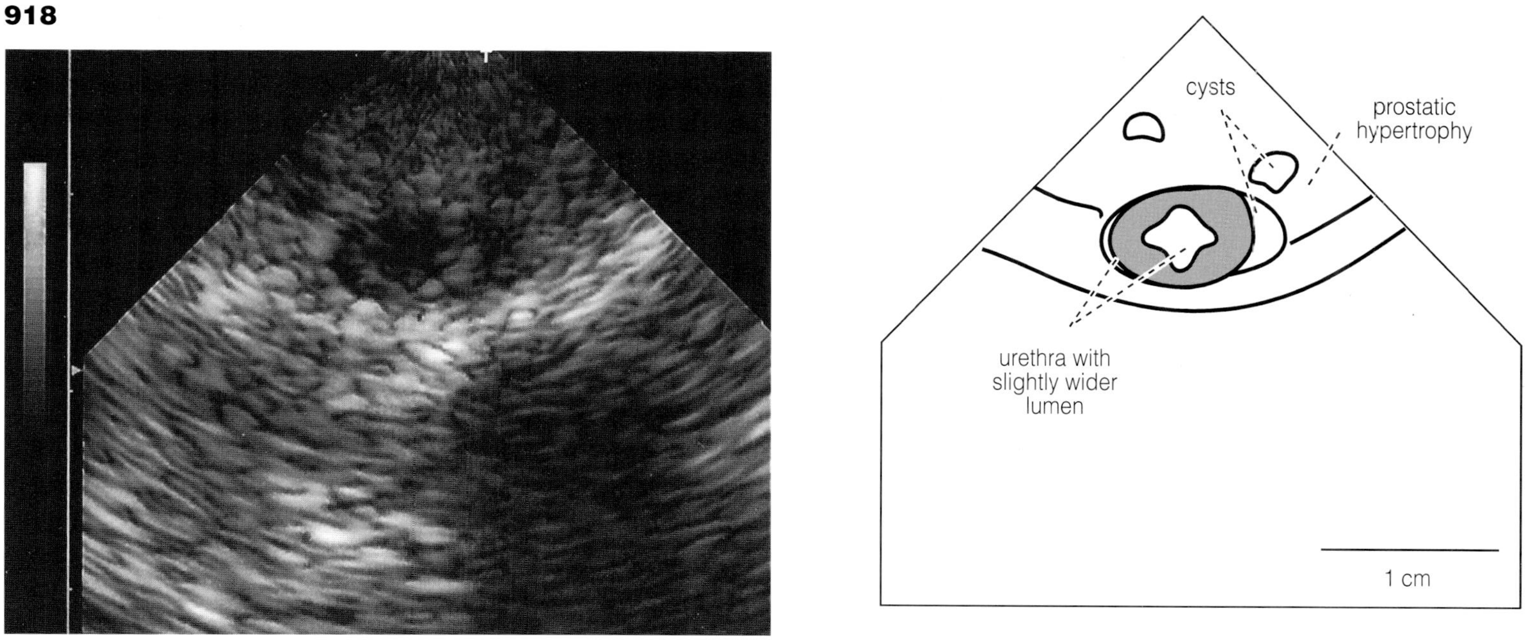

919

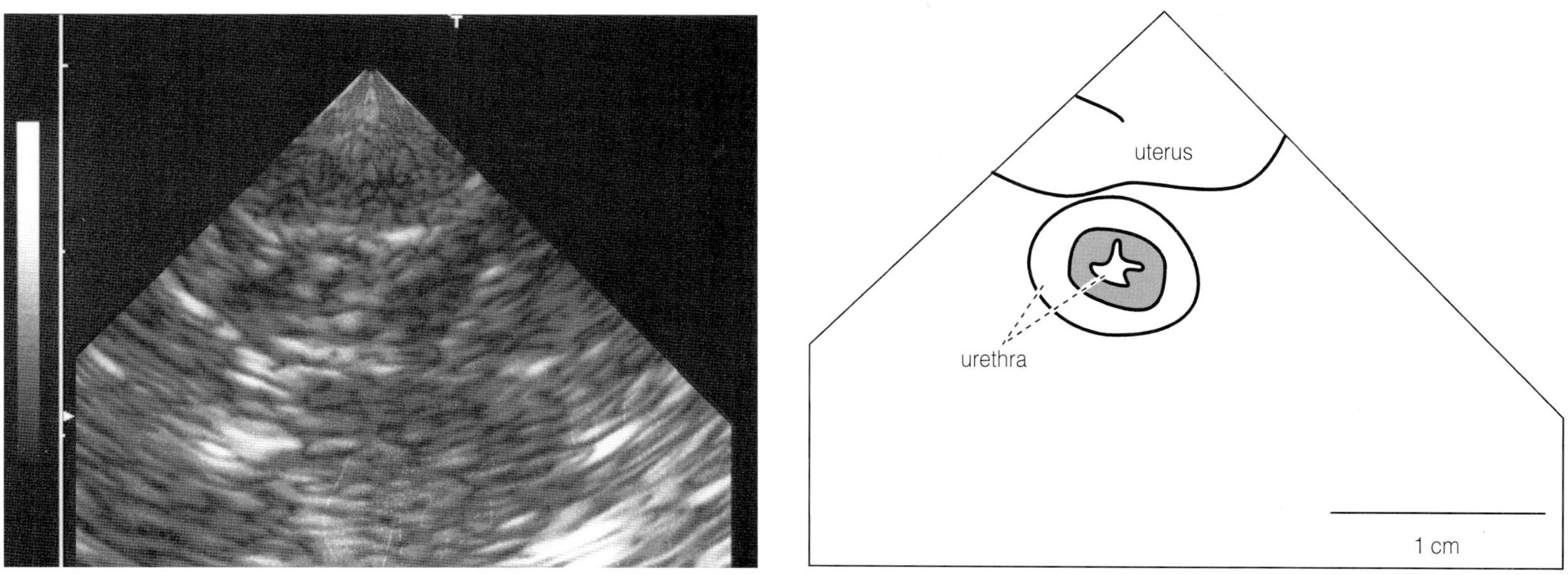

918, 919 Transrectal sonograms, using a TEE probe, of a normal intrapelvic urethra in a male dog (**918**) and a bitch (**919**).

920

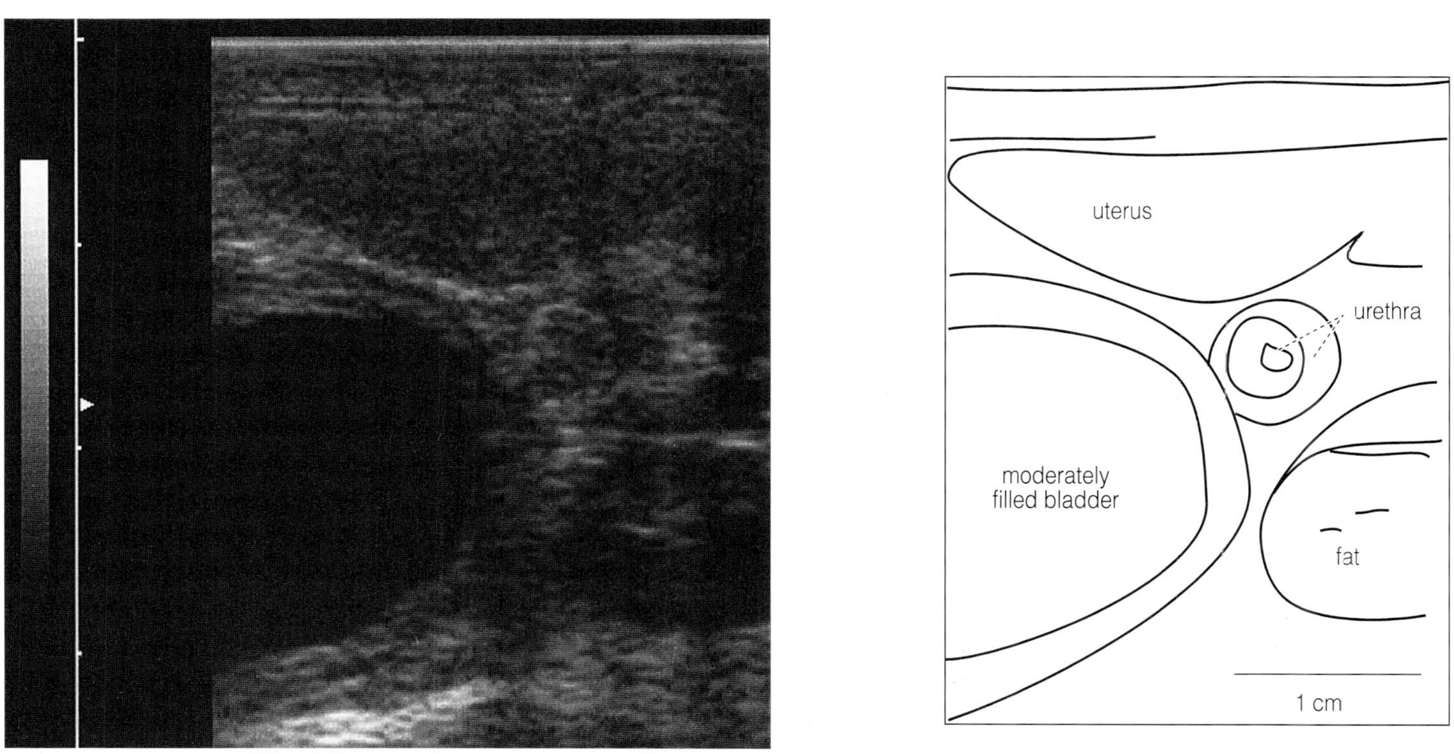

920 Transrectal sonogram, using an ultrasonographic gastroscope, of the bladder, urethra and uterine body in a healthy bitch.

921

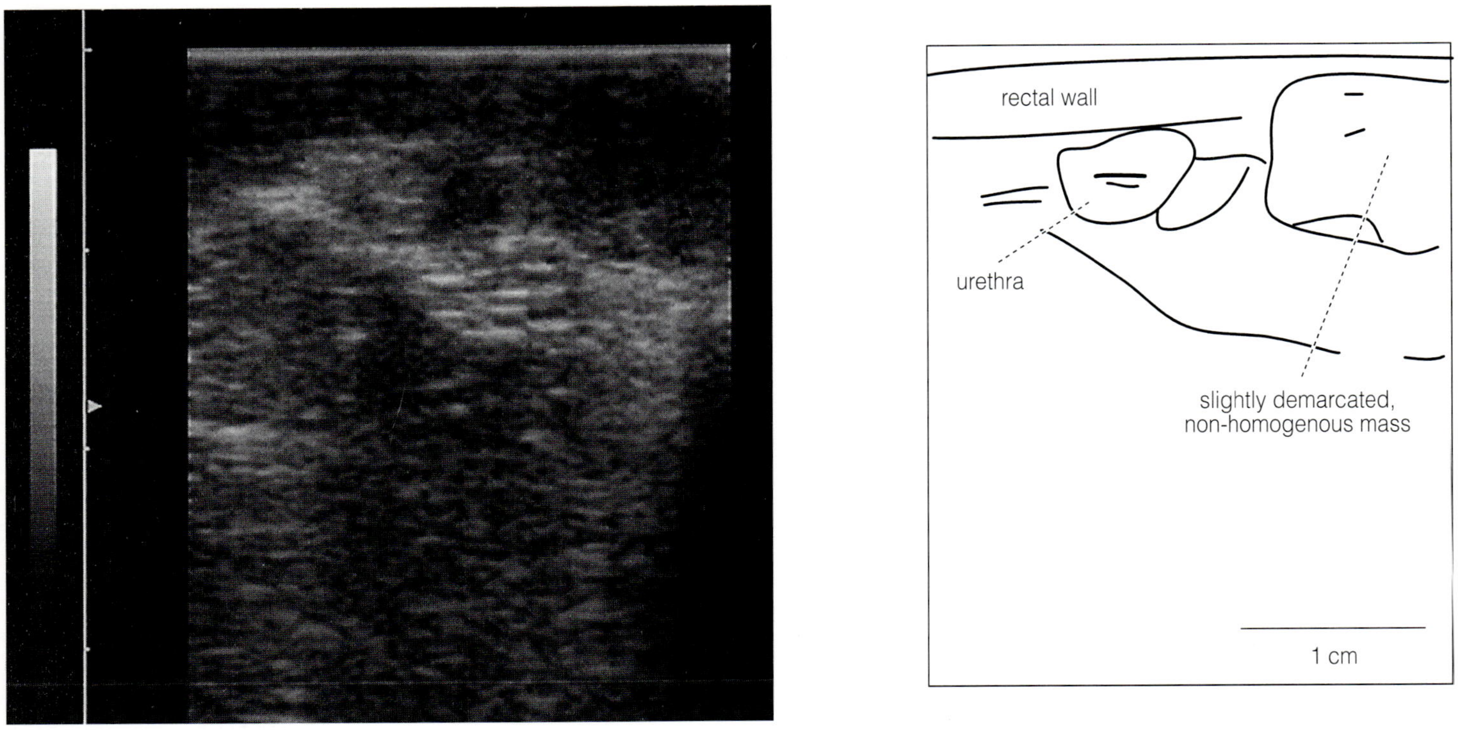

921 Transrectal sonogram, with an ultrasonographic gastroscope, of an anal gland tumour in a male dog.

922

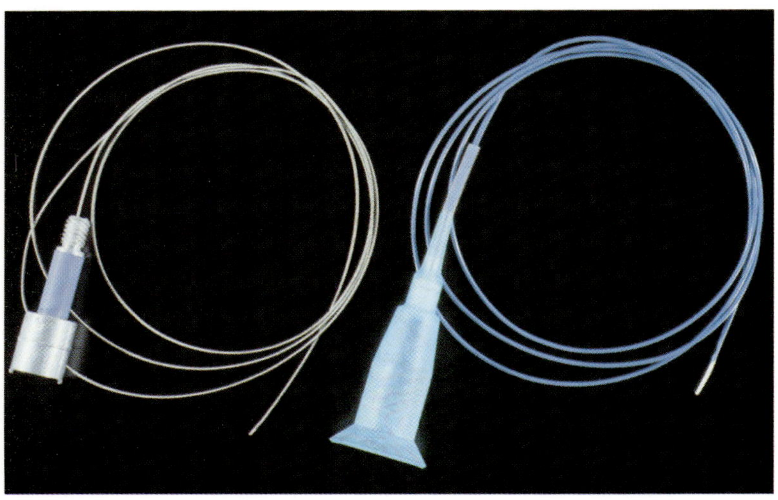

922 Ultrasound probes for intravascular ultrasonography. The metal instrument (left) represents the 'transducer'. To the right is the blue plastic sheath.

Intravascular Ultrasonography

By progressively minimizing the size of transducers, probes have been developed with a diameter of 4.8–3.2 French gauge, which are suitable for intravasal use (**922**). Ultrasound frequencies of 18–30 MHz provide extremely high resolution and sufficient depth penetration to evaluate vessel walls and inner structures. After sedating and positioning the patient, the partially flexible catheter is inserted into the vessel, e.g. jugular vein or femoral artery, with the help of an introducer (Catheter Sheath Introducer System with 6 French gauge, Cordis Co., Miami). The probe can also be used in other narrow tubular structures, such as the uterine neck in the bitch, to evaluate the walls of these organs.

The main indication for intravascular ultrasonography in humans is diagnosis and evaluation of arteriosclerotic vessel wall lesions, especially the coronary arteries. This is of minimal interest in veterinary medicine. Detailed imaging of vessels (**923, 924**) and heart valves is the main use in veterinary medicine. The right atrium up to the tricuspid valve can be imaged from the jugular vein, while the aortic valve is visualized by retrograde insertion of the catheter from the femoral artery.

Normal arterial vessels have a characteristic three-layered appearance with a fine, smooth, hyperechoic interface between the lumen and the intima, a hypoechoic media and an echogenic layer between adventitia and surrounding tissue[1]. These layers are not apparent in veins. Venous valves are very fine and smooth. They are usually found at the junction with smaller vessels.

While the value of intravascular and endovaginal ultrasonography is still in the experimental stage[2], clinical use of transrectal ultrasonography and transoesophageal echocardiography in small animals is more common.

923

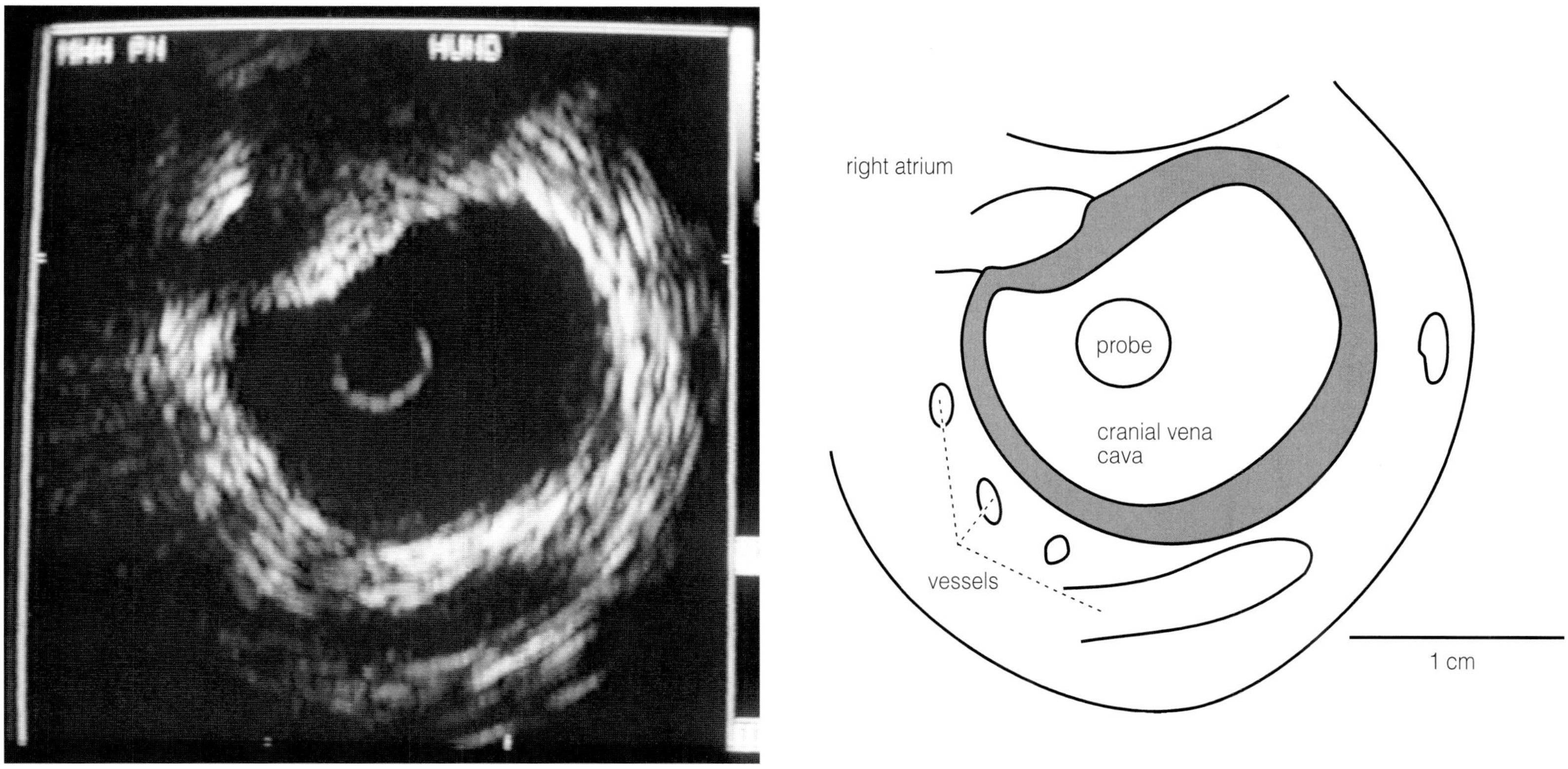

924

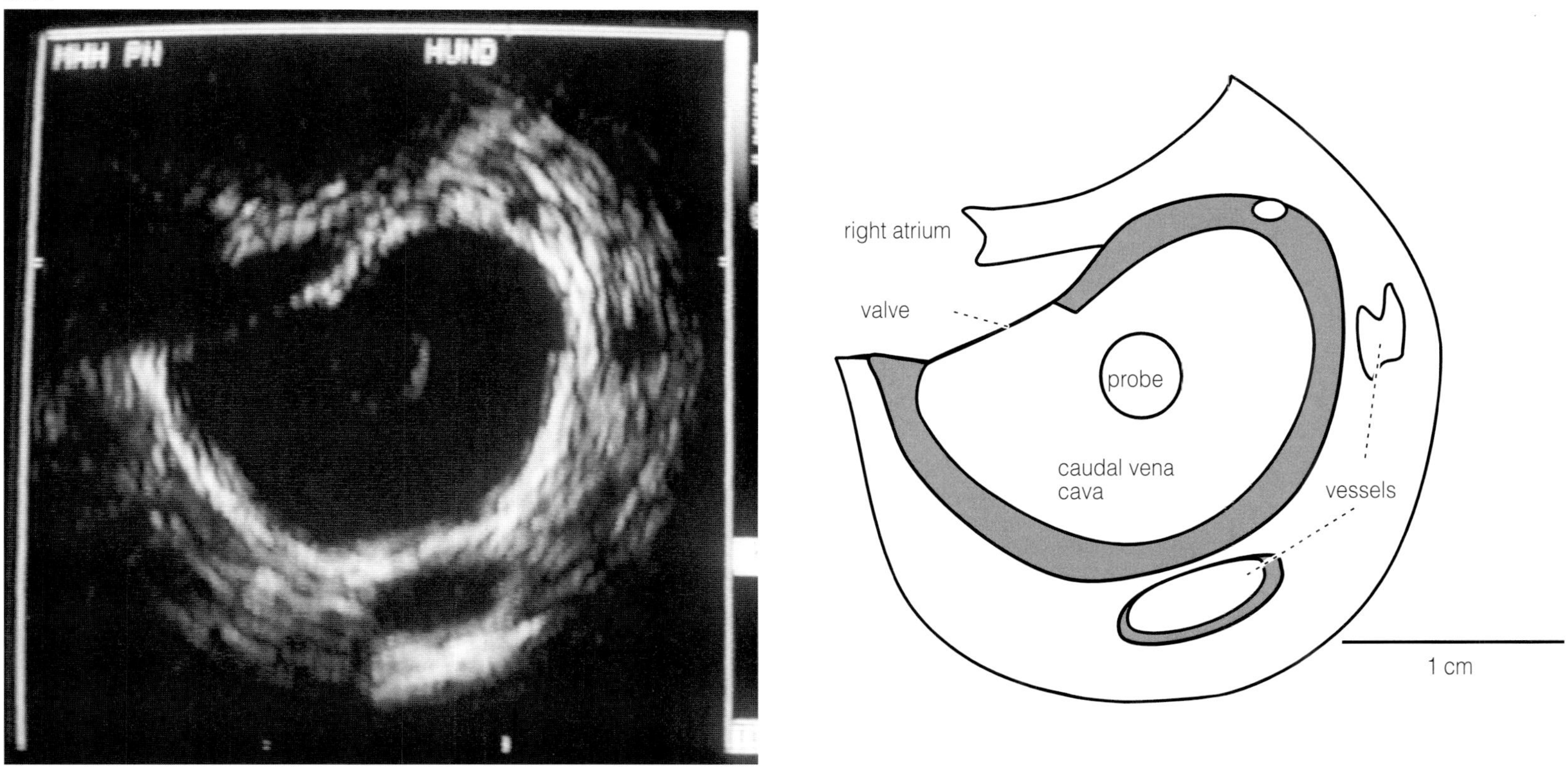

923, 924 Intravascular sonograms of the cranial vena cava slightly cranial to (**923**) and at the level of (**924**) its opening into the right atrium in a healthy dog.

References

1 Köhler E (1992) *Ein- and zweidimensionale Echokardiographie mit Dopplertechnik: Untersuchung, Befandung, Interpretation*. Ferdinand Enke Verlag Stuttgart.

2 Liebson PR and Klein LW (1992) Intravascular ultrasound in coronary atherosclerosis: a new approach to clinical assessment. *Am. Heart J.* **123**, 212–226.

3 Loyer C and Thomas WP (1995) Biplane transesophageal echocardiography in the dog: technique, anatomy and imaging planes. *Vet. Radiol. Ultrasound* **36**, 212–226.

4 Mosca Zohil A and Castellano C (1995) Prepubic and transrectal ultrasonography of the canine prostate: a comparative study. *Vet. Radiol. Ultrasound* **36**, 393–396.

5 Otto K and Matis U (1994) Changes in cardiopulmonary variables and platelet count during anesthesia for total hip replacement in dogs. *Vet. Surg.* **23**, 266–273.

Index

Simple page numbers refer to text; page numbers in *italics* refer to illustrations; page numbers in **bold** type indicate text and illustrations.